Test Drive

India's Most Trusted Practice Resource

AF819720

15 Practice Sets

NEET UG 2025

Exactly as per the Latest Pattern of NTA

Released on 25 Jan 2025

- PHYSICS
- CHEMISTRY
- BIOLOGY

Authors

Ajay Kumar *(Physics)*

Swati Chauhan *(Chemistry)*

Anuksha Arora *(Biology)*

arihant

SUCCESS AND NOTHING LESS

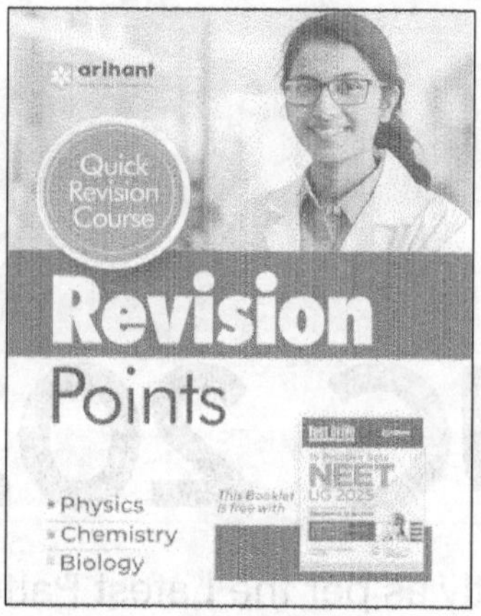

arihant
SUCCESS AND NOTHING LESS

ARIHANT PRAKASHAN (SERIES), MEERUT

Administrative & Production Offices
Regd. Office
'Ramchhaya' 4577/15, Agarwal Road, Darya Ganj, New Delhi -110002
Tele: 011- 47630600, 43518550

Head Office
Kalindi, TP Nagar, Meerut (UP) - 250002
Tel: 0121-7156203, 7156204

Sales & Support Offices
Agra, Ahmedabad, Bengaluru, Bareilly, Chennai, Delhi, Guwahati, Hyderabad, Jaipur, Jhansi, Kolkata, Lucknow, Nagpur & Pune.

PRICE ₹555.00

PO No : TXT-XX-XXXXXXX-X-XX

Published by Arihant Publications (India) Ltd.

For further information about the books published by Arihant, log on to www.arihantbooks.com or e-mail at info@arihantbooks.com

Follow us on

CONTENTS

NEET 2024 Analysis

Physics	No. of Ques in NEET 2024		Chemistry	No. of Ques in NEET 2024		Zoology	No. of Ques in NEET 2024		Botany	No. of Ques in NEET 2024	
	Section A	Section B		Section A	Section B		Section A	Section B		Section A	Section B
Units and Measurements	1	1	Some Basic Concepts of Chemistry	2	1	Animal Kingdom	3	1	The Living World	0	0
Motion in a Straight Line	0	1	Structure of Atom	2	0	Structural Organisation in Animals	2	2	Biological Classifiction	2	0
Motion in a Plane	1	0	Classification of Elements and Periodicity in Properties	2	0	Cell : The Unit of Life	1	1	Plant Kingdom	0	1
Laws of Motion	1	0	Chemical Bonding and Molecular Structure	2	1	Biomolecules	1	1	Morphology of Flowering Plants	3	2
Work, Energy and Power	2	1	Thermodynamics	2	1	Cell Cycle and Cell Division	2	0	Anatomy of Flowering Plants	3	0
System of Particles and Rotational Motion	3	0	Chemical Equilibrium	2	0	Breathing and Exchange of Gases	2	0	Cell : The Unit of Life	1	1
Gravitation	1	1	Ionic Equilibrium	0	1	Body Fluids and Circulation	1	1	Biomolecules	3	1
Mechanical Properties of Solids	1	0	Redox Reactions	1	0	Excretory Products and their Elimination	1	1	Cell Cycle and Cell Division	2	0
Mechanical Properties of Fluids	1	0	*p*-Block Elements-1	0	0	Locomotion and Movements	1	0	Photosynthesis in Flowering Plants	2	1
Thermal Properties of Matter	0	1	Purification and Characterisation of Organic Compounds	1	0	Neural Control and Coordination	1	1	Respirations in Plants	0	2
Thermodynamics	1	0	Some Basic Principles and Techniques of Organic Chemistry	3	0	Chemical Coordination and Integration	2	1	Plant Growth and Development	2	1
Kinetic Theory of Gases	0	1	Hydrocarbons	1	0	Human Reproduction	2	1	Sexual Reproduction in Flowering Plants	1	1
Oscillations	1	1	Solutions	1	1	Reproductive Health	2	0	Inheritance and Variation	4	0
Waves	0	0	Electrochemistry	1	1	Principles of Inheritance and Variation	1	1	Molecular Basis of Inheritance	2	2
Electric Charges and Fields	0	0	Chemical Kinetics	2	1	Molecular Basis of Inheritance	1	1	Biotechnology:Principles and Processes	2	0
Electrostatics Potential and Capacitance	2	1	*p*-Block Elements-2	2	0	Evolution	3	1	Biotechnology and Its Applications	3	1
Current Electricity	3	1	*d*-and *f*- Block Elements	2	1	Human Health and Diseases	5	1	Organisms and Population	1	0
Moving Charges and Magnetism	1	0	Coordination Compounds	2	1	Microbes in Human Welfare	1	0	Ecosystem	0	1
Magnetism and Matter	2	1	Haloalkanes and Haloarenes	1	1	Biotechnology:Principles and Processes	2	0	Biodiversity and Its Conservation	4	1
Electromagnetic Induction	1	1	Alcohols, Phenols & Ethers	1	1	Biotechnology and its Applications	1	0			
Alternating Current	1	1	Aldehydes, Ketones & Carboxylic Acids	2	1	Organisms and Populations	0	1			
Electromagnetic Waves	0	2	Organic Compounds Containing Nitrogen	1	1						
Ray Optics	1	1	Biomolecules	1	0						
Wave Optics	2	0	Principles Related to Practical Chemistry	1	2						
Dual Nature of Radiation and Matter	2	0									
Atoms	2	0									
Nuclei	1	0									
Semiconductor Electronics (Materials,Devices & Simple Circuits)	3	0									
Experimental Physics	1	0									

SYLLABUS

Physics

UNIT 1 Physics & Measurement

Units of measurements, System of Units, , SI Units, fundamental and derived units, **least count**, significant figures, Errors in measurements , Dimensions of Physics quantities, dimensional analysis and its applications.

UNIT 2 Kinematics

The frame of reference, motion in a straight line, Position- time graph, speed and velocity; Uniform and non-uniform motion, average speed and instantaneous velocity. **Uniformly** accelerated motion, velocity-time, position-time graph, relations for uniformly accelerated motion, Scalars and Vectors. Vector addition and subtraction, scalar and vector products. Unit Vector, Resolution of a Vector, Relative Velocity. Motion in a plane, Projectile Motion. Uniform Circular Motion.

UNIT 3 Laws of Motion

Force and inertia, Newton's First law of motion: Momentum, Newton's Second law of motion, Impulses: Newton's third law of motion. Law of conservation of linear momentum and its applications. Equilibrium of concurrent forces.

Static and Kinetic friction, laws of friction, rolling friction.

Dynamics of uniform circular motion: centripetal force and its applications: vehicle on a level circular road. vehicle on a banked road.

UNIT 4 Work, Energy and Power

Work done by a constant force and a variable force; kinetic and potential energies. work-energy theorem, power.

The potential energy of spring conservation of mechanical energy. conservative and non-conservative forces; motion in a vertical circle: Elastic and inelastic collisions in one and two dimensions.

UNIT 5 Rotational Motion

Centre of the mass of a two-particles system, Centre of the mass of a rigid body: Basic concepts of rotational motion; moment of a force; torque, angular momentum, conservation of angular momentum and its applications;

The moment of inertia, the radius of gyration, values of moments of inertia for simple geometrical objects, parallel and perpendicular axes theorems. and their applications. Equilibrium of rigid bodies. rigid body rotation and equations of rotational motion, comparison of linear and rotational motions.

UNIT 6 Gravitation

The universal law of gravitation. Acceleration due to gravity and its variation with altitude and depth. Kepler's law of planetary motion. Gravitational potential energy; gravitational potential.

Escape velocity, Motion of a satellite, orbital velocity, Time period and energy of satellite.

UNIT 7 Properties of Solids and Liquids

Elastic behaviour, Stress-strain relationship, Hooke's law, Young's modulus, bulk modulus, modulus of rigidity. Pressure due to a fluid column; Pascal's law and its applications. Effect of gravity on fluid pressure.

Viscosity, Stokes' law, terminal velocity, streamline, and turbulent flow.critical velocity, Bemoulli's principle and its applications.

Surface energy and surface tension, angle of contact, excess of pressure across a curved surface, application of surface tension - drops, bubbles, and capillary rise. Heat, temperature, thermal expansion; specific heat capacity, calorimetry; change of state, latent heat. Heat transfer-conduction, convection and radiation.

UNIT 8 Thermodynamics

Thermal equilibrium, zeroth law of thermodynamics, the concept of temperature. Heat, work, and internal energy. The first law of thermodynamics, isothermal and adiabatic processes.

The second law of thermodynamics: reversible and irreversible processes.

UNIT 9 Kinetic Theory of Gases

Equation of state of a perfect gas, work done on compressing a gas, Kinetic theory of gases - assumptions, the concept of pressure. Kinetic interpretation of temperature: **RMS speed of gas molecules:** Degrees of freedom. Law of equipartition of energy and applications to specific heat capacities of gases; Mean free path. **Avogadro's number.**

UNIT 10 Oscillations and Waves

Oscillations and periodic motion - time period, frequency, displacement as a function of time.

Periodic functions, Simple Harmonic Motion (SHM) and its equation; phase: oscillations of a spring -restoring force and force constant: energy in SHM - Kinetic and potential energies; Simple pendulum - derivation of expression for its time period:

Wave motion, Longitudinal and transverse waves, speed of travelling wave. Displacement relation for a progressive wave. Principle of superposition of waves, reflection of waves. Standing waves in strings and organ pipes, fundamental mode and harmonics. Beats.

UNIT 11 Electrostatics

Electric charges: Conservation of charge. Coulomb's law forces between two point charges, forces between multiple charges: superposition principle and continuous charge distribution.

Electric field: Electric field due to a point charge, Electric field lines. Electric dipole, Electric field due to a dipole. Torque on a dipole in a uniform electric field.

Electric flux, Gauss's law and its applications to find field due to infinitely long uniformly charged straight wire, uniformly charged infinite plane sheet and uniformly charged thin spherical shell. Electric potential and its calculation for a point charge, electric dipole and system of charges; potential difference, Equipotential surfaces, Electrical potential energy of a system of two point charges and of electric dipole in an electrostatic field.

Conductors and insulators, Dielectrics and electric polarization, capacitors and capacitances, the combination of capacitors in series and parallel, capacitance of a parallel plate capacitor with and without dielectric medium between the plates. Energy stored in a capacitor.

UNIT 12 Current Electricity

Electric current, Drift velocity, mobility and their relation with electric current. Ohm,s law, Electrical resistance, V-I characteristics of Ohmic and non-ohmic conductors. Electrical energy and power, Electrical resistivity and conductivity. Series and parallel combinations of resistors; Temperature dependence of resistance.

Internal resistance, potential difference and emf of a cell, a combination of cells in series and parallel. Kirchhoff's laws and their applications. Wheatstone bridge, Metre Bridge.

UNIT 13 Magnetic Effects of Current and Magnetism

Biot - Savart law and its application to current carrying circular loop. Ampere's law and its applications to infinitely long current carrying straight wire and solenoid. Force on a moving charge in uniform magnetic and electric fields.

Force on a current-carrying conductor in a uniform magnetic field. The force between two parallel currents carrying conductors-definition of ampere. Torque experienced by a current loop in a uniform magnetic field: Moving coil galvanometer, its sensitivity and conversion to ammeter and voltmeter.

Current loop as a magnetic dipole and its magnetic dipole moment. Bar magnet as an equivalent solenoid. magnetic field lines; Magnetic field due to a magnetic dipole (bar magnet) along its axis and perpendicular to its axis. Torque on a magnetic dipole in a uniform magnetic field. Para, dia and ferromagnetic substances with examples, Effect of temperature on magnetic properties.

UNIT 14 Electromagnetic Induction and Alternating Currents

Electromagnetic induction: Faraday's law, Induced emf and current: Lenz's law, Eddy currents, Self and mutual inductance. Alternating currents, peak and RMS value of alternating current/voltage : reactance and impedance: LCR series circuit, resonance : power in AC circuits, wattless current, AC generator and transformer.

UNIT 15 Electromagnetic Waves

Displacement current, Electromagnetic waves and their characteristics, Transverse nature of electromagnetic waves, Electromagnetic spectrum (radio waves, microwaves, infrared, visible, ultraviolet. X-rays. Gamma rays), Applications of e.m. waves.

UNIT 16 Optics

Reflection of light, spherical mirrors, mirror formula. Refraction of light at plane and spherical surfaces, thin lens formula and lens maker formula. Total internal reflection and its applications.

Magnification, power of a lens, Combination of thin lenses in contact, Refraction of light through a prism. Microscope and astronomical telescope (reflecting and refracting) and their magnifying powers.

Wave optics: wavefront and Huygens' principle, Laws of reflection and refraction using Huygens principle, Interference, Young's double-slit experiment and expression for fringe width, coherent sources, and sustained interference of light. Diffraction due to a single slit, width of central maximum.. Polarization, plane-polarized light: Brewster's law, uses of plane-polarized light and Polaroid.

UNIT 17 Dual Nature of Matter and Radiation

Dual nature of radiation. Photoelectric effect. Hertz and Lenard's observations; Einstein's photoelectric equation: particle nature of light. Matter waves-wave nature of particle, de-Broglie relation.

UNIT 18 Atoms and Nuclei

Alpha-particle scattering experiment; Rutherford's model of atom; Bohr model, energy levels, hydrogen spectrum. Composition and size of nucleus, atomic masses, mass-energy relation, mass defect; binding energy per nucleon and its variation with mass number, nuclear fission, and fusion.

UNIT 19 Electronic Devices

Semiconductors; semiconductor diode: I-V characteristics in forward and reverse bias; diode as a rectifier; I-V characteristics of LED. the photodiode, solar cell, and Zener diode; Zener diode as a voltage regulator. Logic gates (OR, AND, NOT, NAND and NOR).

UNIT 20 Experimental Skills

Familiarity with the basic approach and observations of the experiments and activities:

1. Varnier calipers-its use to measure the internal and external diameter and depth of a vessel.
2. Screw gauge-its use to determine thickness/diameter of thin sheet/wire.
3. Simple pendulum-dissipation of energy by plotting a graph between the square of amplitude and time.
4. Metre Scale - the mass of a given object by the principle of moments.
5. Young's modulus of elasticity of the material of a metallic wire.
6. Surface tension of water by capillary rise and effect of detergents,
7. Co-efficient of viscosity of a given viscous liquid by measuring terminal velocity of a given spherical body.
8. Speed of sound in air at room temperature using a resonance tube.
9. Specific heat capacity of a given (i) solid and (ii) liquid by method of mixtures.
10. The resistivity of the material of a given wire using a metre bridge.
11. The resistance of a given wire using Ohm's law.
12. Resistance and figure of merit of a galvanometer by half deflection method.
13. The focal length of;
    (i) Convex mirror
    (ii) Concave mirror and
    (iii) Convex lens, using the parallax method.
14. The plot of the angle of deviation vs angle of incidence for a triangular prism.
15. Refractive index of a glass slab using a travelling microscope.
16. Characteristic curves of a p-n junction diode in forward and reverse bias.
17. Characteristic curves of a Zener diode and finding reverse break down voltage.
18. Identification of Diode, LED,. Resistor. A capacitor from a mixed collection of such items.

Chemistry

Physical Chemistry

UNIT 1 Some Basic Concepts in Chemistry

Matter and its nature, Dalton's atomic theory Concept of atom, molecule, element and compound; laws of chemical combination: Atomic and molecular masses, mole concept, molar mass, percentage composition, empirical and molecular formulae: Chemical equations and stoichiometry.

UNIT 2 Atomic Structure

Nature of electromagnetic radiation, photoelectric effect, Spectrum of the hydrogen atom, Bohr model of a hydrogen atom its postulates, derivation of the relations for the energy of the electron and radii of the different orbits, limitations of Bohr's model. Dual nature of matter, de-Broglie's relationship. Heisenberg uncertainty principle. Elementary ideas of quantum mechanics, quantum mechanics, the quantum mechanical model of the atom, its important features. Concept of atomic orbitals as one-electron wave functions: Variation of Ψ and Ψ^2 with *r* for 1*s* and 2*s* orbitals; various quantum numbers (principal, angular momentum, and magnetic quantum numbers) and their significance; shapes of *s*, *p* and *d* - orbitals, electron spin and spin quantum number: Rules for filling electrons in orbitals-Aufbau principle. Pauli's exclusion principle and Hund's rule. electronic configuration of elements, extra stability of half-filled and completely filled orbitals.

UNIT 3 Chemical Bonding and Molecular Structure

Kossel-Lewis approach to chemical bond formation, the concept of ionic and covalent bonds, Ionic bonding: Formation of ionic bonds, factors affecting the formation of ionic bonds, calculation of lattice enthalpy.
Covalent Bonding: Concept of electronegativity. Fajan's rule, dipole moment: Valence Shell Electron Pair Repulsion (VSEPR) theory and shapes of simple molecules.

Quantum mechanical approach to covalent bonding: Valence bond theory - its important features, the concept of hybridisation involving *s, p* and *d* orbitals; Resonance.

Molecular Orbital Theory-Its important features, LCAOs, types of molecular orbitals (bonding, antibonding), sigma and pi-bonds, molecular orbital electronic configurations of homonuclear diatomic molecules, the concept of bond order, bond length, and bond energy.

Elementary idea of metallic bonding. Hydrogen bonding and its applications.

UNIT 4 Chemical Thermodynamics

Fundamentals of thermodynamics System and surroundings, extensive and intensive properties. state functions, types of processes.

The first law of thermodynamics - Concept of work, heat internal energy and enthalpy, heat capacity, molar heat capacity: Hess's law of constant heat summation: Enthalpies of bond dissociation, combustion, formation, atomisation, sublimation, phase transition, hydration. Ionisation, and solution.

The second law of thermodynamics -
Spontaneity of processes; ΔS of the universe and ΔG of the system as criteria for spontaneity. ΔG° (Standard Gibbs energy change) and equilibrium constant.

UNIT 5 Solutions

Different methods for expressing the concentration of solution - molality, molarity, mole fraction, percentage (by volume and mass both), the vapour pressure of solutions and Raoult's law - Ideal and non-ideal solutions, vapour pressure-composition, plots for ideal and non-ideal solutions: Colligative properties of dilute solutions- a relative lowering of vapour pressure, depression of freezing point, the elevation of boiling point and osmotic pressure, Determination of molecular mass using colligative properties: Abnormal value of molar mass, van't Hoff factor and its significance.

UNIT 6 Equilibrium

Meaning of equilibrium, the concept of dynamic equilibrium.
Equilibria involving physical processes: Solid-liquid, liquid gas and solid-gas equilibria. Henry's law. General characteristics of equilibrium involving physical processes.
Equilibrium involving chemical processes: Law of chemical equilibrium, equilibrium constants (K_p and K_c) and their significance, the significance of ΔG and ΔG° in chemical equilibrium, factors affecting equilibrium concentration, pressure, temperature, the effect of catalyst: Le-Chatelier's principle.

Ionic equilibrium: Weak and strong electrolytes, ionisation of electrolytes, various concepts of acids and bases (Arrhenius. Bronsted - Lowry and Lewis) and their ionisation, acid-base equilibria (including multistage ionisation) and ionisation constants, ionisation of water. pH scale, common ion effect, hydrolysis of salts and pH of their solutions, the solubility of sparingly soluble salts and solubility products, buffer solutions.

UNIT 7 Redox Reactions and Electrochemistry

Electronic concepts of oxidation and reduction, redox reactions, oxidation number, rules for assigning oxidation number, balancing of redox reactions.

Electrolytic and metallic conduction, conductance in electrolytic solutions, molar conductivities and their variation with concentration: Kohlrausch's law and its applications.

Electrochemical cells-Electrolytic and Galvanic cells, different types of electrodes, electrode potentials including standard electrode potential, half-cell and cell reactions, emf of a Galvanic cell and its measurement: Nernst equation and its applications: Relationship between cell potential and Gibbs' energy change: Dry cell and lead accumulator, Fuel cells.

UNIT 8 Chemical Kinetics

Rate of a chemical reaction, factors affecting the rate of reactions: concentration, temperature, pressure and catalyst; elementary and complex reactions, order and molecularity of reactions. rate, law, rate constant and its units, differential and integral forms of zero and first-order reactions, their characteristics and half-lives, the effect of temperature on the rate of reactions, Arrhenius theory, activation energy and its calculation, collision theory of bimolecular gaseous reactions (no derivation).

Inorganic Chemistry

UNIT 9 Classification of Elements and Periodicity in Properties

Modern periodic law and present form of the periodic table, *s*, *p*, *d* and *f* - block elements, periodic trends in properties of elements atomic and ionic radii, ionization enthalpy, electron gain enthalpy, valence, oxidation states, and chemical reactivity.

UNIT 10 *p*-block Elements

Group-13 to Group 18 Elements

General Introduction: Electronic configuration and general trends in physical and chemical properties of elements across the periods and down the groups; unique behaviour of the first element in each group.

UNIT 11 *d*- and *f*- Block Elements

Transition Elements

General introduction, electronic configuration, occurrence and characteristics, general trends in properties of the first-row transition elements- physical properties, ionisation enthalpy, oxidation states, atomic radii, colour, catalytic behaviour, magnetic properties, complex formation. interstitial compounds, alloy formation: Preparation, properties, and uses of $K_2Cr_2O_7$, and $KMnO_4$.

Inner Transition Elements Lanthanoids-Electronic configuration, oxidation states, and lanthanoid contraction.

Actinoids-Electronic configuration and oxidation states.

UNIT 12 Co-ordination Compounds

Introduction to coordination compounds. Werner's theory: ligands. coordination number. denticity, chelation: IUPAC nomenclature of mononuclear co-ordination compounds, isomerism: Bonding-Valence bond approach and basic ideas of Crystal field theory, colour and magnetic properties; Importance of co-ordination compounds (in qualitative analysis, extraction of metals and in biological systems).

Organic Chemistry

UNIT 13 Purification and Characterisation of Organic Compounds

Purification - Crystallisation, sublimation, distillation, differential extraction and chromatography-principles and their applications. Qualitative analysis - Detection of nitrogen, sulphur, phosphorus, and halogens.

Quantitative analysis (basic principles only) Estimation of carbon, hydrogen, nitrogen. halogens, sulphur, phosphorus. Calculations of empirical formulae and molecular formulae: Numerical problems in organic quantitative analysis, New chapter formed from Organic Chemistry : Some Basic Principles and Techniques.

UNIT 14 Some Basic Principles of Organic Chemistry

Tetravalency of carbon: Shapes of simple molecules- hybridisation (*s* and *p*): Classification of organic compounds based on functional groups: and those containing halogens, oxygen, nitrogen, and sulphur, Homologous series: Isomerism - structural and stereoisomerism.

Nomenclature (Trivial and IUPAC) Covalent bond fission - Homolytic and heterolytic: free radicals, carbocations, and carbanions: stability of carbocations and free radicals, electrophiles, and nucleophiles.

Electronic displacement in a covalent bond - Inductive effect, electromeric effect, resonance, and hyperconjugation. Common types of organic reactions- Substitution, addition, elimination, and rearrangement.

UNIT 15 Hydrocarbons

Classification, isomerism, IUPAC nomenclature, general methods of preparation, properties, and reactions.

Alkanes - Conformations: Sawhorse and Newman projections (of ethane): Mechanism of halogenation of alkanes.

Alkenes - Geometrical isomerism: Mechanism of electrophilic addition: addition of hydrogen, halogens, water. hydrogen halides (Markownikoffs and peroxide effect): Ozonolysis and polymerisation.

Alkynes - Acidic character: Addition of hydrogen, halogens, water, and hydrogen halides: Polymerization.

Aromatic hydrocarbons - Nomenclature, benzene structure and aromaticity: Mechanism of electrophilic substitution: halogenation, nitration.

Friedel - Craft's alkylation and acylation, directive influence of the functional group in mono- substituted benzene.

UNIT 16 Organic Compounds Containing Halogens

General methods of preparation, properties, and reactions: Nature of *C—X* bond; Mechanisms of substitution reactions. Uses: Environmental effects of chloroform, iodoform freons, and DDT.

UNIT 17 Organic Compounds Containing Oxygen

General methods of preparation, properties, reactions, and uses.

ALCOHOLS, PHENOLS, AND ETHERS

Alcohols: Identification of primary, secondary, and tertiary alcohols: mechanism of dehydration.

Phenols: Acidic nature, electrophilic substitution reactions: halogenation, nitration and sulphonation. Reimer - Tiemann reaction.

Ethers: Structure.

Aldehyde and Ketones: Nature of carbonyl group. Nucleophilic addition to $>C{=}O$ group. relative reactivities of aldehydes and ketones: Important reactions such as- Nucleophilic addition reactions (addition of HCN, NH_3 and its derivatives), Grignard reagent; oxidation: reduction (Wolff Kishner and Clemmensen); the acidity of α-hydrogen, aldol condensation. Cannizzaro reaction. Haloform reaction. Chemical tests to distinguish between aldehydes and ketones.

Carboxylic Acids acidic strength and factors affecting it.

UNIT 18 Organic Compounds Containing Nitrogen

General methods of preparation. Properties, reactions, and uses.

Amines: Nomenclature, classification, structure, basic character, and identification of primary, secondary and tertiary amines and their basic character.

Diazonium Salts: Importance in synthetic organic chemistry.

UNIT 19 Biomolecules

General introduction and importance of biomolecules.

Carbohydrates - Classification, aldoses and ketoses: monosaccharides (glucose and fructose) and constituent monosaccharides of oligosaccharides (sucrose, lactose, and maltose).

Proteins - Elementary Idea of α-amino acids, peptide bond, polypeptides. Proteins: primary. secondary, tertiary, and quaternary structure (qualitative idea only), denaturation of proteins, enzymes.

Vitamins - Classification and functions.

Nucleic Acids - Chemical constitution of DNA and RNA. Biological functions of nucleic acids. Hormones (General introduction).

UNIT 20 Principles Related To Practical Chemistry

Detection of extra elements (Nitrogen. Sulphur, halogens) in organic compounds: Detection of the following functional groups; hydroxyl (alcoholic and phenolic), carbonyl (aldehyde and ketones) carboxyl, and amino groups in organic compounds.

The chemistry involved in the preparation of the following:

Inorganic compounds; Mohr's salt, potash alum.

Organic compounds: Acetanilide, *p*-nitro acetanilide, aniline yellow, iodoform.

- The chemistry involved in the titrimetric exercises - Acids, bases and the use of indicators, oxalic- acid *vs* $KMnO_4$ Mohr's salt *vs* $KMnO_4$
- Chemical principles involved in the qualitative salt analysis:

Cations–Pb^{2+}, Cu^{2+}, Al^{3+}, Fe^{3+}, Zn^{2+}, Ni^{2+}, Ca^{2+}, Ba^{2+}, Mg^{2+}, NH_4^+

Anions–CO_3^{2-} , S^{2-}, SO_4^{2-} , NO_3^- , NO^{2-}, Cl^-, Br^-, I^-(Insoluble salts excluded).

Chemical principles involved in the following experiments:

1. Enthalpy of solution of $CuSO_4$.
2. Enthalpy of neutralisation of strong acid and strong base.
3. Preparation of lyophilic and lyophobic sols.
4. Kinetic study of the reaction of iodide ions with hydrogen peroxide at room temperature.

Biology

UNIT 1 Diversity in Living World

- What is living?: Biodiversity; Need for classification;: Taxonomy & Systematics: Concept of species and taxonomical hierarchy: Binomial nomenclature:
- Five kingdom classification, salient features and classification of Monera: Protista and Fungi into major groups: Lichens: Viruses and Viroids.
- Salient features and classification of plants into major groups-Algae, Bryophytes, Pteridophytes, Gymnosperms (three to five salient and distinguishing features and at least two examples of each category):
- Salient features and classification of animals non-chordate up to phyla level and chordate up to classes level (three to five salient features and at least two examples).

UNIT 2 Structural Organisation in Animals and Plants

- Morphology and modifications; Tissues; Anatomy and functions of different parts of flowering plants: Root, stem, leaf, inflorescence- cymose and recemose. flower, fruit and seed (To be dealt along with the relevant practical of the Practical Syllabus) Family (Malvaceae, Cruciferae, Leguminoceae, Compositae, Graminae).
- Animal tissues, Morphology, anatomy and functions of different systems (digestive, circulatory, respiratory, nervous and reproductive) of an insect (Frog). (Brief account only).

UNIT 3 Cell Structure and Function

- Cell theory and cell as the basic unit of life: Structure of prokaryotic and eukaryotic cell: Plant cell and animal cell; Cell envelope, cell membrane, cell wall: Cell organelles- structure and function; Endomembrane system-endoplasmic reticulum, Golgi bodies. lysosomes, vacuoles; mitochondria, ribosomes, plastids, micro bodies: Cytoskeleton, cilia, flagella, centrioles (ultra structure and function): Nucleus-nuclear membrane, chromatin, nucleolus.
- Chemical constituents of living cells: Biomolecules-structure and function of proteins, carbodydrates, lipids, nucleic acids; Enzymes-types, properties, enzyme action, classification and nomenclature of enzymes.
- Cell division: Cell cycle, mitosis, meiosis and their significance.

UNIT 4 Plant Physiology

- Photosynthesis: Photosynthesis as a means of Autotrophic nutrition: Site of photosynthesis take place; pigments involved in Photosynthesis (Elementary idea): Photochemical and biosynthetic phases of photosynthesis; Cyclic and non-cyclic and photophosphorylation: Chemiosmotic hypothesis; Photorespiration C_3 and C_4 pathways: Factors affecting photosynthesis.
- Respiration: Exchange gases; Cellular respiration-glycolysis, fermentation (anaerobic), TCA cycle and electron transport system (aerobic), Energy relations- Number of ATP molecules generated; Amphibolic pathways: Respiratory quotient.
- Plant growth and development: Seed germination; Phases of Plant growth and plant growth rate; Conditions of growth; Differentiation, dedifferentiation and redifferentiation; Sequence of developmental process in a plant cell; Growth regulators. auxin, gibberellin, cytokinin, ethylene, ABA.

UNIT 5 Human Physiology

- Breathing and Respiration: Respiratory organs in animals (recall only). Respiratory system in humans; Mechanism of breathing and its regulation in humans-Exchange of gases, transport of gases and regulation of respiration, Respiratory volumes: Disorders related to respiration-Asthma, Emphysema, Occupational respiratory disorders
- Body fluids and circulation: Composition of blood, blood groups, coagulation of blood. Composition of lymph and its function: Human circulatory system-Structure of human heart and blood vessels: Cardiac cycle, cardiac output, ECG, Double circulation: Regulation of cardiac activity; Disorders of circulatory system-Hypertension, Coronary artery disease. Angina pectoris, Heart failure.
- Excretory products and their elimination: Modes of excretion- Ammonotelism, ureotelism, uricotelism: Human excretory system-structure and function: Urine formation, Osmoregulation: Regulation of kidney function-Renin-angiotensin, Atrial Natriuretic Factor. ADH and Diabetes insipidus: Role of other organs in excretion. Disorders: Uraemia, Renal failure. Renal calculi. Nephritis; Dialysis and artificial kidney.
- Locomotion and Movement: Types of movement-ciliary, fiagellar, muscular, Skeletal muscle- contractile proteins and muscle contraction; Skeletal system and its functions (To be dealt with the relevant practical of practical syllabus); Joints; Disorders of muscular and skeletal system-Myasthenia gravis, Tetany, Muscular dystrophy, Arthritis, Osteoporosis, Gout.
- Neural control and coordination: Neuron and nerves; Nervous system in humans central nervous system, peripheral nervous system and visceral nervous system: Generation and conduction of nerve impulse;
- Chemical coordination and regulation: Endocrine glands and hormones: Human endocrine system-Hypothalamus, Pituitary, Pineal. Thyroid, Parathyroid. Adrenal, Pancreas, Gonads; Mechanism of hormone action (Elementary Idea); Role of hormones as messengers and regulators, Hypo-and hyperactivity and related disorders (Common disorders, e.g. Dwarfism. Acromegaly, Cretinism, Goitre, Exopthalmic goitre, Diabetes. Addison's disease).

  (Imp Diseases and disorders mentioned above to be dealt in brief)

UNIT 6 Reproduction

- Sexual reproduction in flowering plants: Flower structure: Development of male and female gametophytes: Pollination-types, agencies and examples, Outbreeding devices: Pollen-Pistil interaction; Double fertilization; Post-fertilization events-Development of endosperm and embryo, Development of seed and formation of fruit; Special modes-apomixis, parthenocarpy. polyembryony; Significance of seed and fruit formation
- Human Reproduction: Male and female reproductive systems; Microscopic anatomy of testis and ovary: Gametogenesis-spermatogenesis & oogenesis: Menstrual cycle: Fertilisation, embryo development upto blastocyst formation, implantation: Pregnancy and placenta formation (Elementary idea); Parturition (Elementary idea); Lactation (Elementary idea).
- Reproductive health: Need for reproductive health and prevention of sexually transmitted diseases (STD); Birth control-Need and Methods, Contraception and Medical Termination of Pregnancy (MTP); Amniocentesis: Infertility and assisted reproductive technologies- IVF, ZIFT, GIFT (Elementary idea for general awareness).

UNIT 7 Genetics and Evolution

- Heredity and variation: Mendelian Inheritance: Deviations from Mendelism- Incomplete dominance. Co-dominance. Multiple alleles and Inheritance of blood groups. Pleiotropy: Elementary idea of polygenic inheritance: Chromosome theory of inheritance; Chromosomes and genes; Sex determination-In humans, birds, honeybee: Linkage and crossing over; Sex linked inheritance-Haemophilia, Colour blindness; Mendelian disorders in humans-Thalassemia; Chromosomal disorders in humans; Down's syndrome, Turner's and Klinefelter's syndromes.
- Molecular basis of Inheritance: Search for genetic material and DNA as genetic material: Structure of DNA and RNA: DNA packaging, DNA replication, Central dogma, Transcription, genetic code, translation; Gene expression and regulation- *Lac* Operon: Genome and human genome project; DNA fingerprinting, protein biosynthesis.
- Evolution: Origin of life; Biological evolution and evidences for biological evolution from Paleontology, comparative anatomy, embryology and molecular evidence); Darwin's contribution, Modern Synthetic theory of Evolution; Mechanism of evolution- Variation (Mutation and Recombination) and Natural Selection with examples, types of natural selection; Gene flow and genetic drift; Hardy-Weinberg's principle: Adaptive Radiation; Human evolution.

UNIT 8 Biology and Human Welfare

- Health and Disease; Pathogens: parasites causing human diseases (Malaria, Filariasis, Ascariasis, Typhoid, Pneumonia, Common cold, Amoebiasis, Ringworm, Dengue, Chikungunya) Basic concepts of immunology-vaccines: Cancer, HIV and AIDS; Adolescence, drug and alcohol abuse. Tobacco abuse.
- Microbes in human welfare: In household food processing, industrial production. sewage treatment, energy generation and as biocontrol agents and biofertilizers.

UNIT 9 Biotechnology and Its Applications

- Principles and process of Biotechnology, Genetic engineering (Recombinant DNA technology).
- Application of Biotechnology in health and agriculture: Human insulin and vaccine production, gene therapy; Genetically modified organisms-*Bt* crops; Transgenic animals; Biosafety issues-Biopiracy and patents.

UNIT 10 Ecology and Environment

- Organisms and environment Population interactions-mutualism, competition, predation, parasitism: Population attributes-growth, birth rate and death rate, age distribution.
- Ecosystem: Patterns, components: productivity and decomposition: Energy flow: Pyramids of number, biomass, energy.
- Biodiversity and its conservation: Concept of Biodiversity; Patterns of Biodiversity; Importance of Biodiversity; Loss of Biodiversity: Biodiversity conservation; Hotspots, endangered organisms, extinction, Red Data Book, hiosphere reserves, National parks and sanctuaries, Sacred Groves.

NEET
TEST DRIVE

SECTION I
Foundation Builders

This section contains **3 Practice Sets** of initial level. The section is structured to strengthen your basics and built foundation for higher level practice.

SECTION I

Foundation Builders

PRACTICE SET 1

Maximum Marks : 720 | Time : 3 hrs | No. of Questions : 180

Instructions

1. This question paper contains **180** multiple-choice questions (four options with a single correct answer) from **Physics, Chemistry** and **Biology**.
2. These questions are distributed as 45 questions, each from Physics and Chemistry and 90 questions in Biology. These are to be compulsorily attempted by the candidate.
3. Each question carries 4 marks. For each correct response, the candidate will get 4 marks. For each incorrect response, one mark will be deducted from the total scores.

PHYSICS

1. A capacitor of capacitance 5 μF is connected as shown in the figure. The internal resistance of the cell is 0.5 Ω. The amount of charge on the capacitor plates is

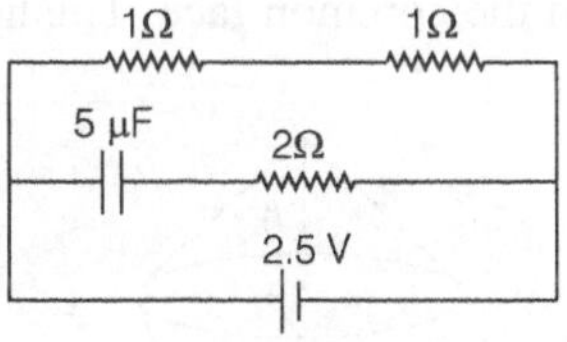

(a) 80 μC (b) 40 μC (c) 20 μC (d) 10 μC

2. The work done in increasing the size of a soap film from 10 cm × 6 cm to 10cm × 11cm is 3×10^{-4} J. The surface tension of film is

(a) 1.5×10^{-2} N/m (b) 3.0×10^{-2} N/m
(c) 6.0×10^{-2} N/m (d) 11.0×10^{-2} N/m

3. In an *L-C-R* circuit, inductance is changed from L to $L/2$. To keep the same resonance frequency, C should be changed to

(a) $2C$ (b) $\frac{C}{2}$
(c) $4C$ (d) $\frac{C}{4}$

4. Output B is given by

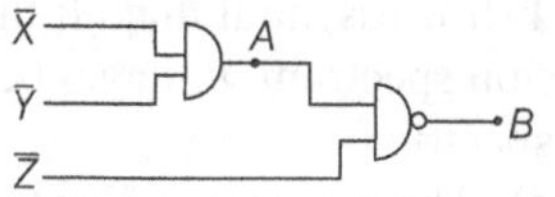

(a) $X + Y + Z$ (b) $\overline{XY} + Z$
(c) $\overline{X} + YZ$ (d) $X + XYZ$

5. A particle moves with uniform acceleration has average velocities v_1, v_2 and v_3 over the successive intervals of 5 s, 10 s and 15 s, respectively. Then, the value of $\frac{v_1 - v_2}{v_2 - v_3}$ will be

(a) $\frac{5}{3}$ (b) 1 (c) $\frac{3}{5}$ (d) $\frac{1}{2}$

6. The density of a solid ball is to be determined in an experiment. The diameter of the ball is measured with a screw gauge, whose pitch is 0.5 mm and there are 50 divisions on the circular scale. The reading on the main scale is 2.5 mm and that on the circular scale is 20 divisions. If the measured mass of the ball has a relative error of 2%, the relative percentage error in the density is

(a) 0.9% (b) 2.4%
(c) 3.1% (d) 4.2%

7. A body is moving with velocity 30 ms^{-1} towards east. After 10s, its velocity becomes 40 ms^{-1} towards north. The average acceleration of the body is

(a) 7 ms^{-2} (b) $\sqrt{7}$ ms^{-2} (c) 5 ms^{-2} (d) 1 ms^{-2}

8. A 500 kg car takes a round turn of radius 50 m with a velocity of 36 kmh^{-1}. The centripetal force is

(a) 250 N (b) 750 N
(c) 1000 N (d) 1200 N

9. A transformer is used on a 800 V line to deliver 20 A at 220 V on the secondary coil. If the efficiency of transformer is 80%, then the current drawn from the line is

(a) 12.875 A (b) 6.875 A
(c) 8.125 A (d) 7.125 A

10. A resonance in an air column of length 40 cm resonates with a tuning fork of frequency 450 Hz. Ignoring end correction, the velocity of sound in air is

(a) 1020 ms^{-1} (b) 720 ms^{-1}
(c) 620 ms^{-1} (d) 820 ms^{-1}

11. Given below are two statements.

Statement I It is essential that all the lines available in the emission spectrum will also be available in the absorption spectrum.

Statement II The spectrum of hydrogen atom is only absorption spectrum.

(a) Both Statement I and Statement II are correct.
(b) Statement I is correct but Statement II is incorrect.
(c) Statement I is incorrect but Statement II is correct.
(d) Both Statement I and Statement II are incorrect.

12. The effective resistance of n number of resistors when connected in parallel is P. If one of the resistor is removed, the effective resistance becomes Q. Then, the resistance of resistor which is removed, is

(a) $\frac{PQ}{P+Q}$ (b) $\frac{PQ}{Q-P}$ (c) $\frac{P^2Q^2}{(Q-P)^2}$ (d) $\frac{PQ}{P-Q}$

13. In the given circuit, the current through the resistor 2 kΩ is

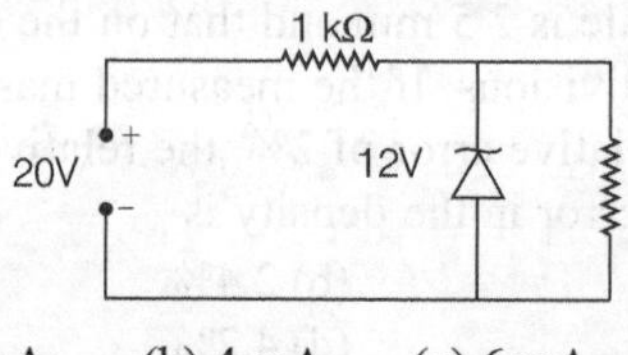

(a) 2 mA (b) 4 mA (c) 6 mA (d) 1 mA

14. In a vernier calipers, 10 divisions of vernier scale is equal to 9 divisions of main scale. One main scale division is equal to 1 mm. While measuring diameter of a spherical body, it is observed that zero of vernier scale lies between 30 and 31 divisions of main scale reading and 6th vernier scale divison exactly coincides with the main scale reading. The diameter of the spherical body is

(a) 3.00 cm (b) 3.06 cm (c) 3.106 cm (d) 3.016 cm

15. A current I flows in an infinitely long wire with cross-section in the form of a semi-circular ring of radius R. The magnitude of the magnetic induction along its axis is

(a) $\frac{\mu_0 I}{\pi^2 R}$ (b) $\frac{\mu_0 I}{2\pi^2 R}$ (c) $\frac{\mu_0 I}{2\pi R}$ (d) $\frac{\mu_0 I}{4\pi R}$

16. The wavelength λ of a photon and the de-Broglie wavelength of an electron have the same value. Find the ratio of energy of photon to the kinetic energy of electron in terms of mass m, speed of light c and Planck's constant h.

(a) $\frac{\lambda mc}{h}$ (b) $\frac{hmc}{\lambda}$ (c) $\frac{2hmc}{\lambda}$ (d) $\frac{2\lambda mc}{h}$

17. A uniform solid right circular cone and a solid hemisphere of same base radius 2 m and same density are placed on each other, so as to have common face. The centre of mass of the compositive solid lies on the common face. The height of the cone is

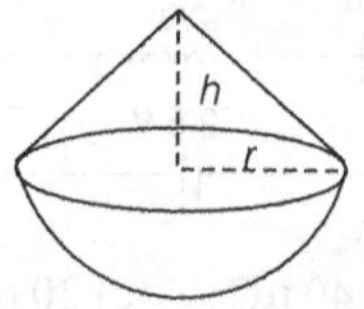

(a) 2 m (b) 6 m (c) $2\sqrt{3}$ m (d) 8 m

18. A billiard ball of mass m and radius r hit by a cue stick at a height h above the centre and it acquires a linear velocity v. The angular velocity ω acquired by the ball is

(a) $\frac{5vr^2}{2h}$ (b) $\frac{5vh}{2r^2}$ (c) $\frac{2vr^2}{5h}$ (d) $\frac{2vh}{5r^2}$

19. Two slits are separated by a distance of 0.5 mm and illuminated with light of $\lambda = 6000$ Å. If the screen is placed 2.5 m from the slits, the distance of the third bright fringe from the centre will be

(a) 1.5 mm (b) 3 mm
(c) 6 mm (d) 9 mm

20. A thin symmetrical double convex lens of refractive index $\mu_2 = 1.5$ is placed between a medium of refractive index $\mu_1 = 1.4$ to the left and another medium of refractive index $\mu_3 = 1.6$ to the right. Then, the system behaves as

(a) a convex lens (b) a concave lens
(c) a glass plate (d) a convex or concave lens

21. When a positive charge particle is moving on equipotential surface, then work done in this process will be

(a) positive (b) negative
(c) zero (d) None of these

22. If 8 dipoles of charges of magnitude $\pm e$ are placed inside the cube. The electric flux coming out of cube will be

(a) $16\,e/E_0$ (b) $8\,e/E_0$ (c) e/E_0 (d) zero

23. A current I flows in a conducting wire of length L. If we bent it in a circular form, its magnetic dipole moment would be

(a) $\frac{IL^2}{4\pi}$ (b) $\frac{IL}{4\pi}$ (c) $\frac{I^2L}{4\pi}$ (d) $\frac{I^2L^2}{4\pi}$

24. A straight conductor of length 2 m moves at right angles to both its length and uniform magnetic field. If the speed of the conductor is 4 ms^{-1} and the strength of magnetic field is 1 G, then the value of induced emf across the conductor is

(a) 0.2 mV (b) 0.6 mV
(c) 0.8 mV (d) 1 mV

25. A light ray from air is incident (as shown in figure) at one end of a glass fibre (refractive index, $\mu = 1.5$) making an incidence angle of 60° on the lateral surface, so that it undergoes a total internal reflection. How much time would it take to traverse the straight fibre of length 1 km ?

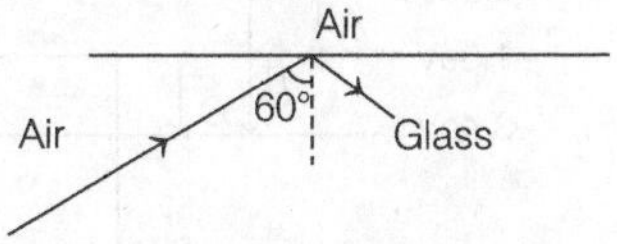

(a) 3.33 μs (b) 6.67 μs
(c) 5.77 μs (d) 3.85 μs

26. A ball is floating on the surface of water with half the volume submerged. If the ball has radius of 12 cm, what is the buoyant force on the ball due to water ?

(a) 33 N (b) 35 N
(c) 25 N (d) 40 N

27. A boy standing at the top of a tower of 20 m height drops a stone. Assuming $g = 10\,ms^{-2}$, the velocity with which it hits the ground is

(a) $20\,ms^{-1}$ (b) $40\,ms^{-1}$
(c) $5\,ms^{-1}$ (d) $10\,ms^{-1}$

28. The speed of a moving object is expressed in terms of time t as $v = \sqrt{PQ} + Qt + \frac{R}{S+t}$, then acceleration is represented by

(a) P (b) Q (c) R (d) S

29. A lift is moving down with acceleration a. A man in the lift drops a ball inside the lift. The acceleration of the ball as observed by the man in the lift is

(a) g (b) $a+g$ (c) $g-a$ (d) $a-g$

30. At room temperature (27°C), a vehicle tyre has pressure of 3 atm. The temperature if the tyre suddenly burst will be (given, $\gamma_{air} = \frac{7}{5}$)

(a) 246K (b) 274K (c) 219K (d) 204K

31. A force of 100 N acts on a charge of 2×10^{-4}C. The intensity of electric field at a point close to charge is

(a) 5×10^5 N/C (b) 4×10^4 N/C
(c) 2×10^{-2} N/C (d) 2×10^5 N/C

32. Given below are two statements.

Statement I The displacement current goes through the gap between the plates of a capacitor when the charge of the capacitor does not change.

Statement II The displacement current arises in the region in which the electric field does not change and hence, the electric flux does not change with time.

(a) Statement I is incorrect but Statement II is correct.
(b) Both Statement I and Statement II are incorrect.
(c) Statement I is correct but Statement II is incorrect.
(d) Both Statement I and Statement II are correct.

33. Three identical metallic uncharged spheres A, B and C of radius a are kept on the corners of an equilateral triangle of side d ($d >> a$). A fourth sphere (radius a) which has charge Q touches A and is then removed to a position for away. B is earthed and then the earth connection is removed. C is then earthed. The charge on C is

(a) $\frac{Qa}{2d}\left(\frac{2d-a}{2d}\right)$ (b) $\frac{Qa}{2d}\left(\frac{2d-a}{d}\right)$
(c) $\frac{Qa}{2d}\left(\frac{a-d}{d}\right)$ (d) $\frac{2Qa}{d}\left(\frac{d-a}{2d}\right)$

34. The variation of magnetic field $B(r)$ due to a thick cable of radius R with the distance r from the axis of cable is shown in figure below. Which of the following statement is correct for current I flowing through cable?

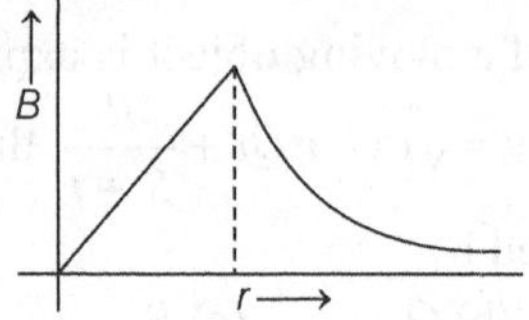

(a) Current I across cross-section increases with distance r.
(b) Current I across cross-section decreases with distance r.
(c) Current I across cross-section is uniformly distributed.
(d) None of the above.

35. Two identical particles each of mass m are interconnected by a light spring of stiffness k, the time period for small oscillation is equal to

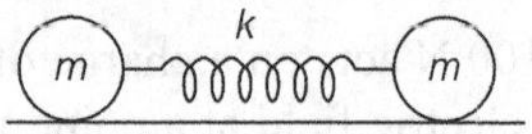

(a) $2\pi\sqrt{\frac{m}{k}}$ (b) $\frac{\pi}{2}\sqrt{\frac{m}{k}}$
(c) $\pi\sqrt{\frac{m}{2k}}$ (d) $\pi\sqrt{\frac{2m}{k}}$

36. In the following circuit diagram, effective resistance between point A and B is

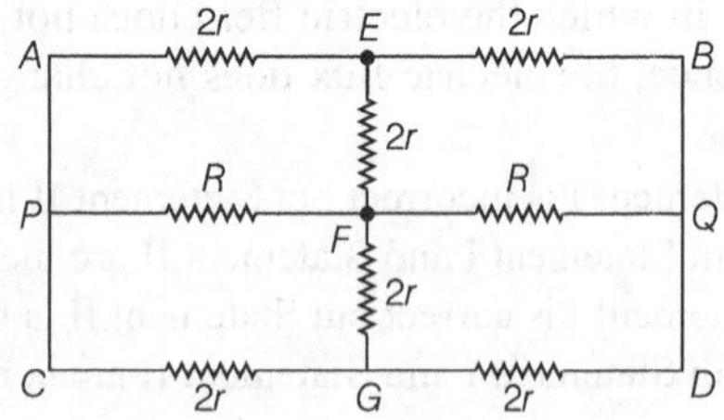

(a) $\frac{Rr}{2(R+r)}$ (b) $\frac{Rr}{(R+r)}$
(c) $2(R+r)$ (d) $\frac{2Rr}{R+r}$

37. In a match, a six is hit by a batsman and the ball touches the ground outside the boundary. Then, which of the following graphs describe the variation of the cricket ball's vertical velocity v with time? (between the time t as it hits the bat and time t', when it touches the ground)

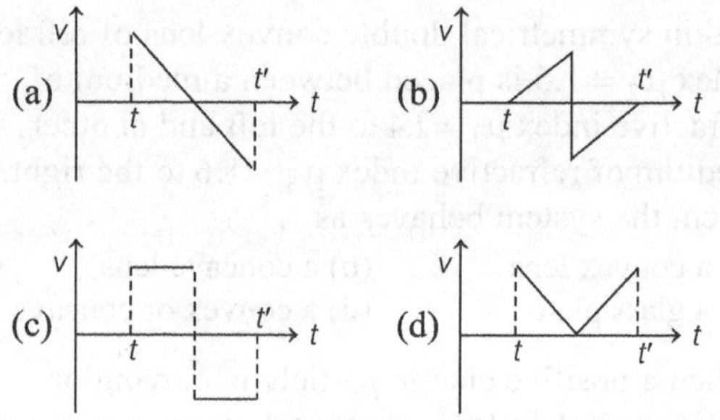

38. A mass M is broken into two parts of masses m_1 and m_2. For the force of attraction or gravitation to be maximum between them, the m_1 and m_2 have value

(a) $m_1 = \frac{M}{3}, m_2 = \frac{2M}{3}$ (b) $m_1 = \frac{2M}{3}, m_2 = \frac{M}{3}$
(c) $m_1 = m_2 = \frac{M}{2}$ (d) $m_1 = \frac{M}{4}, m_2 = \frac{3M}{4}$

39. A rectangular film of liquid is extended from (4 cm × 2 cm) to (5 cm × 4 cm). If the work done is 3×10^{-4} J, the value of the surface tension of the liquid is

(a) 0.250 Nm^{-1} (b) 0.125 Nm^{-1}
(c) 0.2 Nm^{-1} (d) 8.0 Nm^{-1}

40. The heart of an athlete pumps 7 L of blood through the arteries per minute at a pressure of 150 mm of mercury. If the density of mercury be $13.6 \times 10^3 kg/m^3$ and $g = 10 m/s^2$, then power of heart (in W) is

(a) 2.38 (b) 1.50
(c) 1.70 (d) 3.40

41. The energy level diagram of an element is shown below. Which transition corresponds to the emission of a spectral line of wavelength 102.7 nm ? (Take, $h = 6.626 \times 10^{-34}$ Js)

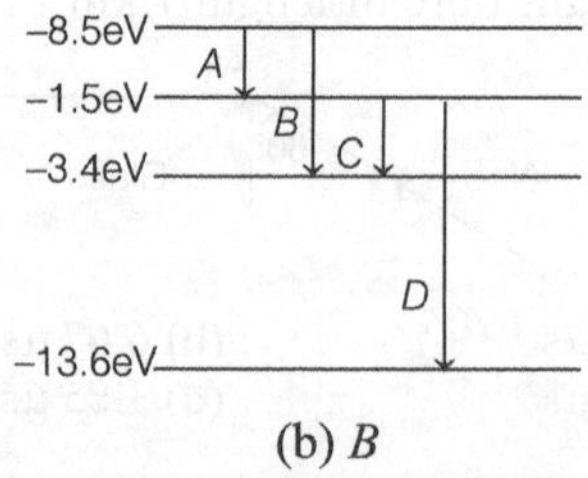

(a) A (b) B
(c) D (d) C

42. If λ_1 and λ_2 are the wavelengths of the first members of the Lyman and Paschen series, respectively. Then $\lambda_1 : \lambda_2$ is

(a) 1 : 3 (b) 1 : 30
(c) 7 : 50 (d) 7 : 108

43. A body weighs 72 kgf on the surface of earth, then its weight on surface of mars, whose mass is $\frac{1}{9}$ and radius is $\frac{1}{2}$ of that of earth is
(Here, kgf = kilogram-force)
(a) 72 kgf (b) 54 kgf
(c) 62 kgf (d) 32 kgf

44. Two plane mirrors of length 24 m each are kept at a distance of 8 cm parallel to each other. A ray of light incident on one end of one mirror at an angle of 53°, then total number of reflections before it reaches the other end is (given, $\tan 53° = \frac{4}{3}$)
(a) 225 (b) 175
(c) 250 (d) 200

45. One mole of monoatomic gas and three moles of diatomic gas are put together in a container. The molar specific heat (in $JK^{-1}\ mol^{-1}$) at constant volume is ($R = 8.3\ JK^{-1}\ mol^{-1}$)
(a) 18.7 (b) 18.9
(c) 19.2 (d) 20.7

CHEMISTRY

46. At 500 K, the half-life period of a gaseous reaction at an initial pressure of 100 kPa is 364 s. When the pressure is 50 kPa, the half-life period is 182 s. The order of the reaction is
(a) zero (b) one
(c) half (d) two

47. Addition of 0.643 g of a compound to 50 mL of benzene (density = 0.879 g mL^{-1}), lowers the freezing point from 50.51°C to 50.03°C. If K_f for benzene is 5.12 K kg mol^{-1}, the molecular mass (in g mol^{-1}) of the compound is
(a) 156.05 (b) 312.00 (c) 78.00 (d) 468.00

48. In Carius method, 0.099 g of organic compound gives 0.287 g of AgCl. The percentage of chlorine in the compound will be
(a) 71.71% (b) 29.39% (c) 53.06% (d) 76.23%

49. In the reaction, $N_2O_4 \rightleftharpoons 2NO_2$, α is that part of N_2O_4 which dissociates, then the number of moles at equilibrium will be
(a) $(1-\alpha)^2$ (b) 3α (c) α (d) $1+\alpha$

50. Which of the following represents the correct order of solubility of the noble gases in water?
(a) Ne > Ar > Kr > He > Xe
(b) He > Ne > Ar > Kr > Xe
(c) Ar > Ne > He > Kr > Xe
(d) Xe > Kr > Ar > Ne > He

51. Product obtained on reaction of 2-methylcyclohexene with *m*-CPBA followed by hydrolysis is

(a) 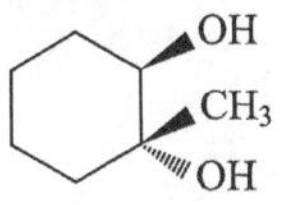
(b) 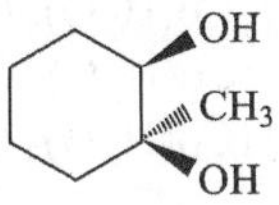
(c) 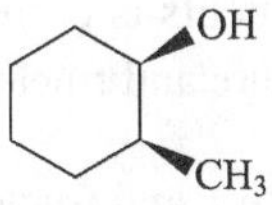
(d) 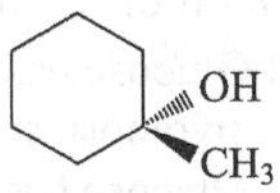

52. The reduction of $>C{=}O$ to $>CH_2$ is done by Wolff-Kishner reduction. The reagent used in Wolff-Kishner reduction is
(a) NH_2—NH_2 followed by heating in presence of base
(b) Zn—Hg in dil. HCl
(c) $Ph_3P{=}CH_2$
(d) None of the above

53. Compound Ph—O—C(=O)—Ph can be prepared by the reaction of
(a) phenol and benzaldehyde in the presence of palladium
(b) phenol and benzoic acid in the presence of NaOH
(c) phenol and benzoyl chloride in the presence of pyridine
(d) phenol and benzoyl chloride in presence of $ZnCl_2$

54. Which of the following would react most readily with nucleophiles?

(a) 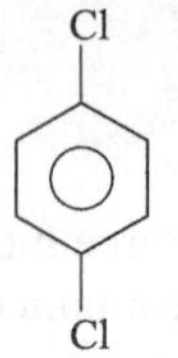
(b) 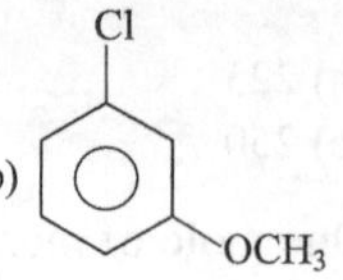
(c) 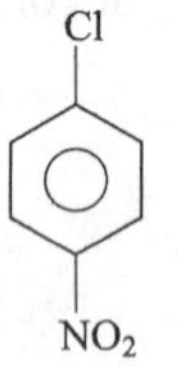
(d) 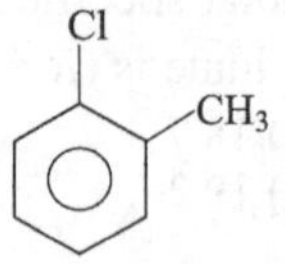

55. One mole of the complex $CoCl_3 \cdot 6H_2O$ on reaction with excess of $AgNO_3$ gives two moles of white precipitate. Thus, complex is

(a) $[Co(H_2O)_6]Cl_3$
(b) $[Co(H_2O)_5Cl]Cl_2 \cdot H_2O$
(c) $[Co(H_2O)_4Cl_2]Cl \cdot 2H_2O$
(d) $[Co(H_2O)_3Cl_3] \cdot 3H_2O$

56. Which of the following statements is correct?

(a) Glucose has furanose structure and fructose has pyranose structure.
(b) Glucose has pyranose structure and fructose has furanose structure.
(c) Both glucose and fructose have furanose structure.
(d) Both glucose and fructose have pyranose structure.

57. The decreasing order of stability of following cation is

(P) 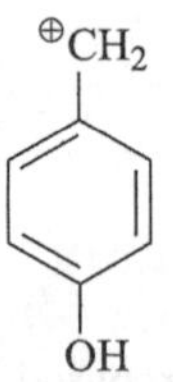
(Q) 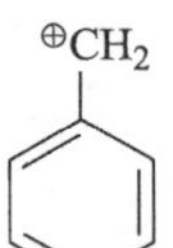
(R) 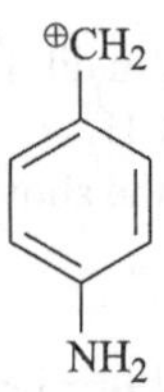
(S) 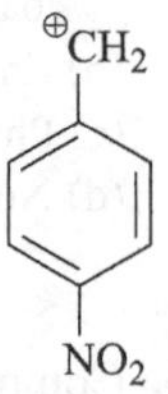

(a) P > Q > R > S (b) R > P > Q > S
(c) S > R > Q > P (d) S > Q > P > R

58. Arrange Cl, F, F^-, Cl^- in increasing order of ionisation potential.

(a) $F^- < Cl^- < Cl < F$ (b) $Cl < F^- < Cl^- < F$
(c) $Cl^- < F^- < F < Cl$ (d) $F^- < Cl^- < F < Cl$

59. What are the possible values of n, l and m for an atomic orbital $4f$?

(a) $n = 4, l = 0, 1, 2, 3, m = -2, -1, 0, +1, +2$
(b) $n = 4, l = 3, m = -3, -2, -1, 0, +1, +2, +3$
(c) $n = 4, l = 2, m = -2, -1, 0, +1, +2, +3$
(d) $n = 4, l = 0, m = -1, 0, +1$

60. 10 mL $C_4H_y(g)$ requires 55 mL $O_2(g)$ for its complete combustion. Find the value of y.

(a) 4 (b) 6 (c) 8 (d) 10

61. For the solution of the gases w, x, y and z in water at 298 K, the Henry's law constants (K_H) are 0.5, 5, 32 and 40 k bar respectively the correct plot for the given data is

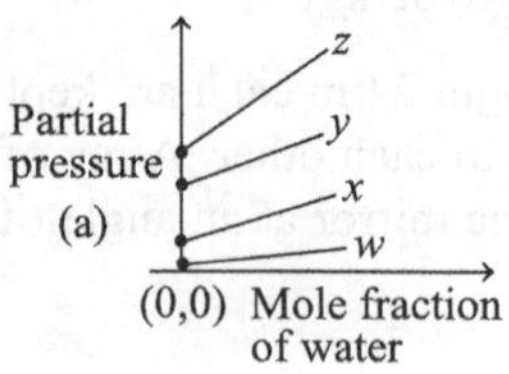

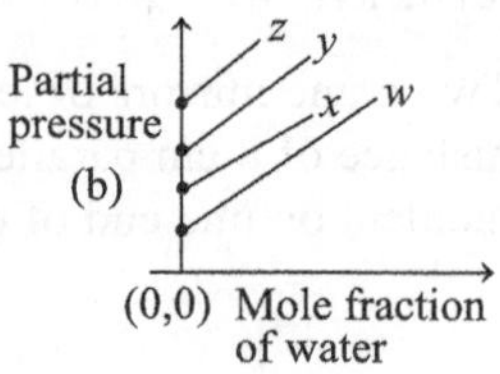

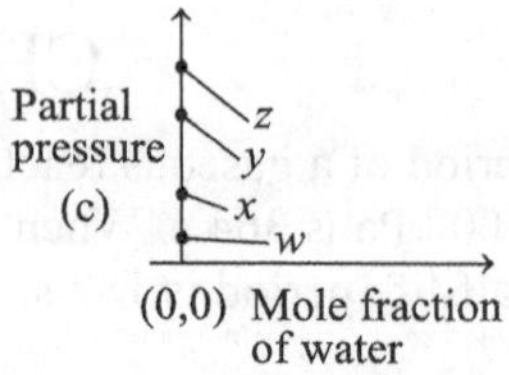

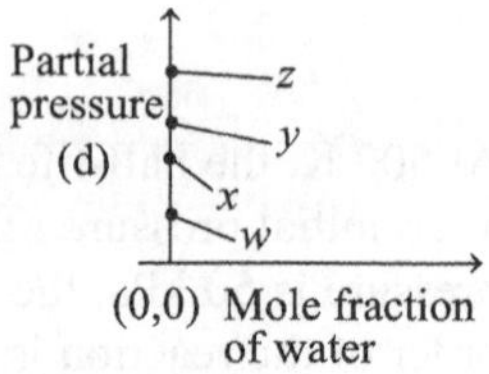

62. Match the List-I with List-II.

List-I (Catalyst)		List-II (Process)	
A.	Ni in presence of hydrogen	(i)	Contact process
B.	Cu_2Cl_2	(ii)	Reduction of vegetable oil to ghee
C.	V_2O_5	(iii)	Sandmeyer reaction
D.	Finely divided iron	(iv)	Haber's process

Choose the correct answer from the options given below.

(a) A-(ii), B-(iii), C-(i), D-(iv)
(b) A-(iii), B-(ii), C-(iv), D-(i)
(c) A-(ii), B-(iii), C-(iv), D-(i)
(d) A-(ii), B-(i), C-(iii), D-(iv)

63. Given below are two statements, one is labelled as Assertion (A) and the other is labelled as Reason (R).

Assertion (A) Transition metal compounds generally exhibit bright colours.

Reason (R) The electrons in the partially filled d-orbitals are easily promoted to excited states

In the light of the above statements, choose the most appropriate answer from the options given below.

(a) Both (A) and (R) are true but (R) is not the correct explanation of (A).
(b) (A) is true but (R) is false.

(c) (A) is false but (R) is true.
(d) Both (A) and (R) are true and (R) is the correct explanation of (A).

64. Match the List-I with List-II.

List-I	List-II
A. $PCl_5(g) \rightleftharpoons PCl_3(g) + Cl_2(g)$	(i) $\Delta H > \Delta U$
B. $2HI(g) \rightleftharpoons H_2(g) + I_2(g)$	(ii) $\Delta H = \Delta U - RT$
C. $N_2(g) + 3H_2(g) \rightleftharpoons 2NH_3(g)$	(iii) $\Delta H = \Delta U \neq 0$
D. $2CO(g) + O_2(g) \rightleftharpoons 2CO_2(g)$	(iv) $\Delta H = \Delta U - 2RT$

Choose the correct answers from the options given below.
(a) A-(i), B-(iii), C-(iv), D-(ii)
(b) A-(i), B-(iii), C-(ii), D-(iv)
(c) A-(iii), B-(i), C-(iv), D-(ii)
(d) A-(i), B-(ii), C-(iv), D-(iii)

65. During nitrogen estimation of an organic compound by Kjeldahl's method, the ammonia evolved by 0.5 g of the compound neutralises 10 mL of 1 M H_2SO_4. Calculate the percentage of nitrogen in the compound.
(a) 56% (b) 75%
(c) 48% (d) 40%

66. Given below are two statements.
Statement I The increasing order of C—O bond length of CO, CO_3^{2-} and CO_2 is $CO < CO_2 < CO_3^{2-}$.
Statement II The bond order for CO, CO_2 and CO_3^{-2} are 3, 2.5 and 1.33 respectively.
In the light of the above statements, choose the correct answer from the options given below.
(a) Both Statement I and Statement II are incorrect.
(b) Statement I is correct but Statement II is incorrect.
(c) Statement I is incorrect but Statement II is correct.
(d) Both Statement I and Statement II are correct.

67. The 'isoelectronic and iso structural' compounds are
A. TeI_2 B. $BeCl_2$ C. IF_3
D. XeF_2 E. IBr_2^-

Chosoe the most appropriate answer from the options given below.
(a) A, C and D
(b) B and E
(c) D and E
(d) A and B

68. Match List-I with List-II.

List-I (Ion + Reagent)	List-II (Colour)
A. $Fe^{3+} + [Fe(CN)_6]^{4-}$	I. Cherry red
B. $Fe^{3+} + CNS^-$	II. Pink
C. Ni^{2+} + DMG	III. Blood red
D. $Mn^{2+} + PbO_2 + H^+$	IV. Prussian blue

Choose the correct answer from the options given below:
(a) A-I, B-IV, C-II, D-III
(b) A-IV, B-III, C-I, D-II
(c) A-III, B-IV, C-II, D-I
(d) A-III, B-I, C-IV, D-II

69. The mixture of concentrated HCl and HNO_3 made in 3 : 1 ratio contains
(a) N_2O_4 (b) NOCl
(c) NCl_3 (d) ClO_2

70. Given below are two statements.
Statement I $[Ni(CO)_4]$ has tetrahedral geometry.
Statement II $[Ni(CO)_4]$ is paramagnetic since nickel is in zero oxidation state.
In the light of the above statements, choose the correct answer from the options given below.
(a) Both Statement I and Statement II are incorrect.
(b) Statement I is correct but Statement II is incorrect.
(c) Statement I is incorrect but Statement II is correct.
(d) Both Statement I and Statement II are correct.

71. In BrF_3 molecule, the lone pairs occupy equatorial positions to minimize
(a) lone-pair-bond pair repulsion.
(b) bond pair-bond pair repulsion.
(c) both lone pair-lone pair and bond pair-bond pair repulsion
(d) lone pair-lone pair repulsion.

72. Given below are two statements.
Statement I F_2 doesn't undergoes disproportionation reaction.
Statement II Fluorine shows both positive and negative oxidation states.
In the light of the above statements, choose the correct answer from the options given below.
(a) Both statement I and statement II are false.
(b) Statement I is true but statement II is false.
(c) Statement I is false but statement II is true.
(d) Both statement I and statement II are true.

73. Given below are two statements, one is labelled as Assertion (A) and the other is labelled as Reason (R).

Assertion (A) Ethylamine is soluble in water whereas aniline is not.

Reason (R) The extent of hydrogen bonding in aniline is more than ethylamine.

In the light of the above statements, choose the most appropriate answer from the options given below.

(a) Both (A) and (R) are correct but (R) is not the correct explanation of (A).
(b) (A) is correct but (R) is not correct.
(c) (A) is not correct but (R) is correct.
(d) Both (A) and (R) are correct and (R) is the correct explanation of (A).

74. A direct iodination of benzene is not possible because

(a) iodine is an oxidising agent.
(b) resulting C_6H_5I is reduced to C_6H_6 by HI.
(c) HI is unstable.
(d) the ring gets deactivated.

75. Which of the following statements is correct in relation to the halogenation of alkane?

(a) The reactivity of chlorine is less than bromine towards alkanes.
(b) For photochemical chlorination of methane, Cl is formed in slowest step.
(c) Free radicals are pyramidal intermediate, stabilised by hyperconjugation and resonance.
(d) Bromine has much higher regioselectivity than chlorine in abstracting 3° hydrogen.

76. MnO_4^{2-} undergoes disproportionation reaction in acidic medium but MnO_4^- does not due to the

(a) highest oxidation state of Mn in MnO_4^{2-}.
(b) highest oxidation state of Mn in MnO_4^-.
(c) exothermic nature of disproportionation reaction.
(d) endothermic nature of disproportionation reaction.

77. The shortest wavelength transition in the Paschen series in hydrogen atom occurs at 821 nm. At what wavelength does it occur in Li^{2+} (isoelectronic to hydrogen)?

(a) 91.2 nm (b) 273.6 nm
(c) 822.0 nm (d) 7389.0 nm

78. If the electron is visualised as a classical charged particle laterally rotating about an axis with angular momentum L and magnetic dipole moment μ, then find the magnetic moment of $K_3[FeF_6]$.

(a) 3.87 BM (b) 4.89 BM
(c) 5.92 BM (d) 6.92 BM

79. A certain current liberates 0.500 g of H_2 in 2.00 hr. How many gram of oxygen can be liberated by the same current in the same time?

(a) 0.500 g (b) 8.00 g (c) 4.00 g (d) 16.00 g

80. Match List I with List II.

	List-I		List-II
A.	16 g of $CH_4(g)$	I.	Weighs 32 g
B.	1 g of $H_2(g)$	II.	60.2×10^{23} electrons
C.	1 mole of $O_2(g)$	III.	Weighs 64 g
D.	1 mol of $SO_2(g)$	IV.	Occupies 11.4 L volume at STP

Choose the correct answer from the options given below.

(a) A-I, B-III, C-II, D-IV (b) A-II, B-IV, C-I, D-III
(c) A-II, B-III, C-IV, D-I (d) A-II, B-IV, C-III, D-I

81. For the reaction, $2SO_{2(g)} + O_{2(g)} \rightleftharpoons 2SO_{3(g)}$, $\Delta H = -57.2$ kJ mol^{-1} and $K_C = 1.7 \times 10^{16}$

Which of the following statements is correct?

I. The equilibrium will shift in forward direction as the pressure increases.
II. The addition of inert gas at constant volume will not affect the equilibrium constant.
III. The equilibrium constant is large suggestive of reaction going to completion and so no catalyst is required.
IV. The equilibrium constant decreases as the temperature increases.
V. The equilibrium will shift in backward direction as the pressure increases.

Choose the correct option.

(a) I, II, III and IV (b) I, II and IV
(c) II, III, IV and V (d) III and IV

82. Given below are two statements.

Statement I pH of pure water is less than 7 at 60°C.

Statement II Ionisation of water into H^+ and OH^- is an endothermic process.

In the light of above statements above the statements, choose the correct answer from the options given below:

(a) Both Statement I and Statement II are incorrect.
(b) Statement I is correct but Statement II is incorrect.
(c) Statement I is incorrect but Statement II is correct.
(d) Both Statement I and Statement II are correct.

83. Dehydrohalogenation of ethyl chloride in presence of alc. KOH produces.
(a) $HC \equiv CH + KCl + H_2O$
(b) $CH_4 + KCl + H_2O$
(c) $CH_2 = CH_2 + KCl + H_2O$
(d) $C_2H_4 + HCl$

84. A first order reaction was commenced with 0.2 M solution of the reactants. If the molarity of the solution falls to 0.02 M after 100 minutes the rate constant of the reaction is
(a) $2 \times 10^{-2}\ min^{-1}$ (b) $2.3 \times 10^{-2}\ min^{-1}$
(c) $4.6 \times 10^{-2}\ min^{-1}$ (d) $2.3 \times 10^{-1}\ min^{-1}$

85. Match the List-I with List-II.

List-I	List-II
A. $Pt \mid Fe^{3+} \mid Fe^{2+}$	(i) Metal sparingly soluble salt half-cell
B. $Pt \mid H_2 \mid H^+$	(ii) Oxidation reduction half-cell
C. $Pt \mid Hg \mid Hg_2^{2+}$	(iii) Gas-gas ion half-cell
D. $Pb \mid PbSO_4 \mid SO_4^{2-}$	(iv) Metal-metal ion half-cell

Choose the correct answer from the options given below.
(a) A-(i), B-(ii), C-(iii), D-(iv)
(b) A-(ii), B-(iii), C-(iv), D-(i)
(c) A-(ii), B-(iii), C-(i), D-(iv)
(d) A-(ii), B-(i), C-(iii), D-(iv)

86. Identify '*X*' in the following reaction.

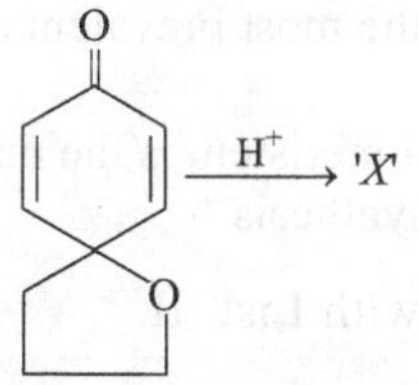

(a) 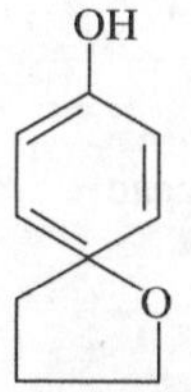 (b) 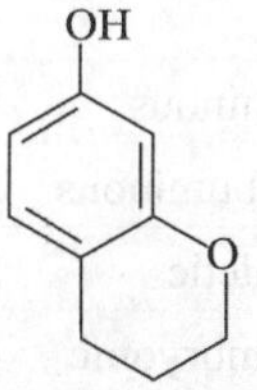

(c) 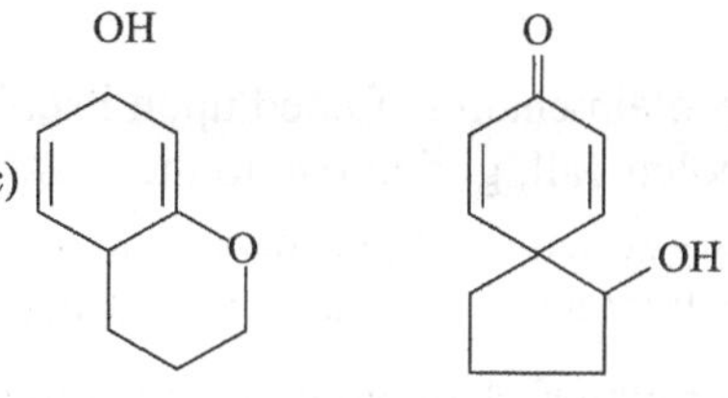

87. Which of the following compounds will give a yellow precipitate with iodine and alkali?
I. 2-hydroxypropane II. Acetophenone
III. Acetamide IV. Methyl acetate
V. Benzyl alcohol
Choose the correct option.
(a) I and IV (b) II and V
(c) I and II (d) IV and V

88. Phenolphtalein act as an indicator in acid-base titration, it exists as
(a) quinonoid form in acid and benzenoid form in basic solution.
(b) benzenoid form in acid and quinonoid form in basic solution.
(c) quinonoid form in both acidic as well as basic solution.
(d) benzenoid form in both acidic as well as basic solution.

89. Arrange the following in correct sequence of basic strength.

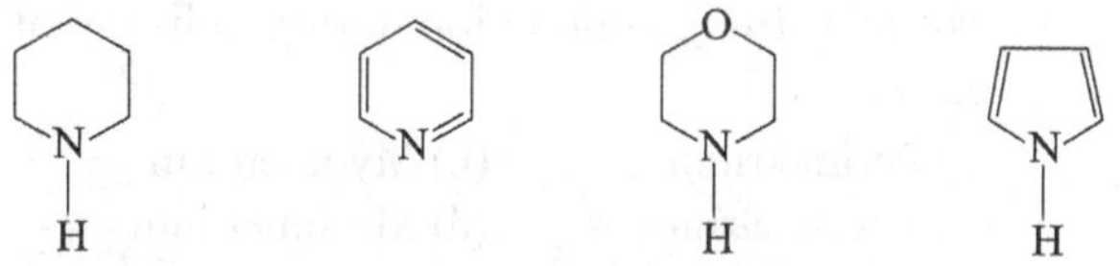

I II III IV

(a) IV > I > III > II (b) III > I > II > IV
(c) II > I > III > IV (d) I > III > II > IV

90. Which of the following reagent is used to convert the given below reaction?

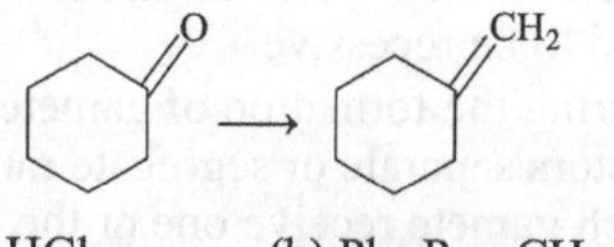

(a) Zn-Hg in HCl (b) $Ph_3P{=}CH_2$
(c) Li/H_2 (d) $LiAlH_4$

BIOLOGY

91. The long protein chain is folded upon itself like a hollow woolen ball, giving rise to the

(a) secondary structure (b) primary structure
(c) tertiary structure (d) quaternary structure

92. Secretion of which gland nourish and activate spermatozoa to swim?

(a) Vasa efferentia (b) Pituitary gland
(c) Prostate gland (d) Cowper's gland

93. Which among the following statements is/are correct regarding meristematic cells?

(a) These cells have the power of division
(b) Their cell wall is thin
(c) Their nuclei are prominent
(d) All of the above

94. Which of the following statements is correct regarding the genetic material?

(a) Both DNA and RNA are able to mutate, but DNA mutate at a faster rate
(b) DNA is not dependent on RNA for the synthesis of proteins
(c) For the transmission of genetic information, RNA is better
(d) Viruses containing RNA genome and having longer lifespan mutate and evolve faster

95. Which of the following layer of the uterine wall exhibits strong contraction during delivery of the baby?

(a) Perimetrium (b) Myometrium
(c) Endometrium (d) Mesometrium

96. Which of the following statement(s) is/are true?

(a) Genetic characters are controlled by unit factors existing in pairs in individual organism
(b) When two unlike unit factors responsible for single character are present in a single individual, one unit factor is dominant to the other, which is said to be recessive
(c) During the formation of gametes, the paired unit factors separate or segregate randomly, so that each gamete receive one or the other with equal likelihood
(d) All are true

97. Given below are two statements; one is labelled as Assertion (A) and the other is labelled as Reason (R).

Assertion (A) A person of 'AB' blood group can donate blood to person of O blood group.

Reason (R) The blood group O has no antigen and have A and B antibodies.

In the light of the above statements, choose the correct answer from the options given below.

(a) A is false, but R is true
(b) Both A and R are true and R is the correct explanation of A
(c) Both A and R are true, but R is not the correct explanation of A
(d) A is true, but R is false

98. Consider the following statements.

I. In frogs, skin acts as aquatic respiratory organ.
II. In frog, during aestivation and hibernation gaseous exchange takes place through lungs.
III. The vascular system in frogs is well-developed and open type.
IV. In frog, RBCs are nucleated and contain red coloured pigment namely haemoglobin.
V. The frog excrete urea and thus is a ureotelic animal.

Choose the correct set of statements from the options given below

(a) I, III and IV (b) I, IV and V
(c) I, III and V (d) II, III and IV

99. Which of the following statements is not true?

(a) Auxin is synthesised from amino acid tryptophan
(b) Methionine is the precursor of ethylene
(c) Kinetin is the most prevalent natural cytokinin in plants
(d) Root apical meristem is the main site for cytokinin synthesis

100. Match List I with List II.

	List I		List II
A.	Albuminous	1.	*Citrus*
B.	Ex- albuminous	2.	Asteraceae
C.	Apomictic	3.	Pea
D.	Polyembryonic	4.	Castor

Codes

	A	B	C	D
(a)	3	4	1	2
(b)	2	3	4	1
(c)	4	3	2	1
(d)	3	2	1	4

101. Match List I with List II.

	List I		List II
A.	Regulator genes	1.	Act as switch
B.	Operator genes	2.	Provide sites for the binding of RNA polymerase
C.	Promoter genes	3.	Codes for repressor proteins
D.	Exon	4.	Coding sequence of DNA

Codes

	A	B	C	D		A	B	C	D
(a)	1	2	3	4	(b)	3	1	2	4
(c)	2	3	1	4	(d)	1	3	2	4

102. The non-staining secondary constriction in a few chromosomes that gives the appearance of small fragment is called
(a) satellite (b) centromere
(c) kinetochores (d) telomere

103. *Taq* polymerase has similar activity to
(a) DNA polymerase-I (b) DNA polymerase-II
(c) DNA polymerase-III (d) RNA polymerase

104. Which one is not allowed by a prudent predator?
(a) Keeps prey population under control
(b) Maintains species diversity
(c) Over exploitation of prey
(d) Allows transfer of energy across trophic levels

105. Identify the incorrect matching regarding pyramid of biomass.
(a) Grassland - Upright (b) Forest - Upright
(c) Pond - Upright (d) None of these

106. Given below are two statements.
Statement I Replication and transcription occur in the nucleus, but translation takes place in the cytoplasm.
Statement II *m*RNA is transferred from the nucleus into cytoplasm, where ribosomes and amino acids are available for protein synthesis.
In the light of the above statements, choose the correct answer from the options given below.
(a) Both statement I and statement II are false
(b) Statement I is true, but statement II is false
(c) Statement I is false, but statement II is true
(d) Both statement I and statement II are true

107. Which of the following phase of the cell cycle is not a part of interphase?
(a) M (b) S (c) G_1 (d) G_2

108. Match List I with List II.

	List I		List II
A.	Vital capacity	1.	500 mL
B.	Tidal volume	2.	3000 mL
C.	Expiratory reserve volume	3.	4800 mL
D.	Inspiratory reserve volume	4.	1000 mL

Choose the correct answer from the options given below.

	A	B	C	D		A	B	C	D
(a)	2	1	4	3	(b)	3	1	4	2
(c)	1	2	4	3	(d)	2	1	3	4

109. Given below are two statements; one is labelled as Assertion (A) and other is labelled as Reason (R).
Assertion (A) STRs are usually considered junk DNA.
Reason (R) They are intron and do not code for protein.
In the light of the above statements, choose the correct answer from the options given below.
(a) Both A and R are true and R is the correct explanation of A
(b) Both A and R are true, but R is not the correct explanation of A
(c) A is true, but R is false
(d) A is false, but R is true

110. Which of the following is an edible fungi?
(a) *Aspergillus* (b) *Agaricus*
(c) *Neurospora* (d) *Claviceps*

111. Which of the following phytohormone inhibits mitosis in vascular cambium?
(a) Gibberellins (b) Abscisic acid
(c) Ethylene (d) Cytokinin

112. Given below are two statements.
Statement I In echinodermates, fertilisation is usually external and development is indirect with free swimming larva.
Statement II Water vascular system is the most distinctive feature of echinoderms which helps in locomotion and digestion.

In the light of the above statements, choose the correct answer from the options given below.
(a) Both statement I and statement II are false
(b) Statement I is true, but statement II is false
(c) Statement I is false, but statement II is true
(d) Both statement I and statement II are true

113. Given below are two statements.
Statement I The ratio of carbon dioxide formation in aerobic and anaerobic respiration is 3 : 1.
Statement II The ratio of ATP in anaerobic respiration and aerobic respiration is 18 : 1.
In the light of the above statements, choose the correct answer from the options given below.
(a) Both statement I and statement II are correct
(b) Both statement I and statement II are incorrect
(c) Statement I is correct, but statement II is incorrect
(d) Statement I is incorrect, but statement II is correct

114. Match List I with List II.

List I	List II
A. Diabetes insipidus	1. Insulin
B. Diabetes mellitus	2. Melatonin
C. Addison's disease	3. ADH
D. Circadian rhythm	4. Adrenal insufficiency

Choose the correct answer from the options given below.

	A	B	C	D
(a)	1	2	3	4
(b)	3	1	4	2
(c)	3	4	1	2
(d)	3	2	4	1

115. Given below are two statements.
Statement I Phloem tissue is composed of sieve tube cells, which form long columns with holes in their end walls called sieve plates.
Statement II The functions of sieve tubes are controlled by the nucleus of the phloem fibres.
In the light of the above statements, choose the correct answer from the options given below.
(a) Both statement I and statement II are correct
(b) Both statement I and statement II are incorrect
(c) Statement I is correct, but statement II is incorrect
(d) Statement I is incorrect, but statement II is correct

116. Given below are two statements.
Statement I During photorespiration, RuBP binds with CO_2 to form one molecule of phosphoglycolate and phosphoglycerate.
Statement II In this pathway, there is neither synthesis of sugars nor of ATP.
In the light of the above statements, choose the correct answer from the options given below.
(a) Both statement I and statement II are correct
(b) Both statement I and statement II are incorrect
(c) Statement I is correct, but statement II is incorrect
(d) Statement I is incorrect, but statement II is correct

117. Which of the following is correct with respect to phenylketonuria?
(a) Phenylketonuria is caused by the mutation in two genes that code for phenylalanine hydroxylase
(b) It is characterised by mental retardation and rise in skin pigmentation
(c) It is an autosomal recessive disorder
(d) The mutated gene can express itself in both homozygous and heterozygous conditions

118. Given below are two statements.
Statement I In *Pila*, body is covered by a calcareous shell and is unsegmented.
Statement II *Limulus* respires with book gills.
In the light of the above statements, choose the correct answer from the options given below
(a) Both statement I and statements II are false
(b) Statements I is true, but statement II is false
(c) Statements I is false, but statement II is true
(d) Both statements I and statements II are true

119. The NADH formed in glycolysis must be recycled to regenerate NAD^+, under anaerobic conditions. Yeast regenerates NAD^+ by
(a) transferring electrons from NADH to pyruvate
(b) transferring electrons from NADH to O_2 in mitochondrial respiration
(c) reducing pyruvate to ethanol and CO_2
(d) none of the above

120. Given below are two statements; one is labelled as Assertion (A) and the other is labelled as Reason (R).

Assertion (A) Most of the enzymes are proteins, which catalyse biochemical reactions.

Reason (R) The enzyme itself remains unchanged in the reaction, its presence allows the reaction to takes place.

(a) Both A and R are true and R is the correct explanation of A
(b) Both A and R are true, but R is not the correct explanation of A
(c) A is correct, but R is not correct
(d) A is not correct, but R is correct

121. Which of the following statement is correct about operon?

(a) A gene sequence that regulates other genes
(b) A protein binding subunit that enhances gene expression
(c) A cluster of structural genes with related functions
(d) A protein that inhibits translation

122. Which of the following set of cell organelles show the endomembrane system?

(a) Mitochondria, endoplasmic reticulum, Golgi apparatus, lysosomes
(b) Lysosomes, plastids, mitochondria, endoplasmic reticulum
(c) Golgi apparatus, endoplasmic reticulum, plastids, vacuoles
(d) Endoplasmic reticulum, Golgi apparatus, lysosomes, vacuole

123. Given below are two statements.

Statement I Mutations are indiscriminate with respect to the adaptive needs of organisms.

Statement II If genes are exchanged between two different population of a species, it is known as gene pool.

In the light of the above statements, choose the correct answer from the options given below

(a) Both statement I and statement II are correct
(b) Both statement I and statement II are incorrect
(c) Statement I is correct, but statement II is incorrect
(d) Statement I is incorrect, but statement II is correct

124. Which one of the following has diploid set of chromosomes?

(a) Secondary spermatocyte
(b) Secondary oocyte
(c) Primary spermatocyte
(d) Second polar body

125. Which one is not related to evil quartet with respect to biodiversity loss?

(a) Fragmentation of habitat
(b) High trophic level in food chain
(c) Over exploitation
(d) Alien species invasion

126. Consider the following statements.

I. During decomposition, decomposers breakdown complex inorganic substances into organic matters.
II. Detritus is the raw material for decomposition.
III. Detritivores breakdown detritus into smaller particles, this process is known as leaching.
IV. In catabolism, bacterial and fungal enzymes degrade raw material into simple inorganic substances.
V. Microbes play an important role in the mineralisation process.

Choose the correct set of statements from the options given below.

(a) I, III and IV (b) II, IV and V
(c) I, IV and V (d) II, III and IV

127. Identify the correct statements.

I. *Albugo* is a parasitic fungi that cause rust disease in mustard.
II. Many members of Ascomycetes such as morels and truffles are highly toxic and considered as non-edible fungi.
III. Mushrooms, bracket fungi or puff balls are commonly known forms of Basidiomycetes.
IV. Ascomycetes are commonly known as imperfect fungi.
V. The deuteromycetes reproduce only by asexual spores known as conidia.

Choose the correct answers from the options given below

(a) I, II and III
(b) I, III and V
(c) II, IV and V
(d) II, III and IV

128. Which of the following is an incorrect statement?

(a) Tobacco contains number of chemical substances including nicotine, an alkaloid
(b) Nicotine stimulates adrenal gland to release adrenaline and nor-adrenaline, which increase blood pressure and heart rate
(c) Tobacco chewing is associated with increased risk of cancer of the oral cavity
(d) Smoking reduces carbon monoxide content in blood and increases the concentration of haem-bound oxygen

129. The dominance of gametophyte is observed in

(a) bryophytes (b) pteridophytes
(c) angiosperms (d) gymnosperms

130. Which of the following techniques is not used for the early diagnosis of diseases?

(a) Recombinant DNA technology
(b) Polymerase chain reaction
(c) Enzyme linked immuno sorbent assay
(d) Serum and urine analysis

131. Consider the following statements with respect to *Rana tigrina* and choose the incorrect set of statements.

I. The vocal sacs help to produce mating calls.
II. Blood capillaries and pigment cells are present in the dermis.
III. Frogs have same method for respiration in land and in water.
IV. The sound producing organ of frog is the laryngotracheal chamber.
V. System for control and coordination is not well-developed.

Choose the correct answer from the options given below.

(a) I, II and IV (b) II, III and V
(c) III and V (d) IV and V

132. Consider the following statements.

I. One species can be distinguished from other closely related species based on the distinct morphological differences.
II. Plant families are characterised on the basis of stem height.
III. All organisms, including those in the plant and animal kingdoms have species as the lowest category.
IV. The process by which anything can be grouped into convenient categories based on easily observable characters is called classification.
V. Based on characteristics, all living organisms can be classified into different taxa.

Choose the correct set of statements from the options given below.

(a) I, II and III (b) I, III, IV and V
(c) III, IV and V (d) I, II and IV

133. Where among the following are the luminal and extra-luminal compartments situated respectively in the cell?

(a) Nucleus, cytoplasm
(b) Cytoplasm, plasma membrane
(c) Cytoplasm, inside ER
(d) Inside ER, cytoplasm

134. The outer layer of nuclear membrane is a part of

(a) mitochondrial membrane
(b) plasma membrane
(c) endoplasmic reticulum
(d) nucleoplasm

135. Which of the following vaccines are inactivated toxins?

(a) Attenuated (b) Conjugated
(c) Toxoids (d) Subunit

136. Myasthenia gravis is a term that describes

(a) a notch lying in the concavity of left lung
(b) an autoimmune disorder affecting neuromuscular junction leading to paralysis of skeletal muscles
(c) change in the ear pressure as we move away from the gravity
(d) joints containing fibrocartilage

137. All eukaryotic cells possess a *criss-cross* network of filamentous structures consisting of microtubules, microfilaments and intermediate filaments. This elaborate network is proteinaceous and is termed as ……… It is involved in ……… .

(a) hub ; cell division
(b) cytoskeleton ; mechanical support
(c) cytoskeleton ; flexibility
(d) axoneme ; motility

138. Read the following statements, choose the incorrect set of statements.

I. The primary structure of protein does not make a protein functional.
II. Due to the formation of hydrogen bonds, polypeptide chains assumes a secondary structure.

III. The unsaturated fatty acids have higher melting points than those of saturated fatty acids.
IV. The manner in which individual folded peptides are arranged with respect to each other is the architecture of a protein.
V. Nicotinamide adenine dinucleotide act as cofactor of oxidising enzymes.

Choose the correct answer from the options given below.
(a) I and IV (b) II and V (c) III and V (d) I and II

139. Given below are two statements.
Statement I After primary treatment of sewage, all solids that settle down form the primary sludge and the supernatant forms the effluent.
Statement II Spent slurry of biogas plant is used as fertiliser.

In the light of the above statements, choose the correct answer from the options given below.
(a) Both statement I and statement II are correct
(b) Both statement I and statement II are incorrect
(c) Statement I is correct, but statement II is incorrect
(d) Statement I is incorrect, but statement II is correct

140. From where did life originate on earth according to Oparin and Haldane?
(a) Thick red hot liquid
(b) Snowball earth
(c) Primordial soup
(d) Earthshake due to Tsunami

141. Of the five names given below, identify the diploid cells.
I. Nucellus II. Egg cell
III. Male gamete IV. Endosperm
V. Polar nuclei

Choose the correct option.
(a) III and V (b) IV and V
(c) I and V (d) All of these

142. Identify the correct statements.
I. Bryophytes are also called amphibians of the plant kingdom.
II. In mosses, the predominant stage of the life cycle is the gametophyte.
III. In bryophytes, sporophyte is free-living and attached to the photosynthetic gametophyte.
IV. Mosses along with fungi are the first organisms to colonise the rocks.
V. Pteridophytes are the first terrestrial plants to possess vascular tissues, i.e. xylem and phloem.

Choose the correct answer from the options given below.
(a) I, II and V (b) I, III and IV
(c) II, III and V (d) I, III and V

143. Which of the following conventions used in human pedigree is not paired correctly?

(a) 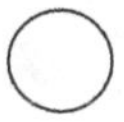 Female

(b)  Male

(c)  5 Unaffected offsprings

(d) 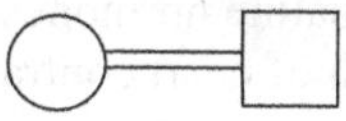 Parents (unrelated)

144. Which of the following represents the correct formula of family-Cruciferae?
(a) $\oplus ⚥ K_{2+2}C_4A_{2+4}\underline{G}_{(2)}$
(b) $\oplus ⚥ K_{3+3}C_4A_{2+4}\underline{G}_{(2)}$
(c) $\oplus ⚥ K_{2+2}C_3A_{2+4}\underline{G}_{(2)}$
(d) $\oplus ⚥ K_{2+2}C_4A_{3+3}G_{(2)}$

145. Puncturing of the diaphragm of a person would result in
(a) sudden unconsciousness which would be revived after some time
(b) stoppage of breathing and would be fatal
(c) diffusion of the residual volume of air
(d) collapse of the intercostal muscles

146. The extrastelar region forms
(a) intrafascicular cambium
(b) periderm
(c) ray initials
(d) all of the above

147. In dicot stem, the vascular bundles are
(a) scattered in ground tissue
(b) arranged in a ring
(c) closed and show bundle sheath
(d) not found at all

148. The region of the nephron found in the renal medulla is
(a) Malpighian corpuscle
(b) Proximal Convoluted Tubule (PCT)
(c) Distal Convoluted Tubule (DCT)
(d) Henle's loop

149. The recent illegal introduction of the African catfish *Clarias gariepinus* for aquaculture purposes is posing a threat to the indigenous catfishes in our rivers. Which of the following options correctly describes the cause of this biodiversity loss?
(a) Habitat loss and fragmentation
(b) Over exploitation
(c) Alien-species invasion
(d) Co-extinctions

150. Which of the following statements is not true with reference to hormones?
(a) Adrenaline and nor-adrenaline hormones increase the heartbeat, the strength of heart contraction and the rate of respiration
(b) Catecholamines stimulate the breakdown of glycogen
(c) Cholecystokinin stimulate gluconeogenesis lipolysis and proteolysis
(d) Gastrin acts on the gastric glands and stimulates the secretion of HCl and pepsinogen

151. Which one of the following pituitary hormones does not stimulate the other endocrine glands?
(a) Thyrotropin (b) Gonadotropin
(c) Somatotropin (d) Adrenocorticotropin

152. The stone cells that possess suberised thick secondary walls are
(a) sclereids (b) aerenchyma
(c) stellate parenchyma (d) angular collenchyma

153. Given below are two statements; one is labelled as Assertion (A) and the other is labelled as Reason (R).

Assertion (A) Mutualism is a type of positive interaction.

Reason (R) In mutualism, one organism is benefitted, while other is harmed.

In the light of the above statements, choose the correct answer from the options given below.
(a) A is false, but R is true
(b) Both A and R are true and R is the correct explanation of A
(c) Both A and R are true, but R is not the correct explanation of A
(d) A is true, but R is false

154. The first heart sound is associated with
(a) opening of the tricuspid and bicuspid valves
(b) closure of the tricuspid and bicuspid valves
(c) opening of pulmonary and tricuspid valves
(d) closure of bicuspid and aortic valves

155. A common disease with symptoms like tremors, rigidity, a stiff shuffling walk and memory loss is observed in an individual. Which part of the brain will thus be affected during the disease?
(a) Medulla (b) Cerebrum
(c) Midbrain (d) Hypothalamus

156. Match List I with List II.

	List I		List II
A.	Zeatin	1.	Ethylene
B.	IBA	2.	Synthetic auxin
C.	NAA	3.	Cytokinin
D.	Ethephon	4.	Natural auxin

Choose the correct answer from the options given below.

	A	B	C	D
(a)	3	4	2	1
(b)	1	2	4	3
(c)	1	4	2	3
(d)	3	2	4	1

157. The portion between two successive 'Z' lines is considered as the functional unit of contraction and is called a
(a) collagen (b) sarcomere
(c) band (d) myofibril

158. How is a eukaryotic genome different from a bacterial genome?
(a) In having enzyme reverse transcriptase
(b) In having start and stop codons
(c) Presence of introns
(d) Having thymine instead of uracil

159. What is the role of water (H_2O) during photosynthesis?
(a) It supplies electrons in the reactions of the light dependent phase
(b) It absorbs the excess light energy
(c) It transports hydrogen ions in Hill reaction
(d) It provides oxygen for Hill reaction

160. Consider the graph given below.

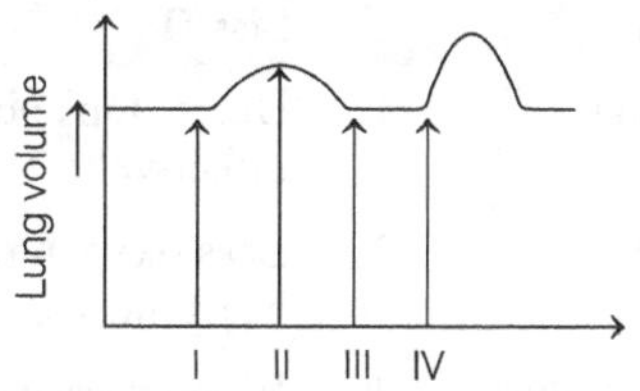

Identify the correct label with its respective characteristic.

(a) IV – Ribs fully expanded
(b) III – Air drawn out of the lungs
(c) I – Lungs completely deflated
(d) II – Contraction of trachea

161. Which of the following does not belong to the super class–Tetrapoda?

(a) Reptilia (b) Amphibia
(c) Osteichthyes (d) Aves

162. In frogs, male reproductive organ consists of a pair of yellowish ovoid testes, which are found adhered to the upper part of kidneys by a double fold of peritonium called

(a) Bidder's canal (b) mesorchium
(c) urinogential duct (d) cloaca

163. Nitrogen-fixation genes can be introduced into non-legumes by which of the following methods?

(a) Incubating *r*DNA with cells in divalent cations
(b) Embryo culture
(c) Gene gun
(d) Hybridisation

164. Given below are two statements; one is labelled as Assertion (A) and the other is labelled as Reason (R).

Assertion (A) In a continuous culture system, cells are maintained in a log/exponential phase.

Reason (R) In this system nutrient availability is unlimited.

In the light of the above statements, choose the correct answers from the options given below.

(a) A is false, but R is true
(b) Both A and R are true and R is the correct explanation of A
(c) Both A and R are true, but R is not the correct explanation of A
(d) A is true, but R is false

165. Which of the following cell organelle principally performs the function of packaging materials, to be delivered either to the intra-cellular targets or secreted outside the cell?

(a) Endoplasmic reticulum (b) Golgi apparatus
(c) Lysosomes (d) Vacuoles

166. The diagram given below, shows various organs that aid in breathing in case of humans.

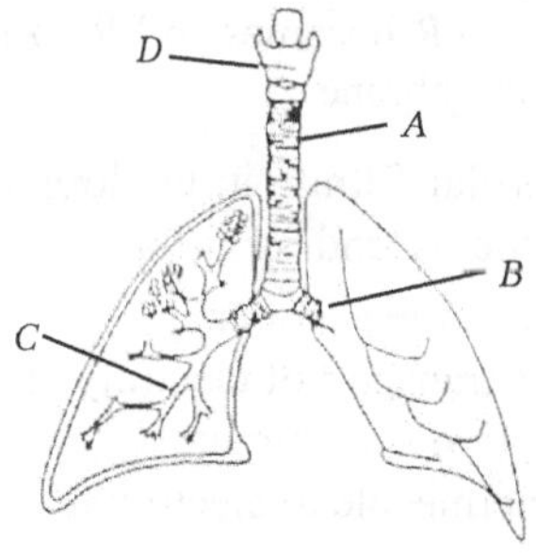

Choose the incorrect statement w.r.t parts labelled as A-D.

(a) A represents trachea, also know as windpipe.
(b) B represents bronchus which are the first branches of trachea.
(c) D represents larynx, found in the posterior neck at the level of 2nd to 5th cervical vertebrae.
(d) C are finer branches of bronchi which eventually form alveolar duct.

167. Which of the following statement is incorrect with respect to the plants showing photorespiraton?

(a) There is enhancement of CO_2 assimilation in light and high concentration of oxygen
(b) In C_3 plants, CO_2 fixation is decreased
(c) It is biologically important pathway
(d) It does not occur in C_4 plants

168. Match List I with List II.

	List I		List II
A.	Red algae	1.	*Spirogyra*
B.	Green algae	2.	*Fucus*
C.	Brown algae	3.	*Porphyra*
D.	Mosses	4.	*Polytrichum*

Choose the correct answer from the options given below.

	A	B	C	D		A	B	C	D
(a)	2	1	3	4	(b)	3	2	4	1
(c)	4	1	2	3	(d)	3	1	2	4

169. Which of the following correctly represents the sequence of cell organelles in secretion of proteins from the cell?

(a) Nucleus → Ribosomes → ER → Golgi apparatus Lysosomes → Plasma membrane
(b) Nucleus → ER → Ribosomes → Golgi apparatus → Lysosomes → Plasma membrane
(c) Nucleus → ER → Ribosomes → Golgi apparatus → Secretory vesicles → Plasma membrane
(d) Nucleus → Ribosomes → ER → Lysosomes → Plasma membrane

170. The glomerular filtrate in the loop of Henle gets diluted in the ascending limb as

(a) it is permeable to water
(b) it allows transport of electrolytes
(c) reabsorption is maximum
(d) it is impermeable to electrolytes

171. Consider the following statements and identify the correct set of statements.

I. The positively charged DNA is wrapped around the negatively charged histone octamer.
II. A typical nucleosome contains 200 bp of DNA helix.
III. The plane of one base pair stacks over the other in double helix.
IV. DNA with higher percentage of A=T have more density than those with higher percentage of G≡C.
V. 1μm of DNA contains about 300 base pairs.

Choose the correct answer from the options given below.

(a) II, III and V (b) I, III and IV
(c) III, IV and V (d) I, II and V

172. Consider the given statements regarding muscle protein.

I. Thick filaments constitute mainly of myosin protein.
II. Myosin is splitted by an enzyme trypsin into LMM and HMM.
III. ATPase requires Na^+ for its functioning.
IV. Sub-fragment S_2 contains ATPase binding sites.
V. Rigor mortis is caused due to incomplete depletion of ATP and phosphocreatine.

Which of the following above statements is/are correct?

(a) Only I (b) I and II
(c) II and III (d) Only IV

173. Match List I with List II.

	List I		List II
A.	Angina	1.	Heart stops pumping blood effectively
B.	CAD	2.	Less oxygen reaching the heart muscle
C.	Heart failure	3.	Blood pressure higher than normal
D.	Hypertension	4.	Deposition of calcium, fat, cholesterol, etc.

Choose the correct answer from the options given below.

	A	B	C	D		A	B	C	D
(a)	2	4	1	3	(b)	1	3	2	4
(c)	3	2	4	1	(d)	4	1	3	2

174. Which of the following statement is not true?

(a) BAC and YAC are the commonly used vectors in human genome sequencing
(b) During HGP, the fragments were sequenced using automated DNA sequences that worked on the principle of a method developed by Marshall Nirenberg
(c) *Caenorhabditis, Drosophila*, and *Arabidopsis* have also been completely sequenced
(d) The human genome contains 3164.7 million nucleotide base

175. Choose the correct identification for the given stage in mitosis.

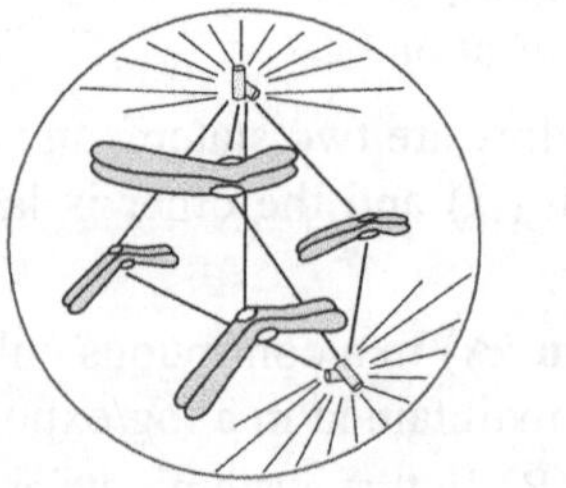

(a) Chromatids moving to opposite poles
(b) Transition to metaphase
(c) Formation of compact mitotic chromosome
(d) Development of nuclear envelope arround chromosome

176. The sequence of events in a nerve conduction is

(a) Threshold → Depolarisation → Repolarisation → Hyperpolarisation
(b) Hyperpolarisation → Repolarisation → Depolarisation

(c) Repolarisation → Threshold → Depolarisation → Hyperpolarisation
(d) Resting potential → Repolarisation → Depolarisation

177. Match List I with List II.

	List I		List II
A.	IUT	1.	Copper releasing IUDs
B.	Multiload 375	2.	Non-medicated IUDs
C.	ZIFT	3.	Embryos with more than 8 blastomeres
D.	Lippes loop	4.	Zygote upto 8 blastomeres

Choose the correct answer from the options given below.

	A	B	C	D
(a)	1	3	2	4
(b)	3	1	4	2
(c)	3	2	4	1
(d)	1	2	3	4

178. Given below are two statements; one is labelled as Assertion (A) and the other is labelled as Reason (R).

Assertion (A) In most ecosystems, all the pyramids of number, energy and biomass are upright.

Reason (R) Energy at higher tropic level is always more than a lower level.

In the light of the above statements, choose the correct answer from the options given below.
(a) A is false, but R is true
(b) Both A and R are true and R is the correct explanation of A
(c) Both A and R are true, but R is not the correct explanation of A
(d) A is true, but R is false

179. Given below are two statements; one is labelled as Assertion (A) and the other labelled as Reason (R).

Assertion (A) Bottled fruit juices are more clearer as compared to home made ones.

Reason (R) The bottled juice are clarified with the help of lipase.

In the light of the above statements, choose the correct answer from the options given below.
(a) Both A and R are true and R is the correct explanation of A
(b) Both A and R are true, but R is not the correct explanation of A
(c) A is true, but R is false
(d) A is false, but R is true

180. Which among the following statements is/are correct regarding J-shaped growth curve?
(a) Minor fluctuations are not observed
(b) Environmental resistance does not operate
(c) Equilibrium phase is rarely reached
(d) All of the above

Explanations

Physics

1. (d) In steady state, there will be no current in the capacitor branch. Net resistance of the first parallel branch and cell,

$$R = 1 + 1 + 0.5 = 2.5\,\Omega$$

Current drawn from the cell, $i = \frac{E}{R} = \frac{2.5}{2.5} = 1\,\text{A}$

Potential drop across two parallel branches,

$$V = E - ir = 2.5 - 1 \times 0.5 = 2.5 - 0.5 = 2.0\,\text{V}$$

So, charge on the capacitor plates

$$q = CV = 5 \times 10^{-6} \times 2 = 10\,\mu\text{C}$$

2. (b) Given, initial area, $A_1 = (10 \times 6)\,\text{cm}^2$

$$= 60 \times 10^{-4}\ \text{m}^2$$

Final area, $A_2 = (10 \times 11)\,\text{cm}^2$

$$= 110 \times 10^{-4}\ \text{m}^2$$

Work done, $W = 3 \times 10^{-4}$ J

As we know that, $W = 2T\Delta A$

$$T = \frac{W}{2(A_2 - A_1)}$$

$$= \frac{3 \times 10^{-4}}{2 \times 50 \times 10^{-4}} = 3 \times 10^{-2}\ \text{N/m}$$

3. (a) Resonance frequency, $f = \frac{1}{\sqrt{LC}}$

For f = constant $C \propto \frac{1}{L}$

When L is changed to $L/2$, C must be changed to $2C$ to keep f same.

4. (a) As, $A = \overline{\overline{X} \cdot \overline{Y}} = \overline{\overline{X + Y}}$ $\quad (\because \overline{A} \cdot \overline{B} = \overline{A + B})$

$B = \overline{\overline{\overline{X + Y}} \cdot \overline{\overline{Z}}}$ $\quad$ (NAND gate)

$= \overline{\overline{\overline{X + Y}}} + \overline{\overline{\overline{Z}}} = X + Y + Z$

5. (c) Let, u be the initial velocity and a be uniform acceleration.

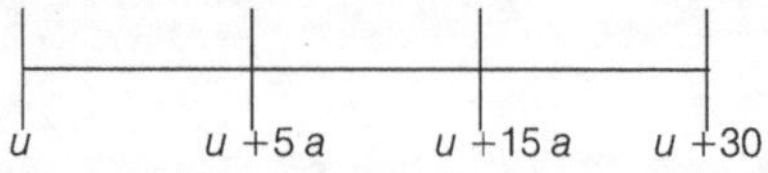

Then, average velocities are,

$$v_1 = \frac{u + u + 5a}{2} = u + \frac{5}{2}a$$

$$v_2 = \frac{u + 5a + u + 15a}{2} = u + 10a$$

$$v_3 = \frac{u + 15a + u + 30a}{2} = u + \frac{45}{2}a$$

$$\therefore \quad \frac{v_1 - v_2}{v_2 - v_3} = \frac{\frac{5}{2}a - 10a}{10a - \frac{45}{2}a} = \frac{-15a}{-25a} = \frac{15}{25} = \frac{3}{5}$$

6. (c) Least count $= \frac{\text{Pitch}}{\text{Number of divisions}} = \frac{0.5\text{mm}}{50}$

$$= 0.01\,\text{mm}$$

Diameter of ball, $D = \text{MSR} + \text{CSR} \times \text{LC}$

$$= 2.5 + 20 \times 0.01 = 2.7\,\text{mm}$$

Density, $\rho = \frac{\text{Mass}}{\text{Volume}} = \frac{M}{\frac{4}{3}\pi\left(\frac{D}{2}\right)^3}$

Percentage error in density, $\frac{\Delta\rho}{\rho} \times 100$

$$= \frac{\Delta M}{M} \times 100 + \frac{3\Delta D}{D} \times 100$$

$$= 2\% + 3 \times \frac{0.01}{2.7} \times 100$$

$$= 2\% + 1.1\% = 3.1\,\%$$

Problem Solving Tactics	Ensure consistent units are used throughout of the calculations to avoid errors.

7. (c) Given, $\mathbf{v}_i = 30\hat{\mathbf{i}}$ m/s

$\mathbf{v}_f = 40\hat{\mathbf{j}}$ m/s

Average acceleration, $\mathbf{a} = \frac{\mathbf{v}_f - \mathbf{v}_i}{\text{Total time}}$

$$\therefore \quad a = \frac{|\mathbf{v}_f - \mathbf{v}_i|}{\Delta t} = \frac{\sqrt{(40)^2 + (30)^2}}{10}$$

$$= \frac{\sqrt{1600 + 900}}{10} = 5\,\text{ms}^{-2}$$

8. (c) Given, $m = 500\,\text{kg}$, $v = 36\,\text{kmh}^{-1}$

$= 36 \times \frac{5}{18}\,\text{ms}^{-1} = 10\,\text{ms}^{-1}$ and $r = 50\,\text{m}$

Now, centripetal force, $F = \frac{mv^2}{r} = \frac{500 \times (10)^2}{50} = 1000\,\text{N}$

9. (b) Given, $V_p = 800\,\text{V}$

$I_s = 20\,\text{A}, V_s = 220\,\text{V}$

Efficiency, $\eta = 80\%$

$I_p = ?$

For a transformer, we know that,

$$\eta = \frac{\text{Output power}}{\text{Input power}}$$

$$\Rightarrow \frac{80}{100} = \frac{V_s I_s}{V_p I_p}$$

$$\Rightarrow \frac{4}{5} = \frac{220 \times 20}{800 \times I_p}$$

$$\Rightarrow \frac{4}{5} = \frac{11}{2I_p} \Rightarrow I_p = \frac{55}{8}$$

$$\Rightarrow I_p = 6.875 \text{ A}$$

10. (b) Given, length of air column,

$$L = 40\text{cm} = 0.4\text{m}$$

Let the air column be closed.

For first harmonic,

$$\Rightarrow \lambda = 4L$$

$$\Rightarrow \lambda = 4 \times (0.4) = 1.6 \text{ m}$$

Velocity of sound in air,

$$v = f\lambda = 450 \times 1.6 = 720 \text{ ms}^{-1}$$

11. (d) Emission transitions can take place between any higher energy level and any energy level below it, while absorption transitions start from the lowest energy level only and may end at any higher energy level. Hence, number of absorptions transitions between two given levels is always less than the number of emission transitions between same two levels.

Since hydrogen shows both absorption spectrum as well as emission spectrum. Hence, both statements are incorrect.

12. (b) When n resistors are connected in parallel, then

$$\frac{1}{P} = \frac{1}{R_1} + \frac{1}{R_2} + \frac{1}{R_3} + \ldots\ldots + \frac{1}{R_n} \quad \ldots\text{(i)}$$

When last resistor is removed, then

$$\frac{1}{Q} = \frac{1}{R_1} + \frac{1}{R_2} + \frac{1}{R_3} + \ldots + \frac{1}{R_{n-1}} \quad \ldots\text{(ii)}$$

Subtracting Eq. (i) from Eq. (ii), then

$$\frac{1}{P} - \frac{1}{Q} = \frac{1}{R_n}$$

$$\frac{Q-P}{PQ} = \frac{1}{R_n} \Rightarrow R_n = \frac{PQ}{Q-P}$$

13. (c) Potential difference across $2\,k\Omega$ resistor,

$$V = V_Z = 12 \text{ V}$$

$\therefore$ Current through resistor $2\,k\Omega$

$$I = \frac{V}{R} = \frac{12}{2 \times 10^3} = 6 \times 10^{-3} \text{ A} = 6 \text{mA}$$

14. (b) Given, 10 VSD = 9 MSD, 1 MSD = 1 mm

$\therefore$ Least count, LC = 1 MSD − 1 VSD

$$= \left(1 - \frac{9}{10}\right) \text{VSD} = \frac{1}{10} \times 1 = 0.01 \text{cm}$$

$\therefore$ The diameter of the spherical body is

$$d = \text{MSR} + \text{VSR} \times \text{LC}$$

$$= 3 + 6 \times 0.01 = 3.06 \text{ cm}$$

15. (a) For a small angle $d\theta$,

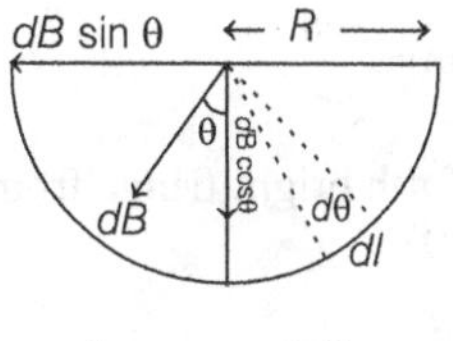

$$dI = \frac{I}{\pi R} R d\theta = \frac{I d\theta}{\pi}$$

$$dB = \frac{\mu_0 dI}{2\pi R} = \frac{\mu_0 I d\theta}{2\pi^2 R}$$

The magnitude of the magnetic induction along its axis,

$$B_a = \int_0^\pi dB \sin\theta$$

So, $$B_a = \frac{\mu_0 I}{\pi^2 R}$$

16. (d) The de-Broglie wavelength of electron

$$\lambda = \frac{h}{mv} \Rightarrow v = \frac{h}{m\lambda} \quad \ldots\text{(i)}$$

Energy of photon, $E_p = \dfrac{hc}{\lambda}$ (Since, λ is same)

So, required ratio, $\dfrac{E_p}{E_e} = \dfrac{hc/\lambda}{\frac{1}{2}mv^2} = \dfrac{2hc}{\lambda mv^2}$

Substituting value of v from Eq. (i), we get

$$\frac{E_p}{E_e} = \frac{2hc}{\lambda m\left(\frac{h}{m\lambda}\right)^2} = \frac{2\lambda mc}{h}$$

17. (c) Mass of hemisphere $= \dfrac{2}{3}\pi r^3 \rho$

Mass of cone $= \dfrac{1}{3}\pi r^2 h\rho$

The mass moments about the centre of mass is zero.

So, $$m_H\left(\frac{3r}{8}\right) = m_C\left(\frac{h}{4}\right)$$

$$\Rightarrow \frac{2}{3}\pi r^3 \rho \times \frac{3r}{8} = \frac{\pi r^2 h\rho}{3} \times \frac{h}{4}$$

$$\Rightarrow h^2 = 3r^2 \text{ or } h = \sqrt{3}\, r = 2\sqrt{3} \text{ m}$$

18. (b) Impulse imparted to ball = Change in linear momentum

$= mv$

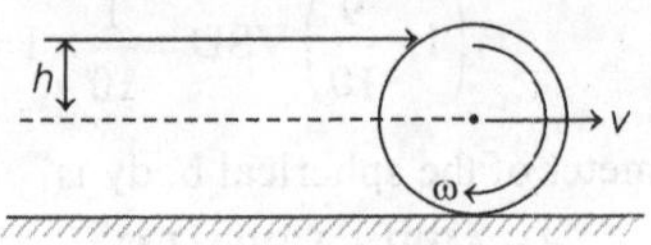

As, angular momentum = moment of linear momentum

$$I\omega = mvh \Rightarrow \frac{2}{5}mr^2\omega = mvh$$

$$\Rightarrow \quad \omega = \frac{5vh}{2r^2}$$

19. (d) Distance of nth bright fringe from the centre,

$$y_n = \frac{nD\lambda}{d}$$

$$y_3 = \frac{3\times 2.5\times 6000\times 10^{-10}}{0.5\times 10^{-3}} = 9\times 10^{-3}\,\text{m} = 9\,\text{mm}$$

20. (c) For first refracting surface,

For parallel beam of light, $u = -\infty$

$$-\frac{\mu_1}{u} + \frac{\mu_2}{v} = \frac{\mu_2 - \mu_1}{R}$$

$$\Rightarrow \quad -\frac{1.4}{-\infty} + \frac{1.5}{v} = \frac{1.5 - 1.4}{R}$$

$$v = 15R$$

For second refracting surface,

$$-\frac{\mu_2}{15R} + \frac{\mu_3}{v'} = \frac{\mu_3 - \mu_2}{-R}$$

$$\Rightarrow \quad -\frac{1.5}{15R} + \frac{1.6}{v'} = \frac{1.6 - 1.5}{-R} \Rightarrow v' = \infty$$

Hence, the combination behaves as glass plate.

21. (c) Work done by moving charge particle on equipotential surface is zero because potential difference is zero.

22. (d) From Gauss' theorem,

$$\phi_E = \frac{q_{\text{in}}}{\varepsilon_0} = \frac{+8e - 8e}{\varepsilon_0} = 0$$

23. (a) Let, a wire of length L is bent in a circular form of radius r

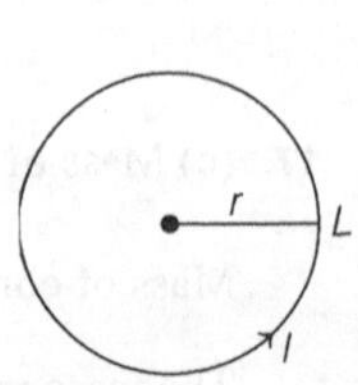

$$2\pi r = L$$

$$\Rightarrow \quad r = \frac{L}{2\pi} \quad \text{...(i)}$$

The magnetic dipole moment of a circular ring,

$$M = IA$$

$$M = I\pi r^2 \quad \text{...(ii)}$$

On putting the the value of r from Eq. (ii), we get

$$\Rightarrow \quad M = I\pi\left(\frac{L}{2\pi}\right)^2 = I\pi\frac{L^2}{4\pi^2} = \frac{IL^2}{4\pi}$$

24. (c) Given, $l = 2\,\text{m}$, $v = 4\,\text{ms}^{-1}$

$$B = 1\,\text{G} = 10^{-4}\,\text{T}$$

$\therefore$ Induced emf, $e = Bvl = 10^{-4}\times 4\times 2$

$$= 8\times 10^{-4}\,\text{V} = 0.8\times 10^{-3}\,\text{V}$$

$$= 0.8\,\text{mV}$$

25. (c) Refractive index of the glass fibre, $\mu = 1.5$

Speed of light in the given medium, $v = \frac{c}{\mu}$

Critical angle for glass-fibre-air

$$i_c = \sin^{-1}\left(\frac{1}{n}\right) = \sin^{-1}\left(\frac{1}{1.5}\right)$$

$$i_c \approx 42^\circ$$

$\because i > i_c$, TIR will take place.

Length of the fibre, $l = 1\,\text{km} = 1000\,\text{m}$

Angle of incidence, $\theta = 60°$

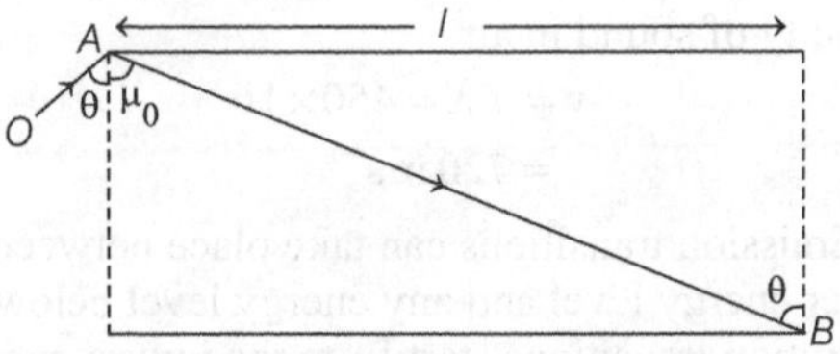

The time taken to cover the length l in the fibre,

$$t = \frac{l}{v} = \frac{l}{(c/\mu)} = \frac{\mu l}{c\sin\theta} \quad \left[\because AB = \frac{l}{\sin\theta}\right]$$

$$= \frac{1.5\times 1000}{(3\times 10^8)\sin 60^\circ}$$

$$t = 5.77\times 10^{-6}\,\text{s} = 5.77\,\mu\text{s}$$

26. (b) Buoyant force, $F = mg$

where, m = mass of water displaced

Given, $V_w = \frac{1}{2}V_b$

where, V_w = volume of water displaced

and V_b = volume of ball.

$$\Rightarrow \quad V_w = \frac{1}{2}\left(\frac{4}{3}\pi r^3\right) = \frac{2}{3}\pi(0.12)^3$$

$[\because r = 12\,\text{cm} = 0.12\,\text{m}]$

$\therefore \quad F = \rho V_w g$ (where, ρ = density of water)

$$= 1000\times\frac{2}{3}\pi(0.12)^3\times 9.8 = 35\,\text{N}$$

27. (a) Given, $g = 10\,\text{ms}^{-2}$

$$h = 20\,\text{m and } u = 0$$

we have, $v = \sqrt{2gh} = \sqrt{2\times 10\times 20}$

$$= \sqrt{400} = 20\,\text{ms}^{-1}$$

28. (b) Given, $v=\sqrt{PQ}+QT+\frac{R}{S+t}$

According to principle of homogeneity

$$[v]=[Q][T]$$

$$\Rightarrow \quad [LT^{-1}]=[Q][T] \Rightarrow Q=[LT^{-2}]$$

Therefore, dimensions of Q are same as dimensions of a acceleration.

Hence, acceleration represented by Q.

29. (c) Acceleration of man in lift, $a_{man}=-a\hat{j}$

Acceleration of ball, $a_{ball}=-g\hat{j}$

Here, $\hat{j}$ represents downward direction.

∴ Relative acceleration,

$$a_{rel}=a_{ball}-a_{man}=-(g-a)\hat{j}$$

∴ Acceleration observed by man in downward direction in lift $=g-a$

30. (c) It is a adiabatic process, so

$$p^{(1-\gamma)}T^{\gamma}=\text{constant}$$

$$\left(\frac{p_2}{p_1}\right)^{\gamma-1}=\left(\frac{T_2}{T_1}\right)^{\gamma}$$

When tyre burst, $p_2=1$ atm

$$\left(\frac{1}{3}\right)^{1.4-1}=\left(\frac{T_2}{300}\right)^{1.4} \qquad \left[\because \gamma_{air}=\frac{7}{5}=1.4\right]$$

$$0.4\,[\log 1-\log 3]=1.4\,[\log T_2-\log 300]$$

$$T_2=219\,K$$

31. (a) Given, $F=100\,N$

$Q=2\times10^{-4}\,C$

$$\therefore \quad E=\frac{F}{Q}=\frac{100}{2\times10^{-4}}=50\times10^{4}$$

$$=5\times10^{5}\ N/C$$

32. (b) The displacement current is given by

$$I_D=\varepsilon_0\frac{d\phi_\varepsilon}{dt}=\varepsilon_0\frac{d}{dt}\left(\frac{q}{\varepsilon_0}\right)$$

Also, $\quad I_D=\varepsilon_0\cdot A\frac{dE}{dt}$

where, A is the area of the plate.

Hence, displacement current goes through the gap between the plates of a capacitor, when charge on capacitor and electric field does not remain constant but changes with time.

33. (c) $q_A=\frac{Q}{2}$

When C is earthed,

$$V_C=0$$

$$\therefore \quad \frac{Kq_C}{a}+\frac{K(Q/2)}{d}-\frac{K(Qa/2d)}{d}=0$$

$$\therefore \quad q_C=\frac{Qa^2}{2d^2}-\frac{Qa}{2d}$$

$$=\frac{Qa}{2d}\left(\frac{a}{d}-1\right)=\frac{Qa}{2d}\left(\frac{a-d}{d}\right)$$

34. (c) When current is uniformly distributed, then

Magnetic field of inside conductor, $B=\frac{\mu_0 I}{2\pi R^2}r$

$$\therefore \quad B\propto r$$

Magnetic field of outside conductor, $B=\frac{\mu_0 I}{2\pi r}$

$$\therefore \quad B\propto\frac{1}{r}$$

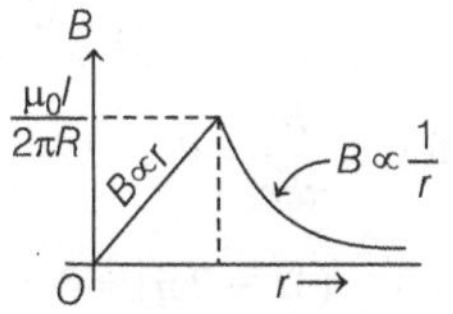

Hence, correct option is (c).

35. (d) Reduced mass, $\mu=\frac{(m)(m)}{m+m}=\frac{m}{2}$

The given system is equivalent to a system of a particle of mass $\frac{m}{2}$ connected to a spring of stiffness k rigidly.

The required period of oscillation,

$$T=2\pi\sqrt{\frac{\mu}{k}}=2\pi\sqrt{\frac{\frac{m}{2}}{k}}=\pi\sqrt{\frac{2m}{k}}$$

36. (d) The closed circuit $ABQP$ and $PQDC$ are balanced Wheatstone bridge circuits, therefore resistance between E and F and between F and G (each equal to $2r$) do not contribute i.e., these are ineffective.

Thus, the circuit simplifies to the figure given below.

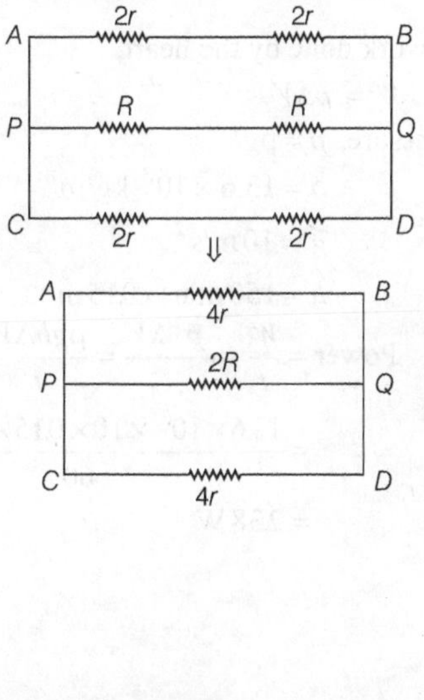

∴ Effective resistance between point A and B is given as

$$\frac{1}{R_{AB}} = \frac{1}{4r} + \frac{1}{2R} + \frac{1}{4r}$$

$$= \frac{R+2r+R}{4Rr} = \frac{R+r}{2Rr}$$

$$\Rightarrow \quad R_{AB} = \frac{2Rr}{R+r}$$

37. (a) At time t, the velocity of the ball will be maximum and it goes on decreasing with respect to time.
At the highest point of path, its velocity beocmes zero, then it increases but direction is reversed.
Thus, the relation between the velocity with time t is represented by the graph (a).

38. (c) Let, $m_1 = m$ and $m_2 = M - m$, then

$$F = \frac{Gm(M-m)}{r^2} = \frac{G}{r^2}(Mm - m^2)$$

For maximum force, $\frac{dF}{dm} = 0$

$$\Rightarrow \quad \frac{G}{r^2}(M - 2m) = 0$$

$$\Rightarrow \quad M = 2m \text{ or } m = \frac{M}{2}$$

$$\therefore \quad m_1 = m_2 = \frac{M}{2}$$

39. (b) Increase in surface energy
= Work done = Increase in area × Surface tension

∴ Increase in surface area,

$$\Delta A = (5\times4 - 4\times2)\times2$$

(∵ film has two surfaces)

$$= (20-8)\times2 = 24\text{ cm}^2$$

$$= 24\times10^{-4}\text{ m}^2$$

So, work done, $W = T\cdot\Delta A$

$$3\times10^{-4} = T\times24\times10^{-4}$$

$$T = \frac{1}{8} = 0.125\text{ N/m}$$

40. (a) Here, work done by the heart,

$$W = p\Delta V$$

where, pressure, $p = \rho gh$

Given, $\rho = 13.6\times10^3\text{ kg/m}^3$

$$g = 10\text{ m/s}^2$$

$$h = 150\text{ mm} = 0.15\text{ m}$$

$$\therefore \quad \text{Power} = \frac{W}{t} = \frac{p\cdot\Delta V}{t} = \frac{\rho gh\Delta V}{t}$$

$$= \frac{13.6\times10^3\times10\times0.15\times7\times10^{-3}}{60}$$

$$= 2.38\text{ W}$$

41. (c) Here, wavelength of spectral line,

$$\lambda = 102.7\text{ nm} = 1.027\times10^{-7}\text{ m}$$

The energy of emitted photon,

$$E = \frac{hc}{\lambda} = \frac{6.626\times10^{-34}\times3\times10^8}{1.027\times10^{-7}}\text{ J}$$

$$= 1.936\times10^{-18}\text{ J}$$

$$= \frac{1.936\times10^{-18}}{1.6\times10^{-19}}\text{ eV}$$

$$= 12.1\text{ eV}$$

This energy corresponds to the transition D for which the energy change

$$= -1.5 - (-13.6) = 12.1\text{ eV}$$

42. (d) For first line of Lyman series, $n_1 = 1$ and $n_2 = 2$

$$\therefore \quad \frac{1}{\lambda_1} = R\left(\frac{1}{1^2} - \frac{1}{2^2}\right) = R\left(1 - \frac{1}{4}\right) = \frac{3R}{4}$$

For first line of Paschen series,

$$n_1 = 3 \text{ and } n_2 = 4$$

$$\therefore \quad \frac{1}{\lambda_2} = R\left(\frac{1}{3^2} - \frac{1}{4^2}\right)$$

$$= R\left(\frac{1}{9} - \frac{1}{16}\right) = \frac{7R}{144}$$

$$\frac{\lambda_1}{\lambda_2} = \frac{7R}{144}\times\frac{4}{3R} = \frac{7}{108}$$

43. (d) The weight of the body on earth is

$$mg = \frac{GMm}{R^2} = 72\text{ kgf}$$

Then, on mars surface, the value of g becomes

$$g' = \frac{GM'}{R'^2} = \frac{GM/9}{(R/2)^2} = \frac{4GM}{9R^2}$$

$$\Rightarrow \quad g' = \frac{4}{9}g$$

The weight of body on mars is

$$mg' = m\times\frac{4}{9}g = \frac{4}{9}mg$$

$$= \frac{4}{9}\times72 = 32\text{ kgf}$$

44. (a) Let, d be the distance travelled by ray in the direction of mirror, then

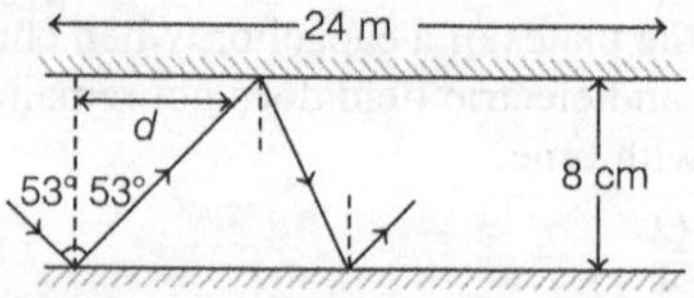

$$\tan 53° = \frac{d}{8\times10^{-2}}$$

$$d = 8\times 10^{-2}\tan 53^\circ = 8\times\frac{4}{3}\times 10^{-2}$$
$$= \frac{0.32}{3}\text{ m}$$

Total number of reflections before it reaches the other end, $N = \frac{24}{d} = \frac{24}{0.32/3} = \frac{24\times 3}{0.32}$
$$= 225$$

45. (a) As, $C_V = \frac{R}{\gamma - 1}$

For monoatomic gas, $C_V = \frac{R}{\frac{5}{3}-1} = \frac{3}{2}R$

For diatomic gas, $C'_V = \frac{R}{\frac{7}{5}-1} = \frac{5}{2}R$

For mixture, $C''_V = \frac{nC_V + n'C'_V}{n+n'}$
$$= \frac{1\times\frac{3}{2}R + 3\times\frac{5}{2}R}{1+3}$$
$$= \frac{9}{4}R = \frac{9}{4}\times 8.3$$
$$= 18.7\text{ JK}^{-1}\text{ mol}^{-1}$$

Chemistry

46. (a) $p_1 = 100\text{ kPa}, (t_{1/2})_1 = 364\text{ s}$
$p_2 = 50\text{ kPa}, (t_{1/2})_2 = 182\text{ s}$
$$(t_{1/2})_1 = \frac{1}{k(p_1)^{n-1}} \text{ and } (t_{1/2})_2 = \frac{1}{k(p_2)^{n-1}}$$

Divide first half-life by second half-life.
$$\frac{(t_{1/2})_1}{(t_{1/2})_2} = \frac{(p_2)^{n-1}}{(p_1)^{n-1}}$$

Now substitute given values in above equation
$$\frac{364}{182} = \left(\frac{50}{100}\right)^{n-1}$$
$$2 = \left(\frac{1}{2}\right)^{n-1}$$
$$n-1 = -1$$
$$n = 0$$

∴ The order of the reaction is zero.

47. (a) Weight of benzene $= V\times d$
$$= 50\times 0.879\text{ g} = 43.95\text{ g}$$

Weight of compound = 0.643 g

$$\Delta T_f = 50.51 - 50.03 = 0.48$$
$$\therefore\ \Delta T_f = K_f\times\frac{w_{\text{compound}}}{M}\times\frac{1000}{w_{\text{benzene}}}$$
$$0.48 = 5.12\times\frac{0.643}{M}\times\frac{1000}{43.95}$$
$$\therefore\ M \approx 156.05\text{ g mol}^{-1}$$

48. (a) Percentage of chlorine
$$= \frac{35.5}{143.5}\times\frac{\text{mass of AgCl}}{\text{mass of the compound}}\times 100$$
$$= \frac{35.5}{143.5}\times\frac{0.287}{0.099}\times 100 \approx 71.71\%$$

Problem Solving Tactics

Halogens are estimated by process known as Carius method. In this method, Percentage of halogen (X) can be calculated as by using the formula
$$= \frac{\text{At. mass of halogen}\times\text{Mass of Ag}X\times 100}{\text{Molar mass of Ag}X\times\text{Mass of compound}}$$

49. (d)

	$N_2O_4 \rightleftharpoons$	$2NO_2$
Initial moles	1	0
Moles at equilibrium	$1-\alpha$	2α

∴ Total number of moles at equilibrium
$$= 1-\alpha+2\alpha = 1+\alpha$$

50. (d) Noble gases are slightly soluble in water and their solubility increases with increase in atomic number on moving down the group. Thus, the correct order of solubility is Xe > Kr > Ar > Ne > He.

51. (a)

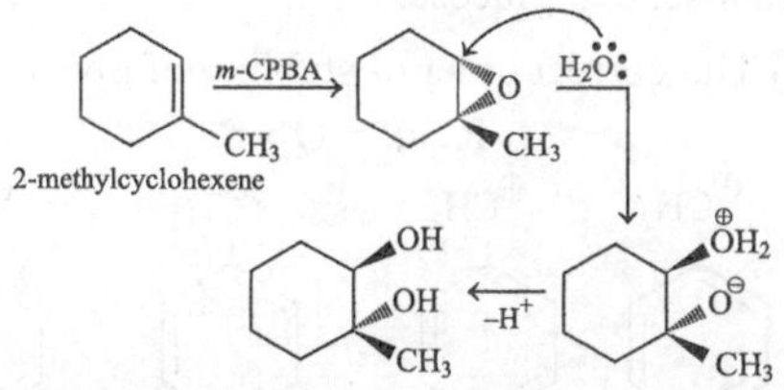

m-CPBA causes formation of epoxide ring and on hydrolysis ring opening will also occur from less hindered side.

52. (a) The Wolff-Kishner reduction reaction is carried out as follows

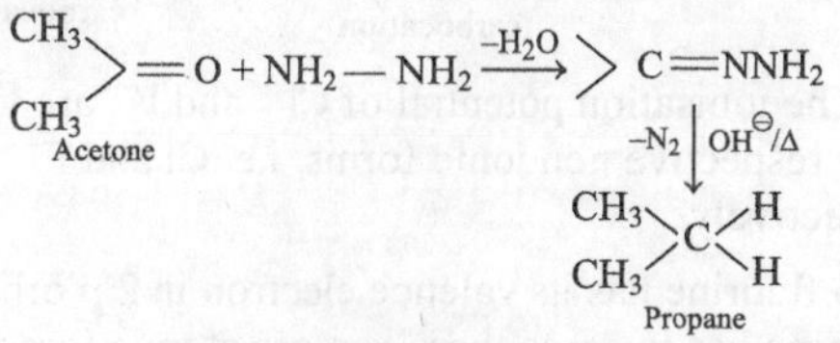

The reagent used in this reaction is $NH_2—NH_2$ followed by heating in the presence of base (OH^-).

53. (c)

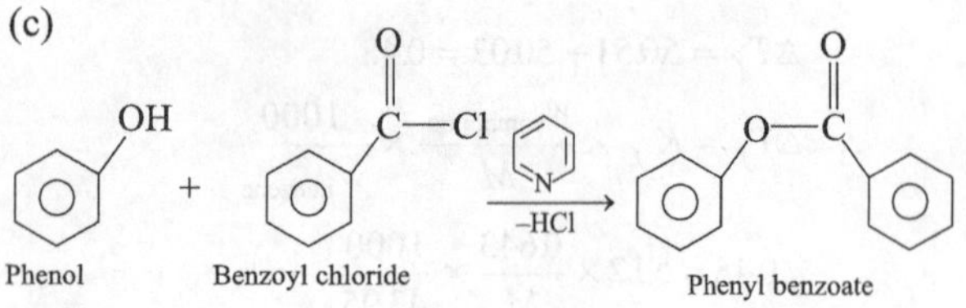

This reaction is an example of Schotten-Baumann reaction.

54. (c) Nucleophile always attack on electron deficient site. Presence of electron withdrawing groups such as NO_2, CHO etc., decreases the electron density on benzene nucleus, hence such groups activate the ring towards nucleophilic attack.

While presence of electron releasing groups such as —*R* or —*OR* increases the electron density, thus deactivates the benzene nucleus toward nucleophilic attack. Hence, NO_2 group activates the ring more than —Cl towards nucleophilic attack.

Thus, 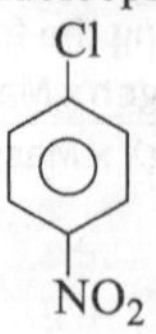 reacts (rapidly) with nucleophiles.

55. (b) $\underset{1\ \text{mol}}{CoCl_3\cdot 6H_2O} + AgNO_3\ (\text{excess}) \longrightarrow \underset{\substack{2\ \text{mol} \\ (\text{white ppt.})}}{2AgCl}$

As two Cl atoms are outside the coordination sphere, so the coordination number of Co = 6. Thus, the complex is $[Co(H_2O)_5Cl]Cl_2 \cdot H_2O$.

56. (b) Cyclic sugars that contain a 5-membered ring are called furanose, e.g. fructose.
Cyclic sugars that contain a 6-membered ring are called pyranose, e.g. glucose.

57. (b) The correct order of stability of given cations is

$$R > P > Q > S.$$

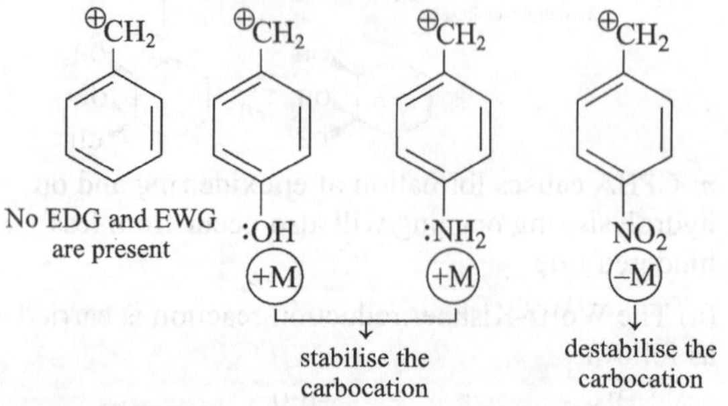

58. (a) The ionisation potential of Cl^- and F^- are less than their respective non ionic forms, i.e. Cl and F respectively.

Also fluorine has its valence electron in 2 *p* orbital while chlorine has in 3*p* so there is more atomic force of attraction in fluorine than chlorine, therefore, the ionisation potential of fluorine, is more than chlorine.

But the ionisation potential of F^- is less than Cl^- as, repulsion occurs in case of F^- thus electrons can easily be remove from it as compared to Cl^-.

Hence, the overall increasing order of ionisation potential is $F^- < Cl^- < Cl < F$.

59. (b) The possible values of *l* and m_l for an atomic orbital 4*f* is $n = 4, l = 3, m = -3, -2, -1, 0, +1, +2, +3$.

60. (b) General equation for combustion is given as

$$\underset{10}{C_xH_y} + \underset{55}{\left(x + \frac{y}{4}\right)O_2} \longrightarrow xCO_2 + \frac{y}{2}H_2O$$

$$1\ \text{mL}\ C_xH_y \equiv \left(x + \frac{y}{4}\right)\text{mL}\ O_2$$

$$10\ \text{mL}\ C_xH_y \equiv \left(x + \frac{y}{4}\right) \times 10\ \text{mL}$$

$$\therefore \left(x + \frac{y}{4}\right)10 = 55$$

$$10x + \frac{10y}{4} = 55$$

$$10 \times 4 + \frac{10y}{4} = 55$$

$$\frac{10y}{4} = 15$$

$$y = 6$$

61. (c) According to Henry's law,

$$p = K_H \chi$$

or $p_{gas} = K_H \cdot \chi_{gas}$

$p_{gas} = K_H(1 - \chi_{H_2O}) = K_H - K_H \cdot \chi_{H_2O}$

On comparing this with $y = mx + c$, we get the plot as given in option (c).

The slope will be negative and $p_{gas} \propto K_H$.

62. (a) The correct match is

A-(ii), B-(iii), C-(i), D-(iv).

A. Ni in the presence of hydrogen is used to reduce vegetable oil to ghee.

B. Cu_2Cl_2 is used in Sandmeyer reaction for the synthesis of aryl halide.

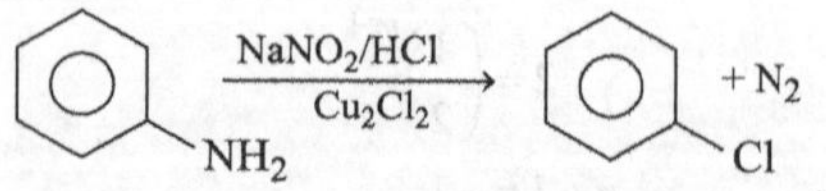

C. V_2O_5 is used in contact process for the oxidation of SO_2 to SO_3

$$2SO_2 + O_2 \xrightarrow{V_2O_5} 2SO_3$$

D. Finely divided iron is used as catalyst in Haber's process.

$$N_2 + 3H_2 \xrightarrow{Fe} 2NH_3$$

63. (d) Transition elements have partially filled *d*-orbitals, the electrons in which can be excited easily and promoted to higher energy levels.
When electrons jump from lower energy orbital to higher energy orbital light is emitted due to which the compounds of transition elements seems to be coloured compounds. Hence, (A) and (R) are true and (R) is correct explanation of (A).

64. (a) The correct match is A-(i), B-(iii), C-(iv), D-(ii).

$$\Delta H = \Delta U + \Delta n_g (RT)$$

$$PCl_5(g) \rightleftharpoons PCl_3(g) + Cl_2(g);\ \Delta n_g = 1$$
$$\Delta H > \Delta U$$

$$2HI(g) \rightleftharpoons H_2(g) + I_2(g);\quad \Delta n_g = 0$$
$$\Delta H = \Delta U \neq 0$$

$$N_2(g) + 3H_2(g) \rightleftharpoons 2NH_3(g);\ \Delta n_g = -2$$
$$\Delta H = \Delta U - 2RT$$

$$2CO(g) + O_2(g) \rightleftharpoons 2CO_2(g);\quad \Delta n_g = -1$$
$$\Delta H = \Delta U - RT$$

65. (a) Mass of organic compound = 0.5 g
Volume of 1 M H_2SO_4 required = 10 mL
$\therefore$ 10 mL of 1 M H_2SO_4 = 20 mL of 1 M NH_3.
Now 1000 mL of 1 M NH_3 contains 14g N

$\therefore$ 20 mL of 1 M NH_3 contains $= \frac{14}{1000} \times 20$ g nitrogen

$$\% \text{ of N} = \frac{14 \times 20}{1000} \times \frac{100}{0.5} = 56\%$$

66. (d) Both statements I and statement II are correct.

67. (b) IBr_2^- and XeF_2 are isoelectronic as they both have 22 electrons. Also, both are isostructural. The structures are shown below.

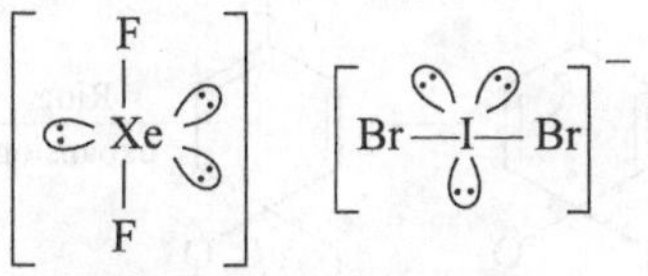

XeF_2 (Linear) IBr_2^- (Linear)

While all other species does not have equal number of electrons and same structure.

68. (b) Correct match is A-IV, B-III, C-I, D-II.

A. $4Fe^{3+} + 3[Fe(CN)_6]^{4-} \longrightarrow \underset{\text{Prussian blue}}{Fe_4[Fe(CN)_6]_3}$

B. $Fe^{3+} + SCN^- \longrightarrow \underset{\text{Blood red}}{[Fe(SCN)]^{2+}}$

C. $Ni^{2+} + 2DMG \longrightarrow \underset{\text{Cherry red}}{[Ni(DMG)_2]}$

D. $2Mn^{2+} + 5PbO_2 + 4H^+ \xrightarrow{H^+} \underset{\text{Pink}}{2MnO_4^-} + 5Pb^{2+} + 2H_2O$

69. (b) The mixture of conc. HCl and HNO_3 made in 3: 1 ratio is called *aqua-regia*.
The reaction is given below.

$$\underset{\text{Conc.}}{HNO_3} + \underset{\text{Conc.}}{3HCl} \longrightarrow NOCl + Cl_2 + 2H_2O$$

70. (b) Statement I is correct but Statement II is incorrect. The correct form of Statement II is as follows
$[Ni(CO)_4]$ is diamagnetic since nickel is in zero oxidation state.

71. (c) The structure of BrF_3 is shown as

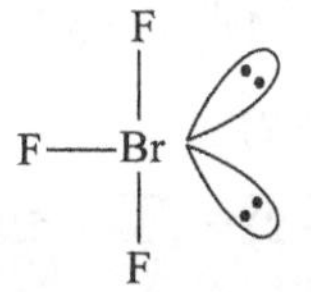

Here, lone pairs occupy equatorial position to minimize repulsion in all direction also from each other.

72. (b) As fluorine shows an oxidation of only − 1 and only has a tendency to reduce. So, it doesn't undergo disproportionation reaction.
Hence, statement I is true but statement II is false.

Problem Solving Tactics	Disproportionation is a specific type of redox reaction in which a species is simultaneously reduced and oxidised to form two different products.

73. (b) (A) is correct but (R) is not correct.
Ethylamine is soluble in water due to hydrogen bonding.
In aniline due to bulky hydrocarbon part the extent of hydrogen bonding is less and it is not soluble in water.

74. (b) The direct iodination reaction of benzene is as follows

$$C_6H_6 + I_2 \rightleftharpoons C_6H_5I + HI$$

This reaction is a reversible reaction. The product HI reacts with iodobenzene to get back benzene.
Hence, direct iodination of benzene is not possible.

75. (d) Br is more region selective in its reactions and prefers to react with the weaker R—H bonds. The strength of R—H varies slightly depending on the hydrogen in primary, secondary or tertiary compound. Bromination is 1640 times more likely to occur at 3° position than 1°. Chlorination is 5.2 times more likely to occur at 3° position than 1°.
Hence, bromine atom has much higher regioselectivity than chlorine in abstracting 3° hydrogen.

76. (b) In its compounds, manganese exhibits oxidation states from +2 to +7.

In MnO_4^-, Mn is in highest oxidation state that is +7. Thus, here manganese cannot undergo oxidation that is why disproportionation is not possible whereas, in MnO_4^{2-}, Mn is in +6 oxidation state which can be oxidised as well as reduced.

77. (a) Wavelength of transition is inversely proportional to the square of atomic number of the atom.

$$\lambda \propto \frac{1}{Z^2}$$

$$\frac{\lambda_{(Li^{2+})}}{\lambda_{(H)}} = \frac{1}{9} \Rightarrow \lambda_{(Li^{2+})} = \frac{821}{9} = 91.2\text{ nm}$$

78. (c) $Fe^{3+} = [Ar]\,3d^5\,4s^0, n = 5$

$$\mu = \sqrt{n(n+2)}$$

$$\mu = \sqrt{5(5+2)} = \sqrt{35} = 5.92\text{ BM}$$

79. (c) According to Faraday's law,

$$w = z \cdot it$$

Given, the value of *it* is same for H_2 and O_2.

Then, $$\frac{w_{H_2}}{w_{O_2}} = \frac{z_{H_2}}{z_{O_2}}$$

$$\frac{w_{H_2}}{w_{O_2}} = \frac{E_{H_2}}{E_{O_2}}$$

$$\frac{0.500}{w_{O_2}} = \frac{2}{16}$$

$$w_{O_2} = \frac{16 \times 0.500}{2} = 4.00\text{ g}$$

80. (b) The correct match is A-II, B-IV, C-I, D-III.

A. 16 g of CH_4 = 1 mole CH_4 contains $10 \times 6.02 \times 10^{23}$ electrons

$= 60.2 \times 10^{23}$

B. 1 g H_2 = 0.5 mole H_2 gas occupy 1 mole contains = 22.7 L

∴ 0.5 mole contains 11.35 (approx 11.4) litre volume at STP.

C. 1 mole of $O_2\,(g)$ = 32 g

D. 1 Mole of SO_2 = 64 g

81. (b) Among the given statements I, II and IV are correct while III and V are incorrect.

The larger value of K_C suggest that the reaction should go almost to completion. However, practically, the oxidation of SO_2 to SO_3 is very slow. Hence, the rate of reaction is increased by adding catalyst.

Also, the equilibrium will shift in forward direction as the pressure increases.

82. (d) Both Statement I and Statement II are correct.

83. (c) The complete reaction can be written as

$$\underset{\text{Ethyl chloride}}{CH_3{-}CH_2Cl} + \underset{\text{(alc.)}}{KOH} \longrightarrow \underset{\text{Ethene}}{CH_2{=}CH_2} + KCl + H_2O$$

In this process, alc. KOH is used for dehydrohalogenation.

84. (b) For a first order reaction,

$$k = \frac{1}{t}\ln\left[\frac{C_0}{C_t}\right]$$

where, C_0 = initial concentration of reactant

C_t = concentration of reactant at time *t*.

$$k = \frac{1}{100}\ln\left[\frac{0.2}{0.02}\right] = \frac{\ln 10}{100}$$

$$= 2.3 \times 10^{-2}\text{ min}^{-1}$$

85. (b) The correct match is A-(ii), B-(iii), C-(iv), D-(i).

A. $Pt|Fe^{3+}|\,Fe^{2+}$ represents oxidation reduction half-cell.

B. $Pt|H_2|H^+$ represents gas-gas ion half-cell.

C. $Pt|Hg|Hg_2^{2+}$ represents metal-metal ion half-cell.

D. $Pb|PbSO_4|SO_4^{2-}$ represents metal sparingly soluble salt half-cell.

86. (b) Compound containing ketone functional group undergoes protonation in acidic medium to oxonium ion. Since, oxonium ion is highly unstable, it undergoes ring expansion. In last step, deprotonation occur to gain aromaticity in the required product.

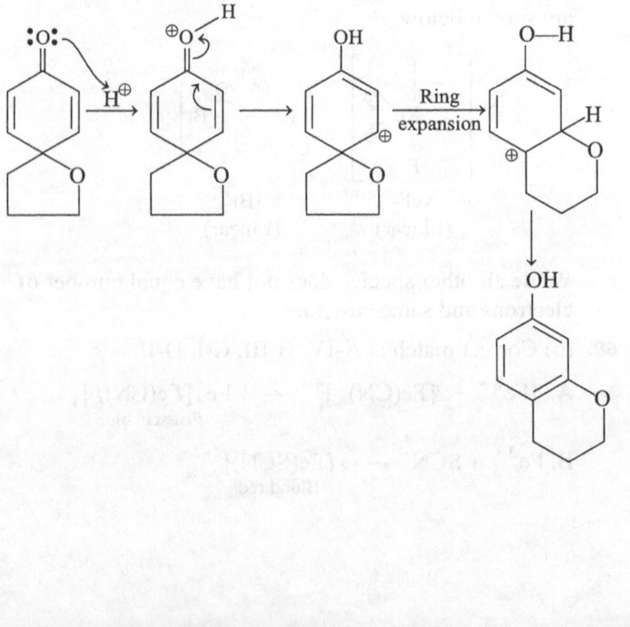

87. (c) Among the given compounds only I and II will give a yellow precipitate with iodine and alkali.

2-hydroxypropane $\left(\begin{array}{c} CH_3\,CH—CH_3 \\ \quad | \\ \quad OH \end{array}\right)$ contains the

$CH_3CH(OH)$ and CH_3CO—is present in acetophenone $\left(\begin{array}{c} \quad O \\ \quad \| \\ C_6H_5—C\,CH_3 \end{array}\right)$ so, both of these compounds will gives, iodoform test, i.e. form iodoform on reaction with I_2 and alkali.

88. (b) Phenolphthalein is colourless in acid solution (benzenoid form) and pink in alkali (basic) solution (quinonoid form).

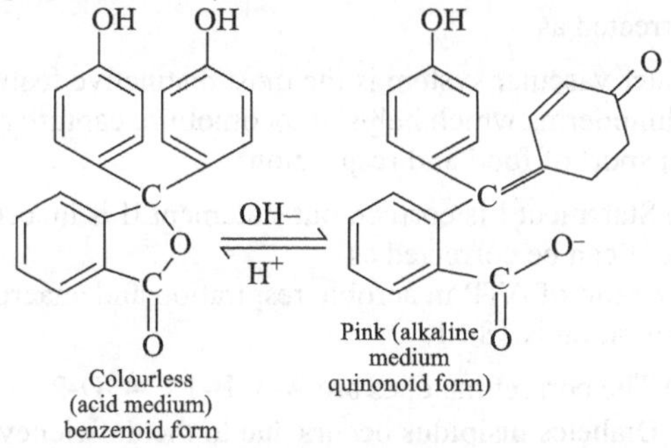

89. (d) Piperidine (I) and morpholine (III) both are non-aromatic and N-atom is sp^3-hybridised in them, so these are more basic as compared to other two (which are aromatic and have sp^2-hybridised N-atom). –I-effect of oxygen-atom in morpholine makes it less basic as compared to piperidine. Now, out of pyridine (II) and pyrrole (IV), pyridine is much stronger base as the lone pair of nitrogen atom in pyridine is not involved in resonance. So, the order of basic strength is I > III > II > IV.

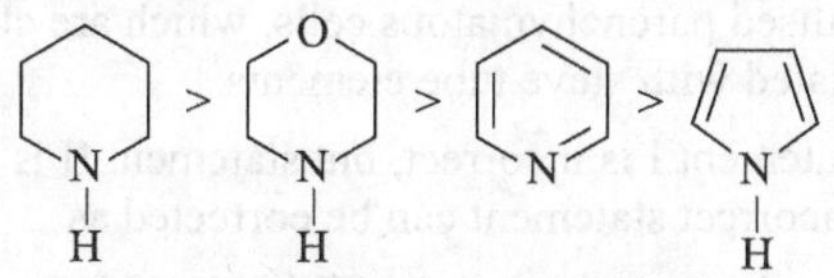

I III II IV

90. (b) Cyclohexanone is converted to methylene cyclohexane by reaction with Wittig reagent.

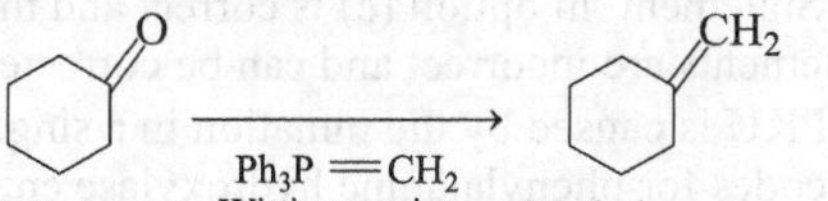

Cyclohexanone Wittig reaction Methylene cyclohexane

Biology

91. (c) The long protein chain is folded upon itself like a hollow woolen ball, giving rise to the tertiary structure. It gives a 3-dimensional view of protein and is absolutely necessary for many biological activities.

92. (c) Secretion of prostate gland nourishes and activates spermatozoa to swim. The sperms along with the fluid called semen is injected into the female body.

93. (d) All the statements are correct regarding meristematic cells. They have the power of division. Their cell wall is thin and nucleus is prominent.

94. (c) Statement in option (c) is correct. Rest of the incorrect statements can be corrected as

- Both DNA and RNA are able to mutate, but RNA mutate at faster rate.
- DNA is dependent on RNA for the synthesis of proteins.
- Consequently, viruses having RNA genome and shorter lifespans mutate and evolve faster.

95. (b) The wall of the uterus has three layers of tissues perimetrium, myometrium and endometrium. The myometrium exhibits strong contraction during child birth while endometrium undergoes cyclical changes during menstrual cycle.

96. (d) All the statements are Mendel's first three postulates. His third postulate states that during gamete formation, segregating pairs of unit factors assort independently of each other.

97. (a) A is false, but R is true. A can be corrected as A person of 'AB' blood group cannot donate blood to person of O blood group because plasma of recipient have antibody-A and anti-B which can cause agglutination of donor's RBCs.

98. (b) Statements I, IV and V are correct and rest of the statements are incorrect and these can be corrected as

- In frogs, during aestivation and hibernation gaseous exchange takes place through skin.
- The vascular system in frogs is well-developed and closed type.

99. (c) The statement in option (c) is incorrect. It can be corrected as
Kinetin (6-furfurylaminopurine) does not occur naturally in plants. It is a synthetic hormone.
Rest all statements are correct.

100. (c) The correct matches are A-4, B-3, C-2, D-1.

- Castor is an example of albuminous seeds. These seeds retain a part of endosperm as it is not completely used during embryo development.
- Pea is an example of ex-albuminous seeds. They do not have residual endosperm as it is completely consumed during embryo development.

- Asteraceae is an example of apomictic seeds, which are produced without fertilisation.
- *Citrus* is an example of polyembryonic seeds in which occurrence of more than one embryo in a seed is seen.

101. (b) The correct matches are A-3, B-1, C-2, D-4.
- Regulator genes code for repressor proteins which regulate transcription of cistron.
- Operator genes act as switch and turn on or off the transcription of structural gene.
- Promoter genes provide sites for the binding of RNA polymerase enzyme.
- Exon are the coding sequence of DNA which codes for certain proteins.

102. (a) Sometimes a few chromosomes have non- staining secondary constrictions at a constant location. This gives the appearance of small satellite DNA consisting of highly repetitive sequences which do not code for any protein.

103. (a) The DNA polymerase from *Thermus aquaticus* is homologous to *E. coli* DNA polymerase-I and likewise has domains responsible for DNA polymerisation and 5′ nuclease activities.

104. (c) Over exploitation of prey is not allowed by a prudent predator. If a predator is too efficient and over exploits its prey, then the prey might become extinct and following it, the predator will also become extinct due to lack of food.

105. (c) The option (c) is incorrectly matched. In a pond ecosystem, the standing crop of phytoplanktons, the mass of major producers will be lower than the mass of heterotrophs such as fish and insects. Thus, the pyramid of biomass will be inverted for pond ecosystem. Rest pairs are correctly matched.

106. (d) Both statement I and statement II are true.
In eukaryotes, replication and transcription take place in the nucleus. The fully processed *hn*RNA now called *m*RNA, is transferred from the nucleus into cytoplasm, where translation occur. This is because all the amino acids, *t*RNA and ribosomes required for translation are present in the cytoplasm.

107. (a) M-phase of the cell cycle is not a part of interphase. The M-phase starts with the nuclear division and ends with the division of cytoplasm. The interphase is divided into three phases
- G_1-phase (Gap 1)
- S-phase (Synthesis)
- G_2-phase (Gap 2)

108. (b) The correct matches are A-3, B-1 C-4, D-2.
- Vital capacity is the total amount of air inhaled after forced expiration. This includes ERV, TV and IRV. The value is about 4800 mL.
- Tidal volume is the volume of air inspired or expired during a normal respiration. It is approx. 500 mL.
- Expiratory resereve volume is the additional volume of air that a person can expire by a forcible expiration. This average 1000 mL to 1100 mL.
- Inspiratory reserve volume is the additional volume of air that a person can inspire by a forcible inspiration. This averages 2500 mL to 3000 mL.

109. (a) Both A and R are true and R is the correct explanation of A.
Short Tandem Repeats (STRs) are introns and do not code for protein. Therefore, they are usually considered as junk DNA.

110. (b) *Agaricus* is an edible fungi. It is commonly known as mushroom. It belongs to class–Basidiomycetes.

111. (b) Abscisic acid is responsible for stoppage of cambial activity. It inhibits mitosis in vascular cambium.

112. (b) Statement I is true, but statement II is false. It can be corrected as

Water vascular system is the most distinctive feature of echinoderms which helps in locomotion, capture and transport of food and respiration.

113. (c) Statement I is correct, but statement II is incorrect and it can be corrected as
The ratio of ATP in aerobic respiration and anaerobic respiration is 18 : 1.

114. (b) The correct matches are A-3, B-1 C-4, D-2.
- Diabetes insipidus occurs due to the deficiency of ADH.
- Diabetes mellitus is associated with insulin hyposecretion.
- Addison's disease is associated with insuffiency of adrenal gland hormones.
- Melatonin hormone is responsible of circadian cycle.

115. (c) Statement I is correct, but statement II is incorrect. It can be corrected as
The functions of sieve tubes are controlled by the nucleus of the companion cells. These cells are specialised parenchymatous cells, which are closely associated with sieve tube elements.

116. (d) Statement I is incorrect, but statement II is correct. The incorrect statement can be corrected as

During photorespiration, RuBP binds with O_2 to form one molecule of phosphoglycerate and phosphoglycolate.

117. (c) Statement in option (c) is correct and the other statements are incorrect and can be corrected as
- PKU is caused by the mutation in a single gene that codes for phenylalanine hydroxylase enzymes.
- It is characterised by the mental retardation and reduction in hair and skin pigmentation.

- The mutated gene can express itself in homozygous condition only.

118. (d) Both statement I and statement II are true.

In *Pila*, body is covered by a calcareous shell and is unsegmented with distinct head, muscular foot and visceral hump, whereas *Limulus* an arthropod, respires with book gills.

119. (c) In anaerobic respiration (fermentation), there is no net oxidation or reduction of the carbons of glucose. The anaerobic regeneration of NAD is called fermentation. In yeast, the regeneration of NAD^+ from NADH takes place under anaerobic conditions. Here, pyruvate is converted into ethanol and CO_2 in a two step reaction.

120. (b) Both A and R are true, but R is not the correct explanation of A.

Enzymes are either proteins or RNA (e.g. ribozyme) that catalyse a specific chemical reaction. These do not affect the equilibrium of the catalysed reaction.

It just enhances the rate of a reaction by providing a reaction path with a lower activation energy. Enzyme itself remains unchanged after reaction.

121. (c) An operon is a cluster of genes whose expression is controlled by a single operator, e.g. *lac* operon. This *lac* operon is required for the transport and metabolism of lactose in *E. coli* and many other enteric bacteria.

122. (d) Many organelles are considered together as an endomembrane system because their functions are coordinated. These include endoplasmic reticulum, Golgi complex, lysosomes and vacuoles. Since, the functions of mitochondria, chloroplast and peroxisomes are not coordinated with the above organelles, these are not considered as part of endomembrane system.

123. (c) Statement I is correct, but statement II is incorrect and it can be corrected as

If genes are exchanged between two different population of a species, it is known as gene flow.

124. (c) Primary spermatocytes have diploid set of chromosomes. A primary spermatocyte completes the first meiotic division leading to the formation of haploid secondary spermatocyte.

125. (b) High trophic level in food chain is not related to evil quartet with respect to biodiversity loss. There are four major causes of biodiversity loss, namely

- habitat loss and fragmentation
- over exploitation
- alien species invasion
- co-extinction

'The Evil Quartet' is the sobriquet used to describe them.

126. (b) Statements II, IV and V are correct and rest of the statements are incorrect. These can be corrected as

- During decomposition, decomposers breakdown complex organic matter into inorganic substances.
- In fragmentation, detritivores breakdown the detritus into smaller particles.

127. (b) Statements I, III and V are correct and statements II and IV are incorrect. The incorrect statements can be corrected as

Many members of Ascomycetes such as morels and truffles are edible and are considered delicacies. Fungal class–Deuteromycetes is commonly known as imperfect fungi because only asexual or vegetative phase of these fungi are known.

128. (d) Statement in option (d) is incorrect and can be corrected as

Smoking increases carbon monoxide content in blood due to which concentration of O_2 decreases in body.

129. (a) The dominance of gametophyte is observed in bryophytes.

This means that the more prominent longer lived state is the haploid gametophyte. The diploid sporophyte appears only occasionally and remains attached to gametophyte. It nutritionally depends on the gametophyte.

130. (d) Serum and urine analysis are conventional methods of diagnosis and are not used for early detection of diseases.

131. (c) Statements III and V are incorrect and can be corrected as

- Frogs respire on land and in water by two different methods.
- System for control and coordination is highly evolved in frogs. It includes both neural system and endocrine glands.

Rest are correct statements.

132. (b) Statements I, III, IV and V are correct. Statement II is incorrect. It can be corrected as

Plant families are characterised on the basis of both vegetative and reproductive features.

133. (d) Endoplasmic reticulum divides the intracellular space into two distinct compartments; luminal and extra-luminal.

The luminal and extra- luminal compartments are situated inside ER and the cytoplasm, respectively.

134. (c) The nuclear envelope consists of two lipid bilayer membranes, i.e. an inner nuclear membrane and an outer nuclear membrane. The outer nuclear membrane is continuous with the endoplasmic reticulum membrane. The space between the membranes is called the perinuclear space.

135. (c) Toxoids are vaccines that are made from toxin produced by a pathogen. These toxins are made harmless.

136. (b) Myasthenia gravis is an autoimmune disease affecting neuromuscular junction, leading to fatigue, weakening and paralysis of skeletal muscles.

137. (b) An elaborate network of filamentous proteinaceous structures consisting of microtubules, microfilaments and intermediate filaments present in the cytoplasm is referred to as cytoskeleton. It is involved in many functions such as mechanical support, motility, etc.

138. (c) Statements III and V are incorrect and can be corrected as
The unsaturated fatty acids have lower melting points than those of saturated fatty acids. Nicotinamides adenine dinucleotide act as coenzyme of oxidising enzymes.

139. (a) Both statement I and statement II are correct.

140. (c) Alexander Oparin and JBS Haldane proposed that the life originated from carbon based molecules in the primordial soup. According to them, UV-rays from sun induced reactions on a mixture of water, CO_2 and ammonia. Organic substances such as sugars and protein components were synthesised and they accumulated till the primitive oceans reached to consistency of hot dilute soup. Thus, the primordial soup from the living things was created.

141. (c) Nucellus and polar nuclei are diploid among the given options. Endosperm is triploid, while others are haploid.

142. (a) Statements I, II and V are correct and statements III and IV are incorrect. The incorrect statements can be corrected as

In bryophytes, sporophyte is not free-living, but attached to the photosynthetic gametophyte and derives nourishment from it. Mosses along with lichens are the first organisms to colonise rocks and hence are of great ecological importance.

143. (d) The option (d) is not paired correctly. It symbolises consanguineous parents (closely related). Rest options are correctly matched.

144. (a) ⊕ ⚥ $K_{2+2}C_4A_{2+4}\underline{G}_{(2)}$ represents the correct formula of family–Cruciferae. Members of the family are distributed all over the world, particularly in mediterranean and temperate regions.

145. (b) Puncturing of the diaphragm of a person would result in stoppage of breathing and can prove fatal. The diaphragm is a muscular structure, which separates the thoracic and abdominal cavities. Most important function of diaphragm in mammals is to aid in respiration and any damage would stop the breathing process and thus prove fatal.

146. (b) The extrastelar region forms the periderm. The periderm includes the phellogen, phellem and phelloderm.

147. (b) In dicot stem, vascular bundles are arranged in a ring surrounding pith. They are open and without bundle sheath.

148. (d) The region of the nephron found in the renal medulla is Henle's loop. Rest are present in the renal cortex.

149. (c) Alien-species invasion correctly describes the cause of this biodiversity loss. When alien species (e.g. *Clarias gariepinus*) are introduced unintentionally or deliberately, some of them turn invasive and cause decline or extinction of indigenous species.

150. (c) Statement in option (c) is incorrect and can be corrected as
Glucocorticoids stimulate gluconeogenesis, lipolysis and proteolysis and inhibit cellular uptake and utilisation of amino acids.

151. (c) Somatotropin or growth hormone plays an important role in the growth of both hard and soft tissues and does not stimulate other endocrine glands. Whereas, all the other three, i.e. thyrotropin stimulates the thyroid gland, gonadotropin stimulates the gonadal activity and adrenocorticotropin stimulates adrenal glands.

152. (a) Sclereids are often called stone cells or sclerotic cells. They are dead cells with small lumen. These are found in hard part of the plants and possess strongly lignified and sometimes even suberised thick secondary walls.

153. (d) A is true, but R is false because Positive interactions are those, in which organisms help one another and either one or both the species (associating) are benefitted. Mutualism is a type of positive interaction in which both organisms are benefitted and neither is harmed.

154. (b) During each cardiac cycle two prominent sounds are produced which can be heard by stethoscope. The first sound (lubb) is associated with the closure of tricuspid and bicuspid valves, whereas the second heart sound (dubb) is associated with the closure of semilunar valves.

155. (b) Cerebrum that forms the major part of the brain, will be affected in the given case. It is associated with memory.

156. (a) The corrected matches are A-3, B-4, C-2, D-1.
- Zeatin is a naturally occurring cytokinin which was found in coconut milk.
- IBA (Indole Butyric Acid) is a natural auxin isolated from plants.
- NAA (Naphthalene Acetic Acid) is a synthetic auxin.
- Ethephon is the most widely used compound as source of ethylene.

157. (b) The portion between two successive 'Z' lines is considered as the functional unit of contraction and is called a sarcomere. It is a multi-protein complex composed of three different filament systems.

158. (c) An eukaryotic genome differs from a bacterial genome in having introns. Eukaryotic genome has introns and exons. Introns are non-coding segments of a gene, whereas exons are coding regions. During the process of RNA splicing, introns are removed and exons are joined.

Bacteria contain a single DNA molecule that makes up the entire genome.

159. (a) The electrons that are moved from PS-II need to be replaced. This is achieved by electrons available due to splitting of water. Water is split into O_2, H^+ and e^-. The electrons needed to replace those removed from photosystem-I are provided by photosystem-II.

160. (b) Correct label with its respective characteristic is represented by option (b).

A decline in the lung volume, as represented by label III shows that a certain amount of air is drawn out of the lungs.

161. (c) Osteichthyes does not belong to the class-Tetrapoda rather it belongs to Pisces. It includes all bony fishes that have paired fins.

162. (b) In frogs, male reproductive organs consist of a pair of yellowish ovoid testes, which are found adhered to the upper part of kidneys by a double fold of peritonium called mesorchium.

163. (c) Nitrogen fixation genes can be introduced into non-legumes by gene gun method. In this method, cells are bombarded with high velocity micro-particles of gold or tungsten coated with DNA. Gene gun is suitable for plants.

164. (b) Both A and R are true and R is the correct explanation of A.

In a continuous culture system, nutrient availability is unlimited. So, the cells are maintained in a continuous log or exponential phase.

165. (b) The Golgi apparatus principally performs the functions of packaging materials, to be delivered either to the intracellular targets or secreted outside the cell.

166. (c) Statement in option (c) is incorrect. The incorrect statement can be corrected as *D* represents larynx, or the sound box. It is found in the anterior neck at the level of 3rd to 6th cervical vertebrae.

167. (c) Incorrect statement with respect to photorespiration is represented by option (c). Photorespiration is a biologically wasteful process because there is neither synthesis of sugars nor of ATP. Rather it results in the release of CO_2 with the utilisation of ATP.

168. (d) The correct matches are A-3, B-1 C-2, D-4.

- *Porphyra* is an example of red algae or Rhodophyceae.
- *Spirogyra* is an example of green algae or Chlorophyceae.
- *Fucus* is an example of brown algae or Phaeophyceae.
- *Polytrichum* is an example of mosses which belongs to bryophytes.

169. (c) Proteins are secreted by the cell organelles in the following sequence

Nucleus $\rightarrow$ ER $\rightarrow$ Ribosomes $\rightarrow$ Golgi apparatus $\rightarrow$ Secretory vesicles $\rightarrow$ Plasma membrane.

After post-transcriptional modification *m*RNA synthesised in nucleus gets released from nucleus. It is then translated with ribosomes attached with ER. The proteins then enter the lumen of ER and eventually the Golgi body where they are processed, packaged and ultimately released as vesicles. These secretory vesicles then fuse with plasma membrane.

170. (b) The ascending limb is impermeable to water, but allows transport of electrolytes actively or passively. Therefore, as the concentrated filtrate is passed through, it gets diluted due to passage of electrolytes to the medullary fluid.

171. (a) Statements II, III and V are correct, while statements I and IV are incorrect and can be corrected as

The negatively charged DNA is wrapped around the positively charged histone octamer to form nucleosome. DNA with higher percentage of $G \equiv C$ have more density than those with higher percentage of $A = T$.

172. (b) Statements I and II are correct, while statements III, IV and V are incorrect and can be corrected as ATPase requires Mg^{2+} for its functioning. HMM consists of two sub-fragments S1 and S2. Each S1 fragment consists of an ATPase site and a binding site for actin. Rigor mortis is caused due to complete depletion of ATP and phosphocreatine.

173. (a) The correct matches are A-2, B-4, C-1, D-3.

- Angina is a symptom of acute chest pain, which appears when not enough oxygen (less oxygen) is reaching the heart muscle.
- CAD, often referred to as atherosclerosis, affects the vessels that supply blood to the heart muscle. It is caused by the deposition of calcium, fat, cholesterol and fibrous tissues, which makes the lumen of arteries narrower.
- Heart failure means the state of heart when it is not pumping blood effectively enough to meet the needs of the body.
- Hypertension means blood pressure higher than the normal (120/80 mm Hg). It leads to heart diseases and also affects vital organs like brain and kidney.

174. (b) Statement in option (b) is incorrect and can be corrected as

During HGP, fragments were sequenced using automated DNA sequences that worked on the principle of a method developed by Frederick Sanger. He is also credited for developing method for determination of amino acid sequence in proteins.

175. (b) The given figure shows the transition to metaphase. In this stage of mitosis, the nucleus disappears and the chromosome appear in the cytoplasm of the cell.

176. (a) The sequence of events in a nerve conduction is

Threshold $\rightarrow$ Depolarisation $\rightarrow$ Repolarisation $\rightarrow$ Hyperpolarisation.

177. (b) The correct matches are A-3, B-1, C-4, D-2.

- Multiload 375 is a copper releasing IUDs that acts as a contraceptive device.
- Lippes loop is a non-medicated IUD that is made of plastic and can be inserted for long periods.
- In IUT, embryos with more than 8 blastomeres are transferred into the uterus to complete further development.
- In ZIFT, zygote or early embryos with upto 8 blastomeres are transferred in the Fallopian tube.

178. (d) A is true, but R is false. R can be corrected as Energy at a lower trophic level is always more than that at higher level.

This is due to the fact that some amount of energy is lost during transfer from one level to another.

179. (c) A is true, but R is false. R can be corrected as The bottled fruit juice are clarified with the help of enzymes, pectinase and protease. Hence, the bottled fruit juice found in the market are clearer as compared to home made juice.

180. (d) All the given statements are correct regarding J-shaped growth curve.

This type of curve represents the population growing exponentially or geometrically until there is a resource limitation or population growth is limited by other factors.

In it, minor fluctuations are not observed. The equilibrium phase is rarely reached and environmental resistances do not operate.

SECTION I
Foundation Builders

PRACTICE SET 2

Maximum Marks : 720 | Time : 3 hrs | No. of Questions : 180

Instructions

1. This question paper contains **180** multiple choice questions (four options with a single correct answer) from **Physics, Chemistry** and **Biology**.
2. These questions are distributed as 45 questions, each from Physics and Chemistry and 90 questions in Biology. These are to be compulsorily attempted by the candidate.
3. Each question carries 4 marks. For each correct response, the candidate will get 4 marks. For each incorrect response, one mark will be deducted from the total scores.

PHYSICS

1. Relation between wavelength of photon and electron of same energy is

(a) $\lambda_{ph} > \lambda_e$ (b) $\lambda_{ph} < \lambda_e$
(c) $\lambda_{ph} = \lambda_e$ (d) $\lambda_e / \lambda_{ph} = \text{constant}$

2. A boat is moving with a velocity $3\hat{i} + 4\hat{j}$ with respect to ground. The water in the river is moving with a velocity $-3\hat{i} - 4\hat{j}$ with respect to ground. The relative velocity of the boat with respect to water is

(a) $6\hat{i} + 8\hat{j}$ (b) $-6\hat{i} - 8\hat{j}$ (c) $8\hat{i} + 6\hat{j}$ (d) $4\hat{i} + 3\hat{j}$

3. Two coherent light beams of intensities I and $4I$ are superposed. The maximum and minimum possible intensities in the resulting beam are

(a) $5I$ and I (b) $5I$ and $3I$
(c) $9I$ and I (d) $9I$ and $3I$

4. Pressure *versus* temperature graph of an ideal gas is shown in the figure. If density of the gas at point A is ρ_0, then density at point B will be

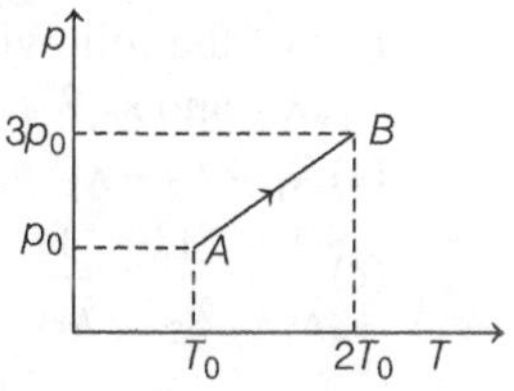

(a) $\frac{3}{4}\rho_0$ (b) $\frac{3}{2}\rho_0$ (c) $\frac{4}{3}\rho_0$ (d) $2\rho_0$

5. The following questions consists of two statements-Assertion (A) and Reason (R).

Assertion (A) During rapid pumping of air in tyres, air inside the tyre is colder than atmospheric air.

Reason (R) Adiabatic process occurs at very high rate.

In the light of above statements, choose the most appropriate answer from the following options.

(a) Both A and R are true and R is correct explanation of A.
(b) Both A and R are true but R is not the correct explanation of A.
(c) A is true but R is false.
(d) A is false but R is true.

6. If Young's double slit experiment is performed in water instead of air, then

(a) no fringes would be seen
(b) fringe width would decrease
(c) fringe width would increase
(d) fringe width would remain unchanged

7. In an experiment for determining the mass of a given body using a meter scale suspended horizontally with a thread and a standard weight of 1.0 kg, the power (mass) arm is adjustable and the weight is fixed. If the unknown mass is kept at a distance 65 cm from the thread, then the given mass (in kg) is

(a) 0.24 (b) 0.35
(c) 0.54 (d) 0.86

8. A projectile P is projected at an angle of 30° with the horizontal. If a second projectile Q is projected such that their speeds are in ratio 3 : 1 for same maximum height, then the angle of projection of Q is

(a) $\sin^{-1}\left(\frac{3}{1}\right)$ (b) $\sin^{-1}\left(\frac{1}{3}\right)$

(c) $\sin^{-1}\left(\frac{3}{2}\right)$ (d) $\sin^{-1}\left(\frac{2}{3}\right)$

9. If c is the speed of electromagnetic waves in vacuum, its speed in a medium of dielectric constant K and relative permeability μ_r is

(a) $v=\frac{K}{\sqrt{\mu_r c}}$ (b) $v=\frac{1}{\sqrt{\mu_r K}}$

(c) $v=c\sqrt{\mu_r K}$ (d) $v=\frac{c}{\sqrt{\mu_r K}}$

10. At what height from the surface of earth, the value of acceleration due to gravity becomes one-fourth to its value present on the surface of earth ?
(Take, R = radius of earth)

(a) $\sqrt{2}R$ (b) $\frac{R}{\sqrt{2}}$

(c) R (d) $\frac{R}{2}$

11. Transitions between the energy levels in a particular atom give rise to three spectral lines of wavelengths, in increasing magnitudes as λ_1, λ_2 and λ_3. Which one of the following equations correctly related to λ_1, λ_2 and λ_3?

(a) $\lambda_1=\lambda_2-\lambda_3$ (b) $\lambda_1=\lambda_3-\lambda_2$

(c) $\frac{1}{\lambda_1}=\frac{1}{\lambda_2}+\frac{1}{\lambda_3}$ (d) $\frac{1}{\lambda_2}=\frac{1}{\lambda_3}+\frac{1}{\lambda_1}$

12. Potential energy of a particle in a force field is given by $U=\frac{A}{x^2}-\frac{B}{x}$, where A and B are positive constants and x is the distance of particle from centre of the field. For stable equilibrium, the distance of particle is

(a) $\frac{A}{B}$ (b) $\frac{B}{A}$

(c) $\frac{2A}{B}$ (d) $\frac{B}{2A}$

13. The excess pressure inside a spherical drop of water is five times that of another drop, then their respective mass ratio is

(a) 5 : 3 (b) 25:137

(c) 125:137 (d) 1:125

14. The mass of jupiter is 1.9×10^{27} kg and that of sun is 1.99×10^{30} kg. The mean distance of the jupiter from the sun is 7.8×10^{11} m. Assume that the jupiter moves in a circular orbit around the sun. Velocity of jupiter is

(a) 1.3×10^4 ms^{-1} (b) 1.5×10^4 ms^{-1}

(c) 1.2×10^4 ms^{-1} (d) 1.6×10^4 ms^{-1}

15. A voltmeter has a resistance of G ohm and range of V volt. The value of resistance used in series to convert it into a voltmeter of range nV volt is

(a) nG (b) $\frac{G}{(n-1)}$ (c) $(n-1)G$ (d) $\frac{G}{n}$

16. Two statements are given below.

Statement I If the phase difference between the two sources varies continuously, then interference pattern disappears.

Statement II If two slits in Young's double slit experiment are illuminated by two different lamps emitting light of the same wavelength, then no interference pattern will be observed.

In the light of above statements, choose the most appropriate answer from the options given below.

(a) Both Statement I and Statement II are correct.
(b) Both Statement I and Statement II are incorrect.
(c) Statement I is correct and Statement II is incorrect.
(d) Statement I is incorrect and Statement I is correct.

17. An α-particle enters into uniform magnetic field perpendicular to its direction, then

(a) momentum and kinetic energy both will remain unchanged
(b) momentum will change but kinetic energy will remain unchanged
(c) momentum and kinetic energy, both will be changed
(d) kinetic energy will change but momentum will remain unchanged

18. The diode shown in the circuit is a silicon diode. The potential difference between the points A and B will be

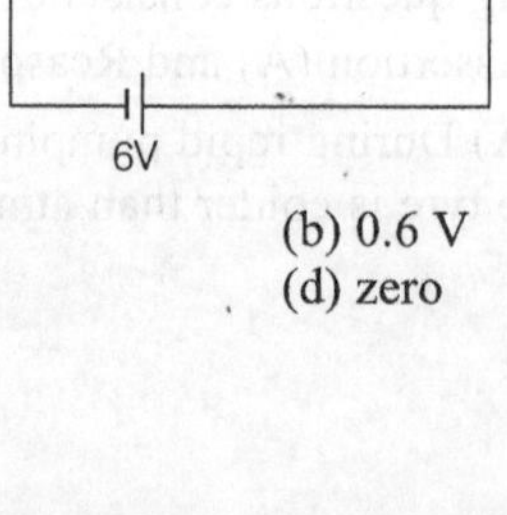

(a) 6 V (b) 0.6 V

(c) 0.7 V (d) zero

19. In the diagram shown below, equivalent resistance between A and B is

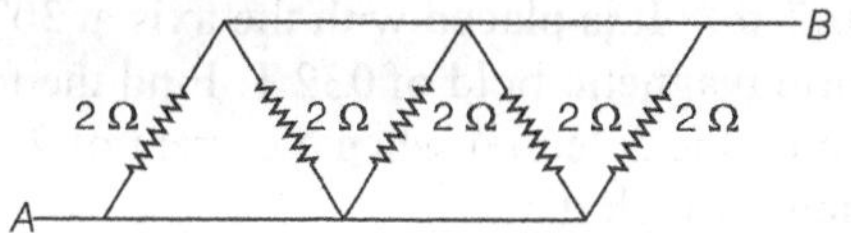

(a) 7.5 Ω (b) 5 Ω (c) 0.4 Ω (d) 10 Ω

20. The ionisation energy of hydrogen is 13.6 eV. The energy of the photon released when an electron jumps from the first excited state ($n=2$) to the ground state of hydrogen atom is

(a) 13.6 eV (b) 10.2 eV (c) 4.53 eV (d) 3.4 eV

21. In the following figure, what is the final value of current in the 10Ω resistor when the plug of key K is inserted ?

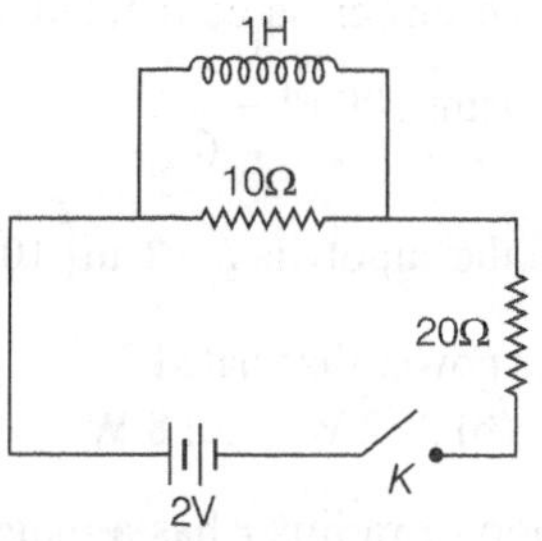

(a) (3/10) A (b) (3/20) A (c) (3/11) A (d) Zero

22. Given below are two statements

Statement I n-type semiconductor is electrically neutral.

Statement II n-type semiconductor has an excess of negative charge carriers.

In the above statements, choose the most appropriate answer from the options given below

(a) Statement I is incorrect but Statement II is correct.
(b) Both Statement I and Statement II are correct.
(c) Statement II is incorrect but Statement I is correct.
(d) Both statement I and Statement II are incorrect.

23. A. The maximum value of the photoelectric current is called saturation current.

B. If the frequency of the incident radiation and potential is fixed, then photocurrent decreases linearly with intensity of incident light.

C. For a given frequency of incident radiation, the stopping potential is independent of the intensity.

Choose the correct option from the following for the statements which are true.

(a) A and B (b) A and C
(c) B and C (d) Only A

24. The frequency f of a stretched string depends upon the tension force F, length l of the string and the mass per unit length μ of the string. The formula for frequency is (k = constant)

(a) $f=\frac{k}{l}\sqrt{\frac{\mu}{F}}$ (b) $f=\frac{k}{l}\sqrt{\frac{F}{\mu}}$

(c) $f=kl\sqrt{\frac{\mu}{F}}$ (d) $f=kl\sqrt{\frac{F}{\mu}}$

25. The magnetic flux linked with coil varies with time as $\phi_B=4t^2+3t-4$. The magnitude of induced emf at 2 s is

(a) 12 V (b) 17 V (c) 19 V (d) 21 V

26. In an experiment, three quantities a, b and c are measured with percentage error of 2%, 4% and 6%, respectively. A quantity P is calculated as follows $P=\frac{a^2b^{1/2}}{c^{3/2}}$. Percentage error in P will be

(a) 5% (b) 10% (c) 20% (d) 15%

27. Two bodies of masses of 2 kg and 8 kg are tied to the ends of a massless string. The string passes over a frictionless pulley. The acceleration of the system is

(a) $\frac{g}{5}$ (b) $\frac{3g}{5}$ (c) $\frac{g}{10}$ (d) $\frac{g}{4}$

28. Moment of inertia of a circular wire of mass $2M$ and radius $2R$ about its diameter is

(a) $8MR^2$ (b) $4MR^2$ (c) $2MR^2$ (d) $\frac{MR^2}{2}$

29. The equivalent capacitance between point A and B is

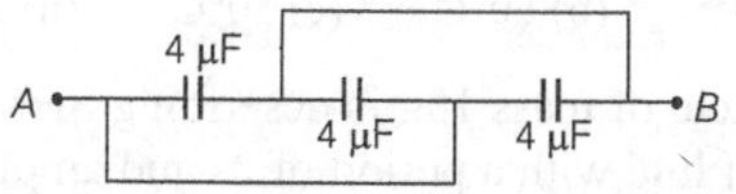

(a) 6μF (b) 12μF (c) 4μF (d) 18μF

30. The velocity of an object is changing with time and relation is given by the following equation $v=2t+3t^2$. Calculate the position of the object from the origin at $t=2$ s, assume particle to be at origin at $t=0$.

(a) 16 m (b) 12 m (c) 18 m (d) 22 m

31. Charge on a free pith-ball of mass 8 g is 5×10^{-8} C. The magnitude of charge on second pith-ball fixed 5 cm below the former ball, so that upper ball is stationary will be

(a) 0.44 μC (b) 1.25 μC (c) 2.36 μC (d) 7.15 μC

32. Force required to move a train of 1500 quintals up an incline of 1 in 75 (a slope that has a rise of 1 unit for every 75 unit of displacement) with an acceleration of 4 ms^{-2} is
(where, force of friction = 0.2 newton per quintal)
(a) 650000 N (b) 690000 N
(c) 619900 N (d) 625000 N

33. A hammer is placed on a plane surface. Two forces, each of magnitude F, are applied on it, as shown in the figure. The hammer will have

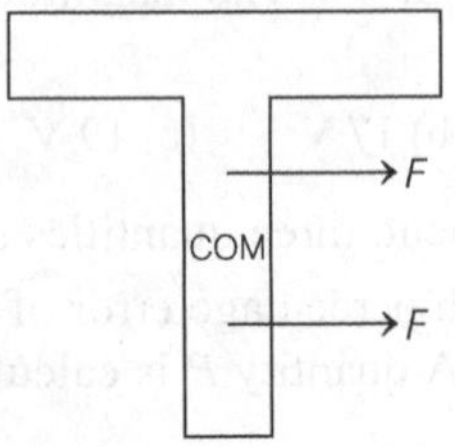

(a) only translational motion
(b) only rotational motion
(c) both translational and rotational motion
(d) No motion

34. Three rods made of the same material and having the same cross-section have been joined as shown in the figure. Each rod is of the same length. The left and right ends are kept at 0°C and 90°C, respectively. The temperature of the junction of the three rods will be

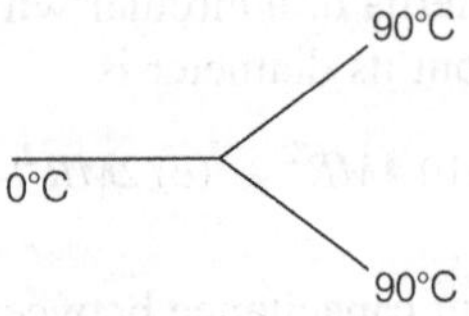

(a) 45°C (b) 60°C (c) 30°C (d) 20°C

35. A particle of mass 10g is describing SHM along a straight line with a period of 2s and amplitude of 10 cm. The difference in kinetic energy, when it is 2 cm and 5 cm from its equilibrium position is
(a) $100\pi^2$ erg (b) $105\pi^2$ erg
(c) $480\pi^2$ erg (d) $375\pi^2$ erg

36. Two soap bubbles of diameter d_A and d_B combine under isothermal conditions in space outside international space station at lower earth orbit. Now, find the new radius of bubble, if lower earth orbit is at a distance of 37000 km from earth.
(a) $\frac{d_A + d_B}{2}$ (b) $\frac{d_A d_B}{d_A + d_B}$
(c) $\sqrt{d_A d_B}$ (d) $\sqrt{d_A^2 + d_B^2}$

37. A straight solenoid of length 50 cm has 1000 turns per metre and mean cross-sectional area of 2×10^{-4} m^2. It is placed with the axis at 30° with uniform magnetic field of 0.32 T. Find the torque acting on the solenoid when a current of 2 A is passing through it.
(a) 0.022 N-m (b) 0.02 N-m
(c) 0.032 N-m (d) 0.15 N-m

38. An air bubble inside a cubical block of glass of side 7 cm appears to be at 3.5 cm from one face and 1.5 cm from the other face opposite to the first when viewed normally, then the real depth of the bubble from the opposite face is [take, refractive index of glass, $\mu = 1.5$]
(a) 3 cm (b) 2.5 cm (c) 2.1 cm (d) 2 cm

39. A series L-C-R circuit is connected across an AC source $E = 10\sin\left(100\pi t - \frac{\pi}{6}\right)$.
Current from the supply is $I = 2\sin\left(100\pi t + \frac{\pi}{12}\right)$, what is the average power dissipated ?
(a) $5\sqrt{2}$ W (b) $2\sqrt{2}$ W (c) 8 W (d) 16 W

40. A current loop of radius r has a magnetic field induction B_1, at a point on its axis at a distance r from its centre and B_2 at its centre, then $B_1 : B_2$ is
(a) $1 : 2\sqrt{2}$ (b) $2\sqrt{2} : \sqrt{3}$ (c) $1 : \sqrt{2}$ (d) $\sqrt{3} : 2\sqrt{2}$

41. A train of 150 m length is going towards north direction at a speed of 10 ms^{-1}. A parrot flies at a speed of 5 ms^{-1} towards south direction parallel to the railway track. The time taken by parrot to cross the train is equal to
(a) 12 s (b) 8 s (c) 15 s (d) 10 s

42. Five equal resistors, each of 5Ω are connected in a network as shown in the following figure, then equivalent resistance between P and Q is

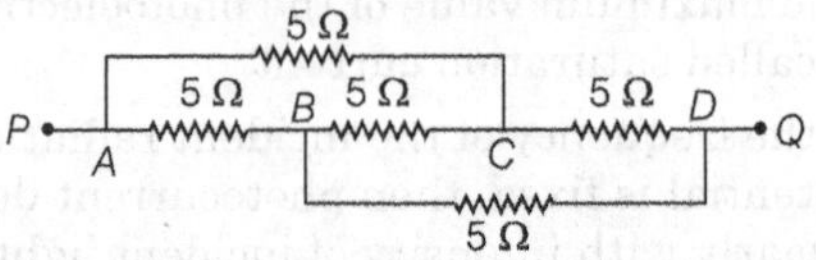

(a) 5Ω (b) 10Ω (c) 25Ω (d) 20Ω

43. The Q-value of the reaction
$${}^1_1H + {}^3_1H \longrightarrow {}^2_1H + {}^2_1H$$
is [atomic masses are $m({}^1_1H) = 1.007825$ amu
$m({}^2_1H) = 2.014102$ amu

$m(^3_1H) = 3.016049$ amu)

(a) – 4.03 MeV (b) – 2.01MeV
(c) 2.01 MeV (d) 4.03 MeV

44. Two condensers, one of capacity C and the other of capacity $\frac{C}{2}$, are connected to V volt battery, as shown in the figure.

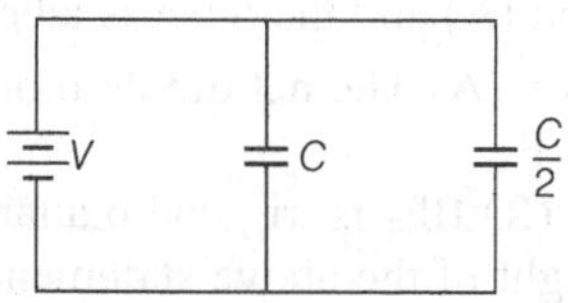

The work done in charging fully both the condensers is

(a) CV^2 (b) $\frac{1}{4}CV^2$
(c) $\frac{3}{4}CV^2$ (d) $\frac{1}{2}CV^2$

45. If a source is transmitting electromagnetic wave of frequency 8.2×10^6 Hz, the wavelength of the electromagnetic wave transmitted from the source will be

(a) 42.3 m (b) 36.6 m
(c) 50.9 m (d) 40.5 m

CHEMISTRY

46. Match the List-I with List-II.

List-I	List-II
A. Victor-Meyer's test	I. distinguish the presence of acetaldehyde and methyl ketone
B. Iodoform test	II. distinguish only aldehyde not ketone
C. Tollen's test	III. distinguish between 1°, 2° and 3° alcohols
D. Fehling test	IV. distinguish the both aliphatic and aromatic aldehyde.

Choose the correct answer from the options given below:

(a) A-III, B-I, C-II, D-IV (b) A-I, B-III, C-IV, D-II
(c) A-II, B-I, C-III, D-IV (d) A-IV, B-II, C-I, D-III

47. The value of n in

$MnO_4^- + 8H^+ + ne^- \longrightarrow Mn^{2+} + 4H_2O$, is

(a) 5 (b) 4 (c) 2 (d) 3

48. Given below are two statements.

Statement I $SiCl_4$ is easily hydrolysed.

Statement II PbF_4 is covalent in nature.

In the light of the above statements, choose the correct answer from the options given below.

(a) Both statement I and Statement II are false.
(b) Statement I is true but Statement II is false.
(c) Statement I is false but Statement II is true.
(d) Both statement I and Statement II are true.

49. Consider the following

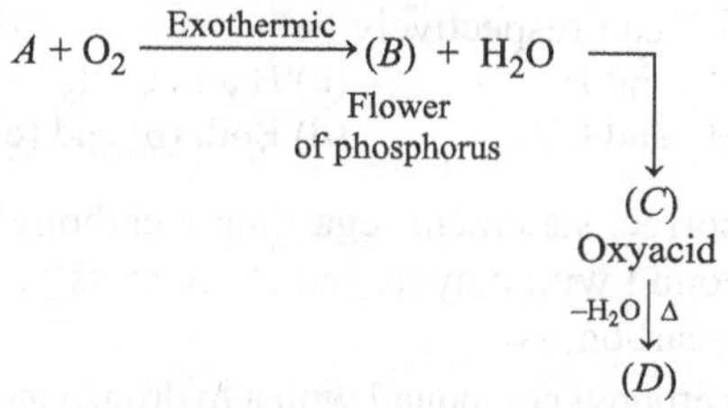

then A, B, C, D respectively are

(a) B_2H_6, P_4, H_3PO_4, P_2O_5
(b) P_4, P_4O_{10}, H_3PO_4, P_2O_5
(c) PCl_5, H_3PO_4, HPO_3, P_4O_{10}
(d) P_2O_5, P_4O_{10}, H_3PO_4, P_4

50. A graph of log $[A]$ *vs* t for first order reaction is given below.

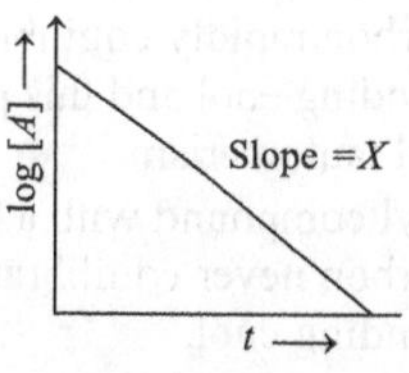

X is equal to

(a) $\frac{0.693}{k}$ (b) $\frac{k}{2.303}$
(c) $-\frac{k}{2.303}$ (d) log $[A_0]$

51. Aniline dissolves in HCl due to formation of

(a) anilinium chloride
(b) *o*-chloroaniline
(c) azo dye
(d) diazonium chloride

52. What is the activation energy for a reaction if its rate doubles when the temperature is raised from 20°C to 35°C? ($R = 8.314$ J mol^{-1}K^{-1} $\log 2 = 0.3010$)

(a) 342 kJ mol^{-1} (b) 269 kJ mol^{-1}
(c) 34.7 kJ mol^{-1} (d) 15.1 kJ mol^{-1}

53. In the Newman projection for

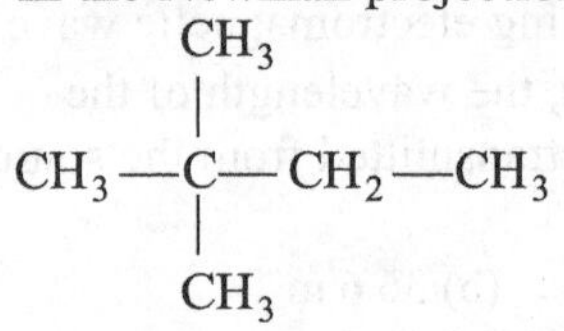

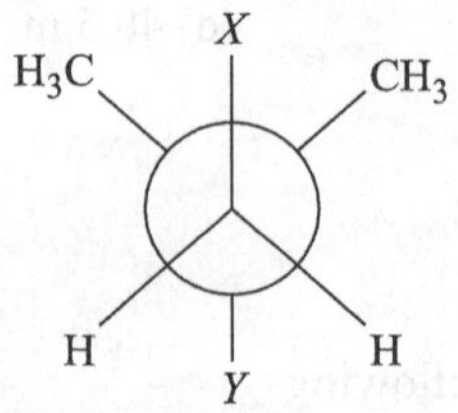

X and *Y* can respectively be

(a) CH_3 and H (b) H and C_2H_5
(c) CH_3 and CH_3 (d) Both (b) and (c)

54. The correct statement regarding a carbonyl compound with a hydrogen atom on its alpha-carbon, is

(a) a carbonyl compound with a hydrogen atom on its alpha-carbon rapidly equilibrates with its corresponding enol and this process is known as aldehyde-ketone equilibration.
(b) a carbonyl compound with a hydrogen atom on its alpha-carbon rapidly equilibrates with its corresponding enol and this process is known as carbonylation.
(c) a carbonyl compound with a hydrogen atom on its alpha-carbon rapidly equilibrates with its corresponding enol and this process is known as keto-enol tautomerism.
(d) a carbonyl compound with a hydrogen atom on its alpha-carbon never equilibrates with its corresponding enol.

55. An electrochemical cell consists of two half-cell reactions

$$AgCl(s) + e^- \longrightarrow Ag(s) + Cl^-(aq)$$
$$Cu(s) \longrightarrow Cu^{2+}(aq) + 2e^-$$

The mass of copper (in grams) dissolved on passing 0.5 A current for 1 hour is (Given : Atomic mass of Cu is 63.6; $F = 96500$ C mol^{-1})

(a) 0.88 g (b) 1.18 g
(c) 0.29 g (d) 0.59 g

56. Consider the given reaction,

$BX_3 + NH_3 \longrightarrow BX_3 \cdot NH_3$ + Heat of adduct (ΔH).

The numerical value of ΔH is found to be maximum for

(a) BF_3 (b) BCl_3
(c) BBr_3 (d) BI_3

57. Given below are two statements, one is labelled as Assertion (A) and the other is labelled as Reason (R).

Assertion (A) The net dipole moment of BF_3 is zero B.M.

Reason (R) BF_3 is trigonal planar in structure.

In the light of the above statements, choose the most appropriate answer from the options given below.

(a) Both (A) and (R) are true but (R) is not the correct explanation of (A).
(b) (A) is true but (R) is false.
(c) (A) is false but (R) is true.
(d) Both (A) and (R) are true and (R) is the correct explanation of (A).

58. Given below are two statements.

Statement I The first ionisation energy (I.E) of N is more than that of oxygen while 2nd I.E. of oxygen is more than that of nitrogen.

Statement II Nitrogen has half-filled *p*-orbitals which is stable as compared to oxygen.

In the light of the above statements, choose the correct answer from the options given below:

(a) Both statement I and Statement II are false.
(b) Statement I is true but Statement II is false.
(c) Statement I is false but Statement II is true.
(d) Both statement I and Statement II are true.

59. Consider the reactions,

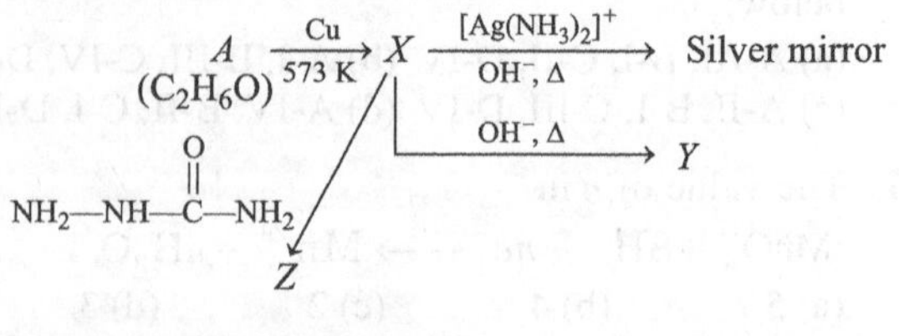

Identify *A*, *X*, *Y* and *Z*.

(a) *A*-methoxymethane, *X*-ethanoic acid, *Y*-acetate ion, *Z*-hydrazine
(b) *A*-methoxymethane, *X*-ethanol, *Y*-ethanoic acid, *Z*-semicarbazide
(c) *A*-ethanol, *X*-acetaldehyde, *Y*-but-2-en-1-al, *Z*-semicarbazone
(d) *A*-ethanol, *X*-acetaldehyde, *Y*-butanone, *Z*-hydrazone

60. Given below are two statements.

Statement I To a solution of potassium chromate, if a strong acid is added, it changes its colour from yellow to orange.

Statement II The colour change is due to the change in oxidation state of potassium chromate.

In the light of the above statements, choose the correct answer from the options given below.

(a) Both Statement I and Statement II are false.
(b) Statement I is true Statement II is false.
(c) Statement I is false but Statement II is true.
(d) Both Statement I and Statement II are true.

61. Basic strength of $CH \equiv \bar{C}$(I); $CH_2 = \bar{C}H$ (II) and $CH_3\bar{C}H_2$ (III) will be in order

(a) I <II<III
(b) II <III< I
(c) III <II<I
(d) III <I<II

62. Among Pb^{2+}, Ba^{2+}, Mn^{2+}, Zn^{2+}, Ag^{+} and Hg_2^{2+}, the number of cations that give white precipitate in dil. HCl is ....

(a) 1 (b) 2
(c) 3 (d) 4

63. Match the List-I with List-II.

	List-I	List-II
A.	PCl_5	(i) Square pyramidal
B.	SF_6	(ii) Trigonal planar
C.	BrF_5	(iii) Octahedral
D	BF_3	(iv) Trigonal bipyramidal

Choose the correct answer from the options given below.

(a) A-(iv), B-(ii), C-(iii), D-(i)
(b) A-(iv), B-(iii), C-(i), D-(ii)
(c) A-(iii), B-(iv), C-(i), D-(ii)
(d) A-(iii), B-(i), C-(ii), D-(iv)

64. Which of the following statement(s) regarding actinides is/are correct?

(a) Pu^{4+} disproportionates to Pu^{3+} and PuO_2^{2+} in acidic medium.
(b) Maximum oxidation state of Np is +7.
(c) UO_2^{2+} is stable.
(d) All of the above statements are correct.

65. pH of 0.5 M aqueous solution of HF ($K_a = 2 \times 10^{-4}$) is

(a) 2 (b) 4
(c) 6 (d) 10

66. The correct order of dipole moment is

(a) $CH_4 < NF_3 < NH_3 < H_2O$
(b) $NF_3 < CH_4 < NH_3 < H_2O$
(c) $NH_3 < NF_3 < CH_4 < H_2O$
(d) $H_2O < NH_3 < NF_3 < CH_4$

67. A solution containing 2.665 g of $CrCl_3 \cdot 6H_2O$ is passed through a cation exchanger. The chloride ions obtained in solution were treated with excess of $AgNO_3$ to give 2.87 g of AgCl. The formula of compound is

(a) $[CrCl\cdot(H_2O)_5]Cl_2 \cdot H_2O$
(b) $[CrCl_2 \cdot (H_2O)_4]Cl\cdot 2H_2O$
(c) $[CrCl_3 \cdot (H_2O)_3] H_2O$
(d) $[Cr\cdot(H_2O)_6]Cl_3$

68. Match the List-I with List-II.

List-I	List-II
A. $n=6 \rightarrow n=3$	(i) 3 lines in spectra
B. $n=5 \rightarrow n=3$	(ii) 10 lines in spectra
C. $n=5 \rightarrow n=1$	(iii) 6 lines in spectra
D. $n=4 \rightarrow n=3$	(iv) 1 line in spectra

Choose the correct answer from the options given below.

(a) A-(iii), B-(i), C-(ii), D-(iv)
(b) A-(i), B-(ii), C-(iii), D-(iv)
(c) A-(iv), B-(iii), C-(ii), D-(i)
(d) A-(i), B-(iv), C-(ii), D-(iii)

69. Given below are two statements.

Statement I S_N2 reaction always proceeds with inversion of configuration.

Statement II $CHCl_3$ is stored in dark bottles as it will reduce in sunlight.

In the light of the above statements, choose the correct answer from the options given below.

(a) Both statement I and Statement II are false.
(b) Statement I is true but Statement II is false.
(c) Statement I is false but Statement II is true.
(d) Both statements I and Statement II are true.

70. Match the List-I with List-II.

	List-I (Oxide)	List-II (Nature)
A.	CO	(i) Basic
B.	BaO	(ii) Neutral
C.	Al_2O_3	(iii) Acidic
D.	Cl_2O_7	(iv) Amphoteric

Choose the correct answer from the options given below.
(a) A-(ii), B-(i), C-(iv), D-(iii)
(b) A-(iii), B-(iv), C-(i), D-(ii)
(c) A-(iv), B-(iii), C-(ii), D-(i)
(d) A-(i), B-(ii), C-(iii), D-(iv)

71. Which of the following ether react with conc. HBr according to S_N2 mechanism?

(a) 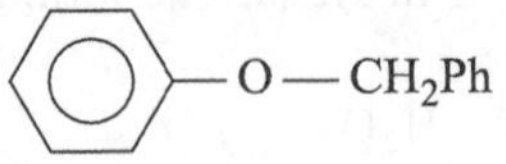

(b) 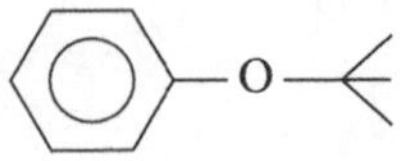

(c) 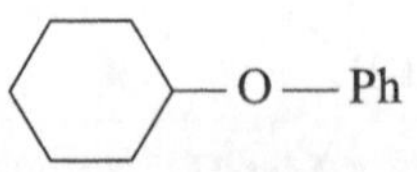

(d) 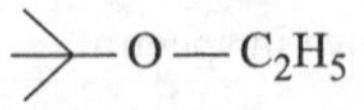

72. Which of the following does not show optical isomerism?
(a) $[Co(ox)_3]^{-3}$ (b) $[Cr(en)_2(NH_3)_2]^{+3}$
(c) $[Co(NH_3)_3Cl_3]$ (d) $[Co(en)Cl_2(NH_3)_2]^+$

73. Which of the following statements is not true for halogens?
(a) All form monobasic oxyacids.
(b) All halogen except fluorine show positive oxidation states.
(c) All are oxidising agents.
(d) Chlorine has the highest electron-gain enthalpy.

74. Consider the following equation.
$2SO_2(g) + O_2(g) \rightleftharpoons 2SO_3(g), \Delta H = -190$ kJ
A. increasing temperature
B. increasing pressure
C. adding more SO_2
D. adding more O_2
E. addition of catalyst
Which of the following factors will increase the yield of SO_2 at equilibrium?
(a) A and E only (b) A and B only
(c) B, C and D (d) A, B and C

75. The correct statement regarding the comparison of staggered and eclipsed conformations of ethane is
(a) the staggered conformation of ethane is less stable than eclipsed conformation, because staggered conformation has torsional strain.
(b) the eclipsed conformation of ethane is more stable than staggered conformation, because eclipsed conformation has no torsional strain.
(c) the eclipsed conformation of ethane is more stable than staggered conformation even though the eclipsed conformation has torsional strain.
(d) the staggered conformation of ethane is more stable than eclipsed conformation, because staggered conformation has no torsional strain.

76. Given below are two statements.
Statement I Alcohols on dehydration can produce ether as well as alkene under different conditions.
Statement II Dehydration of alcohol proceeds through the formation of carbonium ion.
In the light of the above statements, choose the correct answer from the options given below.
(a) Both Statement I and Statement II are false.
(b) Statement I is true but Statement II is false.
(c) Statement I is false but Statement II is true.
(d) Both Statement I and Statement II are true.

77. The correct statement regarding hydrolysis of a nitrile to a carboxylic acid is (are)

$$RCN + H_2O \longrightarrow RCOOH$$

(a) the reaction passes through an amide intermediate.
(b) acid catalyses the hydrolysis reaction.
(c) intermediate product is impractical to separate.
(d) the reaction does not work for the preparation of an aromatic acid.

78. Perkin's condensation is an example of chemical properties of aromatic aldehydes only. In this reaction, aromatic aldehydes condense with an acid anhydride to yield α,β-unsaturated acids. Intermediate involved in Perkin reaction is
(a) carbocation (b) carbanion
(c) free radical (d) carbene

79. In the reaction,

$$Ar\overset{+}{N}_2Cl^- \xrightarrow{Cu/HCl} ArCl + N_2 + CuCl \text{ is}$$

(a) Sandmeyer reaction
(b) Gattermann reaction
(c) Claisen reaction
(d) Carbylamine reaction

80. For a given reaction, $\Delta H = 40$ kJ mol^{-1} and $\Delta S = 80$ JK^{-1} mol^{-1}. The reaction is spontaneous at (assume that ΔH and ΔS does not vary with temperature)
(a) $T > 500$ K (b) $T < 500$ K
(c) At all temperatures (d) $T > 298$ K

81. Calculate $E°$ for the reaction

$$Cu(s) + 2Ag^{+}(aq) \longrightarrow Cu^{+2}(aq) + 2Ag(s)$$

If equilibrium constant for the reaction is 4×10^{15} at 298 K.

(a) 0.23 V (b) – 0.46 V
(c) 0.46 V (d) – 0.23 V

82. At a certain temperature, the vapour pressure of water is 90 mm. At the same temperature the vapour pressure of a solution containing a non-volatile solute is 81 mm. The relative lowering of vapour pressure is

(a) 9 (b) 0.9 (c) 10 (d) 0.1

83. Which of the following statements is/are correct?

I. During the decomposition of an oxide into oxygen and metal vapour, entropy increases.
II. Decomposition of an oxide is an endothermic change.
III. To make $\Delta G°$ negative, temperature should be high enough so that $T\Delta S° > \Delta H°$.
IV Decomposition of an oxide is exothermic change.
V. During the decomposition process, entropy decreases.

Choose the correct answer from the options given below.

(a) I, III and IV (b) II,III and V
(c) IV and V (d) I, II and III

84. The correct order of stability of the halous acids in aqueous solution is

(a) HClO < HBrO < HIO (b) HClO > HBrO < HIO
(c) HClO>HBrO > HIO (d) HClO < HBrO > HIO

85. Consider the following compounds.

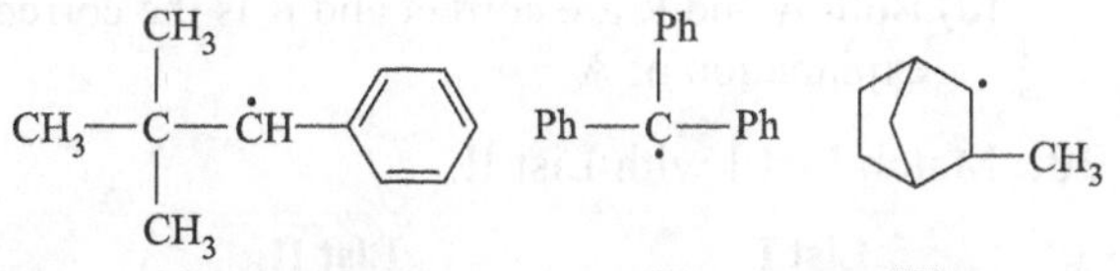

(I) (II) (III)

hyperconjugation occurs in

(a) Only I (b) Only II
(c) Only III (d) I and III

86. The coordination entity formed when excess of KCN is added to an aqueous solution of $CuSO_4$ is

(a) $[Cu(CN)_2]^{+}$ (b) $[Cu(CN)_6]^{4-}$
(c) $[Cu(CN)_4]^{3-}$ (d) $[Cu(CN)_4]^{3+}$

87. Which one of the following pairs of pyrimidine bases are present in DNA?

(a) Cytosine and uracil (b) Adenine and guanine
(c) Cytosine and adenine (d) Cytosine and thymine

88. Match the List-I with List-II.

	List-I		List-II
A.	Fructose	I.	Aldopentose
B.	Ribose	II.	Ketohexose
C.	Glucose	III.	Aldotetrose
D.	Erythrose	IV.	Aldohexose

Choose the correct answer from the options given below:

(a) A-IV, B-I, C-III, D-II
(b) A-III, B-IV, C-I, D-II
(c) A-I, B-II, C-III, D-IV
(d) A-II, B-I, C-IV, D-III

89. When 20g of naphthoic acid ($C_{11}H_8O_2$) is dissolved in 50g of benzene ($K_f = 1.72$ K kg mol^{-1}) freezing point depression of 2K is observed. The van't Hoff factor (i) is

(a) 0.5 (b) 1
(c) 2 (d) 3

90. In sulphur estimation, 0.157 grams of an organic compound gave 0.4813 gram of barium sulphate. What is the percentage of sulphur in the compound?

(a) 52.10% (b) 42.10%
(c) 38.11% (d) 11.01%

BIOLOGY

91. Productivity at the second trophic level is always
(a) greater than the productivity at the first trophic level
(b) less than the productivity at the first trophic level
(c) equal to the productivity at the first trophic level
(d) extremely variable compared to the productivity at the first trophic level

92. Given below are two statements.
Statement I Mutations are non-directional.
Statement II Darwin's small variations are directional.
In the light of the above statements, choose the correct answer from the options given below.
(a) Both statement I and statement II are true
(b) Both statement I and statement II are false
(c) Statement I is true, but statement II is false
(d) Statement I is false, but statement II is true

93. Given below are two statements.
Statement I Stolon is a subterranean long lateral branch arising from base of stem.
Statement II Offset arises from the axillary bud of underground part of stem.
In the light of the above statements, choose the correct answer from the options given below.
(a) Both statement I and statement II are false
(b) Statement I is true, but statement II is false
(c) Statement I is false, but statement II is true
(d) Both statement I and statement II are true

94. Which one of the following method is used to introduce alien DNA into host cells in animal cell?
(a) Micro-injection (b) Biolistics
(c) Gene gun (d) Insertional inactivation

95. Consider the following statements and choose the correct set of statements.
I. The axoneme usually has nine pairs of doublets in an arrangement of 9+2 array.
II. In animal cells, lipid-like steroidal hormones are synthesised in SER.
III. The cytoplasmic ribosomes are smaller than the ribosomes of chloroplasts.
IV. Mesosomes of eukaryotes perform function similar to mitochondria.
V. Cyanophycean granules are not membrane bound and lie free in the cytoplasm.

Choose the correct answer from the options given below.
(a) I, IV and V
(b) I and V
(c) II, III, IV and V
(d) I, II and V

96. Which one of the following is a correct statement?
(a) *Bt* in *Bt*-cotton indicates that it is a genetically modified organism produced through biotechnology
(b) Somatic hybridisation involves fusion of two complete plant cells carrying desired genes
(c) The human protein alpha-lactalbumin is being obtained from transgenic cow
(d) "Golden rice" variety of tomato has enhanced the production of vitamin-A, which improves its taste

97. Given below are two statements; one is labelled as Assertion (A) and the other is labelled as Reason (R).
Assertion (A) The axonal membrane of a neuron is polarised.
Reason (R) The membrane is negatively charged from outside.
In the light of above statements choose the correct answer from the options given below.
(a) Both A and R are true, but R is not the correct explanation of A
(b) A is true, but R is false
(c) A is false, but R is true
(d) Both A and R are correct and R is the correct explanation of A

98. Match List I with List II.

	List I		List II
A.	PCT	1.	Urine concentration
B.	Vasa recta	2.	Reabsorption
C.	Glomerulus	3.	Ultrafiltration
D.	DCT	4.	Selective secretion

Choose the correct answer from the options given below.

	A	B	C	D
(a)	2	4	3	1
(b)	4	1	3	2
(c)	2	1	3	4
(d)	1	2	3	4

99. Identify the incorrectly matched pair.
(a) J-shaped curve - Logistic growth
(b) S-shaped curve - Represented under limited resource conditions
(c) Mortality - Death rate
(d) Natality - Birth rate

100. Which of the following statements are incorrect?
I. Synaptic cleft of neurons secrete adrenaline.
II. Myelinated nerve fibres are enveloped with Schwann cells, which form a myelin sheath around the axon.
III. Non-myelinated nerve fibre is enclosed by a Schwann cell that does not form a myelin sheath.
IV. Spinal cord and cranial nerves are made of non-myelinated nerve fibres.
V. Short fibres, which branch repeatedly and project out of the cell body also contains Nissl's granules.

Codes
(a) I, II and III (b) II and III
(c) I and IV (d) I, IV and V

101. During eukaryotic transcription, what is the role or function of an enhancer ?
(a) Increases *m*RNA stability
(b) Elongation of transcript
(c) Transcription initiation
(d) Stimulates the rate of transcription

102. A series of genes in which transcription is regulated by DNA binding proteins is
(a) promoter (b) operator
(c) operon (d) terminator

103. Match List I with List II.

List I	List II
A. Insulin	1. δ - cells
B. Glucagon	2. α - cells
C. Somatostatin	3. F - cells
D. Pancreatic polypeptide	4. β - cells

Choose the correct answer from the options given below.

	A	B	C	D
(a)	4	2	1	3
(b)	1	3	4	2
(c)	4	2	3	1
(d)	1	3	2	4

104. A boy whose metabolic rate is abnormally high and has protruding eyeball is suffering from which of the following diseases?
(a) Goitre (b) Grave's disease
(c) Hashimoto's disease (d) Addison's disease

105. Which of the following is an example of family–Cruciferae and is useful in bronchitis and fever?
(a) *Raphanus sativus* (b) *Vetiveria zizanoides*
(c) *Iberis amara* (d) *Cheiranthus cheiri*

106. Match List I with List II.

List I		List II	
A.	Endangered species	1.	Facing a very high risk of extinction in near future
B.	Threatened species	2.	Liable to become extinct
C.	Extinct species	3.	Species that no longer exist
D.	Vulnerable species	4.	Not critically endangered

Choose the correct answer from the options given below.

	A	B	C	D
(a)	1	3	2	4
(b)	4	3	2	1
(c)	3	4	2	1
(d)	1	2	3	4

107. Name the antibody produced in response to the allergens.
(a) IgM (b) IgE (c) IgG (d) IgA

108. Read the following statements with respect to regulation of respiration and choose the correct option.
Statement I Respiratory rhythm centre present in the medulla region of brain is primarily responsible for regulation of normal rhythm of breathing.
Statement II The role of oxygen in the regulation of respiratory rhythm is very significant.
In the light of the above statements, choose the correct answer from the options given below.
(a) Both statement I and statement II are incorrect
(b) Statement I is incorrect, but statement II is correct
(c) Statement I is correct, but statement II is incorrect
(d) Both statement I and statement II are correct

109. Consider the following statements and select the correct statements from the options given below.

I. In dicotyledonous plants the cotyledon is known as scutellum.
II. Among animals, insects particularly birds are the dominant biotic pollinating agents.
III. Some flowers secrete foul odours to attract the animals for pollination.
IV. Castor prevents autogamy, but not geitonogamy.
V. Eggs are deposited in the locule of the *Yucca* plant by moth.

Choose the correct answer from the options given below.

(a) I, II, III and V (b) IV and V only
(c) III, IV and V (d) I, III, IV and V

110. Which of the following is true?

(a) Endosperm in angiosperm is a polyploid structure and form before fertilisation
(b) Triple fusion leads to the formation of a triploid Primary Endosperm Nucleus (PEN)
(c) The cylindrical portion below the level of cotyledon is called epicotyl
(d) Cotyledon of pea family is called scutellum

111. The maximum transportation of oxygen in the blood occurs

(a) in dissolved form (b) as bicarbonate
(c) as oxyhaemoglobin (d) both (a) and (b)

112. Diuretic drugs that promote secretion of excess urine from the body, are commonly used in the treatment of

(a) high blood pressure (b) renal failure
(c) renal calculi (d) glomerulonephritis

113. The two kingdom system of classification was discarded because of the fact that

(a) the plant kingdom comprised of photosynthetic and non photosynthetic organisms
(b) it did not distinguish between prokaryotes and eukaryotes
(c) it did not distinguish between unicellular and multicellular
(d) all of the above

114. In garden pea, yellow colour of cotyledons is dominant over green and round shape of seed is dominant over wrinkled. When a plant with yellow and round seed is crossed with a plant having yellow and wrinkled seeds, the progeny showed segregation for all the four characters. The probability of obtaining green round seeds in the progeny of this cross, is

(a) 1/4 (b) 1/8 (c) 1/16 (d) 3/16

115. Acquired Immuno Deficiency syndrome is caused by

(a) DNA containing arbovirus
(b) RNA containing arbovirus
(c) RNA containing retrovirus
(d) DNA containing retrovirus

116. The circulatory system of frog is well-developed and closed type. Some features of frog vascular system are given below. Read them carefully and identify the incorrect one.

(a) Heart is muscular, situated in the upper part of the body cavity
(b) A triangular structure called sinus venosus joins the left ventricle. It receives blood through the major vein called vena cava
(c) Special venous connections between liver and intestine as well as the kidney and lower part of the body are present in frogs
(d) RBCs are nucleated and contain red coloured pigment namely haemoglobin

117. Which among the following is not an example of biopiracy ?

(a) Basmati rice (*Oryza sativa*)
(b) Turmeric (*Curcuma longa*)
(c) Neem (*Azadirachta indica*)
(d) *Bacillus anthracis*

118. CAM (Crassulacean Acid Metabolism) plants have adapted in a way, that allows them to

(a) function better in humid conditions
(b) fix CO_2 during the day
(c) save enzyme RuBisCO from denaturation
(d) survive in arid conditions

119. Given below are two statements.

Statement I Rheumatoid arthritis is an auto-immune disease.

Statement II In rheumatoid arthritis the body attacks the foreign cells and protects itself against disease.

In the light of the above statements, choose the correct answer from the options given below.

(a) Both statement I and statement II are false
(b) Statement I is true, but statement II is false
(c) Statement I is false, but statement II is true
(d) Both statement I and statement II are true

120. Which of the following represents the correct sequence for the transport of sperms?
(a) Rete testis→ Vasa efferentia→ Seminiferous tubules→ Ejaculatory duct→ Epididymis→ Urethra→ Vas deferens
(b) Seminiferous tubules→ Rete testis→ Vasa efferentia→ Epididymis→ Vas deferens→ Ejaculatory duct→ Urethra
(c) Epididymis→ Seminiferous tubules→ Vasa efferentia→ Vas deferens→ Ejaculatory duct→ Urethra→ Rete testis
(d) Vasa efferentia→ Vas deferens→ Seminiferous tubules→ Epididymis→ Rete testis→ Ejaculatory duct→ Urethra

121. Match List I with List II.

	List I		List II
A.	Deuteromycetes	1.	Gametes are similar in morphology
B.	Ascomycetes	2.	Sexual spores are produced endogenously
C.	Basidiomycetes	3.	Imperfect fungi
D.	Phycomycetes	4.	Sex organ are absent

Codes

	A	B	C	D		A	B	C	D
(a)	3	4	1	2	(b)	4	1	3	2
(c)	4	3	1	2	(d)	3	2	4	1

122. What is the primary mechanism of action for a copper IUD?
(a) Prevents ovulation
(b) Creates a hostile environment for sperm
(c) Thickens cervical mucus
(d) Prevents implantation of a fertilised egg

123. Given below are two statements.
Statement I ATP synthesis is linked to the development of proton gradient across the membrane of thylakoid.
Statement II Protons in the stroma increase in number, while in thylakoid lumen there is decrease in protons when sunlight is received by the chloroplast.
In the light of the above statements, choose the correct answer from the options given below.
(a) Both statement I and statement II are false
(b) Statement I is true, but statement II is false
(c) Statement I is false, but statement II is true
(d) Both statement I and statement II are true

124. The host cells are made competent to take up DNA by treating them with ....
(a) potassium (b) bromine
(c) sodium (d) calcium

125. Match List I with List II.

	List I		List II
A.	Commensalism	1.	+, +
B.	Parasitism	2.	+, 0
C.	Mutualism	3.	+, –
D.	Predation	4.	+, –

Choose the correct answer from the options given below.

	A	B	C	D		A	B	C	D
(a)	3	2	1	4	(b)	4	3	1	2
(c)	1	2	3	4	(d)	2	3	1	4

126. Which of the following belongs to Leguminosae and have imbricate aestivation?
(a) Gobhi, *Labularia*
(b) Gulmohar, *Cassia*
(c) Aloe vera, *Pisum sativum*
(d) Khuskhus, *Cymbopogon flexuosus*

127. With respect to plant growth, which of the following statements is correct?
(a) In coriander, leaves of the juvenile plant are different in shape from the mature plants
(b) Due to the presence of tracheids the plants retain the capacity of unlimited growth throughout their life
(c) Auxin is used to speed up the malting process in brewing industry
(d) Natural cytokinins like kinetin are synthesised in the root apices

128. Choose the correct organism showing A type of symmetry, B type of embryonic layer arrangement and C type of coelom from the following options.

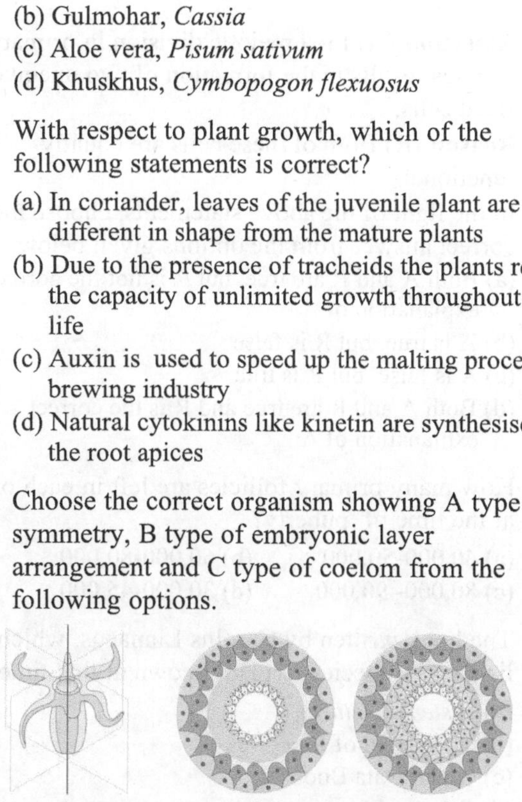

(a) *Fasciola* (b) *Pennatula*
(c) *Ancylostoma* (d) *Hirudinaria*

129. Which of the following statement is correct for *Mycoplasma*?
(a) It is a prokaryote and lacks cell wall
(b) Smallest living cells
(c) They can survive without oxygen
(d) All of the above

130. A cell examined during prophase of cell cycle contained 100 chromatids and 50 chromosomes. What would be the number of chromatids and chromosomes in anaphase of this cell cycle?
(a) 200 chromatids and 100 chromosomes
(b) 100 chromatids and 50 chromosomes
(c) 100 chromatids and 100 chromosomes
(d) 50 chromatids and 25 chromosomes

131. Name the phenomenon in which the living cells regain the capacity of division.
(a) Redifferentiation (b) Dedifferentiation
(c) Differentiation (d) None of these

132. Given below are two statements; one is labelled as Assertion (A) and the other is labelled as Reason (R).
Assertion (A) First meiotic division in primary oocytes results in the formation of two unequal sized cells.
Reason (R) Both of these cells are equally functional.
In the light of the above statements, choose the correct answer from the options given below.
(a) Both A and R are true, but R is not the correct explanation of A
(b) A is true, but R is false
(c) A is false, but R is true
(d) Both A and R are true and R is the correct explanation of A

133. How many primary follicles are left in each ovary at the time of puberty?
(a) 40,000-50,000 (b) 60,000-80,000
(c) 80,000- 90,000 (d) 30,000-45,000

134. The book written by Carolus Linnaeus, which lists every species of plant known at that time is
(a) *Systema Naturae*
(b) The origin of life
(c) Green Data Book
(d) *Species Plantarum*

135. Give below are two statements; one is labelled as Assertion (A) and the other is labelled as Reason (R).
Assertion (A) AV node present near the groove separates auricles from ventricle.
Reason (R) The left auricle receives deoxygenated blood from the lungs.
In the light of the above statements, choose the correct answer the options given below.
(a) Both A and R are true, but R is not the correct explanation of A
(b) A is true, but R is false
(c) A is false, but R is true
(d) Both A and R are true and R is the correct explanation of A

136. Identify the correct statements(s) regarding bulliform cells.
(a) Bulliform cells are found in monocot leaves
(b) They help in rolling of leaves in dry weather
(c) They are also known as motor cells
(d) All of the above

137. The vital capacity includes
(a) inspiratory reserve volume + tidal volume
(b) tidal volume + inspiratory reserve volume + expiratory reserve volume
(c) expiratory reserve volume + tidal volumé
(d) expiratory reserve volume + inspiratory reserve volume

138. Which one of the following statements is false with respect to the condition phenylketonuria?
(a) It is the result of pleiotropy
(b) It is an autosomal recessive trait
(c) It is a metabolic error
(d) It is a case of aneuploidy

139. In which of the following species, food is stored in the form of laminarin?
(a) *Dictyota* (b) *Spirogyra*
(c) *Gracilaria* (d) *Polytrichum*

140. Select the correct statements with reference to recombinant DNA technology.
I. Lysozyme acts as a cell wall degrading enzyme for plant cells.
II. Agarose gel electrophoresis is used to check the progression of restriction enzyme digestion.

III. DNA polymerase is isolated from a bacterium *Thermus aquaticus*.
IV. When a protein encoding gene is expressed in a homologous host it is known as recombinant protein.
V. DNA being negatively charged moves towards the anode.

Choose the correct answer from the options given below.
(a) I, II, III and IV
(b) I, III, IV and V
(c) II, III and V
(d) I, II and V

141. The first clinical gene therapy to a 4 year old girl was given in which year?
(a) 1989 (b) 1990
(c) 1995 (d) 1991

142. Given below are two statements, one is labelled as Assertion (A) and the other is labelled as Reason (R).
Assertion (A) Two turns of Krebs' cycle occur per glucose molecule used.
Reason (R) Each turn of Krebs' cycle produces 3 NADH, 1 $FADH_2$ and 1 ATP molecule.
In the light of the above statements, choose the correct answer from the options given below.
(a) Both A and R are true, but R is not the correct explanation of A
(b) A is true, but R is false
(c) A is false, but R is true
(d) Both A and R are true and R is the correct explanation of A

143. Select the correct statement with respect to bundle sheath cells of C_4-plants.
I. Cell wall is permeable to atmospheric gases.
II. Small sized chloroplast with well developed grana.
III. Glucose formation takes place by C_4 cycle.
IV. Photorespiration is absent.
V. PEP synthetase is present.

Codes
(a) I, II, III and IV
(b) II, III, IV and V
(c) III, IV and V
(d) IV only

144. Match List I with List II.

	List I		List II
A.	Dicot stem	1.	Hypodermis is sclerenchymatous
B.	Monocot stem	2.	Pericycle gives rise to lateral roots only
C.	Monocot root	3.	Pericycle gives rise to lateral roots and secondary meristem
D.	Dicot root	4.	Hypodermis is collenchymatous

Choose the correct answer form the options given below.

	A	B	C	D
(a)	1	2	3	4
(b)	1	4	3	2
(c)	1	4	2	3
(d)	4	1	2	3

145. Identify the correct statement about the structure labelled as '*A*' in the given figure.

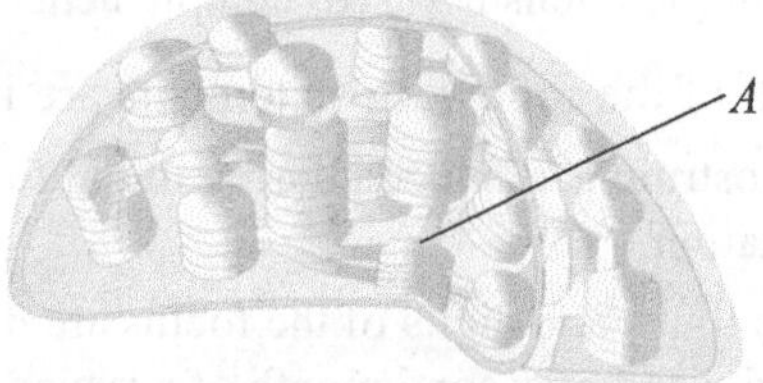

(a) These are flattened membranous sacs present in granum
(b) These are arranged in stacks called stroma lamella
(c) Their membrane encloses a space which is called as lumen.
(d) They connect stroma of different grama by flat membranous tubules

146. If a person has 'B' blood group, the type of antibodies present in the plasma of the person will be
(a) anti-B (b) anti- A, B
(c) anti-A (d) nil

147. Given below are two statements.
Statement I A flat bone called sternum is present on the ventral midline of thorax.
Statement II The progressive degeneration of skeletal muscle is known as myasthenia gravis.

In the light of the above statements, choose the correct answer from the options given below.
(a) Both statement I and statement II are false
(b) Statement I is true, but statement II is false
(c) Statement I is false, but statement II is true
(d) Both statement I and statement II are true

148. In collenchyma, the corners of cells are deposited with
(a) cellulose
(b) pectin substances
(c) Both (a) and (b)
(d) none of these

149. Heavy Mero-Myosin (HMM) contains
(a) globular head
(b) tail
(c) globular head with a short arm
(d) long arm and a tail

150. When a gene has two or more alleles that are common in a population, the phenomenon is known as
(a) polyploidy (b) polygenic inheritance
(c) multiple allelism (d) complementary genes

151. Which of the following statements are incorrect?
I. Colostrum is produced during initial few days of lactation.
II. The limbs and digits of the foetus are developed by the end of second month of pregnancy.
III. The transformation of spermatids to sperms is termed as spermatogenesis.
IV. Excess of testosterone inhibits LH/ICSH.
V. The progesterone level in blood increases resulting in strong sex urge in the female.
Choose the incorrect answer from the options given below.
(a) I and II (b) III and V
(c) I and III (d) IV and V

152. Match List I with List II.

	List I		List II
A.	Invertebrates	1.	350 mya
B.	*Ichthyosaurus*	2.	200 mya
C.	Jawless fish	3.	320 mya
D.	Sea weeds	4.	500 mya

Choose the correct answer from the options given below.

	A	B	C	D		A	B	C	D
(a)	1	2	4	3	(b)	3	2	1	4
(c)	4	2	1	3	(d)	4	1	2	3

153. How many gram per litre of human protein enriched milk was produced by the first transgenic cow, Rosie?
(a) 1.5 grams per litre
(b) 2.4 grams per litre
(c) 3 grams per litre
(d) 2 grams per litre

154. Which of the following fungi is used for the production of antibiotic penicillin?
(a) *S. griesus* (b) *P. butylicum*
(c) *S. cerevisiae* (d) *P. notatum*

155. Given below are two statements; one is labelled as Assertion (A) and the other is labelled Reason (R).

Assertion (A) In arithmetic growth, following mitotic cell division, only one daughter cell continues to divide, while other differentiate and matures.

Reason (R) The simplest expression of arithmetic growth is exemplified by a root elongating at a constant rate.

In the light of above statement, choose the correct answer from the options given below.
(a) Both A and R are true, but R is not the correct explanation of A
(b) A is correct, but R is incorrect
(c) A is incorrect, but R is correct
(d) Both A and R are correct and R is the correct explanation of A

156. Which of the following correctly differentiates prosthetic group from co-enzyme?
(a) Prosthetic group require metal ions for their activity
(b) Prosthetic groups are tightly bound to apoenzymes
(c) Prosthetic groups are associated with apoenzymes in transient
(d) Prosthetic group can serve as cofactors in a number of enzyme catalysed reactions

157. Match List I with List II.

	List I		List II
A.	Turner's syndrome	1.	Autosomal recessive disorder
B.	Down's syndrome	2.	Additional copy of X-chromosome
C.	Klinefelter's syndromes	3.	Trisomy of 21 chromosome
D.	Phenylketonuria	4.	Absence of one X-chromosome

Choose the correct answer from the options given below

	A	B	C	D		A	B	C	D
(a)	4	3	2	1	(b)	4	3	1	2
(c)	3	4	2	1	(d)	1	4	3	2

158. The enzyme DNA polymerase works in which direction?

(a) 5′–3′ direction (b) 3′–5′ direction
(c) 3′–3′ direction (c) 5′–5′ direction

159. Read the following statements and choose the correct set of statements.

I. Cellulose is a homopolymer consisting of one type of monosaccharide.
II. The first and last amino acids are also called C-terminal and N- terminal amino acids, respectively.
III. The exoskeleton of arthropods contains chitin, are heteropolymer.
IV. Starch is a heteropolymer and not homopolymer.
V. Gingely oil has low melting point due to which it remains as oil in winters.

Choose the most appropriate answer from the options given below.

(a) I, II and V (b) I and V only
(c) III and IV only (d) I, II, III and V

160. Given below are two statements.

Statement I Cleistogamous flowers are invariably autogamous.

Statement II Cleistogamous flowers do not open at all.

In the light of the above statements, choose the correct answer from the options given below.

(a) Both statement I and statement II are false
(b) Statement I is true, but statement II is false
(c) Statement I is false, but statement II is true
(d) Both statement I and statement II are true

161. Read the following statements and choose the correct set of statements.

I. Cyclosporin has antibacterial properties.
II. Statins are the products of fermentation activity of yeast *Monascus purpureus*.
III. Gluconic acid was the first acid to be produced by industrial fermentation.
IV. Bottled juices are clarified using proteases and pectinase.
V. The large holes in Swiss cheese are due to production of large amount of CO_2.

Choose the correct answer from the options given below.

(a) II, IV and V
(b) I, II and III
(c) II, III and IV
(d) I, II and V

162. Which of the following directs the formation of the bipolar spindle fibres during cell division?

(a) Golgi body (b) Centriole
(c) Ribosome (d) Cilia

163. Genetically Modified Organisms (GMOs) are developed by *r*DNA technology and genetic engineering. They are useful in

(a) enhancing food's nutritional value
(b) reducing in the post-harvest losses
(c) increasing the tolerance power of crops against the abiotic stresses
(d) all of the above

164. Which of the following represents the correct sequence for the transmission of an electrical impulse through a neuron?

(a) Cell body→ Axon→ Axon terminal→ Dendrites
(b) Dendrites→ Cell body→ Axon→ Axon terminal
(c) Axon→ Axon terminal→ Dendrites→ Cell body
(d) Axon→ Cell body→ Dendrites→ Axon terminal

165. The species which shows bioluminescence is
(a) *Pleurobrachia* (b) *Taenia*
(c) *Obelia* (d) *Gorgonia*

166. To produce 104 pollen grains, how many meiotic divisions are required ?
(a) 25 (b) 26
(c) 25.5 (d) 27

167. The logistic model is given as

$$\frac{dN}{dt} = rN(1 - N/K)$$

When does the growth rate of a population following the logistic model equal zero? .
(a) When N nears the carrying capacity of the habitat
(b) When N/K equal to zero
(c) When death rate is greater than birth rate
(d) When N/K is exactly one

168. The five kingdom system of classification is based on
(a) cell structure (b) body structure
(c) nutrition and lifestyle (d) all of these

169. Which of the following techniques is/are highly effective for birth control?
I. Vasectomy II. Tubectomy
III. Periodic abstinence
IV. Coitus interruptus
V. Condoms
Choose the correct answer from the options given below.
(a) I and II (b) III and IV
(c) II and III (d) Only IV

170. Consider the following statements and select the correct set of option.
I. The UTRs are present at both 3′ end before start codon and 5′ end after stop codon.
II. Mg^{2+} is essential during activation of amino acids.
III. Poly-A is added to 3′ end of newly formed *hn*RNA by poly-A polymerase.
IV. Non-formylated methionine is attached with *t*RNA in eukaryotes.
V. Release factor bind to the stop codon, resulting in termination of translation.

Codes
(a) I, II and III
(b) III, IV and V
(c) II, III, IV and V
(d) I and III

171. Identify the incorrectly matched pair.
(a) Virus - Take over cellular machinery of the host cell
(b) Prions - Modified hydrophobic glycoproteins
(c) Viroids-RNA entities consist of 250-370 nucleotides
(d) Creutzfeldt Jacob disease-Viral disease

172. The condition where the anthers do not dehisce and the germinated pollen tube pierces anther wall and enters the stigma of same flower, is known as
(a) geitonogamy (b) cleistogamy
(c) herkogamy (d) dicliny

173. Match List I with List II.

	List I		List II
A.	Neanderthal man	1.	900 cc
B.	*Homo habilis*	2.	1600 cc
C.	*Homo erectus*	3.	1400 cc
D.	Cro-Magnon man	4.	650 cc

Choose the correct answer from the options given below.

	A	B	C	D
(a)	1	2	3	4
(b)	2	3	4	1
(c)	3	4	1	2
(d)	4	1	2	3

174. The Nile perch was introduced in lake Victoria which led to the extinction of cichlid fish in the lake. This cause is best explained by
(a) overexploitation
(b) alien species invasion
(c) co-extinction
(d) habitat loss and fragmentation

175. Arrange the number of chromosomes in antipodal cells, embryo, integuments, endosperm and nucellus sequentially, if the haploid number in flowering plant is 20.

(a) 40, 40, 10, 60, 20 (b) 20, 40, 20, 60, 20
(c) 40, 10, 20, 60, 20 (d) 20, 40, 40, 60, 40

176. Which one among the following statements correctly describes a tracheid?

(a) Lignin is deposited in the cellulose wall to form annular or spiral thickenings
(b) Dead, single cells with hard and lignified walls
(c) Both (a) and (b)
(d) None of the above

177. Give below are two statements.

Statement I The chorionic villi and uterine tissue interlink to form the placenta.

Statement II Placenta acts as an endocrine tissue and produces several hormones.

In the light of the above statements, choose the correct answer from the options given below.

(a) Both statement I and statement II are false
(b) Statement I is true, but statement II is false
(c) Statement I is false, but statement II is true
(d) Both statement I and statement II are true

178. Which among the following has isogamous and non- flagellated gametes?

(a) *Spirogyra* (b) *Volvox*
(c) *Chlamydomonas* (d) *Ulothrix*

179. In protein structure, the strongest bonds are

(a) ionic bonds
(b) covalent bonds
(c) hydrogen bonds
(d) Van der Waals interactions

180. *Calotropis* shows

(a) whorled phyllotaxy (b) alternate phyllotaxy
(c) opposite phyllotaxy (d) parallel phyllotaxy

Explanations

Physics

1. (a) For electron,

$$\lambda_e = \frac{h}{p} = \frac{h}{mv} = \frac{h}{\frac{2mv^2}{2v}} = \frac{hv}{2E_e}$$

For photon, $\lambda_{ph} = \frac{hc}{E_{ph}}$

Now, $\frac{\lambda_{ph}}{\lambda_e} = \frac{\frac{hc}{E_{ph}}}{\frac{hv}{2E_e}} = \frac{2c}{v}$ $[\because E_{ph} = E_e]$

Since, $c >> v$

$\therefore$ $\frac{\lambda_{ph}}{\lambda_e} > 1$

$\Rightarrow$ $\lambda_{ph} > \lambda_e$

2. (a) Here,

$$\mathbf{v}_{BG} = 3\hat{\mathbf{i}} + 4\hat{\mathbf{j}}$$
$$\mathbf{v}_{WG} = -3\hat{\mathbf{i}} - 4\hat{\mathbf{j}}$$

$\therefore$
$$\mathbf{v}_{BW} = \mathbf{v}_{BG} - \mathbf{v}_{WG} = (3\hat{\mathbf{i}} + 4\hat{\mathbf{j}}) - (-3\hat{\mathbf{i}} - 4\hat{\mathbf{j}}) = 6\hat{\mathbf{i}} + 8\hat{\mathbf{j}}$$

3. (c) Given, $I_1 = I, I_2 = 4I$

$$I_{\max} = (\sqrt{I_1} + \sqrt{I_2})^2 = (\sqrt{I} + \sqrt{4I})^2 = (3\sqrt{I})^2 = 9I$$
$$I_{\min} = (\sqrt{I_2} - \sqrt{I_1})^2 = (\sqrt{4I} - \sqrt{I})^2 = (\sqrt{I})^2 = I$$

4. (b) Here, $\rho_A = \rho_0$

From $pV = \frac{m}{M}RT$, we get

$$\frac{m}{V} = \frac{pM}{RT}$$

and $\rho = \frac{m}{V} = \frac{pM}{RT}$

$\therefore$ $\frac{\rho_B}{\rho_A} = \frac{p_B T_A}{T_B\, p_A} = \frac{3p_0 \cdot T_0}{2T_0 \cdot p_0} = \frac{3}{2}$

$$\rho_B = \frac{3}{2}\rho_0$$

5. (d) During rapid pumping of air in tyres, air inside the tyre is hotter than atmospheric air.
Hence, Assertion is false but Reason is true.

6. (b) Fringe width, $\beta = \frac{D\lambda}{d}$

or $\beta \propto \lambda$

If the experiment is performed in water, wavelength λ decreases, so fringe width also decreases.

7. (c)

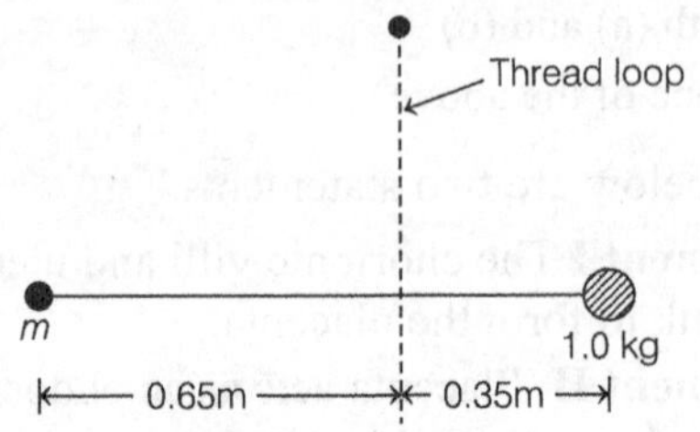

Using the principle of moments of masses,

$$mg \times 0.65 = 1g \times 0.35$$
$$m = \frac{35}{65} = 0.54 \text{ kg}$$

8. (c) As heights are same,

i.e. $H_P = H_Q$

$\Rightarrow$ $\frac{u_P^2 \sin^2 30^\circ}{2g} = \frac{u_Q^2 \sin^2\theta}{2g}$

$\Rightarrow$ $\frac{\sin^2\theta}{\sin^2 30^\circ} = \left(\frac{u_P}{u_Q}\right)^2 = \frac{9}{1}$

or $\sin^2\theta = \frac{9}{1} \times \sin^2 30^\circ = \frac{9}{4}$

$\Rightarrow$ $\theta = \sin^{-1}\left(\frac{3}{2}\right)$

9. (d) Speed of light in vacuum, $c = \frac{1}{\sqrt{\mu_0 \varepsilon_0}}$

and in another medium, $v = \frac{1}{\sqrt{\mu\varepsilon}}$

$\therefore$ $\frac{c}{v} = \sqrt{\frac{\mu\varepsilon}{\mu_0\varepsilon_0}} = \sqrt{\mu_r K} \Rightarrow v = \frac{c}{\sqrt{\mu_r K}}$

10. (c) On going above the surface of earth at height h, the value of acceleration due to gravity (g_h) is given as

$$g_h = \frac{g}{\left(1 + \frac{h}{R}\right)^2}$$

$$\Rightarrow \quad \frac{g}{4} = \frac{g}{\left(1+\frac{h}{R}\right)^2} \quad \left[\text{Given}, g_h = \frac{g}{4}\right]$$

$$\Rightarrow \quad \left(\frac{1}{2}\right)^2 = \frac{1}{\left(1+\frac{h}{R}\right)^2}$$

$$\Rightarrow \quad \frac{1}{2} = \frac{1}{1+\frac{h}{R}} \Rightarrow 1+\frac{h}{R} = 2$$

$$\Rightarrow \quad h = R$$

11. (c) As, $\lambda_1 < \lambda_2 < \lambda_3$

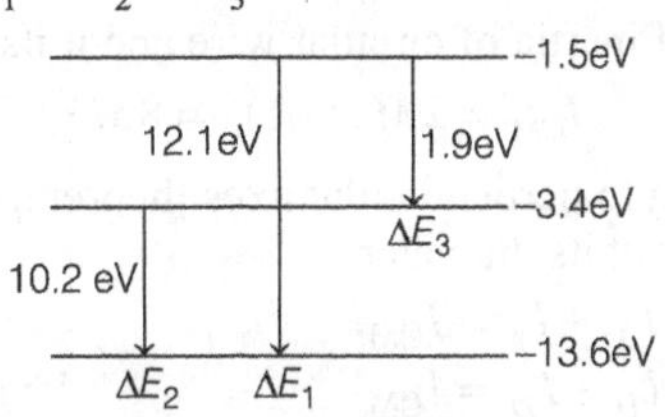

$$\Delta E_1 = \Delta E_2 + \Delta E_3$$

$$\therefore \quad \frac{hc}{\lambda_1} = \frac{hc}{\lambda_2} + \frac{hc}{\lambda_3}$$

$$\Rightarrow \quad \frac{1}{\lambda_1} = \frac{1}{\lambda_2} + \frac{1}{\lambda_3}$$

12. (c) As, $U = \frac{A}{x^2} - \frac{B}{x}$

For equilibrium, $\frac{dU}{dx} = 0$

$$\Rightarrow \quad \frac{d}{dx}\left(\frac{A}{x^2} - \frac{B}{x}\right) = -\frac{2A}{x^3} + \frac{B}{x^2} = 0$$

$$\Rightarrow \quad x = \frac{2A}{B}$$

For stable equilibrium, $\frac{d^2U}{dx^2} > 0$

$$\therefore \quad \frac{d^2U}{dx^2} = \frac{d}{dx}\left(-\frac{2A}{x^3} + \frac{B}{x^2}\right) = \frac{6A}{x^4} - \frac{2B}{x^3}$$

$$\therefore \quad \left(\frac{d^2U}{dx^2}\right)_{x=\frac{2A}{B}} = \frac{B^4}{8A^3} > 0$$

The distance at which both the particles will be in stable equilibrium is $x = \frac{2A}{B}$

13. (d) Pressure in spherical drop, $p = \frac{2T}{R}$

$$\frac{2T}{R_1} = 5 \times \frac{2T}{R_2} \quad (\because \text{Given}, \ p_1 = 5p_2)$$

$$\Rightarrow \quad R_2 = 5R_1$$

and

$$\frac{m_1}{m_2} = \frac{(4/3)\pi R_1^3 d_1}{(4/3)\pi R_2^3 d_2} = \frac{1}{125} \quad [\because d_1 = d_2]$$

14. (a) As the gravitational force of attraction between sun and jupiter provide the necessary centripetal force to jupiter to move in a circular orbit.

So, $$F = \frac{mv^2}{r} = \frac{GMm}{r^2} \Rightarrow v = \sqrt{\frac{GM}{r}}$$

$$= \sqrt{\frac{6.67 \times 10^{-11} \times 1.99 \times 10^{30}}{7.8 \times 10^{11}}}$$

$$= 1.3 \times 10^4 \text{ ms}^{-1}$$

15. (c) $I_g = \frac{V}{G}$

and $$R = \frac{nV}{I_g} - G = \frac{nV}{V/G} - G = (n-1)G$$

16. (a) When the phase difference between the two sources varies continuously, then positions of bright and dark fringes will change rapidly. Such rapid changes cannot be detected by our eyes. Thus, a uniform illumination is seen on the screen, i.e., interference pattern disappears. Hence, Statement I is correct.

The light waves emitted by two different lamps cannot be coherent. So the conditions of maxima and minima of intensity will change rapidly on the screen, producing uniform illumination and thus, no interference pattern will be observed. Hence, Statement II is also correct.

17. (b) When an α-particle enters into a uniform magnetic field perpendicular to its direction, then it moves on circular path in magnetic field i.e., it performs uniform circular motion in magnetic field.

In uniform circular motion of α-particle, its momentum changes due to change in its velocity but kinetic energy remains unchanged because magnitude of velocity (i.e, speed) always remains constant.

18. (a) In the given circuit, diode is in reverse biasing, so it acts as open circuit. Hence, potential difference between A and B is 6V.

19. (c) Given, resistance is in a parallel combination

So, $$\frac{1}{R_{AB}} = \frac{1}{2} + \frac{1}{2} + \frac{1}{2} + \frac{1}{2} + \frac{1}{2} = \frac{5}{2}$$

$$\therefore \quad R_{AB} = 0.4\ \Omega$$

20. (b) The energy of the photon

$$= Rhc\left(\frac{1}{1} - \frac{1}{n^2}\right) = 13.6\left(\frac{1}{1} - \frac{1}{4}\right) \quad (\because n = 2)$$

$$= 13.6\left(\frac{4-1}{4}\right)$$

$$= 13.6 \times \frac{3}{4} = \frac{40.8}{4} = 10.2 \text{ eV}$$

Problem Solving Tactics To better understand this concept, review the Bohr's model of the hydrogen atom and the energy levels associated with different quantum number (n).

21. (d) At steady state, the inductor behaves as a closed circuit. So, whole current will pass through the inductor and current in $10\,\Omega$ resistor is zero.

22. (b) In n-type semiconductor, the pentavalent impurity atom shares four of its valence electrons with four Si or Ge atoms, while its fifth electron remains free. Thus, n-type semiconductor has an excess of negative charge carriers (electrons). Since, amount of positive and negative charges in n-type semiconductor are equal, thus net charge on n-type semiconductor is zero. Hence, n-type semiconductor is electrically neutral.

23. (b) Statement B is incorrect because photocurrent increases linearly with intensity of incident light.

24. (b) Speed of wave over string, $v = \sqrt{\dfrac{F}{\mu}}$

$$f \cdot \lambda = \sqrt{\frac{F}{\mu}} \Rightarrow f = \frac{1}{\lambda}\sqrt{\frac{F}{\mu}}$$

As for a string, $\lambda = \dfrac{2l}{n}$

where, n = number of harmonic = 1,2,3, ...

So, $$f = \frac{n}{2l}\sqrt{\frac{F}{\mu}} = \frac{k}{l}\sqrt{\frac{F}{\mu}} \qquad \left[\because k = \frac{n}{2}\right]$$

25. (c) Given, $\phi = 4t^2 + 3t - 4$

$$\therefore \quad |e| = \left|\frac{d\phi}{dt}\right| = \frac{d}{dt}(4t^2 + 3t - 4) = 8t + 3$$

At $\quad t = 2\text{s}, |e| = 8 \times 2 + 3 = 19\text{ V}$

26. (d) Given, $\quad P = \dfrac{a^2 b^{1/2}}{c^{3/2}}$

$$\Rightarrow \frac{\Delta P}{P} \times 100 = 2\frac{\Delta a}{a} \times 100 + \frac{1}{2} \times \frac{\Delta b}{b} \times 100 + \frac{3}{2} \times \frac{\Delta c}{c} \times 100$$

$$= 2 \times 2\% + \frac{1}{2} \times 4\% + \frac{3}{2} \times 6\% = 4\% + 2\% + 9\% = 15\%$$

27. (b) From the figure,

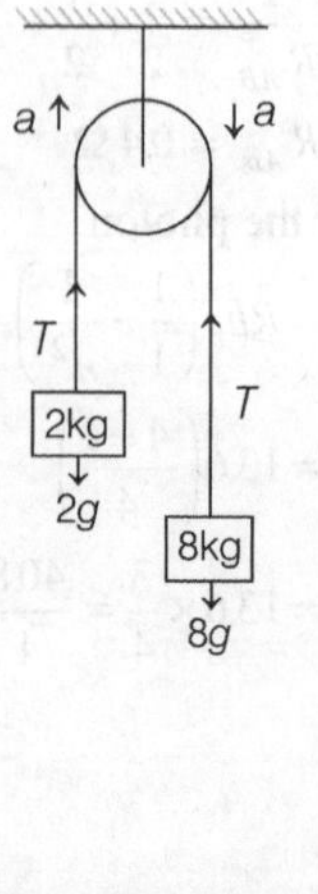

For mass 2 kg, $\quad T - 2g = 2a \quad$ ...(i)

For mass 8kg, $\quad 8g - T = 8a \quad$ ...(ii)

From Eqs.(i) and (ii), we get

$$6g = 10a \Rightarrow a = \frac{6g}{10} = \frac{3g}{5}$$

28. (b)

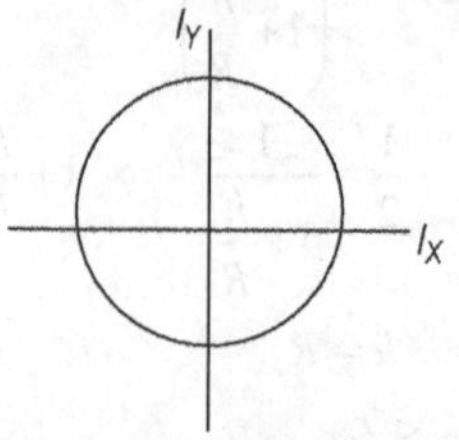

Moment of inertia of circular wire about its axis,

$$I_{CM} = 2M \cdot (2R)^2 = 8MR^2$$

According to perpendicular axes theorem, moment of inertia about its diameter,

$$I_X + I_Y = I_{CM}$$

$$\Rightarrow \quad I_D + I_D = I_{CM} \qquad [\because I_X = I_Y = I_D]$$

$$\Rightarrow \quad I_D = \frac{I_{CM}}{2} = \frac{8MR^2}{2} = 4MR^2$$

29. (b) The given circuit diagram can be represented as

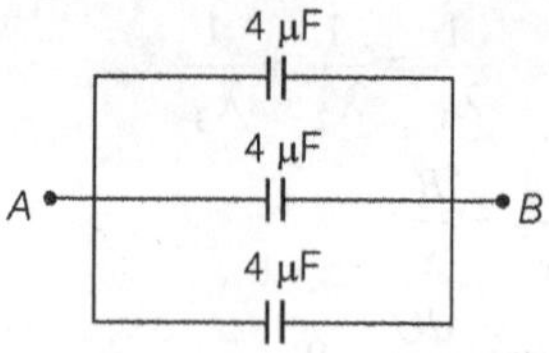

$$\therefore \quad C_{AB} = 4 + 4 + 4 = 12\mu\text{F}$$

30. (b) We know that, $v = \dfrac{dx}{dt}$

So, position x is given by $x = \int v\,dt$

$$= \int_{t=0}^{t=2} (2t + 3t^2)\,dt = \left[\frac{2t^2}{2} + \frac{3t^3}{3}\right]_{t=0}^{t=2} = [t^2 + t^3]_{t=0}^{t=2}$$

$$x = (2)^2 + (2)^3 = 4 + 8 = 12\text{ m}$$

Position of object is 12 m from the origin at $t = 2$ s

31. (a) The given situation is shown below

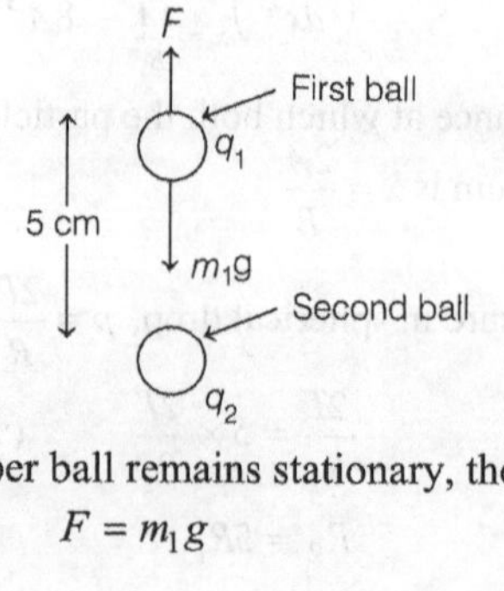

When the upper ball remains stationary, then

$$F = m_1 g$$

$$\Rightarrow \quad \frac{1}{4\pi\varepsilon_0}\cdot\frac{q_1 q_2}{r^2} = m_1 g$$

Here, $m_1 = 8\text{g} = 8\times10^{-3}$ kg

$q_1 = 5\times10^{-8}$C

$r = 5\text{ cm} = 5\times10^{-2}$ m

$$\therefore \quad \frac{9\times10^9\times5\times10^{-8}\times q_2}{(5\times10^{-2})^2} = 8\times10^{-3}\times9.8$$

$$\Rightarrow \quad q_2 = 0.44\times10^{-6}\text{ C} = 0.44\,\mu\text{C}$$

32. (c) Given, $m = 1500$ quintals $= 15\times10^4$ kg,

$$\sin\theta = \frac{1}{75},\ a = 4\text{ms}^{-2}$$

Total force of friction = $0.2\times1500 = 300$ N

Force required against gravity in moving the train up the inclined plane = $mg\sin\theta$

$$= 15\times10^4\times9.8\times\frac{1}{75} = 19600\text{ N}$$

Force required to produce an acceleration of 4 ms^{-2}

$$= ma = 15\times10^4\times4 = 600000\text{ N}$$

Total force required

$$= 300 + 19600 + 600000 = 619900\text{ N}$$

33. (b) The hammer will have both translational and rotational motion as the two forces acting on the hammer create a net force that results in translational motion, while the forces also create a torque about the hammer's centre of mass, leading of rotational motion.

34. (b) Rate of heat flow,

$$H = \frac{\text{Temperature difference}}{\text{Thermal resistance}}$$

where, $R = \dfrac{l}{KA}$

here, K = thermal conductivity of the rod,

l = length of the rod

and A = area of cross-section.

Let x be the temperature of the junction

$$\frac{90-x}{R} + \frac{90-x}{R} = \frac{x}{R}$$

$$180 - 2x = x \Rightarrow x = 60°\text{C}$$

35. (b) Velocity at displacement y,

$$v = \omega\sqrt{A^2 - y^2}$$

Angular frequency,

$$\omega = \frac{2\pi}{T} = \frac{2\pi}{2} = \pi\text{ rad s}^{-1}$$

When $y = 2$ cm,

$$v = \omega\sqrt{10^2 - 2^2} = \sqrt{96}\,\pi\text{ cms}^{-1}$$

$$\text{KE} = \frac{1}{2}mv^2 = \frac{1}{2}\times10\times96\times\pi^2 = 480\,\pi^2\text{ erg}$$

When $y = 5$ cm,

$$v = \omega\sqrt{10^2 - 5^2} = \sqrt{75}\pi\text{cms}^{-1}$$

$$\text{KE} = \frac{1}{2}mv^2 = \frac{1}{2}\times10\times75\times\pi^2 = 375\,\pi^2\text{ erg}$$

Difference in KE = $480\pi^2 - 375\pi^2 = 105\pi^2$ erg

36. (d) For first bubble, $p_1 = \dfrac{8T}{d_A}$ and $p_2 = \dfrac{8T}{d_B}$

where, T = surface tension.

Under isothermal condition, temperature remains constant.

So, equating number of moles,

$$pV = p_1V_1 + p_2V_2$$

$$\frac{8T}{D}\left[\frac{4}{3}\pi\left(\frac{D}{2}\right)^3\right] = \frac{8T}{d_A}\left[\frac{4}{3}\pi\left(\frac{d_A}{2}\right)^3\right] + \frac{8T}{d_B}\left[\frac{4}{3}\pi\left(\frac{d_B}{2}\right)^3\right]$$

$$D^2 = d_A^2 + d_B^2$$

$$\Rightarrow \quad D = \sqrt{d_A^2 + d_B^2}$$

Problem Solving Tactics To find the new radius of the combined bubble after they merge, the law of conservation of volume is applied which states that the total volume of the combined bubbles remains constant.

37. (c) Torque of solenoid is given by

$$\tau = MB\sin\theta$$

$$= (NiA)B\sin\theta\left(\because N = nl = 1000\times\frac{50}{100} = 500\right)$$

$$= 500\times2\times2\times10^{-4}\times0.32\times\frac{1}{2}$$

$$= 0.032\text{ N-m}$$

38. (c)

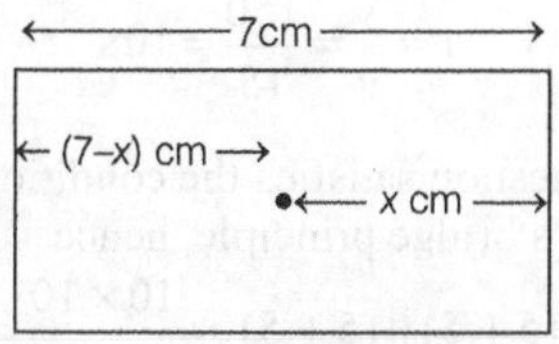

Refractive index, $\mu = \dfrac{\text{Real depth}}{\text{Apparent depth}}$

$$\mu = \frac{7-x}{3.5} \quad \text{... (i) [For first face]}$$

and $\mu = \frac{x}{1.5}$ ... (ii) [For opposite face]

From Eqs. (i) and (ii), we get

$$\frac{7-x}{3.5} = \frac{x}{1.5}$$

$\Rightarrow$ $1.5(7-x) = 3.5x$

$\Rightarrow$ $10.5 - 1.5x = 3.5x$

$\Rightarrow$ $10.5 = 3.5x + 1.5x$

$\Rightarrow$ $10.5 = 5x$

$\Rightarrow$ $x = \frac{10.5}{5} = 2.1\,\text{cm}$

39. (a) Phase difference between voltage and current,

$$\phi = \frac{\pi}{12} - \left(-\frac{\pi}{6}\right) = \frac{\pi}{4}$$

$\Rightarrow$ Power factor $= \cos\phi = \frac{1}{\sqrt{2}}$

Average power dissipated $= \frac{E_m I_m}{2}\cos\phi$

$$= \frac{10 \times 2}{2} \times \frac{1}{\sqrt{2}}$$

$$= 5\sqrt{2}\,\text{W}$$

40. (a) As we know that, magnetic field at the axis,

$$B_1 = \frac{\mu_0}{4\pi} \cdot \frac{2\pi I r^2}{(r^2 + r^2)^{3/2}}$$

$$= \frac{\mu_0}{4} \cdot \frac{I}{\sqrt{2}r} = \frac{\mu_0 I}{4\sqrt{2}r}$$

Magnetic field at the centre, $B_2 = \frac{\mu_0 I}{2r}$

So, $B_1 : B_2 = 1 : 2\sqrt{2}$

41. (d) Given, $l = 150\,\text{m}$, $v_1 = 10\,\text{ms}^{-1}$

and $v_2 = 5\,\text{ms}^{-1}$

Relative velocity of the parrot w.r.t. the train

$$= [10 - (-5)]\,\text{ms}^{-1} = 15\,\text{ms}^{-1}$$

Time taken by the parrot to cross the train,

$$t = \frac{s}{v} = \frac{150}{15} = 10\,\text{s}$$

42. (a) Given question satisfies the condition of Wheatstone's bridge principle, hence

$$R_{PQ} = (5+5)\,||\,(5+5) = \frac{10 \times 10}{10 + 10} = 5\,\Omega$$

43. (a) ${}_1\text{H}^1 + {}_1\text{H}^3 \longrightarrow {}_1\text{H}^2 + {}_1\text{H}^2 + Q$

$$Q = \Delta M \times 931.5\,\text{MeV}$$

$$\Delta M = [m({}_1\text{H}^1) + m({}_1\text{H}^3) - 2m({}_1\text{H}^2)]$$

$$\Delta M = [4.023874 - 2 \times 2.014102]\,\text{u}$$

$$= -4.03\,\text{MeV}$$

44. (c) The two condensers in the circuit are in parallel combination, hence $C' = C + \frac{C}{2} = \frac{3C}{2}$

The work done in charging the equivalent capacitor is stored in the form of potential energy.

Hence, $W = U = \frac{1}{2}C'V^2$

$$= \frac{1}{2}\left(\frac{3C}{2}\right)V^2 = \frac{3}{4}CV^2$$

45. (b) Here, $\lambda = \frac{c}{v} = \frac{3 \times 10^8}{8.2 \times 10^6} = 36.6\,\text{m}$

Chemistry

46. (a) The correct option is (a) A-III, B-I, C-II, D-IV.

47. (a) $\overset{+7}{\text{Mn}}\text{O}_4^- + 8\text{H}^+ + 5e^- \longrightarrow \text{Mn}^{2+} + 4\text{H}_2\text{O}$ ($5e^{\ominus}$)

$\therefore$ $n = 5$

48. (b) All the tetrahalides of group 14 elements are covalent in nature and sp^3-hybridised with tetrahedral geometry. Exception are SnF_4 and PbF_4 which are ionic in nature. Thus, statement II is false while statement I is true.

49. (b)

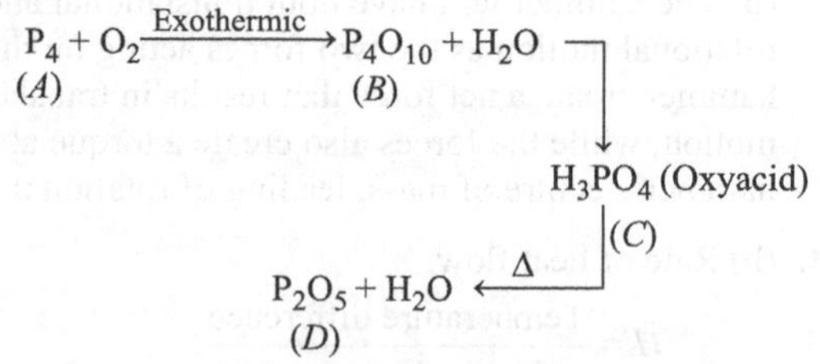

So, option (b) is correct.

50. (c) From first order equation,

$$\log[A] = \log[A_0] - \frac{kt}{2.303}$$

On comparing this equation with equation of straight line.

$$y = mx + c \text{ and } m = \frac{-k}{2.303} = X$$

$\therefore$ Slope $(X) = \frac{-k}{2.303}$

Intercept $(c) = \log[A_0]$.

51. (a) Aniline is basic in nature and HCl is acidic in nature.

So, acid-base reaction will take place.

52. (c) Given, initial temperature,

$$T_1 = 20 + 273 = 293\text{ K}$$

Final temperature,

$$T_2 = 35 + 273 = 308\text{ K}$$

$$R = 8.314\text{ J mol}^{-1}\text{ K}^{-1}$$

Since, rate becomes double on raising temperature,

$$\therefore \quad r_2 = 2r_1 \text{ or } \frac{r_2}{r_1} = 2$$

As rate constant, $k \propto r$

$$\therefore \quad \frac{k_2}{k_1} = 2$$

From Arrhenius equation, we know that

$$\log\frac{k_2}{k_1} = -\frac{E_a}{2.303\,R}\left[\frac{T_1 - T_2}{T_1T_2}\right]$$

$$\log 2 = -\frac{E_a}{2.303 \times 8.314}\left[\frac{293 - 308}{293 \times 308}\right]$$

$$0.3010 = -\frac{E_a}{2.303 \times 8.314}\left[\frac{-15}{293 \times 308}\right]$$

$$\therefore \quad E_a = \frac{0.3010 \times 2.303 \times 8.314 \times 293 \times 308}{15}$$

$$= 34673.48\text{ J mol}^{-1}$$

$$\simeq 34.7\text{ kJ mol}^{-1}$$

53. (d) Correct options are (b) and (c), i.e. (d) is the answer. There are two cases possible in this question:

(b) On C_1—C_2 bond axis 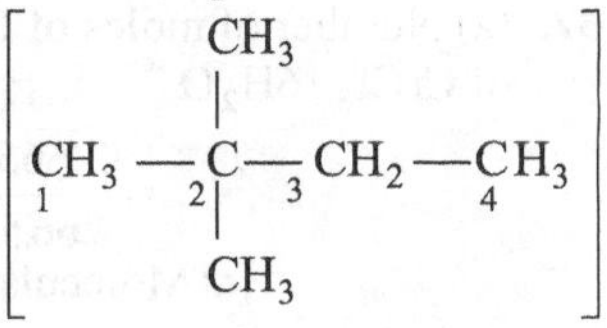

$X = H, Y = C_2H_5$

(c) On C_2—C_3 bond axis

$X = CH_3$, $Y = CH_3$

54. (c) In keto-enol tautomerism, a carbonyl compound with a hydrogen atom on its alpha-carbon rapidly equilibrates with its corresponding enol.

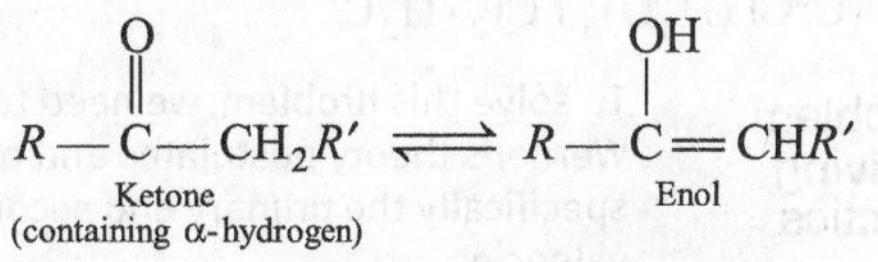

55. (d) From Faraday's second law of electrolysis,

$W = Z \times i \times t$

where, Z = electrochemical equivalent

i = current (Amp)

t = time (sec)

$$W = \frac{63.6}{2 \times 96500} \times 0.5 \times 60 \times 60$$

$$W = 0.59\text{ g}$$

56. (d) Order of adduct formation

$$BI_3 > BBr_3 > BCl_3 > BF_3$$

As in BF_3, strong back-bonding is present which decreases the rate of adduct formation.

i.e. $\quad$ Back-bonding $\propto \dfrac{1}{\text{adduct formation}}$

Hence, for BI_3 ΔH will be maximum.

57. (d) BF_3 molecule has a symmetrical trigonal planar geometry. In such a structure, the resultant moment of any two B—F dipoles is equal in magnitude but opposite in direction to the moment of the third one. Hence, the net dipole moment of BF_3 molecule is zero.

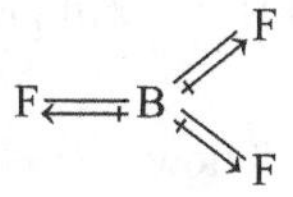

58. (d) E.C of N = $1s^2\,2s^2\,2p^3$

↓

More stable

E.C of O = $1s^2\,2s^2\,2p^4$

↓

Less stable

E.C of N (After 1st I.E) = $1s^2\,2s^2\,2p^2$

↓

Less stable

E.C of O (After 1st I.E)

= $1s^2\,2s^2\,2p^3$

↓

More stable

More stable the electronic configuration, higher the ionisation energy. Hence, both statements I and II are true.

59. (c)

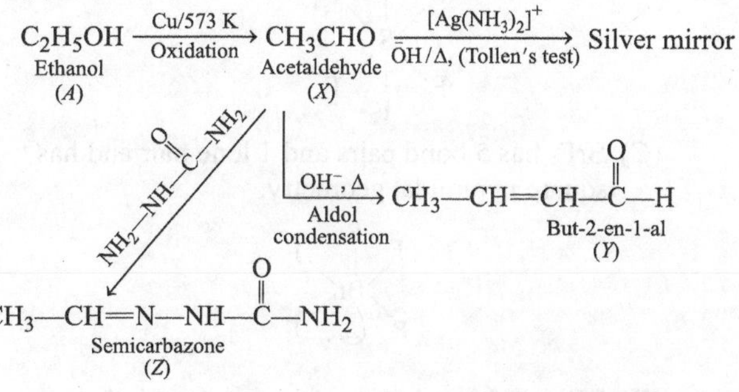

60. (b) When dilute acid is added to an aqueous solution of potassium chromate (VI). Colour changes are observed,

$$\underset{\text{(Yellow)}}{2\overset{+6}{Cr}O_4^{2-}(aq)} + 2H^+(aq) \longrightarrow \underset{\text{(Orange)}}{\overset{+6}{Cr_2}O_7^{2-}(aq)} + H_2O(l)$$

61. (a) $\underset{sp}{CH} \equiv \underset{sp}{CH}$, $\underset{sp^2}{CH_2} = \underset{sp^2}{CH_2}$, $\underset{sp^3}{CH_3} - \underset{sp^3}{CH_3}$

Order of electronegativity of carbon atom is

$$sp > sp^2 > sp^3.$$

∴ Acidic character follows the order

$$CH \equiv CH > CH_2 = CH_2 > CH_3 - CH_3$$

Hence, order of basic strength is

$$\underset{(I)}{CH \equiv \bar{C}} < \underset{(II)}{CH_2 = \bar{C}H} < \underset{(III)}{CH_3 - \bar{C}H_2}$$

62. (c) Pb^{2+}, Ag^+ and Hg_2^{2+} will give white precipitate in dil. HCl.

The reaction are as follow

$$Pb^{2+} + 2HCl \longrightarrow \underset{\text{(White ppt.)}}{PbCl_2 \downarrow} + 2H^+$$

$$Hg_2^{2+} + 2HCl \longrightarrow \underset{\text{(White ppt.)}}{Hg_2Cl_2 \downarrow} + 2H^+$$

$$Ag^+ + HCl \longrightarrow \underset{\text{(White ppt.)}}{AgCl \downarrow} + H^+$$

63. (b) The correct match is A-(iv), B-(iii), C-(i), D-(ii).

(A) PCl_5 has 5 bond pairs. It has trigonal bipyramidal geometry and shape.

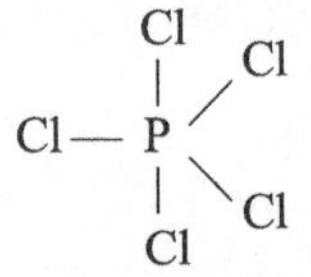

(B) SF_6 has 6 bond pairs and has octahedral geometry and shape.

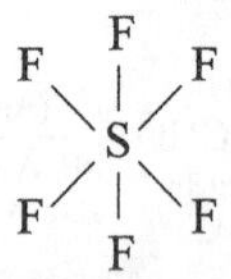

(C) BrF_5 has 5 bond pairs and 1 lone pair and has square pyramidal geometry.

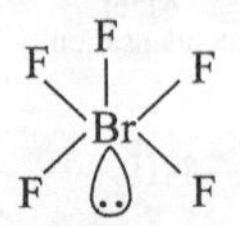

(D) BF_3 has 3 bond pairs and has trigonal planar geometry and shape.

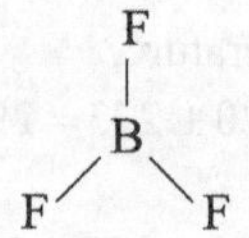

64. (d)

(a) Pu^{4+} disproportionates to Pu^{3+} and PuO_2^{2+} in acidic medium. In strongly acidic mediums it stabilizes by forming complex with H^+ ions.

(b) Np shows oxidation states ranging between +3 and +7, +7 being the maximum.

(c) UO_2^{2+}, uranium dioxide, is a linear shaped stable oxide which exists in a powdered crystalline form.

All given statements are correct.

65. (a) $[H^+] = \sqrt{CK_a} = \sqrt{0.5 \times 2 \times 10^{-4}} = \sqrt{1.0 \times 10^{-2}}$

$$[H^+] = 10^{-2}$$

$$pH = -\log[H^+] = -\log(10^{-2}) = +2$$

66. (a) CH_4 is regular tetrahedral and the electronegativity (EN) difference between C and H is negligible, which cancel out. Hence, dipole moment of CH_4 is zero.

NF_3 has less EN difference between N and F as compared to N and H in NH_3, therefore will have a lower dipole moment.

H_2O has maximum EN difference between H and O therefore will have a maximum dipole moment.

$$CH_4(0) < NF_3(0.24) < NH_3(1.46) < H_2O(1.85)$$

67. (a) Number of moles of Cl^- ions ionised from one mole of $CrCl_3 \cdot 6H_2O$.

$$= \frac{2.665}{266.5} = 0.01$$

[∵ Molecular mass of $CrCl_3 \cdot 6H_2O = 266.5$]

∴ Moles of AgCl obtained = Moles of Cl^- ionised

$$= \frac{2.87}{143.5} = 0.02$$

∴ 0.01 mole of complex $CrCl_3 \cdot 6H_2O$ gives 0.02 moles of Cl on ionisation.

Thus, the formula of the complex is

$$[CrCl(H_2O)_5]Cl_2 \cdot H_2O.$$

Problem Solving Tactics To solve this problem, we need to recall Werner's theory postulates and observe specifically the primary and secondary valencies.

68. (a) The number of lines in transition $n_2 \rightarrow n_1$ will be

$$\frac{(n_2 - n_1)(n_2 - n_1 + 1)}{2}$$

The transition $n = 6 \rightarrow n = 3$ corresponds to 6 lines in the spectrum.

$n = 5 \rightarrow n = 3$ corresponds to 3 lines in the spectrum.
$n = 5 \rightarrow n = 1$ corresponds to 10 lines in the spectrum.
$n = 4 \rightarrow n = 3$ corresponds to 1 line in the spectrum.
Hence, the correct match is A-(iii), B-(i), C-(ii), D-(iv).

69. (b) $CHCl_3$ undergoes oxidation in presence of sunlight. Hence, Statement I is true but Statement II is false.

70. (a) Generally metal oxides are basic in nature while non-metal oxides are acidic in nature.
Thus, BaO is basic and Cl_2O_7 is acidic in nature.
Neutral oxides are oxides which are neither acidic nor basic. CO is neutral oxide.
Amphoteric oxide, i.e. Al_2O_3 reacts with both acids and alkalis to form salt and water.
Hence, the correct match is A-(ii), B-(i), C-(iv), D-(iii).

71. (c) 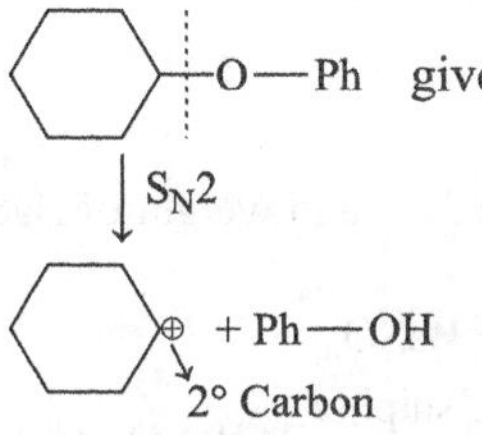

gives S_N2 mechanism with concentrated HBr.

Hence, by the formation of secondary carbocation which is more stable it gives S_N2 reaction.

72. (c) $[Co(NH_3)_3Cl_3]$ is a $[MA_3B_3]$ type complex which, do not show optical isomerism, because this compound has symmetrical geometry (octahedral), co-ordination number is 6. It also does not contain any bidentate ligand.

73. (b) Due to high electronegativity and small size, F only forms one oxyacid that is HOF. Only in HOF, F is in +1 oxidation state.
All show oxidising properties. Chlorine has the highest electron gain enthalpy. Hence, only (b) is false.

74. (c) $2SO_2(g) + O_2(g) \rightleftharpoons 2SO_3(g), \Delta H = -190\,kJ$
The reaction is exothermic in nature. On increasing pressure, equilibrium will shift in forward direction. Apart from addition of more SO_2 and O_2 will also increase the yield of SO_3 and O_2 will also increase the yield of SO_3 at equilibrium while other factors decreases the yield of SO_3.

75. (d) The staggered conformation of ethane is more stable than eclipsed conformation. Since, eclipsed conformation has greater potential energy due to torsional strain, it is less stable than the staggered conformation.

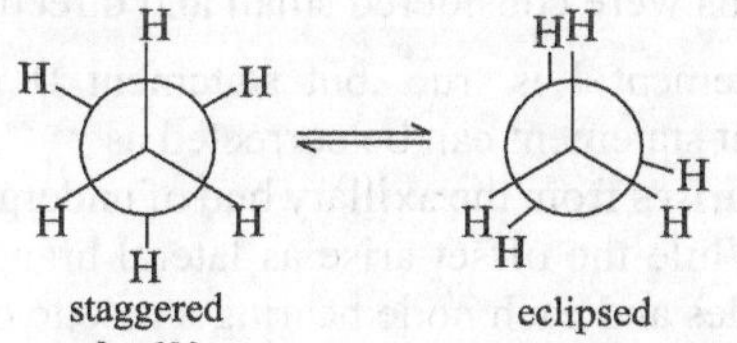
staggered $\theta = 60°$ eclipsed $\theta = 0°$

76. (d) Alcohols on dehydration can produce ether as well as alkene under different conditions.
Dehydration of alcohol proceeds through the formation of carbonium ion. The carbonium ion can lose a proton to form alkene. The carbonium ion may be attacked by a fresh molecule of alcohol and form an oxonium ion which can then lose a proton to form ether. Usually, secondary and tertiary alcohols form alkene.

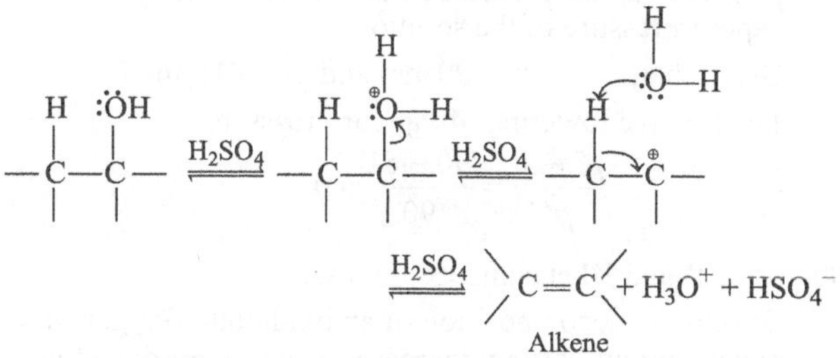

Alkene

77. (a) Hydrolysis of a nitrile to a carboxylic acid involves the formation of amide intermediate.

78. (b) Base catalysed condensation of acid anhydride and aromatic aldehyde is known as Perkin reaction.

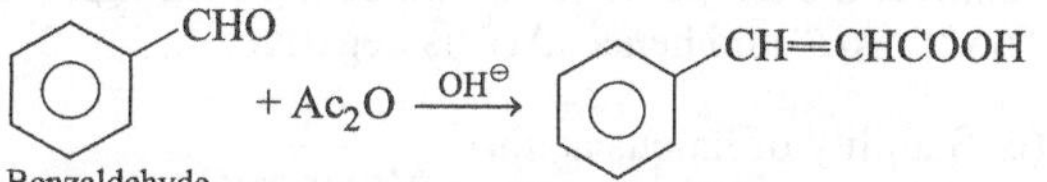

Benzaldehyde Cinnamic acid

Reaction starts with the formation of carbanion.

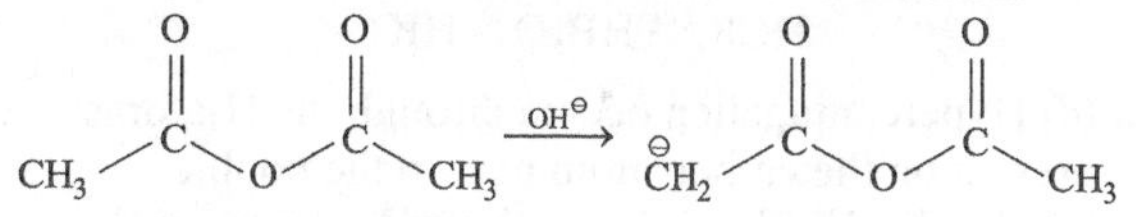

Carbanion

79. (a) 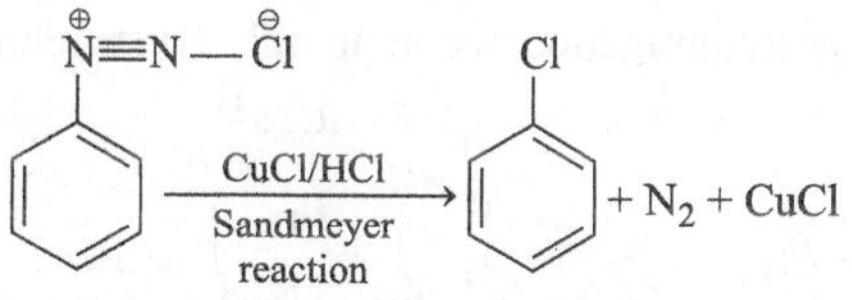

This reaction is known as Sandmeyer reaction. In this reaction diazonium group is replaced by chloro group.

80. (a) $\Delta G = \Delta H - T\Delta S$
Temperature is constant $\Delta G = 0$
$\Delta H = T\Delta S$
$40000 = T \times 80$ $\left[\begin{array}{l}\Delta H = 40\,kJ = 40 \times 10^3\ J \\ \Delta S = 80\,JK^{-1}\ mol^{-1}\end{array}\right]$
$T = 500\,K$
So, $T > 500$ so that ΔG value comes (– ve) and reaction becomes spontaneous.

81. (c) $Cu(s) + 2Ag^+(aq) \longrightarrow Cu^{+2}(aq) + 2Ag(s)$
Equilibrium constant $(K) = 4 \times 10^{15}$
$$E^{\circ}_{cell} = \frac{0.0591}{2} \log K$$

$$= \frac{0.0591}{2} \log [4 \times 10^{15}]$$

$$E^{\circ}_{cell} = 0.46\,V$$

82. (d) The relative lowering of vapour pressure

$$= \frac{p^{\circ} - p}{p^{\circ}}$$

p° is the vapour pressure of pure solvent and p is the vapour pressure of the solution.

Given that, $p^{\circ} = 90\,mm$ and $p = 81\,mm$

The relative lowering of vapour pressure

$$\frac{p^{\circ} - p}{p^{\circ}} = \frac{90 - 81}{90} = 0.1$$

83. (d) I, II and III statements are true.

During the decomposition of an oxide into oxygen and metal vapour, entropy increases as gas is produced in the reaction. Decomposition of an oxide is an endothermic change. This is because it is reverse of combustion reaction and all combustion reactions are exothermic in nature. Since both ΔH° and ΔS° are positive, the temperature should be high enough so that $T\Delta S^{\circ} > \Delta H^{\circ}$ and hence, ΔG° is negative.

84. (c) Stability of halous acids $\propto \frac{1}{\text{Molar mass}}$

So, as the molar mass increases, the stability decreases .

$\therefore$ $HClO > HBrO > HIO$

85. (c) Hyperconjugation occurs through the H-atoms present on the carbon atom next to the double bond/radical/carbonium ion, i.e. α-hydrogen atoms. There is no α-H in the structures I and II.

So, hyperconjugation occurs in only III structure, i.e.

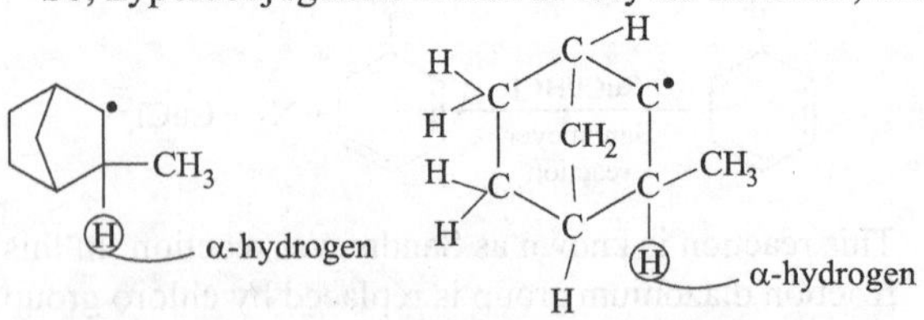

Problem Solving Tactics

Hyperconjugation is the stabilising interaction that results from the interaction of the electrons in a σ-bond (usually C—H or C—C) with an adjacent empty or partially filled *p*-orbital or π-orbital to give an extended molecular orbital that increases the stability of the system.

86. (c) $\underset{\text{Excess}}{CuSO_4 + 4KCN} \longrightarrow 2CuCN + (CN)_2 + K_2SO_4$

$$CuCN + 3KCN \longrightarrow K_3[Cu(CN)_4]$$

87. (d) The two most common pyrimidines of DNA are cytosine (C) and thymine (T) and the two most common purines of DNA are adenine (A) and guanine (G).

88. (d) The correct option is (d) A-II, B-I, C-IV, D-III.

89. (a) Depression in freezing point, $\Delta T_f = i \times K_f \times m$

where, K_f = cryoscopic constant

m = molality of solution and, i is van't Hoff factor

$$\Delta T_f = iK_f \times \frac{\text{Weight of naphthoic acid}}{\text{Molar mass of naphthoic acid}} \times \frac{1000}{\text{Weight of benzene}}$$

$$2 = i \times 1.72 \times \frac{20}{(12 \times 11 + 1 \times 8 + 16 \times 2)} \times \frac{1000}{50}$$

$$2 = i \times \frac{34.4}{172} \times \frac{1000}{50},\ 2 = i \times 4$$

$$\frac{2}{4} = i$$

$$0.5 = i$$

90. (b) Weight of sulphur is 32 u and weight of $BaSO_4$ is 233 u.

So, weight of sulphur in $BaSO_4$

$$= \frac{\text{Weight of sulphur}}{\text{Weight of } BaSO_4} \times BaSO_4 \text{ in organic compound}$$

$$= \frac{32}{233} \times 0.4813 = 0.0661$$

Percentage of sulphur

$$= \frac{\text{Weight of sulphur in } BaSO_4}{\text{Weight of organic compound}} \times 100$$

$$= \frac{0.0661}{0.157} \times 100 = 42.10\,\%$$

Biology

91. (b) Productivity at second trophic level is always less than the productivity at first trophic level. This is because only 10% of energy is transferred from one trophic level to another. Thus, decrease in energy would result in decrease in productivity too.

92. (a) Both statement I and statement II are true.

Hugo de Vries, based on his work on *Oenthera lamarckiana,* proposed the mutation theory. In this theory, he explained that new species evolve by sudden and distinct heritable changes called mutations. These mutations can occur at any time, hence are random and can be useful, harmful or have no effects at all, hence are directionless. On the other hand, Darwinian variations were considered small and directional.

93. (b) Statement I is true, but statement II is false. The incorrect statement can be corrected as

Sucker arises from the axillary bud of underground part of stem. While the offset arise as lateral branch with short internodes and each node bearing a rosette of leaves

94. (a) Micro-injection is the method used to introduce alien DNA into host cells in animals, while biolistics or gene gun method is suitable for plants.

95. (d) Statements I, II and V are correct, whereas statements III and IV are incorrect. These can be corrected as

- The ribosomes of chloroplasts (70S) are smaller than the cytoplasmic ribosomes (80S).
- The mesosomes are the specialised differentiated form of cell membrane which is the characteristic of prokaryotes.

96. (a) Statement in option (a) is correct. Other statements are incorrect and can be corrected as

- In somatic hybridisation, the isolated protoplasts from two different varieties of plants (each having a desired character) are fused to get hybrid protoplasts.
- The milk obtained from transgenic cow contained human alpha lactalbumin which was nutritionally more enhanced.
- Golden rice is a genetically modified rice variety with enhanced production of vitamin-A.

97. (b) A is true, but R is false. R can be corrected as

The axonal membrane is more permeable to potassium ions and it moves from higher concentration to lower concentration. Since, the membrane loses its positive ions, it becomes more negatively charged inside, while outside the axonal membrane becomes positively charged. This state of the axonal membrane is called the polarised state.

98. (c) The correct matches are A-2, B-1, C-3, D-4.

- PCT (Proximal Convoluted Tubule) is responsible for reabsorption of significant substances like glucose, amino acids, water, ions, etc.
- The vasa recta and Henle's loop plays a significant role in production of concentrated urine.
- The initial step of urine formation starts at glomerulus. This filtration is called ultrafiltration.
- Selective secretion of hydrogen and potassium ions takes place in DCT (Distal Convoluted Tubule).

99. (a) Matched pair in option (a) is not correct, it can be corrected as

J-shaped curve is called exponential growth curve. It occurs when the resources are unlimited. This type of curve represents the population growing exponentially or geometrically until there is a resource limitation or limitation of population growth by other factors. Growth of the population declines rapidly until a favourable period is restored.

100. (c) Statements I and IV are incorrect and these can be corrected as

- Synaptic cleft of neurons secrete chemicals called neurotransmitters, which are involved in the transmission of impulses.
- Spinal cord and cranial nerves are made of myelinated nerve fibres.

101. (d) An enhancer is a short sequence of segment of DNA that can be bound to activators to stimulate the transcription of a particular gene. They are usually referred to as transcription factors.

102. (c) An operon is a unit of genetic expression consisting of one or more related genes including the operator and promoter sequences that have regulatory function.

103. (a) The correct matches are A-4, B-2, C-1, D-3.

- β-cells are cells that make insulin which controls the level of glucose in the blood.
- α-cells release glucagon, which elevates blood glucose.
- δ-cells produce somatostation which is a strong inhibitor of somatotropin, insulin and glucagon.
- F-cells secrete pancreatic polypeptide (PP) which is an endogenous peptide hormone.

104. (b) The boy is suffering from exophthalmic goitre or Grave's disease. The signs of this disease include hyperthyroidism, exophthalmos, i.e. protrusion of eyeball due to the deposition of fat behind the eyes.

105. (d) *Cheiranthus cheiri* also called as wall flower belong to family–Cruciferae. These flowers are very useful in bronchitis and fever.

Other options can be corrected as

- *Raphanus sativus* (muli) belongs to family–Cruciferae also known as Brassicaceae. It is consumed as vegetable.
- *Vetiveria zizanoides* belongs to family–Graminea (Poaceae). It produce volatile scented oil used in perfumes.
- *Iberis amara* (chandni) belongs to family–Cruciferae. It also has medicinal property. It is useful for patient suffering from gout and rheumatism.

106. (d) The correct matches are A-1, B-2, C-3, D-4.

- Endangered species are species facing a very high risk of extinction in the wild in near future.
- A threatened species is one which is liable to become extinct if not allowed to realise its full biotic potential.
- Extinct species are ones with no surviving individual on earth.
- Vulnerable species are the ones which are not critically endangered, but are facing a high risk of extinction in the wild.

107. (b) The antibodies produced in response to allergens like dust, pollens, animal dander, etc., is IgE type.

108. (c) Statement I is correct, but statement II is incorrect and can be corrected as

The role of oxygen in the regulation of respiratory rhythm is quite insignificant.

Instead, the chemosensitive area situated adjacent to the rhythm centre are highly sensitive to CO_2 and hydrogen ions. Increase in these substances can activate this centre, which in turn can signal the rhythm centre to make necessary adjustments in the respiratory process by which these substances can be eliminated.

109. (c) Statements III, IV and V are correct. Rest statements are incorrect and can be corrected as

- In monocots (grass family) the cotyledon is called scutellum and is situated on the lateral side of embryonal axis.
- Among animals, insects particularly bees are the dominant biotic pollinating agents.

110. (b) Statement in option (b) is correct, while rest of the other statements are false and can be corrected as

Endosperm in angiosperm is triploid in nature and form after fertilisation.

The cylindrical portion below the level of cotyledons is hypocotyl that terminates at its lower end in the radicle or root tip.

The cotyledon of gram family is called scutellum.

111. (c) About 97% of oxygen is carried in combination with haemoglobin of erythrocytes. Thus, the maximum transportation of O_2 in blood occurs as oxyhaemoglobin.

112. (a) Diuretic drugs like acetozolamide, mannitol, etc, are frequently used in the treatment of high blood pressure as they increase the removal of excess fluid from the body.

113. (d) The two kingdom system of classification was discarded because this system did not distinguish between the eukaryotes and prokaryotes, unicellular and multicellular and photosynthetic and non-photosynthetic organisms.

114. (b) The probability of obtaining progeny containing green round seeds from a cross between a parent with yellow round seeds and another parent with yellow wrinkled seeds is 1/8.

YyRr (Yellow round) × Yyrr (Yellow wrinkled)

↓

♂ / ♀	YR	Yr	yR	yr
Yr	YYRr	YYrr	YyRr	Yyrr
yr	YyRr	Yyrr	yyRr	yyrr
Yr	YYRr	YYrr	YyRr	Yyrr
yr	YyRr	Yyrr	yyRr	yyrr

Thus, progeny with green round seeds is 2/16 = 1/8.

115. (c) AIDS is caused by the human immunodeficiency Virus (HIV), a member of a group of virus called retro virus which have an envelope enclosing the RNA genome.

116. (b) Statement in option (b) is incorrect and can be corrected as

The triangular structure called sinus venosus joins the right atrium in frog's heart. It receives blood through the major veins called vena cava.

117. (d) Some organisations exploit biological resources of other nations without proper authorisation from the countries concerned. This is known as biopiracy. The plants such as basmati rice, turmeric, neem, etc., are related with biopiracy. However, *Bacillus anthracis* is the only organism which is not linked with biopiracy.

118. (d) In CAM plants, the stomata remain close during the day in order to reduce evaporation. CAM or Crassulacean Acid Metabolism, is a carbon-fixation pathway that is evolved in some plants as an adaptation to arid conditions.

119. (b) Statement I is true, but statement II is false and can be corrected as ; Due to genetic and other unknown reasons in arthritis the body attacks self-cells, which results in damage to the body.

120. (b) The correct sequence for the transport of sperms is as follows

Seminiferous tubules→ Rete testis→ Vasa efferentia→ Epididymis→ Vas deferens→ Ejaculatory duct→ Urethra

121. (d) The correct matches are A-3, B-2, C-4, D-1

- Deuteromycetes are commonly known as imperfect fungi because only the asexual or vegetative phases of these fungi are known.
- Ascomycetes are commonly known as sac-fungi. Here the sexual spores are called ascospores, which are produced endogenously in sac like asci.
- Basidiomycetes include mushrooms. Members of this group lack sex organs, but plasmogamy is brought about by fusion of two vegetative or somatic cells of different strains or genotypes.
- Phycomycetes are commonly found in aquatic habitats and on decaying wood in moist and damp places. Gametes of these can be similar in morphology (isogamous) or dissimilar (anisogamous or oogamous).

122. (b) Copper IUDs work primarily by releasing copper ions, which suppress sperm motility and the fertilising capacity of sperms.

123. (b) Statement I is true, but statement II is false and it can be corrected as

Protons in thylakoid lumen increases in number when sunlight is received by the chloroplast.

124. (d) The host cells are treated with a specific concentration of divalent cations, such as calcium to increase the efficiency with which DNA enters the bacterium (host).

125. (d) The correct matches are A-2, B-3, C-1, D-4.
- '+' sign indicates beneficial interaction and '–' sign use for detrimental and 0 for neutral interaction.
- In commensalism, one species is benefitted (+) and other is neither benefitted nor harmed (0).
- In both parasitism and predation, only one species benefitted (+) and the interaction is detrimental (–) to other species.
- Both the species are benefitted in mutualism.

126. (b) Gulmohar and *Cassia* belong to Leguminosae family and have imbricate aestivation.

Imbricate aestivation is the arrangement of five petals in such a way that one petal is completely external and other one petal is completely internal, while three petals are partially external and partially internal.

127. (a) Statement in option (a) is correct, rest incorrect statements can be corrected as
- The ability of unlimited growth in plant is due to the presence of meristems.
- GA_3 is used to speed up the malting process in brewing industry.
- Kinetin does not occur naturally in plants.

128. (b) The given figures, A, B and C show radial symmetry, diploblastic organisation of embryonic layers and acoelomate body organisation, respectively.
Out of the given organisms, *Pennatula* or sea-pen (coelenterate/cnidarian) is the only one that is radially symmetrical, diploblastic and acoelomate.
Fasciola belong to platyhelminthes and are bilaterally symmetrical, triploblastic and acoelomates.
Ancylostoma belong to Aschelminthes and are bilaterally symmetrical, triploblastic and pseudocoelomate animals.
Hirudinaria belong to Annelida and are bilaterally symmetrical, triploblastic and coelomate.

129. (d) *Mycoplasma* are organisms that completely lack a cell wall. They are smallest living cells known and can survive without oxygen.

130. (c) The number of chromosomes are equal to the number of functional centromere and the number of chromatids are equal to the number of DNA molecules.
During prophase, the number of chromatids are 100 and the number of chromosomes are 50.

But during anaphase the chromosomes separate from each other, thus the number of chromatids will be 100 and number of chromosome will also become 100.

Hence, option (c) is correct.

131. (b) The living differentiated cells, that have lost the capacity to divide can regain the capacity of division under certain conditions. This phenomenon is known as dedifferentiation.

132. (b) A is true, but R is false. R can be corrected as
The primary oocyte gives rise to two unequal sized cells by first meiotic division. One of the daughter cells of the secondary oocytes, is large and receives most of the cytoplasm, while the other is small called polar body. Both of these cells are not equally functional. The secondary oocyte divides by second meiotic division and form ovum or egg cell, which plays an important role in fertilisation. The role of polar body is unidentified, but do not play any role in fertilisation.

133. (b) A large number of primary follicles degenerate during the phase from birth to puberty. Therefore, at puberty only 60,000 to 80,000 primary follicles are left in each ovary.

134. (d) Carolus Linnaeus was a Swedish naturalist. He is considered as the father of taxonomy. *Species Plantarum* is a famous publication of Linnaeus (1753), which lists every species of plant known at that time, classified into genera. It is also the first work to consistently apply binomial names.

135. (b) A is true, but R is false. R can be corrected as

The left auricle receives oxygenated blood from the lungs.

136. (d) Bulliform cells are found in monocot leaves. They are also known as motor cells and help in rolling of leaves in dry weather. Hence, all the statements are correct regarding bulliform cells.

137. (b) The maximum volume of air a person can breathe in after a forced expiration or the maximum volume of air a person can breathe out after a forced inspiration is called vital capacity. This includes Tidal Volume, Inspiratory Reserve Volume and Expiratory Reserve volume (TV+ IRV+ ERV).

138. (d) Statement in option (d) is incorrect about phenylketonuria. It can be corrected as
It is an inborn error of metabolism that results in decreased metabolism of the amino acid phenylalanine.

139. (a) In the members of Phaeophyceae or brown algae food is stored as complex carbohydrates, in the form of laminarin, e.g. *Dictyota*, *Ectocarpus*, etc.

140. (c) Statements II, III and V are correct. Rest statements are incorrect and can be corrected as
- Lysozyme acts as a cell wall degrading enzyme for bacteria.
- When a protein encoding gene is expressed in a heterologous host, it is known as recombinant protein.

141. (b) The first clinical gene therapy was given in 1990 to a 4 year old girl with Adenosine Deaminase (ADA) deficiency. This enzyme is crucial for the immune system to function.

142. (a) Both A and R are true, but R is not the correct explanation of A.
Two Krebs' cycles occur per glucose molecule because glycolysis results in the formation of 2 pyruvic acid molecules by glucose breakdown. Each turn of Krebs' cycle produces 3 NADH, 1 $FADH_2$ and 1 ATP molecule. On oxidation, NADH produces 3 ATP molecules and 1 $FADH_2$ produces 2 ATP molecules. Thus, in each turn of Krebs' cycle 12 ATP molecules are produced.

143. (d) Statement IV is correct, while the other statements are incorrect and can be corrected as
- The bundle sheath of C_4 plants has thick cell walls impervious to gaseous exchange.
- These plants have large agranal chloroplasts which fix carbon dioxide into sugar with the help of RuBisCO enzyme.
- The glucose formation in C_4 plant takes place by Calvin cycle.
- These cells lack PEP carboxylase.

144. (d) The correct matches are A-4, B-1, C-2, D-3.
- Dicot stem have an outer epidermis followed by a layer of collenchymatous cells called hypodermis.
- Hypodermis is made up of a few layers of sclerenchymatous cells in monocot stem.
- In monocot roots, the pericycle give rise to lateral roots only.
- In dicot root, the pericycle gives rise to lateral roots and secondary meristem.

145. (b) Structure '*A*' represents a structure known as thylakoid. The membrane of thylakoids enclose a space called lumen. Other statements are incorrect and can be corrected as
- Thylakoids are flattened membranous sacs present in the stroma.
- Thylakoids are arranged in stacks like the piles of coins called grana.
- Thylakoids of different grana are connected by a flat membranous tubule called the stroma lamella.

146. (c) For person with blood group 'B' the antigens on RBCs would be B type, while the antibodies in the plasma would be anti-A type.

147. (b) Statement I is true, but statement II is false and it can be corrected as
Muscular dystrophy is the progressive degeneration of skeletal muscle mostly due to genetic disorder.

148. (c) In collenchyma, the corners of cells are deposited with cellulose and pectin substances. It is mechanical tissue which provides support, flexibility and elasticity to the plant organs.

149. (c) Myosin filaments are constituted by monomeric proteins 'meromyosin', which has two important parts, a globular head with short arm (HMM) and a tail (LMM).

150. (c) In addition to having more than one allele at a specific locus, each allele must also occur in the population at a rate of at least 1% to generally be considered multiple allelism.

151. (b) Statements III and V are incorrect. These can be corrected as
- The transformation of spermatids into sperms is termed as spermiogenesis.
- The oestrogen level in blood increases, resulting in strong sex urge in the female.

Rest statements are correct.

152. (c) The correct matches are A-4, B-2, C-1, D-3.
- By the end of 500 mya invertebrates were formed.
- Fish like reptile, i.e *Ichthyosaurs* evolved around 200 mya.
- Jawless fish probably evolved around 350 mya.
- Sea weeds and few plants existed probably around 320 mya.

153. (b) In 1997, the first transgenic cow, Rosie, produced human protein enriched milk (2.4 grams per litre). The milk contained the human alpha-lactalbumin and was nutritionally a more balanced product for human babies.

154. (d) In 1928, Sir Alexander Fleming extracted penicillin from the fungus *P. notatum*. This fungus is extensively used for the production of penicillin.

155. (a) Both A and R are true, but R is not the correct explanation of A.
The growth rate shows an increase that may be arithmetic or geometrical. In arithmetic growth, following mitotic cell division, only one daughter cell continues to divide while the other differentiates and matures. The simplest expression of arithmetic growth is exemplified by a root elongating at a constant rate.

156. (b) The prosthetic groups are organic compounds, they differ from other co-factors, because they are tightly bound to apoenzymes whereas coenzymes are associated with the apoenzyme for a short period of time and do not remain attached to enzyme.

157. (a) The correct matches are A-4, B-3, C-2, D-1.
- Turner's syndrome is caused due to the absence of one of the X-chromosome, leading to 45 with XO. People suffering from this syndrome are short statured and have webbed neck.
- Down's syndrome also called trisomy of 21, is a genetic disorder causing slow motor development.

- Klinefelter's syndrome is also called XXY syndrome, since the affected male is born with an additional copy of X-chromosome.
- Phenylketonuria is an autosomal recessive disorder. This disorder is caused due to the presence of defective gene of phenylalanine hydroxylase.

158. (a) The DNA-dependent DNA polymerases catalyse polymerisation only in one direction, i.e. $5' - 3'$ direction.

159. (b) Statements I and V are correct and statements II, III and IV are incorrect. They can be corrected as
- The first amino acid is also called N- terminal amino acid, whereas the last amino acid is also called C-terminal amino acid.
- The exoskeleton of arthropods containing polysaccharide chitin are mostly homopolymers.
- Starch is a homopolymer and not a heteropolymer.

160. (d) Both statement I and statement II are true.

The cleistogamous flowers do not open at all. These flowers are invariably autogamous as there is no chance of pollen from different flower landing on the stigma.

161. (a) Statements II, IV and V are correct. Rest statement are incorrect and can be corrected as
- Cyclosporin-A has immunosuppressive property and it is commonly used in organ transplants to prevent rejections.
- Lactic acid was the first acid to be produced by industrial fermentation.

162. (b) The structure involved in the formation of spindle fibres are centrioles. They exist in a pair close to the nucleus and are present only in the animal cell.

163. (d) GMOs developed by *r*DNA technology and genetic engineering are useful in enhancing the nutritional value of food. They reduce the post-harvest losses. They are also useful in increasing the tolerance power of crops against the abiotic stresses.

164. (b) The correct sequence for the transmission of an electrical impulse through a neuron is as follows Dendrites→ Cell body→ Axon→ Axon terminal
- The dendrites receive the signals.
- The cell body integrates the signals.
- The axon conducts the impulses.
- The axon terminal releases neurotransmitters for signal transmission.

165. (a) Bioluminescence is the production and emission of light by some living organisms. It is well marked in ctenophores, e.g. *Pleurobrachia* and *Ctenoplana*.

166. (b) To produce 104 pollen grains, 26 meiotic divisions are required.

Formation of n number of pollen grain $= \frac{n}{4}$

$$n = 104 \Rightarrow \frac{104}{4} = 26$$

167. (d) When N/K is exactly one, the growth rate of a population following the logistic growth model is equal to zero.

The logistic model is given as $\frac{dN}{dt} = rN\left(\frac{1-N}{K}\right)$

Where, N = population density at time 't'

r = intrinsic rate of natural increase

K = carrying capacity

when, $\frac{N}{K} = 1$, then $\frac{1-N}{K} = 0$

Therefore, $\frac{dN}{dt} = 0$

168. (d) The five kingdom system of classification is based on cell structure (prokaryotic or eukaryotic), body structure (unicellular or multicellular), nutrition (autotrophic or heterotrophic) and lifestyle (producers, consumers or decomposers).

169. (a) The techniques vasectomy and tubectomy are highly effective for birth control. In vasectomy, a small part of the vas deferens is removed or cut tied up in males. In tubectomy, a small part of the Fallopian tube is removed or tied up in female.

170. (c) Statements II, III, IV and V are correct statements whereas statement I is incorrect and can be corrected as

The UTRs are present at both $5'$ end before start codon and $3'$ end after stop codon.

171. (d) Option (d) is incorrectly matched pair. It can be corrected as
Creutzfeldt-Jacob disease is caused by prions.
Virus is a nucleoprotein entity. It is capable of multiplication by taking over cellular machinery of the host cell. Prions are modified hydrophobic glycoproteins. Viroids are RNA entities consisting of 250-370 nucleotides.

172. (b) The given condition is known as cleistogamy. It is an adaptation for self-pollination in which the flowers never open. The pollen grains from anther lobe pollinates the stigma of same flower, e.g. *Commelina benghalensis*.

173. (c) The correct matches areA-3, B-4, C-1, D-2.
- Neanderthal man lived in Eurasia until about 40,000 years ago. They had a cranial capacity of 1400 cc.
- *Homo habilis* had a cranial capacity of 650-800 cc.
- *Homo erectus* had a cranial capacity of 900 cc.
- Cro-Magnon man are evolved 10,000 years ago and had a cranial capacity of 1600 cc.

174. (b) When alien species (Nile perch) was introduced deliberately for whatever purpose, some of them turned invasive and caused extinction of indigenous species (cichlid fish). This is known as alien species invasions.

175. (d) The correct option is (d) as When the number of chromosome in flowering plant is $20 = n$ Antipodal cell $\Rightarrow n = 20$, Embryo $\Rightarrow 2n = 40$

Integuments $\Rightarrow 2n = 40$, Endosperms $\Rightarrow 3n = 60$

Nucellus $\Rightarrow 2n = 40$

176. (b) Statement in option (b) correctly describes a tracheid. Tracheid is a type of cell in the xylem. Their main function is conduction of sap. These are elongated or tube-like cells with thick and lignified walls and tapering ends. These are dead and the inner layer of the cell walls have thickenings.

177. (d) Both statement I and statement II are true.

The chorionic villi and uterine tissue interlink with each other and jointly form a structural and functional unit between developing embryo (foetus) and maternal body called placenta. It helps in the transport of substances to and from the embryo. It also acts as an endocrine tissue and produces several hormones like human chorionic Gonadotropin (hCG), human Placental Lactogen (hPL), oestrogen, progestogens, etc.

178. (a) *Spirogyra* isogamous and non-flagellated (non-motile) gametes. *Spirogyra*, commonly known as water silk, possess non-flagellated gametes. Thus, the gametes are non-motile.

179. (b) In protein structure, covalent bonds are the strongest. They are of two types, peptide bonds and -S - S (disulphide) bonds.

180. (c) *Calotropis* shows opposite type of phyllotaxy, where a pair of leaves arise at each node and lie opposite to each other.

SECTION I
Foundation Builders

PRACTICE SET 3

Maximum Marks : 720	Time : 3 hrs	No. of Questions : 180

Instructions

1. This question paper contains **180** multiple-choice questions (four options with a single correct answer) from **Physics**, **Chemistry** and **Biology**.
2. These questions are distributed as 45 questions, each from Physics and Chemistry and 90 questions in Biology. These are to be compulsorily attempted by the candidate.
3. Each question carries 4 marks. For each correct response, the candidate will get 4 marks. For each incorrect response, one mark will be deducted from the total scores.

PHYSICS

1. A wire has density $7.5 \times 10^3\ kg/m^3$. If the stress in the wire is $3 \times 10^8\ Nm^{-2}$, then the speed of transverse wave in the wire, is

(a) $225\ ms^{-1}$ (b) $250\ ms^{-1}$
(c) $200\ ms^{-1}$ (d) $100\ ms^{-1}$

2. A particle of mass 10g is kept on the surface of a uniform sphere of mass 100 kg and radius 10 cm, then the work to be done to take the particle far away from the sphere is
(take, $G = 6.67 \times 10^{-11}\ N\text{-}m^2kg^{-2}$)

(a) 3.33×10^{-10} J (b) 6.67×10^{-10} J
(c) 13.34×10^{-10} J (d) 3.67×10^{-9} J

3. What is the current through an ideal *p-n* junction diode shown in figure below ?

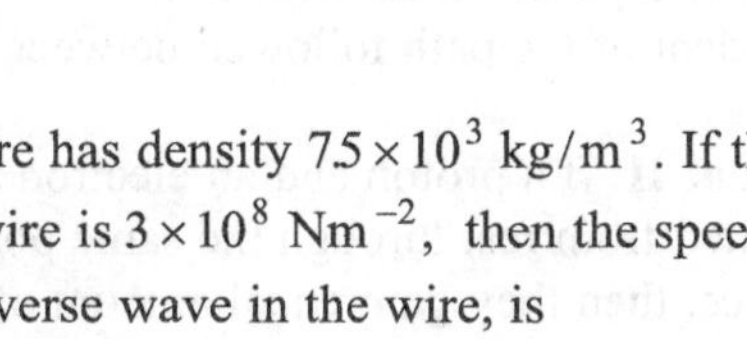

(a) Zero (b) 10 mA
(c) 20 mA (d) 40 mA

4. A rectangular coil having 20 turns carries a current of 15 A. The coil is oriented with respect to uniform magnetic field of $0.2\ \hat{i}$ T, such that its area vector is $-0.05\ \hat{i}\ m^2$. The potential energy of coil in the given orientation is

(a) 0 (b) 7.5 J
(c) 4 J (d) 3 J

5. In an adiabatic compression of a monoatomic gas and its volume reduces to one-third of initial volume, then its final pressure would be, if gas has initial pressure p

(a) $3^{1/2}p$ (b) $3^{3/2}p$ (c) $3^{5/3}p$ (d) $3^{3/5}p$

6. Nuclear fission experiments show that the neutrons split the uranium nuclei into two fragments of about same size. This process is accompanied by the emission of several

(a) protons and positrons (b) α-particles
(c) neutrons (d) protons and α-particles

7. If the expression of electric field vector and magnetic field vector of an electromagnetic wave are $E = E_0 \sin(kx - \omega t)$ and $B = B_0 \sin(kx - \omega t)$, then

(a) $E_0 B_0 = \omega k$ (b) $E_0 k = B_0 \omega$
(c) $E_0 \omega = B_0 k$ (d) $E_0 B_0 = \sqrt{\frac{\omega}{k}}$

8. Two similar coils of radius r and number of turns N are lying concentrically with their planes at right angles to each other. The current flowing in them are $\sqrt{6}I$ and $\sqrt{3}I$ respectively, then the magnetic field induction at centre of the coils is

(a) $\frac{3\mu_0 NI}{4r}$ (b) $\frac{\mu_0 NI}{4r}$ (c) $\frac{3\mu_0 NI}{2r}$ (d) $\frac{\mu_0 NI}{2r}$

9. An aluminium sphere of radius 10 cm is heated from 0° to 100°C. Its volume changes by (given that, coefficient of linear expansion for aluminium $= 23 \times 10^{-6}$/°C)

(a) 28.9 cc (b) 2.89 cc (c) 9.28 cc (d) 49.8 cc

10. The output Y, when all the three inputs are first high and then low, will respectively be

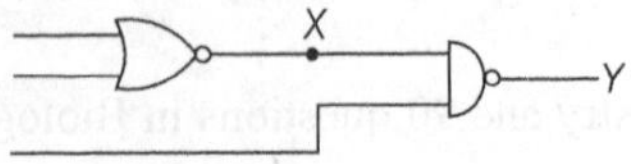

(a) 1, 1 (b) 1, 0 (c) 0, 1 (d) 0, 0

11. The ionisation energy of hydrogen atom is 13.6 eV. An electron in the ground state of a hydrogen atom absorbs a photon of energy 12.75 eV. How many different spectral lines can one expect when the electron makes a downward transition?

(a) 1 (b) 4 (c) 2 (d) 6

12. A copper wire has a mass (0.3 ± 0.003) g, radius (0.5 ± 0.005) mm and length $(6 \pm 0.06$ cm). The maximum percentage error in the measurement of its density is

(a) 2% (b) 3% (c) 6% (d) 4%

13. During an adiabatic process, the pressure of a gas is found to be proportional to the cube of its temperature. The ratio of $\frac{C_p}{C_V}$ for the gas is

(a) $\frac{3}{2}$ (b) 2 (c) $\frac{5}{3}$ (d) $\frac{4}{3}$

14. Which of the following graphs shows correct variation between capacitive reactance (X_C) and angular frequency (ω) of AC source?

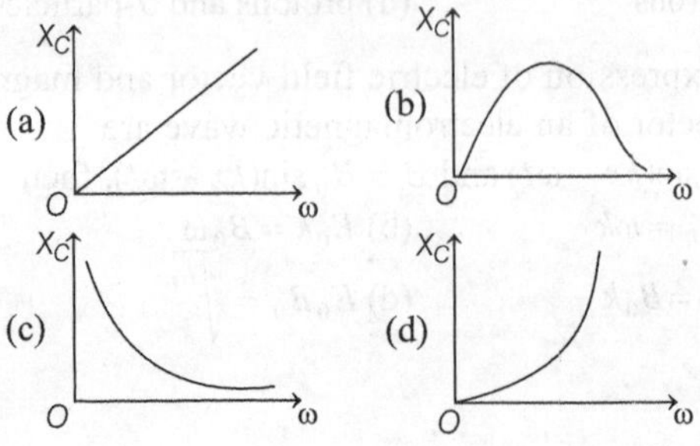

15. Four balls each of mass 2 kg are placed at the corners of a square of side 10 cm. If mass m_3 is removed as shown in the figure, then the shift in the centre of mass of the system is

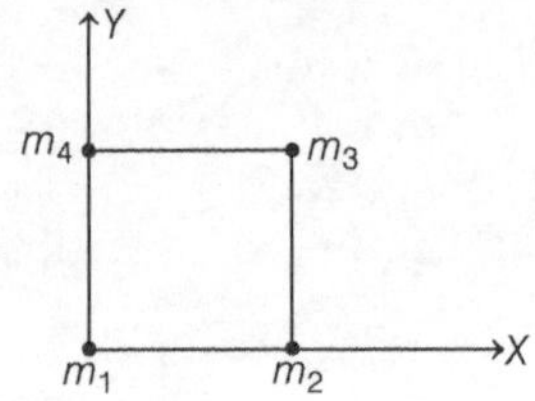

(a) $(5\hat{i} + 5\hat{j})$ (b) $-\left(\frac{10}{3}\hat{i} + \frac{10}{3}\hat{j}\right)$

(c) $-\left(\frac{5}{3}\hat{i} + \frac{5}{3}\hat{j}\right)$ (d) $(3\hat{i} + 3\hat{j})$

16. The total energy of the electron in the first excited state of hydrogen is –3.4 eV. The kinetic energy of the electron in this state is

(a) +1.7 eV
(b) +3.4 eV
(c) +6.8 eV
(d) +13.4 eV

17. Two statements are given below.

Statement I The work done in a moving charge between two points in an electric field is independent of the path followed between these two points.

Statement II If a proton and an electron are accelerated from rest through the same potential difference, then they gain equal amount of kinetic energy.

In light of above statements, choose the most appropriate answer from the options given below.

(a) Both Statement I and Statement II are correct.
(b) Both Statement I and Statement II are incorrect.
(c) Statement I is correct and Statement II is incorrect.
(d) Statement I is incorrect and Statement II is correct.

18. A convex lens of refractive index 1.5 and focal length 18 cm in air is immersed in water. The change in focal length of the lens will be .... (Given, refractive index of water = 4 / 3)

(a) 54 cm (b) 36 cm
(c) 27 cm (d) 72 cm

19. A capacitor is charged in such a manner that it stores energy of 2 J. Now, potential energy is increased to 8 J, it is done by

(a) double the potential difference across the capacitor without changing the charge
(b) double both the potential difference and charge
(c) double the charge without changing the potential difference
(d) quadruple the potential difference across the capacitor without changing the charge

20. A ray falls on a prism $ABC(AB = BC)$ and travels as shown in the figure. The minimum refractive index of the prism material should be

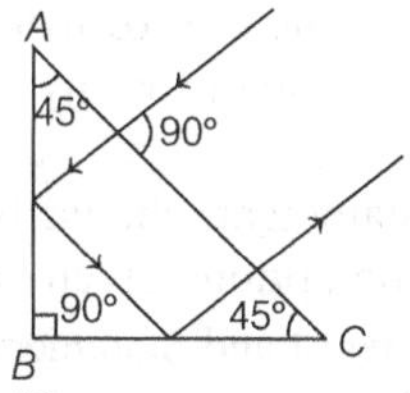

(a) 4/3 (b) $\sqrt{2}$ (c) 1.5 (d) $\sqrt{3}$

21. A linearly polarised electromagnetic wave given as $\mathbf{E} = E_0\hat{\mathbf{i}} \cos(kz - \omega t)$ is incident normally on a perfectly reflecting infinite wall at $z = a$. Assuming, that the material of the wall is optically inactive, the reflected wave will be given as

(a) $\mathbf{E}_r = E_0\hat{\mathbf{i}}(kz - \omega t)$
(b) $\mathbf{E}_r = E_0\hat{\mathbf{i}} \cos(kz + \omega t)$
(c) $\mathbf{E}_r = -E_0\hat{\mathbf{i}} \cos(kz + \omega t)$
(d) $\mathbf{E}_r = E_0\hat{\mathbf{i}} \sin(kz - \omega t)$

22. A copper wire of length 2 m and radius 0.1cm is joined in series with an iron wire of length 4 m and radius 0.4 cm and a current is passed through the wires. The ratio of the current density in iron and copper wires is

(a) 1 : 2 (b) 4 : 1
(c) 1 : 16 (d) 16 : 1

23. A student performs meter bridge experiment to determine specific resistance of a conducting wire of length 10 cm and diameter 1 mm. When a standard resistance of 6 Ω is connected on left gap and the given conducting wire is connected on the right gap, the balance point is obtained for 60 cm length of the meter bridge wire.
The specific resistance (in Ω-m) for the material of the given wire is

(a) 3.14×10^{-5} (b) 6.28×10^{-2}
(c) 3.14×10^{-4} (d) 6.28×10^{-4}

24. A body of mass 4 kg is acted upon by a force which causes a displacement in it given by $x = t^2$ m, where t is time in second. The work done by force in 4s is

(a) 64 J (b) 128 J
(c) 200 J (d) 240 J

25. If a wire is stretched to make it 0.2% longer, then percentage increase in its resistance will be

(a) increase by 0.4% (b) decrease by 0.4%
(c) increase by 0.1% (d) decrease by 0.1%

26. By sucking through a straw, a man can reduce the pressure in his lungs to 750 mm of Hg (density $= 13.6\ \text{g/cm}^3$). Using the straw, he can drink water from a glass up to a maximum depth of

(a) 75 cm (b) 13.6 cm (c) 1.36 cm (d) 10 cm

27. In a non-uniform electric field, an electric dipole experiences

(a) torque only
(b) force only
(c) torque as well as net force
(d) None of the above

28. The primary and secondary coils of a transformer have 50 and 1500 turns, respectively. If the magnetic flux ϕ linked with the primary coil is given by $\phi = \phi_0 + 4t$, where ϕ is in weber, t is in second and ϕ_0 is a constant, the output voltage across the secondary coil is

(a) 90 V (b) 120 V (c) 220 V (d) 30 V

29. Two bodies of masses 2 kg and 4 kg are connected to the ends of a string which passes over a massless, frictionless pulley. The total downward thrust on the pulley is (take, $g = 10\ \text{m/s}^2$)

(a) 53.3 N (b) 26.7 N
(c) 72.5 N (d) 46.7 N

30. In photoelectric emission from a metallic surface, wavelength of incident light is 2×10^{-7} m and stopping potential is 2.5 V. The threshold frequency of the metal in Hz approximately
(charge on electron, $e = 1.6 \times 10^{-19}$ C and Planck's constant, $h = 6.6 \times 10^{-34}$ J-s)

(a) 12×10^{16} (b) 9×10^{15} (c) 9×10^{14} (d) 9×10^{16}

31. A man crosses a 320 m wide river perpendicular to the current of water in 4 min. If in still water he can swim with a speed 5/3 times that of the current of water, then the speed of the current (in m/min) is

(a) 30 (b) 60 (c) 40 (d) 50

32. There are 20 cells connected in series, each having emf E and internal resistance r. Some of cells are connected wrongly, a battery of emf $3E$ with internal resistance $5r$ and an ammeter are connected in series with above arrangement. The ammeter reads 5A when both add each other and 3A when both oppose each other. Then, number of cells wrongly connected is

(a) 2 (b) 3
(c) 5 (d) 4

33. A particle is projected vertically upwards with a velocity $\sqrt{gR}$, where R denotes the radius of the earth and g the acceleration due to gravity on the surface of the earth. Then, the maximum height ascended by the particle is

(a) $\frac{5R}{4}$ (b) $2R$ (c) $\frac{R}{2}$ (d) R

34. A disc of mass 40 g is kept floating horizontally by throwing 20 marbles per second against it from below. If the mass of each marble is 4.9 g, then the velocity with which the marbles are striking the disc is
(Assume that, the marbles strike normally and rebound downward with same speed)

(a) 9.8 ms^{-1} (b) 4.9 ms^{-1} (c) 5 ms^{-1} (d) 2 ms^{-1}

35. An object is projected at an angle of 45° with the horizontal at a speed of 12 ms^{-1}. A second object is simultaneously released from a point on the vertical line along maximum height of first object, where they collide. The initial height of second object is ($g = 10\ m/s^2$)

(a) 3.6 m (b) 7.2 m (c) 2.5 m (d) 5 m

36. A circular disc rolls down an inclined plane without slipping. What fraction of its total energy is translational?

(a) $\frac{1}{2}$ (b) $\frac{1}{\sqrt{2}}$
(c) $\frac{2}{3}$ (d) $\frac{1}{\sqrt{3}}$

37. Object distance, $u = (50.1 \pm 0.5)$ cm and image distance, $v = (20.1 \pm 0.2)$ cm, then focal length is $\left(\frac{1}{f} = \frac{1}{u} + \frac{1}{v}\right.$, where u and v are positive$\left.\right)$

(a) (12.4 ± 0.4) cm (b) (12.4 ± 0.1) cm
(c) (14.3 ± 0.4) cm (d) (14.3 ± 0.1) cm

38. In the given circuit (as shown in the figure) neglecting source resistance, then voltmeter and ammeter reading will be

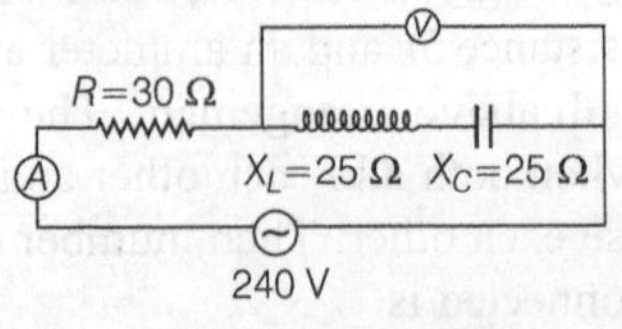

(a) 120V, 3A (b) 120 V, 6A
(c) 0V, 8A (d) 0V, 3A

39. Given below are two statements

Statement I A zener diode is used to protect meters from burning.

Statement II At the breakdown, voltage across zener diode remains constant for any current flowing through it.

In the above statement, choose the most appropriate answer from the options given below.

(a) Both Statement I and Statement II are incorrect.
(b) Statement I is incorrect but Statement II is correct.
(c) Both Statement I and Statement II are correct.
(d) Statement II is incorrect but Statement I is correct.

40. A charged particle q is shot with speed v towards another fixed charged particle Q. It approaches Q upto a closest distance r and then returns. If q was given a speed $2v$, the closest distance of approach would be

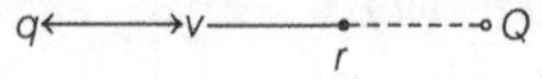

(a) r (b) $2r$
(c) $r/2$ (d) $r/4$

41. Two rods of copper and aluminium of length L_1 and L_2 and the coefficient of linear expansion of both metal rods are α_1 and α_2, respectively. If they are joined together and $(L_1 + L_2)$ is maintained same at all temperatures, which one of the following relations holds good?

(a) $\alpha_1 L_2^2 = \alpha_2 L_1^2$ (b) $\alpha_1^2 L_2 = \alpha_2^2 L_1$
(c) $-\alpha_1 L_1 = \alpha_2 L_2$ (d) $\alpha_1 L_2 = \alpha_2 L_1$

42. A block of mass m and charge q is attached to an unstretched spring of spring constant k. When a horizontal electric field E is switched ON, the block performs simple harmonic motion, whose amplitude of oscillation is

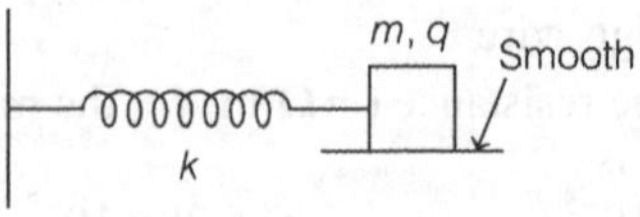

(a) $\frac{qE}{k}$ (b) $\frac{2qE}{k}$
(c) $\frac{qE}{m}$ (d) $\frac{2qE}{m}$

43. In an ammeter, 0.4% of main current passes through galvanometer. If resistance of galvanometer is R_g, then shunt resistance of ammeter will be

(a) $\frac{R_g}{299}$ (b) $\frac{R_g}{120}$
(c) $\frac{R_g}{200}$ (d) $\frac{R_g}{249}$

44. In Young's double slit experiment, the 5th bright fringe from central maxima due to wavelength λ_1 coincides with 8th bright fringe from central maxima due to wavelength λ_2, then the wavelengths of visible lights are
(a) 500 nm and 800 nm (b) 480 nm and 400 nm
(c) 640 nm and 400 nm (d) 640 nm and 560 nm

45. Electron in hydrogen atom first jumps from third excited state to second excited state and then from second excited state to first excited state, then the ratio of wavelengths $\lambda_1 : \lambda_2$ emitted in two cases is
(a) 27 : 5
(b) 7 : 5
(c) 20 : 7
(d) 27 : 20

CHEMISTRY

46. Consider the following reactions,

$$A \longrightarrow X,\ k_A = 10^{18}\ e^{-8000/T}$$
$$B \longrightarrow X,\ k_B = 10^{17}\ e^{-4000/T}$$

Temperature (T/K) at which $k_A = k_B$ is
(a) 4000 K (b) 8000 K (c) $\frac{4000}{2.303}$ K (d) $\frac{8000}{2.303}$ K

47. The entropy values (in $JK^{-1}\ mol^{-1}$) of $H_2 = 130.6$, $Cl_2(g) = 223.0$ and $HCl(g) = 186.7$ at 298 K and 1 atm, then entropy change for the reaction,

$$H_2(g) + Cl_2(g) \longrightarrow 2HCl(g), \text{ is}$$

(a) $+540.3\ JK^{-1}mol^{-1}$ (b) $-166.9\ JK^{-1}mol^{-1}$
(c) $+727.3\ JK^{-1}mol^{-1}$ (d) $+19.8\ JK^{-1}mol^{-1}$

48. 4 moles of X and 4 moles of Y are mixed together. For the reaction $X + Y \rightleftharpoons P + Q$, 2 moles of P and Q are formed at equilibrium. The equilibrium constant for the reaction will be
(a) $\frac{1}{4}$ (b) $\frac{1}{2}$ (c) 1 (d) 4

49. Normality and molarity changes with temperature because they involve volumes. The normality of 0.3 M phosphorus acid, H_3PO_3 is
(a) 0.9 N (b) 0.1 N
(c) 0.3 N (d) 0.6 N

50. The product P in the following reaction is

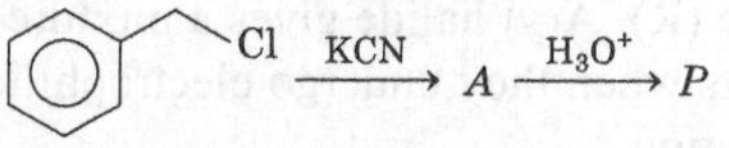

(a) 2-phenylpropanoic acid
(b) benzoic acid
(c) 2-phenylethanoic acid
(d) phenylmethanoic acid

51. In the given reaction, products A and B are

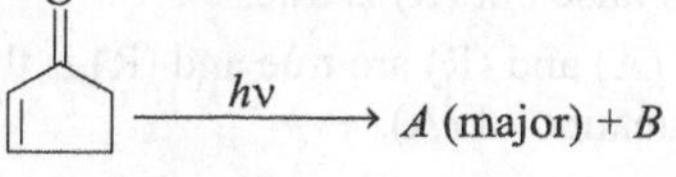

(a) 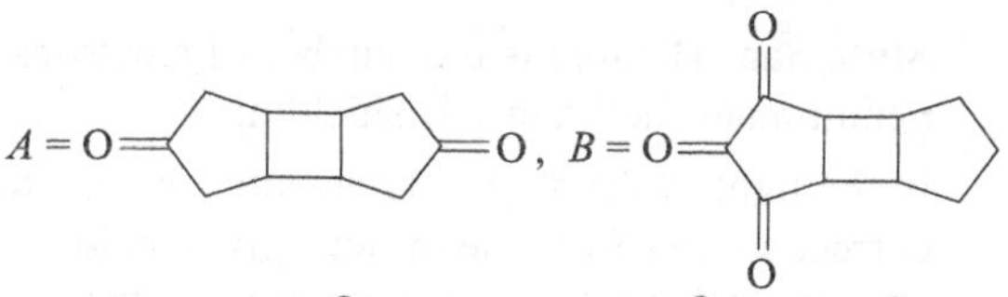

(b) 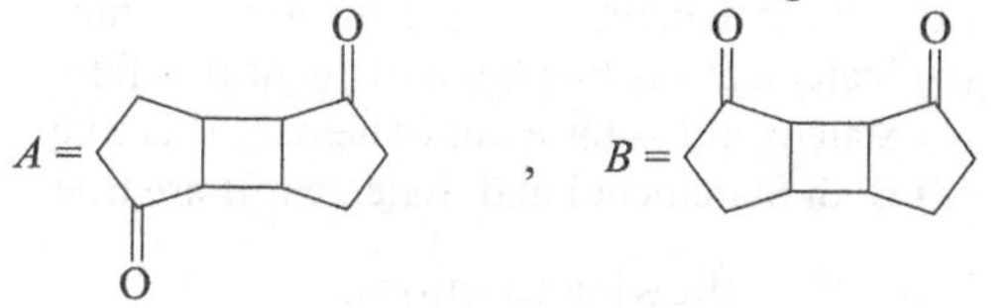

(c) 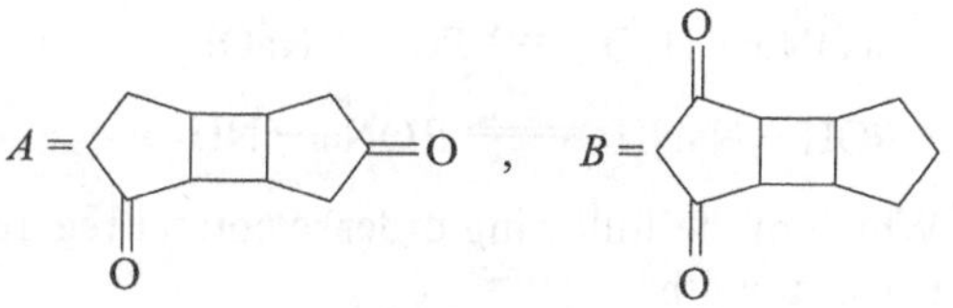

(d) 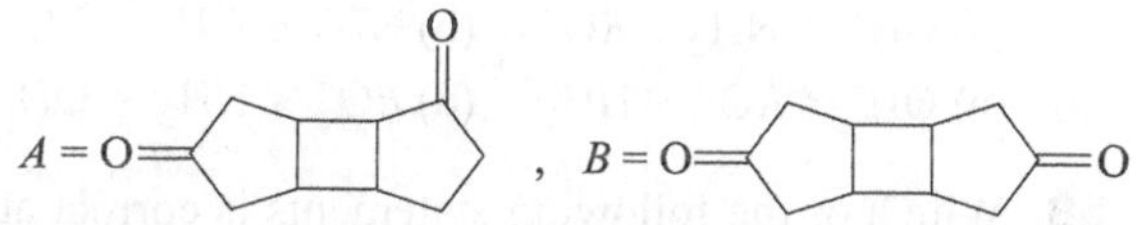

52. $CH \equiv CH \xrightarrow{O_3/NaOH} X \xrightarrow{Zn/CH_3COOH} Y$, Y is
(a) CH_2OH—CH_2OH (b) CH_3CH_2OH
(c) CH_3COOH (d) CH_3OH

53. Although +3 is the characteristic oxidation state for lanthanoid yet cerium also shows +4 oxidation state because it
(a) has tendency to attain noble gas configuration.
(b) has variable ionisation enthalpy.
(c) resembles Pb^{4+}.
(d) has tendency to attain f^7 configuration.

54. The C— C bond length of the following molecules is in the order
(a) $C_2H_6 > C_2H_4 > C_6H_6 > C_2H_2$
(b) $C_2H_2 < C_2H_4 < C_6H_6 < C_2H_6$
(c) $C_6H_6 > C_2H_2 > C_2H_6 > C_2H_4$
(d) $C_2H_4 > C_2H_6 > C_2H_2 > C_6H_6$

55. Suppose the elements P and Q combine to form two compounds PQ and PQ_2. When 0.05 mole of PQ weighs 5 g and 0.03 mole of PQ_2 weighs 4.5 g then atomic weights of P and Q are respectively:
(a) 50, 75
(b) 75, 50
(c) 50, 50
(d) 25, 25

56. Given below are two statements.
Statement I Shielding effect increases as we go down the group.
Statement II More is the number of electrons in the penultimate shell, more is shielding.
In the light of the above statements, choose the correct answer from the options given below:
(a) Both Statement I and Statement II are false.
(b) Statement I is true but Statement II is false.
(c) Statement I is false but Statement II is true.
(d) Both Statement I and Statement II are true.

57. From the following reactions,

$$R\overset{-}{O}\overset{+}{Na} + H_2O \rightleftharpoons ROH + NaOH$$

$$ROH + NaNH_2 \rightleftharpoons R\overset{-}{O}\overset{+}{Na} + NH_3$$

Which of the following order is correct regarding basic strength?
(a) $OH^- < NH_2^- < RO^-$ (b) $NH_2^- < OH^- < RO^-$
(c) $OH^- < RO^- < NH_2^-$ (d) $RO^- < NH_2^- < OH^-$

58. Which of the following statements is correct about resonance?
(a) Resonating structures are more stable than hybrid-resonance.
(b) Equivalent resonating structures do not contribute equally.
(c) Resonance affects bond lengths but not bond angles.
(d) Resonating structures indicate that the molecule has no real existence.

59. The number of radial node present in $4d$-orbital is
(a) 3 (b) 2 (c) 1 (d) 0

60. The ions O^{2-}, F^-, Na^+, Mg^{2+} and Al^{3+} are isoelectronic. Their ionic radii show
(a) an increase from Na^+ to Al^{3+} and then decreases from O^{2-} to F^-.
(b) a decrease from Na^+ to Al^{3+} and then increases from O^{2-} to F^-.
(c) a significant increase from Al^{3+} to O^{2-}.
(d) a significant decrease from Al^{3+} to O^{2-}.

61. Match List-I with List-II.

List-I (Compounds)	List-II (Oxidation number)
A. N_2H_4	I. -1
B. NH_2OH	II. -2
C. HNO_2	III. $+5$
D. HNO_3	IV. $+3$

Choose the correct answer from the options given below:
(a) A-IV, B-I, C-II, D-III
(b) A-II, B-I, C-IV, D-III
(c) A-II, B-III, C-IV, D-I
(d) A-I, B-IV, C-II, D-III

62. Which of the following method can be used to synthesize fluorobenzene in the laboratory?
(a) Heating phenol with HF and KF.
(b) Reacting bromobenzene with NaF solution.
(c) Diazotisation of aniline follows by heating the diazonium salt with HBF_4.
(d) Direct fluorination of benzene with F_2 gas.

63. Given below are two statements.
Statement I Use of *cis*-platin in cancer treatment can cause severe kidney damage.
Statement II The d_{xy}, d_{yz} and d_{xz} orbitals lie between the axes and collectively called t_{2g} orbitals.
In the light of the above statements choose the correct answer from the options given below.
(a) Both statement I and Statement II are false.
(b) Statement I is true but Statement II is false.
(c) Statement I is false but Statement II is true.
(d) Both statement I and Statement II are true.

64. Given below are two statements, one is labelled as Assertion (A) and the other is labelled as Reason (R).
Assertion (A) Aryl halides undergo electrophilic substitution more readily than benzene.
Reason (R) Aryl halide gives a mixture of o-, p-products when they undergo electrophilic substitution.
In the light of the above statements choose the most appropriate answer from the options given below.
(a) Both (A) and (R) are true but (R) is not the correct explanation of (A).
(b) (A) is true but (R) is false.
(c) (A) is false but (R) is true.
(d) Both (A) and (R) are true and (R) is the correct explanation of (A).

65. X, Y and Z in the given graph are

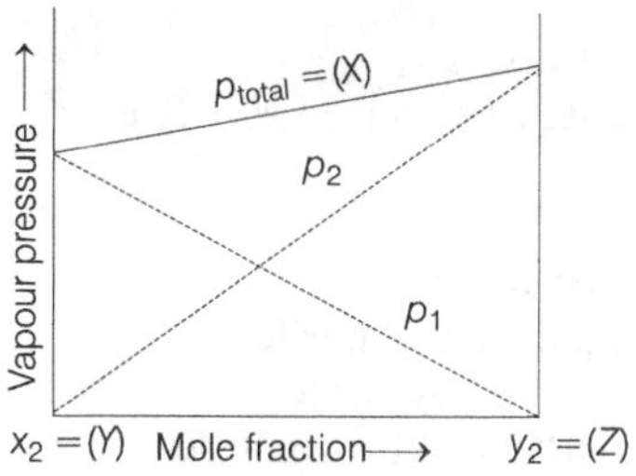

(a) $X = p_1 + p_2, Y = 1, Z = 0$
(b) $X = p_1 + p_2, Y = 0, Z = 0$
(c) $X = p_1 \times p_2, Y = 0, Z = 0$
(d) $X = p_1 - p_2, Y = 1, Z = 0$

66. Given below are two statements.
Statement I 2-methyl-1, 3-cyclohexanedione is more acidic than cyclohexanone.
Statement II Aldehyde and ketone undergoes nucleophilic addition reaction but acyl group undergoes nucleophilic substitution reaction.
In the light of the above statements, choose the correct answer from the options given below.
(a) Both statement I and Statement II are false.
(b) Statement I is true but Statement II is false.
(c) Statement I is false but Statement II is true.
(d) Both statement I and Statement II are true.

67. Match the List-I with List-II.

	List-I		List-II
A.	Ammonium chloride	(i)	Rechargeable
B.	Sulphuric acid	(ii)	Strong electrolytes
C.	Zinc chloride	(iii)	Lead storage batteries
D.	Secondary batteries	(iv)	Dry cell

Choose the correct answer from the options given below.
(a) A-(iv), B-(iii), C-(ii), D-(i)
(b) A-(iv), B-(ii), C-(iii), D-(i)
(c) A-(i), B-(iii), C-(ii), D-(iv)
(d) A-(i), B-(ii), C-(iii), D-(iv)

68. Which of the following is the correct statement regarding a solution exhibiting positive deviation from ideal behaviour?
(a) Intermolecular force of attraction between A—A and B—B are stronger than A—B.
(b) $\Delta H_{mix} = 0$ at constant T and P.
(c) $\Delta V_{mix} < 0$ at constant T and P.
(d) It will obeys Raoult's law.

69. Given below are two statements.
Statement I An alcohol does not react with Cl^- ion in aqueous medium, but reacts with concentrated HCl solution to form alkyl chloride,
Statement II The strong acid (HCl) accelerates the removal of proton from —OH group of alcohol.
In the light of the above statements, choose the correct answer from the options given below.
(a) Both statement I and Statement II are false.
(b) Statement I is true but Statement II is false.
(c) Statement I is false but Statement II is true.
(d) Both statement I and Statement II are true.

70. The partial hydrolysis of one mole of peroxydisulphuric acid produces
I. two moles of sulphuric acid.
II. one mole of sulphuric acid.
III. one mole of peroxymono-sulphuric acid.
IV. one mole of hydrogen peroxide.
V. one mole of hydrogen gas.
Choose the correct answers from the options given below.
(a) Only I (b) I and IV
(c) II and III (d) I, II and III

71. Reversible expansion of an ideal gas under isothermal and adiabatic conditions are as shown in the figure.

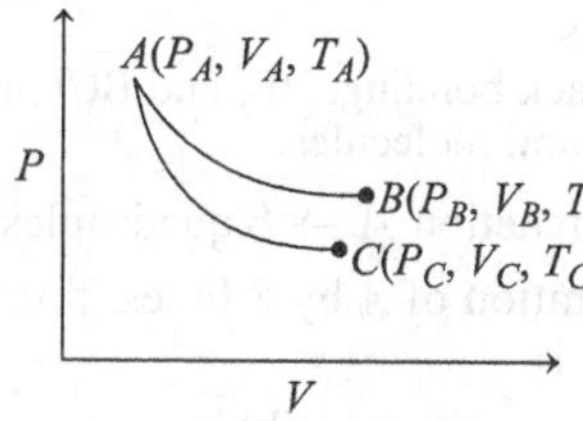

$AB \longrightarrow$ Isothermal expansion
$AC \longrightarrow$ Adiabatic expansion
Which of the following is correct?
(a) $\Delta S_{\text{Isothermal}} > \Delta S_{\text{Adiabatic}}$
(b) $T_C = T_A$
(c) $W_{\text{Isothermal}} < W_{\text{Adiabatic}}$
(d) $T_A < T_B$

72. Solubility of $AlCl_3$ in pure water is 10^{-5} M, then find out it's solubility in presence of 0.1 M NaCl.
(a) 2.7×10^{-16} M (b) 2.7×10^{-17} M
(c) 5.4×10^{-17} M (d) 9×10^{-17} M

73. Which of the following compounds will give silver mirror with ammoniacal silver nitrate?
A. Benzophenone B. Formaldehyde
C. Benzaldehyde D. Acetone
E. Formic Acid

Choose the most appropriate answer from the options given below.

(a) B, C and D (b) A, B and C

(c) B, C and E (d) C, D and E

74. Three types of solutions are prepared and labelled as A, B and C.

A : 5 g of 15 M NaOH ($d = 1 \text{ g mL}^{-1}$)

B : 5 mL of 50% (w/V) NaOH

C : 5 g of 40% (w/V) NaOH ($d = 1.25 \text{ g mL}^{-1}$)

Increasing order of mass of NaOH in the above solution is

(a) A < B < C (b) C < B < A

(c) B < C < A (d) B < A < C

75. The complex that absorbs light of shortest wavelength is

(a) $[CoF_6]^{3-}$

(b) $[Co(H_2O)_6]^{3+}$

(c) $[Co(NH_3)_6]^{3+}$

(d) $[Co(Ox)_3]^{3-}$ $(Ox = C_2O_4^{2-})$

76. Which one of the following statements is incorrect about the structural properties of BF_3?

(a) The unsual shortness of B—F bonds is due to $p\pi$ - $p\pi$ interaction between B and F atoms.

(b) All the three B—F bond lengths are equal.

(c) Double bond is delocalised giving three resonance structures.

(d) Due to back bonding, BF_3 and BCl_3 are not isostructural molecules.

77. The rate of reaction $A \rightarrow B$ quadruples on increasing the concentration of A by 8 times, thus the order of the reaction is

(a) 4 (b) 2/3

(c) 2 (d) 1

78. Match List-I with List-II.

	List-I	List-II
A.	λ_m	I. Intensive property
B.	E°_{cell}	II. Depends on number of ions/volume
C.	κ	III. Extensive property
D.	$\Delta_r G_{cell}$	IV. Increases with dilution.

Choose the correct answer from the options given below:

(a) A-III, B-IV, C-I, D-II

(b) A-I, B-II, C-IV, D-III

(c) A-IV, B-I, C-II, D-III

(d) A-IV, B-I, C-III, D-II

79.

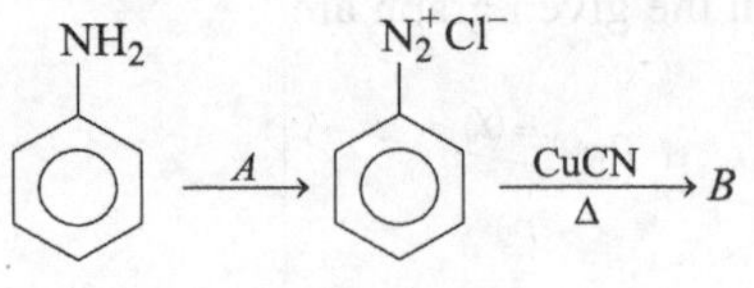

A and B respectively are

(a) phenol and methyl nitrile

(b) HNO_3 and benzonitrile

(c) $NaNO_2/HCl$ and benzonitrile

(d) HNO_3/H^+ and methyl cyanide

80. Maximum number of unpaired electrons are present in which ion?

(a) Sm^{3+} (b) Eu^{3+} (c) Ho^{3+} (d) Gd^{3+}

81. For the reaction, the major product is

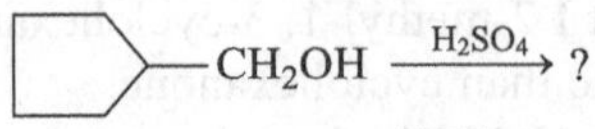

(a) 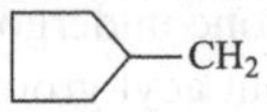

(b) 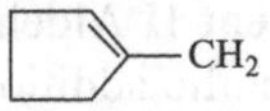

(c) 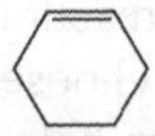

(d) 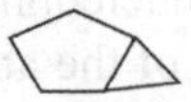

82. Sodium carbonate cannot be used in place of $(NH_4)_2CO_3$ for the identification of Ca^{2+} and Ba^{2+} (in group V) during mixture analysis because

(a) Na^+ ions will react with acid radicals

(b) Na^+ ions will interfere with the detection of Ca^{2+} and Ba^{2+} ions

(c) Concentration of CO_3^{2-} ions is very low

(d) Mg^{2+} ions will also be precipitated

83. Which of the following species behave both as a nucleophile as well as an electrophile?

(i) $CH_3C{\equiv}N:$ (ii) $H_2C{=}O$ (iii) H_2O

(iv) H_2 (v) BF_3

Choose the most appropriate answer from the options given below.

(a) (i), (ii) and (v) (b) (i), (ii) and (iii)

(c) (ii), (iii) and (v) (d) (iii), (iv) and (v)

84. Consider the following ions:

I. Fe^{2+} $(Z = 26)$ II. Cu^+ $(Z = 29)$

III. Ni^{2+} $(Z = 28)$ IV. Mn^{2+} $(Z = 25)$

V. Zn^{2+} $(Z = 30)$

Select paramagnetic and coloured ions out of

(a) II and III

(b) II, III, IV and V

(c) II, III and IV

(d) I, III and IV

85. What is the standard electrode potential for the electrode MnO_4^- / MnO_2 in solution?

(Given: $E^\circ\ MnO_4^- / Mn^{2+} = 1.51$ volt,

$E^\circ\ MnO_2 / Mn^{2+} = 1.23$ volt).

(a) 1.70V (b) – 1.70 V
(c) 5.10V (d) – 5.10 V

86. Which one of the following represents correct order of basic strength?

(a) $NH_2OH < NH_3 < N_2H_4$
(b) $NH_3 < N_2H_4 < NH_4OH$
(c) $NH_2OH < N_2H_4 < NH_3$
(d) $N_2H_4 < NH_2OH < NH_3$

87. The technique which is used to separate chloroform and aniline is

(a) column chromatography
(b) distillation
(c) sublimation
(d) crystallisation

88. Match the reactions given in Column I with the product given in Column II.

	Column-I		Column-II
A.	$CH_3CH_2CH_2OH \xrightarrow[443\ K]{H_2SO_4 \cdot \Delta}$	I.	Acetaldehyde
B.	$CH_3—CH═CH—CH_2—OH \xrightarrow{PCC}$	II.	But-2-one
C.	$CH_3—CH(OH)—CH_2CH_3 \xrightarrow{CrO_3}$	III.	But-2-en-al
D.	$CH_3CH_2—OH \xrightarrow[573\ K]{Cu}$	IV.	Propene

Choose the correct answer from the options given below.

(a) A-IV, B-III, C-II, D-I
(b) A-II, B-I, C-IV, D-III
(c) A-III, B-IV, C-I, D-II
(d) A-IV, B-II, C-I, D-III

89. The dipole moment of hydrogen chloride with bond distance 127 pm is 1.03 D. The percent ionic character of its bond is about

(a) 16% (b) 17%
(c) 16.9% (d) 16.5%

90. Match the List-I with List-II.

List-I	List-II
A. $N_2 \longrightarrow N_2^+$	(i) Bonds order increases and magnetic property changes
B. $O_2^+ \longrightarrow O_2^{2+}$	(ii) Bond order decreases and magnetic property not changes
C. $B_2 \longrightarrow B_2^+$	(iii) Bond order increases and magnetic property not changes
D. $NO^- \longrightarrow NO$	(iv) Bond order decreases magnetic property changes.

Choose the correct answer from the options given below.

(a) A-(iv), B-(i), C-(iii), D-(ii)
(b) A-(iv), B-(i), C-(ii), D-(iii)
(c) A-(iii), B-(ii), C-(iv), D-(iv)
(d) A-(i), B-(iv), C-(iii), D-(iii)

BIOLOGY

91. In succulents like *Opuntia* and *Bryophyllum*, the value of RQ is zero because of
(a) incomplete oxidation of fats
(b) complete oxidation of carbohydrates
(c) incomplete oxidation of carbohydrates
(d) incomplete oxidation of proteins

92. Which of the following is not an area of biotechnology?
(a) Provide the best catalyst
(b) Create optimal conditions
(c) Down stream processing technology
(d) Creating evolutionary mapping

93. The anatomy of heart wood shows some particular features. Identify the correct set of statements about heart wood.
I. It is composed of dead cells.
II. It is mechanically strong.
III. It is less easily penetrated by wood preservative chemicals.
IV. Its cells contain tannins that make it light in colour.
V. It is also called alburnum.
Choose the correct answer from the options given below.
(a) I, II and IV (b) I, II and III
(c) II, III and V (d) III, IV and V

94. Among the following venereal diseases which one is non-curable even if detected early?
(a) Syphilis (b) Trichomoniasis
(c) Genital herpes (d) Chlamydiasis

95. Given below are two statements; one is labelled as Assertion (A) and the other is labelled as Reason (R).
Assertion (A) Lysosomes are single membrane bound organelles that are capable of digesting the own substances of cell.
Reason (R) Lysosomes have hydrolytic enzymes in them.
In the light of the above statements, choose the correct answer from the options given below.
(a) A is false, but R is true
(b) Both A and R are true and R is the correct explanation of A
(c) Both A and R are true and R is not the correct explanation of A
(d) A is true, but R is false

96. Which is wrong about nucleic acid?
(a) Nucleotide is the building block
(b) RNA is double-stranded occasionally
(c) The skeletal homocyclic ring is purine and pyrimidine
(d) DNA is single-stranded in some viruses

97. Observe the given diagram of TS of sunflower stem and identify *X* in the same.

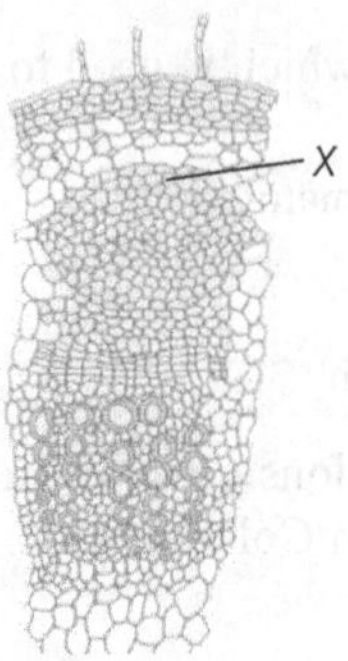

(a) Medullary rays
(b) Starch sheath
(c) Sclerenchymatous pericycle
(d) Hypodermis

98. Identify the incorrect statement.
(a) In *Opuntia*, stem is modified into flattened structure
(b) In leaves, veins provide rigidity to the leaf blade and act as channels of transport for water, minerals and food materials
(c) In peas, leaves are converted into tendrils for storage of food materials
(d) In *Euphorbia*, stem is modified into a cylindrical structure

99. Match List I with List II.

	List I		List II
A.	Annelida	1.	*Laccifer*
B.	Arthropoda	2.	*Cucumaria*
C.	Echinodermata	3.	*Pheretima*
D.	Cephalochordata	4.	*Branchiostoma*

Choose the correct answer from the options given below.

	A	B	C	D
(a)	1	2	3	4
(b)	3	1	4	2
(c)	3	2	1	4
(d)	3	1	2	4

100. Which organism shows female heterogamety?
(a) Grasshopper (b) *Drosophila*
(c) Humans (d) Birds

101. .... type of excretion occurs in frog.
(a) Uricotelic (b) Amphotelic
(c) Ureotelic (d) Ammonotelic

102. Which one of the following process produce four ATP and two NADH?
(a) Electron transport (b) Citric acid cycle
(c) Glycolysis
(d) Oxidation of pyruvic acid

103. Which of the following is used to initiate flowering and for synchronising fruit set in pineapples?
(a) Ethylene (b) Abscisic acid
(c) Cytokinins (d) Auxins

104. Which of the following microbes flourish in hot springs and deep sea hydrothermal vents where temperatures far exceed 100°C?
(a) Eubacteria (b) Fungi
(c) Algae (d) Archaebacteria

105. Columnar cells bearing cilia on their surface are known as
(a) columnar epithelium
(b) cuboidal epithelium
(c) ciliated epithelium
(d) squamous epithelium

106. Given below are two statements.
Statement I Colour blindness occurs due to recessive gene on X-chromosome.
Statement II The genes for colour blindness are present on the X-chromosome.
In the light of the above statements, choose the correct answer from the options given below.
(a) Statement I is incorrect, but statement II is correct
(b) Both statement I and statement II are correct
(c) Both statement I and statement II are incorrect
(d) Statement I is true, but statement II is incorrect

107. Which of the following options contains all the three stop or terminator codons?
(a) UGA, UUU, UAA (b) UGA, UAG, UAA
(c) AUG, UAG, UUU (d) AUC, UAG, AUG

108. CO_2 is carried by haemoglobin as carbamino-haemoglobin, whose enzyme activity is represented as

(a) $CO_2 + H_2O \xrightleftharpoons[\text{acid}]{\text{Carbonic}} HCO_3 \xrightleftharpoons[\text{anhydrase}]{\text{Carbonic}} HCO_3^- + H^+$

(b) $CO_2 + H_2O \xrightleftharpoons[\text{acid}]{\text{Carbonic}} H_2CO_3 \xrightleftharpoons{\text{Anhydrase}} HO_3^- + H^+$

(c) $CO_2 + H_2O \xrightleftharpoons[\text{anhydrase}]{\text{Carbonic}} H_2CO_3 \xrightleftharpoons[\text{anhydrase}]{\text{Carbonic}} HCO_3^- + H^+$

(d) $CO_2 + OH \xrightleftharpoons[\text{anhydrase}]{\text{Carbonic}} H_2CO_3 \xrightleftharpoons[\text{acid}]{\text{Carbonic}} HCO_3^- + H^+$

109. Identify the correct pair.
(a) Endangered species – *Clarias gariepinus* and catfishes
(b) Extinct species – Steler's sea cow and passenger pigeon
(c) Co-extinct species – Catfish and passenger pigeon
(d) Both (a) and (c)

110. The regulator gene - *R* produces a repressor protein which prevents transcription of structural gene, when
(a) lactose is absent (b) lactose is present
(c) glucose is absent (d) glucose is present

111. In the context of the given figure, identify the correct observation from the given statements

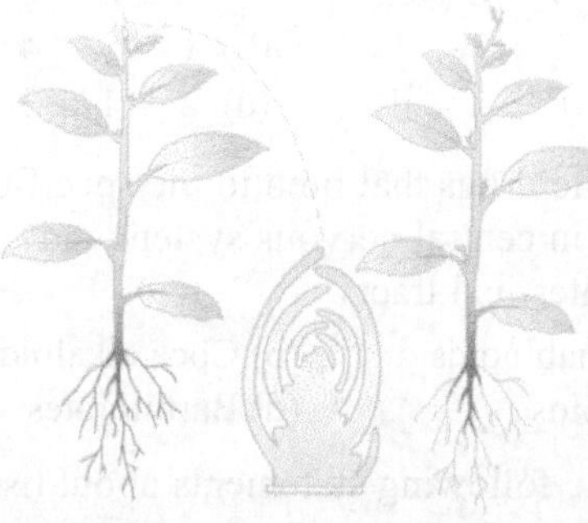

(a) (b)

(a) Plant (a) shows internodal elongation just prior to flowering
(b) Plant (b) shows alternate phyllotaxy
(c) Plant (b) shows growth of lateral buds into branches after decapitation
(d) Plant (a) represents heterophyllous conditions

112. Match List I with List II.

	List I		List II
A.	Hilum	1.	Mass of cells
B.	Nucellus	2.	Small opening
C.	Micropyle	3.	Region of fusion
D.	Pericarp	4.	Thick wall of fruit

Choose the correct answer from the options given below.

	A	B	C	D		A	B	C	D
(a)	4	2	3	1	(b)	1	2	3	4
(c)	3	1	2	4	(d)	3	4	1	2

113. The double walled cup-like structure, which encloses the glomerular is called

(a) columns of Bertini (b) Bowman's capsule
(c) hilum (d) nephrons

114. Match List I with List II.

	List I		List II
A.	Cuticle	1.	Monocot stem
B.	Radial vascular bundles	2.	Root system
C.	Trichomes	3.	Epidermal tissue system
D.	Conjoint and closed vascular bundles	4.	Prevents water loss

Choose the correct answer from the options given below.

	A	B	C	D		A	B	C	D
(a)	4	2	3	1	(b)	1	3	4	2
(c)	3	1	2	4	(d)	2	1	3	4

115. Name the drugs that bind to the specific receptors present in central nervous system and gastrointestinal tract.

(a) Cannabinoids (b) Coca alkaloid
(c) Opioids (d) Barbiturates

116. Read the following statements about tissue system.

I. In the monocotyledons, the vascular bundles have no cambium present in them.
II. The conjoint vascular bundles usually have the xylem located only on the outer side of phloem.
III. In dicot roots, epiblema is the outermost layer.
IV. Walls of endodermal cells have a deposition of water-impermeable waxy material suberin.
V. Tissues such as pericycle, vascular bundles and cortex constitute the stele.

Choose the correct statements from the options given below.

(a) I, IV and V only (b) II, IV and V only
(c) I, III and IV only (d) I and V only

117. Which of the following statements is incorrect about human respiratory system?

(a) Pharynx acts as a common passage for food and air
(b) Larynx helps in sound production
(c) The pleural fluid reduces friction on the lung surface
(d) The inner pleural membrane is close to the thoracic lining

118. Which of the following is not a protein in composition?

(a) Trypsin (b) Antibody
(c) GLUT-4 (d) Lecithin

119. Which of the following chromosome contains one extremely short and one very long arm?

(a) Metacentric chromosome
(b) Sub-metacentric chromosome
(c) Acrocentric chromosome
(d) Telocentric chromosome

120. Auxins are responsible for initiating and promoting cell division in tissues like

(a) hypodermis (b) cambium
(c) cortex (d) epidermis

121. Given below are two statements; one is labelled as Assertion (A) and the other is labelled as Reason (R).

Assertion (A) All amino acids are essential for our body.

Reason (R) Proteins like antibody fight infectious organisms.

In the light of the above statements, choose the correct answer from the options given below.

(a) A is false, but R is true
(b) Both A and R are true and R is the correct explanation of A
(c) Both A and R are true, but R is not the correct explanation of A
(d) A is true, but R is false

122. Consider the given diagrammatic presentation of a standard ECG, and identify which part represents the return of the ventricles from excited to normal state.

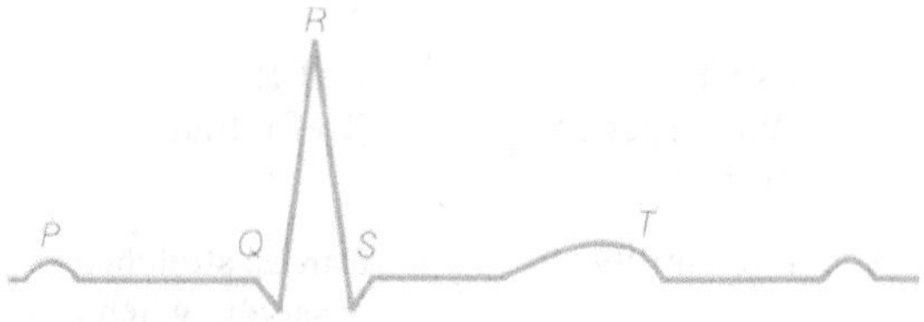

(a) *P* (b) *T* (c) *R* (d) *S*

123. Which of the following functions is not related to posterior pituitary hormones?
(a) Helps in milk ejection
(b) Regulates basal metabolic rate
(c) It reduces the volume of urine
(d) It influences body temperature, pigmentation, etc.

124. Which of the following statements cannot be connected to mitosis?
(a) It helps in maintaining uniformity within a species
(b) It restores the surface volume ratio of the cell
(c) Growth takes place by increase in the size of cells rather than increase in the number of cells
(d) Repair of the body takes place by the addition of new cells by mitosis

125. Select the incorrect statement regarding restriction enzymes.
(a) *Hind* II was the first discovered restriction endonuclease
(b) Today we know more than 900 restriction enzymes isolated from 230 strains
(c) Each exonuclease function by inspecting the length of DNA sequence
(d) The restriction endonuclease recognises a specific palindromic nucleotide sequences

126. Match List I with List II.

	List I		List II
A.	Liverworts	1.	Fragmentation
B.	Mosses	2.	Starch
C.	Chlorophyceae	3.	Mannitol
D.	Phaeophyceae	4.	Gemmae

Codes

	A	B	C	D		A	B	C	D
(a)	2	4	3	1	(b)	4	1	2	3
(c)	2	3	1	4	(d)	1	3	2	4

127. The alien species introduced into lake Victoria that was responsible for the extinction of cichlid fishes is
(a) African fish (b) Water hyacinth
(c) Carrot grass (d) Nile perch

128. Which of the following is not floral character of family–Fabaceae?
(a) Calyx – 5 fused sepals
(b) Corolla – Polypetalous
(c) Androecium – Diadelphous condition
(d) Gynoecium – Inferior ovary

129. When a pure tall plant (TT) is crossed with a pure dwarf plant (tt) the ratio of pure tall plants to pure dwarf plants in F_2-generation will be
(a) 1 : 4 (b) 3 : 1 (c) 1 : 1 (d) 2 : 3

130. The pair of helminths, which are pathogenic to man is
(a) *Ascaris* and *Wuchereria*
(b) *Entamoeba histolytica* and *Ascaris*
(c) *Wuchereria* and *Plasmodium*
(d) *Salmonella typhi* and *P. vivax*

131. Given below are two statements.
Statement I All the chambers of the heart are in relaxed state in joint diastole.
Statement II The cardiac output of atheletes will be less compared to ordinary man.
In the light of the above statements, choose the correct answer from the options given below.
(a) Statement I is correct, but statement II is correct
(b) Both statement I and statement II are correct
(c) Both statement I and statement II are incorrect
(d) Statement I is correct, but statement II is incorrect

132. In eukaryotes, the cistrons are split into several coding units separated by
(a) non-coding base sequence
(b) non-coding polycistronic gene
(c) exons
(d) *m*RNA

133. Compared to mitosis, which is the longer and more complex phase of first meiotic division?
(a) Anaphase-I (b) Metaphase-I
(c) Prophase-I (d) Telophase-I

134. The part of pituitary gland that consists of two portions, pars distalis and pars intermedia is called
(a) neurohypophysis
(b) adenohypophysis
(c) sella turcica
(d) pars intermedia

135. Thalamus contributes to fruit formation in which of the following options?
(a) Apple, guava and groundnut
(b) Mustard, orange and banana
(c) Apple, strawberry and cashew
(d) Orange, mustard and groundnut

136. Identify the incorrect statement.
(a) Erythroblastosis foetalis can be prevented if the (anti-Rh) antibodies are administered to the mother
(b) Most of the substances released by thrombocytes are involved in coagulation
(c) Plasma along with the clotting factor is called serum
(d) The impulse of contraction of the heart originates in the SA node

137. Plants such as mulethi and caesarweed having medicinal value, belong to the which of the families of plants?
(a) Fabaceae and Cruciferae
(b) Fabaceae and Malvaceae
(c) Malvaceae and Graminae
(d) Leguminoceae and Liliaceae

138. Given below are two statements.
Statement I In *Cycas*, small specialised coralloid roots are associated with N_2- fixing bacteria.
Statement II In gymnosperms, male and female gametophytes have an independent free-living existence.
In the light of the above statements, choose the correct answer from the options given below.
(a) Statement I is incorrect, but statement II is correct
(b) Both statement I and statement II are correct
(c) Both statement I and statement II are incorrect
(d) Statement I is correct, but statement II is incorrect

139. Match List I with List II

	List I (Properties of muscles)		List II (Definition)
A.	Excitability	1.	Can be stretched passively when relaxed.
B.	Contractility	2.	Returns to their original shape after contraction and extension.
C.	Extensibility	3.	Shortens and thickens to do work.
D.	Elasticity	4.	Receives and responds to stimuli.

Choose the correct answer from the options given below.

	A	B	C	D		A	B	C	D
(a)	4	3	1	2	(b)	1	2	3	4
(c)	4	1	2	3	(d)	3	1	4	2

140. Which one of the following statements is incorrect?
(a) Organisms like pacific salmon fish breed only once in their life time
(b) Oysters and pelagic fishes produce a large number of small sized offsprings
(c) some species of insects and frogs are cryptically coloured to avoid being detected by predator
(d) Lichens represent a relationship wherein the algae suffers due to the fugal partner

141. Given below are two statements.
Statement I Anaerobiosis increases the decomposition and causes piling up of detritus.
Statement II Primary consumers are also known as transducers.
In the light of the above statements, choose the correct answer from the options given below.
(a) Statement I is incorrect, but statement II is correct
(b) Both statement I and statement II are correct
(c) Both statement I and statement II are incorrect
(d) Statement I is correct, but statement II is incorrect

142. Which of the following sequences correctly represents central dogma?
(a) Translation → DNA replication → *m*RNA transcription
(b) DNA replication → *m*RNA transcription → Translation
(c) *m*RNA transcription → Translation → DNA replication
(d) DNA replication → DNA transcription → Translation

143. Identify the incorrect match.
(a) *ECoRI* – sticky ends
(b) *Hind* II – blunt ends
(c) *Hind* II – Cuts DNA at 5 base pair sequence
(d) Plasmid –Autonomously replicating DNA

144. Which of the following statements are not correct w.r.t the nerve impulse?
I. Nerve cells have polarised membrane.
II. The resting membrane has high permeability for Na^+.
III. The stimulus of threshold value causes stoppage of K^+ – Cl^-ATPase pump.
IV. The membrane potential which sets in a wave of depolarisation is called action potential.
V. With the pumping out of K^+ ions, the neuron interior become positive.
Choose the correct answer from the options given below.
(a) II, III and IV (b) I, III and V
(c) II, III and V (d) IV and V

145. Given below are two statements.
Statement I Endosperm is absent in the mature seeds of groundnut and beans.
Statement II In black pepper and beet, remnants of nucellus are also present.
In the light of the above statements, choose the correct answer from the options given below.
(a) Statement I is incorrect, but statement II is correct
(b) Both statement I and statement II are correct
(c) Both statement I and statement II are incorrect
(d) Statement I is correct, but statement II is incorrect

146. Stirred tank bioreactor has advantages over shake flask culture method. Which of the following is false regarding the stirred tank bioreactor?
(a) Cultures can be prepared on large scale
(b) Large volume of cultures can be withdrawn periodically for sampling
(c) Culture medium can be renewed from time to time
(d) Temperature and pH of culture medium can be maintained

147. When nucleic acids behaves like an enzyme it is termed as
(a) ribonucleotidase (b) ribozymes
(c) nucleotidase (d) nucleases

148. Given below are two statements.
Statement I α-thalassemia is controlled by HBA1 and HBA2 genes.
Statement II Thalassemia is a qualitative problem.
In the light of the above statements, choose the correct answer from the options given below.
(a) Statement I is correct, but statement II is correct
(b) Both statement I and statement II are correct
(c) Both statement I and statement II are incorrect
(d) Statement I is correct, but statement II is incorrect

149. Which of the following antibodies transfers from the mother to her foetus through placenta?
(a) IgG (b) IgA
(c) IgD (d) IgM

150. Which of the following two RNAs initiate the process of RNA interference in eukaryotic organisms?
(a) *t*RNA and *m*RNA
(b) *r*RNA and *t*RNA
(c) *sn*RNA and *hn*RNA
(d) Sense RNA and antisense RNA

151. Raceme, corymb, ebracteate, hermaphrodite and actinomorphic type of inflorescence is found in family
(a) Malvaceae (b) Leguminoceae
(c) Graminae (d) Brassicaceae

152. Read the following statements on gel electrophoresis and choose the correct set of statements.

I. DNA fragments are negatively charged molecules.
II. It is a technique of separation of DNA and RNA only.
III. The most commonly used matrix is agarose which is a monosaccharide extracted from sea weeds.
IV. DNA fragments separate according to size through the pore of agarose gel.
V. The separated DNA fragments can be seen only after staining the DNA with ethidium bromide (EtBr).

Choose the correct answer from the options given below.

(a) I, II and III (b) II and IV
(c) I, IV and V (d) III, IV and V

153. In winter, the cambium is less active and forms fewer xylary elements. This wood is called

(a) early wood (b) autumn wood
(c) heart wood (d) sapwood

154. Match List I with List II.

List I	List II
A. Capacitation	1. Progesterone
B. Colostrum	2. Sperm activation
C. Placenta	3. Mammary gland
D. Corpus luteum	4. hCG

Choose the correct answer from the options given below.

	A	B	C	D		A	B	C	D
(a)	2	3	1	4	(b)	1	2	3	4
(c)	2	3	4	1	(d)	3	4	2	1

155. Select the mismatched pair.

(a) *Bt* cotton - Pest-resistant
(b) Golden rice - Vitamin-A rich
(c) *cry* II Ab-Corn borer
(d) Wheat - High protein content

156. Given below are two statements; one is labelled as Assertion (A) and other is labelled as Reason (R).

Assertion (A) Dehydration and dormancy of mature seeds are crucial for storage of seeds.

Reason (R) Dehydration maintain physiological activity and dormancy helps overcome drought conditions.

In the light of the above statements, choose the correct answer from the options given below.

(a) A is false, but R is true
(b) Both A and R are true and R is the correct explanation of A
(c) Both A and R are true, but R is not the correct explanation of A
(d) A is true, but R is false

157. *Mangifera indica* belongs to the order

(a) Primata
(b) Diptera
(c) Sapindales
(d) Poales

158. Match List I with List II.

List I	List II
A. Mutualism	1. Nematode and fish
B. Predation	2. *Balanus* and *Chathamalus*
C. Parasitism	3. Pitcher Plant and insects
D. Competition	4. Fig and wasp

Choose the correct answer from the options given below.

	A	B	C	D
(a)	4	3	1	2
(b)	3	1	2	4
(c)	4	2	1	3
(d)	2	1	3	4

159. Which of the following is an example of flagellated protozoans?

(a) *Paramecium* (b) *Trypanosoma*
(c) *Plasmodium* (d) *Entamoeba*

160. Read the following statements and choose the incorrect set of statements.

I. Bacteria live in extreme habitats such as hot springs, deserts, snow and deep oceans.
II. Methanogens are present in the gut of several ruminant animals.
III. The colonies of Archaebacteria are surrounded by gelatinous sheath.
IV. The bacteria that live in salty areas are known as thermoacidophils.
V. Bacteria reproduce mainly by fission.

Choose the correct answer from the options given below.

(a) I and V (b) II, IV and V
(c) III and IV (d) I, II and III

161. In which of the following, zygote undergoes dormancy after its formation to tide over adverse condition?

(a) Algae only
(b) Only fungi
(c) Pteridophytes and bryophytes
(d) Both Algae and fungi

162. Identify the correct set of statements.

I. Earth summit at Rio de Janeiro, Brazil promoted Convention on biological diversity which was signed by 152 nations.
II. Tropical rainforests are inhabited by evergreen forest.
III. Amazon rainforest was so large that it used to be called lungs of the planet.
IV. Eastern ghats have a greater amphibian species diversity than the Western ghats.
V. The first national park to be established in India was Kaziranga National Park.

Choose the correct answer from the options given below.

(a) I, III and V only
(b) II, IV and V only
(c) I, II and III only
(d) I and IV only

163. The TCA cycle starts with the condensation of acetyl group with OAA and water to yield

(a) citric acid
(b) pyruvic acid
(c) carbonic acid
(d) acetic acid

164. Match List I with List II.

	List I		List II
A.	Innate immunity	1.	Transferred from mother to child
B.	Natural passive immunity	2.	Antirabies serum
C.	Artificial passive immunity	3.	Develops due to vaccination
D.	Artificial active immunity	4.	PMNL-neutrophils

Choose the correct answer from the options given below

	A	B	C	D		A	B	C	D
(a)	1	4	3	2	(b)	3	1	2	4
(c)	4	1	2	3	(d)	4	2	1	3

165. Given below are two statements; one is labelled as Assertion (A) and the other is labelled as Reason (R).

Assertion (A) The human placenta is called the chorionic placenta.

Reason (R) The chorion takes part in the formation of placenta.

In the light of the above statements, choose the correct answer from the options given below.

(a) A is false, but R is true
(b) Both A and R are true and R is the correct explanation of A
(c) Both A and R are true, but R is not the correct explanation of A
(d) A is true, but R is false

166. A plasmid is considered suitable as cloning vector because it

I. can be easily isolated.
II. has sites for restriction enzymes.
III. is easily reintroduced into bacterial cell.
IV. has selectable marker.
V. has no cloning site.

Choose the correct answer from the options given below.

(a) I, II and V (b) II and III
(c) I, II, III and IV (d) I and III

167. Given below are two statements; one is labelled as Assertion (A) and the other is labelled as Reason (R).

Assertion (A) In some organisms multinucleate condition arises leading to the formation of syncytium.

Reason (R) In these organisms karyokinesis is not followed by cytokinesis.

In the light of the above statements, choose the correct answer from the options given below.

(a) A is false, but R is true
(b) Both A and R are true and R is the correct explanation of A
(c) Both A and R are true, but R is not the correct explanation of A
(d) A is true, but R is false

168. Given below are two statements.

Statement I The LHC are made up of hundreds of pigment molecules bound to proteins.

Statement II Each photosystem has few special pigments forming a light harvesting system, reaction centre.

(a) Statement I is incorrect, but statement II is correct
(b) Both statement I and statement II are correct
(c) Both statement I and statement II are incorrect
(d) Statement I is correct, but statement II is incorrect

169. Bioluminescence is described as
(a) the property of living organism to reflect light
(b) the property of living organism to emit light
(c) the property of living organism to absorb light
(d) None of the above

170. Given below are two statements; one is labelled as Assertion (A) and the other is labelled as Reason (R).

Assertion (A) Genetic drift is a random change in gene frequencies.

Reason (R) Bottle neck event reduce genetic diversity.

In the light of the above statements, choose the correct answer from the options given below.
(a) A is false, but R is true
(b) Both A and R are true and R is the correct explanation of A
(c) Both A and R are true, but R is not the correct explanation of A
(d) A is true, but R is false

171. The epididymis leads to
(a) vas deferens (b) rete testis
(c) ejaculatory duct (d) seminal vesicle

172. Read the following statements and choose the set of correct statements.

I. Louis Pasteur by his experiment demonstrated that life comes from outer space.
II. Oparin and Haldane proposed that the first form of life could have come from pre-existing non-living organic molecules.
III. The universe is almost 100 billion years old.
IV. The first non-cellular forms of life could have originated 3 billion years back.
V. SL Miller observed formation of amino acid during his experiment.

Choose the correct answer from the options given below.
(a) I, II and III (b) II, IV and V
(c) I, III and IV (d) II, III and V

173. Given below are two statements; one is labelled as Assertion (A) and the other is labelled as Reason (R).

Assertion (A) Vital capacity is the maximum volume of air that can be moved in and out of lungs.

Reason (R) It is the sum of RV, ERV, IRV and TV.

In the light of the above statements, choose the correct answer from the options given below.
(a) A is false, but R is true
(b) Both A and R are true and R is the correct explanation of A
(c) Both A and R are true and R is not the correct explanation of A
(d) A is true, but R is false

174. In which kind of inhibition, the V_{max} remains constant and K_m increases?
(a) Allosteric inhibition
(b) Competitive inhibition
(c) Non-competitive inhibition
(d) None of the above

175. Read the following statements and choose the correct set of statements.

I. When more than one pistils are fused together the condition is called apocarpous.
II. The placenta is located inside the ovarian cavity.
III. The gynoecium that consist of a single pistil known as monocarpellary.
IV. Gynoecium consisting of more than one pistil is called multicarpellary.
V. The ovary serves as a landing platform for pollen grains.

Choose the correct answer from the options given below.
(a) I, II and III (b) II, IV and V
(c) II, III and IV (d) I, III and V

176. Given below are two statements.

Statement I In *Obelia* the polyp form produces medusae form asexually.

Statement II In cnidarians like *Pleurobrachia* the skeleton is composed of calcium carbonate.

In the light of the above statements, choose the correct answer from the options given below.
(a) Statement I is incorrect, but statement II is correct
(b) Both statement I and statement II are correct
(c) Both statement I and statement II are incorrect
(d) Statement I is correct, but statement II is incorrect

177. Match List I with List II.

	List I		List II
A.	DNA polymerase	1.	*t*RNA
B.	RNA polymerase-II	2.	DNA
C.	RNA polymerase-I	3.	*r*RNA
D.	RNA polymerase-III	4.	*hn*RNA

Choose the correct answer from the options given below.

	A	B	C	D
(a)	2	4	3	1
(b)	2	3	4	1
(c)	2	1	3	4
(d)	1	2	4	3

178. Given below are two statements.

Statement I Parapodia is present in aquatic annelids.

Statement II *Nereis*, an aquatic form of annelids is monoecious.

In the light of the above statements, choose the correct answer from the options given below.
(a) Statement I is incorrect, but statement II is correct
(b) Both statement I and statement II are correct
(c) Both statement I and statement II are incorrect
(d) Statement I is correct, but statement II is incorrect

179. Analogous structures are anatomically .... and perform .... functions.
(a) different; similar
(b) different; different
(c) similar; similar
(d) similar; different

180. Identify the correct set of statements.

I. Mammary glands begin to develop under the influence of human chorionic gonadotropin.
II. Second polar body and ovum are formed after second mitotic division.
III. Endometrium is maintained by corpus luteum.
IV. LH acts on the Leydig cells and stimulates androgens synthesis.
V. The signals for parturition are originated from the fully developed foetus and the placenta.

Choose the correct answer from the options given below.
(a) I, II, III and V
(b) III, IV and V
(c) I, III, IV and V
(d) I, II, III, IV and V

Explanations

Physics

1. (c) Tension in wire, $T = \text{Stress} \times \text{Area} = 3 \times 10^8 \times A$

Mass per unit length, $m = A \times \rho = A \times 7.5 \times 10^3$

Speed of transverse wave,

$$v = \sqrt{\frac{T}{m}} = \sqrt{\frac{3 \times 10^8 \times A}{A \times 7.5 \times 10^3}} = 200 \text{ ms}^{-1}$$

2. (b) Initial PE of the body,

$$U_i = -\frac{GMm}{R} = \frac{-6.67 \times 10^{-11} \times 100 \times 10^{-2}}{0.1}$$

$$= -6.67 \times 10^{-10} \text{ J}$$

When the particle is far away from the sphere, the PE of the system will be zero, i.e.,

$$U_f = 0$$

$$\therefore \quad W = U_f - U_i = +6.67 \times 10^{-10} \text{ J}$$

3. (d) It is clear from below diagram that given diode will be forward biased.

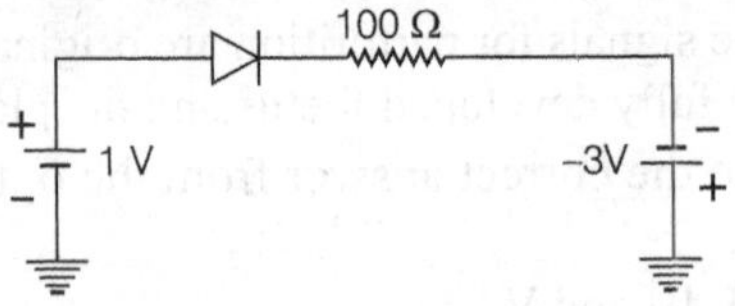

Hence, $I = \frac{1-(-3)}{100} = \frac{4}{100} \text{ A} = 40 \text{ mA}$

4. (d) Potential energy of coil,

$$U = -\mathbf{M} \cdot \mathbf{B} = -NI \cdot [\mathbf{A} \cdot \mathbf{B}]$$

$$= -20 \times 15 \, [-0.05\hat{i} \cdot 0.2\hat{i}] = 3\text{J}$$

5. (c) For monoatomic gas, $\gamma = \frac{5}{3}$

So, $pV^{5/3} = p'\left(\frac{V}{3}\right)^{5/3} \Rightarrow p' = p(3)^{5/3}$

6. (c) In nuclear fission, neutrons are released.

7. (b) We know that, in EM-waves amplitude of electric field vector E_0 and magnetic field vector B_0 are related as

$$E_0 = B_0 c \quad \text{...(i)}$$

where, c is speed of light.

$\because$ the magnetic field at the centre of a coil,

$$c = \nu\lambda$$

$$= \frac{\omega}{2\pi} \cdot \frac{2\pi}{k} \quad \left[\because \nu = \frac{\omega}{2\pi} \text{ and } k = \frac{2\pi}{\lambda}\right]$$

$$\Rightarrow \quad c = \frac{\omega}{k} \quad \text{...(ii)}$$

From Eqs. (i) and (ii), we get

$$E_0 = B_0 \cdot \frac{\omega}{k}$$

$$\Rightarrow \quad E_0 k = B_0 \omega$$

8. (c) As we know, $B = \sqrt{B_1^2 + B_2^2}$ $\quad (\because \cos 90° = 0)$

$\because$ The magnetic field at the centre of a coil,

$$B = \frac{\mu_0 NI}{2r}$$

$$B_1 = \frac{\mu_0 N\sqrt{3I}}{2r}$$

$$B_2 = \frac{\mu_0 N\sqrt{6I}}{2r}$$

$$\therefore \quad B = \frac{\mu_0 NI}{2r}\sqrt{3+6} = \frac{3\mu_0 NI}{2r}$$

9. (a) Cubical expansion,

$$\Delta V = \gamma V \Delta T = 3\alpha V \Delta T \quad [\because \gamma = 3\alpha]$$

$$= 3 \times 23 \times 10^{-6} \times \left(\frac{4}{3}\pi \times 10^3\right) \times 100 = 28.9 \text{ cc}$$

10. (a) When all inputs are high

NOR (1, 1) = 0 = X

and NAND (X = 0, 1) = 1

$\therefore$ $Y = 1$

When all inputs are low

NOR (0, 0) = 1 = X

and NAND (X = 1, 0) = 1

$\therefore$ $Y = 1$

11. (d)

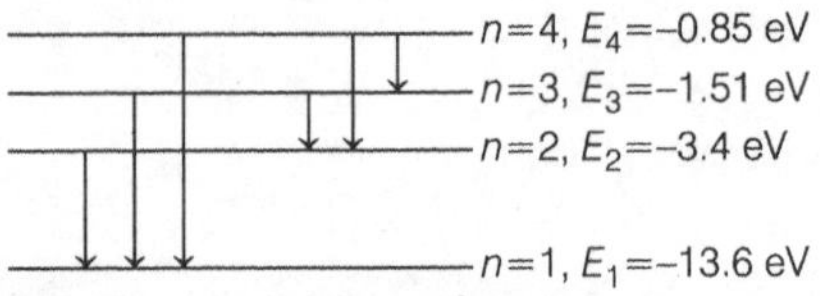

Energy used for excitation is 12.75 eV,

i.e. $(-13.6 + 12.75)\text{eV} = -0.85\text{eV}$

The photons of energy 12.75 eV can excite the fourth level of H-atom.

where, $n = 4$

So, number of spectral lines $= \frac{n(n-1)}{2} = \frac{4\,(4-1)}{2}$

$$= \frac{4(3)}{2} = 6$$

Therefore, six lines will be emitted.

12. (d) As we know, density, $\rho = \dfrac{m}{\pi r^2 L}$

$$\therefore \quad \frac{\Delta\rho}{\rho} \times 100 = \left[\frac{\Delta m}{m} + \frac{2\Delta r}{r} + \frac{\Delta L}{L}\right] \times 100$$

$$= \left[\frac{0.003}{0.3} + \frac{2 \times 0.005}{0.5} + \frac{0.06}{6}\right] \times 100 = 4\%$$

13. (a) According to the question, $p \propto T^3$

Since, $pV = nRT$

$\therefore \quad p \propto (pV)^3$

$\Rightarrow \quad p^2V^3 = \text{constant}$

$\Rightarrow \quad pV^{3/2} = \text{constant} \qquad (\because pV^{\gamma} = \text{constant})$

$\therefore \quad \gamma = \dfrac{3}{2} \Rightarrow \gamma = \dfrac{C_p}{C_V} = \dfrac{3}{2}$

14. (c) We know that, capacitive reactance of AC circuit having capacitor only,

$$X_C = \frac{1}{\omega C} \Rightarrow X_C \propto \frac{1}{\omega}$$

Hence, graph shown in option (c) is correct.

15. (c) The coordinates of centre of mass are

$$X_{CM} = \frac{2\times0 + 2\times10 + 2\times10 + 2\times0}{2+2+2+2} = \frac{40}{8} = 5\text{ cm}$$

$$Y_{CM} = \frac{2\times0 + 2\times0 + 2\times10 + 2\times10}{2+2+2+2} = \frac{40}{8} = 5\text{ cm}$$

$\therefore \quad \vec{\mathbf{r}}_{CM_1} = 5\hat{\mathbf{i}} + 5\hat{\mathbf{j}}$

When m_3 is removed, then the new coordinates of centre of mass are

$$X'_{CM} = \frac{2\times0 + 2\times10 + 2\times0}{2+2+2} = \frac{20}{6} = \frac{10}{3}\text{ cm}$$

$$Y'_{CM} = \frac{2\times0 + 2\times0 + 2\times10}{2+2+2} = \frac{10}{3}\text{ cm}$$

$\therefore \quad \mathbf{r}_{CM_2} = \dfrac{10}{3}\hat{\mathbf{i}} + \dfrac{10}{3}\hat{\mathbf{j}}$

$\therefore$ Shift, $\Delta\mathbf{r}_{CM} = \mathbf{r}_{CM_2} - \mathbf{r}_{CM_1}$

$$= \left(\frac{10}{3}\hat{\mathbf{i}} + \frac{10}{3}\hat{\mathbf{j}}\right) - (5\hat{\mathbf{i}} + 5\hat{\mathbf{j}}) = -\left(\frac{5}{3}\hat{\mathbf{i}} + \frac{5}{3}\hat{\mathbf{j}}\right).$$

16. (b) Total energy of the electron, $E = -3.4$ eV

Kinetic energy of the electron is equal to the negative of the total energy

$$K = -E = -(-3.4) = +3.4\text{ eV}$$

Hence, the kinetic energy of the electron in the given state is +3.4 eV.

17. (a) Since, electrostatic force is conservative in nature, hence work done by electrostatic force in a moving charge between two points in an electric field is independent of the path followed between these two points.

We know that amount of charge on electron and proton is equal, thus they gain equal amount of kinetic energy when they accelerated through same potential difference.

18. (a) Focal length of a lens in a liquid f_l can be determined by

$$\frac{f_l}{f_a} = \frac{{}_a\mu_g - 1}{{}_l\mu_g - 1} = \frac{\dfrac{\mu_g}{\mu_a} - 1}{\dfrac{\mu_g}{\mu_l} - 1}$$

Here, f_a = focal length of lens in air

= 18 cm

$\mu_g = 1.5, \ \mu_l = \dfrac{4}{3}$

$$\text{So,} \quad f_l = \frac{f_a\left(\dfrac{\mu_g}{\mu_a} - 1\right)}{\left(\dfrac{\mu_g}{\mu_l} - 1\right)} = \frac{18 \times \left(\dfrac{3}{2} - 1\right)}{\left(\dfrac{3/2}{4/3} - 1\right)} = 72\text{ cm}$$

$\therefore$ Change in focal length

= 72 − 18 = 54 cm

19. (b) $U_{\text{initial}} = 2\text{ J}, U_{\text{final}} = 8\text{ J}, U_{\text{final}} = 4 \times U_{\text{initial}}$

The potential energy stored in capacitor in terms of potential difference V and charge Q is

$$U = \frac{1}{2}QV \Rightarrow U \propto QV$$

Hence, to increase U by four times, both Q and V are increased by two times.

20. (b) Angle of incidence (i) for both surfaces AB and BC will be 45°. For total internal reflection to take place,

$i \geq \theta_c$ or $\sin i \geq \sin\theta_c$

$$\therefore \quad \frac{1}{\sqrt{2}} \geq \frac{1}{\mu} \text{ or } \mu \geq \sqrt{2}$$

So, $\mu_{\min} = \sqrt{2}$

21. (b) When a wave is reflected from denser medium, then the type of wave doesn't change but only its phase changes by 180° or π radian.

Thus, for the reflected wave $\hat{\mathbf{z}} = -\hat{\mathbf{z}}, \hat{\mathbf{i}} = -\hat{\mathbf{i}}$ and additional phase of π in the incident wave.

Given, here the incident electromagnetic wave,

$$\mathbf{E} = E_0\hat{\mathbf{i}}\cos(kz - \omega t)$$

The reflected electromagnetic wave is given by

$$\mathbf{E}_r = E_0(-\hat{\mathbf{i}})\cos[k(-z) - \omega t + \pi]$$

$$= -E_0\hat{\mathbf{i}}\cos[-(kz + \omega t) + \pi]$$

$$= E_0\hat{\mathbf{i}}\cos(kz + \omega t)]$$

$\cos(\pi - \theta) = -\cos\theta$

22. (c) In series combination, electric current is same through both wires.

Hence, currect density $J \propto \frac{I}{A}$

$$\frac{J_{\text{copper}}}{J_{\text{iron}}} = \frac{r_{\text{iron}}^2}{r_{\text{copper}}^2} = \frac{(0.4)^2}{(0.1)^2} = 16$$

$$\therefore \quad \frac{J_{\text{iron}}}{J_{\text{copper}}} = \frac{1}{16}$$

23. (a) Resistance of the given wire,

$$x = \frac{(100-l)}{l} \times R = \frac{100-60}{60} \times 6\,\Omega = 4\,\Omega$$

Specific resistance for the material of given wire,

$$\rho = \frac{x \cdot \pi D^2}{4L} = \frac{4 \times 3.14 \times (10^{-3})^2}{4 \times 0.1} = 3.14 \times 10^{-5}\ \Omega\text{-m}$$

24. (b) Velocity of body at time t is given by

$$v = \frac{dx}{dt} = \frac{d}{dt}(t^2) = 2t$$

Now, at $t = 0$ s, initial velocity $v_i = 0$

at $t = 4$ s, final velocity $v_f = 8$ m/s

Work done = Increase in KE

$$= \frac{1}{2}mv_f^2 - \frac{1}{2}mv_i^2 = \frac{1}{2}m(v_f^2 - v_i^2)$$

$$= \frac{1}{2} \times 4 \times (8^2 - 0^2) = 128\,\text{J}$$

25. (a) For given volume of wire, $R = \rho\frac{l^2}{V} \Rightarrow R \propto l^2$

Resistance of a wire increases with increase in length.

$$\frac{\Delta R}{R} = 2\frac{\Delta l}{l} = 2 \times 0.2\% = 0.4\%$$

26. (b) Pressure difference between lungs and atmosphere = 760 − 750 = 10 mm of Hg or 1 cm of Hg

$$\rho_w g h_w = \rho_m g h_m$$
$$\rho_w h_w = \rho_m h_m$$
$$1 \times h_w = 13.6 \times 1$$
$$h_w = 13.6\,\text{cm}$$

27. (c) In a non-uniform electric field, an electric dipole experiences net force as well as torque.

28. (b) The magnetic flux linked with the primary coil is given by $\phi = \phi_0 + 4t$

So, voltage across primary,

$$V_p = \frac{d\phi}{dt} = \frac{d}{dt}(\phi_0 + 4t) = 4\,\text{V} \text{ (as } \phi_0 = \text{constant)}$$

Also, we have $N_P = 50$ and $N_S = 1500$

From relation, $\frac{V_S}{V_P} = \frac{N_S}{N_P}$

or $V_S = V_P \cdot \frac{N_S}{N_P} = 4\left(\frac{1500}{50}\right) = 120\,\text{V}$

29. (a) Given, $m_1 = 2$ kg, $m_2 = 4$ kg

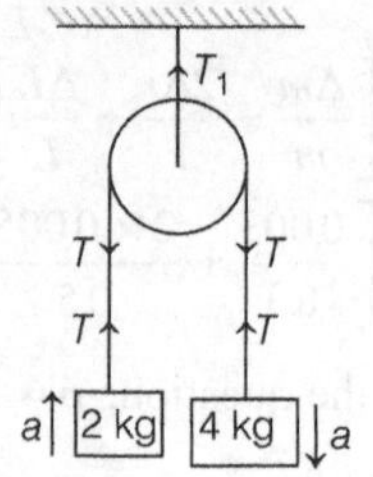

∴ Tension in the string,

$$T = \frac{2m_1 m_2}{m_1 + m_2} g = 2 \times \frac{2 \times 4}{2+4} \times 10 = 26.67\,\text{N}$$

∴ Total downward thrust on the pulley

$$T_1 = 2T = 2 \times 26.67 = 53.34\,\text{N} \approx 53.3\,\text{N}$$

30. (c) By Einstein's photoelectric equation,

$$hc\left(\frac{1}{\lambda} - \frac{1}{\lambda_0}\right) = eV_0$$

$$h\left(\frac{c}{\lambda} - \nu_0\right) = eV_0$$

$$\Rightarrow \quad \nu_0 = \frac{1}{h}\left(\frac{hc}{\lambda} - eV_0\right)$$

$$= \frac{1}{6.6 \times 10^{-34}}\left(\frac{6.6 \times 10^{-34} \times 3 \times 10^8}{2 \times 10^{-7}} - 1.6 \times 10^{-19} \times 2.5\right)$$

$$= 8.94 \times 10^{14}\ \text{Hz} \simeq 9 \times 10^{14}\ \text{Hz}$$

31. (b)

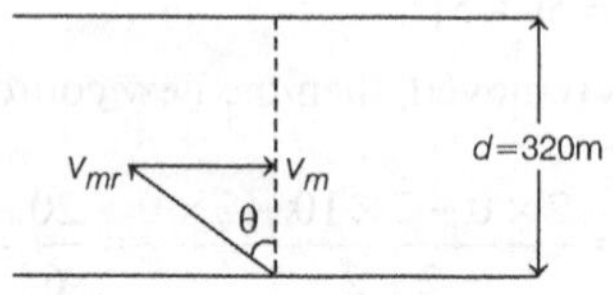

Given, $v_{mr} = \frac{5}{3}v_r$ ...(i)

Time to cross the river, $t = 4$ min

$$\therefore \quad v_m = \frac{d}{t} = \frac{320}{4} = 80\,\text{m/min}$$

Now, $\sin\theta = \frac{v_r}{v_{mr}} = \frac{3}{5}$

$$\therefore \quad \cos\theta = \frac{4}{5}$$

Also, $v_m = v_{mr}\cos\theta$

$$\Rightarrow \quad 80 = \frac{5}{3}v_r \times \frac{4}{5}$$ [from Eq. (i)]

$\therefore v_r$ = Speed of river current $= \frac{80 \times 3}{4} = 60$ m/min

32. (d) Let, n cells are connected with wrong polarity.

∴ Effective emf of the battery

$$= (20-n)E - nE = (20-2n)E$$

Current in the above two cases must be proportional to the emf in the two cases, i.e.,

$$\frac{(20-2n)E+3E}{(20-2n)E-3E}=\frac{5}{3}$$

$$\Rightarrow \quad \frac{20-2n+3}{20-2n-3}=\frac{5}{3}$$

$$\Rightarrow \quad n=4$$

33. (d) Applying conservation of energy,

$$\frac{1}{2}mv^2-\frac{GMm}{R}=-\frac{GMm}{R+h}$$

$$\frac{1}{2}m\cdot gR=GMm\left(\frac{1}{R}-\frac{1}{R+h}\right) \quad (\because v=\sqrt{gr})$$

$$\Rightarrow \quad \frac{1}{2}mgR=mgR^2\left(\frac{h}{R(R+h)}\right) \quad (\because GM=gR^2)$$

$$\frac{1}{2}=\frac{h}{R+h}\Rightarrow h=R$$

34. (d) Let, velocity of each marble = v
Change in momentum per second

$$=20[mv-(-mv)]=40mv$$

$\therefore$ Force exerted by marble on the disc = 40 mv
To keep the disc, floating the force must balances the weight of disc, i.e.,

$$40\,mv=Mg$$

$$\Rightarrow \quad 40\times 4.9\times 10^{-3}\times v=40\times 10^{-3}\times 9.8$$

$$\Rightarrow \quad v=\frac{9.8}{4.9}=2\text{ ms}^{-1}$$

35. (b) Maximum height of first object,

$$h_0=\frac{u^2\sin^2\theta}{2g}=\frac{(12)^2\sin^2 45^\circ}{2\times 10}=3.6\text{ m}$$

Time of attaining maximum height,

$$t=\frac{u\sin\theta}{g}=\frac{12\times\sin 45^\circ}{10}=\frac{3\sqrt{2}}{5}\text{ s}$$

Distance of vertical fall by second object in $\frac{3\sqrt{2}}{5}$ s,

$$s=\frac{1}{2}gt^2=\frac{1}{2}\times 10\times\left(\frac{3\sqrt{2}}{5}\right)^2=3.6\text{ m}$$

$\therefore$ Initial height of second object

$$=3.6+3.6=7.2\text{ m}$$

36. (c) Rotational kinetic energy,

$$(\text{KE})_R=\frac{1}{2}I\omega^2=\frac{1}{2}\times\frac{1}{2}(mR^2)\omega^2$$

$$=\frac{1}{4}mR^2\omega^2$$

Translational kinetic energy, (In pure rolling, $v=R\omega$)

$$(\text{KE})_T=\frac{1}{2}mv^2=\frac{1}{2}m(R\omega)^2=\frac{1}{2}mR^2\omega^2$$

Total energy,

$$\text{KE}=(\text{KE})_R+(\text{KE})_T=\frac{3}{4}mR^2\omega^2$$

$$\therefore \quad \frac{(\text{KE})_T}{\text{KE}}=\frac{(1/2)mR^2\omega^2}{(3/4)mR^2\omega^2}=\frac{2}{3}$$

37. (c) As, $\frac{1}{f}=\frac{1}{u}+\frac{1}{v}$ or $f=\frac{uv}{u+v}$

$$\Rightarrow \quad f=\frac{(50.1)(20.1)}{50.1+20.1}=14.3\text{ cm}$$

$$\frac{\Delta f}{f}=\pm\left[\frac{\Delta u}{u}+\frac{\Delta v}{v}+\frac{\Delta u+\Delta v}{u+v}\right]$$

$$=\pm\left[\frac{0.5}{50.1}+\frac{0.2}{20.1}+\frac{0.5+0.2}{50.1+20.1}\right]=\pm 0.0299$$

$$\Rightarrow \quad \Delta f=\pm 0.0299\times 14.3=\pm 0.4\text{ cm}$$

$$\therefore \quad f=(14.3\pm 0.4)\text{ cm}$$

38. (c) Since, $X_L=X_C=25\,\Omega$, so, V_L and V_C are equal and opposite in phase, i.e. volmeter reading = 0 V.
$\therefore$ Ammeter reading,

$$I=\frac{V}{\sqrt{R^2+(X_L-X_C)^2}}=\frac{240}{30}=8\text{A}$$

39. (c) At the breakdown situation, voltage across zener diode remains constant for any current flowing through it, hence it is used to protect meters from burning due to overloading.

40. (d) At closest distance r, its whole KE is converted into PE.

$$\therefore \quad \frac{1}{2}mv^2=\frac{1}{4\pi\varepsilon_0}\frac{Q\cdot q}{r}$$

$$\Rightarrow \quad r=\frac{1}{4\pi\varepsilon_0}\frac{Q\cdot q\cdot 2}{mv^2}$$

In next case, $$r'=\frac{1}{4\pi\varepsilon_0}\frac{Qq\cdot 2}{m(2v)^2}$$

$$\Rightarrow \quad r'=\frac{1}{4}\left(\frac{1}{4\pi\varepsilon_0}\cdot\frac{Qq\cdot 2}{mv^2}\right)$$

$$\Rightarrow \quad r'=r/4$$

41. (c) Given that, lengths of copper and aluminum are L_1 and L_2.
The length change with temperature,

$$L_1'+L_2'=L_1(1+\alpha_1\Delta\theta)+L_2(1+\alpha_2\Delta\theta)$$

$$\because \quad \text{Given, } L_1+L_2=L_1'+L_2'$$

$$\Rightarrow \quad L_1\alpha_1\Delta\theta+L_2\alpha_2\Delta\theta=0$$

So, $$L_1\alpha_1\Delta\theta=-L_2\alpha_2\Delta\theta$$

$$\Rightarrow \quad -L_1\alpha_1=L_2\alpha_2$$

42. (a) This problem is based on the oscillations of a charged mass and spring system in an external electric field.

In an electric field E, the block of charge q experience an electric force qE. Due to this force, if the spring stretches by a distance x, work done by the electric force is qEx. This is stored in the spring as potential energy, given by $\frac{1}{2}kx^2$.

$$\therefore \quad \frac{1}{2}kx^2 = qEx \Rightarrow x = \frac{2qE}{k}$$

Thus, the amplitude of oscillation, $A = \frac{x}{2} = \frac{qE}{k}$

43. (d) Here, $I_g = 0.4\%$ of $I = 0.004\,I$

Shunt current, $I_S = I - I_g = 0.996\,I$

$\therefore$ Shunt resistance, $R_s = \frac{I_g \cdot R_g}{I_s} = \frac{0.004IR_g}{0.996I} = \frac{R_g}{249}$

44. (c) Position of n th bright fringe from central, $x_n = \frac{nD\lambda}{d}$

i.e., $x_{n_1} = x_{n_2}$

$$\frac{n_1 D\lambda_1}{d} = \frac{n_2 D\lambda_2}{d} = \frac{\lambda_1}{\lambda_2} = \frac{n_2}{n_1} = \frac{8}{5} = \frac{640\,\text{nm}}{400\,\text{nm}}$$

Hence, only option (c) satisfies.

45. (c) We know that, $\frac{1}{\lambda} = R\left(\frac{1}{n_1^2} - \frac{1}{n_2^2}\right)$

For first case, $\frac{1}{\lambda_1} = R\left(\frac{1}{3^2} - \frac{1}{4^2}\right)$

$$\frac{1}{\lambda_1} = \frac{7R}{144} \quad \ldots\text{(i)}$$

For second case, $\frac{1}{\lambda_2} = R\left(\frac{1}{2^2} - \frac{1}{3^2}\right) = \frac{5}{36}R$

$$\frac{1}{\lambda_2} = \frac{5R}{36} \quad \ldots\text{(ii)}$$

From Eqs. (i) and (ii), we get

$$\therefore \quad \frac{\frac{1}{\lambda_1}}{\frac{1}{\lambda_2}} = \frac{\frac{7R}{144}}{\frac{5R}{36}} = \frac{7}{20} \Rightarrow \frac{\lambda_1}{\lambda_2} = \frac{20}{7}$$

Chemistry

46. (c) As $k_A = k_B$,

$$\therefore \quad 10^{18} e^{-8000/T} = 10^{17} e^{-4000/T}$$

$$10 = e^{4000/T}$$

$$\ln 10 = \frac{4000}{T}$$

$$\therefore \quad T = \frac{4000}{\ln 10} = \frac{4000}{2.303}\,\text{K}$$

47. (d) $\Delta S^\circ = 2S^\circ_{HCl} - (S^\circ_{H_2} + S^\circ_{Cl_2})$

$= 2 \times 186.7 - (130.6 + 223.0) = 19.8\,\text{JK}^{-1}\,\text{mol}^{-1}$

48. (c)

	X	+ Y ⇌	P	+ Q
No. of moles initially	4	4	0	0
No. of moles at equilibrium	(4 − 2)	(4 − 2)	2	2

Equilibrium constant is,

$$K_C = \frac{[P][Q]}{[X][Y]} = 1$$

49. (d) Since, H_3PO_3 is a diprotic acid.

$\therefore N = M \times n \Rightarrow N = M \times 2 \qquad (\because n = 2)$

$N = 2 \times 0.3 = 0.6\,\text{N}$

50. (c) The complete reaction sequence is as follows

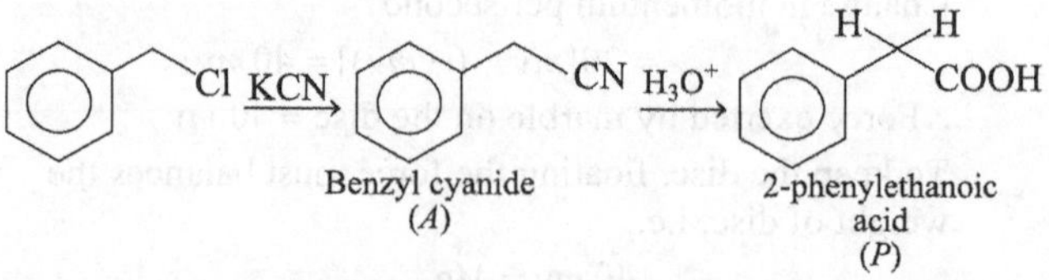

51. (b) The completed reaction is as follows

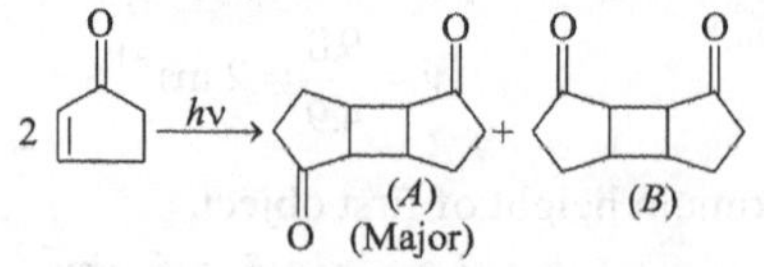

52. (a) The complete reaction can be written as

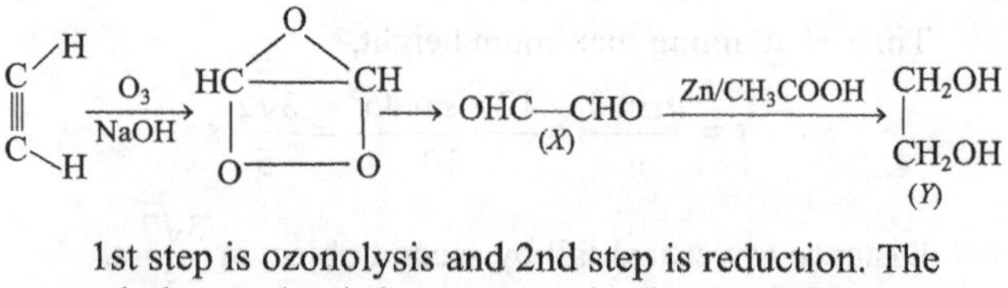

1st step is ozonolysis and 2nd step is reduction. The whole reaction is known as reductive ozonolysis. The final product (Y) formed is $(CH_2OH)_2$.

53. (a) Ce shows (+4) oxidation state because it attains noble gas configuration and moreover, it has tendency to attain f^0 configuration.

54. (b) C—C, C$=$C and C$\equiv$C bond lengths are 1.54 Å, 1.34 Å and 1.20 Å respectively. In benzene, C$=$C is 1.40 Å. So, the correct order of their C—C bond length is $C_2H_2 < C_2H_4 < C_6H_6 < C_2H_6$.

Hence, correct option is (b).

55. (c) Let atomic weight of P is P_x and Q is Q_y.

$$n_{PQ} = 0.05 = \frac{5}{P_x + Q_y}$$

$$P_x + Q_y = 100 \quad ...(i)$$

$$n_{PQ_2} = 0.03 = \frac{4.5}{P_x + 2Q_y}$$

$$P_x + 2Q_y = 150 \quad ...(ii)$$

On solving Eqs. (i) and (ii)

$$P_x = 50, Q_y = 50$$

56. (d) Both Statement I and Statement II are true.

57. (c) The acidic character of conjugate acids is $H_2O > ROH > NH_3$. A stronger acid has weak conjugate base and *vice-versa*. Hence, the correct order of basic strength is : $\bar{O}H < R\bar{O} < \bar{N}H_2$.

58. (c) Statement (c) is correct for resonance because resonance affects bond lengths but not bond angles while (a), (b) and (d) are false statements.

Due to resonance, delocalisation of electrons in every bond which is participating in resonance attains partial double character. Thus, their bond length decreases but causes no effect on bond angle.

59. (c) Radial node $= n - l - 1$

For $4d$-orbital, $n = 4$, $l = 2$,

i.e. $4 - 2 - 1 = 1$.

60. (c) Within a series of isoelectronic ions, as the nuclear charge increases, the force of attraction by the nucleus on the electrons also increases. As a result, ionic radii decreases. Thus, their ionic radii increases in the order

$$Al^{3+} < Mg^{2+} < Na^+ < F^- < O^{2-}$$

61. (b) The correct match is A-II, B-I, C-IV, D-III.

62. (c) Aniline undergoes diazotisation reaction in presence of $NaNO_2$ / HCl to give benzene diazonium chloride which further on heating with HBF_4 to give fluorobenzene as product.

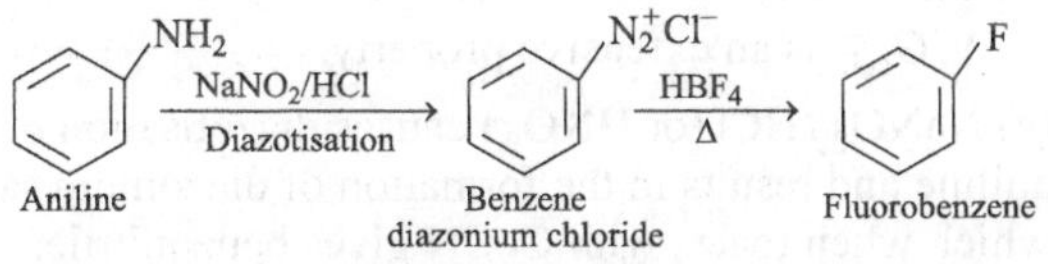

63. (d) *cis*-platin is used to treat testicular, bladder, and ovarian cancers that have spread. It can also be used to treat several other cancers, such as lung cancer. Possible side effects are kidney damage, decreased blood levels of magnesium, potassium, and calcium, nausea etc. Hence, statement I is true.

In octahedral complexes, the three d -orbitals (d_{xy}, d_{yz} and d_{xz}) experience less repulsion from the ligands and lie between the axes and collectively called t_{2g} orbitals. Hence, Statement II is also true.

64. (c) X-(halogen group) has two effects, i.e. $-I$ and $+M$. Due to $-I$ effect of X-group, it reduces electron density of benzene, so halobenzene is less reactive than benzene for electrophilic substitution reaction.

But due to $+M$ effect, it is *ortho*, *para*-directing and in halobenzene, further substitution takes place at *ortho* and *para*-positions.

Hence, (A) is false but (R) is true.

65. (b) Here, $X = p_T = p_1 + p_2 =$ Total pressure of the solution.

where, p_1 and p_2 is the partial pressure of component 1 and 2 respectively.

$Y = x_2 =$ mole fraction of component 2 in the liquid phase.

$Z = y_2 =$ mole fraction of component 2 in the vapour phase.

When mole fraction of component 2 in the liquid phase is 0 then mole fraction of component 2 in the vapour phase is also 0 which means the liquid is pure of component 1 only. Hence, $Y = 0$, $Z = 0$.

66. (d) Statement I is true as more number of carbonyl group, more will be the acidic strength. This is because the carbonyl carbon is electron withdrawing group.

In both aldehydes and ketones, C-atom is double bonded with oxygen atom.

Since, electronegativity of O-atom is more than that of the C-atom, it pulls the shared pair of electron towards itself. Due to which C-atom acquires partial positive charge and O-atom acquires partial negative charge.

Hence, nucleophile can easily attack on the C-atom to neutralize the positive charge and makes it stable. In case of acyl group, nucleophilic addition does not occur as it occur in electron deficient, double or triple bond but acyl group is electron rich in nature. So, statement II is true.

67. (a) The dry cell consists of a paste of manganese dioxide, ammonium chloride and carbon.

The lead storage battery is formed by dipping lead peroxide plate in dilute sulphuric acid.

Zinc chloride is a strong electrolyte.

The secondary battery is a rechargeable battery which can be charged and recharged many times.

68. (a) Solution exhibiting positive deviation, does not obey Raoult's law.

$$\Delta H_{mix} > 0$$

$$\Delta V_{mix} > 0$$

A—A and B—B interaction > A—B interaction

Problem Solving Tactics Positive deviation occurs when the solution is said to have strong interactions between solute-solute and solvent-solvent molecule than solution.

69. (b) HCl is a strong acid and protonates the oxygen atom of alcohol.

$$R\text{—OH} + HCl \rightleftharpoons R\text{—}\overset{+}{O}H_2 + Cl^-$$

Water is a better leaving group than chloride ion. Hence alkyl chloride is formed along with a molecule of water.

$$R—\overset{+}{O}H_2 + Cl^- \longrightarrow R—Cl + H_2O$$

70. (c) The reaction for the hydrolysis of 1 mol of peroxydisulphuric acid is

$$\underset{\text{Peroxydi-sulphuric acid}}{H_2S_2O_8} + H_2O \longrightarrow \underset{\text{Peroxymono sulphuric acid}}{H_2SO_5} + \underset{\text{Sulphuric acid}}{H_2SO_4}$$

71. (a) The entropy change in isothermal process will be greater than in an adiabatic process. Hence, option (a) is correct.

72. (a) $AlCl_3 \rightleftharpoons \underset{S}{Al^{3+}} + \underset{3S}{3Cl^-}$

$$K_{sp} = [S][3S]^3 = 27S^4 = 27 \times (10^{-5})^4 = 27 \times 10^{-20}$$

In presence of 0.1 M NaCl

$$AlCl_3 \rightleftharpoons \underset{S'}{Al^{3+}} + \underset{3S'+0.1}{3Cl^-}$$

$$K_{sp} = [S'][3S' + 0.1]^3$$

(3S′ is negligible as compare to 0.1)

$$27 \times 10^{-20} = [S'][10^{-3}]$$

$$[S'] = \frac{27 \times 10^{-20}}{10^{-3}} = 27 \times 10^{-17} \text{ M}$$

$$= 2.7 \times 10^{-16} \text{ M}$$

73. (b) Compound containing aldehyde, alpha hydroxy ketones or formic acid gives silver mirror with ammonical silver nitrate.

74. (b) A : $15 \times 40 \text{ gL}^{-1} \Rightarrow 15 \times 40 \text{ g in } 1000 \text{ g}$

$(d = 1 \text{ g mL}^{-1})$

$$= \frac{15 \times 40}{1000} \times 5g \text{ solution}$$

$$= 3 \text{ g NaOH}$$

B : Mass of 5 mL NaOH solution $= \frac{50}{100} \times 5 = 2.5$ g

C : 5 g of NaOH $= \frac{5}{1.25}$ mL = 4 mL

Thus, 5g of 40% NaOH is 4 mL = 1.6 g

Hence, C < B < A.

75. (c) According to the spectrochemical series

$$NH_3 > H_2O > C_2O_4^{2-} > F^-$$

NH_3 is stronger ligand in comparison to other. So, there will be large splitting. Therefore, it will absorb high energy or shorter wavelength.

76. (d) BF_3 has a trigonal planar structure, all three B—F bonds lie in the same plane. Thus, the *p*-orbitals of boron and fluorine become parallel.

p-orbital of boron is empty while fluorine has a lone pair. Fluorine donates its lone pair and this is called back bonding, or $p\pi$ - $p\pi$ bond. Resonating structures can be obtained.

Since, BF_3 molecule is highly symmetrical, it has no dipole moment. All bonds are of equal length.

In Boron trihalides, the length of B—F bond would be shorter than expected for a single bond, due to $p\pi$ - $p\pi$ bonding.

BCl_3 is also a trigonal planar molecule.

Back bonding does not change the structure of the molecule.

It simply decreases bond length B—*X* and decreases Lewis acidity of BX_3.

77. (b) For the reaction $A \rightarrow B$, on increasing the concentration of reactant by 8, rate becomes 4 times.

$$\text{rate } (r) = k[A]^x \quad \ldots \text{(i)}$$

$$4r = k[8A]^x \quad \ldots \text{(ii)}$$

Divide Eq. (ii) by Eq. (i)

$$\frac{4r}{r} = \frac{k[8A]^x}{k[A]^x} \Rightarrow 4 = \frac{[8A]^x}{[A]^x}$$

$$(2)^{3x} = (2)^2$$

$$3x = 2$$

$$x = \frac{2}{3}$$

78. (c) The correct match is A-IV, B-I, C-II, D-III.

- λ_m increases with dilution due to increase in number of ions and volume of the solution.
- E°_{cell} is an intensive property.
- Specific conductivity depends on number of ions per unit volume.
- $\Delta_r G_{cell}$ is an extensive property.

79. (c) $NaNO_2/HCl$ (or HNO_2) causes diazotisation of aniline and results in the formation of diazonium salt which when reacts with CuCN gives benzonitrile.

The reaction is as follow

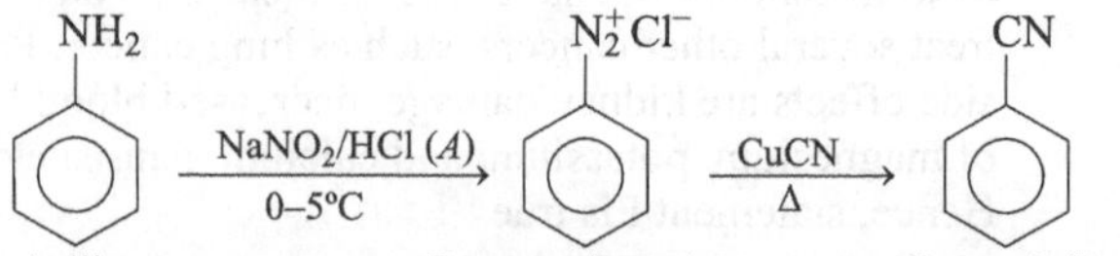

Aniline Benzene diazonium chloride Benzonitrile (*B*)

80. (d) The electronic configuration of the given ion are as follows

$Sm^{3+} = [Xe]\, 4f^5$; | 1 | 1 | 1 | 1 | 1 | | | = 5 unpaired electron

$Eu^{3+} = [Xe]\, 4f^6$; | 1 | 1 | 1 | 1 | 1 | 1 | | = 6 unpaired electron

$Ho^{3+} = [Xe]4f^{10}$; | ⥮ | ⥮ | ⥮ | 1 | 1 | 1 | 1 | = 4 unpaired electron

$Gd^{3+} = [Xe]4f^{7}$; | 1 | 1 | 1 | 1 | 1 | 1 | 1 | = 7 unpaired electron

So, Gd^{3+} has maximum number of unpaired electrons, i.e. 7.

81. (c) A ring expansion creates the six membered carbocation intermediate which is more stable than cyclopentyl methyl membered carbocation.

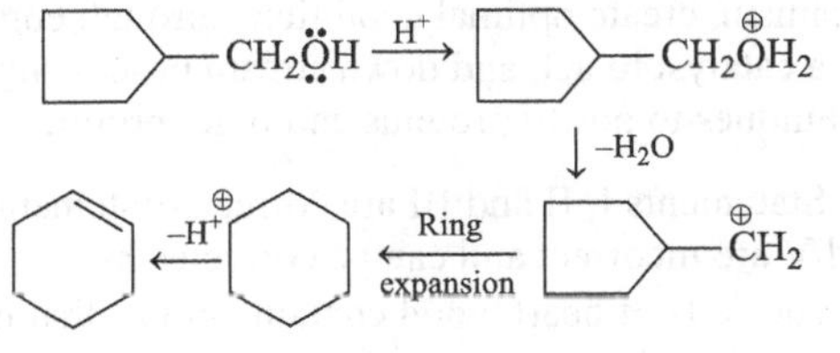

82. (d) If Na_2CO_3 is used in place of $(NH_4)_2CO_3$. It will precipitate group V radicals as well as magnesium radical. The reason for this is the high ionisation of Na_2CO_3 in water into Na^+ and CO_3^{2-}. So, the higher concentration of CO_3^{2-} is available which exceeds the solubility product of group V radicals as well as that of magnesium radical.

83. (b) CH_3CN and H_2CO act as both nucleophile and electrophile because C atom in each of these species in pi-bonded to a highly electronegative atom N and O respectively.

- Water can act as both an electrophile and a nucleophile because it has a partial negative charge on oxygen, indicating its function as a nucleophile and a partially positive charge on hydrogen which indicates its function as an electrophile
- .H_2 and BF_3 can only act as electrophile.

84. (d) Ion is paramagnetic, if it has unpaired electron. It is also coloured ion if it has unpaired electrons in *d*-orbitals.

		Magnetic behaviour	Coloured
I.	$Fe^{2+}[Ar]3d^6$	unpaired $e^- = 4$ (paramagnetic)	Yes
II.	$Cu^+ [Ar]3d^{10}$	unpaired $e^- = 0$ (diamagnetic)	No
III.	$Ni^{2+} [Ar] 3d^8$	unpaired $e^- = 2$ (paramagnetic)	Yes
IV.	$Mn^{2+} [Ar]3d^5$	unpaired $e^- = 5$ (paramagnetic)	Yes
V.	$Zn^{2+}[Ar]3d^{10}$	unpaired $e^- = 0$ (diamagnetic)	No

85. (a) The reactions involved are

$$MnO_4^- + 8H^+ + 5e^- \longrightarrow Mn^{2+} + 4H_2O \quad \ldots(i)$$

$$MnO_2 + 4H^+ + 2e^- \longrightarrow Mn^{2+} + 2H_2O \quad \ldots(ii)$$

On subtracting equation (ii) from (i), we get

$$MnO_4^- + 4H^+ + 3e^- \longrightarrow MnO_2 + 2H_2O$$

The relationship between standard Gibbs energy change for a reaction and its cell potential is

$$\Delta G^\circ = -nFE^\circ_{cell}$$

For manganese electrodes,

$$\Delta G^\circ_{MnO_4^-|Mn^{2+}} = \Delta G^\circ_{MnO_4^-|MnO_2} + \Delta G^\circ_{MnO_2|Mn^{2+}}$$

$$-nFE^\circ_{MnO_4^-|Mn^{2+}} = -nFE^\circ_{MnO_4^-|MnO_2} - nFE^\circ_{MnO_2|Mn^{2+}}$$

$$5E^\circ_{MnO_4^-|Mn^{2+}} = 3\times E^\circ_{MnO_4^-|MnO_2} + 2\times E^\circ_{MnO_2|Mn^{2+}}$$

Substitute values in the above equation,

$$5\times 1.51\text{ V} = 3\times E^\circ_{MnO_4^-|MnO_2} + 2\times 1.23\text{ V}$$

$$E^\circ_{MnO_4^-|MnO_2} \simeq 1.70\text{ V}$$

86. (c) NH_2OH and NH_2 — NH_2 may be considered as NH_3 derivatives in which H is replaced by—OH and — NH_2 respectively. Due to their electron withdrawing nature, these groups decreases electron density over nitrogen making them less basic. The effect of —OH group is stronger than —NH_2.

Problem Solving Tactics When comparing basicity of species central atom is important. More electronegative elements are always less basic. Electron donating groups increases basicity, while electron-withdrawing groups decreases · basicity.

87. (b) Mixture of aniline and water can be separated by simple distillation as they have sufficiently high difference in their boiling point.

Boiling point of chloroform = 334 K

Boiling point of aniline = 457 K

89. (a) The correct match is as:

A-IV, B-III, C-II, D-I

99. (c) Observed dipole moment = 1.03 D.

$$\mu_{theoritical} = q\times d = 1.6\times 10^{-19}\text{ C}\times 1.27\times 10^{-10}\text{ m}$$

$$= 2.032\times 10^{-29}\text{ Cm}$$

$$= 6.10\text{ D (as 1D} = 3.33\times 10^{-30}\text{ Cm)}$$

$$\%\text{ ionic character} = \frac{\text{Observed dipole moment}}{\text{Theoritical dipole moment}}\times 100$$

$$= \frac{1.03}{6.1}\times 100 = 16.88\%$$

$$\approx 16.9\%$$

90. (b) (A) $N_2 = \sigma 1s^2, \sigma^* 1s^2, \sigma 2s^2, \sigma^* 2s^2,$

$$\pi 2p_x^2 \approx \pi 2p_y^2, \sigma 2p_z^2$$

$$B.O = \frac{\text{Bonding } e^- - \text{Antibonding } e^-}{2} = \frac{10-4}{2} = 3$$

No. of unpaired electron = 0 = Diamagnetic

$N_2^+ = \sigma 1s^2, \sigma^* 1s^2, \sigma 2s^2, \sigma^* 2s^2, \pi 2p_x^2 \approx \pi 2p_y^2, \sigma 2p_z^1$

$$B.O = \frac{9-4}{2} = 2.5$$

No. of unpaired electron (n) = 1 = Paramagnetic

∴ (A) matches with (iv).

(B) $O_2^+ = \sigma 1s^2, \sigma^* 1s^2, \sigma 2s^2, \sigma^* 2s^2, \sigma 2p_z^2,$

$$\pi 2p_x^2 \approx \pi 2p_y^2, \pi^* 2p_x^1 \approx \pi^* 2p_y^0$$

$$B.O = \frac{10-5}{2} = 2.5, \ n = 1 = \text{Paramagnetic}$$

$O_2^{2+} = \sigma 1s^2, \sigma^* 1s^2, \sigma 2s^2, \sigma^* 2s^2,$

$$\sigma 2p_z^2, \pi 2p_x^2 \approx \pi 2p_y^2$$

$$B.O = \frac{10-4}{2} = 3, \ n = 0 = \text{Diamagnetic}$$

∴ (B) matches with (i).

(C) $B_2 = \sigma 1s^2, \sigma^* 1s^2, \sigma 2s^2, \sigma^* 2s^2, \pi 2p_x^1 \approx \pi 2p_y^1$

$$B.O = \frac{6-4}{2} = 1, \ n = 2 = \text{Paramagnetic}$$

$B_2^+ = \sigma 1s^2, \sigma^* 1s^2, \sigma 2s^2, \sigma^* 2s^2, \pi 2p_x^1 \approx \pi 2p_y^0$

$$B.O = \frac{5-4}{2} = \frac{1}{2}, \ n = 1 = \text{Paramagnetic}$$

∴ (C) matches with (ii).

(D) $NO^- = \sigma 1s^2, \sigma^* 1s^2, \sigma 2s^2, \sigma^* 2s^2, \sigma 2p_z^2, \pi 2p_x^2$

$$\approx \pi 2p_y^2, \pi^* 2p_x^1 \approx \pi^* 2p_y^1$$

$$B.O = \frac{10-6}{2} = 2, \ n = 2 = \text{Paramagnetic}$$

$NO = \sigma 1s^2, \sigma^* 1s^2, \sigma 2s^2, \sigma^* 2s^2, \sigma 2p_z^2, \pi 2p_x^2$
$\approx \pi 2p_y^2, \ \pi^* 2p_x^1 \approx \pi^* 2p_y^0$

$$B.O = \frac{10-5}{2} = 2.5, \ n = 1 = \text{Paramagnetic}$$

∴ (D) matches (iii).

Biology

91. (c) In succulent plants like *Opuntia* and *Bryophyllum* respiration occurs at night time. This results in the consumption of O_2 without evolvement of CO_2.

This results in incomplete oxidation of food, containing carbohydrates resulting in the formation of organic acids. CO_2 is not released.

$$2C_6H_{12}O_6 + 3O_2 \rightarrow 3C_4H_6O_5 + 3H_2O + 386 \text{ kcal}$$

Thus, the value of RQ is zero as

$$RQ = \frac{\text{Volume of } CO_2 \text{ evolved}}{\text{Volume of } O_2 \text{ consumed}} = \frac{0}{3} = 0$$

92. (d) Creating evolutionary mapping is not an area of biotechnology whereas rest of the options are considered under biotechnology. For example, providing best catalyst in the form of improved organism, create optimal conditions through engineering for a catalyst to act, and down stream processing techniques to purify proteins and other products.

93. (b) Statements I, II and III are correct. Statements IV and V are incorrect and can be corrected as

- The cells of heart wood contain tannins that make it dark in colour.
- It is also called duramen.

94. (c) Except genital herpes, hepatitis-B and HIV infections, other veneral diseases are completely curable if detected early.

95. (b) Both A and R are true and R is the correct explanation of A.

Lysosomes are single membrane bound small spherical organelles that contain hydrolytic enzymes in them. Due to the presence of such enzymes, they are capable of digesting the own substances of cell. Hence, they are called suicidal bags.

96. (c) All the statements are correct except statement in option (c). It can be corrected as,

The skeletal heterocyclic ring is called purine and pyrimidine.

97. (b) The endodermal cells of dicot stem consist of starch grain as a food reserve. Therefore, the stem endodermis is also called starch sheath.

98. (c) Statement in option (c) is incorrect and it can be corrected as

In peas, leaves are converted into tendrils for climbing whereas fleshy leaves of onion and garlic store food. Rest of the statements are correct.

99. (d) The correct matches are A-3; B-1, C-2, D-4.

- *Pheretima* (Earthworm) is an example of annelids.
- *Laccifer* (Lac insect) an economically important insect is the member of phylum–Arthropoda.
- *Cucumaria* (Sea cucumber) is an example of echinoderms.
- *Branchiostoma* (Lancelet) belongs to the subphyla–Cephalochordata.

100. (d) In birds, fishes, insects, etc. female heterogamety is observed. In birds the male have a pair of Z-chromosomes besides the autosomes, while the females have Z and W chromosomes.

101. (c) Frog excretes urea and thus is a ureotelic animal, while fishes excrete ammonia and are ammonotelic.

Reptiles, birds and insects excrete uric acid in the form of pellet and are uricotelic in nature.

102. (c) The process of glycolysis starts with one molecule of glucose and produces two pyruvate molecules, four ATP and two NADH. Electron transport chain forms 34 ATP, citric acid cycle produces 2 ATP, 6 NADH and 2 $FADH_2$ and oxidation of pyruvic acid releases 2 NADH.

103. (a) Ethylene is a simple gaseous Plant Growth Regulator (PGR). It is synthesised in large amounts by tissues undergoing senescence and ripening fruits. It is used to initiate flowering and synchronising fruit set in pineapples.

104. (d) Archaebacteria are found in hot water springs and deep sea hydrothermal vents. They are able to survive in high temperatures because their bodies have adapted to such environmental conditions.

105. (c) When the columnar or cuboidal cells bear cilia on their free surface they are known as ciliated epithelium. Their function is to move particles in a specific direction.

106. (b) Both statement I and statement II are correct.

Colour blindness is a sex-linked recessive disorder. This defect occurs due to mutation in certain genes present on the X-chromosome.

107. (b) UAA, UAG, UGA are the terminator codons, which stop the protein synthesis in a cell.

108. (c) The reaction in option (c) shows the correct enzyme activity. CO_2 is carried by haemoglobin as carbamino haemoglobin and this binding is related to the partial pressure of CO_2. The related enzymes facilitate in both the direction.

109. (b) Matched pair in option (b) is correct. Both steler's sea cow and passenger pigeon are extinct species which suffered extinction due to overexploitation by human beings.

Rest incorrect pairs can be corrected as

The illegal introduction of the African catfish *Clarias gariepinus* for aquaculture purposes is posing threat to the indigenous catfishes in our rivers. This represents the example of alien species invasion.

The catfish and passenger pigeon are not co-extinct species. They do not possess any association, as the catfish is still found in various parts of ecosystem and the passenger pigeon is an extinct species.

110. (a) In the absence of lactose, the regulator gene-*R* produces a repressor protein which binds to operator site and prevents transcription of structural genes.

111. (c) Statement (c) is correct, as plant (b) shows growth of lateral buds into branches after decapitation i.e., apical dominance. It is a phenomenon where the main central stem grows more dominantly than the side branches. This occurs due to the production of auxin by apical bud which suppresses the growth of lateral buds. if apical buds is removed auxin levels drop, allowing lateral buds to grow.

112. (c) The correct matches are A-3, B-1, C-2, D-4.

- The body of the ovule fuses with funicle in the region called hilum.
- Enclosed within the integument is a mass of cells called nucellus.
- Integuments encircle the nucellus except at the tip where a small opening called micropyle is present.
- Fruit develops a thick covering or wall called pericarp. It is protective in nature.

113. (b) The renal tubule begins with a double walled cup-like structure, called Bowman's capsule. It encloses the glomerular.

114. (a) The correct matches are A-4, B-2, C-3, D-1.

- Cuticle is a waxy thick layer that prevents water loss from epidermis.
- Radial vascular bundles with xylem and phloem arranged alternatively at different radii are found in both monocot and dicot roots.
- Epidermal hair on the stem are called trichomes. They are multicellular in shoot system.
- In monocot stem, vascular bundles are conjoint and closed. These are closed due to absence of secondary growth.

115. (c) The opioids are the drugs, that bind to specific opioid receptors present in our central nervous system and gastrointestinal tract.

These are some of the commonly abused drugs.

116. (c) Statements I, III and IV are correct. Rest of the statements are incorrect. These can be corrected as.

- The conjoint vascular bundles usually have the phloem located on the outer side of the xylem.
- All tissues on the innerside of endodermis such as pericycle, vascular bundles and pith constitute the stele.

117. (d) Statement in option (d) is incorrect and can be corrected as

The outer pleural membrane is in close contact with the thoracic lining, whereas the inner pleural membrane is in contact with the lung surface.

118. (d) Lecithin is not a protein. It is an example of lipids which contain phosphorous and a phosphorylated organic compound in them.

119. (c) In case of acrocentric chromosome the centromere is situated close to its end, forming one extremely short and one very long arm.

120. (b) Auxins are responsible for initiating and promoting cell division in tissues like cambium. They are generally produced by the growing apices of the stems and roots, from where they migrate to the regions of their action.

121. (a) A is false, but R is true. A can be corrected as Amino acids can be essential or non-essential. The non-essential amino acids can be made by our body while we get essential amino acids through our diet/food.

122. (b) ECG is a graphical representation of the electrical activity of the heart during a cardiac cycle. Each peak in the ECG is identified with a letter from P to T that corresponds to a specific electrical activity of the heart. The T wave represents the return of the ventricles from excited to normal state.

123. (d) All the functions are related to hormones of posterior pituitary except option (d). It is related to pineal gland and melatonin which influences body temperature, pigmentation, etc.

124. (c) All the options are correct except option (c). It can be corrected as
Growth takes place by increase in the number of cells rather than increase in the size of cells.

125. (c) All statements are correct regarding restriction enzymes except (c). It can be corrected as
Restriction endonuclease functions by inspecting the length of DNA sequence. It recognises a specific palindromic nucleotide sequence within the DNA and cuts each of the two strands of the double helix at specific point in their sugar-phosphate backbones.

126. (b) The correct matches are A-4, B-1, C-2, D-3.
- Liverworts reproduce asexually by fragmentation of thalli, or by the formation of specialised structure called gemmae.
- Vegetative reproduction in mosses is by fragmentation.
- The food is stored as starch in Chlorophyceae and as mannitol in Phaeophyceae.

127. (d) When Nile perch was introduced in lake Victoria of South Africa, it killed and eliminated over 200 species of small cichlid fish.

128. (d) Inferior ovary is not related to Fabaceae family. In such plants the gynoecium is monocarpellary with a superior ovary.

129. (c) Ratio of pure tall (TT) to pure dwarf (tt) plants in F_2-generation will be 1 : 1.
Following diagram can explain the expected ratio of F_2-generation.

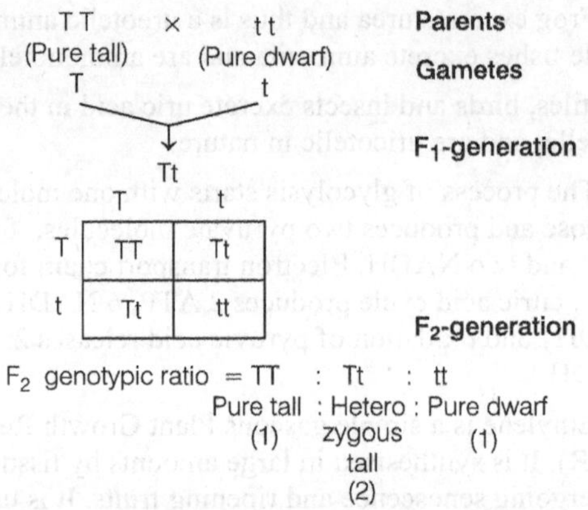

Thus, the ratio of pure tall to pure dwarf plants will be 1 : 1.

130. (a) *Ascaris,* the common roundworm and *Wuchereria*, the filarial worm are helminths, which are known to be pathogenic to man.

131. (d) Statement I is correct, but statement II is incorrect and it can be corrected as
The cardiac output of atheletes will be much higher compared to ordinary man.

132. (a) In eukaryotes, the cistrons are split into several coding units separated by non-coding base sequence called introns.

133. (c) Prophase-I of meiotic division is typically longer and more complex in comparison to mitosis.
It is subdivided into 5 phases leptotene, zygotene, pachytene, diplotene and diakinesis.

134. (b) Adenohypophysis also known as anterior pituitary consists of two portions, i.e. pars distalis and pars intermedia.

135. (c) The thalamus contributes to fruit formation and such fruits are called false fruits. The example includes apple, strawberry, cashew, etc. Most fruits however develop only from the ovary and are called true fruits.

136. (c) Statement in option (c) is incorrect and it can be corrected as
Plasma without the clotting factors is called serum.
Rest all the statements are correct.

137. (b) *Liquorice*, commonly known as mulethi, is a medicinal plant of the bean family–Fabaceae.
Urena lobata commonly known as caesarweed are used as a cure for skin problems. It is member of family-Malvaceae.

138. (d) Statement I is correct, but statement II is incorrect. It can be corrected as
In gymnosperms, male and female gametophytes do not have an independent free-living existence. They remain within the sporangia retained on the sporophytes.

139. (a) The correct matches are A-4, B-3, C-1, D-2.
- Excitability is the property of muscle in which it receives and responds to stimuli.
- Muscles shorten and thicken to do work, this property is known as contractility.
- Muscles can be stretched passively when relaxed and this property is known as extensibility.
- Muscles have a property to return to their original shape after contraction and extension, this property of muscle called elasticity.

140. (d) Statement in option (d) is incorrect and can be corrected as

Lichens represent an intimate mutualistic relationship wherein the fungus provides water, minerals and shelter to the algae and in return, receive food prepared by the algae.

141. (c) Both statement I and statement II are incorrect and can be corrected as
- Anaerobiosis reduces the decomposition and causes piling up of detritus.
- Producers are also known as transducers. Since, they convert energy from one form to another.

142. (b) Francis Crick proposed the central dogma in molecular biology, which states that the genetic information flows from DNA $\rightarrow$ RNA $\rightarrow$ protein.

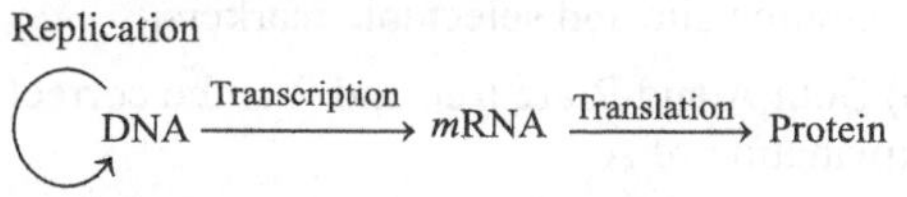

143. (c) Matched pair in option (c) is incorrect. It can be corrected as
Hind II is a restriction endonuclease that always cuts DNA molecules at a particular point by recognising a specific sequence of 6 base pairs.
All other matches are correct.

144. (c) Statements II, III and V are not correct w.r.t nerve impulse. These can be corrected as
- The resting membrane has high permeability for K^+.
- The stimulus of threshold value causes stoppage of $Na^+ - K^+$ ATPase pump.
- With the pumping out of K^+ ions, interior of the neuron becomes negative.

145. (b) Both statement I and statement II are correct.
In groundnut and beans, endosperm is completely consumed by the developing embryo before seed maturation. Whereas, in some seeds such as black pepper and beet, remnants of nucellus are also present. This residual, persistent nucellus is the perisperm.

146. (b) All the given options are true regarding the stirred tank bioreactor except option (b) and it can be corrected as
Small volume of cultures can be withdrawn periodically for sampling.

147. (b) Some nucleic acids that behave like enzymes are called as ribozymes. These are molecules of ribonucleic acid with catalytic activity.

148. (d) Statement I is correct but statement II is incorrect. Incorrect statement can be corrected as

α-thalassemia is controlled by two closely linked genes HBA1 and HBA2 on chromosome 16 of each parent.
Thalassemia is a quantitative problem due to less synthesis of globin molecules.

149. (a) IgG antibodies transfer from the maternal blood to her foetus through placenta. It is the only antibody which passes through the placenta.

150. (d) RNA interference is a method of cellular defence which takes place in all eukaryotic organisms.

This method involves silencing of specific *m*RNA due to both sense and antisense RNA, which form a complementary *ds*RNA molecule that binds and prevents translation of *m*RNA.

151. (d) Brassicaceae family, also known as Cruciferae have floral characters such as raceme, corymb, flower pedicellate, ebracteate, hermaphrodite and actinomorphic.

152. (c) Statements I, IV and V are correct. Statements II and III are incorrect and can be corrected as
- It is a technique of separation of DNA, RNA and protein.
- The most commonly used matrix is agarose which is a polysaccharide extracted from sea weeds.

153. (b) In autumn wood or late wood, the cambium is less active and forms fewer xylary elements that have narrow vessels.

154. (c) The correct matches are A-2, B-3, C-4, D-1.
- Sperms undergo physiological maturation acquiring increased motility and fertilising capacity. This phenomenon is called capacitation.
- Colostrum is the first mother milk produced by the mammary glands of humans.
- Placenta releases several hormones like human Chorionic Gonadotropin (hCG), human Placental Lactogen (hPL), oestrogen, progesterone, etc.
- The corpus luteum secretes large amount of progesterone which is essential for maintenance of the endometrium.

155. (c) All the pairs are correctly matched except option (c).
The correct match for it is *Bt* toxin is coded by *cry* gene in which *cry* IAb controls corn borer insect and *cry* II Ab controls cotton bollworms.

156. (b) Both A and R are true and R is the correct explanation of A.
In order to store seeds for a long time, it is important that activities inside the cell are stopped. This becomes possible under lesser water conditions, when the seed undergoes dormancy. This also helps the seed overcome extreme stressful conditions like drought. This results in easy transportation and storage of seeds for longer.

157. (c) *Mangifera indica* commonly known as mango belongs to the order–Sapindales.

158. (a) The correct matches are A-4, B-3, C-1, D-2.
- Fig and wasp show mutualism interaction. In this both the organisms get benefitted.
- Predation involves an interaction in which one species (predator) captures, kills and eats up the other (prey), e.g. Pitcher plant eats up insects to fulfill its Nitrogen deficiency.
- Nimatodes live as parasite in numerous species of fishes.
- *Balanus* and *Chathamalus* show competition in which *Balanus* dominates the intertidal area and excludes the smaller barnacle *Chathamalus* from that zone.

159. (b) *Trypanosoma* is an example of flagellated protozoan which causes sleeping sickness diseases in humans. Other options can be explained as
Paramecium - Ciliated protozoans
Plasmodium - Sporozoans
Entamoeba - Amoeboid protozoans

160. (c) Statements III and IV are incorrect. Incorrect statements can be corrected as
The colonies of cyanobacteria are generally surrounded by gelatinous sheath.
The bacteria that live in salty areas are known as halophiles, whereas those who live in hot springs are known as thermoacidophiles.
Rest statements are correct.

161. (d) In algae and fungi, zygote after its formation undergoes a period of rest or dormancy to tide over adverse conditions.

162. (c) I, II and III statements are correct. Rest statements are incorrect and can be corrected as
- Western ghats have a greater primitive amphibian species diversity than the Eastern ghats.
- The first national park to be established in India was Jim Corbett National Park.

163. (a) The Tricarboxylic Acid (TCA) cycle starts with the condensation of acetyl group with Oxaloacetic Acid (OAA) and water to yield citric acid.

164. (c) The correct matches are A–4, B–1, C–2, D–3.
- Innate immunity is a non-specific type of defence which involves various barriers like physical, physiological, cytokine and cellular barriers like PMNL-neutrophils.
- Natural passive immunity is the immunity conferred by antibodies and are transferred by mother to the child.
- Artifical passive immunity is the type of immunity provided by giving antibodies in the form of injection, e.g. antirabies serum.
- Artifical active immunity is the immunity which develops by vaccination.

165. (b) Both A and R are true and R is the correct explanation of A.
In humans, the chroionic villi and uterine tissue become interdigitated with each other and jointly form a structural and functional unit between developing embryo (foetus) and maternal body called placenta. As the chorion is involved in the formation of placenta, it is known as chorionic placenta.

166. (c) I, II, III and IV are the features that contributes to make a plasmid a suitable cloning vector. Other features include,
- It should be of a small size.
- It must be self-replicating inside the host cell.
- The vector DNA must have *ori*, restriction site, cloning site and selectable markers.

167. (b) Both A and R are true and R is the correct explanation of A.
In some organisms karyokinesis is not followed by cytokinesis. As a result of this, multinucleate condition arises leading to the formation of syncytium, e.g. liquid endosperm in coconut.

168. (d) Statement I is correct, but statement II is incorrect. It can be corrected as
Each photosystem has all the pigments, (except one molecule of chlorophyll-*a*) forming a light harvesting system called as antennae.

169. (b) Bioluminescence, i.e. the property of living organism to emit light is the characteristic feature of ctenophores.

170. (c) Both A and R are true, but R is not the correct explanation of A. Genetic drift is the change in allele frequencies in a population from generation to generation that occurs due to chance events.
It operates in small population sizes, serve reductions in population size called bottle necks, and founder events where a new population starts from a small number of individuals.
Genetic drift leads to fixation of alleles or genotypes in population. It increases the inbreeding coefficient and increases homozygosity as a result of removing alleles.

171. (a)The epididymis located along the posterior surface of each testis leads to vas deferens that ascends to the abdomen.

172. (b) Statements II, IV and V are correct.

Other statements are incorrect and these can be corrected as

- Louis Pasteur by his experiment demonstrated that life comes only from pre-existing life.
- The universe is vast and very old almost 20 billion years old.

173. (d) A is true, but R is false. R can be corrected as

Vital capacity is the maximum volume of air that can be moved in and out of lungs. It is the sum total of TV, IRV and ERV and equals to about 3500-4500 mL.

174. (b) Competitive inhibition is the kind of inhibition in which the inhibitor competes with the substrate for binding to the active site of enzyme.

With increase in substrate concentration, a constant V_{max} can be acheived. However, K_m increases as the reaction reaches half the $V_{\max}$ at increased substrate concentration.

In non-competitive inhibition, the $V_{\max}$ is lowered and Km is changed.

175. (c) Statements II, III and IV are correct, whereas statements I and V are incorrect. These can be corrected as

- When there are more than one pistils fused together the condition is called syncarpous.
- The stigma serves as a landing platform for pollen grains.

176. (d) Statement I is correct, but statement II is incorrect. It can be corrected as

In some cnidarians like corals the skeleton is composed of calcium carbonate. The cnidarians exhibit two basic body forms called polyp and medusae.
Pleurobrachia belongs to phylum-Ctenophora.

177. (a) The correct matches are A-2, B-4, C-3, D-1.

- The DNA polymerase enzyme uses a DNA template to catalyse the polymerisation of deoxynucleotides.
- RNA polymerase-I transcribes *r*RNA. Whereas RNA polymerase-II transcribes *hn*RNA and RNA polymerase-III transcribes *t*RNA, 5*sr*RNA and *sn*RNA.

178. (d) Statement I is correct, but statement II is incorrect. It can be corrected as
Nereis, which is an aquatic form of annelids is dioecious, i.e. both the male and female reproductive organs are present in separate individuals. While earthworm and leeches are monoecious, i.e. both male and female reproductive organs are present in single individual.

179. (a) Analogous structures are anatomically different and perform similar functions, e.g. flippers of dolphin and penguins.

180. (b) Statements III, IV and V are correct. Statements I and II are incorrect and can be corrected as

- Mammary glands begin to develop under the influence of oestrogen and progesterone.
- The second polar body and ovum are formed after second meiotic division.

NEET

TEST DRIVE

SECTION II

Mastery Builders

This section contains **10 Practice Sets** designed to match the exact difficulty level of NEET. These practice papers will simulate the real exam experience, preparing you to tackle any question that comes your way.

SECTION II

Mastery Builders

PRACTICE SET 4

Maximum Marks : 720	Time : 3 hrs	No. of Questions : 180

Instructions

1. This question paper contains **180** multiple-choice questions (four options with a single correct answer) from **Physics**, **Chemistry** and **Biology**.
2. These questions are distributed as 45 questions, each from Physics and Chemistry and 90 questions in Biology. These are to be compulsorily attempted by the candidate.
3. Each question carries 4 marks. For each correct response, the candidate will get 4 marks. For each incorrect response, one mark will be deducted from the total scores.

PHYSICS

1. Three lenses of focal length +15 cm, +150 cm and +250 cm are available for making an astronomical telescope. To produce the largest magnification, the focal length of the eyepiece should be

(a) +15 cm (b) +150 cm
(c) + 250 cm (d) None of these

2. In the third orbit of hydrogen atom, de-Broglie wavelength of an electron is λ, then radius of third orbit is

(a) 3λ (b) λ
(c) $\frac{3\lambda}{2\pi}$ (d) $\frac{\lambda}{2\pi}$

3. Work done by 3 mole of gas at 47° C to triple its volume at constant pressure is ($R = 2$ cal mol^{-1} °C^{-1})

(a) 3402 cal (b) 3428 cal
(c) 3832 cal (d) 3840 cal

4. A transformer of 100% efficiency has 200 turns in the primary winding and 40000 turns in secondary winding. It is connected to a 220 V main supply and secondary feeds to a 100 kΩ resistance. The potential difference per turn is

(a) 1.1 V (b) 11 V
(c) 25 V (d) 18 V

5. A particle is executing SHM of amplitude 8 cm. At what displacement from the mean position, the energy is half-kinetic and half-potential?

(a) 4 cm (b) $2\sqrt{2}$ cm (c) $4\sqrt{2}$ cm (d) $8\sqrt{2}$ cm

6. Three particles each of mass m are placed at the corners of an equilateral triangle of side d. If the side of the triangle is changed from d to $2d$, then work done on this sytem is

(a) $-\frac{3Gm^2}{2d}$ (b) $\frac{3Gm^2}{2d}$
(c) $\frac{Gm^2}{2d}$ (d) $-\frac{3Gm^2}{d}$

7. A wooden block floats in water, where 50% of its volume is outside water. When the same block floats in alcohol 70% of its volume remains outside the alcohol, the relative density of alcohol is

(a) 1.78 (b) 1.50 (c) 1.66 (d) 2.1

8. Light from two coherent sources of the same amplitude A and wavelength λ illuminate the screen. The intensity of the central maximum is I_0. If the sources are incoherent, then the intensity at the same point will be

(a) $4I_0$ (b) $2I_0$ (c) I_0 (d) $\frac{I_0}{2}$

9. A body A is thrown up vertically from the ground with a velocity v_0 and another body B is simultaneously dropped from a height H. They meet at a height $\frac{H}{2}$, if v_0 is equal to

(a) $\sqrt{2gH}$ (b) $\sqrt{gH}$ (c) $\frac{1}{2}\sqrt{gH}$ (d) $\sqrt{\frac{2g}{H}}$

10. In an experiment of Ohm's law, a potential difference of 5.0 V is applied across the end of a conductor of length 10.0 cm and diameter of 5.00 mm. The measured current in the conductor is 2.00 A. The maximum permissible percentage error in the resistivity of the conductor is

(a) 3.9 % (b) 8.4 % (c) 7.5 % (d) 3.0 %

11. In the Rutherford experiment, α-particles are scattered from a nucleus as shown. Out of the four paths, which path is not possible ?

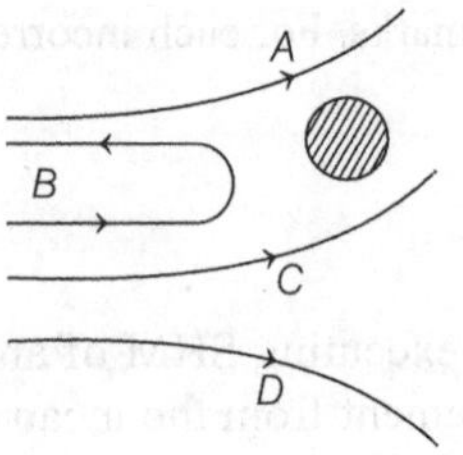

(a) D (b) B (c) C (d) A

12. The diode used in the circuit shown in the figure has a constant voltage drop of 0.5 V at all current and a maximum power rating of 200 mW. What should be the value of the resistor R, connected in series with the diode, for obtaining maximum current ?

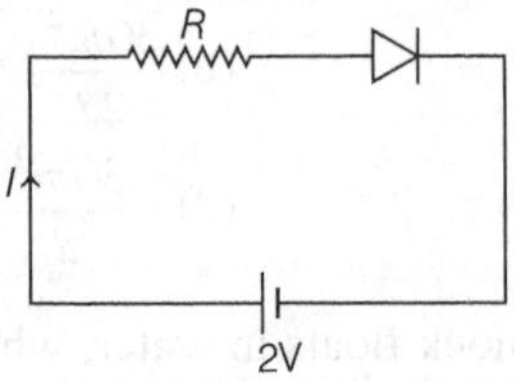

(a) 3.75 Ω (b) 215Ω (c) 1.75 Ω (d) 7.25 Ω

13. The power dissipated in the 9Ω resistor in the circuit shown is 36W. The potential difference across the 2Ω resistor is

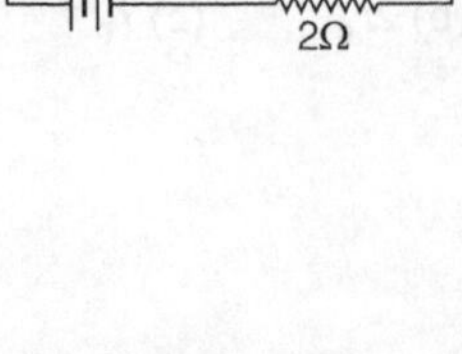

(a) 4 V (b) 8 V
(c) 10 V (d) 2 V

14. Consider the circular loop having current i and with central point O. The magnetic field at the central point O is

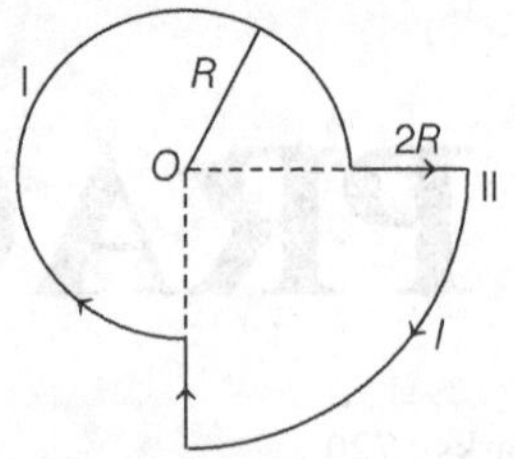

(a) $\frac{2\mu_0 i}{3\pi R}$ acting downward.
(b) $\frac{5\mu_0 i}{12R}$ acting downward.
(c) $\frac{6\mu_0 i}{11R}$ acting downward.
(d) $\frac{3\mu_0 i}{7R}$ acting upward.

15. Two bodies of masses 2 kg and 5 kg are located at (1, – 2) and (1, 3) respectively, then the centre of mass have co-ordinates at

(a) $\left(1, \frac{11}{7}\right)$ (b) $\left(\frac{11}{7}, 1\right)$
(c) $\left(\frac{1}{7}, \frac{11}{7}\right)$ (d) $\left(\frac{11}{7}, \frac{1}{7}\right)$

16. If one of the slits in Young's double slit experiment is covered with a black opaque paper, then
(a) the fringe width decreases.
(b) the bright fringes become fainter.
(c) there will be uniform illumination all over the screen.
(d) diffraction pattern will be observed.

17. The equivalent resistance between A and B as shown in the figure, is

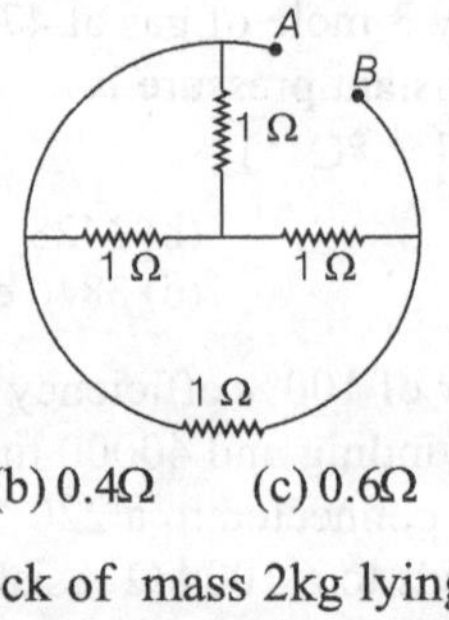

(a) 0.2 Ω (b) 0.4Ω (c) 0.6Ω (d) None of these

18. A marble block of mass 2kg lying on ice when given a velocity of 6 m/s is stopped by a friction force in 20s. The coefficient of friction is

(a) 30.0 (b) 0.03 (c) 0.3 (d) 3.0

19. The graph between applied potential difference V and electric current I for a metallic wire having length l and area of cross-section A is given in figure. The slope of the curve becomes

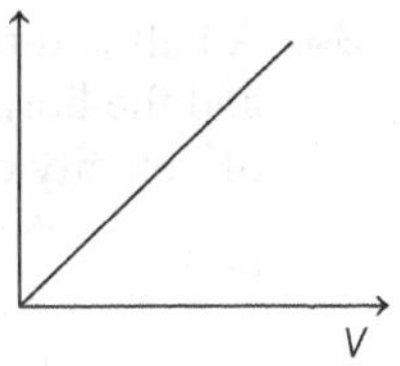

(a) more if the length of the wire is increased.
(b) more if the area of cross-section is decreased.
(c) less if the length of the wire is increased.
(d) more if temperature of the wire is increased.

20. In X-ray tube, the accelerating potential applied at the anode is V volt. The minimum wavelength of the emitted X-ray will be

(a) hc/eV (b) eV/ch (c) h/eV (d) eV/h

21. Molecules of an ideal gas are known to have three translational degrees of freedom and two rotational degrees of freedom. The gas is maintained at a temperature of T. The total internal energy U of one mole of this gas and the value of $\gamma\left(=\frac{C_p}{C_V}\right)$ are given respectively, by

(a) $U=\frac{5}{2}RT$ and $\gamma=\frac{6}{5}$ (b) $U=5RT$ and $\gamma=\frac{7}{5}$
(c) $U=\frac{5}{2}RT$ and $\gamma=\frac{7}{5}$ (d) $U=5RT$ and $\gamma=\frac{6}{5}$

22. A particle of mass m and charge $-q$ enters the region between the two charged plates of a condenser. The charge is initially moving along the positive X-axis with a speed v. If the length of each plate is L and E is the uniform electric field between the plates, the vertical deflection of the particle at the far edge of the plate is

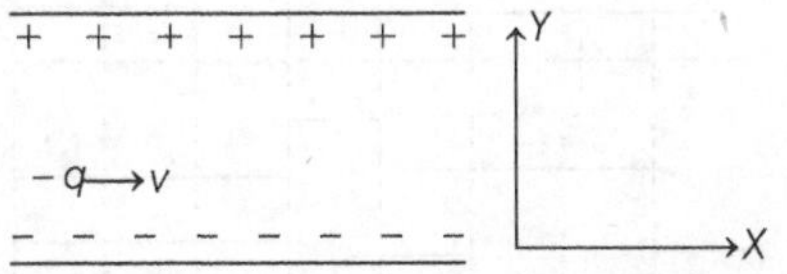

(a) $\frac{qEL^2}{mv^2}$ (b) $\frac{qEL^2}{2mv^2}$ (c) $\frac{q}{m}\left(\frac{EL}{v}\right)^2$ (d) $\frac{q^2EL^2}{2mv^2}$

23. A battery of emf E and internal resistance r is first connected to an external resistance r_1 and then connected to another external resistance r_2 for the same time. The value of r for which heats dissipated in r_1 and r_2 will be same, is

(a) $\frac{r_1}{r_2}$ (b) $\sqrt{r_1r_2}$ (c) r_1r_2 (d) $\frac{r_2}{r_1}$

24. Electric field in the space is given by $3\hat{i}-2\hat{j}+4\hat{k}$, then the value of electric flux passing through an area 36 unit lying in the XY-plane is

(a) 180 unit (b) 108 unit
(c) 144 unit (d) 72 unit

25. A long solenoid has 1000 turns. When current of 4A flows through it, the magnetic flux linked with each turn of the solenoid is 4×10^{-3} Wb. The self-inductance of the solenoid is

(a) 4H (b) 1H
(c) 3H (d) 2H

26. A block is dragged on a smooth plane with the help of a rope which moves with velocity v as shown in the figure. The horizontal velocity of the block is

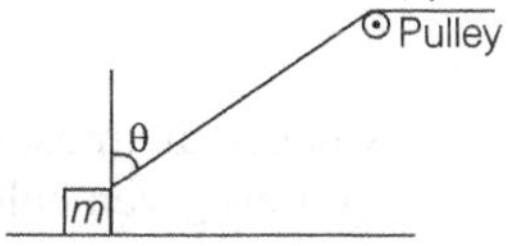

(a) v (b) $v\sin\theta$
(c) $\frac{v}{\sin\theta}$ (d) $\frac{v}{\cos\theta}$

27. A 220 V input is supplied to a transformer. The output circuit draws a current of 2.0 A at 440 V. If efficiency of transformer is 80%, the current drawn by the primary winding of the transformer is

(a) 3.6 A (b) 2.8 A
(c) 2.5 A (d) 5.0A

28. A satellite is launched into a circular orbit of radius R around the earth. A second satellite is launched into an orbit of radius 1.01 R. The period of the second satellite is larger than that of the first one by

(a) 0.5% (b) 1%
(c) 1.5% (d) 3%

29. A position dependence force $F=(7-2x+3x^2)$N, acts on a small body of mass 2 kg and displaces it from $x=0$ to $x=5$ m, work done (in J) is

(a) 35 (b) 70
(c) 135 (d) 270

30. A particle moves in a straight line with a uniform acceleration a, initial velocity of the particle is zero. Find the average velocity of the particle in first s distance.

(a) $\sqrt{\frac{a}{2s}}$ (b) $\sqrt{\frac{2s}{a}}$
(c) $\sqrt{\frac{as}{2}}$ (d) $\frac{as}{2}$

31. Match the different parts of electromagnetic spectrum in column I with their uses in column II.

	Column I		Column II
A.	Radiowaves	I.	In fibre optic communication system to transmit data.
B.	Visible Light	II.	In radar and airport body scanners to detect objects.
C.	Ultraviolet Light	III.	In the manufacture of polythene from ethylene.
D.	γ-rays	IV.	In the study of invisible writings.

Choose the most appropriate answer from the options given below.
(a) A-II, B-I, C-IV, D-III
(b) A-I, B-II, C-III, D-IV
(c) A-III, B-II, C-IV, D-I
(d) A-IV, B-II, C-III, D-I

32. For an aircraft, a force F on wing span depend on its speed v, density of air ρ and area of wing span s. If the force F is proportional to $\rho^m v^n s^p$, then
(a) $m=1, n=1, p=1$ (b) $m=1, n=2, p=1$
(c) $m=2, n=2, p=1$ (d) $m=1, n=2, p=2$

33. Students I, II and III perform an experiment for measuring the acceleration due to gravity (g) using a simple pendulum. They use different lengths of the pendulum and/or record time for different number of oscillations. The observations are shown in the table.
Least count for length = 0.1 cm, Least count for time = 0.1 s

Student	Length of the pendulum (cm)	Number of oscillations (n)	Total time for n oscillations (s)	Time period (s)
I	64.0	8	128.0	16.0
II	64.0	4	64.0	16.0
III	20.0	4	36.0	9.0

If E_{I}, E_{II} and E_{III} are the percentage errors in g, i.e. $\left(\frac{\Delta g}{g} \times 100\right)$ for students I, II and III, respectively, then
(a) $E_{\text{I}} = 0$ (b) E_{I} is minimum
(c) $E_{\text{I}} = E_{\text{II}}$ (d) E_{II} is maximum

34. A ball is thrown such that the time of flight is 5s and the horizontal range is 200 m. Find the direction of velocity of projection.
(a) $\tan^{-1}\left(\frac{5}{8}\right)$ (b) $\tan^{-1}\left(\frac{2}{3}\right)$
(c) $\sin^{-1}\left(\frac{1}{2}\right)$ (d) $\tan^{-1}\left(\frac{4}{5}\right)$

35. The value of R for which, current through 7 V battery is zero, is

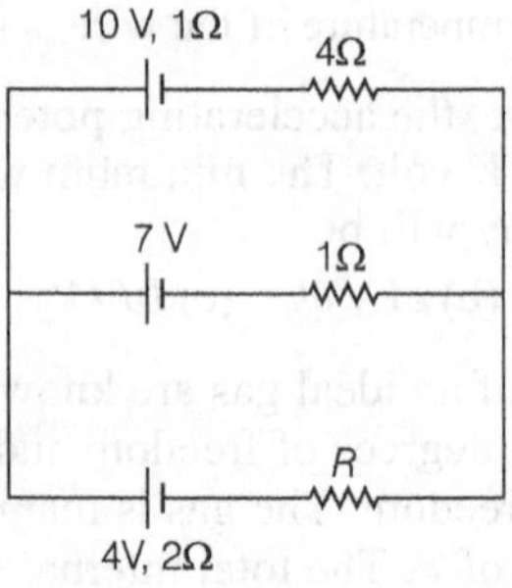

(a) 3Ω (b) 4Ω (c) 5Ω (d) 6Ω

36. The logic circuit shown below has the input waveforms A and B as shown in the figure. Pick out the correct output waveform.

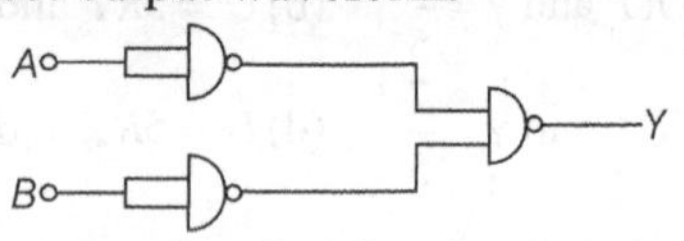

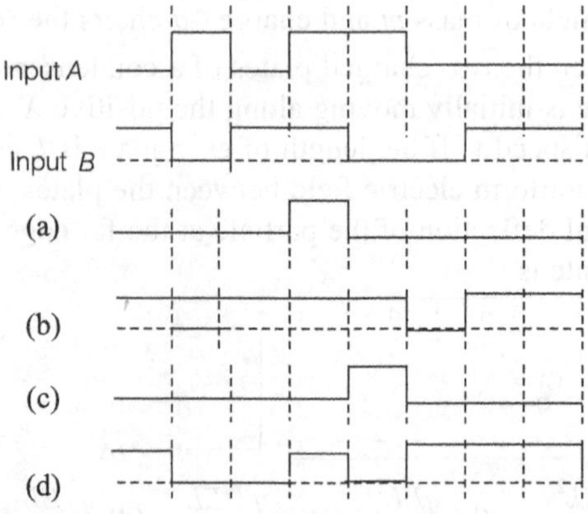

37. If a biconvex lens is cut into identical parts by a horizontal plane XY as shown in the figure, then which of the following statement is correct?

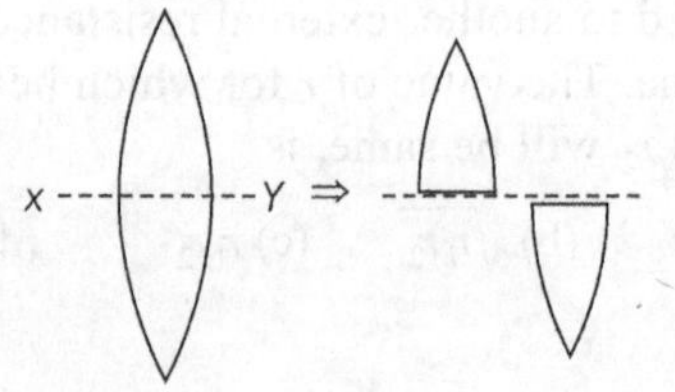

(a) Focal length of each part will be same and forms image with same intensity.
(b) Focal length of each part will be same and forms image with reduced intensity.
(c) Focal length of each part will be different and forms image with reduced intensity.
(d) None of the above.

38. A mass m hangs with the help of a string wrapped around a pulley on a frictionless bearing. The pulley has mass m and radius R. Assuming pulley to be perfect uniform circular disc, the acceleration of the mass m, if the string does not slip on the pulley is

(a) $\frac{3}{2}g$ (b) $\frac{2}{3}g$
(c) $\frac{g}{3}$ (d) g

39. Total energy stored in the system given in figure is

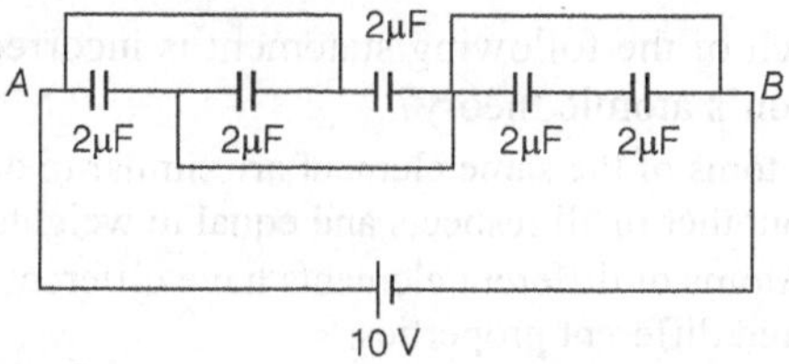

(a) 3×10^{-4} J
(b) 2.4×10^{-4} J
(c) 12×10^{-6} J
(d) 2.4×10^{-6} J

40. Given below are two statements.
Statement I Conductors having equal positive charge and volume, must also have same potential.
Statement II Potential depends only on charge and volume of conductor.
In the light of above statements, choose the most appropriate answer the options given below.
(a) Both Statement I and Statement II are correct.
(b) Statement I is incorrect but Statement II is correct.
(c) Both Statement I and Statement II are incorrect.
(d) Statement I is correct but Statement II is incorrect.

41. In the following circuit, current through 2Ω resistor just after switch closed is

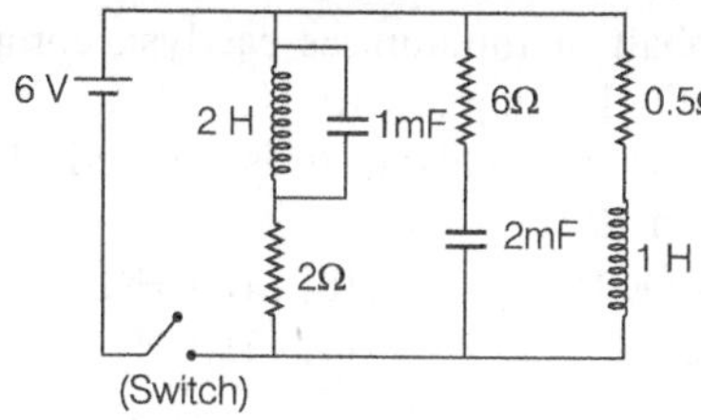

(a) 3A (b) 2.25 A (c) 0.71 A (d) 0A

42. Two glass capillary tubes of length L and $3L$ and radii R and $\frac{3R}{2}$ are connected in series. The net rate of flow of liquid through them will be (given, rate of the flow through single glass capillary, $Q=\frac{\pi pR^4}{8\eta L}$)

(a) $0.62Q$ (b) $1.73Q$ (c) $11.6Q$ (d) $1.38Q$

43. The work function of metal is in the range of 2eV to 5eV, then which of the following wavelength of light cannot be used for photoelectric effect? (Take, $h=4\times10^{-15}$ eV, $c=3\times10^8$ m/s)

(a) 510 nm (b) 650 nm (c) 400 nm (d) 570 nm

44. A mass m attached to a spring oscillates with a period of 3 s. If the mass is increased by 1 kg, the time period increases by 1s. The initial mass m is

(a) $\frac{18}{7}$ kg (b) $\frac{9}{7}$ kg (c) $\frac{7}{9}$ kg (d) $\frac{14}{7}$ kg

45. A parallel plate capacitor with square plates, each of side 20 cm has a capacitance of 1 μF. At time $t=0$, it is connected for charging to a 2V battery through a series resistance of 1 kΩ. The charge on the capacitor varies with time t (in second) as $q(t)=q_0[1-e^{-t/\tau}]$, where $q_0=CV$ and $\tau=CR$ is the time constant of CR circuit. The displacement current between the plates at $t=10^{-3}$ s is

(a) 7.4×10^{-5} A (b) 7.36×10^{-4} A
(c) 7.63×10^{-4} A (d) 7×10^{-5} A

CHEMISTRY

46. Methyl alcohol when reacted with carbon monoxide using cobalt or rhodium as catalyst, compound *A* is formed. On heating *A* with HI in the presence of red phosphorus as catalyst, *B* is formed. Identify the compound '*B*'.

(a) CH_3COOH (b) CH_3CHO
(c) CH_3CH_2I (d) CH_3CH_3

47. Consider the following sequence of reaction,

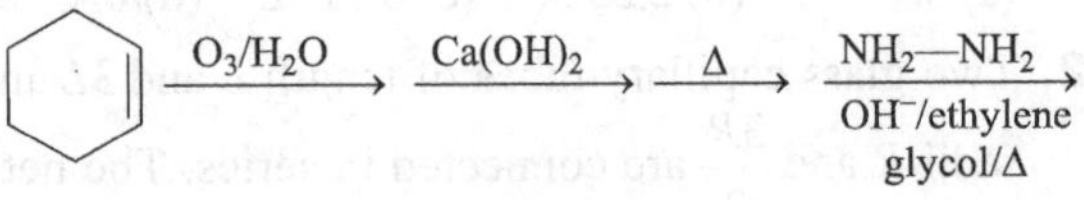

The end product of the given reaction is

(a) 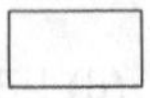 (b) 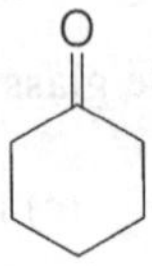 (c) 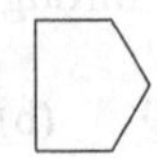 (d) 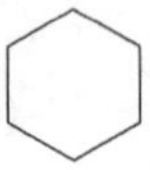

48. Which one of the following equations does not correctly represent the first law of thermodynamics for the given process involving an ideal gas? (Assume non-expansion work is zero)

(a) Adiabatic process: $\Delta U = -W$
(b) Isochoric process : $\Delta U = q$
(c) Isothermal process : $q = -W$
(d) Cyclic process : $q = -W$

49. Match List-I with List-II.

	List-I		List-II
A.	$[Cr(NH_3)_4 Cl_2]Cl$	I.	Paramagnetic and exhibits ionisation isomerism
B.	$[Ti(H_2O)_5 Cl](NO_3)_2$	II.	Diamagnetic and exhibits *cis-trans*-isomerism
C.	$[Pt(en)(NH_3)Cl]NO_3$	III.	Paramagnetic and exhibits *cis-trans* isomerism
D.	$[Co(NH_3)_4(NO_3)_2]NO_3$	IV.	Diamagnetic and exhibits ionisation isomerism

Choose the correct answer from the following options.

(a) A-IV, B-II, C-III, D-I
(b) A-III, B-I, C-IV, D-II
(c) A-II, B-I, C-III, D-IV
(d) A-I, B-III, C-IV, D-II

50. Select the correct statements.

I. Heat and work are path dependent function.
II. Mass and internal energy are intensive properties.
III. Internal energy of an ideal gas is function of temperature only.
IV. Mass and density are extensive property.
V. Enthalpy of graphite is lower than that of diamond.

Choose the correct answer from the options given below.

(a) I and V (b) II and IV
(c) I, III and V (d) I, II and III

51. 1 mole of FeC_2O_4 is oxidised by *x* mole of $Cr_2O_7^{2-}$ in acidic medium. Here, *x* is

(a) 3 (b) 1.5 (c) 0.5 (d) 1.0

52. Which of the following statement is incorrect about Dalton's atomic theory?

(a) Atoms of the same element are similar to one another in all respects and equal to weights.
(b) Atoms of different elements have different masses and different properties.
(c) Matter is made up of tiny indivisible particle called atom.
(d) The relative number and kinds of atoms in a given compound is variable in nature.

53. Which of the following alkenes can exhibit cis-trans isomerism?

(i) 1-propene (ii) 1-butene
(iii) 2-butene (iv) 1-chlorobutene
(v) 1-pentene

Choose the correct answer from the options given below.

(a) (i) and (ii) (b) (ii), (iii) and (v)
(c) (iii) and (iv) (d) (i) and (iv)

54. Given below are two statements.

Statement I O_2 and F_2 both stabilise higher oxidation states of metals but the higher oxidation state of metal with O_2 is more stable.

Statement II Structure of xenon fluorides can't be explained by valence bond theory.

In the light of the above statements, choose the correct answer from the options given below.

(a) Both statement I and statement II are false.
(b) Statement I is true but statement II is false.
(c) Statement I is false but statement II is true.
(d) Both statement I and statement II are true.

55. If the rate constant of a reaction with virus is $4.8\times 10^{-4}\ s^{-1}$, then the time required for the virus to become 80% inactivated is

[Given : log 5= 0.699]

(a) 48 min (b) 62 min (c) 39 min (d) 56 min

56. $10\,Cl^-(aq)+2MnO_4^-(aq)+16H^+(aq) \rightleftharpoons 5Cl_2(g)+2Mn^{2+}(aq)+8H_2O(l)$

The value of $E°$ for this reaction is 0.15 V. What is the value of the equilibrium constant (K_C) for this reaction ?

(a) Antilog [25.42] (b) Antilog [2.542]
(c) Antilog [24.52] (d) Antilog [254.2]

57. $(NH_4)_2CO_3$ is added to precipitate out the carbonates of group V cations. Na_2CO_3 is not added because

(a) $CaCO_3$ is soluble in Na_2CO_3.
(b) Na_2CO_3 increases the solubility of group V cations.
(c) $MgCO_3$ will be precipitated out in group V.
(d) Na_2CO_3 is weaker electrolyte than $(NH_4)_2CO_3$.

58. Match the List-I with List-II.

List-I (Metal complex)		List-II (Unpaired electrons)
A. $[Cr(H_2O)_6]^{3+}$	(i)	3
B. $[Fe(H_2O)_6]^{2+}$	(ii)	4
C. $[Zn(H_2O)_6]^{2+}$	(iii)	0
D. $[Fe(CN)_6]^{3-}$	(iv)	5

Choose the correct answer from the options given below.

(a) A-(i), B-(ii), C-(iii), D-(iv)
(b) A-(iii), B-(iv), C-(i), D-(ii)
(c) A-(ii), B-(i), C-(iv), D-(iii)
(d) A-(iv), B-(iii), C-(i), D-(ii)

59. In $[Ni(CO)_4]$, $[Ni(CN)_4]^{2-}$, $[NiCl_4]^{2-}$ species, the hybridisation state of Ni atom in all the complexes are respectively

(a) sp^3, dsp^2, dsp^2 (b) sp^3, dsp^2, sp^3
(c) $sp^3, sp^3\ dsp^2$ (d) dsp^2, sp^3, sp^3

60. Turnbull's blue and Prussian blue respectively are

(a) $Fe^{II}[Fe^{II}(CN)_6]$ and $Fe^{III}[Fe^{III}(CN)_6]$
(b) $Fe^{III}[Fe^{III}(CN)_6]$ and $Fe^{II}[Fe^{II}(CN)_6]$
(c) $Fe_3^{II}[Fe^{III}(CN)_6]_2$ and $Fe_4^{III}[Fe^{II}(CN)_6]_3$
(d) $Fe_4^{II}[Fe^{II}(CN)_6]_3$ and $Fe_3^{II}[Fe^{III}(CN)_6]_2$

61. Match the List-I with List-II.

List-I (Molecule)		List-II (Geometry)
A. XeO_3	I.	Square pyramidal
B. SF_6	II.	Trigonal planar
C. BrF_5	III.	Octahedral
D. SO_3	IV.	Trigonal pyramidal

Choose the correct answer from the options given below.

(a) A-IV, B-II, C-III, D-I
(b) A-IV, B-III, C-I, D-II
(c) A-III, B-IV, C-I, D-II
(d) A-III, B-I, C-II, D-IV

62. Uncertainty in position of minute particle of mass 2.5 g in space is 10^{-5} m. What is the uncertainty in its velocity (in ms^{-1})? ($h=6.6\times10^{-34}$ Js)

(a) 2.1×10^{-34} (b) 0.5×10^{-34}
(c) 2.1×10^{-27} (d) 0.5×10^{-23}

63. Glucose on reaction with ammoniacal silver nitrate gives silver mirror because it has

(a) alcoholic silver nitrate
(b) ester group
(c) aldehyde group
(d) ketone group

64. If an ideal solution is made by mixing 2 moles of benzene ($p°=266$ mm of Hg) and 3 moles of another liquid ($p°=236$ mm of Hg). The total vapour pressure of the solution at the same temperature would be

(a) 502 mm Hg (b) 248 mm Hg
(c) 600 mm Hg (d) 250.6 mm Hg

65. In Lassaigne's test, the organic compound is fused with a piece of sodium metal in order to

(a) increase the ionisation of the compound.
(b) decrease the melting point of the compound.
(c) increase the reactivity of the compound.
(d) convert the covalent compound into a mixture of ionic compounds.

66. Given that the standard potential of Cu^{2+}/Cu and Cu^+/Cu are 0.34 V and 0.522 V respectively, $E°$ of Cu^{2+}/Cu^+ is

(a) 0.182 V (b) 0.158 V
(c) −0.182 V (d) −0.158 V

67. Choose the incorrect statement according to the Arrhenius equation.

(a) A high activation energy usually implies a fast reaction.

(b) Rate constant increases with increase in temperature this is due to greater number of collision whose energy exceeds the activation energy.

(c) Higher the magnitude of activation energy, stronger is the temperature dependence of the rate constant.

(d) The pre-exponential factor is a measure of the rate at which collisions occur, irrespective of their energy.

68. Match the List-I with List-II.

	List-I		List-II
A.	$TiCl_4$	(i)	Adams catalyst in reduction
B.	$PdCl_2$	(ii)	In preparation of $(CH_3)_2SiCl_2$
C.	PtO_2	(iii)	Used as a Ziegler-Natta catalyst in polythene production
D.	Cu	(iv)	Wacker's process for converting C_2H_4 to CH_3CHO

Choose the correct answer from the options given below.

(a) A-(iii), B-(iv), C-(i), D-(ii)
(b) A-(iii), B-(iv), C-(ii), D-(i)
(c) A-(iv), B-(iii), C-(i), D-(ii)
(d) A-(ii), B-(i), C-(iii), D-(iv)

69. Given below are two statements, one is labelled as Assertion (A) and the other is labelled as Reason (R).

Assertion (A) Dipositive zinc exhibits diamagnetism due to loss of two electrons from 3*d*-orbital of neutral atom.

Reason (R) The electronic configuration of zinc is [Ar] $3d^{10}4s^2$.

In the light of the above statements, choose the most appropriate answer from the options given below.

(a) Both (A) and (R) are true but (R) is not the correct explanation of (A).
(b) (A) is true but (R) is not true.
(c) (A) is false but (R) is true.
(d) Both (A) and (R) are true and (R) is the correct explanation of (A).

70. Match the List-I with List-II.

List-I	List-II
A. $R'NH_2 \xrightarrow{NaNO_2 + HCl}$	(i) $RR'N{-}N{=}O$
B. $PhNH_2 \xrightarrow{NaNO_2 + HCl}$	(ii) $Ph{-}N^+{\equiv}NCl^-$
C. $PhN(CH_3)_2 \xrightarrow{NaNO_2 + HCl}$	(iii) $(CH_3)_2NPh(NO)$
D. $RR'NH \xrightarrow{NaNO_2 + HCl}$	(iv) $R'OH + N_2$

Choose the correct answer from the options given below.

(a) A-(iv), B-(ii), C-(i), D-(iii)
(b) A-(iv), B-(ii), C-(iii), D-(i)
(c) A-(i), B-(ii), C-(iv), D-(iii)
(d) A-(iv), B-(i), C-(ii), D-(iii)

71. Correct statement about reaction and related graph is

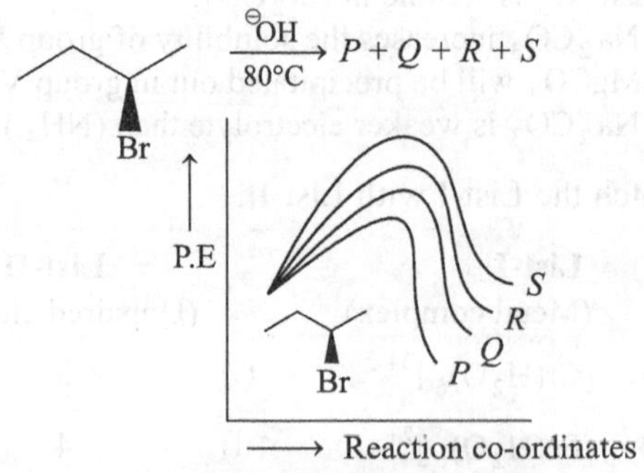

(a) *P* and *Q* are nucleophilic substitution products by S_N2 reaction mechanism.

(b) only *R* and *S* are elimination products by E_2 reaction mechanism.

(c) *P* is nucleophilic substitution product by S_N2 reaction mechanism and *Q*, *R*, *S* are elimination products by E_2 reaction mechanism.

(d) *P* is nucleophilic substitution product by E_2 reaction mechanism and *Q*, *R*, *S* are elimination products by S_N2 reaction mechanism.

72. Among Al_2O_3, SiO_2, P_2O_3 and SO_2 the correct order of acid strength is

(a) $Al_2O_3 < SiO_2 < SO_2 < P_2O_3$
(b) $SiO_2 < SO_2 < Al_2O_3 < P_2O_3$
(c) $SO_2 < P_2O_3 < SiO_2 < Al_2O_3$
(d) $Al_2O_3 < SiO_2 < P_2O_3 < SO_2$

73. Given below are two statements.

Statement I When Al is added to potassium hydroxide solution, hydrogen gas is evolved.

Statement II H_2SiF_6 is formed when silica reacts with hydrogen fluoride followed by hydrolysis.

In the light of the above statements, choose the correct answer from the options given below.

(a) Both statement I and statement II are false.
(b) Statement I is true but statement II is false.
(c) Statement I is false but statement II is true.
(d) Both statement I and statement II are true.

74. The dipole moments of halo compounds are in the order

(a) $CH_3Cl > CCl_4 > CH_2Cl_2 > CHCl_3$
(b) $CHCl_3 > CH_3Cl > CH_2Cl_2 > CCl_4$
(c) $CH_3Cl > CH_2Cl_2 > CHCl_3 > CCl_4$
(d) $CHCl_3 > CCl_4 > CH_3Cl > CH_2Cl_2$

75. Given below are two statements.

Statement I Zn^{2+} salts are white while Cu^{2+} salts are blue in colour.

Statement II Fluorine and chlorine gives only one oxide.

In the light of the statements, choose the correct answer from the options given below.

(a) Both statement I and statement II are false.
(b) Statement I is true but statement II is false.
(c) Statement I is false but statement II is true.
(d) Both statement I and statement II are true.

76. The bond dissociation energy of B—F in BF_3 is 646 kJ mol^{-1} whereas that of C—F in CF_4 is 515 kJ mol^{-1}. The correct reason for higher B—F bond dissociation energy as compared to that of C—F is

(a) significant $p\pi$ - $p\pi$ interaction between B and F in BF_3 whereas there is no possibility of such interaction between C and F in CF_4.
(b) lower degree of $p\pi$ - $p\pi$ interaction between B and F in BF_3 than that between C and F in CF_4.
(c) smaller size of B-atom as compared to that of C-atom.
(d) stronger bond between B and F in BF_3 as compared to that between C and F in CF_4.

77. Given below are two statements.

Statement I Perfectly ideal solution is not possible with respect to binary solution of two liquids.

Statement II No two substances can have exactly the same nature of intermolecular forces and also of the same magnitude.

In the light of the above statements, choose the correct answer from the options given below.

(a) Both statement I and statement II are false.
(b) Statement I is true but statement II is false.
(c) Statement I is false but statement II is true.
(d) Both statement I and statement II are true.

78. Consider the reaction,

$$2N_2O_5(g) \longrightarrow 4NO_2(g) + O_2(g)$$

If the concentration of NO_2 increases by 8.5×10^{-3} M in 100 s, then the rate of reaction will be

(a) 1.3×10^{-5} Ms^{-1}
(b) 2.8×10^{-5} Ms^{-1}
(c) 7.6×10^{-4} Ms^{-1}
(d) 2.13×10^{-5} Ms^{-1}

79. If the shortest wavelength in Lyman series of hydrogen atom is *A*, then the longest wavelength in Paschen series of He^+ is

(a) 36A/7 (b) 5A/9
(c) 36A/5 (d) 9A/5

80. There are four elements *p*, *q*, *r* and *s* having atomic numbers $Z-1$, Z, $Z+1$ and $Z+2$ respectively. If the element *q* is an inert gas, select the correct statements

(i) *p* has most negative electron gain enthalpy in the respective period.
(ii) *r* is an alkali metal.
(iii) *s* exists in + 2 oxidation state.

Choose the correct answer from the options given below.

(a) (i) and (ii) (b) (ii) and (iii)
(c) (i) and (iii) (d) (i), (ii) and (iii)

81. Hydrolysis of which of the following compound will give carbolic acid?

(a) Cumene
(b) Benzene diazonium chloride
(c) Benzal chloride
(d) Ethylene glycol ketal

82. If at 350K the concentration of $[H_3O^+]$ is 10^{-6} M, then the value of K_w at this temperature will be

(a) 10^{-13} M^2 (b) 10^{-6} M^2
(c) 10^{-12} M^2 (d) 10^{-14} M^2

83. Which of the following compound is most stable ?

(a) 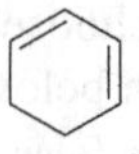 (b) 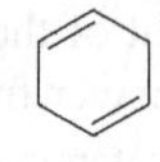

(c) 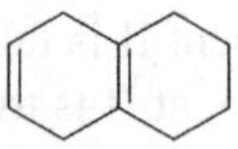 (d) 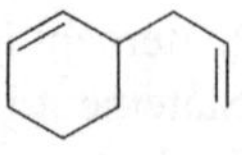

84. Which one of the following is likely to give a precipitate with $AgNO_3$ solution?

(a) $(CH_3)_3CCl$ (b) $CHCl_3$
(c) $CH_2=CH-Cl$ (d) CCl_4

85. Match the List-I with List-II.

List-I (Compound)	List-II (Oxidation by HIO_4)
A. CH_3COCHO	(i) $PhCH=O+HCOOH$
B. 1, 2-cyclohexanedione	(ii) $CH_3CH_2CHO+HOOCCH_3$
C. PhCH(OH)CHO	(iii) $HOOC(CH_2)_4COOH$
D. $CH_3CH_2CH(OH)COCH_3$	(iv) $CH_3COOH+HCOOH$

Choose the correct answer from the options given below.

(a) A-(iv), B-(i), C-(iii), D-(ii)
(b) A-(iv), B-(i), C-(ii), D-(iii)
(c) A-(iv), B-(iii), C-(i), D-(ii)
(d) A-(i), B-(ii), C-(iii), D-(iv)

86. In the given reaction, the product (*B*) is

$$CH_3CHO \xrightarrow[\text{(ii) } H_2O/H^{\oplus}/\Delta]{\text{(i) NaCN/HCl}} (A) \xrightarrow[\text{reagent}]{\text{Fenton}} (B)$$

(a) Acetic acid (b) Oxalic acid
(c) Pyruvic acid (d) Citric acid

87. Give the major organic product of the following reaction

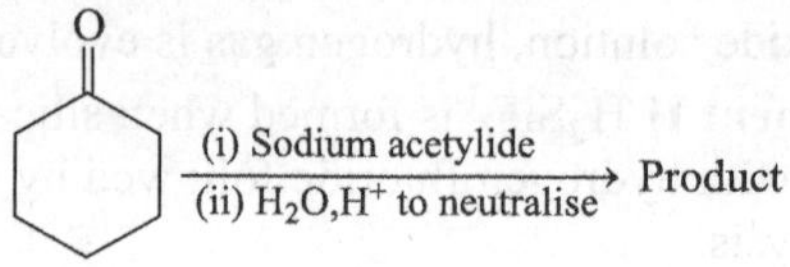

(a) 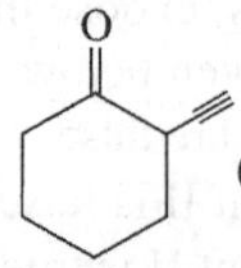

(b) 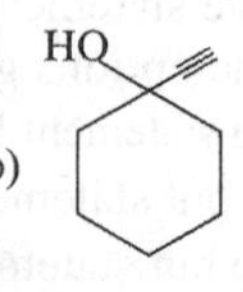

(c) 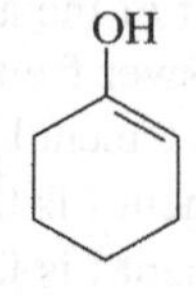

(d) 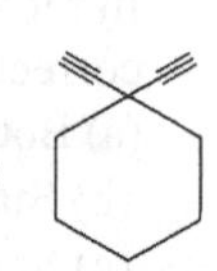

88. Given below are two statements.

Statement I The solubility of *n*-alcohol in water decreases with an increase in molecular weight.

Statement II The reactive proportion of the hydrocarbon part in alcohols increases with increasing molecular weight which permits enhanced hydrogen bonding with water.

In the light of the above statements, choose the correct answer from the options given below.

(a) Both statement I and statement II are false.
(b) Statement I is true but statement II is false.
(c) Statement I is false but statement II is true.
(b) Both statement I and statement II are true.

89. In an aprotic solvent, which relative order best describes the nucleophilicity of the halide ions?

(a) Iodide > Bromide > Fluoride >> Chloride
(b) Iodide > Bromide > Fluoride > Chloride
(c) Iodide < Bromide < Chloride < Fluoride
(d) Iodide < Bromide > Chloride > Fluoride

90. A 0.001 molal solution of $[Pt(NH_3)_4Cl_4]$ in water had a freezing point depression of 0.0054°C. If K_f for water is 1.80, the correct formulation of the above molecule is

(a) $[Pt(NH_3)_4Cl_3]Cl$ (b) $[Pt(NH_3)_4Cl_2]Cl_2$
(c) $[Pt(NH_3)_4Cl]Cl_2$ (d) $[Pt(NH_3)_4Cl_4]$

BIOLOGY

91. A nematode *Meloidegyne incognita* infects the roots of tobacco plants and causes a great yield reduction. A novel strategy is adopted to prevent this infestation which involves

(a) silencing of specific *m*RNA of nematode
(b) inhibition of DNA replication in nematode
(c) inhibition of transcription in nematode
(d) silencing of specific *m*RNA of tobacco plant

92. In frog vasa efferentia entering the kidney opens into ………… .

(a) mesorchium (b) bidder's canal
(c) cloaca (d) ovary

93. Match List I with List II.

List I	List II
A. Deoxyribonucleoside triphosphate	1. Unwinds DNA double helix
B. DNA helicase	2. Chromatin packaging
C. NHC protein	3. Translation
D. UTR	4. Provide energy for polymerisation reaction

Choose the correct answer from the options given below.

	A	B	C	D
(a)	1	2	3	4
(b)	4	1	2	3
(c)	3	2	1	4
(d)	4	1	3	2

94. When we conserve and protect the whole ecosystem, its biodiversity at all level is protected. We save the entire forest to save the tiger, this approach is called

(a) *in situ* conservation
(b) *ex situ* conservation
(c) *in vivo* conservation
(d) *in vitro* conservation

95. Given below are two statements; one is labelled as Assertion (A) and the other is labelled as Reason (R).

Assertion (A) DNA polymorphism is used to develop the DNA fingerprinting technique.

Reason (R) It is based upon variation in the number of tandemly repeated sequence.

In the light of the above statements, choose the correct answer from the options given below.

(a) A is false, but R is true
(b) Both A and R are true and R is the correct explanation of A
(c) Both A and R are true, but R is not the correct explanation of A
(d) A is true, but R is false

96. Given below are two statements; one is labelled as Assertion (A) and the other is labelled as Reason (R).

Assertion (A) The trophic level represent a functional level, not a species as such.

Reason (R) A given species may occupy more than one trophic level in the same ecosystem at the same time.

In the light of above statements, choose the correct answer from the options given below.

(a) A is false, but R is true
(b) Both A and R are true and R is the correct explanation of A
(c) Both A and R are true, but R is not the correct explanation of A
(d) A is true, but R is false

97. The resultant DNA formed when a foreign gene is introduced into the bacterial plasmid by using restriction enzyme and ligase is known as

(a) complementary DNA (b) palindromic DNA
(c) recombinant DNA (d) plasmid DNA

98. In lungs, air is separated from venous body by

(a) squamous epithelium and tunica externa of blood vessel
(b) transitional epithelium and tunica media of blood
(c) columnar epithelium and 3 layered wall of blood vessel
(d) squamous epithelium and endothelium of blood vessel

99. Given below are two statements.

Statement I Krebs' cycle involves eight steps to oxidise one molecule of acetyl Co-A.

Statement II Each turn of Krebs' cycle produces 3 NADH, 1 $FADH_2$ and 1 ATP molecules.

In the light of the above statements, choose the correct answer from the options given below.
(a) Statement I is incorrect, but statement II is correct
(b) Both statement I and statement II are correct
(c) Both statement I and statement II are incorrect
(d) Statement I is correct, but statement II is incorrect

100. In which of the following species, male and female gametophytes do not have an independent free living existence?
(a) *Pteris* (b) *Wolffia* (c) *Cedrus* (d) *Adiantum*

101. Match List I with List II.

	List I		List II
A.	Hashish	1.	Dried unfertilised female inflorescense
B.	Ganja	2.	Dried leaves and flowering shoots
C.	Marijuana	3.	Resinous exudate from the flowering tops of female plants
D.	Bhang	4.	Dried flower and top leaves of female *Cannabis* plant

Choose the correct answer from the options given below.

	A	B	C	D
(a)	1	2	4	3
(b)	3	1	4	2
(c)	2	1	4	3
(d)	4	3	2	1

102. The anaphase-II of meiosis-II begins with the simultaneous splitting of the centromere of each chromosome allowing them to move towards opposite poles of the cell by
(a) shortening of microtubules attached to kinetochores
(b) shortening of microtubules attached to centromere
(c) cytokinesis followed by karyokinesis
(d) karyokinesis followed by cytokinesis

103. Smack a colourless, odourless, bitter compound is obtained by
(a) alkylation of morphine.
(b) acetylation of morphine
(c) methylation of benzodiazepines
(d) hydroxylation of *Papaver somniferum*

104. Read the following statements and find out the incorrect statement.
(a) Long bones of the legs serve weight bearing functions
(b) The intercellular material of cartilage is semi-fluid and pliable
(c) Areolar tissue contain fibroblasts, macrophage and mast cells
(d) Blood is a fluid connective tissue

105. Match List I with List II.

	List I		List II
A.	Natality	1.	Number of deaths in the population during a given period
B.	Mortality	2.	Number of births during a given period
C.	Immigration	3.	Number of individuals of the population who left the habitat
D.	Emigration	4.	Number of individuals of the same species that have come into the habitat

Choose the correct answer from the options given below.

	A	B	C	D		A	B	C	D
(a)	1	2	3	4	(b)	2	1	4	3
(c)	3	2	1	4	(d)	4	2	3	1

106. Given below are two statements.
Statement I Chemosensitive area is situated adjacent to the rhythm centre which is highly sensitive to CO_2 and hydrogen ions.
Statement II Receptors associated with aortic arch and carotid artery can recognise changes in O_2 and H^+ concentration and send necessary signals to the rhythm centre for remedial actions.
It the light of above stantements, choose the correct answer from the options given below.
(a) Statement I is incorrect, but statement II is correct
(b) Both statement I and statement II are correct
(c) Both statement I and statement II are incorrect
(d) Statement I is correct, but statement II is incorrect

107. Read the following statements.
I. Ethylene and ABA hormones accelerate the process of senescence.
II. Zeatin is physiologically active cytokinin in maize kernels.

III. Gibberellins cause fruits like apple to elongate and improve its shape.
IV. F Skoog introduced the term kinetin.
Choose the correct set of statements from the options given below.
(a) I, II and III
(b) II, III and IV
(c) II, III and IV
(d) I and IV

108. Given below are two statements.
Statement I Sexual spores called conidiophores are produced endogenously in asci.
Statement II *Neurospora* is used extensively in biochemical and genetic work.
In the light of the above statements, choose the correct answer from the options given below.
(a) Statement I is incorrect, but statement II is correct.
(b) Both statement I and statement II are correct.
(c) Both statement I and statement II are incorrect.
(d) Statement I is correct, but statement II is incorrect.

109. The genetic defect adenosine deaminase (ADA) deficiency may be cured permanently by
(a) introducing bone marrow cells producing ADA into cells at an early embryonic stage
(b) administrating adenosine deaminase activators
(c) periodic infusion of genetically engineered lymphocytes having functional ADA DNA
(d) enzyme replacement therapy

110. A structure *X* connects the cytoplasm of neighbouring cells and another structure *Y* holds and glues the different neighbouring cells together: Identify these structures from the options given below
(a) Cell wall and middle lamella, respectively
(b) Plasmodesmata and middle lamella, respectively
(c) Middle lamella and desmosomes, respectively
(d) Middle lamella and plasmodesmata, respectively

111. Which of the following is responsible for controlling the copy number of the linked DNA in a plasmid?
(a) Cloning sites
(b) *ori*
(c) Restriction endonuclease
(d) Insertional inactivation

112. Match List I with List II.

	List I		List II
A.	PCR	1.	Restriction endonuclease
B.	*Taq* polymerase	2.	To amplify the gene of interest
C.	*Eco*RI	3.	*Thermus aquaticus*
D.	Chilled ethanol	4.	DNA precipitation

Choose the correct answer from the options given below.

	A	B	C	D		A	B	C	D
(a)	3	4	1	2	(b)	2	3	1	4
(c)	1	4	3	2	(d)	3	2	1	4

113. Vascularisation in plants occurs through
(a) differentiation of procambium followed by primary phloem and then primary xylem
(b) simultaneous differentiation of procambium, xylem and phloem
(c) differentiation of procambium followed by development of xylem and phloem
(d) differentiation of procambium which is immediately followed by the development of secondary xylem and secondary phloem

114. Given below are two statements.
Statement I Based on their location, the three type of muscles are identified as skeletal, smooth and cardiac.
Statement II Cardiac muscles are striated in appearance and are voluntary in nature as the nervous system controls their activity directly.
In the light of the above statements, choose the correct answer from the options given below.
(a) Statement I is incorrect, but statement II is correct.
(b) Both statement I and statement II are correct.
(c) Both statement I and statement II are incorrect.
(d) Statement I is correct, but statement II is incorrect.

115. Read the following statements about ETC.
I. Cytochrome - a_3 donates the electrons to free molecular oxygen.
II. Oxygen acts as the last electron acceptor at the end of respiratory chain.

III. Oxygen also receives two protons directly from the aqueous medium to form one molecule of water.
IV. NADH and $FADH_2$ bring electrons to the electron transport system.
V. Enzyme complex-I accepts electrons and H^+ from NADH and $FADH_2$

Choose the correct set of statements from the options given below.
(a) I and II (b) II and III
(c) I, II, III and V (d) I, II, III and IV

116. In a laboratory there were 40 fruit flies last week and during experiment 4 fruits flies died in a week. Calculate the death rate.
(a) 0.4 individual per fruits flies per week
(b) 0.36 individual per fruits flies per week
(c) 0.4 individual per fruits flies per week
(d) 0.1 individual per fruit flies per week

117. Given below are two statements.
Statement I Bacterial flagellum is composed of filament, hook and basal body.
Statement II The pili are small bristle like fibres sprouting out of the cell.
In the light of the above statements, choose the correct answer from the options given below.
(a) Statement I is incorrect, but statement II is correct
(b) Both statement I and statement II are correct
(c) Both statement I and statement II are incorrect
(d) Statement I is correct, but statement II is incorrect

118. Which of the following statements are correct?
I. Arthropods are characterised by the presence of statocysts.
II. Presence of parapodia is a unique characteristic of *Ascaris*.
III. In *Wuchereria* and *Ancylostoma* the mesoderm is scattered in between the ectoderm and endoderm.
IV. The flame cells of *Planaria* are responsible for digestion.
V. Skeleton in the *Sycon* is composed of spicules.
Choose the correct answer from the options given below.
(a) I, III and V (b) I, II, III and IV
(c) I, II, III and V (d) I, II and V

119. The tangential as well as radial walls of the endodermal cells have a deposition of water-impermeable, waxy material, suberin in the form of
(a) starch sheath (b) casparian strips
(c) conjuctive tissue (d) bundle sheath

120. The action of an inhibitor which diminishes the catalysis *via* reverse binding at the active site of enzyme is best described as
(a) competitive (b) allosteric
(c) facultative (d) non-competitive

121. Some mutations are harmful but do not get eliminated from the gene pool. Which of the following statements correctly explain the above situation ?
(a) They have future survival value
(b) They are recessive and carried by heterozygous individuals
(c) They are dominant and show up more frequently
(d) Genetic drift occurs because of a small population

122. Which of the following is expected to have the highest value in a grassland ecosystem ?
(a) Tertiary production
(b) Gross production
(c) Net production
(d) Secondary production

123. Match List I with List II.

	List I		List II
A.	Strobili	1.	First stage
B.	*Sphagnum*	2.	Sporophylls
C.	Gemma cups	3.	Fuel
D.	Protonema	4.	Thalli

Codes

	A	B	C	D		A	B	C	D
(a)	2	3	4	1	(b)	3	2	1	4
(c)	3	1	2	4	(d)	1	2	4	3

124. Vasopressin is mainly responsible for
(a) obligatory reabsorption of water through Bowman's capsule
(b) facultative reabsorption of water from DCT
(c) facultative reabsorption of water from Henle's loop
(d) obligatory reabsorption of water from PCT

125. Read the following statements.

I. Embryo develops at the chalazal end of the embryo sac.
II. The portion of embryonal axis above the level of cotyledons is the hypocotyl.
III. In the grass family scutellum is situated towards lateral side of the embryonal axis.
IV. All seeds have remnants of persistent nucellus.
V. Epicotyl has a shoot apex and a leaf primordia enclosed in a hollow structure.

Choose the correct set of statements from the options given below.

(a) I, III and V (b) II, IV and V
(c) I, III and IV (d) III and V only

126. Given below are two statements; one is labelled as Assertion (A) and the other is labelled as Reason (R).

Assertion (A) The sequence of amino acids providing the positional information in a protein is its primary structure.

Reason (R) The assembly of more than one polypeptide as individual subunits functioning together represents the secondary structure of protein.

In the light of the above statements, choose the correct answer from the options given below.

(a) A is false, but R is true
(b) Both A and R are true and R is the correct explanation of A
(c) Both A and R are true, but R is not the correct explanation of A
(d) A is true, but R is false

127. Given below are two statements.

Statement I Sewage contains large amounts of inorganic matter and microbes, many of which are pathogenic.

Statement II Before disposal, sewage is treated in Sewage Treatment Plants (STPs) to make it less polluting.

In the light of the above statements, choose the correct answer from the options given below.

(a) Statement I is incorrect, but statement II is correct
(b) Both statement I and statement II are correct
(c) Both statement I and statement II are incorrect
(d) Statement I is correct, but statement II is incorrect

128. Refer to the given equation and answer the question.

$$2(C_{51}H_{98}O_6) + 145\,O_2 \rightarrow 102\,CO_2 + 98\,H_2O + \text{Energy}$$

The RQ of above equation is

(a) 1 (b) 0.7
(c) 1.75 (d) 1.62

129. The aestivation found in pea, which have five petals in which largest one overlaps the two lateral petals, which in turn overlaps the two smallest anterior petals is called

(a) valvate
(b) twisted
(c) imbricate
(d) vexillary

130. Which of the following conditions is correct for resting neurons?

(a) Axonal membrane is impermeable to K^+
(b) Axonal membrane is impermeable to Na^+
(c) Axonal membrane is permeable to negatively charged proteins
(d) Axonal membrane is permeable to Na^+

131. Given below are two statements.

Statement I In monocot seed, the outer covering of endosperm separates the embryo by a proteinous layer called aleurone layer.

Statement II The plumule is enclosed in a sheath, which is called coleorrhiza.

In the light of the above statements, choose the correct answer from the options given below.

(a) Statement I is incorrect, but statement II is correct
(b) Both statement I and statement II are correct
(c) Both statement I and statement II are incorrect
(d) Statement I is correct, but statement II is incorrect

132. Given below are two statements; one is labelled as Assertion (A) and the other is labelled as Reason (R).

Assertion (A) Hemichordata earlier considered as sub-phylum under phylum–Chordata now is placed as a separate phylum under non- Chordata.

Reason (R) Hemichordates have open type of circulatory system and show indirect development.

In the light of the above statements, choose the correct answer from the options given below.
(a) A is false, but R is true
(b) Both A and R are true and R is the correct explanation of A
(c) Both A and R are true, but R is not the correct explanation of A
(d) A is true, but R is false

133. Flowers that are bisexual, bracteate, actinomorphic, hypogynous are characteristics of family
(a) Fabaceae (b) Malvaceae
(c) Graminae (d) Cruciferae

134. The scientist who confirmed the release of a volatile substance from ripened oranges that hastened the ripening of stored unripened bananas is
(a) E Kurosawa (b) F Skoog
(c) Miller (d) H H Cousins

135. Identify the correct matched pair.

(a)	MSH	→	Darkening of skin
(b)	STH	→	Micturition
(c)	ACTH	→	Controls blood glucose level
(d)	FSH	→	Inhibits RBC production

136. In which of the following steps of muscle contraction energy is utilised in the form of ATP?
(a) Release of calcium ion into the sacroplasm
(b) Formation of cross bridge
(c) Breaking of cross bridge
(d) Shortening of sarcomere

137. While the membrane of grana have both PS-I and PS-II. The stroma lamellae membranes lack .... as well as ....
(a) PS-I, PS-II
(b) PS-I, NADP reductase enzyme
(c) PS-II, NADP reductase enzyme
(d) PS-I, ATP reductase enzyme

138. Select the correct statement about protein synthesis.
(a) Translation begins when *m*RNA attaches to small subunit of ribosomes
(b) Peptidase catalyses formation of peptide bond
(c) UTRs are present between start and stop codons
(d) At the end of translation, release factor binds to intiation codon

139. Consider the graph given below.

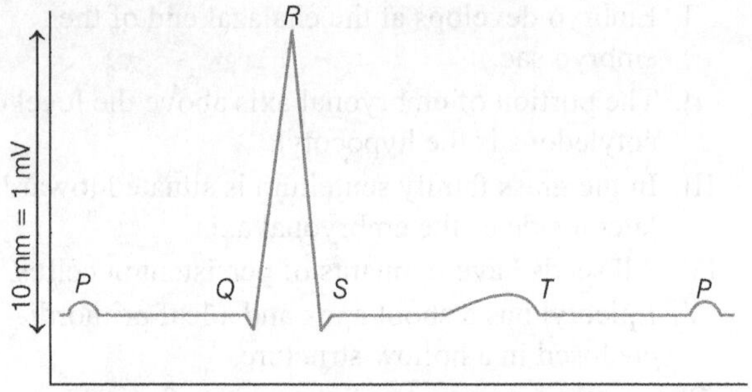

Which of the following is incorrectly matched ?
(a) P wave - Depolarisation of the atria
(b) Q wave - Beginning of systole
(c) QRS wave - Depolarisation of the atria
(d) T wave - End of diastole

140. Electrons from excited chlorophyll of PS-II are first accepted by
(a) quinone
(b) ferredoxin
(c) cytochrome-*b*
(d) cytochrome-*f*

141. Consider the following figure slowing a stage of meiosis.

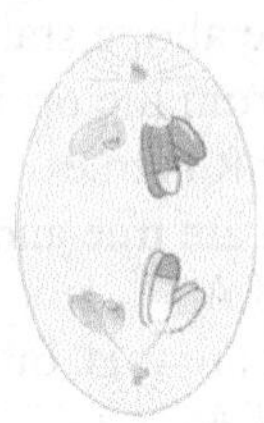

Choose the correct statement w.r.t. the given figure.
(a) The microtubules from the opposite poles of the spindle attach to the pair of homologous chromosomes
(b) The homologous chromosomes separate, while sister chromatids remain associated at their centromeres
(c) It involves simultaneous splitting of the centromere of each chromosome allowing them to move towards opposite poles of the cell
(d) It involves splitting of centromere and separation of chromatids

142. First child of normal couple is sickle-cell anaemic. The possibility of a second child being a sickle-cell anaemic is
(a) 25 % (b) 50 %
(c) 75 % (d) 100 %

143. Next to endodermis lies a few layers of thick-walled parenchymatous cells called
(a) casparian strips (b) stele
(c) pericycle (d) pith

144. *E. coli* with mutated *z* gene of *lac* operon cannot grow in medium containing only lactose as the source of energy because
(a) *lac* operon is constitutively active in these cells
(b) they cannot synthesise functional beta-galactosidase
(c) in the presence of glucose, *E. coli* cannot utilise lactose
(d) the bacterium cannot transport lactose from the medium into cell

145. Tasmanian wolf is a marsupial while wolf is a placental mammal. This shows
(a) convergent evolution
(b) divergent evolution
(c) parallelism
(d) inheritance of acquired characteristics

146. There are three major ways in which different cells handle pyruvic acid produced by glycolysis. These include the following, except
(a) lactic acid fermentation
(b) alcoholic fermentation
(c) aerobic respiration
(d) glucose oxidation

147. Water is a regular mode of transport for the male gametes among all the plants given below, except
(a) algae (b) gymnosperms
(c) bryophytes (d) pteridophytes

148. Given below are two statements; one is labelled as Assertion (A) and the other is labelled as Reason (R).

Assertion (A) Placenta facilitates the supply of oxygen and nutrients. Along with this, it acts as an endocrine tissue.

Reason (R) It produces hormones like hCG, hPL, oxytocin, progestogens and oestrogen.

In the light of the above statements, choose the correct answer from the options given below.
(a) A is false, but R is true
(b) Both A and R are true and R is the correct explanation of A
(c) Both A and R are true, but R is not the correct explanation of A
(d) A is true, but R is false

149. Which of the following pairs shows basal placentation?
(a) Tomato; maize
(b) Pea; maize
(c) Mustard; marigold
(d) Marigold; maize

150. Which one of the following is used as clot buster for removing clots from blood vessels of patients who have undergone myocardial infarction?
(a) Ethanol (b) Statins
(c) Cyclosporin-A (d) Streptokinase

151. The correct sequence of embryogeny in dicot seed is
(a) zygote, proembryo, globular, heart-shaped and mature embryo
(b) zygote, globular, proembryo, heart-shaped and mature embryo
(c) zygote, proembryo, heart-shaped, globular and mature embryo
(d) zygote, globular, heart-shaped, proembryo and mature embryo

152. In glycolysis, which of the following reactions is catalysed by enzyme aldolase ?
(a) Fructose - 6 - phosphate → Fructose 1, 6-bisphosphate
(b) Dihydroxyacetone phosphate → Glyceraldehyde 3-phosphate
(c) Fructose 1, 6- bisphosphate → Glyceraldehyde 3-phosphate + Dihydroxyacetone phosphate
(d) 2- phosphoglycerate → Phosphoenol pyruvate

153. The glandular layer that undergoes cyclical changes during menstrual cycle is termed as
(a) myometrium (b) perimetrium
(c) endometrium (d) exometrium

154. Identify the incorrect match pair.
(a) *Ctenoplana*– Both extracellular and intracellular digestion
(b) *Fasciola*– Flame cell for osmoregulation
(c) *Meandrina*– Cnidoblasts for anchorage
(d) *Taenia*– Body marked out into metamere

155. Given below are two statements.

Statement I Each plant bears flowers on shoot in a specific arrangement.

Statement II Shoot bears flowers when its apical meristem changes into floral meristem.

In the light of the above statements, choose the correct answer from the options given below.
(a) Statement I is incorrect, but statement II is correct
(b) Both statement I and statement II are correct
(c) Both statement I and statement II are incorrect
(d) Statement I is correct, but statement II is incorrect

156. Given below are two statements.
Statement I Life arising from non-living things only, was explained by the theory of spontaneous generation.
Statement II Louis Pasteur's experiment clearly demonstrated the theory of spontaneous generation. In the light of the above statements, choose the correct answer from the options given below.
(a) Statement I is incorrect, but statement II is correct
(b) Both statement I and statement II are correct
(c) Both statement I and statement II are incorrect
(d) Statement I is correct, but statement II is incorrect

157. In assisted reproductive technology after *in vitro* fertilisation, what is transferred in Fallopian tube?
(a) Blastula is transplanted
(b) Only zygote is transplanted
(c) Morula in 8-24 celled stage is transplanted
(d) Embryo upto 8 blastomeres

158. Match List I with List II.

List I (Class)	List II (Feature)
A. Cyclostomata	1. All living members are ectoparasites
B. Chondrichthyes	2. Cartilaginous endoskeleton
C. Osteichthyes	3. Bony endoskeleton
D. Amphibia	4. Most have two pairs of limbs

Choose the correct answer from the options given below.

	A	B	C	D		A	B	C	D
(a)	1	2	3	4	(b)	2	1	3	4
(c)	1	2	4	3	(d)	3	2	4	1

159. Among the following, select the tools of recombinant DNA technology.
(A) Restriction enzymes
(B) Polymerase enzymes
(C) Ligases
(D) Vector
(a) A, B, C and D (b) A, C and D
(c) A, B and D (d) A, B and C

160. Which of the following statements is incorrect?
(a) Ribozymes are nucleic acids that behave like enzymes
(b) Enzymes isolated from halophilic organisms are highly stable at high temperature
(c) Low temperature preserves the enzyme in a temporarily inactive state
(d) Competitive inhibitor closely resembles the substrate in its molecular structure and inhibits the activity of enzyme

161. The organ that is large bean-shaped and mainly consists of lymphocytes and phagocytes is called
(a) thymus
(b) spleen
(c) lymphatic nodes
(d) lymphatic vessels

162. Significance of the 'heat shock' in bacterial transformation is to facilitate
(a) expression of the antibiotic resistance gene in the vector
(b) ligation of DNA to the cell membrane
(c) uptake the DNA through membrane transport protein
(d) uptake of DNA through pores in the bacteria cell wall

163. Match List I with List II.

List I	List II
A. Hypothalamus	1. Stores oxytocin
B. Neurohypophysis	2. Neurosecretory cells
C. LH and FSH	3. Stimulate gonadal activity
D. Somatostatin	4. Growth hormone

Codes

	A	B	C	D		A	B	C	D
(a)	2	4	3	1	(b)	2	1	3	4
(c)	2	3	1	4	(d)	4	3	1	2

164. Which of the following ideas was not a part of Charles Darwin's theory of 'origin of species by natural selection'?
(a) More offsprings are produced by organism than the number an environment can support
(b) Gene mutation is responsible for variation among individuals
(c) Individuals best adapted to environment can successfully survive and reproduce
(d) Individuals of an area tend to compete for scarce resources

165. Read the following statements about the member of kingdom–Monera. Identify the correct set of statements.

I. Bacteria are the sole members of kingdom–Monera.
II. The genetic material is surrounded by nuclear membrane.
III. Chemosynthetic autotrophic bacteria play a great role in recycling nutrients like nitrogen, phosphorous, iron and sulphur.
IV. Majority of the heterotrophic bacteria are important decomposers.

Choose the correct answer from the options given below.

(a) I, II and IV (b) II and III
(c) II only (d) I, III and IV

166. Read the following statements and choose the set of incorrect statements.

I. Each testicular tubules contains one to three highly coiled seminiferous tubules in which sperms are produced.
II. Each semniferous tubule is lined on its inside by two type of cells called Leydig cells and Sertoli cells.
III. In testis immunologically competent cells are also present.
IV. The seminiferous tubules of the testis open into the rete testis through vasa efferentia.
V. The region outside the seminiferous tubules called interstitial space, contains small blood vessels and male germ cells which lead to sperm formation.

Choose the correct answer from the options given below.

(a) I, II and IV (b) III, IV and V
(c) II, IV and V (d) II and III

167. Find the wrongly matched pair.

(a) Har Gobind Khorana - Synthesised RNA molecules
(b) George Gamow - Codon is triplet
(c) Meselson and Stahl - Regulation of gene expression
(d) Alec Jeffreys - DNA fingerprinting

168. Which of the following is incorrect about sex determination?

(a) In grasshoppers, besides autosomes, males have only one X-chromosome whereas females have a pair of X-chromosome
(b) In *Drosophila*, males have one X and one Y-chromosome whereas females have a pair of X-chromosomes besides autosomes
(c) In birds females have one Z and one W-chromosome, whereas males have a pair of Z-chromosomes beside autosomes
(d) In insects with XO type of sex determination, all sperms have X-chromosomes besides autosomes.

169. The packaging of chromatin at higher levels requires an additional set of proteins that are collectively referred to as

(a) basic proteins (b) histone proteins
(c) acidic packaging proteins
(d) non-histone proteins

170. The arrangement of microtubules in a flagellum and a centriole is respectively.

(a) 9 + 2 and 9 + 1 (b) 9 + 1 and 9 + 0
(c) 9 + 0 and 9 + 2 (d) 9 + 2 and 9 + 0

171. Match List I with List II.

	List I		List II
A.	Father of bacteriology	1.	Bacterial food reserve
B.	Glycogen	2.	Bind virus at host surface
C.	Spikes	3.	Single-stranded RNA
D.	Viroids	4.	Louis Pasteur

Choose the correct answer from the options given below.

	A	B	C	D		A	B	C	D
(a)	2	3	4	1	(b)	1	3	2	4
(c)	4	1	2	3	(d)	3	2	1	4

172. The important step of decomposition, by which water-soluble inorganic nutrients go down into the soil and get precipitated is called

(a) fragmentation (b) leaching
(c) humification (d) mineralisation

173. Identify the correct statement.

(a) DNA fingerprinting is the production of living organisms, which are genetically identical to their parents
(b) The satellite DNA forms the major peak and the bulk DNA forms the minor peak
(c) The technique of cloning was developed by Sir Alec Jeffrey
(d) Satellite DNA shows high degree of polymorphism

174. Read the following statements and choose the correct set of statements.

I. Promoter is located towards 5′ end (upstream) of the structural gene.
II. Promoter provides the site for binding of RNA polymerase.
III. The template and coding strands of DNA are defined by the promoter site.
IV. Amino acids are activated in the presence of ATP and linked to *t*RNA.
V. Methyl guanosine triphosphate is added at 5′ end of hnRNA in a process of splicing.

Choose the correct answer from the options given below.

(a) I and II (b) III and V
(c) I and IV (d) I, II, III and IV

175. Observe the diagram given below. Identify the option that correctly represents the labelled part along with its function.

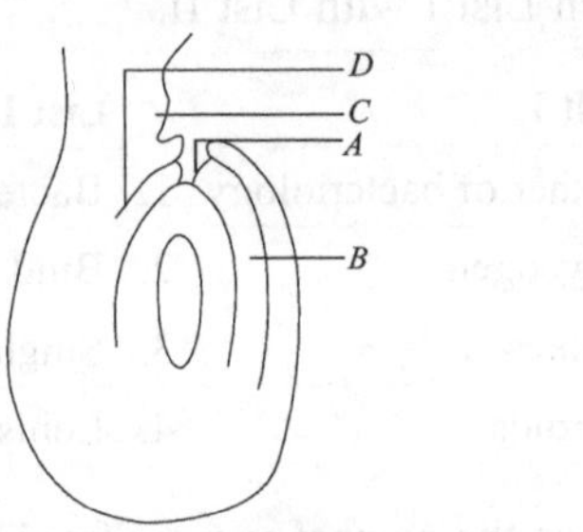

(a) *A* – Chalaza – Allows entry of pollen tube
(b) *C* – Funicle – Helps in attachment of ovule to placenta
(c) *B* – Inner integument – Gives rise to testa
(d) *D* – Outer integument – Gives rise to tegmen

176. Given below are two statements; one is labelled as Assertion (A) and the other is labelled as Reason (R).

Assertion (A) Biodiversity exists at all the levels of biological organisations ranging from macromolecules within cell to biomes.

Reason (R) The term 'biodiversity' describes the combined diversity at all the levels of biological organisation.

In the light of the above statements, choose the correct answer from the options given below.

(a) A is false, but R is true
(b) Both A and R are true and R is the correct explanation of A
(c) Both A and R are true, but R is not the correct explanation of A
(d) A is true, but R is false

177. In some plants a slender lateral branch arises from the base of the main axis and after growing aerially for some time it bends downwards to touch the ground. Among the given options which plants fulfill the above mentioned conditions?

(a) *Pistia* and *Eichhornia*
(b) Mint and jasmine
(c) Banana, pineapple and *Chrysanthemum*
(d) *Opuntia* and *Euphorbia*

178. In frogs, the lungs are characterised as

(a) circular, red-coloured structures
(b) elongated, pink-coloured sac-like structures
(c) cylindrical, bag-like structures
(d) single, bag like structures

179. Match List I with List II.

	List I	List II
A.	*Homo sapiens*	1. Sapindales
B.	*Musca domestica*	2. Primata
C.	*Mangifera indica*	3. Poales
D.	*Triticum aestivum*	4. Diptera

Codes

	A	B	C	D		A	B	C	D
(a)	2	4	1	3	(b)	1	3	4	2
(c)	2	1	3	4	(d)	3	4	2	1

180. Read the following statements and choose the set of incorrect statements about synergids.

I. They are generally two in number and occur laterally to egg cell.
II. These are characterised by the presence of finger-like filiform apparatus towards chalazal pole.
III. They secrete chemotactic substances to keep the egg cell safe.
IV. They have polarised protoplasm where nuclei occur towards the micropylar pole and vacuoles towards the central cell.
V. Synergids degenerate before the entry of the pollen tube into the embryo sac.

Choose the correct answer from the options given below.

(a) II and III (b) II, IV and V
(c) I, IV and V (d) All of these

Explanations

Physics

1. (a) As, magnification, $|m| = \frac{f_o}{f_e}\left(1+\frac{f_e}{D}\right)$

So, $$|m| \propto \frac{1}{f_e}$$

∴ In order to produce largest magnification, the focal length of eyepiece should be small, i.e. +15 cm lens is used.

2. (c) Bohr's second postulate, $mvr = \frac{3h}{2\pi}$

$$\Rightarrow \quad \frac{h}{mv} = \frac{2\pi r}{3}$$

$$\Rightarrow \quad \lambda = \frac{2\pi r}{3}$$

$$\Rightarrow \quad r = \frac{3\lambda}{2\pi}$$

3. (d) As we know, $\frac{V_1}{V_2} = \frac{T_1}{T_2}$

$$\Rightarrow \quad \frac{V}{3V} = \frac{320}{T_2} \quad [\because T_1 = 273 + 47 = 320\,\text{K}]$$

$$\Rightarrow \quad T_2 = 960\,\text{K} \Rightarrow \Delta T = 640\,\text{K}$$

$$W = p\Delta V = nR\Delta T$$
$$= 3 \times 2 \times 640 = 3840\,\text{cal}$$

4. (a) From transformer ratio,

$$\frac{V_s}{V_p} = \frac{N_s}{N_p}$$

$$\Rightarrow \quad V_s = \frac{V_p \times N_s}{N_p} = \frac{220 \times 40000}{200} = 44000\,\text{V}$$

Potential difference per turn is

$$\frac{V_s}{N_s} = \frac{44000}{40000} = 1.1\,\text{V}$$

5. (c) According to question, KE = PE

$$\frac{1}{2}mv^2 = \frac{1}{2}m\omega^2 y^2$$

$$\Rightarrow \quad \frac{1}{2}m\omega^2(A^2 - y^2) = \frac{1}{2}m\omega^2 y^2$$

$$\Rightarrow \quad A^2 - y^2 = y^2 \text{ or } 2y^2 = A^2$$

$$\Rightarrow \quad y = \frac{A}{\sqrt{2}} = \frac{8}{\sqrt{2}} = 4\sqrt{2}\,\text{cm}$$

6. (b) Here, mass of each particle is m.

For two particles system, potential energy,

$$U = -\frac{Gm_1 m_2}{r}$$

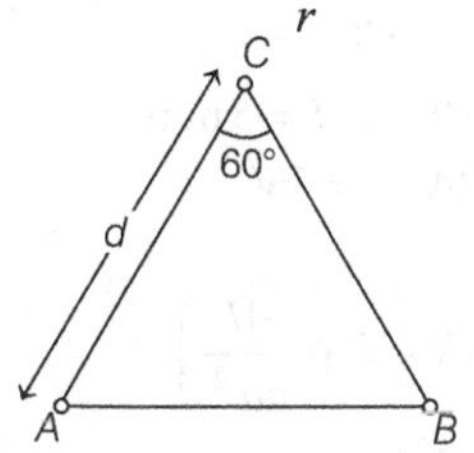

So, $U_a = U_{AB} + U_{BC} + U_{CA}$

$$= -3\frac{Gmm}{d} = -3\frac{Gm^2}{d}$$

When $d = 2d$, $U_b = -\frac{3Gm^2}{2d}$

Work done $= U_b - U_a = \frac{3Gm^2}{2d}$

7. (c) We know that, $V\sigma g = (0.5V)\sigma_w g$ ...(i) [for water]

and $V\sigma g = (0.3V)\sigma_a g$ ...(ii) [for alcohol]

On dividing Eq. (i) with Eq. (ii), we get

$$1 = \frac{5}{3}\cdot\frac{\sigma_w}{\sigma_a}$$

So, $$\frac{\sigma_a}{\sigma_w} = \frac{5}{3} = 1.66$$

8. (d) Let intensity of each source is I, then intensity at central maxima $= 4I = I_0$ (given).

So, $$I = \frac{I_0}{4}$$

When sources are incoherent, intensity at any point on screen

$$= I + I = 2I = 2\left(\frac{I_0}{4}\right) = \frac{I_0}{2}$$

9. (b) For body A, $s = ut + \frac{1}{2}at^2$

$$\Rightarrow \quad \frac{H}{2} = v_0 t - \frac{1}{2}gt^2 \quad \text{...(i)}$$

For body B, $\frac{H}{2} = 0 + \frac{1}{2}gt^2$ ...(ii)

From Eqs (i) and (ii), we get

$$\Rightarrow \quad v_0 t - \frac{1}{2}gt^2 = \frac{1}{2}gt^2$$

$$\Rightarrow \quad t = \frac{v_0}{g}$$

From Eq. (i),

$$\therefore \quad \frac{H}{2} = v_0 \times \frac{v_0}{g} - \frac{1}{2} g \frac{v_0^2}{g^2}$$

$$\Rightarrow \quad \frac{H}{2} = \frac{v_0^2}{g} - \frac{v_0^2}{2g} = \frac{v_0^2}{2g} \Rightarrow v_0 = \sqrt{gH}$$

10. (a) Given, $l = 10\,\text{cm}$, $d = 5\,\text{mm}$

$I = 2\text{A}, V = 5\text{V}$

By Ohm's law,

$$V = IR = I\left(\rho \frac{4l}{\pi d^2}\right)$$

$$\therefore \quad \rho = \frac{\pi d^2 V}{4Il}$$

$\therefore$ Percentage error in resistivity,

$$\left(\frac{\Delta\rho}{\rho} \times 100\right) = \left[2\left(\frac{\Delta d}{d}\right) + \frac{\Delta V}{V} + \frac{\Delta I}{I} + \frac{\Delta l}{l}\right] \times 100\,\%$$

$$= \left[2\left(\frac{0.01}{5}\right) + \frac{0.1}{5} + \frac{0.01}{2} + \frac{0.1}{10}\right] \times 100\,\%$$

$$= 3.9\,\%$$

11. (c) In the Rutherford experiment, α-particles always repel by the nucleus.

The path C shows attractive nature towards nucleus, so path C is not possible.

12. (a) Current through diode (or circuit), $I = \dfrac{\text{Power}}{\text{Voltage}}$

$$\therefore \quad I = \frac{200 \times 10^{-3}\,\text{W}}{0.5\text{V}} = 0.4\,\text{A}$$

and resistance $R = \dfrac{\text{Net voltage}}{\text{Current}}$

$$= \frac{2 - 0.5}{0.4} = 3.75\,\Omega$$

13. (c) Here, $9\,\Omega$ and $6\,\Omega$ are in parallel.

$$\Rightarrow \quad R_p = R_1 = \frac{9 \times 6}{15} = 3.6\,\Omega$$

The potential difference across R_1 is

$$V_1 = \sqrt{PR_1} = \sqrt{36 \times 9}$$

$$= 18\,\text{V}$$

$3.6\,\Omega$ and 2Ω are in series.

$$\Rightarrow \quad \frac{V_1}{V_2} = \frac{R_1}{R_2}$$

$$\Rightarrow \quad \frac{18}{V_2} = \frac{3.6}{2}$$

$\Rightarrow$ Potential difference across 2Ω resistor, $V_2 = 10\,\text{V}$

14. (b) From figure, magnetic field at O due to straight wires AB and $CD = 0$

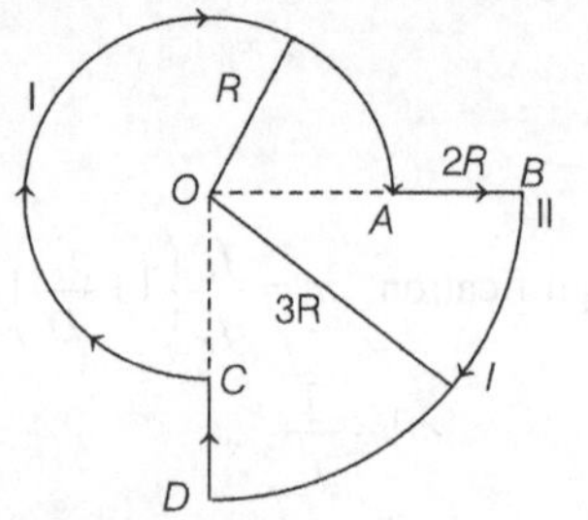

Hence, total magnetic field at O due to circular arc having radii R and $3R$

$$\mathbf{B} = \left[\frac{\mu_0 i}{2R}\left(\frac{270^\circ}{360^\circ}\right) + \frac{\mu_0 i}{2 \times 3R}\left(\frac{90^\circ}{360^\circ}\right)\right](-\hat{\mathbf{k}})$$

$$= \left(\frac{3\mu_0 i}{8R} + \frac{\mu_0 i}{24R}\right)(-\hat{\mathbf{k}}) = \frac{5\mu_0 i}{12R}(-\hat{\mathbf{k}})$$

$$\therefore \quad B = \frac{5\mu_0 i}{12R}, \text{ acting downward}$$

15. (a) Centre of mass, $x_{\text{CM}} = \dfrac{m_1 x_1 + m_2 x_2}{m_1 + m_2} = \dfrac{2 \times 1 + 5 \times 1}{2 + 5} = 1$

and $y_{\text{CM}} = \dfrac{m_1 y_1 + m_2 y_2}{m_1 + m_2} = \dfrac{2 \times -2 + 5 \times 3}{2 + 5} = \dfrac{11}{7}$

$\therefore$ Centre of mass is at $\left(1, \dfrac{11}{7}\right)$

16. (d) If one of the slits in Young's double slit experiment is covered with a black opaque paper, then we will obtain a single slit diffraction pattern on the screen.

17. (c) Equivalent circuit is shown in the figure.

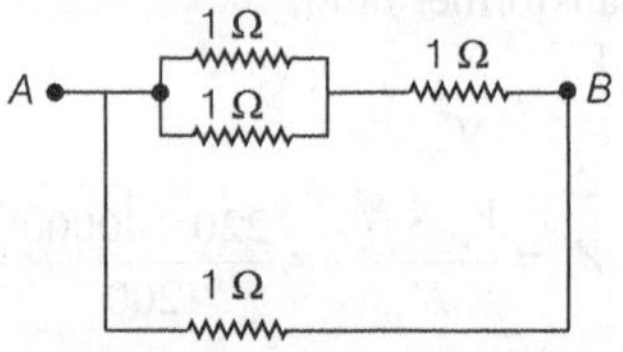

On further solving, we will have following equivalent figures

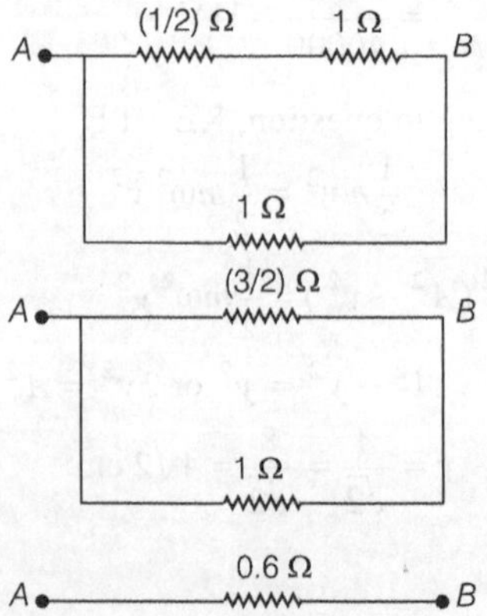

$$\therefore \quad R_{\text{eq}} = 0.6\,\Omega$$

18. (b) $F = ma, \ \mu_{mg} = ma, \ \mu = \frac{a}{g}$

Now, $v = u + at$ or

$0 = 6 + 20a$

$a = \frac{-6}{20} = -0.3 \text{ m/s}^2$

So, $\mu = \frac{a}{g} = \frac{0.3}{10} = 0.03$

19. (c) From the given V-I graph of metallic wire,

$\frac{I}{V}$ = slope of graph = Conductance = $\frac{1}{\text{Resistance}(R)}$

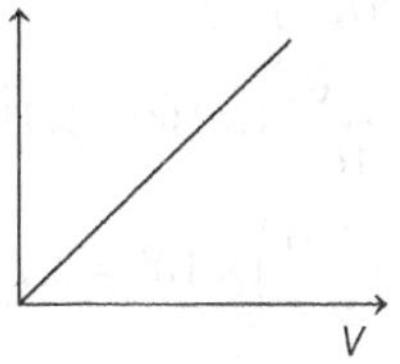

$\because \quad R \propto l$

Hence, on increasing the length of the wire, its resistance increases, thus slope of the curve decreases.

20. (a) $eV = h\nu = \frac{hc}{\lambda} \quad \therefore \ \lambda = \frac{hc}{eV}$

21. (c) Given, translational degree of freedom,

$f_{\text{trans}} = 3$

Rotational degree of freedom, $f_{\text{rot}} = 2$

Total degree of freedom, $f = f_{\text{trans}} + f_{\text{rot}} = 3 + 2 = 5$

At temperature T, total internal energy of an ideal gas is given by $U = \frac{f}{2}\mu RT$

$U = \frac{5}{2}RT \quad (\because \mu = 1)$

$\gamma = \frac{C_p}{C_V} = 1 + \frac{2}{f} = 1 + \frac{2}{5} = \frac{7}{5}$

22. (b) Here, magnitude of the uniform electric field between plates = E

So, acceleration, $a = \frac{F}{m} = \frac{qE}{m}$

Time taken, $t = \frac{\text{Length of the plate}}{\text{Velocity of the particle}} = \frac{L}{v}$

But in vertical direction, initial velocity = 0

By using, $s = ut + \frac{1}{2}at^2 = 0 + \frac{1}{2}\left(\frac{qE}{m}\right)\left(\frac{L}{v}\right)^2$

$s = \frac{qE}{2m}\frac{L^2}{v^2}$

Thus, vertical deflection of the particle at the far edge of the plate is $\frac{qE}{2m}\frac{L^2}{v^2}$.

23. (b) Heat dissipated in r_1 in time t = Heat dissipated in r_2 in time t

$I_1^2 r_1 t = I_2^2 r_2 t$

$\left(\frac{E}{r_1 + r}\right)^2 \cdot r_1 t = \left(\frac{E}{r_2 + r}\right)^2 \cdot r_2 t \Rightarrow r = \sqrt{r_1 r_2}$

24. (c) Since, area lying in XY-plane, hence

$\mathbf{A} = 36\hat{\mathbf{k}}$

$\therefore$ Electric flux, $\phi = \mathbf{E} \cdot \mathbf{A}$

$= (3\hat{\mathbf{i}} - 2\hat{\mathbf{j}} + 4\hat{\mathbf{k}}) \cdot (36\hat{\mathbf{k}}) = 144$ unit

Problem Solving Tactics

In this problem, already given that area lying in the XY- plane, so the normal to the plane of area is along Z-axis. That's why area, $\mathbf{A} = 36\hat{\mathbf{k}}$. Use the proper dot product rule $(\hat{\mathbf{k}} \cdot \hat{\mathbf{k}} = 1), (\hat{\mathbf{i}} \cdot \hat{\mathbf{k}} = 0), (\hat{\mathbf{i}} \cdot \hat{\mathbf{i}} = 1)$ etc., for calculating the electric flux.

25. (b) Given, number of turns of solenoid,

$N = 1000$ turns

Current, $I = 4\text{A}$

Magnetic flux for each turn, $\phi_B = 4 \times 10^{-3}$ Wb

Self-inductance of solenoid is given by

$$L = \frac{N\phi_B}{I} \quad \text{...(i)}$$

Substitute the given value in Eq. (i), we get

$$L = \frac{1000 \times 4 \times 10^{-3}}{4} = 1 \text{ H}$$

26. (c)

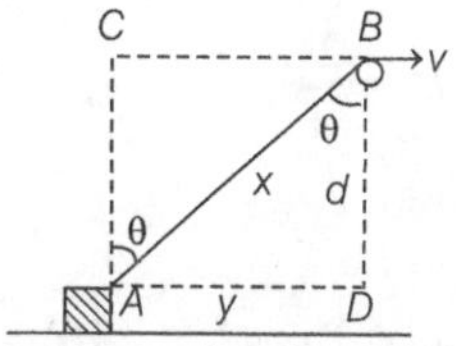

On applying pythagoras theorem in ΔABD, we get

$x^2 = y^2 + d^2$

Now, differentiate both sides with respect to t, we get

$$2x\frac{dx}{dt} = 2y\frac{dy}{dt} + 0 \quad \text{...(i)}$$

From the figure, we see that time rate of change of y is horizontal velocity of the block to be found.

$\frac{dy}{dt} = v'$

From Eq. (i), we have $v' = \frac{2x}{2y}\frac{dx}{dt} = \frac{x}{y}v \quad$ ...(ii)

where, v is the velocity at which the rope is moving.

$\sin\theta = \frac{y}{x} \quad$ [from the figure]

Therefore, $v' = \frac{v}{\sin\theta} \quad$ [from Eq. (ii)]

27. (d) Given, input voltage, $V_p = 220\text{V}$

Output voltage, $V_s = 440\text{ V}$

Input current, $I_p = ?$

Output current, $I_s = 2\text{A}$

Efficiency of the transformer, $\eta = 80\%$

Efficiency of the transformer is given by

$$\eta = \frac{\text{Output power}}{\text{Input power}} = \frac{V_s I_s}{V_p I_p}$$

$$\text{or } I_p = \frac{V_s I_s}{\eta V_p} = \frac{(440)(2)}{(220)\left(\frac{80}{100}\right)} = 5\text{ A}$$

28. (c) The percentage increase in the radius

$$= \frac{1.01-1}{1} \times 100 = 1\%$$

Time period of satellite, $T \propto r^{3/2}$

Percentage change in time period

$$= \frac{3}{2}(\text{Percentage change in radius})$$

$$= \frac{3}{2} \times 1\% = 1.5\%$$

29. (c) Work done,

$$W = \int_{x_1}^{x_2} F dx = \int_0^5 (7 - 2x + 3x^2)dx$$

$$= [7x - x^2 + x^3]_0^5 = 135\text{ J}$$

30. (c) $\because s = 0 + \frac{1}{2}at^2$

$$\Rightarrow 2s = at^2 \Rightarrow t^2 = \frac{2s}{a}$$

$$\therefore \quad t = \sqrt{\frac{2s}{a}}$$

$$\text{Average velocity} = \frac{s}{t} = \frac{s}{\sqrt{\frac{2s}{a}}} = \sqrt{\frac{as}{2}}$$

31. (a) A. Radiowaves are used in radar and airport body scanners to detect objects.

B. Visible light used in fibre optic communication system to transmit data.

C. Ultraviolet light used in the study of invisible writings.

D. γ-rays are used in the manufacture of polythene from ethylene.

Hence, A-II, B-I, C-IV, D-III.

32. (b) From the given situation

$$F = Ks^p v^n \rho^m$$

Writting the dimensions of each term, we get

$$[\text{MLT}^{-2}] = [\text{L}^2]^p[\text{LT}^{-1}]^n[\text{ML}^{-3}]^m$$

$$= [\text{M}^m \text{L}^{2p+n-3m}\text{T}^{-n}]$$

$$m = 1, n = 2$$

and $\quad 2p + n - 3m = 1$

$$\Rightarrow \quad 2p + 2 - 3 \times 1 = 1 \Rightarrow p = 1$$

33. (c) $T = 2\pi\sqrt{\frac{l}{g}}$ or $\frac{t}{n} = 2\pi\sqrt{\frac{l}{g}}$

$$\therefore \quad g = \frac{(4\pi^2)(n^2)l}{t^2}$$

$$\text{Percentage error in } g = \frac{\Delta g}{g} \times 100 = \left(\frac{\Delta l}{l} + \frac{2\Delta t}{t}\right) \times 100$$

$$E_{\text{I}} = \left(\frac{0.1}{64} + \frac{2 \times 0.1}{16}\right) \times 100 = 1.41\%$$

$$E_{\text{II}} = \left(\frac{0.1}{64} + \frac{2 \times 0.1}{16}\right) \times 100 = 1.41\%$$

$$E_{\text{III}} = \left(\frac{0.1}{20} + \frac{2 \times 0.1}{9}\right) \times 100 = 2.7\%$$

Hence, $E_{\text{I}} = E_{\text{II}}$

34. (a) $T = \frac{2u \sin\theta}{g} \Rightarrow 5 = \frac{2}{10} u \sin\theta \Rightarrow u \sin\theta = 25$

$$R = u\cos\theta T$$

$$\Rightarrow \quad 200 = u\cos\theta \times 5 \Rightarrow u\cos\theta = 40$$

$$\tan\theta = \frac{u\sin\theta}{u\cos\theta} = \frac{25}{40} \Rightarrow \theta = \tan^{-1}\left(\frac{5}{8}\right)$$

35. (a) From given circuit,

Current, $I = \frac{V}{R}$

So, $I = \frac{10-4}{4+1+2+R} = \frac{6}{7+R}$ ...(i)

Also, $\quad 4 + I(R+2) = 7$ ...(ii)

On solving Eqs. (i) and (ii), we get $R = 3\ \Omega$

36. (b)

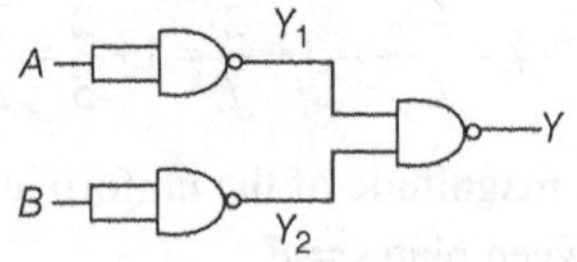

Truth table of given circuit is

A	B	Y_1	Y_2	Y
0	1	1	0	1
1	0	0	1	1
0	1	1	0	1
1	1	0	0	1
1	0	0	1	1
0	0	1	1	0
0	1	1	0	1
0	1	1	0	1

So, output is (b).

37. (b) When the lens is cut along XY, then its focal length remains constant but its aperture will decrease.
Since, intensity $\propto$ (aperture)^2
Hence, intensity will be reduced.

38. (b) From Newton's second law,
Net force = mass × acceleration

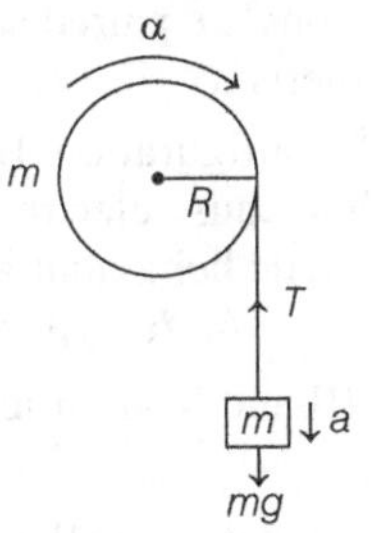

we have, $mg - T = ma$ ...(i)

and $\tau = T \cdot R = \frac{1}{2} mR^2 \alpha$

$\Rightarrow \quad T = \frac{1}{2} mR\alpha = \frac{1}{2} ma \quad [\because a = R\alpha]$

From Eq. (i), we get

$\Rightarrow \quad mg - \frac{1}{2} ma = ma \Rightarrow a = \frac{2}{3} g$

39. (a) Equivalent circuit diagram is

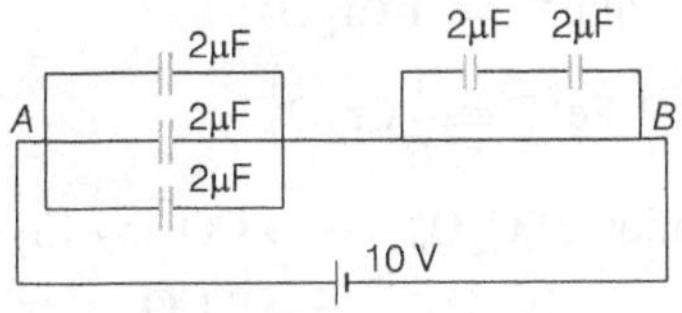

Equivalent capacitance between A and B is

$$C' = (2 + 2 + 2) = 6\mu F$$

So, energy stored, $E = \frac{1}{2} C' V^2 = 3 \times 10^{-4}$ J

40. (c) Electric potential of a charged conductor depends not only on the amount of charge and volume but also on the shape of the conductor. Hence, if their shapes are different , they may have different electric potential.

41. (a) Just after switch is closed, inductor acts like an open switch and capacitor acts like closed switch. Hence, equivalent circuit will be

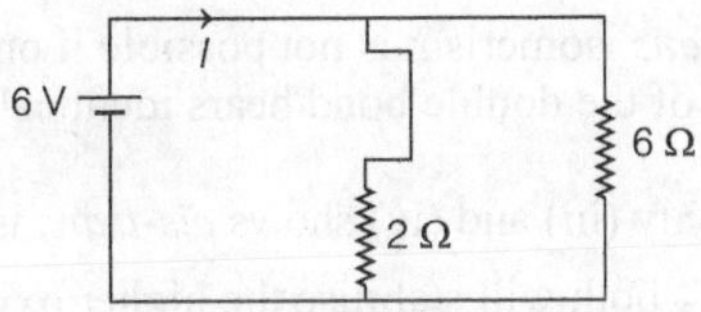

$\therefore \quad R_{eq} = \frac{2 \times 6}{2 + 6} = 1.5\Omega$

$\therefore \quad$ Current, $I = \frac{6}{1.5} = 4$A

$\therefore$ Current through 2Ω resistor

$$= \frac{6}{2+6} \times I = \frac{6}{8} \times 4 = 3 \text{ A}$$

42. (a) Fluid resistance is given by $f = \frac{p}{Q} = \frac{8\eta L}{\pi R^4}$

$$\left[\because Q = \frac{\pi p R^4}{8\eta L}\right]$$

If two capillary tubes are joined together in series,

$$f_{eq} = f_1 + f_2 = \frac{8\eta L}{\pi R^4} + \frac{8\eta 3L}{\pi\left(\frac{3}{2}R\right)^4}$$

$$= \frac{8\eta L}{\pi R^4}\left[1 + \frac{3 \times 2^4}{3^4}\right] = f \times 1.59 \simeq 1.6 f$$

$$\because \quad Q' = \frac{p}{f_{eq}} = \frac{p}{1.6f} = \frac{p}{1.6(8\eta L/\pi R^4)}$$

$$= \frac{\pi R^4 p}{8\eta L} \times \frac{1}{1.6} = \frac{Q}{1.6} = 0.62\,Q$$

43. (b) $\lambda_{min} = \frac{1242\,\text{eV} \times \text{nm}}{5\,\text{eV}} = 248.4$ nm

$$\lambda_{max} = \frac{1242\,\text{eV} \times \text{nm}}{2\,\text{eV}} = 621\,\text{nm}$$

Thus, 650 nm cannot be used.

44. (b) $T = 3 = 2\pi\sqrt{\frac{m}{k}}$

$$T' = 3 + 1 = 2\pi\sqrt{\frac{m+1}{k}}$$

$$\frac{3}{3+1} = \sqrt{\frac{m}{m+1}}$$

$$\Rightarrow \quad \frac{m+1}{m} = \left(\frac{4}{3}\right)^2 = \frac{16}{9} \Rightarrow 9m + 9 = 16m$$

$$\Rightarrow \quad 7m = 9$$

$$\Rightarrow \quad m = \frac{9}{7}\text{ kg}$$

45. (b) As we know, $q = CV = \frac{\varepsilon_0 A}{d} V$

$$= \varepsilon_0 AE \quad \left(\because \frac{V}{d} = E\right)$$

$$\Rightarrow \quad E = \frac{q(t)}{\varepsilon_0 A}$$

A = Area of the plate = 20× 20 cm = 400 = 4×10^{-2} m^2

Electric flux through the capacitor,

$$\phi_E = E \times A = \frac{q(t)}{\varepsilon_0}$$

where, $q_0 = CV = 10^{-6} \times 2 = 2\times10^{-6}$ C

$$\tau = CR = 10^{-6} \times 10^3 = 10^{-3}\text{s}$$

$$\phi_E = \frac{q(t)}{\varepsilon_0} = \frac{q_0[1-e^{-t/\tau}]}{\varepsilon_0}$$

Displacement current, $i_d = \varepsilon_0 \frac{d\phi_E}{dt}$

$$i_d = \varepsilon_0 \frac{d}{dt}\left[\frac{q_0[1-e^{-t/\tau}]}{\varepsilon_0}\right]$$

$$= \frac{q_0}{\tau} e^{-t/\tau} = \frac{2\times10^{-6}}{10^{-3}} e^{-t/10^{-3}}$$

At, $t = 10^{-3}$s,

$$i_d = 2\times10^{-3} e^{-1} = \frac{2\times10^{-3}}{e} = \frac{2\times10^{-3}}{2.718}$$

$$= 7.36\times10^{-4} \text{ A}$$

Chemistry

46. (d) Methyl alcohol reacts with carbon monoxide to give ethanoic acid (*A*) which further reacts with red phosphorus in acidic medium to give ethane (*B*) as final product.

$$\underset{\text{Methyl alcohol}}{CH_3OH} + CO \xrightarrow{\text{Co or Rh-catalyst}}$$

$$\underset{A\text{ (Ethanoic acid)}}{CH_3COOH} \xrightarrow[\text{Red P}]{\text{HI}} \underset{B\text{ (Ethane)}}{CH_3—CH_3}$$

47. (c) The complete sequence of reaction is as follows

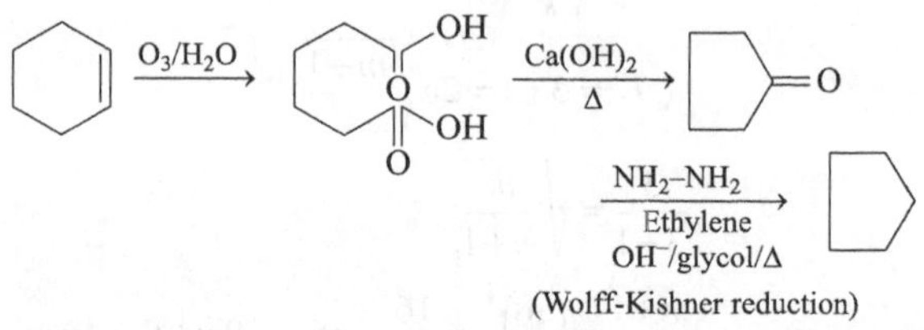

Due to ozonolysis, H_2O_2 is also formed which oxidise —CHO to —COOH.

48. (a) According to first law of thermodynamics,

$$\Delta U = q + W$$

For adiabatic process, $q = 0$; $\Delta U = W$

For isochoric process, $\Delta V = 0$, $W = 0$

Thus, $\Delta U = q$

For isothermal process, $\Delta U = 0$

Thus, $q = -W$

For cyclic process, $\Delta U = 0$; thus, $q = -W$.

49. (b)The correct match is A-III, B-I, C-IV, D-II.

A. Cr^{3+} has $3d^3$ configuration, with 3 unpaired electrons. Hence, it shows paramagnetic behaviour. Complex of the type Ma_4b_2 shows *cis-trans* isomerism.

B. Ti^{3+} has $3d^1$ configuration, hence shows paramagnetic behaviour. Complex gives Cl^- and NO_3^- ions in solution. Hence, it shows ionisation isomerism.

C. Pt^{2+} has $3d^8$ configuration but ligands are strong field ligands hence, it forms square planar complex. Thus, all electrons are paired and it also exhibits ionisation isomerism.

D. Co^{3+} has $3d^6$ configuration. But, ligands present are strong enough to cause electron pairing. Hence, it shows diamagnetic behaviour and exhibits *cis-trans* isomerism as it is Ma_4b_2 type complex.

50. (c) Statements I, III and V are true, while II and IV are false statement.

The correct form of statement II and IV are written as

Mass and internal energy are extensive properties.

Mass is extensive but density is intensive property.

51. (c) $FeC_2O_4 \rightleftharpoons Fe^{2+} + C_2O_4^{2-}$

Fe^{2+} is oxidised to Fe^{3+} and $C_2O_4^{2-}$ to CO_2 by $Cr_2O_7^{2-}$.

(i) Oxidation of $Fe^{2+} \longrightarrow Fe^{3+}$ by $Cr_2O_7^{2-}$

$$[Fe^{2+} \longrightarrow Fe^{3+} + e^-] \times 6$$

$$Cr_2O_7^{2-} + 14H^+ + 6e^- \longrightarrow 2Cr^{3+} + 7H_2O$$

Thus, $6Fe^{2+} \equiv 1\ Cr_2O_7^{2-}$

$$1\ Fe^{2+} \equiv \frac{1}{6} Cr_2O_7^{2-}$$

(ii) Oxidation of $C_2O_4^{2-} \longrightarrow CO_2$ by $Cr_2O_7^{2-}$

$$[C_2O_4^{2-} \longrightarrow 2\ CO_2 + 2e^-] \times 3$$

$$Cr_2O_7^{2-} + 14H^+ + 6e^- \longrightarrow 2Cr^{3+} + 7H_2O$$

$$3C_2O_4^{2-} \equiv Cr_2O_7^{2-}$$

$$1\ C_2O_4^{2-} \equiv \frac{1}{3} Cr_2O_7^{2-}$$

Thus, total $Cr_2O_7^{2-}$ required

$$= \frac{1}{6} + \frac{1}{3} = \frac{1}{2} = 0.5 \text{ mol}$$

52. (d) Statement (d) is incorrect. The correct form is The relative number and kinds of atoms in a given compound remains constant.

53. (c) *cis-trans* isomerism is not possible if one of the C-atoms of the double bond bears identical atoms or groups.

Hence, only (iii) and (iv) shows *cis-trans* isomerism.

54. (d) O_2, F_2 both will stabilise the higher oxidation states but the higher oxidation state of metal with O_2 is more stable because oxygen will gain 2 electrons from metal atom but the fluorine gains only 1 electron leading to the formation of O^{2-}, F^-. The bond between metal and non-metal will be strong when the metal is able to lose more electrons to non metal so the higher oxidation state stabilizes the compound. Hence, statement I is true.

The compounds of xenon fluorides like XeF_2, XeF_4, XeF_6 cannot be explained using valence bond theory because in valence bond theory we take valence electrons into consideration but in compounds of xenon we have lone pair of electrons which affect the shape of a molecule. So, the compounds of xenon are explained by valence shell electron pair repulsion theory. Hence, statement II is true.

55. (d) Given, $k = 4.8 \times 10^{-4} s^{-1}$

Since, it indicates first order reaction,

$$\therefore \quad k = \frac{2.303}{t} \log \frac{a}{a-x}$$

$$4.8 \times 10^{-4} = \frac{2.303}{t} \log \left(\frac{100}{20}\right)$$

$$4.8 \times 10^{-4} = \frac{2.303}{t} \log 5$$

$$t = 3353.7\text{s} = \frac{3353.7}{60} \text{min} = 55.895 \text{min.}$$

$$t \approx 56 \text{min}$$

56. (a) For the given reaction,

$$10Cl^-(aq) + 2MnO_4^-(aq) + 16H^+(aq) \rightleftharpoons 5Cl_2(g) + 2Mn^{2+}(aq) + 8H_2O(l)$$

The number of electrons exchanged $(n) = 10$

From Nernst equation, $E° = \frac{0.059}{n} \log K_C$

$$\therefore K_C = \text{antilog}\left[\frac{nE°}{0.059}\right] = \text{antilog}\left[\frac{10 \times 0.15}{0.059}\right]$$

$$= \text{Antilog } [25.42]$$

57. (c) Na_2CO_3 produces a large number of CO_3^{2-} ions which can precipitate out $MgCO_3$ along with group V cations. Hence, it interferes in the detection of group V cation.

58. (a) The correct match is A-(i), B-(ii), C-(iii), D-(iv).

Metal Complex	Electronic configuration of metal ion		Unpaired electrons
A. $[Cr(H_2O)_6]^{3+}$:	$3d^3 4s^0$	(i)	3
B. $[Fe(H_2O)_6]^{2+}$:	$3d^6 4s^0$	(ii)	4
C. $[Zn(H_2O)_6]^{2+}$:	$3d^{10} 4s^0$	(iii)	0
D. $[Fe(CN)_6]^{3-}$:	$3d^5 4s^0$	(iv)	5

59. (b) In $[Ni(CO)_4]$, Ni is in zero oxidation state Ni(0) has outer electronic configuration $= [Ar]\, 3d^8 4s^2$

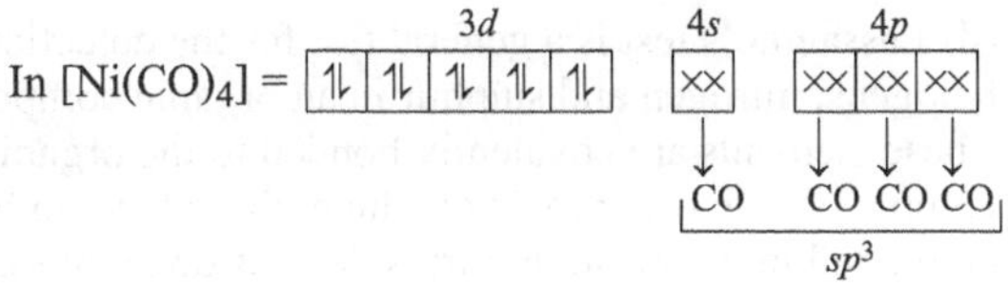

It is sp^3-hybridised.

In $[Ni(CN)_4]^{2-}$, Ni is in +2 oxidation state.

Electronic configuration of $Ni^{2+} = [Ar]3d^8$

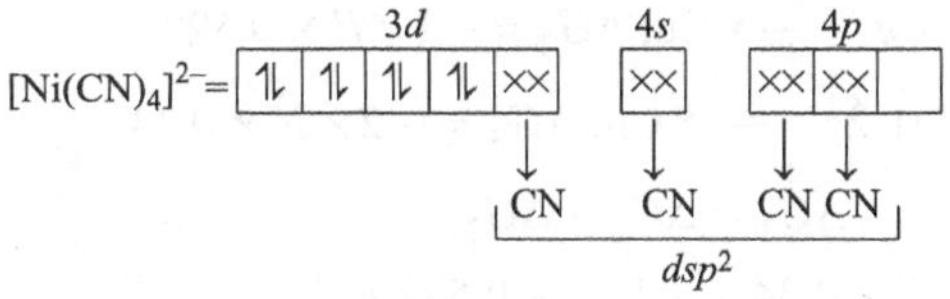

It is dsp^2-hybridised.

In $[NiCl_4]^{2-}$, Ni is in +2 oxidation state.

Electronic configuration of $Ni^{2+} = [Ar]3d^8$

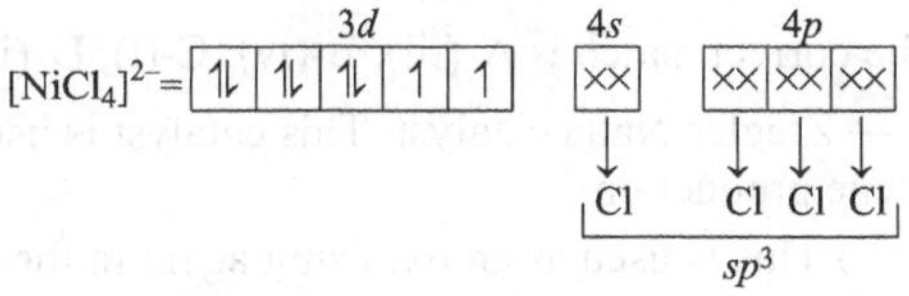

It is sp^3-hybridised.

Problem Solving Tactics

CO and CN are strong field ligands and cause pairing of electrons while Cl is weak field ligand and does not cause pairing.

60. (c) Formation of the compounds are as follows

$$3Fe^{2+} + 2[Fe^{III}(CN)_6]^{2-} \longrightarrow Fe_3^{II}[Fe^{III}(CN)_6]_2$$

Ferrocyanide → (Turnbull's blue)

$$4Fe^{3+} + 3[Fe^{II}(CN)_6]^{4-} \longrightarrow Fe_4^{II}[Fe^{III}(CN)_6]_3$$

(Ferricyanide) → Prussian's blue (Ferriferrocyanide)

61. (b) The correct match is A-IV, B-III, C-I, D-II.

62. (c) According to Heisenberg uncertainty principle

$$\Delta x \cdot m\Delta v = \frac{h}{4\pi}$$

$$\Delta v = \frac{6.6 \times 10^{-34} \times 1000}{4 \times 3.14 \times 2.5 \times 10^{-5}} = 2.1 \times 10^{-27} \text{ m/s}$$

63. (c) Glucose gives silver mirror with ammoniacal silver nitrate because of the presence of —CHO group (aldehyde group) in the structure of glucose.

64. (b) As $P_{total} = P_A^\circ \chi_A + P_B^\circ \chi_B$

$$= 266 \times \frac{2}{2+3} + 236 \times \frac{3}{3+2}$$

$$= 266 \times \frac{2}{5} + 236 \times \frac{3}{5} = 106.4 + 141.6$$

$$= 248 \text{ mm Hg}$$

65. (d) Lassaigne's test is a general test for the detection of halogens, nitrogen and sulphur in an organic compound. These elements are covalently bonded to the organic compounds. In order to detect them, these have to be converted into their ionic forms. This is done by fusing the organic compound with sodium metal.

66. (b) $Cu^{2+} + e^- \longrightarrow Cu^+$;

$$\Delta G_1 = -nFE_1^\circ = -1 \times F \times E_1^\circ$$

$Cu^+ + e^- \longrightarrow Cu$; $\Delta G_2 = -1 \times F \times 0.522$

$Cu^{2+} + 2e^- \longrightarrow Cu$; $\Delta G_3 = -2 \times F \times 0.34$

Now, $\Delta G_3 = \Delta G_1 + \Delta G_2$

$-2 \times F \times 0.34 = -FE_1^\circ - 0.522\,F$

$$E_1^\circ = +0.158\,V$$

67. (a) Among the given statements (a) is incorrect as higher activation energy usually implies a slow reaction.

68. (a) The correct match is A-(iii), B-(iv), C-(i), D-(ii).

$TiCl_4 \rightarrow$ Ziegler-Natta catalyst. This catalyst is used in polythene production.

$PdCl_2 \rightarrow$ This is used as an oxidising agent in the Wacker's process to oxidise alkene to aldehyde.

$PtO_2 \rightarrow$ Adams catalyst. It is used in reduction reactions to convert nitro compounds to amines.

Cu is used in the preparation of $(CH_3)_2SiCl_2$.

69. (c) Dipositive zinc exhibits diamagnetism as its configuration is $[Ar]3d^{10}$ (electrons are removed from outermost shell, i.e. $4s^2$ (from isolated gaseous atom) with no unpaired electron. So, due to the unavailability of the unpaired electron, it shows diamagnetism.

70. (b) The correct match is A-(iv), B-(ii), C-(iii), D-(i).

A. The reaction of aliphatic primary amines with a mixture of sodium nitrite and HCl forms aliphatic alcohols and nitrogen.

$$R'NH_2 \xrightarrow{NaNO_2 + HCl} R'OH + N_2$$

B. The reaction of aniline (aromatic primary amine) with a mixture of sodium nitrite and HCl forms benzene diazonium chloride.This reaction is called diazotisation.

$$PhNH_2 \xrightarrow{NaNO_2 + HCl} Ph{-}N^+{\equiv}NCl^-$$

C. The reaction of N ,N-dimethylaniline (aromatic tertiary amine) with a mixture of sodium nitrite and HCl forms 4-nitroso-N,N-dimethylamine.

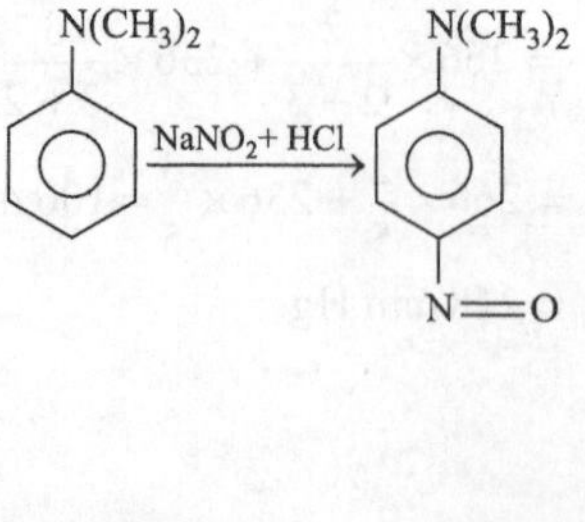

D. The reaction of aliphatic secondary amine with a mixture of sodium nitrite and HCl forms yellow oily N-nitroso amine.

$$RR'NH \xrightarrow{NaNO_2 + HCl} RR'N{-}N{=}O$$

71. (c) 2° halide give both S_N2 and elimination reaction. Here, nucleophile is OH^- ion which is not a bulky group, so it will prefer S_N2. Therefore, P is S_N2 product and Q, R, S are elimination products by E_2 reaction mechanism. An elimination reaction involves the cleavage of two bonds, whereas a substitution reaction requires only one bond to break. Thus, an elimination reaction is more energy-intensive, and it is more likely to occur at higher temperatures.

72. (d) In general, as non-metallic character increases across the period, the acidic character of their oxides increases. Thus, the correct order of acidic strength can be given as

$$Al_2O_3 < SiO_2 < P_2O_3 < SO_2$$

73. (d) When Al is added to potassium hydroxide solution, hydrogen gas is evolved.

$$2Al + 2KOH + 2H_2O \longrightarrow 2KAlO_2 + 3H_2$$

H_2SiF_6 is formed when silica reacts with hydrogen fluoride followed by hydrolysis.

$$SiO_2 \xrightarrow[\text{(ii) Hydrolysis}]{\text{(i) HF}} H_2SiF_6$$

74. (c)

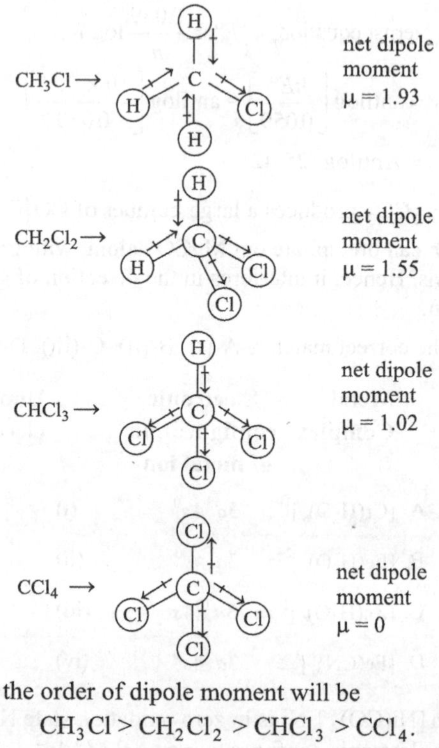

So, the order of dipole moment will be

$$CH_3Cl > CH_2Cl_2 > CHCl_3 > CCl_4.$$

Problem Solving Tactics Dipole moment tells about the charge separation in a molecule. Larger the difference in electronegativity of bonded atoms, larger the dipole moment.

75. (b) Statement I is true but statement II is false.

I. Zinc and copper are transition metals and their ions are generally coloured due to $d-d$ transition of unpaired electron. But in case of Zn^{2+}, $3d$ is completely filled and no unpaired electrons are available for transition. So, light falling on these ions gets completely transmitted and their salts appear white.

However, ion Cu^{2+} ($3d^9$) has 1 unpaired electron. The unpaired electron absorbs particular wavelengths in visible region of light and the transmitted light shows the complementary colour 'blue'.

II. Fluorine has only two orbits. In 2nd orbit, it has $2s^2 2p^5$ configuration with no vacant 'd' orbitals. So it cannot form more than one oxide, i.e. OF_2.

Chlorine, on the other hand, has 3 orbitals in its atoms and $3d$ is lying vacant in it. Therefore it can show variable valency and gives a series of oxides. Like Cl_2O, ClO_2 etc.

76. (a) The reason for higher B—F bond dissociation energy as compared to that of C—F is $p\pi - p\pi$ back bonding in BF_3 molecule, all B—F bonds have partial double bond character whereas such bonding is not possible between C and F in CF_4.

77. (d) In any two substances, the nature and magnitude of the intermolecular forces are not the same.

Hence, the binary solution of two liquids can never form a perfectly ideal solution.

Thus, both statements I and II are correct.

78. (d) For, the reaction

$$2N_2O_5(g) \rightleftharpoons 4NO_2(g) + O_2(g)$$

Rate of reaction

$$= \frac{1}{4}\frac{d[NO_2]}{dt} = \frac{8.5\times10^{-3}}{4\times100}$$

$$= 2.13\times10^{-5}\ Ms^{-1}$$

79. (a) Lyman series hydrogen atom, the shortest wavelength corresponds to : $n_1 = 1$ and $n_2 = \infty$.

$$\frac{1}{\lambda} = RZ^2\left[\frac{1}{n_1^2} - \frac{1}{n_2^2}\right]$$

$$\Rightarrow \quad \frac{1}{A} = R\left[\frac{1}{1^2} - \frac{1}{\infty^2}\right]$$

$$\frac{1}{A} = R \qquad \ldots \text{(i)}$$

For Paschen series of He^+ ion, the longest wavelength corresponds to

$n_1 = 3$ and $n_2 = 4$

$$\frac{1}{\lambda} = RZ^2\left[\frac{1}{n_1^2} - \frac{1}{n_2^2}\right]$$

$$\frac{1}{\lambda} = \frac{1}{A}\times 2^2 \times\left[\frac{1}{3^2} - \frac{1}{4^2}\right]$$

$$\Rightarrow \quad \lambda = \frac{36A}{7}$$

80. (d) As q is a noble gas, p, r and s having atomic number $Z-1, Z+1$ and $Z+2$ should belong to halogen, alkali metal and alkaline earth metal respectively.

As halogen has one electron less than stable noble gas configuration, it has a greater tendency to accept an additional electron forming an anion.

Alkaline earth metal having valence shell configuration ns^2 exists in +2 oxidation state.

81. (b) Hydrolysis of benzene diazonium chloride will give carbolic acid.

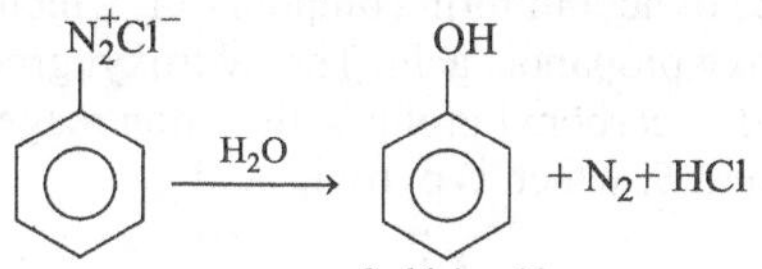

Carbloic acid

82. (c) The ionic product of water is given by

$$[H_3O^+][OH^-] = K_w$$

$$\because \quad [H_3O^+] = [OH^-] = 10^{-6}\ M$$

$$\therefore \quad K_w = 10^{-6}\times10^{-6} = 10^{-12}\ M^2$$

83. (a)

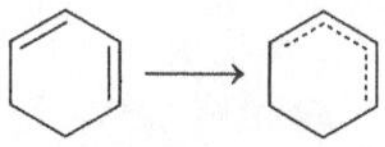

Among the given compounds (a) is the most stable compound as it is a conjugated diene.

Problem Solving Tactics Conjugated dienes are more stable than non-conjugated dienes (both isolated and cumulated) due to factors such as delocalisation of charge through resonance and hybridisation energy.

84. (a) *Tert*-butyl chloride forms most stable 3° carbocation, hence will give white precipitate of AgCl with $AgNO_3$ solution immediately.

85. (c) The correct match is A-(iv), B-(iii), C-(i), D-(ii).

(A) Oxidation of CH_3COCHO.

$$CH_3-\overset{O}{\overset{\|}{C}}-\overset{O}{\overset{\|}{C}}-H \xrightarrow{HIO_4} CH_3COOH + HCOOH$$

(B) Oxidation of 1, 2-cyclohexanedione.

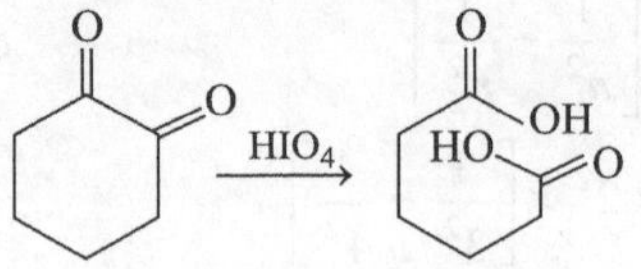

or $HOOC(CH_2)_4COOH$

(C) Oxidation of PhCH(OH)CHO

$Ph—CH(OH)—CHO \xrightarrow{HIO_4} PhCHO + HCOOH$

(D) Oxidation of $CH_3CH_2CH(OH)COCH_3$

$CH_3—CH_2—CH(OH)—C(=O)—CH_3 \xrightarrow{HIO_4}$

$CH_3CH_2CHO + CH_3COOH$

86. (c) Treatment of acetaldehyde with sodium cyanide in the presence of HCl gives acetaldehyde cyanohydrin. This is followed by hydrolysis of cyano group in the presence of acid to form compound *A*, which is 2-hydroxy propanoic acid. The hydroxyl group is then oxidised to carbonyl group with fenton reagent to obtain compound *B*, which is pyruvic acid.

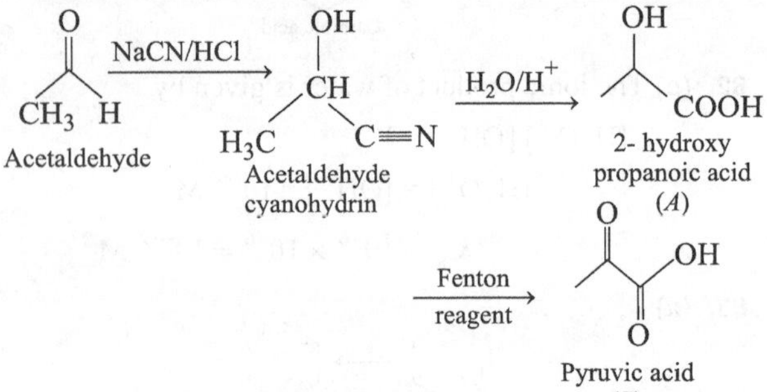

87. (b) Sodium acetylide is a nucleophile which attacks on electrophilic carbons like carbonyl carbons followed by protonation in acidic medium.

Sodium acetylide $\Rightarrow \overset{+}{Na}\overset{-}{C}\equiv CH$

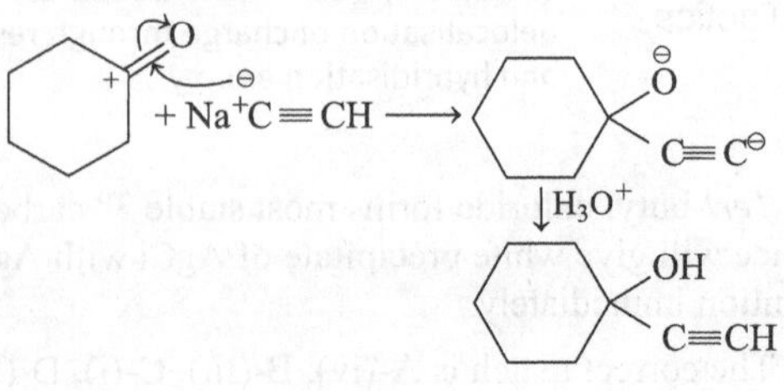

88. (b) As the molecular weight increases, non-polar part increases and solubility decreases. So, statement I is correct. Statement II is incorrect because hydrogen bonding is not affected by an increase in the non-polar part.

89. (c) In an aprotic solvent, the increasing order for the nucleophilicity of the halide ions is iodide < bromide < chloride < flouride.

A polar aprotic solvent does not form hydrogen bond with nucleophiles to a significant extent, meaning that the nucleophiles have greater freedom in solution. Under these conditions, nucleophilicity correlates well with basicity and fluoride ion, being the most unstable of the halide ions, reacts fastest with electrophiles.

90. (b) $\Delta T_f = i \times K_f \times m \Rightarrow 0.0054 = i \times 1.80 \times 0.001$

The van't Hoff factor, $i = 3$

This suggests that 1 molecule of $[Pt(NH_3)_4Cl_4]$ dissociates in solution to produce 3 ions. Hence, the correct formula of the complex is $[Pt(NH_3)_4Cl_2]Cl_2$

$[Pt(NH_3)_4Cl_2]Cl_2 \longrightarrow [Pt(NH_3)_4Cl_2]^{2+} + 2Cl^-$

Problem Solving Tactics All the salts and complexes which can form ions upon the dissolution in the solvent can give abnormal molar masses and this is due to their dissociation into ions.

Biology

91. (a) The strategy used was based on the process of RNA interference which involves silencing of specific *m*RNA of nematode. In RNA silencing, sense and antisense RNA in the host are complementary to each other and form double-stranded RNA. This *ds*RNA prevents translation of *m*RNA and hence prevent the infection.

92. (b) The vasa efferentia (10-12 in number) arise from testes and enter kidneys on their side and open into bidder's canal.

93. (b) The correct matches are A-4, B-1, C-2, D-3.

Deoxyribonucleoside triphosphate act as substrates and provide energy for polymerisation reaction. DNA helicase unwinds the DNA double helix by breaking the hydrogen bonds between two strands at the replicating fork.

NHC proteins or Non-Histone Chromosomal proteins are a set of proteins required for chromatin packaging. UTRs or Untranslated Regions are required for efficient translation process.

94. (a) When we conserve and protect the whole ecosystem, its biodiversity at all level is protected. For example, we save the entire forest to save the tiger this approach is called *in situ* conservation.

95. (b) Both A and R are true, and R is not the correct explanation A.

DNA polymorphism used to develop the DNA fingerprinting technology is based on variation in the number of tandemly repeated sequence.

96. (b) Both A and R are true and R is the correct explanation of A. The trophic level represents a functional level, not a species as such. This is because, a given species may occupy more than one trophic level in the same ecosystem at the same time.

97. (c) The technique of genetic engineering includes the formation of a recombinant DNA, which allows the introduction of a desirable foreign gene into the host plasmid by using the restriction enzyme and ligase.

98. (d) In lungs, the separation of air from venous body occurs through diffusion membrane which is made of squamous epithelium and endothelium of the blood vessels.

99. (b) Both statement I and statement II are correct.

Krebs' cycle is also called the citric acid cycle which has series of eight reactions, i.e. oxidative decarboxylation, oxidation, hydration, dehydration, etc. to oxidise one molecule of acetyl Co-A.

Each turn of Krebs' cycle produces 1 ATP, 3 NADH and 1 $FADH_2$ molecules, which is used for the process of cellular respiration to occur and produce energy.

100. (c) *Cedrus* is an example of gymnosperms. In these plants, male and female gametophytes do not have an independent free living existence.

101. (b) The correct matches are A-3, B-1, C-4, D-2.
- Hashish is a cannabinoid. It is obtained from the resinous exudate, from the flowering top of female plants.
- Ganja is obtained from dried unfertilised female inflorescence of *Cannabis*.
- Marijuana is obtained from dried flower and top leaves of female *Cannabis* plant.
- Bhang is obtained from dried leaves and flowering shoots of both male and female plants of *Cannabis*.

102. (a) The anaphase-II of meiosis-II begins with the simultaneous splitting of the centromere of each chromosome allowing them to move towards opposite poles of the cell by shortening of microtubules attached to kinetochores.

103. (b) Smack also known as heroine is chemically diacetylmorphine as it is obtained by the acetylation of morphine. It is extracted from the latex of *Papaver somniferum*.

104. (b) Statement in option (b) is incorrect and can be corrected as

The inter-cellular material of cartilage is solid and pliable. Rest all the statements are correct.

105. (b) The correct matches are A-2, B-1, C-4, D-3.
- Natality refers to the number of births during a given period in the population that are added to the initial density.
- Mortality is the number of deaths in the population during a given period.
- Immigration is the number of individuals of the same species that have come into the habitat from elsewhere during the time period under consideration.
- Emigration is the number of individuals of the population who left the habitat and gone elsewhere during the time period under consideration.

106. (d) Statement I is correct, but statement II is incorrect and can be corrected as

Receptors associated with aortic arch and carotid artery can recognise changes in CO_2 and H^+ concentration and send signals to the rhythm centre for remedial actions.

107. (a) Statements I, II and III are correct whereas, statement IV is incorrect and can be corrected as
Miller identified and crystalised the cytokinesis promoting active substance and termed them as kinetin.

108. (a) Statement I is incorrect, but statement II is correct.
Incorrect statement can be corrected as
Sexual spores are called ascospores, which are produced endogenously in sac like asci whereas the asexual spores are conidia which are produced exogenously on the special mycelium called conidiophore.

109. (a) The genetic defect adenosine deaminase (ADA) deficiency may be cured permanently by introducing bone marrow cells producing ADA into cells at an early embryonic stages.

110. (b) A structure that connects the cytoplasm of neighbouring cells, is called plasmodesmata and the another structure which holds or glues the different neighbouring cells together is middle lamella.

111. (b) *ori* is responsible for controlling the copy number of the linked DNA in plasmid.
It is a sequence from where DNA replication starts. Any piece of DNA when linked to it, can be made to replicate within the host cells.

112. (b) The correct matches are A-2, B-3, C-1, D-4.
- PCR is the procedure used to amplify gene of interest.
- *Taq* polymerase is extracted from the bacterium *Thermus aquaticus*.
- *Eco*RI is a type of restriction endonuclease that cleaves DNA into smaller fragments by making cuts at specific sites.
- In recombinant DNA technology, during isolation of DNA, purified DNA is precipitated using chilled ethanol.

113. (c) Vascularisation in plants occur through differentiation of procambium followed by the development of xylem and the phloem tissue.

114. (d) Statement I is correct, but statement II is incorrect and can be corrected as
The cardiac muscles are striated in appearance and involuntary in nature as the nervous system does not control their activity directly.

115. (d) All the statements are correct, except statement V and it can be corrected as
There are four proteins complexes, i.e. complex I-IV in the electron transfer chain, which are involved in moving electrons from NADH and $FADH_2$ to molecular oxygen. Complex-I accepts electrons and H^+ from NADH while complex-II accepts from $FADH_2$.

116. (d) Death rate refers to the number of deaths per thousand per year. It can be calculated as

$$\text{Rate} = \frac{\text{change in population}}{\text{original population}}$$

$$\Rightarrow \frac{40-36}{40}$$

$$\Rightarrow \frac{4}{40}$$

$$\Rightarrow \frac{1}{10} = 0.1 \text{ individual per fruit flies per week}$$

117. (d) Statement I is correct, but statement II is incorrect. It can be corrected as
The pili are elongated tubular structures made of a special protein. The fimbrae are small bristle like fibres sprouting out of the cell.

118. (a) Statements I, III and V are correct while the rest of the statements are incorrect. The incorrect statements can be corrected as
Parapodia helps in swimming. It is the characteristic feature of members of phylum–Annelida like *Nereis, Pheretima*, etc.
The flame cells are responsible for excretion in members of Platyhelminthes e.g. *Planaria*.

119. (b) The tangential as well as radial walls of the endodermal cells have a deposition of water-impermeable, waxy material-suberin, in the form of casparian strips.

120. (a) In competitive inhibition of enzymatic catalysis, binding of an inhibitor to active site prevents binding of the specific substrate. This inhibition can be reversed by increasing the substrate concentration in the reaction.

121. (b) Statement in option (b) is correct. Some harmful mutations are not eliminated from the gene pool because they are probably recessive and carried in a heterozygous state and, cannot be detected by selection. Though these are harmful, but they might not contribute to reducing the fitness as they are in recessive state.

122. (b) Gross production will have the highest value in a grassland ecosystem as the producers, (grass) will be in abundance. GPP of an ecosystem is the rate of production of organic matter during photosynthesis, while NPP = GPP–R.

123. (a) The correct matches are A-2, B-3, C-4, D-1.
- Sporophylls in pteridophytes form distinct compact structures called strobili or cones.
- *Sphagnum* is a moss that provide peat that have been long used as a fuel.
- Gemma are green, multicellular, asexual buds, which develop in small receptacles called gemma cups located in thalli.
- Protonema stage is the first stage of mosses' life cycle.

124. (b) Vasopressin is mainly responsible for facultative reabsorption of water from DCT. It maintains the blood volume by retaining the water by kidney during dehydration.

125. (d) The statements III and V are correct. Rest statements are incorrect and can be corrected as
- Embryo develops at the micropylar end of the embryo sac where the zygote is situated.
- The portion of embryonal axis above the level of cotyledons is epicotyl, which terminates with the plumule.
- In some seeds like black pepper and beet, remnants of nucellus are persistent. This is called perisperm.

126. (d) A is true, but R is false. R can be corrected as
The assembly of more than one polypeptides as individual subunit functioning together represents the quaternary structure of protein.

127. (a) Statement I is incorrect, but statement II is correct. Incorrect statement can be corrected as
Sewage contain large amounts of organic matter and microbes. Many of these are pathogenic.

128. (b) $2(C_{51}H_{98}O_6) + 145\,O_2 \rightarrow 102\,CO_2 + 98\,H_2O + \text{Energy}$

$$RQ = \frac{\text{Volume of } CO_2 \text{ evolved}}{\text{Volume of } O_2 \text{ consumed}} = \frac{102\,CO_2}{145\,O_2}$$

$$= \frac{102\,CO_2}{145\,O_2} = 0.7$$

129. (d) Vexillary aestivation is found in pea and bean flowers. In this, there are five petals, the largest one overlaps the two lateral petals, which in turn overlaps the two smallest anterior petals.

130. (b) When a neuron is not conducting any impulse, i.e. resting, the axonal membrane is comparatively more permeable to potassium ions (K^+) and nearly impermeable to sodium ions (Na^+).

131. (d) Statement I is correct, but statement II is incorrect. It can be corrected as

The plumule is enclosed in a sheath, which is called coleoptile whereas coleorrhiza is a sheath which encloses the radicle.

132. (c) Both A and R are true, but R is not the correct explanation of A.

Hemichordates was earlier considered as sub-phylum under Chordata, but now it is placed as separated phylum under Non-chordata. They have a rudimentary structure in the collar region called stomochord, a structure similar to notochord.
Hemichordates have open type of circulatory system and show indirect development.

133. (b) The flowers of Malvaceae family are bisexual, bracteate, actinomorphic, hypogynous and completely pentamerous, e.g. cotton.

134. (d) HH Cousins confirmed the release of a volatile substance which was identified as ethylene, a gaseous plant growth hormone.

135. (a) Match pair in option (a) is correct.

MSH is the only hormone secreted by the intermediate lobe of pituitary, i.e. pars intermedia. It aids in the distribution of melanin granules so that skin colour darkens. Incorrect matched pairs can be corrected as

- STH (Somato Tropin Hormone) is also called growth hormone.
- ACTH (Adreno Cortico Tropic Hormone) regulates release of cortisol.
  FSH (Follicle Stimulating Hormone) is responsible for growth and development of ovarian follicle.

136. (b) A neural signal reaching neuromuscular junction releases a neurotransmitter which generates an action potential in the sarcolemma.
This spread through the muscle fibre and cause the release of calcium ions into the sarcoplasm.

Increase in Ca^{++} level leads to the binding of calcium with a subunit of troponin or actin filaments and there by remove the masking of active sites for myosin.
Utilising the energy from ATP hydrolysis, the myosin head binds to the exposed active sites on actin to form a cross bridge

137. (c) The stroma lamellae membranes lack PS-II as well as NADP reductase enzyme. So, the excited electron does not pass on to $NADP^+$, but is cycled back to the PS-I complex through the ETC.

138. (a) Statement in option (a) is correct for protein synthesis as

The ribosome consist of structural RNA. In its inactive state, it exists as two subunit, a large subunit and a small subunit. When the small subunit encounters an *m*RNA, the translation of the *m*RNA to proteins begins.
Other statements are incorrect and can be corrected as

- Peptidase catalyse breaking of peptide bond.
- UTRs are present before the strart and after stop codons.
- At the end of translation release factor binds to stop condon.

139. (c) Match pair represented by option (c) is incorrect and can be corrected as
QRS wave represents the depolarisation of the ventricles which initiates the ventricular contraction. The contraction starts slowly after Q and marks the beginning of the systole.

140. (a) Electrons from excited chlorophyll of PS-II are first accepted by quinone or plastoquinone. Other options can explained as
Ferredoxin functions as an electron carrier.
Cytochrome-*b* and *f* are the part of the electron transport chain.

141. (b) The given figure represents anaphase - I of meiosis - I.
In this phase, the homologous chromosomes separate, while sister chromatids remain associated at their centromeres.

142. (a) First child of a normal couple is having sickle-cell anaemia. It is autosomal linked recessive disease. Then the genotype of parent can be

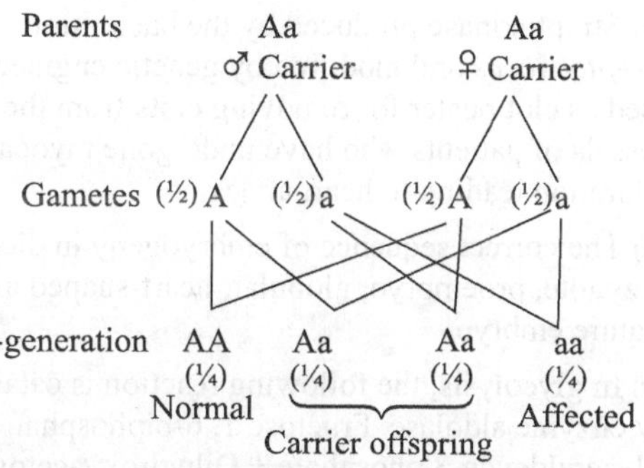

Thus, the 25% offspring will be affected.

143. (c) Pericycle located next to endodermis, is a few layers of thick-walled parenchymatous cells. Initiation of lateral roots and vascular cambium during secondary growth takes place in these cells.

144. (b) *E.coli* with mutated z gene of *lac* operon cannot grow in medium containing only lactose as the source of energy because they cannot synthesise functional beta galactosidase. It is responsible for the hydrolysis of the disaccharide, lactose into its monomeric units galactose and glucose.

145. (a) Convergent evolution refers to the formation of similar traits by unrelated groups of organisms . Tasmanian wolf is a marsupial while wolf is a placental mammal. This shows convergent evolution. They are distantly related and occupy similar natural surroundings, frequently grow autonomously similar morphological characters that make them appear to be similar.

146. (d) Lactic acid fermentation, alcoholic fermentation and aerobic respiration are the three major ways in which different cells handle pyruvic acid produced by glycolysis.
Glucose oxidation is not a part of the process.

147. (b) Water is a regular mode of transport for the male gametes among the lower plant groups such as algae, bryophytes and pteridophytes.

148. (d) A is true, but R is false. It can be corrected as Placenta facilitate the supply of oxygen and nutrients to the embryo. Along with this it also acts as endocrine tissue as it produces hormones like hCG, hPL, progesterons, oestrogen, etc. Oxytocin is released by hypothalamus.

149. (d) The type of placentation where the ovules are attached to the base of the ovary is called basal placentation, e.g. marigold and maize.

Pea shows marginal placentation, where as tomato shows axile type of placentation.

Mustard shows parietal placentation.

150. (d) Streptokinase produced by the bacterium *Streptococcus* and modified by genetic engineering is used as clot buster for removing clots from the blood vessels of patients who have undergone myocardial infarction leading to heart attack.

151. (a) The correct sequence of embryogeny in dicot seed is zygote, proembryo, globular, heart-shaped and mature embryo.

152. (c) In glycolysis, the following reaction is catalysed by enzyme aldolase. Fructose 1, 6-biphosphate $\rightarrow$ Glyceraldeyde-3 phosphate + Dihydroxyacetone phosphate. The 6 carbon molecule is splitted into two 3-carbon molecules-one G3P, another DHAP that is converted into G3P in another reaction.

153. (c) The inner glandular layer called endometrium lines the uterine cavity. This layer undergoes cyclical changes during the menstrual cycle.

154. (d) Match pair in option (d) is incorrect, while rest are correct. The incorrect match can be corrected as

The body surface is distinctly marked out into segments or metameres in the members of phylum–Annelida, e.g. *Nereis, Pheretima*, etc.

155. (b) Both statement I and statement II are correct.

A flower is considered as a modified shoot. Each plant bears flower on shoot in a specific arrangement. The arrangement of flowers on shoot is called inflorescence. Shoot bears flowers when its apical meristem changes into floral meristem.

156. (d) Statement I is correct, but statement II is incorrect and can be corrected as

Louis Pasteur experiment demonstrated that life comes only from pre-existing life, which was a drawback to the theory of spontaneous generation.

157. (d) In assisted reproductive technology after *in vitro* fertilisation, the zygote or early embryo (up to 8 blastomeres) is then transfered into the Fallopian tube. This technique is named as Zygote Intra Fallopian Transfer (ZIFT).

158. (a) The correct matches are A-1, B-2, C-3, D-4.

All living members of the class Cyclostomata are ectoparasites on some fishes. Chondrichthyes and Osteichthyes have cartilaginous and bony endoskeletons, respectively. Most of amphibians have two pairs of limbs.

159. (a) Recombinant DNA technology can be accomplished only if we have the key tools, i.e. restriction enzymes, polymerase enzyme, ligases and vectors. Restriction enzymes are molecular scissors that cut the DNA. Ligase is used as molecular glue to facilitate joining of DNA strands together. DNA polymerase is responsible for forming new copies of DNA in the form of nucleic acid molecules. Vectors act as vehicles of DNA transfer.

160. (b) Statement in option (b) is incorrect and can be corrected as
Enzymes isolated from thermophillic organism are highly stable at high temperature and retain their catalytic power even at temperatures upto 80°-90°C.

161. (b) Spleen is a large bean-shaped organ that mainly contains lymphocytes and phagocytes. It acts as a filter of the blood by trapping blood-borne microorganisms.

162. (d) The significance of the 'heat shock' in bacterial transformation is to facilitate uptake of DNA through pores in the bacterial cell membrane.

In this method bivalent cation like Ca^{2+} is used, which causes greater transient pores in the cell wall, allowing the uptake of foreign DNA.

163. (b) The correct matches are A-2, B-1, C-3, D-4.

- Hypothalamus contains several groups of neurosecretory cells, which produce hormones.
- Neurohypophysis also known as posterior pituitary stores and release oxytocin.
- LH and FSH stimulate gonadal activity and hence are called gonadotropin.
- Somatostatin inhibits the release of growth hormone.

164. (b) Darwin's theory of natural selection did not encompass the role of genetic variation between individuals produced due to genomic mutation.

165. (d) Statements I, III and IV are correct and statement II is incorrect. It can be corrected as

- The genetic material found in the members of kingdom–Monera is without nuclear membrane.

166. (c) Statements II, IV and V are incorrect and can be corrected as

- Each seminiferous tubule is lined on its inside by two type of cells called male germ cells and Sertoli cells. The Sertoli cells are supporting cells.
- The seminiferous tubules of the testis open into the vasa efferentia through rete testis.
- The regions outside the seminiferous tubules called interstitial spaces, contain small blood vessels and interstitial cells or Leydig cells. These synthesise and secrete testicular hormones called androgens.

167. (c) Match pair in option (c) is incorrect and it can be corrected as ; Meselson and Stahl first demonstrated the semi-conservation nature of DNA replication.

168. (d) Statement in option (d) is incorrect and can be corrected as

In insects the mechanism of sex determination is of the XO type, i.e. all eggs bear an additional X-chromosome besides the other chromosomes. On the other hand, some sperms bear the X-chromosome whereas some do not.

169. (d) The packaging of chromatin at higher level requires an additional set of proteins that are collectively called non-histone proteins.

170. (d) Flagellum contains an axoneme of a peripheral doublet fibrils and 2 central singlet fibrils. This arrangement is called 9+2 or 11 strands. A centriole possesses a whorl of nine peripheral fibrils. These fibrils are absent in the centre. The arrangement is therefore, called 9+0.

171. (c) The correct matches are A-4, B-1, C-2, D-3.

- Louis Pasteur is known as the father of bacteriology.
- Reserved food in bacteria is in the form of lipids and glycogen.
- Surface of envelope in case of viruses can be smooth or have outgrowths called spikes. These aid in attachment of virus to host surface.
- Viroids are small, circular, single-stranded RNA molecules that are considered as the smallest known pathogens.

172. (b) By the process of leaching, water soluble inorganic nutrients go down into the soil horizon and get precipitated as unavailable salts.

173. (d) Only statement in option (d) is correct. Rest are incorrect statements and can be corrected as

The technique of DNA fingerprinting was developed by Sir Alec Jeffreys. This technique is used to identify a person's identity on the basis of their DNA specificity. The satellite DNA forms the minor peak, while the bulk DNA forms the major peak.

174. (d) Statements I, II, III and IV are correct whereas statement V is incorrect and can be corrected as

Methyl guanosine triphosphate is added at 5′ end of hnRNA in the process of capping.

175. (b) In the given figure *A*, *B*, *C* and *D* represent the following

A- Micropyle   *B* - Inner integument
C - Funicle   *D* - Hilum

The function of funicle is to attach ovule to the placenta of the plant.

176. (c) Both A and R are true, but R is not the correct explanation of A.

The term biodiversity describes the combined diversity at all the levels of biological organisation.

It ranges from macromolecules within cells to biomes.

177. (b) Plants like mint and jasmine fulfill the given conditions. Here, a slender lateral branch arises from the base of the main axis and after growing aerially for some time arch downwards to touch the ground.

178. (b) In frogs, the lungs are a pair of elongated, pink-coloured sac-like structures present in the upper part of the trunk region (thorax).

179. (a) The correct matches are A-2, B-4, C-1, D-3.

- *Homo sapiens*, common name-man, belongs to order–Primata.
- *Musca domestica*, common name-housefly, belongs to order-Diptera.
- *Mangifera indica*, common name-mango, belongs to order-Sapindales.
- *Triticum aestivum,* common name-wheat, belongs to order-Poales.

180. (a) Statements II and III are incorrect and can be corrected as Synergids are specialised cells lying adjacent to the egg cell. They secrete chemotactic substance for attraction of pollen tube during fertilisation. Synergids form a highly thickened structure called filiform apparatus towards the micropylar pole.

SECTION II
Mastery Builders

PRACTICE SET 5

Maximum Marks : 720	Time : 3 hrs	No. of Questions : 180

Instructions

1. This question paper contains **180** multiple-choice questions (four options with a single correct answer) from **Physics, Chemistry** and **Biology**.
2. These questions are distributed as 45 questions, each from Physics and Chemistry and 90 questions in Biology. These are to be compulsorily attempted by the candidate.
3. Each question carries 4 marks. For each correct response, the candidate will get 4 marks. For each incorrect response, one mark will be deducted from the total scores.

PHYSICS

1. In the cyclic process shown in the p - V diagram, magnitude of the work done is found to be $\frac{\pi p_0 V_0}{m}$, then the value of m is

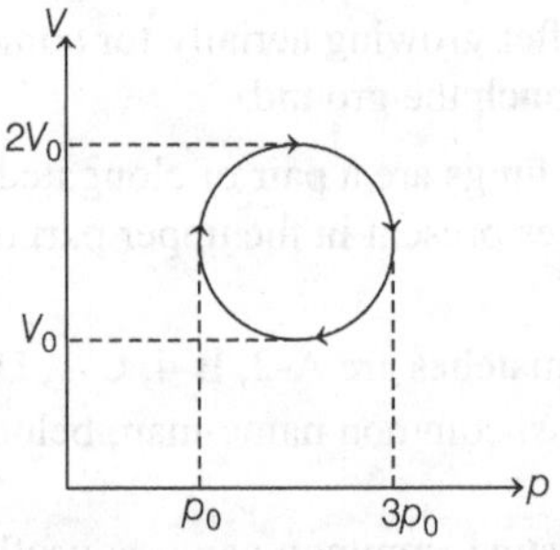

(a) 1 (b) 2 (c) 3 (d) 4

2. A ball of mass 2 kg moving with a speed of 100 ms^{-1} strikes a wall at an angle of 30°. The ball rebounds at the same speed and same angle and remains in contact with the wall for 0.4 s, then the force exerted by the ball on the wall is

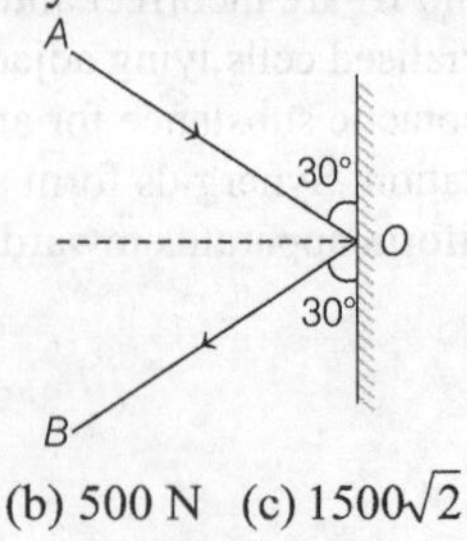

(a) 1500 N (b) 500 N (c) $1500\sqrt{2}$ N (d) 700 N

3. In the following arrangement as shown in figure, the magnetic field at O is given by

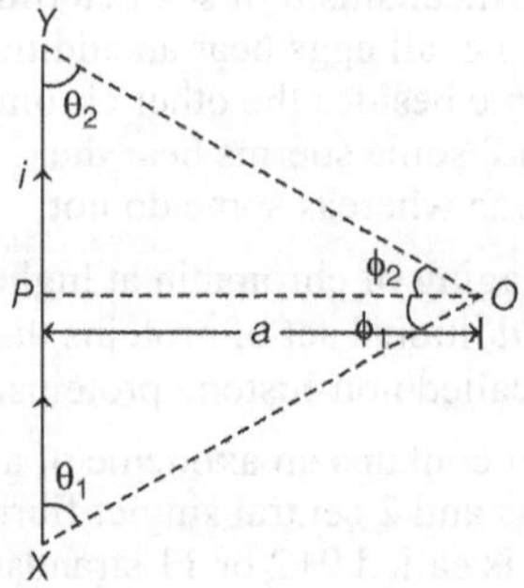

(a) $\frac{\mu_0}{4\pi} \cdot \frac{i}{a} (\cos \theta_1 + \cos \theta_2)$

(b) $\frac{\mu_0}{4\pi} \cdot \frac{i}{a} (\sin \phi_1 + \sin \phi_2)$

(c) Both (a) and (b)

(d) None of the above

4. A ray of light passes from a glass of refractive index 1.6 to air. The angle of incidence for which the angle of refraction is twice the angle of incidence is given by

(a) $\sin^{-1}\left(\frac{2}{5}\right)$ (b) $\sin^{-1}\left(\frac{3}{5}\right)$

(c) $\sin^{-1}\left(\frac{5}{8}\right)$ (d) $\sin^{-1}\left(\frac{4}{5}\right)$

5. Ratio of minimum kinetic energies of two projectiles of same mass is 4 : 1. The ratio of the maximum height attained by them is also 4 : 1. The ratio of their ranges would be

(a) 16 : 1 (b) 4 : 1
(c) 8 : 1 (d) 2 : 1

6. A ball is thrown up with a speed of half the escape velocity from earth's surface. It reaches to the height h above the earth's surface. If the radius of the earth is R, then the ratio of $\frac{h}{R}$ is given by

(a) $\frac{1}{2}$ (b) $\frac{1}{3}$ (c) 2 (d) 3

7. In a biprism experiment, fringes are obtained on the screen at a distance of 2 m from the source, when a monochromatic light of wavelength 400 nm used. When a convex lens is placed between the source and screen, images of the slits in two position 0.03 mm and 0.12 mm respectively, then fringe width on the screen will be

(a) 0.0013 mm (b) 13.3 mm
(c) 0.013 m (d) 1.33 mm

8. A metal rod having a coefficient of linear expansion of 2×10^{-5}/°C has a length of 100 cm at 20°C. The temperature at which it is shortened by 1 mm is

(a) – 40°C (b) – 30°C
(c) – 20°C (d) – 10°C

9. An insulated box containing a diatomic gas of molar mass M moving with a speed v_0 is suddenly stopped. The increase in gas temperature as a result of stopping the box is

(a) zero (b) $\frac{Mv_0^2}{2R}$ (c) $\frac{Mv_0^2}{3R}$ (d) $\frac{Mv_0^2}{5R}$

10. The radius of the first permitted Bohr orbit for the electron in a hydrogen atom equals 0.53 Å and its ground state energy equals –13.6 eV. If the electron in the hydrogen atom is replaced by muon (μ^-) [charge same as electron and mass 207 m_e], then the first Bohr radius and ground state energy will be

(a) 0.53×10^{-13} m, –3.6 eV (b) 25.6×10^{-13} m, –2.8 eV
(c) 2.56×10^{-13} m, –2.8 keV (d) 2.56×10^{-13} m, –13.6 eV

11. The coordinates of a moving particle at any time t are given by $x=\alpha t^3$ and $y=\beta t^3$. The speed of the particle at time t is given by

(a) $\sqrt{\alpha^2+\beta^2}$ (b) $3t\sqrt{\alpha^2+\beta^2}$
(c) $3t^2\sqrt{\alpha^2+\beta^2}$ (d) $t^2\sqrt{\alpha^2+\beta^2}$

12. In which of the following case of spherical lenses (as shown in the figure), the emergent ray is parallel to incident ray ?

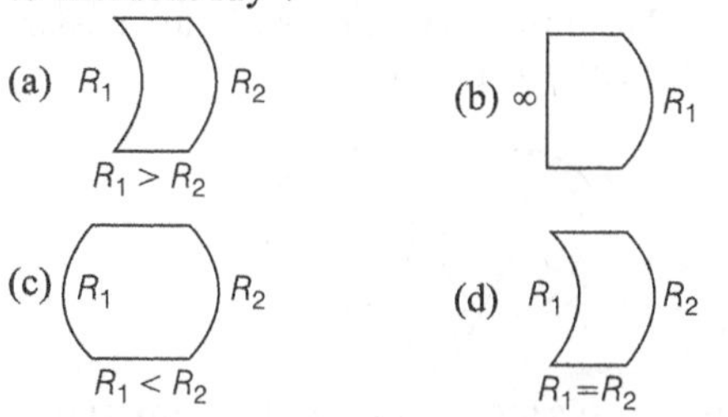

13. A conducting ring of mass 2 kg and radius 0.5 m is placed on a horizontal plane with current 4A. A magnetic field of 10 T is switched on horizontally at $t=0$. The initial angular acceleration of the ring will be

(a) 40π rad/s^2 (b) 15π rad/s^2
(c) 20π rad/s^2 (d) 10π rad/s^2

14. A charge of q μC is placed at the centre of the line joining two exactly equal positive charges of 60 μC. The system of the three charges will be in equilibrium, if the value of charge q is

(a) 45 μC (b) 60 μC (c) 15 μC (d) –15μC

15. A body of mass 4 kg moves in one direction in the presence of a force described by the potential energy graph. If the body is released from rest at $x=2$ m, then its speed when it crosses $x=6$ m is.

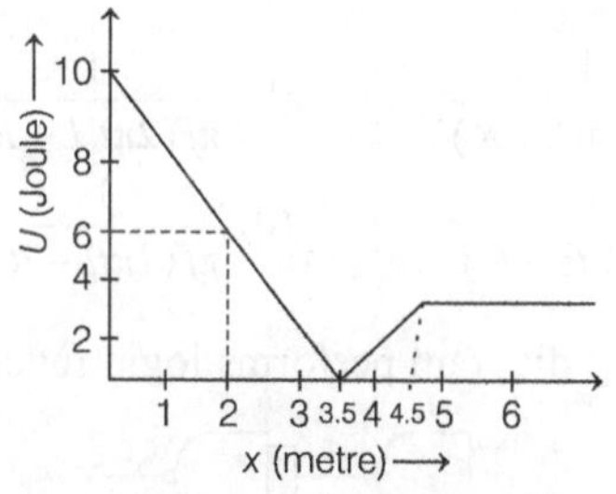

(a) 2 m/s (b) $\frac{1}{\sqrt{2}}$ m/s (c) $\sqrt{2}$ m/s (d) $\frac{1}{2}$ m/s

16. Given below are two statements

Statement I Electromagnetic waves are self-sustaining oscillations of electric and magnetic fields in free space or vacuum.

Statement II No material medium is involved in the vibrations of the electric and magnetic fields.

In the light of above statements, choose the correct option given below

(a) Both Statement I and Statement II are incorrect.
(b) Both Statement I and Statement II are correct.
(c) Statement I is correct but Statement II is incorrect.
(d) Statement I is incorrect but Statement II is correct.

17. Two thin discs of radius R and mass M are attached to each other as shown in the figure. The rotational moment of inertia of this body about its axis perpendicular to the plane of disc B and passing through its centre is given by

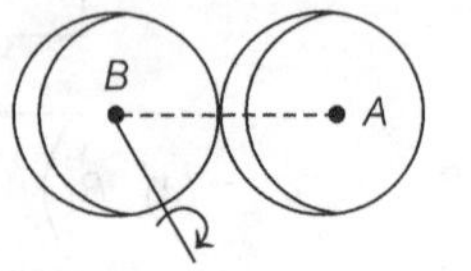

(a) $2MR^2$ (b) $3MR^2$ (c) $4MR^2$ (d) $5MR^2$

18. An experiment is performed to find the refractive index of glass using a travelling microscope. In this experiment, distances are measured by
(a) a vernier scale provided on the microscope
(b) a standard laboratory scale
(c) a meter scale provided on the microscope
(d) a screw gauge provided on the microscope

19. An electric dipole is placed in a uniform electric field, then its potential energy will be minimum, when the angle between its axis and direction of electric field is
(a) $\frac{\pi}{2}$ (b) π (c) $\frac{\pi}{4}$ (d) zero

20. R, L and C are connected in series in a circuit with an AC voltage source of frequency f. The current in the circuit leads the voltage by 45°. The value of C will be
(a) $\frac{1}{2\pi f(2\pi fL+R)}$ (b) $\frac{1}{\pi f(2\pi f L+R)}$
(c) $\frac{1}{2\pi f(2\pi fL-R)}$ (d) $\frac{1}{\pi f(2\pi fL-R)}$

21. Following diagram performs logic function of

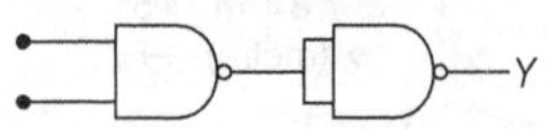

(a) AND gate (b) NAND gate
(c) NOR gate (d) OR gate

22. A block shown in figure slides on a semi-circular frictionless track. If it starts from rest at position A, what is its speed at the point B ?

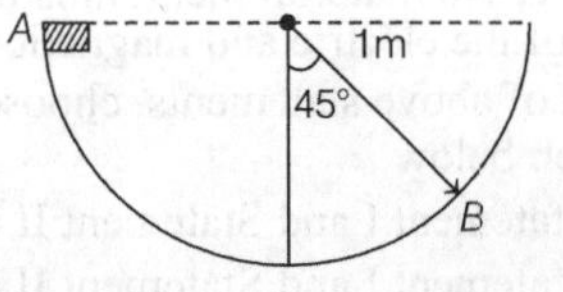

(a) 3 ms^{-1} (b) 3.5 ms^{-1}
(c) 3.76 ms^{-1} (d) 2.75 ms^{-1}

23. A set of n identical resistors, each of resistance $R\ \Omega$, when connected in series have an effective resistance of $A\ \Omega$ and when connected in parallel, the effective resistance is $B\ \Omega$, then the value of R is
(a) $\sqrt{AB}$ (b) AB
(c) $\sqrt{\frac{A^2-B^2}{A^2}}$ (d) $\sqrt{\frac{A^2+B^2}{B^2}}$

24. The total charge induced in a conducting loop, when it is moved in magnetic field depends on
(a) the rate of change of magnetic flux
(b) initial magnetic flux only
(c) the total change in magnetic flux
(d) final magnetic flux only

25. The dimensional formula of $\frac{LI^2}{CV^2}$ is [where, L = inductance, C = capacitance, I = current, V = voltage]
(a) $[M^2L^2T^{-2}A^1]$ (b) $[M^0L^0T^{-3}A^{-2}]$
(c) $[M^0L^0T^0A^0]$ (d) $[M^1L^0T^{-3}A^1]$

26. If loop A of radius $r << R$ moves towards loop B with a constant velocity v in such a way that their planes are always parallel, the distance between the two loops is x, then induced emf in loop A is maximum when x will be

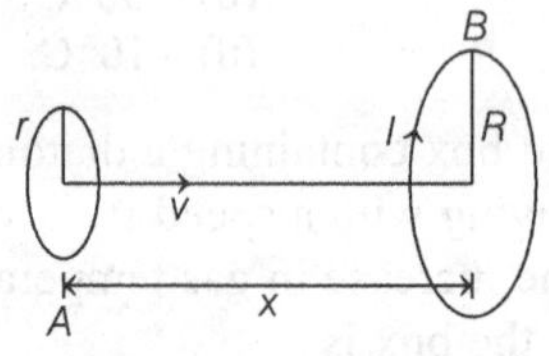

(a) $R/\sqrt{2}$ (b) $R/2$ (c) $2R$ (d) $\sqrt{2}R$

27. In the given circuit, current through the zener diode of breakdown voltage of 12 V, is

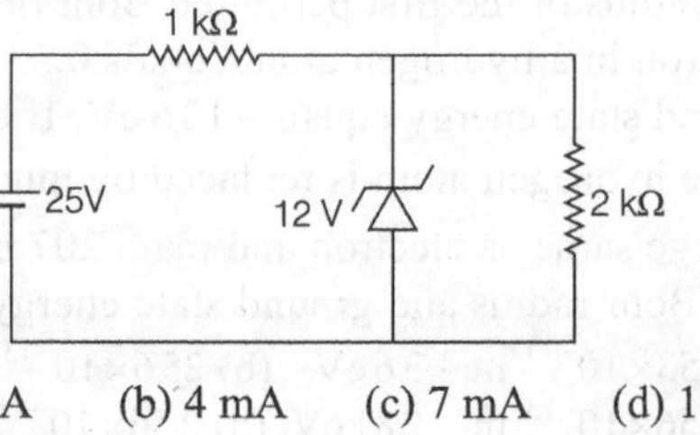

(a) 6 mA (b) 4 mA (c) 7 mA (d) 10 mA

28. The magnetic force acting on a charged particle of charge $-2\ \mu C$ in a magnetic field of 2T acting in y-direction, when the particle velocity is $(2\hat{i}+3\hat{j})\times 10^6 \text{ms}^{-1}$, is
(a) 4N in y- direction (b) 8N in $-z$-direction
(c) 4N in z-direction (d) 8N in y-direction

29. A particle executes linear simple harmonic motion with an amplitude of 3 cm. When the particle is at 2 cm from the mean position, the magnitude of its velocity is equal to that of its acceleration. Then, its time period (in s) is

(a) $\frac{\sqrt{5}}{\pi}$ (c) $\frac{\sqrt{5}}{2\pi}$ (c) $\frac{4\pi}{\sqrt{5}}$ (d) $\frac{2\pi}{\sqrt{3}}$

30. Given below are two statements

Statement I A conductor has large number of free electrons moving with thermal velocity but in the absence of external electric field, net current flowing through it is zero.

Statement II Due to random motion of electron, net flow of charge through any cross-section of conductor is zero.

(a) Both Statement I and Statement II are incorrect.
(b) Statement I is correct but Statement II is incorrect.
(c) Both Statement I and Statement II are correct.
(d) Statement I is incorrect but Statement II is correct.

31. Which of the following transitions gives photon of maximum energy?

(a) $n = 2$ to $n = 1$ (b) $n = 1$ to $n = 2$
(c) $n = 2$ to $n = 6$ (d) $n = 6$ to $n = 2$

32. The radius of earth is 6400 km and $g = 9.8 \text{ m/s}^2$. If the body placed at the equator has to become weightless, then the earth should make one complete rotation in

(a) 12 h (b) 1.4 h (c) 6 h (d) 24 h

33. A boat is moving with a velocity $3\hat{i} + 4\hat{j}$ with respect to the ground. The water in the river is moving with a velocity $-3\hat{i} - 4\hat{j}$ with respect to the ground. The relative velocity of the boat with respect to water is

(a) $8\hat{j}$ (b) $5\sqrt{2}\hat{i}$ (c) $-6\hat{i} - 8\hat{j}$ (d) $6\hat{i} + 8\hat{j}$

34. A zener diode having breakdown voltage equal to 15 V, is used in a voltage regulator. Circuit as shown in the figure, the current through the diode is

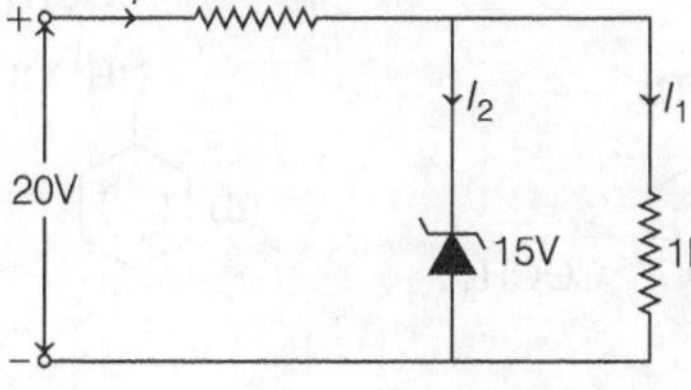

(a) 5 mA (b) 10 mA
(c) 15 mA (d) 20 mA

35. A pipe of length 85 cm is closed from one end. The number of possible natural oscillations of air column in the pipe whose frequencies lie below 1250 Hz are (take, velocity of sound in air $= 340 \text{ ms}^{-1}$)

(a) 5 (b) 4
(c) 6 (d) 10

36. A uniform cylinder has a radius R and length L. If the moment of inertia of this cylinder, about an axis passing through its centre and normal to its circular face is equal to the moment of inertia of the same cylinder about an axis passing through its centre and perpendicular to its length, then

(a) $L = R$ (b) $L = \sqrt{3}R$ (c) $L = \frac{R}{\sqrt{3}}$ (d) $L = \sqrt{\frac{3}{2}}R$

37. The value of electric field inside the capacitor is 50 V/m. If a dielectric material of dielectric constant 6.5 is filled between the plates of capacitor, then the magnitude of polarisation is

(a) 300 (b) 375
(c) 275 (d) 325

38. Three blocks of masses 5 kg, 4 kg and 1 kg, respectively are in contact on a frictionless table as shown in the figure. If a force of 25 N is applied on the 5 kg block, the contact force between 5 kg and 4 kg block will be

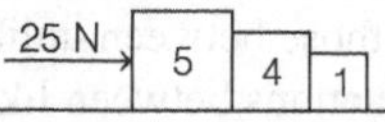

(a) 12.5 N (b) 12 N
(c) 2.5 N (d) 10 N

39. In an experiment, the length of a simple pendulum is about 100 cm known to an accuracy of 1 mm. Its period of oscillation is 2s, determined by measuring the time for 100 oscillations using a clock of 0.1 s resolution. What is the accuracy in the determined value of g ?

(a) 0.5% (b) 0.25%
(c) 0.2% (d) 1.0%

40. de-Broglie wavelength of two particles moving perpendicular to each other are λ_1 and λ_2 respectively. If both the particle suffers perfectly inelastic collision, then de-Broglie wavelength of the final particle will be

(a) $\frac{\lambda_1\lambda_2}{\sqrt{\lambda_1^2 + \lambda_2^2}}$ (b) $\frac{\lambda_1^2\lambda_2^2}{\lambda_1^2 + \lambda_2^2}$

(c) $\frac{\lambda_1\lambda_2}{\lambda_1 + \lambda_2}$ (d) $\frac{\lambda_1\lambda_2}{\sqrt{\lambda_1 + \lambda_2}}$

41. A car accelerates from rest at a constant rate α for sometime after which it decelerates at constant rate β and finally comes to rest. If total time elapsed is T, then maximum velocity attained by car is

(a) $\frac{\alpha+\beta}{\alpha\beta}T$ (b) $\frac{\alpha\beta}{\alpha+\beta}T$ (c) $\frac{\alpha}{\alpha+\beta}T$ (d) $\frac{\beta}{\alpha+\beta}T$

42. An uncharged capacitor with a solid dielectric is connected to a similar air capacitor charged to a potential of 50 V. If the common potential after sharing the charges becomes 2V, then the dielectric constant of dielectric must be

(a) 16 (b) 24 (c) 36 (d) 20

43. Two water drops combine to form a single drop, then what is the ratio of surface energy of bigger drop to smaller one, if both have equal radius?

(a) $2^{\frac{1}{2}}:1$ (b) $2^{\frac{2}{3}}:1$ (c) $1:1$ (d) $2^{\frac{3}{2}}:1$

44. When a conductor is connected to a battery of supply voltage of 220V, then drift velocity of electron across the conductor is 3.6 m/s. If the length of conductor is stretched to double and same potential difference is applied, then drift velocity of electrons will be

(a) 2.4 m/s (b) 1.8 m/s
(c) 4 m/s (d) 7.2 m/s

45. Two polaroids P_1 and P_2 are placed with their axis perpendicular to each other. Unpolarised light of intensity I_0 is incident on P_1. A third polaroid P_3 is kept between P_1 and P_2, such that its axis makes an angle 45° with that of P_1. The ratio of intensity of transmitted light to unpolarised light is

(a) $\frac{1}{4}$ (b) $\frac{1}{2}$
(c) $\frac{1}{8}$ (d) $\frac{1}{16}$

CHEMISTRY

46. Raoult's law is obeyed by each constituent of a binary liquid solution when the

(a) forces of attractions between like molecules are greater than those between unlike molecules.
(b) forces of attractions between like molecules are smaller than those between unlike molecules.
(c) forces of attractions between like molecules are identical with those between unlike molecules.
(d) volume occupied by unlike molecules are different.

47. The reagent and condition required for the following reaction is

$$\underset{\text{Glucose}}{CHO-(CHOH)_4-CH_2OH} \xrightarrow[n\text{-hexane}]{} CH_3-(CH_2)_4-CH_3$$

(a) HI, Δ (b) HBr, Δ
(c) HF, Δ (d) HCl, Δ

48. The product of the following reaction,

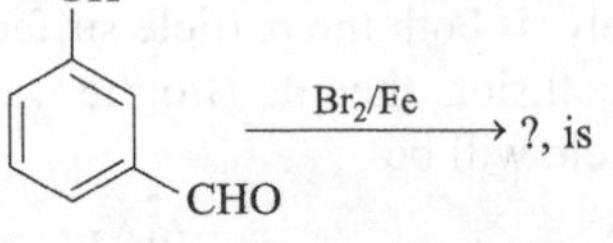

(a) 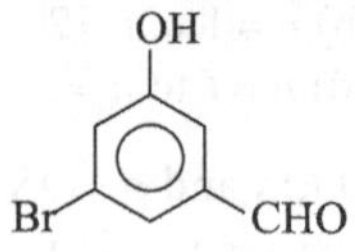

(b) 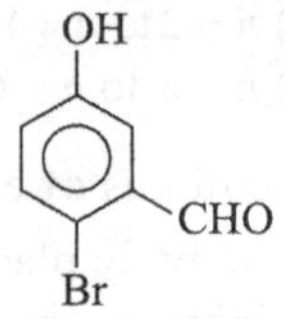

(c) 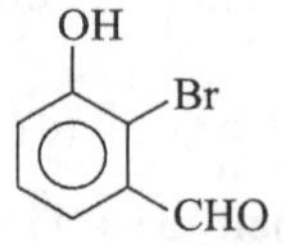

(d) 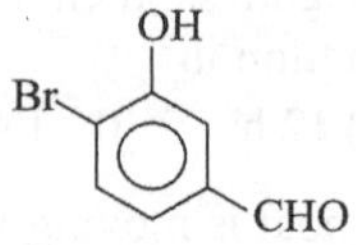

49. Product of the following reaction is

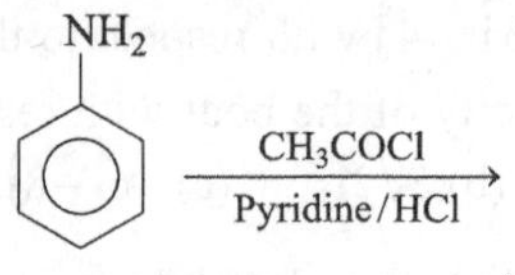

(a) 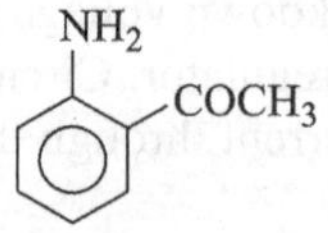

(b) 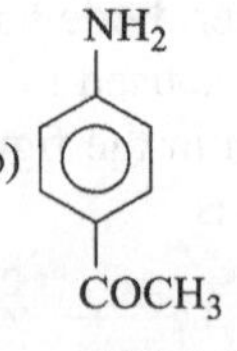

(c) 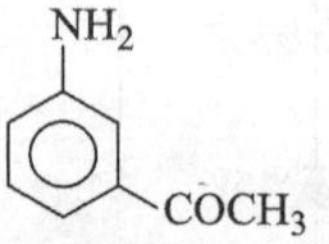

(d) 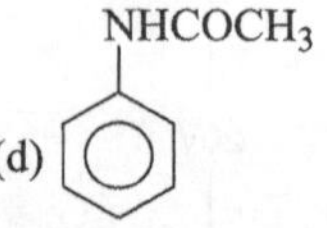

50. Match List-I with List-II.

	List-I		List-II
A.	Saturated solution	I.	Solution having the same osmotic pressure at a given temperature as that of the given solution.
B.	Binary solution	II.	A solution whose osmotic pressure is less than that of another.
C.	Isotonic solution	III.	Solution with two components.
D.	Hypotonic solution	IV.	Solution which contains the maximum amount of solute at a given temperature.

Choose the correct answer from the options given below.

(a) A-I, B-II, C-III, D-IV (b) A-IV, B-III, C-I, D-II
(c) A-II, B-I, C-IV, D-III (d) A-III, B-IV, C-II, D-I

51. α-D-(+)-glucose and β-D-(+)-glucose are

(a) anomers (b) epimers
(c) enantiomers (d) geometrical isomers

52. The half-life time of a first order reaction is 1.26×10^{14} s, then rate constant of this reaction will be

(a) $5.5\times 10^{-10}\ s^{-1}$ (b) $5.5\times 10^{-15}\ s^{-1}$
(c) $6.6\times 10^{-14}\ s^{-1}$ (d) $7.9\times 10^{-13}\ s^{-1}$

53. Here is the graph of the reaction of crystal violet with sodium hydroxide, a first-order reaction (ln *A* vs time)

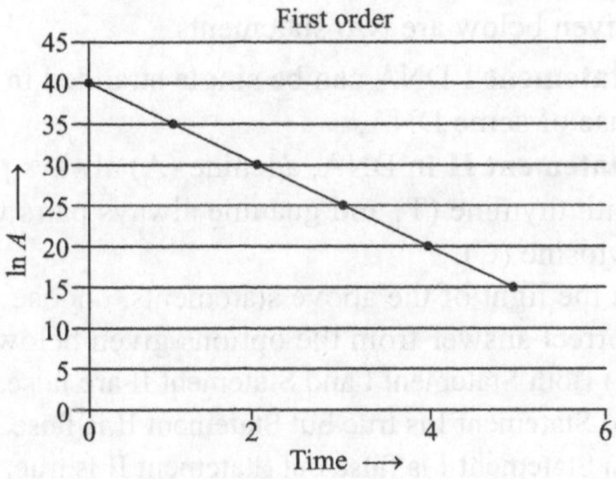

What is the significance of the slope?

(a) The slope represents the change in concentration over time.
(b) The slope represents the inverse of change in concentration over time.
(c) The slope represents the negative value of the rate constant.
(d) The slope represents the negative rate of product concentration over time.

54. Within each transition series, the oxidation state

(a) first decreases till the middle of the period and then increases.
(b) first increases till the middle of the period and then decreases.
(c) decreases regularly on moving from left to right.
(d) increases regularly on moving from left to right.

55. The pair of compounds that illustrate the law of multiple proportion are

A. C_2H_6, C_6H_6
B. H_2O_2, CH_4
C. $MgCl_2$, CaO
D. $SnCl_2$, $SnCl_4$
E. HNO_2, CH_3OH

Choose the correct answer from the options given below.

(a) B and C (b) A and D
(c) D and E (d) C and D

56. For the kinetic study of reaction of iodide ion with hydrogen peroxide, a known volume of sodium thiosulphate solution is added to

(a) oxidise iodine to iodide ion
(b) reduce iodine to iodide ion
(c) form an insoluble blue complex
(d) retard the reaction rate

57. For the reaction, $X_2O_4(l) \longrightarrow 2XO_2(g)$

$\Delta U = 2.1$ kcal, $\Delta S = 20$ cal K^{-1} at 300 K.

Hence, ΔG is

(a) 2.7 kcal
(b) −2.7 kcal
(c) 9.3 kcal
(d) −9.3 kcal

58. Which of the following pair of solution is expected to be isotonic at same temperature?

(a) 0.2 M urea and 0.2 M KCl
(b) 0.1 M urea and 0.2 M $CaCl_2$
(c) 0.1 M KCl and 0.1 M Na_2SO_4
(d) 0.1 M $Ca(NO_3)_2$ and 0.1 M Na_2SO_4

59. Match List I with List II.

	List-I		List-II
(A)	PCl_5	(I)	5 bond pairs and 0 lone pair on central atom
(B)	H_2S	(II)	2 bond pairs and 2 lone pairs on central atom
(C)	ClF_3	(III)	3 bond pairs and 2 lone pair on central atom
(D)	SO_3	(IV)	6 bond pairs and no lone pair on central atom

Choose the correct answer from the options given below.

(a) A-I, B-II, C-III, D-IV (b) A-II, B-III, C-I, D-IV
(c) A-IV, B-II, C-III, D-I (d) A-III, B-IV, C-I, D-II

60. Given below are two statements, one is labelled as Assertion (A) and the other is labelled as Reason (R).

Assertion (A) $E^\circ_{Fe^{2+}/Fe}$ (−0.44 V) < $E^\circ_{Ni^{2+}/Ni}$ (−0.24 V), Fe electrode act as cathode and Ni electrode act as anode.

Reason (R) Because $\Delta G^\circ < 0$ and $E^\circ_{cell} > 0$, cell is possible.

In the light of the above statements, choose the correct answer from the options given below.

(a) Both (A) and (R) are true but (R) is not the correct explanation of (A).
(b) (A) is true but (R) is false.
(c) (A) is false but (R) is true.
(d) Both (A) and (R) are true and (R) is the correct explanation of (A).

61. If ΔG° for the half-cell $MnO_4^-|MnO_2$ in an acid solution is xF, then find the value of x.
(Given : $E^\circ_{MnO_4^-/Mn^{2+}} = 1.5$ V; $E^\circ_{MnO_2/Mn^{2+}} = 1.25$ V)

(a) − 0.75 (b) − 0.95 (c) − 0.85 (d) − 1.15

62. The pK_a of a weak acid HA is 4.92. The pK_b of a weak base BOH is 4.81. The pH of an aqueous solution of the corresponding salt, BA, will be

(a) 7.05 (b) 8.29 (c) 9.58 (d) 4.79

63. Dilute HCl precipitated only group I cations and not other cations. This is because of the fact that

(a) solubility product of first group chloride is less than the chlorides of other metals.
(b) solubility product of group I chlorides is maximum among all metals chlorides.
(c) all metal chlorides are soluble whereas only group I metal chlorides are insoluble.
(d) all metal chlorides are insoluble whereas only group I metal chlorides are soluble.

64. The maximum number of stereoisomer possible for the ion $[Pd(NH_3)_2(H_2O)_2Br_2]^{2+}$ is

(a) 5 (b) 6 (c) 4 (d) 8

65. Given below are two statements, one is labelled as Assertion (A) and the other is labelled as Reason (R).

Assertion (A) *trans*-pent-2-ene is polar but *trans*-but-2-ene is non-polar.

Reason (R) The polarity of *cis*-isomer is more than *trans* which are either non-polar or less polar.

In the light of the above statements, choose the correct answer from the options given below.

(a) Both (A) and (R) are true but (R) is the not the correct explanation of (A).
(b) (A) is true but (R) is false.
(c) (A) is false but (R) is true.
(d) Both (A) and (R) are true and (R) is the correct explanation of (A).

66. In the combustion of 0.4 g of CH_4, 0.25 kcal of heat is liberated. The heat of combustion of CH_4 is

(a) − 20 kcal (b) − 10 kcal (c) − 2.5 kcal (d) − 5 kcal

67. Which of the following order is correct for the acidic nature of the compounds?

(a) $CH_3OH < CH_3SH < CH_3NH_2$
(b) $CH_3NH_2 < CH_3OH < CH_3SH$
(c) $CH_3SH < CH_3OH < CH_3NH_2$
(d) $CH_3SH < CH_3NH_2 < CH_3OH$

68. Which of the following statement(s) is incorrect for oxides of chlorine?

(a) ClO_3 forms dimer due to unpaired electron.
(b) Cl_2O_6 is the anhydride of only $HClO_3$.
(c) ClO_3 is paramagnetic and exists in liquid state.
(d) Cl_2O_6 is diamagnetic in solid state.

69. Given below are two statements.

Statement I DNA can be single stranded in the case of some DNA.

Statement II In DNA, adenine (A) always pairs with thymine (T) and guanine always pairs with cytosine (C).

In the light of the above statements, choose the correct answer from the options given below.

(a) Both Statement I and Statement II are false.
(b) Statement I is true but Statement II is false.
(c) Statement I is false but Statement II is true.
(d) Both Statement I and Statement II are true.

70. When conc. H_2SO_4 is heated with P_2O_5, the acid is converted to
(a) a mixture of sulphur dioxide and sulphur trioxide
(b) sulphur
(c) sulphur dioxide
(d) sulphur trioxide

71. Given below are two statements.

Statement I K_2SO_4 and $CuSO_4$ are added in Kjeldahl's method. K_2SO_4 acts as a catalyst while $CuSO_4$ raises the boiling point of H_2SO_4.

Statement II Baeyer test is used to distinguish Cl^- and Br^- ions.

In the light of the above statements, choose the correct answer from the options given below.
(a) Both Statement I and Statement II are false.
(b) Statement I is true but Statement II is false.
(c) Statement I is false but Statement II is true.
(d) Both Statement I and Statement II are true.

72. Match the List-I with List-II.

List-I	List-II
A. Wurtz reaction	(i) Electrophilic addition reaction
B. Hydration of alkenes	(ii) Nucleophillic substitution reaction
C. Nitration of alkanes	(iii) Free radical substitution
D. Reaction of alkene with NBS	(iv) Electrophilic substitution reaction

Choose the correct answer from the options given below.
(a) A-(i), B-(ii), C-(iv), D-(iii)
(b) A-(iii), B-(i), C-(iv), D-(ii)
(c) A-(ii), B-(i), C-(iv), D-(iii)
(d) A-(iv), B-(i), C-(ii), D-(iii)

73. Which of the following statement is correct?
(a) σ-bond is weaker than π-bond.
(b) HF is less polar than HI.
(c) In NH_4^+ ions, four coordinate bonds are present.
(d) In SF_6, all S—F bond lengths are same.

74. Given below are two statements.

Statement I If a molecule has polar bond, then it is always polar.

Statement II XeF_5^+ has distorted octahedral structure.

In the light of the above statements, choose the correct answer from the options given below.
(a) Both Statement I and Statement II are false.
(b) Statement I is true but Statement II is false.
(c) Statement I is false but Statement II is true.
(d) Both Statement I and Statement II are true.

75. The incorrect statement about the oxoacids, $HClO_4$ and HClO, is
(a) the central atom in both $HClO_4$ and HClO is sp^3 hybridised.
(b) the conjugate base of $HClO_4$ is weaker base than H_2O.
(c) $HClO_4$ is formed in the reaction between Cl_2 and H_2O.
(d) $HClO_4$ is more acidic than HClO because of the resonance stabilisation of its anion.

76. Match the List-I with List-II.

List-I (Name of compounds)	List-II (Structure)
A. *p, p*-dihydroxy benzophenone	(i) 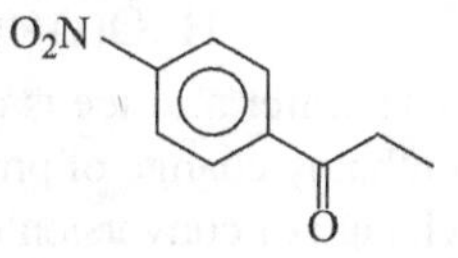
B. 3-bromo-4-phenylpentanoic acid	(ii) 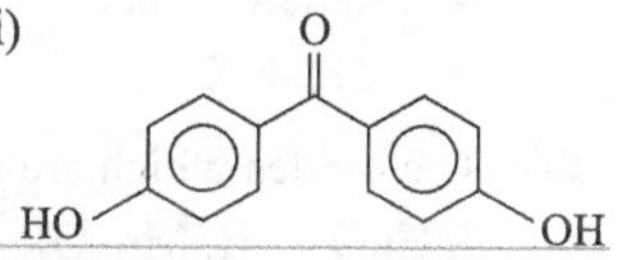
C. *p*-nitropropiophenone	(iii) 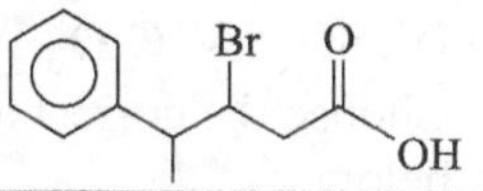
D. Hex-2-en-4-ynoic acid	(iv) 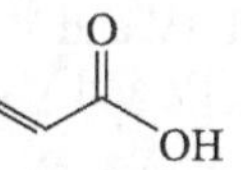

Choose the correct answer from the options given below.
(a) A-(iv), B-(iii), C-(ii), D-(i)
(b) A-(i), B-(iii), C-(iv), D-(ii)
(c) A-(ii), B-(iii), C-(iv), D-(i)
(d) A-(ii), B-(iii), C-(i), D-(iv)

77. Given below are two statements.

Statement I Aromatic aldehydes and formaldehyde undergo Cannizzaro reaction.

Statement II Aromatic aldehydes are almost as reactive as formaldehyde in nucleophilic addition reactions.

In the light of above statement, choose the correct answer from the options given below.
(a) Both Statement I and Statement II are false.
(b) Statement I is true but Statement II is false.
(c) Statement I is false but Statement II is true.
(d) Both Statement I and Statement II are true.

78. Consider the following statements about chelating ligands.

I. They have more than one donor atom.
II. They are non-linear and they must form bonds with reasonable angles at the metal atom.
III. Ethylenediamine is a bidentate chelating ligand.
IV. They have low affinity for a metal ion than monodentate ligands.
V. They form less stable complex than monodentate ligand.

The correct statement is/are
(a) III and V (b) Both I and IV
(c) Both II and III (d) I, II and III

79. Consider the following reaction,

$$H_2O(s) \rightleftharpoons H_2O(l)$$

The water and ice is at equilibrium at 273 K and enthalpy change of process is 6 kJ mol^{-1}. The entropy change of conversion of ice into liquid water is
(a) 21.98 JK^{-1} mol^{-1} (b) – 21.98 JK^{-1} mol^{-1}
(c) – 21.98 JK^{-1} (d) + 21.98 kJ K^{-1}

80. The oxides which are acidic in nature are
I. CuO II. Mn_2O_7 III. CO
IV. SO_2 V. CrO_3
Choose the correct answer from the options given below.
(a) III, IV and V (b) II and V only
(c) II, IV and V (d) Only III

81. For a hydrogen atom, the energies that an electron can have are given by the expression, $E = -13.58 / n^2$ eV, where n is an integer. The smallest amount of energy that a hydrogen atom in the ground state can absorb is
(a) 1.00 eV (b) 3.39 eV
(c) 6.79 eV (d) 10.19 eV

82. The IUPAC nomenclature of an element with electronic configuration $[Rn]5f^{14}6d^1 7s^2$ is
(a) Unnilhexium
(b) Unnilunium
(c) Unnilquadium
(d) Unniltrium

83. A white sodium salt dissolves readily in water to give a solution which is neutral to litmus. When silver nitrate solution is added to the aforementioned solution, a white precipitate is obtained which does not dissolve in dil. nitric acid. The anion is
(a) CO_3^{2-} (b) NO_3^-
(c) S^{2-} (d) Cl^-

84. Which of the following sequence is correct with reference to the oxidation number of iodine?
(a) $I_2 < ICl < HI < HIO_4$
(b) $HIO_4 < ICl < I_2 < HI$
(c) $I_2 < HI < ICl < HIO_4$
(d) $HI < I_2 < ICl < HIO_4$

85. Consider the following statements.
Statement I In Daniell cell, when E_{ext} is less than 1.1 V then Zn dissolves at anode and copper deposits at cathode.
Statement II The potential of individual half-cell can not be measured.
In the light of above statements, choose the most appropriate answer from the options given below.
(a) Statement I is correct but Statement II is incorrect.
(b) Both Statement I and Statement II are correct.
(c) Statement I is incorrect but Statement II is correct.
(d) Both Statement I and Statement II are incorrect.

86.

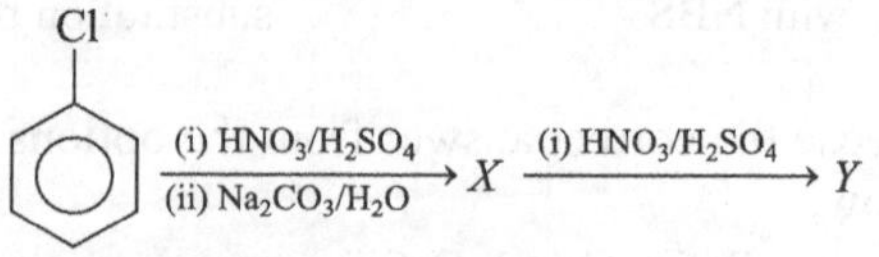

In the above reaction, the product '*Y*' is
(a) phenol
(b) nitrobenzene
(c) 2, 4-dinitrophenol
(d) picric acid

87. The product formed when acetone is treated with phenyl magnesium bromide followed by acidic hydrolysis is

(a) 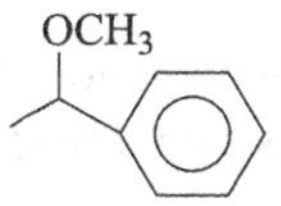

(b) 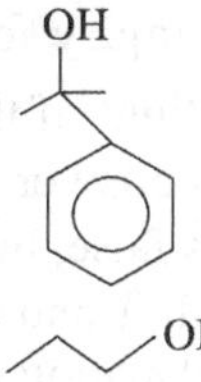

(c) 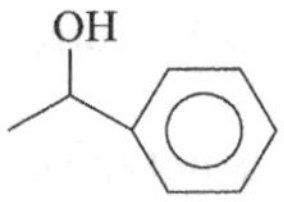

(d) 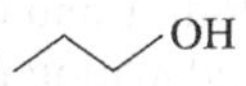

88. Which of the following species does not exist?
(a) Be^+ (b) Be_2 (c) B_2 (d) N_2

89. Which of the following reactants are used to obtain methylphenyl ether?
(a) Phenolate ions and methyl iodide
(b) Methoxide ions and bromobenzene
(c) Methanol and phenol
(d) Bromobenzene and methylbromide

90. Match the List-I with List-II.

List-I (Species)		List-II (Number of lone pairs of electrons on the central atom)	
A.	XeF_2	(i)	0
B.	XeO_2F_2	(ii)	1
C.	XeO_3F_2	(iii)	2
D.	XeF_4	(iv)	3

Choose the correct answer from the options given below.
(a) A-(iv), B-(ii), C-(i), D-(iii)
(b) A-(i), B-(ii), C-(iii), D-(iv)
(c) A-(ii), B-(i), C-(iv), D-(iii)
(d) A-(iii), B-(iv), C-(ii), D-(i)

BIOLOGY

91. The maximum number of trophic levels in an ecosystem is limited by
(a) decomposer activity
(b) nutrient availability
(c) predator-prey relationship
(d) energy availability

92. The biological name of the organism that belongs to family–Anacardiaceae and class–Dicotyledonae is
(a) *Triticum aestivum* (b) *Mangifera indica*
(c) *Solanum tuberosum* (d) *Indica nigrum*

93. The number of haemoglobin subunits found in adult human are
(a) 2 subunits (b) 4 subunits
(c) 3 subunits (d) 4 + 2 subunits

94. The protozoans that have the presence of thousands of cilia and a cavity that opens to the outside of the cell surface is
(a) flagellated (b) sporozoans
(c) amoeboid (d) ciliated

95. Given below are two statements.

Statement I Biopatent is the philosophy and social commentary that deals with the biological sciences and their potential impact on society.

Statement II Biopatents permit private, monopoly right over cells, genes, animals and plants.

In the light of the above statements, choose the correct answer from the options given below.
(a) Statement I is incorrect, but statement II is correct
(b) Both statement I and statement II are correct
(c) Both statement I and statement II are incorrect
(d) Statement I is correct, but statement II is incorrect

96. With respect to eukaryotic gene regulation, which of the following statements is not true for enhancers?
(a) They function in tissue specific manner
(b) They function in any orientation
(c) They function as promoters
(d) They function even when are at a distant from the gene.

97. Given below are two statements.

Statement I Golgian vacuole is formed by budding of the terminal end of maturing face of Golgi apparatus.

Statement II Glycosylation is the formation of lipid from glycolipid.

In the light of the above statements, choose the correct answer from the options given below.
(a) Statement I is incorrect, but statement II is correct
(b) Both statement I and statement II are correct
(c) Both statement I and statement II are incorrect
(d) Statement I is correct, but statement II is incorrect

98. The marine organisms that have a stiff cellulosic cell wall and release toxins that are harmful to other marine animals is

(a) euglenoids (b) slime moulds
(c) dinoflagellates (d) chrysophytes

99. The ABO blood group in humans is an example of

(a) partial dominance
(b) codominance
(c) incomplete dominance
(d) epistasis

100. An organism that belongs to algae which has cell wall made of cellulose and algin. In it the food is stored as laminarin. It belongs to class

(a) Chlorophyceae (b) Phaeophyceae
(c) Rhodophyceae (d) Florophyceae

101. The pair of organisms that have flagellated and pyriform shaped gametes are

(a) *Ulothrix* and *Volvox*
(b) *Porphyra* and *Ectocarpus*
(c) *Laminaria* and *Fucus*
(d) *Sargassum* and *Chlamydomonas*

102. Thyroxine is produced from which of the following amino acids?

(a) Tryptophan (b) Alanine
(c) Glycine (d) Tyrosine

103. Identify the correct set of statements.

I. UTR (Untranslated Regions) are sequences of DNA before the start codon and after the stop codon.
II. Promoter sequences are present downstream of structural genes of a transcription unit.
III. The nascent RNA is synthesised by DNA polymerase-II
IV. In the presence of amino acyl- *t*RNA synthetase, specific amino acid bind with GTP.
V. In genomics, the function of gene is identified by using the technique of reverse genetics.

Choose the correct answer from the options given below.

(a) I, II and IV (b) II, III and V
(c) II, IV and V (d) I, IV and V

104. Given below are two statements; one is labelled as Assertion (A) and the other is labelled as Reason (R).

Assertion (A) White collagen fibres and yellow elastin fibres are two types of areolar fibres.

Reason (R) White collagen fibres are found at the site of injury for repair.

In the light of the above statements, choose the correct answer from the options given below.

(a) A is false, but R is true
(b) Both A and R are true and R is the correct explanation of A
(c) Both A and R are true, but R is not the correct explanation of A
(d) A is true, but R is false

105. The seeds of *Cheiranthus cheiri*, which are useful in bronchitis and fever belongs to family

(a) Cruciferae (b) Leguminosae
(c) Malvaceae (d) Graminae

106. Given below are two statements, one is labelled as Assertion (A) and the other is labelled as Reason (R).

Assertion (A) Vessel is a long, cylindrical tube-like structure made up of many cells called vessel members, they are interconnected through perforations in their common walls.

Reason (R) Vessels form efficient system for transporting food from leaves to root and other parts of plant.

In the light of the above statements, choose the correct answer from the options given below.

(a) A is false, but R is true
(b) Both A and R are true and R is the correct explanation of A
(c) Both A and R are true, but R is not the correct explanation of A
(d) A is true, but R is false

107. Frog shows two types of venous connection *A* between liver and intestine.

B between kidney and lower part of body.

Choose the correct option for *A* and *B*, respectively.

(a) Renal portal system and hepatic portal system
(b) Hepatic portal system and renal portal system
(c) Renal portal system and articular portal system
(d) Sympathetic system and hepatic portal system

108. Total volume of air a person can inspire after a normal expiration is called

(a) RV (b) EC (c) IC (d) FRC

109. Which of the following statements are true?

I. Auxin translocation is non-polar.
II. Abscisic acid is transported through phloem only.
III. Turgidity of cells helps in extension growth.
IV. During the formation of tracheary element the cell losing protoplasm is an example of redifferentiation.
V. IAA is a natural auxin.

Choose the correct answer from the options given below.

(a) I and III (b) III and V
(c) II and III (d) I and IV

110. Given below are two statements.

Statement I In mustard and *Argemone*, ovary becomes two chambered due to the formation of false septum.

Statement II In basal placentation, the placenta develops at the base of ovary and two ovules are attached to it.

In the light of the above statements, choose the correct answer from the options given below.

(a) Statement I is incorrect, but statement II is correct
(b) Both statement I and statement II are correct
(c) Both statement I and statement II are incorrect
(d) Statement I is correct, but statement II is incorrect

111. Read the following statements and choose the correct set of statements.

I. Vectors, whose origin support high copy number, produces many copies of cloned DNA.
II. Transformation is a process by which bacteriophage transfers a piece of DNA into a host bacterium.
III. Hybridisation procedure allows us to isolate and introduce a desirable gene without introducing undesirable genes into the target organism.
IV. More than one recognition sites within a vector will generate several fragments, which will complicate the gene cloning.
V. During insertional inactivation method, non recombinant bacterial cells produce blue coloured colonies on agar medium.

Choose the correct answer from the options given below.

(a) I, II and V (b) I, III and IV
(c) I, IV and V (d) II, IV and V

112. Which factor maintains the distinctive traits of species?

(a) Specific niche
(b) Reproductive isolation
(c) Cooperative interaction
(d) Continuous inter - communication

113 *Bt* toxin gene encoded by *cry IAc*, *cry IAb* and *cry IIAb* genes was isolated from

(a) *Meloidegyne incognitia*
(b) *Bacillus thuringiensis*
(c) *Agrobacterium tumefaciens*
(d) *Bacillus coagulens*

114. The final stage of meiotic prophase-I is known as diakinesis. This is marked by

(a) compaction of chromosomes
(b) terminalisation of chiasmata
(c) recombination between homologous chromosomes
(d) formation of the homologous chromosome

115. Given below are two statements, one is labelled as Assertion (A) and other is labelled as Reason (R).

Assertion (A) Sewage treatment is essential for maintaining public health and protecting the environment.

Reason (R) Sewage contains harmful pollutants that can contaminate water bodies and spread diseases.

In the light of the above statements, choose the correct answer from the options given below.

(a) A is false, but R is true.
(b) Both A and R are true and R is the correct explanation of A.
(c) Both A and R are true but R is not the correct explanation of A.
(d) A is true, but R is false

116. The virus of AIDS is different from hepatitis-C virus as it contains

(a) *ds*DNA (b) *ss*RNA
(c) *ss*DNA (d) *ds*RNA

117. The stroke volume multiplied by the heart rate gives the

(a) articular output
(b) cardiac output
(c) ventricular output
(d) ECG value

118. Given below are two statements.

Statement I *Sorghum* plants show Hatch-Slack pathway.

Statement II In C_4 plants, Calvin cycle does not take place in the mesophyll cells, but only in the bundle sheath cells.

In the light of the above statements, choose the correct answer from the options given below.

(a) Statement I is incorrect, but statement II is correct
(b) Both statement I and statement II are correct
(c) Both statement I and statement II are incorrect
(d) Statement I is correct, but statement II is incorrect

119. Consider the following statements about the structure of ovule and select the one which is incorrect.

(a) Paddy, mango and wheat possess single ovule in each ovary, whereas papaya, watermelon and orchids contain many
(b) Ovule is a small structure attached to the placenta by means of a stalk called hilum
(c) Each ovule is encircled by one or two protective envelopes called integuments
(d) Enclosed within the integuments is a mass of cells called nucellus

120. Which of the following statements is /are incorrect?

I. During fertilisation, changes occur in the zona pellucida.
II. The sperm lysins in the acrosome dissolve the egg envelope facilitating fertilisation.
III. Mitochondria in the head region produces energy for the mobility of sperm.
IV. Corpus luteum secretes large amount of oestrogen for the maintenance of endometrium.
V. Fine hairs and eyelashes are formed in the foetus around 168 days of conception.

Choose the correct answer from the options given below.

(a) I, II and IV (b) I, II, III and IV
(c) III and IV (d) III, IV and V

121 Identify the incorrect statement(s).

I. Amniotic fluid test is used for diagnosing chromosomal abnormalities.
II. In ultrasound imaging, visible images are produced by the pattern of echos made by organs.
III. MTPs are considered safe upto 14 weeks of pregnancy.
IV. Amniocentesis can cause premature labor.
V. MTP was legalised by the goverment of India with some rules in the year 1971.

Choose the correct answer from the options given below.

(a) I and IV (b) Only III
(c) II and IV (d) III and V

122. At the micropylar end, three cells are grouped together and constitute the egg apparatus. This group consists of

(a) one ovum and two antipodals
(b) one ovum and two synergids
(c) ovum, synergids and polar nuclei
(d) ovum, antipodal and synergids

123. Which of the following cells have special cellular thickenings and play an important role in guiding the pollen tube ?

(a) Antipodals (b) Synergids
(c) Egg cell (d) Filiform apparatus

124. Which among the following is not included in brain stem ?

(a) Hypothalamus (b) Medulla
(c) Pons (d) Midbrain

125. The descending limb of loop of Henle is permeable to ...., but almost impermeable to ....

(a) electrolytes, water
(b) water, electrolytes
(c) urea, water
(d) electrolytes, urea

126. Consider the given figure and identify the correct observation about it.

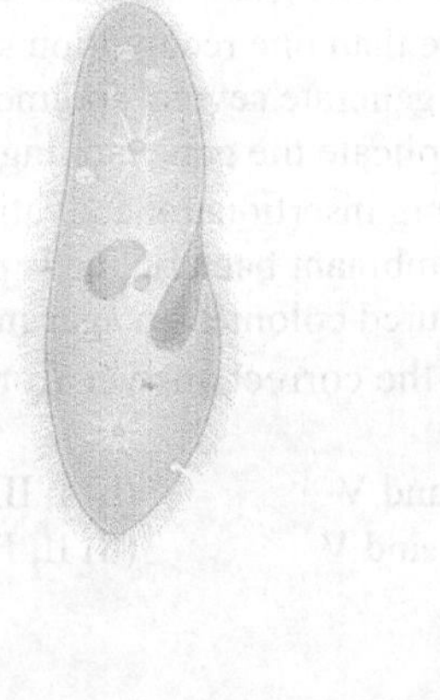

(a) They use their pseudopodia to engulf food particles
(b) They absorb nutrients directly through their cell membrane
(c) They use coordinated movement of cilia to direct food - laden water into the gullet
(d) They depend on photosynthesis for food production

127. Fibres of the tracts are covered with the myelin sheath, which gives an opaque white appearance and are called
(a) white matter
(b) grey matter
(c) pia mater
(d) arachnoid

128. Match List-I with List-II.

List I	List II
A. Intrafascicular cambium	1. Cambium between xylem and phloem
B. Interfascicular cambium	2. Parenchymatous cells of medullary rays
C. Monocot root	3. Polyarch xylem bundles
D. Heartwood	4. Physiologically inactive

Choose the correct answer from the options given below.

	A	B	C	D
(a)	1	3	2	4
(b)	3	1	2	4
(c)	1	2	3	4
(d)	4	1	2	3

129. ...... part of the brain is involved in loss of control when a person consumes alcohol.
(a) Thalamus
(b) Cerebellum
(c) Pons
(d) Cerebrum

130. .... are present below hypodermis that consist of rounded thin walled parenchymatous cells.
(a) Starch sheath
(b) Cortical layers
(c) Vascular bundles
(d) Pith

131. The ring arrangement of vascular bundles is a characteristic of ...... along with ....
(a) dicot stem ; endarch protoxylem
(b) monocot stem ; exarch protoxylem
(c) dicot root ; endarch protoxylem
(d) monocot root ; exarch protoxylem

132. In sodium and potassium pumps exchange of K^+ and Na^+ occurs in .... ratio.
(a) 2 : 3 (b) 3 : 2
(c) 1 : 2 (d) 1 : 3

133. Even when there is no air in lungs, human trachea does not collapse due to the presence of
(a) cartilaginous rings
(b) bony rings
(c) chitinous rings
(d) turgid pressure

134. Given below are two statements; one is labelled as Assertion (A) and the other is labelled as Reason (R).
Assertion (A) The bioresources are being analysed for the identification of valuable biomolecules.
Reason (R) Useful genes are isolated from the bioresources and patented.
In the light of the above statements, choose the correct answer from the options given below.
(a) A is false, but R is true
(b) Both A and R are true and R is the correct explanation of A
(c) Both A and R are true, but R is not the correct explanation of A
(d) A is true, but R is false

135. Choose the character studied by Mendel in *Pisum sativum*, which was dominant ?
(a) Round seed shape (b) Yellow pod colour
(c) Dwarf stem height (d) Green seed colour

136. Read the following statements and choose the correct option.
I. Algae have cell wall made up of cellulose, galactans, mannans.
II. Cell wall only provides shape to the cell.
III. The primary cell wall is capable of growth.
IV. The middle lamella is a layer of calcium carbonate.
V. The cell wall and middle lamella may be transversed by plasmodesmata.

Choose the correct answer from the options given below.
(a) I and II (b) II, IV and V
(c) I, III and V (d) II and V

137. Prosthetic group is a part of holoenzyme. It is
(a) an accessory protein substance attached firmly.
(b) loosely attached organic part
(c) loosely attached inorganic part
(d) tightly bound organic compound

138. Select the incorrect statement from the options given below.
(a) Ecological pyramids cannot explain all vital functions of any ecosystem
(b) Removal of most of the carnivores results in an increased population of consumers.
(c) The length of food chains is generally limited to 3-4 trophic levels due to energy loss
(d) In parasitic food chains, the size of parasites gradually increases in successive trophic levels

139. At the end of which phase, cells when viewed under the microscope, do not show Golgi complexes, endoplasmic reticulum, nucleolus and the nuclear envelope?
(a) Prophase (b) Telophase
(c) Cytokinesis (d) Anaphase

140. Given below are two statements.
Statement I In juxtamedullary nephrons, the blood first passes through vasa recta and then through the capillaries of glomerulus.
Statement II The glomeruli of juxtamedullary nephrons are placed close to the inner margin of the cortex.
In the light of the above statements, choose the correct answer from the options given below.
(a) Statement I is incorrect, but statement II is correct
(b) Both statement I and statement II are correct
(c) Both statement I and statement II are incorrect
(d) Statement I is correct, but statement II is incorrect

141. Given below are two statements; one is labelled as Assertion (A) and the other is labelled as Reason (R).
Assertion (A) Decomposition is the process of physical and chemical breakdown of complex substances.
Reason (R) Decomposers produce organic raw materials for recycling.
In the light of the above statements, choose the correct answer from the options given below.
(a) A is false, but R is true
(b) Both A and R are true and R is the correct explanation of A
(c) Both A and R are true, but R is not the correct explanation of A
(d) A is true, but R is false

142. Which of the following pairs of contrasting traits studied in pea plant by Mendel constitutes recessive characters ?
(a) Dwarf plant and green pod
(b) Yellow seed and yellow pod
(c) Green seed and constricted pod
(d) Yellow seed and white flower

143. In the absence of preferred carbon source such as glucose, if lactose is provided in the growth medium of bacteria, which of the following events would occur ?
(a) The repressor protein binds to RNA polymerase and prevents translation
(b) The structural genes fail to produce polycistronic *m*RNA
(c) The repressor protein attaches to the promoter sequence and depresses the operator
(d) The inducer molecules bind to the repressor protein and RNA polymerase binds to the promoter sequence

144. Given below is a figure showing frontal view of right pectoral girdle and upper arm.

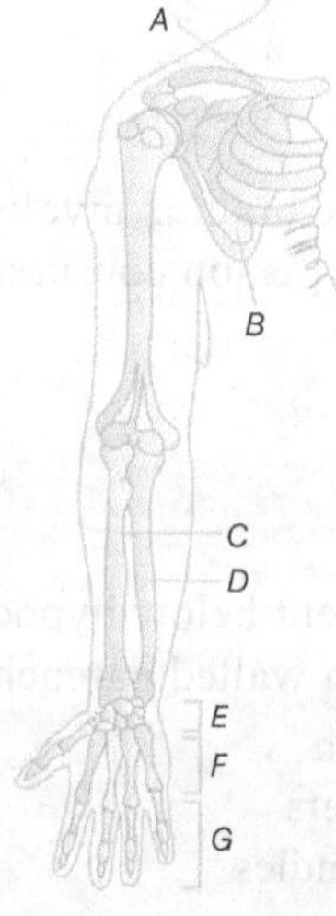

Choose the correct part that possesses spine which projects as acromion.

(a) D (b) A (c) B (d) F

145. The life history traits of organisms have evolved in relation to all of the following, except

(a) Darwinian fitness
(b) organisms evolving under selection pressure developed by environmental factors
(c) organisms achieving most efficient reproductive strategy
(d) loss of energy from one trophic level to another.

146. Match List I with List II.

List I	List II
A. Typhoid	1. Blue fingernails
B. Pneumonia	2. Internal bleeding
C. Ascariasis	3. Gross deformities of genital organs
D. Filariasis	4. Sustained high fever

Choose the correct answer from the options given below.

	A	B	C	D		A	B	C	D
(a)	4	2	1	3	(b)	1	2	4	3
(c)	4	1	2	3	(d)	3	1	2	4

147. If we use DNA polymerase, isolated from normal soil bacterium in PCR, then what would happen?

(a) We cannot obtain even a single copy of DNA
(b) We can obtain millions of copies of DNA within sometime
(c) We have to run PCR for many cycles
(d) We only obtain 15-20 copies of DNA

148. The final product of glycolysis, pyruvate, is transported to .... for aerobic respiration to take place.

(a) nucleus (b) mitochondria
(c) cytoplasm (d) cell membrane

149. Match List I with List II.

List I	List II
A. Pineal gland	1. T-lymphocytes
B. Thyroid gland	2. Melatonin
C. Parathyroid gland	3. Stromal tissue
D. Thymus	4. Ca^{2+}

Codes

	A	B	C	D
(a)	2	3	4	1
(b)	3	4	2	1
(c)	1	3	2	4
(d)	1	2	4	3

150. Given below are two statements.

Statement I In *Salpa*, notochord extends from head to tail and is present throughout the life.

Statement II In *Branchiostoma*, notochord is present only in larval tail.

In the light of the above statements, choose the correct answer from the options given below.

(a) Statement I is incorrect, but statement II is correct
(b) Both statement I and statement II are correct
(c) Both statement I and statement II are incorrect
(d) Statement I is correct, but statement II is incorrect

151. Which of the following statements is not true for *Spirogyra*?

(a) They are usually green due to the presence of pigments chlorophyll-*a* and chlorophyll-*b*
(b) They have one or more storage bodies called pyrenoid which contain protein
(c) Vegetative reproduction usually takes place by bud formation
(d) Sexual reproduction may be isogamous, anisogamous or oogamous type

152. Given below are two statements.

Statement I TSH represents thyroxine stimulating hormone.

Statement II Excessive production of thyroid hormones causes nervousness, irregular hearbeat and weight loss.

In the light of the above statements, choose the correct answer from the options given below.

(a) Statement I is incorrect, but statement II is correct
(b) Both statement I and statement II are correct
(c) Both statement I and statement II are incorrect
(d) Statement I is correct, but statement II is incorrect

153. Which of the following correctly represents the zygotene phase of meiosis-I?
(a) Formation of chiasmata
(b) Formation of synaptonemal complex
(c) Terminalisation of chiasmata
(d) Appearance of recombination nodules

154. Which of the following processes takes place during the formation of both glycosidic bonds and peptide bonds ?
(a) Esterification (b) Acidification
(c) Hydration (d) Dehydration

155. Which of the following metabolic waste is found in land snails?
(a) Urea (b) Uric acid
(c) Hippuric acid (d) Ammonia

156. Saheli is a new oral contraceptive pill for females with
(a) low side effects and minimal monetary value
(b) high side effects and high contraceptive value
(c) low side effects and high contraceptive value
(d) high side effects and low contraceptive value

157. Read the following statements and choose the incorrect set of statements.
I. Columnar or cuboidal cells bearing microvilli on their free surface are called ciliated epithelium.
II. Blood vessels are absent in the epithelial tissue.
III. Intercellular bridges are minute projections that arise from adjacent cell membrane.
IV. Columnar epithelium lines salivary gland and pancreatic ducts.
V. The simple squamous epithelium are not transformed into brush bordered epithelium.
Choose the correct answer from the options given below.
(a) I and V
(b) I and IV
(c) I, II and V
(d) I, III, IV and V

158. 'Transfer of pollen grains from anther to the stigma of a different plant'. This type of pollination is termed as *A* and is found in *B*
A *B*
(a) autogamy ; rose (b) geitonogamy ; China rose
(c) cleistogamy ; *Viola* (d) xenogamy ; grasses

159. What is the ratio of CO_2, ATP and NADPH used in the Calvin cycle ?
(a) 1 : 2 : 3 (b) 1 : 3 : 2
(c) 1 : 3 : 6 (d) 1 : 2 : 4

160. Some strains of *Bacillus thuringiensis* produce proteins that kill certain insects such as coleopterans like
(a) tobacco budworm (b) beetles
(c) flies (d) mosquitoes

161. Find the set of analogous organs.
(a) Wings of parrot and hands of man
(b) Forelimbs of frog, rabbit and wing of bird
(c) Eye of mammals and octopus
(d) Thorn of *Bougainvillea* and tendrils of *Cucurbita*

162. Which of the following statements is incorrect?
(a) Each trophic level has a certain mass of living material at a particular time called standing crop
(b) Standing crop is measured as the mass of living organisms only
(c) GFC is the major conduit for energy flow
(d) DFC begins with dead organic matter

163. In the glomerulus of nephron, the afferent arteriole is
(a) longer than efferent arteriole
(b) of same diameter as efferent arteriole
(c) wider than efferent arteriole
(d) narrower than efferent arteriole

164. Oxidative phosphorylation refers to
(a) formation of ATP by transfer of phosphate group from substrate to ADP
(b) oxidation of phosphate group in ATP
(c) reduction of phosphate group to ATP
(d) ATP formation by energy released from electrons removed during substrate oxidation

165. Read the following statements and identify the correct set of statements.
I. Eastern ghats have greater amphibian species diversity.
II. Norway has a greater ecosystem diversity than mangroves, coral reefs, wetlands and alpine meadows of India.
III. India has more than 50,000 genetically different strains of rice.

IV. A single species might show high diversity at the genetic level over its distributional range.
V. India has more than 1,000 varieties of mango.

Choose the correct answer from the options given below.

(a) I and II (b) III, IV and V
(c) IV and V (d) III and V

166. Match List I with List II.

	List I		List II
A.	Golden rice	1.	Emphysema
B.	α-1- antitrypsin	2.	Protein-enriched milk
C.	*Flavr Savr*	3.	Enriched with vitamin -A
D.	Rosie cow	4.	Increased shelf life

Choose the correct answer from the options given below.

	A	B	C	D
(a)	1	2	4	3
(b)	3	4	1	2
(c)	3	1	2	4
(d)	3	1	4	2

167. Match List I with List II.

	List I		List II
A.	Golden rice	1.	Army worm
B.	*Bt* toxin	2.	Rich in vitamin-A
C.	RNAi	3.	cry protein
D.	Lepidopteran	4.	Gene silencing

Choose the correct answer from the options given below.

	A	B	C	D
(a)	2	3	4	1
(b)	3	4	1	2
(c)	4	1	2	3
(d)	2	1	3	4

168. Which among the following is correct w.r.t . cardiac cycle?

(a) The volume of blood pumped out by the right and left ventricles are same
(b) The volume of blood pumped out by the right and left ventricles is different
(c) The volume of blood received by each atrium is different
(d) The volume of blood received by the aorta and pulmonary artery is different

169. Given below are two statements; one is labelled as Assertion (A) and the other is labelled as Reason (R).

Assertion (A) The chromosomal size is measured during metaphase.

Reason (R) Maximum coiling occurs during this phase.

In the light of the above statements, choose the correct answer from the options given below.

(a) A is false, but R is true
(b) Both A and R are true and R is the correct explanation of A
(c) Both A and R are true, but R is not the correct explanation of A
(d) A is true, but R is false

170. Read the following statements and choose the incorrect set of statements.

I. The nuclear matrix or the nucleoplasm contains nucleolus and chromatin.
II. Duplication of centrioles takes place during interkinesis.
III. The centrosomes are surrounded by a non-amorphous pericentriolar material.
IV. The gas vacuoles are the membrane bound system and lie in the cytoplasm.
V. The humans erythrocyte membrane has 52 per cent protein and 40 per cent lipids.

Choose the correct answer from the options given below.

(a) III and IV (b) I, III and IV
(c) I, III IV and V (d) II, III, IV and V

171. Given below are two statements; one is labelled as Assertion (A) and the other is labelled as Reason (R).

Assertion (A) Specific *Bt* toxin genes are isolated from *Bacillus thuringiensis* and incorporated into several crop plants such as cotton.

Reason (R) The choice of genes depends upon the crop and the targeted pest.

In the light of the above statements, choose the correct answer from the options given below.

(a) A is false, but R is true
(b) Both A and R are true and R is the correct explanation of A
(c) Both A and R are true, but R is not the correct explanation of A
(d) A is true, but R is false

172. The secondary follicle soon transforms into a tertiary follicle, which is characterised by a fluid-filled cavity called

(a) colostrum (b) antrum
(c) Graafian follicle (d) zona pellucida

173. XX/XY type of sex-determination is seen in

(a) birds (b) *Drosophila*
(c) grasshopper (d) peacock

174. Match List I with List II.

	List I		List II
A.	Green algae	1.	*Marchantia*
B.	Liverworts	2.	*Polytrichum*
C.	Mosses	3.	*Dictyota*
D.	Brown algae	4.	*Spirogyra*

Choose the correct answer from the options given below.

	A	B	C	D		A	B	C	D
(a)	4	1	2	3	(b)	3	1	2	4
(c)	4	3	2	1	(d)	3	2	1	4

175. Select the correct sequence of vertebrae as we proceed down the spine from the skull.

(a) Thoracic, Cervical, Lumbar, Sacral, Coccygeal
(b) Coccygeal, Lumbar, Thoracic, Sacral, Cervical
(c) Cervical, Thoracic, Lumbar, Sacral, Coccygeal
(d) Cervical, Thoracic, Coccygeal, Sacral, Lumbar

176. .... is a pathogenic bacterium, which causes typhoid fever and generally enter the small intestines through food and water.

(a) *Streptococcus pneumoniae*
(b) *Haemophilus influenzae*
(c) *Salmonella typhi*
(d) *Plasmodium malariae*

177. Anabolic steroids in females causes

(a) masculinisation, excessive hairs on face, mood swings and enlargement of clitoris
(b) masculinisation, breast enlargement, premature baldness and enlargement of prostate gland
(c) ulcers, mental illness and reduced size of testicles
(d) hypertension, vitamin deficiency and enlargement of prostate gland

178. Refer to the diagram given below and choose the option that indicates incorrect labelling.

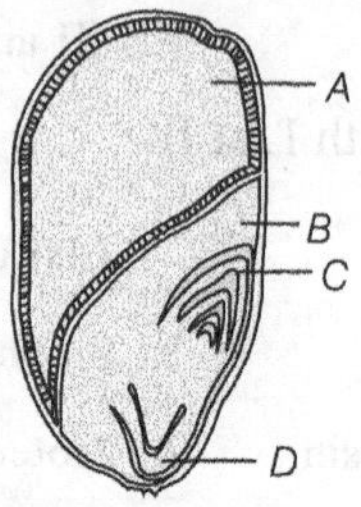

(a) *A* represents the storage tissue rich in starch
(b) *B* represents scutellum
(c) *C* represents coleorrhiza
(d) *D* represents the protective covering of radicle

179. Identify the incorrectly matched pair.

(a) Widal test – Typhoid
(b) Common cold – Rhinoviruses
(c) Cytokine barriers – Interferons
(d) Dengue – *W. malayi*

180. Match List I with List II.

	List I (Hormones)		List II (Functions)
A.	Human chorionic gonadotrophin	1.	Promotes growth of myometrium
B.	Progesterone	2.	Maintains corpus luteum
C.	Oestrogen	3.	Suppress uterine contractions
D.	Relaxin	4.	Softens cervix to prepare for dilation

Choose the correct answer from the options given below.

	A	B	C	D
(a)	2	3	1	4
(b)	3	2	4	1
(c)	4	1	3	2
(d)	1	4	2	3

Explanations

Physics

1. (b) $\Delta W_{cyclic} = \pi\left(\frac{3p_0 - p_0}{2}\right)\left(\frac{2V_0 - V_0}{2}\right)$

$$= \frac{\pi p_0 V_0}{2} = \frac{\pi\, p_0 V_0}{m} \text{ (given)}$$

$\therefore \quad m = 2$

2. (b) Change in momentum,

$$\Delta p = p_f - p_i$$
$$= -\, mv\sin 30^\circ - mv\sin 30^\circ$$

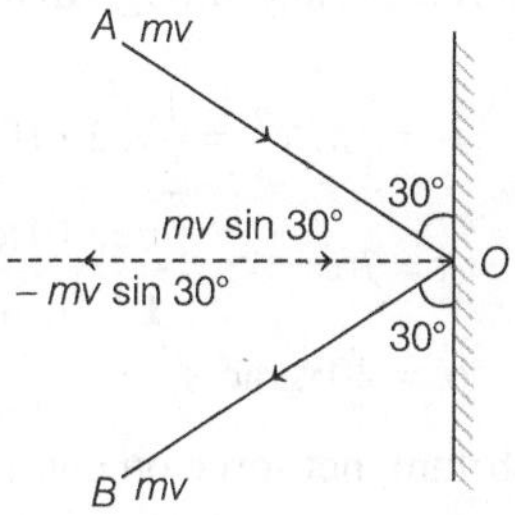

or $\quad \Delta p = -\,2mv\sin 30^\circ$

$$= -\,2\times 2\times 100\times \frac{1}{2} = -\,200 \text{ kg ms}^{-1}$$

The force exerted by the ball on the wall,

$$F = \frac{-\,\Delta p}{\Delta t} = \frac{200}{0.4} = 500\text{N}$$

3. (c) Magnetic field at O,

$$B = \frac{\mu_0}{4\pi}\cdot\frac{i}{a}(\sin\phi_1 + \sin\phi_2)$$

But $\phi_1 = 90^\circ - \theta_1$

and $\phi_2 = 90^\circ - \theta_2$

$\therefore \quad B = \frac{\mu_0\, i}{4\pi\, a}[\sin(90^\circ - \theta_1) + \sin(90^\circ - \theta_2)]$

$$= \frac{\mu_0}{4\pi}\cdot\frac{i}{a}(\cos\theta_1 + \cos\theta_2)$$

4. (b) Refractive index is given by

$${}_g\mu_a = \frac{\sin i}{\sin r}$$

$\Rightarrow \quad \frac{1}{{}_a\mu_g} = \frac{\sin i}{\sin 2i} \qquad (\because 2i = r)$

$\Rightarrow \quad \frac{1}{1.6} = \frac{\sin i}{2\sin i\cos i}$

$\Rightarrow \quad \frac{1}{1.6} = \frac{1}{2\cos i}$

$$\frac{1}{\cos i} = \frac{5}{4}$$

$\Rightarrow \quad \cos i = \frac{4}{5}$

Now, $\quad \sin i = \sqrt{1 - \cos^2 i}$

$\Rightarrow \quad \sin i = \sqrt{1 - \frac{16}{25}} = \frac{3}{5}$

$\Rightarrow \quad i = \sin^{-1}\left(\frac{3}{5}\right)$

5. (b) Minimum kinetic energies are at highest point,

$$\frac{\frac{1}{2}mu_1^2\cos^2\theta_1}{\frac{1}{2}mu_2^2\cos^2\theta_2} = \frac{4}{1} \Rightarrow \frac{u_1\cos\theta_1}{u_2\cos\theta_2} = 2 \quad \text{...(i)}$$

and ratio of the maximum height,

$$\frac{u_1^2\sin^2\theta_1}{u_2^2\sin^2\theta_2} = \frac{4}{1} \Rightarrow \frac{u_1\sin\theta_1}{u_2\sin\theta_2} = \frac{2}{1} \quad \text{...(ii)}$$

From Eqs. (i) and (ii), we get

$$\frac{u_1\sin\theta_1\cdot u_1\cos\theta_1}{u_2\sin\theta_2\cdot u_2\cos\theta_2} = \frac{4}{1}$$

$$\frac{\left(\frac{gR_1}{2}\right)}{\left(\frac{gR_2}{2}\right)} = \frac{4}{1} \Rightarrow \frac{R_1}{R_2} = \frac{4}{1}$$

6. (b) $\frac{1}{2}mv^2 - \frac{GMm}{R} = -\frac{GMm}{(R+h)}$

$\Rightarrow \quad v^2 = \frac{2GM}{R}\left(\frac{h}{R+h}\right) \quad \text{...(i)}$

Now, escape velocity, $v_e = \left(\frac{2GM}{R}\right)^{1/2}$

Also $\quad v = \frac{v_e}{2}$

So, from Eq. (i),we get

$$\frac{1}{4}\frac{2GM}{R} = \frac{2GM}{R}\left(\frac{h}{R+h}\right)$$

$\Rightarrow \quad h = \frac{R}{3}$

$\Rightarrow \quad \frac{h}{R} = \frac{1}{3}$

Problem Solving Tactics	If a body is thrown up from the surface of the earth, then $K_i + U_i = K_f + U_f$

7. (b) Here, $d = \sqrt{d_1 d_2}$

$$= \sqrt{0.03 \times 0.12} = 0.06\,\text{mm} = 6 \times 10^{-5}\,\text{m}$$

$\therefore$ Fringe width, $\beta = \dfrac{D\lambda}{d} = \dfrac{2 \times 400 \times 10^{-9}}{6 \times 10^{-5}}$

$$= 1.33 \times 10^{-2}\,\text{m} = 13.3\,\text{mm}$$

8. (b) We know that, $\alpha = \dfrac{dl}{l \times dt}$

where, dl = change in length, l = initial length and dt = change in temperature.

So, $dt = \dfrac{dl}{l \times \alpha}$

In this case, $\alpha = 2 \times 10^{-5}\,/°\text{C}$,

$l = 1\text{m},\ t = 20°\text{C}$

$dl = 1\,\text{mm} = 1 \times 10^{-3}\,\text{m}$

$$dt = \frac{1 \times 10^{-3}}{1 \times 2 \times 10^{-5}}$$

We get, $dt = 50°\text{ C}$

Since, present temperature = 20° C

The final temperature should be −30° C.

9. (d) Decrease in kinetic energy = Increase in internal energy of the gas

$$\frac{1}{2} m v_0^2 = n C_V \Delta T = \frac{m}{M}\left(\frac{5}{2} R\right)\Delta T \Rightarrow \Delta T = \frac{M v_0^2}{5R}$$

10. (c) Given, radius of first Bohr orbit for electron in a hydrogen atom, $r = 0.53\,\text{Å}$

and its ground state energy, $E_0 = -13.6\,\text{eV}$

Charge of muon = Charge of electron

Mass of muon = 207× (Mass of electron)

$\therefore$ When electron is replaced by muon, then first Bohr radius, $r_1{}' = \dfrac{0.530\,\text{Å}}{207} = 2.56 \times 10^{-13}\,\text{m}$

and ground state energy, $E_1{}' = -13.6 \times 207$

$$= -2815.2\,\text{eV} = -2.815\,\text{keV}$$

$$\simeq -2.8\,\text{keV}$$

11. (c) $x = \alpha t^3 \Rightarrow v_x = \dfrac{dx}{dt} = 3\alpha t^2$

$$y = \beta t^3 \Rightarrow v_y = \frac{dy}{dt} = 3\beta t^2$$

$$v = \sqrt{v_x^2 + v_y^2} = 3t^2\sqrt{\alpha^2 + \beta^2}$$

12. (d) In option (d), the radii of two curvature of two faces (convex and concave) of a lens are equal. i.e., $R_1 = R_2$

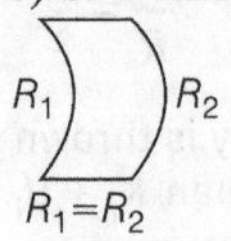

So, the incident and emergent rays will be parallel.

13. (a) Magnetic moment of the ring is given by

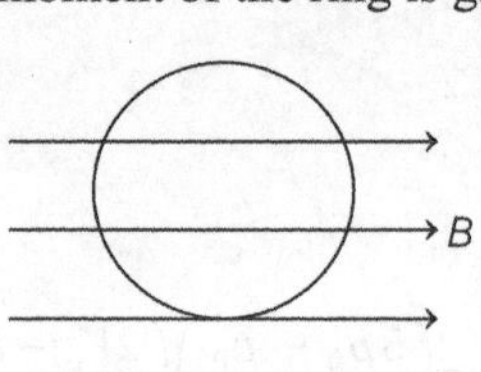

$$\mathbf{M} = \mathbf{I} \cdot \mathbf{A}$$

$$= 4 \times \pi (0.5)^2 (-\hat{\mathbf{k}}) = -\pi \hat{\mathbf{k}}\,\text{A-m}^2$$

Torque acting on the ring,

$$\tau = \mathbf{M} \times \mathbf{B} = (-\pi \hat{\mathbf{k}}) \times (10\hat{\mathbf{i}}) = -10\pi \hat{\mathbf{j}}$$

So, axis of rotation is along τ, i.e., negative Y-axis.

Due to torque of magnetic field, ring will rotate about its diameter.

Moment of inertia of ring through diameter about Y-axis,

$$I = \frac{1}{2} MR^2 = \frac{1}{2} \times 2 \times (0.5)^2 = \frac{1}{4}\,\text{kg-m}^2$$

$$\tau = I\alpha \Rightarrow \alpha = \frac{\tau}{I} = \frac{10\pi}{1/4}$$

$$\alpha = 40\pi\,\text{rad/s}^2$$

14. (d) For equilibrium, net force on charge A must be zero,

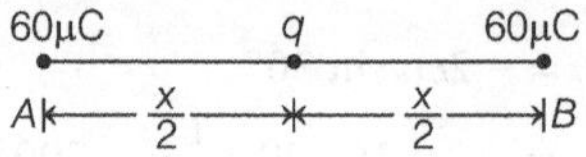

i.e. $$\frac{1}{4\pi\varepsilon_0} \cdot \frac{60 \times 10^{-6} \cdot q}{\left(\frac{x}{2}\right)^2} + \frac{1}{4\pi\varepsilon_0} \cdot \frac{(60 \times 10^{-6})^2}{x^2} = 0$$

$\Rightarrow$ $4q = -60 \times 10^{-6}$

$\Rightarrow$ $q = -15 \times 10^{-6}$

$\Rightarrow$ $q = -15\,\mu\text{C}$

15. (c) At $x = 2\,\text{m}, U = 6\,\text{J}$

At $x = 5\,\text{m}, U = 2\,\text{J}$

$\because$ $\Delta U = \Delta \text{KE}$

$$6 - 2 = \frac{1}{2}(4) v^2$$

$\Rightarrow$ $4 = 2v^2$

$$v = \sqrt{2}\,\text{m/s}$$

16. (b) Electromagnetic waves are self-sustaining oscillation of electric and magnetic fields in free space or vacuum. They differ from all other waves we have studied so far, in respect that no material medium is involved in the vibration of electric and magnetic fields.

17. (d) Moment of inertia of each disc about the axis through the centre is given by

$$I_A = I_B = \frac{1}{2} MR^2$$

From theorem of parallel axes,

$$I'_A = \frac{1}{2}MR^2 + M(2R)^2 = \frac{9}{2}MR^2$$

$$\therefore \quad I = I'_A + I_B = \frac{9}{2}MR^2 + \frac{1}{2}MR^2$$

$$I = 5MR^2$$

18. (a) If an experiment is performed to find the refractive index of glass using a travelling microscope, distances are measured by a vernier scale which is provided on the microscope.

19. (d) When axis of dipole is parallel to the direction of electric field, then potential energy is minimum.

i.e., $\phi = 0°$

$\therefore \quad U = -pE\cos 0° = -pE$

20. (a) $\tan\phi = \dfrac{\frac{1}{\omega C} - \omega L}{R}$

$\therefore \quad \phi = 45°$

$$\tan 45° = \frac{\frac{1}{\omega C} - \omega L}{R} \Rightarrow 1 = \frac{\frac{1}{\omega C} - \omega L}{R}$$

$$\Rightarrow R = \frac{1}{\omega C} - \omega L \Rightarrow \omega C = \frac{1}{\omega L + R}$$

$$\Rightarrow C = \frac{1}{\omega(\omega L + R)} \quad (\because \omega = 2\pi f)$$

$$= \frac{1}{2\pi f(2\pi f L + R)}$$

21. (a) Truth table of given combination is

A	B	Y'	Y
0	0	1	0
0	1	1	0
1	0	1	0
1	1	0	1

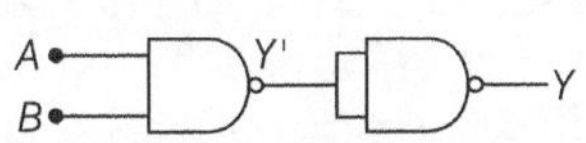

The diagram performs logic function of AND gate.

22. (c) Total energy at point A = Total energy at point B

$$0 + mgR = \frac{1}{2}mv_B^2 + mgR\left(1 - \frac{1}{\sqrt{2}}\right)$$

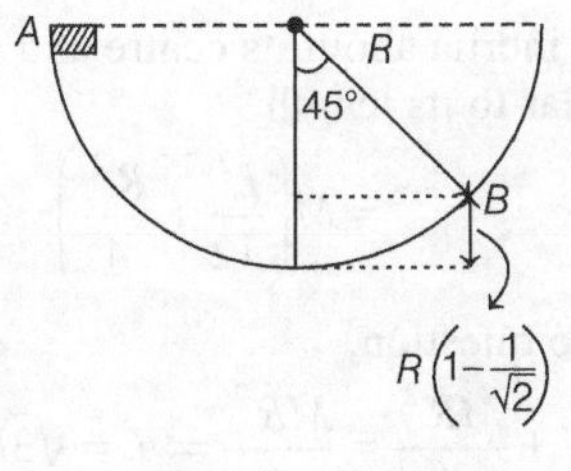

$$\therefore \quad v_B = \sqrt{\sqrt{2}gR} = 3.76\,\text{ms}^{-1} \; (\because R = 1\,\text{m, given})$$

23. (a) When n resistors are connected in series, then

$$A = nR \quad \ldots\text{(i)}$$

When n resistors are connected in parallel, then

$$B = \frac{R}{n} \quad \ldots\text{(ii)}$$

From Eqs. (i) and (ii), we get

$$AB = R^2$$

$$\Rightarrow \quad R = \sqrt{AB}$$

24. (c) Induced emf is given by $e = -\dfrac{d\phi}{dt}$

As, $i = \dfrac{e}{R} = -\dfrac{1}{R}\dfrac{d\phi}{dt}$

$\therefore$ Total charge induced $= \int i\,dt$

$$= -\int \frac{1}{R}\frac{d\phi}{dt}dt = -\frac{1}{R}\int_{\phi_1}^{\phi_2} d\phi$$

$$= -\frac{1}{R}[\phi_2 - \phi_1] = \frac{1}{R}(\phi_1 - \phi_2)$$

Thus, the induced charge in a conducting loop, moving in a magnetic field depends on the total change in magnetic flux.

25. (c) We know that, energy stored in capacitor,

$$E_C = \frac{1}{2}CV^2$$

and energy stored in inductor,

$$E_L = \frac{1}{2}LI^2$$

$$\text{Thus,} \quad \frac{LI^2}{CV^2} = \frac{\frac{1}{2}LI^2}{\frac{1}{2}CV^2} = \frac{E_L}{E_C} = \frac{[\text{ML}^2\text{T}^{-2}]}{[\text{ML}^2\text{T}^{-2}]}$$

$$= [\text{M}^0\text{L}^0\text{T}^0\text{A}^0]$$

26. (b) Magnetic field at A due to current carrying loop B,

$$B_A = \frac{\mu_0 IR^2}{2(R^2 + x^2)^{\frac{3}{2}}}$$

Magnetic flux passing through loop A,

$$\phi_A = B_A \cdot \pi r^2 \text{ and } e_A = -\frac{d\phi_A}{dt}$$

Induced emf will be maximum, if

$$\frac{d}{dx}e_A = \frac{d}{dx}\left(\frac{-d\phi_A}{dt}\right) = 0$$

[where, e_A = Induced emf in loop A]

On solving, we get $x = \dfrac{R}{2}$

27. (c) Current through resistance of 1 kΩ,

$$i = \frac{25 - 12}{1 \times 10^3}\,\text{A} = 13\,\text{mA}$$

But current through 2kΩ

$$= \frac{V_{2k\Omega}}{(2\times10^3)} = \frac{12}{2\times10^3}\text{ A} = 6\text{ mA}$$

$\therefore$ Current through zener diode = 13 mA − 6 mA = 7 mA

28. (b) Given $q = -2\mu C$

$$v = (2\hat{i} + 3\hat{j})\times10^6\text{ ms}^{-1}$$

$B = 2$ T along y-direction

$$B = 2\hat{j}\text{ T}$$

$\because$ Magnetic force, $\mathbf{F} = q(\mathbf{v}\times\mathbf{B})$

$$= [-2\times10^{-6}][(2\hat{i}+3\hat{j})\times10^6\times2\hat{j}]$$

$$= (-2\times10^{-6})[4(\hat{i}\times\hat{j})\times10^6] \quad [\because \hat{j}\times\hat{j} = 0]$$

$$= -8\hat{k} = 8\text{ N in } -z\text{-direction.}$$

29. (c) Magnitude of velocity of particle, when it is at displacement x from mean position

$$= \omega\sqrt{A^2 - x^2}$$

Also, magnitude of acceleration of particle in SHM $= \omega^2 x$

Given, when $x = 2$ cm, $|v| = |a|$

$$\Rightarrow \omega\sqrt{A^2 - x^2} = \omega^2 x$$

$$\Rightarrow \quad \omega = \frac{\sqrt{A^2-(2)^2}}{2} = \frac{\sqrt{9-4}}{2}$$

$\Rightarrow$ Angular velocity, $\omega = \frac{\sqrt{5}}{2}$ rad/s

$\therefore$ Time period of motion, $T = \frac{2\pi}{\omega} = \frac{4\pi}{\sqrt{5}}$ s

30. (c) Due to random motion of thermal electrons, net flow of charge through any cross-section of conducting wire is zero, hence in the absence of external electric field, net current flowing through it is zero.

31. (a) Energy level of H-atom is given by

$$E_n = \frac{-13.6}{n^2}\text{ eV}$$

Photons are emitted only when electron jumps from higher energy level to lower energy level.

Hence, options (b) and (c) are wrong.

$$\Delta E_{2\to1} = 13.6\left(\frac{1}{1^2} - \frac{1}{2^2}\right)\text{ eV} = 10.2\text{ eV}$$

$$\Delta E_{6\to2} = 13.6\left(\frac{1}{2^2} - \frac{1}{6^2}\right) = 3.02\text{ eV}$$

Hence, $\Delta E_{2\to1}$ is maximum.

32. (b) The body will be weightless if weight is balanced by centrifugal force.

i.e. $\quad mR\omega^2 = mg \Rightarrow \quad \omega = \sqrt{\frac{g}{R}}$

$$T = 2\pi\sqrt{\frac{R}{g}} = 2\times\frac{22}{7}\times\sqrt{\frac{6400\times10^3}{9.8}}$$

$$\simeq 5080\text{ s} \simeq 1.4\text{ h}$$

33. (d) $\mathbf{v}_{b/g} = 3\mathbf{i} + 4\mathbf{j}$

$$\mathbf{v}_{w/g} = -3\mathbf{i} - 4\mathbf{j}$$

$$\mathbf{v}_{b/w} = \mathbf{v}_{b/g} - \mathbf{v}_{w/g} = 6\mathbf{i} + 8\mathbf{j}$$

34. (a) The voltage drop across 1 kΩ, $V_2 = 15$ V

The current through 1 kΩ,

$$I_1 = \frac{15\text{ V}}{1\times10^3\ \Omega} = 15\times10^{-3}\text{ A} = 15\text{ mA}$$

The voltage drop across 250 Ω

$$= 20\text{ V} - 15\text{ V} = 5\text{ V}$$

The current through 250 Ω,

$$I = \frac{5\text{ V}}{250\ \Omega} = 0.02\text{ A} = 20\text{ mA}$$

The current through zener diode,

$$I_2 = I - I_1 = (20 - 15)\text{ mA} = 5\text{ mA}$$

35. (c) For closed organ pipe, frequency of closed organ pipe is given by

$$f = \frac{v}{4L} \quad (f = \text{fundamental frequency})$$

$$f = \frac{340}{(4\times0.85)} = 100\text{ Hz}$$

Natural frequency of closed organ is

$f_n = (2n-1)f \Rightarrow$ for $n = 1, 2, 3, 4, 5, 6, \ldots\ldots$

$f_n = 100$ Hz, 300 Hz, 500 Hz, 700 Hz, 900 Hz, 1100 Hz

So, number of possible natural oscillations below 1250 Hz are 6.

36. (b) Moment of inertia of a cylinder about an axis passing through its centre and parallel to its length

$$= \frac{MR^2}{2}$$

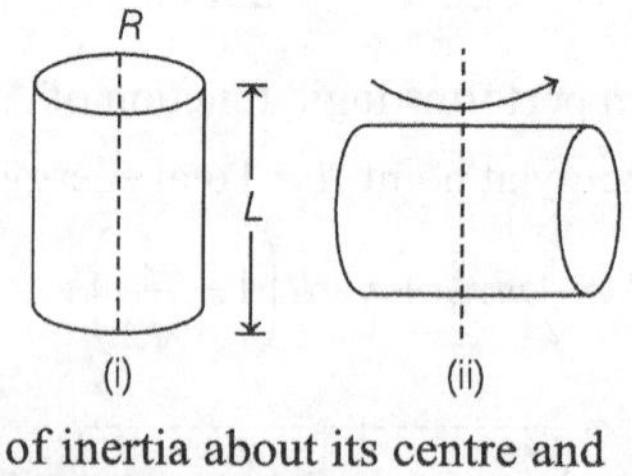

Moment of inertia about its centre and perpendicular to its length

$$= M\left(\frac{L^2}{12} + \frac{R^2}{4}\right)$$

According to question,

$$\frac{ML^2}{12} + \frac{MR^2}{4} = \frac{MR^2}{2} \Rightarrow L = \sqrt{3}R$$

37. (c) Given, $E = 50$ V/m

$\therefore \quad \varepsilon_r = 1+\chi$

where, χ is electrical susceptibility and ε_r is dielectric constant.

$$6.5 = 1+\chi \Rightarrow \chi = 5.5$$

$\therefore$ Polarisation, $P = \chi E = 5.5\times 50 = 275$

38. (a) $a = \dfrac{25}{5+4+1} = 2.5\,\text{ms}^{-2}$

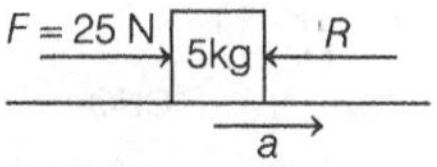

The equation of motion is

$$F - R = ma$$
$$25 - R = 5\times 2.5$$
$$\Rightarrow \quad R = 12.5\,\text{N}$$

39. (c) For a pendulum, the time period,

$$T = 2\pi\sqrt{\frac{l}{g}}$$

$$g = \frac{4\pi^2 l}{T^2} \Rightarrow \frac{\Delta g}{g} = \frac{\Delta l}{l} + 2\frac{\Delta T}{T}$$

$$= \frac{0.1}{100} + \frac{2(0.1)}{2(100)} = 0.002$$

Therefore, the accuracy in the value of

$$g = \frac{\Delta g}{g}\times 100 = 0.2\%$$

40. (a) According to given situation,

$$\lambda_1 = \frac{h}{p_1} \text{ and } \lambda_2 = \frac{h}{p_2}$$

$$\Rightarrow p_1 = \frac{h}{\lambda_1} \text{ and } p_2 = \frac{h}{\lambda_2}$$

where, p_1 and p_2 are momentum of the particle.

Given that, particles are moving perpendicular to each other and collide inelastically. So, they move as a single particle.

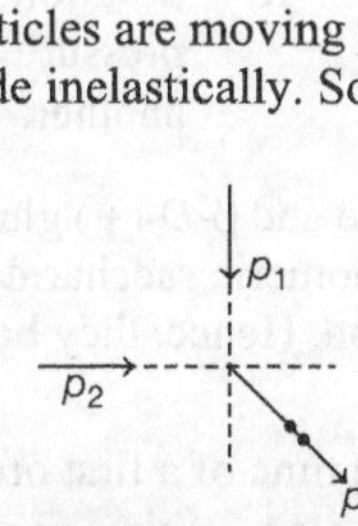

So, by conservation of momentum and vector addition law, net momentum after collision,

$$p_{\text{net}} = p' = \sqrt{p_1^2 + p_2^2 + 2p_1p_2\cos 90^\circ}$$
$$= \sqrt{p_1^2 + p_2^2}$$

Since, $p_1 = \dfrac{h}{\lambda_1}$ and $p_2 = \dfrac{h}{\lambda_2}$

$$\therefore \quad p' = \sqrt{\frac{h^2}{\lambda_1^2} + \frac{h^2}{\lambda_2^2}} \quad \ldots\text{(i)}$$

$\therefore$ de-Broglie wavelength of final particle after collision,

$$\lambda' = \frac{h}{p'} = \frac{h}{\sqrt{\dfrac{h^2}{\lambda_1^2} + \dfrac{h^2}{\lambda_2^2}}} = \frac{\lambda_1\lambda_2}{\sqrt{\lambda_1^2 + \lambda_2^2}}$$

41. (b) Let, T_1 be the time of acceleration and T_2 for deceleration, then

$$T_1 + T_2 = T$$

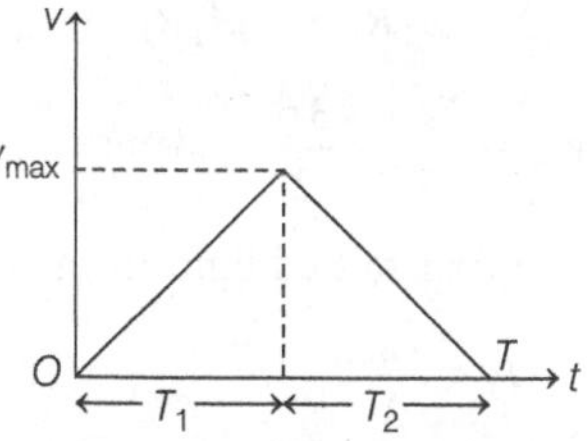

From figure, $\alpha = \dfrac{v_{\text{max}}}{T_1} \Rightarrow T_1 = \dfrac{v_{\text{max}}}{\alpha}$

and $\quad \beta = \dfrac{v_{\text{max}}}{T_2} \Rightarrow T_2 = \dfrac{v_{\text{max}}}{\beta}$

$$\therefore \quad \frac{v_{\text{max}}}{\alpha} + \frac{v_{\text{max}}}{\beta} = T \Rightarrow v_{\text{max}} = \frac{\alpha\beta T}{\alpha+\beta}$$

42. (b) Common potential,

$$V = \frac{C_1V_1 + C_2V_2}{C_1 + C_2}$$

$$\Rightarrow \quad 2 = \frac{C_0K\times 0 + C_0\times 50}{C_0K + C_0}$$

$$\Rightarrow \quad 2 = \frac{50}{K+1} \Rightarrow 2K + 2 = 50$$

$$\Rightarrow \quad K = 24$$

43. (b) Let, radius of larger drop be R and each of small drop is r.

As per given condition,

$$\frac{4}{3}\pi R^3 = 2\cdot\frac{4}{3}\pi r^3$$

So, $\quad R = 2^{\frac{1}{3}} r$

Surface energy,

$$W_1 = T\cdot A = 4\pi R^2 T = 4\pi\, 2^{\frac{2}{3}} r^2 T$$

$$W_2 = 4\pi r^2 T \Rightarrow \frac{W_1}{W_2} = \frac{2^{\frac{2}{3}}}{1}$$

$$\Rightarrow W_1 : W_2 = 2^{2/3} : 1$$

44. (b) When the conductor is stretched to double, then its resistance becomes 4 times and area becomes half.

$$I = neAv_d$$

$$\Rightarrow \quad \frac{V}{R} = neAv_d$$

$$\Rightarrow \quad v_d = \frac{V}{neAR}$$

$$\Rightarrow \quad v_d \propto \frac{1}{AR}$$

$$\Rightarrow \quad \frac{v_{d_1}}{v_{d_2}} = \frac{A_2R_2}{A_1R_1} = \frac{\frac{A_1}{2}\cdot 4R_1}{A_1R_1} = 2$$

$$\Rightarrow \quad v_{d_2} = \frac{v_{d_1}}{2} = \frac{3.6}{2} = 1.8\,\text{m/s}$$

45. (c) Intensity of transmitted light from polaroid P_1,

$$I_1 = \frac{I_0}{2}$$

Intensity of transmitted light from polaroid P_3,

$$I_3 = I_1 \cos^2 45° = \frac{I_0}{2} \times \frac{1}{2} \Rightarrow I_3 = \frac{I_0}{4}$$

Intensity of transmitted light from polaroid P_2,

$$I_2 = I_3 \cos^2 45° = \frac{I_0}{4}\cdot\frac{1}{2}$$

$$I_2 = \frac{I_0}{8}$$

$$\therefore \quad \frac{I_2}{I_0} = \frac{1}{8}$$

Chemistry

46. (c) When the forces of attractions between like molecules are identical with those between unlike molecules, Raoult's law is obeyed by each constituent of a binary liquid solution.

In such case, the total vapour pressure of the solution is the sum of the partial vapour pressures of components of the solution.

47. (a) On prolonged heating with HI, glucose forms *n*-hexane, suggesting that all 6 carbon atoms are linked in a straight chain.

$$\underset{\text{Glucose}}{\overset{\text{CHO}}{\underset{\text{CH}_2\text{OH}}{(\text{CHOH})_4}}} \xrightarrow[\Delta]{\text{HI}} \underset{n\text{-hexane}}{CH_3CH_2CH_2CH_2CH_2CH_3}$$

Problem Solving Tactics

Firstly, consider the role of given reagents. HI is a reducing agent. It reduces primary alcohol, secondary alcohol and aldehyde group.

48. (b) The complete reaction can be written as

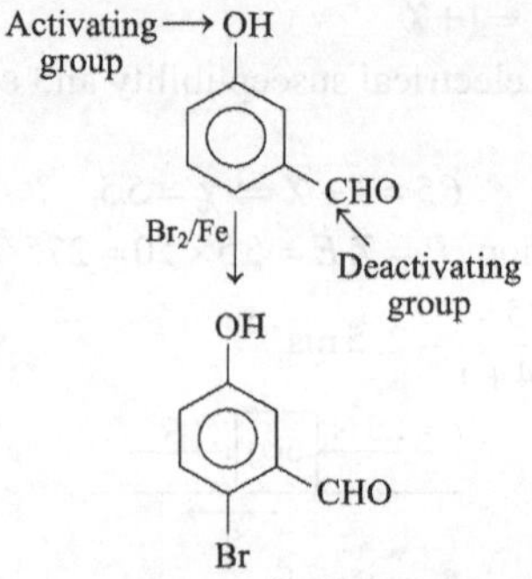

$\therefore$ Strongly activating group generally dominates over the deactivating group and —OH is *ortho/para*-directing group and *p*-product predominants.

49. (d)

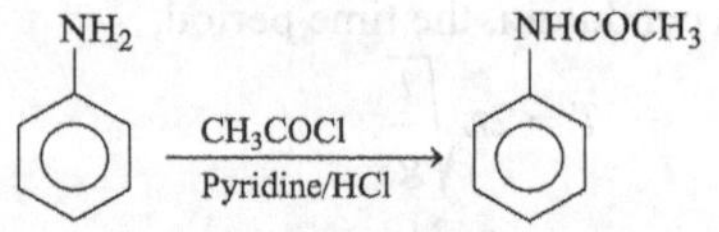

Formation of N-acetylated product is due to presence of lone pair of electrons on nitrogen atom.

50. (b) The correct option is A-IV, B-III, C-I, D-II.

A.	Saturated solution	IV.	Solution which contains the maximum amount of solute at a given temperature.
B.	Binary solution	III.	Solution with two components.
C.	Isotonic solution	I.	Solution having the same osmotic pressure at a given temperature as that of the given solution.
D.	Hypotonic solution	II.	Solution whose osmotic pressure is less than that of another.

51. (a) α-*D*-(+)-glucose and β-*D*-(+)-glucose are anomers. The structure of anomeric saccharide changes at only the anomeric carbon. Hence, they both differ at carbon-1 only.

52. (b) Given, half-life time of a first order reaction $= 1.26 \times 10^{14}$ s

Half-life for a first order reaction is given by,

$$t_{1/2} = \frac{0.693}{k}$$

where, k = rate constant, $t_{1/2}$ = half-life time

$$k = \frac{0.693}{1.26 \times 10^{14}}$$

$$= 5.5 \times 10^{-15}\ \text{s}^{-1}$$

53. (a) By graph, $\ln [A_t] = -kt + \ln[A_0]$

$$\therefore \quad \ln\left[\frac{A_t}{A_0}\right] = -kt \quad \ldots \text{(i)}$$

$k \rightarrow$ Rate constant = slope of graph $[A_t], [A_0] \rightarrow$ concentrations of reactant at time t and at $t = 0$.

It is a first order reaction.

$\therefore$ The slope represents change in concentration over time. [from (i)]

54. (b) In transition series, oxidation state first increases from Sc to Mn due to increase in number of unpaired electrons and then decreases because pairing takes place.

55. (b) Among the given pair of compounds only A and D illustrate the law of multiple proportions because all these contain the same atoms in the given compounds.

56. (b) In the above experiment, the reaction occurs

$$H_2O_2 + 2I^- + 2H^+ \longrightarrow 2H_2O + I_2$$

I_2 liberates in this reaction and it reacts with sodium thiosulhpate solution and is reduced to iodide ions.

$$I_2 + 2S_2O_3^{2-} \xrightarrow{\text{Fast}} S_4O_6^{2-} + 2I^-$$

57. (b) The change in Gibbs free energy is given by

$$\Delta H = \Delta U + \Delta n_g RT$$

Here, R = gas constant taken as = 2 cal.mol^{-1}K^{-1}

But, $\Delta H = (2.1 \times 10^3) + (2 \times 2 \times 300) = 3300$ cal

Hence, $\Delta G = \Delta H - T\Delta S$

$$\Delta G = 3300 - (300 \times 20)$$

$$\Delta G = -2700 \text{ cal} = -2.7 \text{ kcal}$$

58. (d) Solutions having same number of ions will exert equal osmotic pressure and expected to be isotonic.

$$Ca(NO_3)_2 \rightleftharpoons Ca^{2+} + 2NO_3^-, i = 3$$

$$Na_2SO_4 \rightleftharpoons 2Na^+ + SO_4^{2-}, i = 3$$

Osmotic pressure of $Ca(NO_3)_2 = i \times CRT = 3 \times CRT$

Osmotic pressure of $Na_2SO_4 = i \times CRT = 3 \times CRT$

As osmotic pressure are equal, so they are isotonic. While in other options value of i is different, so value of osmotic pressure is also different. Hence, they are not isotonic.

Problem Solving Tactics

The solutions having the same concentration of salts are known as isotonic solutions.

Due to same concentrations the isotonic solutions have the same osmotic pressure.

59. (a) The correct match is A-I, B-II, C-III, D-V

60. (c) $E^\circ_{Ni^{2+}|Ni} = -0.24$ V $E^\circ_{Fe^{2+}|Fe} = -0.44$ V

$$E^\circ_{cell} = E^\circ_{Ni^{2+}/Ni} - E^\circ_{Fe^{2+}/Fe}$$

$$= -0.24 + 0.44 = 0.20 \text{ V}$$

Fe electrode is anode, Ni electrode is cathode.

$\Delta G^\circ < 0$ and $E^\circ_{cell} > 0$ for working of cell.

Hence, (A) is false but (R) is true.

61. (a) The expression for the standard free energy change is $\Delta G^\circ = -nFE^\circ$ but it is equal to xF.

Hence, $x = \dfrac{-nFE^\circ}{F} = -nE^\circ$

But for the given half reaction, $n = 3$ and

$E^\circ = E^\circ_{MnO_4^- | Mn^{2+}} - E^\circ_{MnO_2 | Mn^{2+}} = 1.5 - 1.25 = 0.25$ V

Hence, $x = -nE^\circ = -3 \times 0.25 = -0.75$

62. (a) For a salt of weak acid and weak base.

$$pH = \frac{1}{2}[\log K_a + \log K_w - \log K_b]$$

$$= \frac{1}{2}pK_a + \frac{1}{2}pK_w - \frac{1}{2}pK_b$$

$$= \frac{1}{2} \times 4.92 + 7 - \frac{1}{2} \times 4.81 = 7.055 \approx 7.05$$

63. (a) K_{sp} of group I metal chlorides is $\leq 10^{-4}$, K_{sp} of other metal chloride is more than 10^{-4}.

Hence, other metal chlorides are not precipitated by dil. HCl.

64. (b) Six stereoisomers are possible for $[Pd(NH_3)_2(H_2O)_2Br_2]^{2+}$.

They are as follows

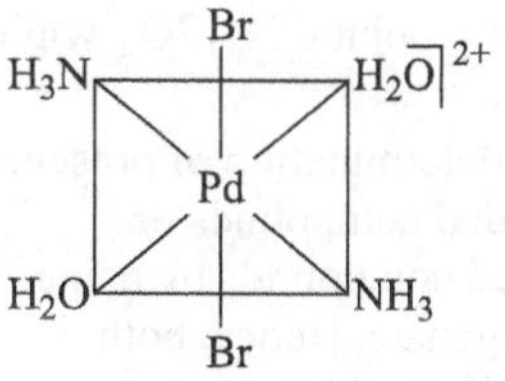

(1)

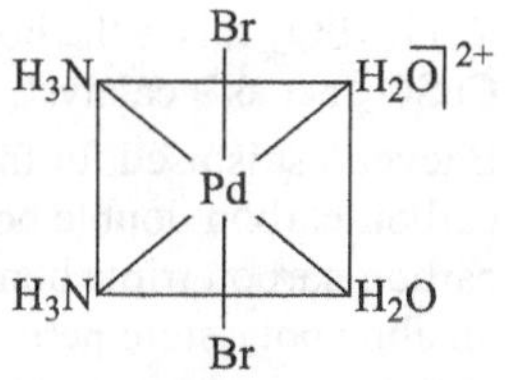

(2)

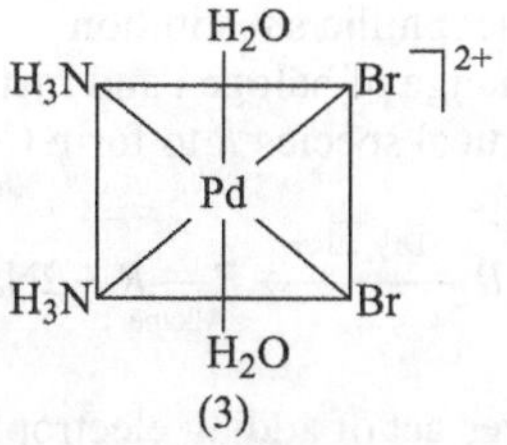

(3)

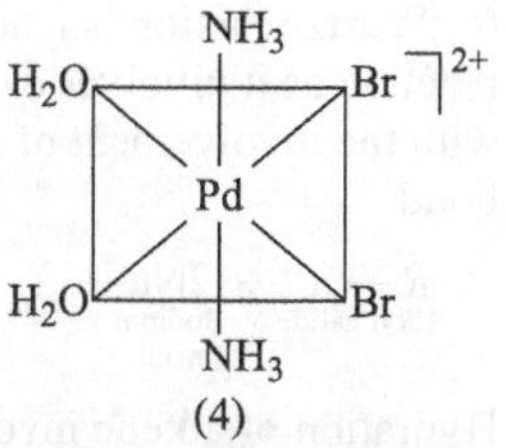

(4)

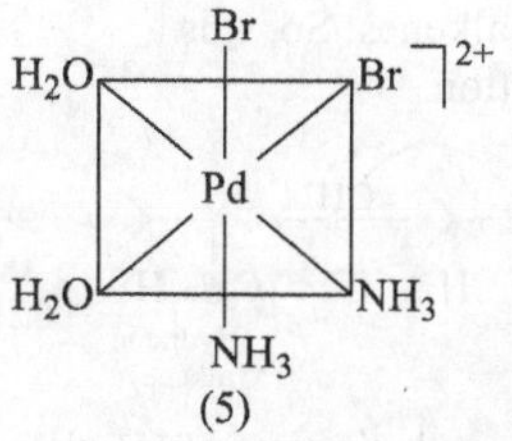

(5)

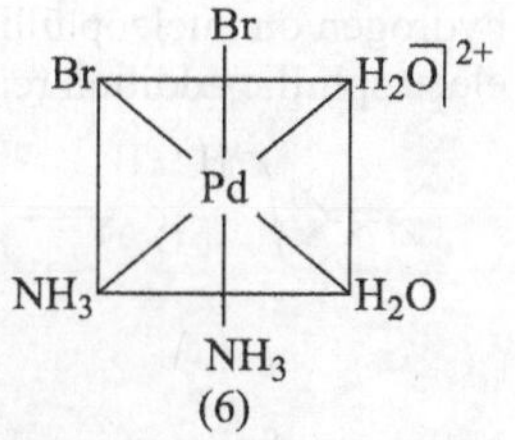

(6)

(1) to (5) are geometrical isomers; (5) and (6) are optical isomers.

65. (a) The vector sum of all polar bonds in *trans*-pent-2-ene is not zero but the vector sum is zero in *trans*-but-2-ene.

66. (b) Molecular weight of $CH_4 = 16\,g$

Heat liberated in the combustion of 0.4 g of $CH_4 = -0.25$ kcal

So, in the combustion of 16 g CH_4 heat liberated

$$= -\frac{0.25}{0.4} \times 16 = -10\,kcal$$

Hence, the heat of combustion of CH_4 is 10 kcal where the (– ve) sign showing that heat is liberated.

67. (b) Greater is the electronegativity difference of *M*—H bond greater will be acidic nature. Strong acid has weak conjugate base and *vice-versa*, so the correct order will be

$$CH_3NH_2 < CH_3OH < CH_3SH$$

68. (b) Cl_2O_6 (dimer of ClO_3) is a mixed anhydride of $HClO_3$ and $HClO_4$.

$$Cl_2O_6 + H_2O \longrightarrow HClO_3 + HClO_4$$

69. (d) Both Statement I and Statement II are true.

70. (d) When conc. H_2SO_4 is heated with P_2O_5, the acid is converted to sulphur trioxide. The reaction is as follows

$$\underset{\text{Sulphuric acid (conc.)}}{2H_2SO_4} + \underset{\text{Phosphorus pentoxide}}{2P_2O_5} \xrightarrow{\Delta} \underset{\text{Sulphur trioxide}}{2SO_3} + \underset{\text{Metaphosphoric acid}}{4HPO_3}$$

71. (a) K_2SO_4 raises the boiling point of H_2SO_4 while $CuSO_4$ act as a catalyst.

Baeyer test is used for the determination of presence of carbon-carbon double bonded compounds or carbon-carbon triple bonded compounds by using alkaline potassium permanganate. Hence, both Statement I and Statement II are false.

72. (c) Wurtz reaction is a nucleophillic substitution reaction as it involves exchange of halogen and metal with the involvement of radical species *R* to form C—C bond.

$$\underset{\text{Alkyl halide}}{R{-}X} + \underset{\text{Sodium metal}}{2Na} + X{-}R \xrightarrow{\text{Dry ether}} \underset{\text{Alkane}}{R{-}R} + 2NaX$$

Hydration of alkene involves act of adding electrophillic hydrogen on nucleophillic alkenes. So, it is a electrophillic addition reaction.

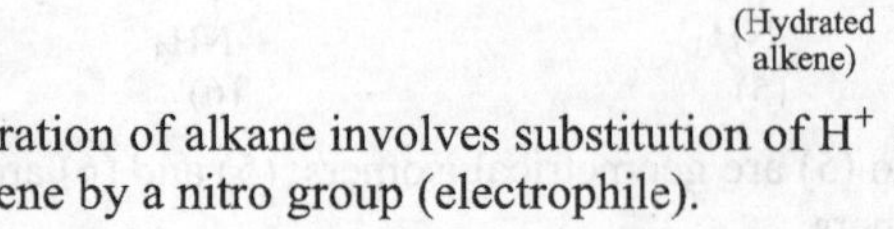

(Hydrated alkene)

Nitration of alkane involves substitution of H^+ from alkene by a nitro group (electrophile).

So, it is a electrophillic substitution reaction.

Reaction of alkene with NBS involves formation of free radical $\dot{Br}$ from NBS reagent and hydrogen atom at allylic position will get substitution by bromine radical. So, it is a type of free radical substitution reaction.

Hence, the correct match is A-(ii), B-(i), C-(iv), D-(iii).

73. (d) The σ-bond is stronger than π-bond as in σ-bond co-axial bonding overlap of orbital takes place whereas in π-bond lateral overlapping of orbital takes place. Hence, (a) is incorrect.

HF is more polar than HI as electronegativity between H and F is more than H and I. Hence, (b) is incorrect.

In NH_4^+, there is only one coordinate bond as shown below.

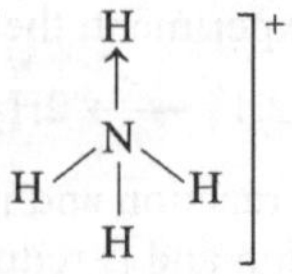

Hence, (c) is also incorrect.

In SF_6 all S—F bond are equivalent and of same length in octahedral geometry.

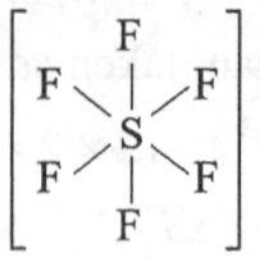

Hence, (d) is the correct statement.

74. (c) Even though the molecule contains polar bond but it will be non-polar if net dipole moment is zero.

XeF_5^+ undergoes sp^3d^2-hybridisation with one lone pair. Thus, due to lone pair on Xe, it creates lone pair-bond pair repulsion, which distorts the shape.

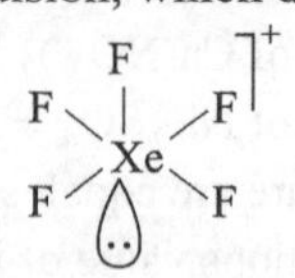

(Distorted octahedral)

Hence, Statement I is false but Statement II is true.

75. (c) $HClO_4$ is not formed in the reaction between Cl_2 and H_2O.

Instead, the following reaction is used to form $HClO_4$.

$$NaClO_4 + HCl \longrightarrow NaCl + HClO_4$$

76. (d) (A) *p*, *p*-dihydroxy benzophenone

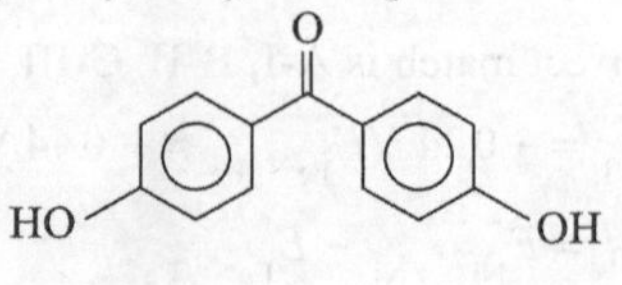

(B) 3-bromo-4-phenylpentanoic acid

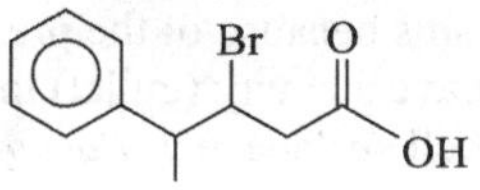

(C) *p*-nitropropiophenone

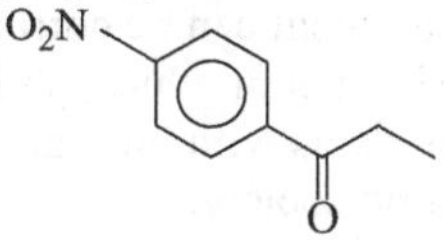

(D) Hex-2-en-4-ynoic acid

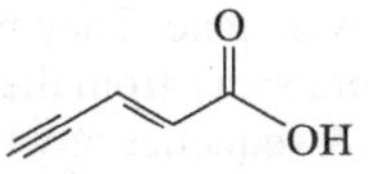

Hence, the correct match is A-(ii), B-(iii), C-(i), D-(iv).

77. (b) Aromatic aldehydes and formaldehydes don't contain α-hydrogen and thus undergo Cannizzaro reaction. Formaldehyde is more reactive than aromatic aldehyde in nucleophilic addition reactions. This is due to electron-donating resonance effect of aromatic ring which makes carbon less electrophilic.
Hence, Statement I is true but Statement II is false.

Problem Solving Tactics Cannizzaro reaction involves the base-induced disproportionation of two molecules of aldehyde (which does not contain α-hydrogen) to yield a carboxylic acid and a primary alcohol.

78. (d) Statements given in I, II and III are correct while IV and V are incorrect. Chelating ligands have more than one donor atom. They are non-linear and they must form bonds with reasonable angles at the metal atom.
Ethylene diamine is a bidentate chelating ligand.
They have higher affinity for a metal ion than monodentate ligands also they form more stable complex than monodentate ligand.

79. (a) We know that, $\Delta S_{\text{fus}} = \dfrac{\Delta H_{\text{fus}}}{T_{\text{fus}}}$

$$= \frac{6000 \text{ J mol}^{-1}}{273 \text{ K}} = 21.98 \text{ JK}^{-1} \text{ mol}^{-1}$$

80. (c) Among the given oxides II, IV and V are acidic. I is basic and III is neutral.

81. (d) For a hydrogen atom, the energies that an electron can have are given by the expression,
$E = -13.58/n^2$ eV, where n is an integer.

For first energy level,

$$E_1 = -13.58/1^2 \text{ eV}$$
$$= -13.58 \text{ eV}$$

For second energy level,

$$E_2 = -13.58/2^2 \text{ eV}$$
$$= -3.395 \text{ eV}$$

The difference $E_2 - E_1 = -3.395 \text{ eV} - (-13.58 \text{ eV})$
$= 10.185$
≈ 10.19 eV

82. (d) Atomic number of the element.
$[\text{Rn}]\, 5f^{14} 6d^1 7s^2 = 86 + 14 + 1 + 2$
$= 103$
So, IUPAC name = Unniltrium.

83. (d) $Cl^- + Na^+ \longrightarrow \underset{\text{(Neutral)}}{NaCl} \xrightarrow{AgNO_3} \underset{\text{(Insoluble in dil. } HNO_3)}{AgCl}$ (white ppt.)

84. (d)

Compound	Calculation	Oxidation state of iodine
I_2		0
ICl	$x - 1 = 0; x = +1$	+1
HI	$+1 + x = 0; x = -1$	−1
HIO_4	$+1 + x + (-2)4 = 0; x = +7$	+7

Hence, correct sequence is $HI < I_2 < ICl < HIO_4$.

85. (b) Both Statement I and Statement II are correct.

86. (d) Chlorobenzene undergoes nitration reaction. It gives 2-4-dinitrochlorobenzene which further reacts with sodium carbonate to form *X*, i.e. 2, 4-dinitrophenol.
'*X*' further undergoes nitration reaction to form 2, 4, 6-trinitrophenol '*Y*'.
The given reaction is

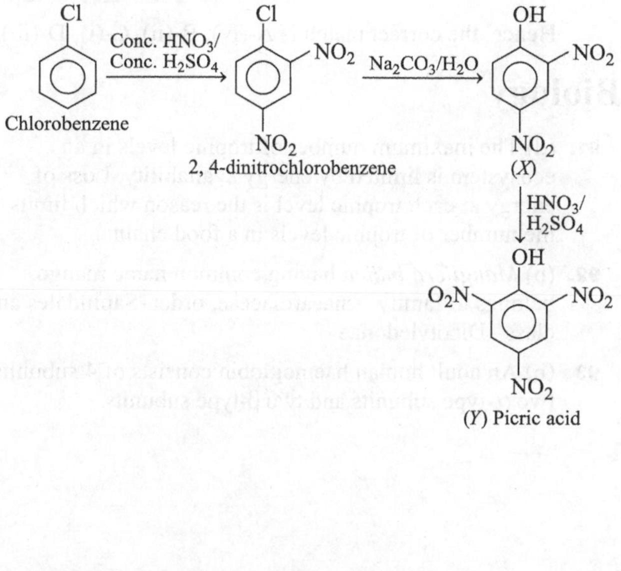

87. (b) Acetone reacts with phenyl magnesium bromide followed by acidic hydrolysis to give 2-phenyl propan-2-ol.

The given reaction is as follows

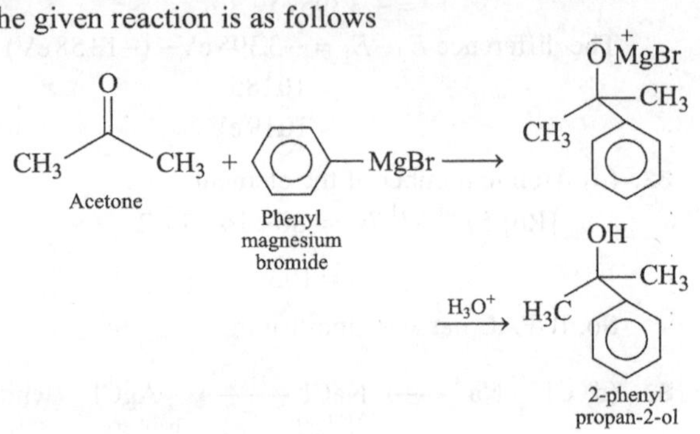

88. (b) Be_2 having bond order zero does not exist in nature.

89. (a) Methylphenylether is obtained by the reaction of phenolate ions and methyl iodide.

$$\underset{\text{Phenolate}}{C_6H_5O^-} + \underset{\text{Methyl iodide}}{CH_3I} \longrightarrow \underset{\text{Methyl phenyl ether}}{C_6H_5OCH_3} + \underset{\text{Iodide ion}}{I^-}$$

90. (a) Number of lone pair of electrons on the central atom

$$= \frac{\text{Number of valence electrons on central atom} - 2\,(\text{Number of bivalent atoms}) - (\text{Number of monovalent atoms})}{2}$$

Species	No. of lone pair
XeF_2	$n = (8-2)/2 = 3$
XeO_2F_2	$n = \dfrac{8-(2\times 2)-2}{2} = 1$
XeO_3F_2	$n = \dfrac{8-(2\times 3)-2}{2} = 0$
XeF_4	$n = \dfrac{8-4}{2} = 2$

Hence, the correct match is A-(iv), B-(ii), C-(i), D-(iii).

Biology

91. (d) The maximum number of trophic levels in an ecosystem is limited by energy availability. Loss of energy at each trophic level is the reason which limits the number of trophic levels in a food chain.

92. (b) *Mangifera indica* having common name mango, belongs to family–Anacardiaceae, order–Sapindales and class– Dicotyledonae.

93. (b) An adult human haemoglobin consists of 4 subunits, two α-type subunits and two β-type subunits.

94. (d) Ciliated protozoans are aquatic and are actively moving organisms because of the presence of thousands of cilia. They have a cavity (gullet) that opens to the outside of the cell surface, e.g. *Paramecium*.

95. (a) Statement I is incorrect, but statement II is correct. The incorrect statement can be corrected as Bioethics is the branch of ethics, philosophy and social commentary that deals with biological sciences and their potential impact on society.

96. (c) Enhancers are DNA sequences that facilitate the expression of a given gene. They may be located few hundreds base pairs away from the gene. Whereas, promoter is a DNA sequence at which RNA polymerase may bind, leading to the initiation of transcription.

97. (d) Statement I is correct, but statement II is incorrect and can be corrected as

Glycosylation is the formation of glycolipid from lipid and glycoprotein from protein.

98. (c) Dinoflagellates are mostly marine and photosynthetic. Their cell wall has stiff cellulosic plates on the outer surface. They release toxins that may even kill other marine animals.

99. (b) The ABO blood group in humans is an example of codominance. In codominance, there is joint expression of both alleles in a heterozygote. In this situation, alleles of a single gene are responsible for producing distinct and detectable gene products.

100. (b) The members of Phaeophyceae or brown algae have a cellulosic wall usually covered on the outside by a gelatinous coating of algin. The food is stored as laminarin.

101. (c) *Laminaria* and *Fucus* belong to Phaeophyceae. They have pyriform (pear-shaped) gametes and bear two laterally attached flagella.

102. (d) Thyroxine is formed by the amino acid tyrosine.

103. (d) Statements I, IV and V are correct, while statements II and III are incorrect and these can be corrected as

- Promoter sequences are present upstream of structural gene (towards the 5′ region of sense strand).
- The nascent RNA is synthesised by the RNA polymerase-II and is called *hn*RNA.

104. (c) Both A and R are true, but R is not the correct explanation of A.

Three types of cells are present in aerolar tissue namely mast cell, macrophages and fibroblasts. Aerolar tissue consists of two types of fibre, i.e. yellow elastin fibres and white collagen fibres.

White collagen fibres are found at the site of injury during tissue repair.

105. (a) The seeds of *Cheiranthus cheiri* belong to family Cruciferae also known as Brassicaceae. They are useful in bronchitis and fever.

106. (d) A is true, but R is false. R can be corrected as Vessels form an efficient system for transporting water and minerals from root to the leaves and other parts of the plant.

107. (b) Hepatic portal system (*A*) is a special venous connection between the liver and intestine.

Renal portal system (*B*) is a special venous connection between kidney and lower part of the body.

108. (c) Total volume of air a person can inspire after a normal expiration is called Inspiratory Capacity (IC). This includes Tidal Volume and Inspiratory Reserve Volume (TV + IRV).

109. (b) Statements III and V are correct. Rest statements are incorrect and can be corrected as

- Auxin translocation is polar.
- Abscisic acid is transported through xylem.
- During differentiation cells undergo few to major structural changes both in their cell walls and protoplasm. For example, to form a tracheary element, the cells would lose their protoplasm.

110. (d) Statement I is correct, but statement II is incorrect. It can be corrected as

In basal placentation, the placenta develops at the base of ovary and a single ovule is attached to it, as in sunflower and marigold.

111. (c) Statements I, IV and V are correct. Rest of the statements are incorrect and can be corrected as

- Transformation is a process in which a piece of DNA is directly introduced in a host bacterium, whereas transduction is the process by which a virus transfers the genetic material from one bacterium to another.
- The techniques of genetic engineering such as gene cloning and gene transfer allow us to isolate and introduce desirable genes without introducing undesirable genes into target organism.

112. (b) A species is a group of individuals, which resemble each other in morphological, physiological, biochemical and behavioural characters.
These individuals are capable of breeding, feeding on between themselves under natural conditions, but are incapable of breeding with members of other species. This is referred to as reproductive isolation.

113. (b) The *Bt* toxin genes are produced by a bacterium called *Bacillus thuringiensis*. The toxin is coded by *cry* gene. *cry IAc* and *cry II Ab* control the cotton bollworms and *cry I Ab* controls the corn borer.

114. (b) The final stage of meiotic prophase-I is diakinesis. This is marked by terminalisation of chiasmata. During this phase the chromosomes are fully condensed and meiotic spindle is assembled to prepare the homologous chromosomes for separation.

115. (b) Both A and R are true and R is the correct explanation of A.
Sewage contains large amount of organic matter and microbes many of which are pathogenic and can spread diseases so the treatment of sewage is essential to maintain public health and to protect environment.

116. (b) The virus of AIDS contains a single-strand of RNA enclosed in an envelope.

117. (b) The stroke volume multiplied by the heart rate (no. of beats per minute) gives the cardiac output.

118. (b) Both statement I and statement II are correct.

To fix CO_2 Hatch and Slack pathway is the alternate to the C_3 cycle. This pathway is slightly common in several grasses, maize, sugarcane and *Sorghum*.

Whereas, Calvin pathway is common to both C_3 and C_4 plants. In C_3 plants, it occurs in all mesophyll cells while in C_4 plant it takes place in bundle sheath cells only.

119. (b) Statement is option (b) is incorrect and can be corrected as
Ovule is a small structure attached to the placenta by means of a stalk called funicle. The body of the ovule fuses with funicle in the region called hilum.
Rest are correct statements.

120. (c) Statements III and IV are incorrect.

The incorrect statements can be corrected as

- Mitochondria in the middle piece produces energy for the mobility of sperm.
- The corpus luteum secretes large amount of progesterone for the maintenance of endometrium.

Rest other statements are correct.

121. (b) Statement III is incorrect. It can be corrected as MTP are considered relatively safe during the first trimester, i.e. upto 12 weeks of pregnancy.

122. (b) There is a characteristic distribution of the cells within the embryo sac. Three cells are grouped together at the micropylar end and constitute the egg apparatus. The egg apparatus consists of two synergids and one egg cell (ovum).

123. (b) The synergids have special cellular thickenings at the micropylar tip called filliform apparatus, which play an important role in guiding the pollen tubes into the synergids.

124. (a) The midbrain and hindbrain (Pons and Medulla oblongata) together form the brain stem. Hypothalamus forms a part of forebrain.

125. (b) The descending limb of loop of Henle is permeable to water, but almost impermeable to electrolytes. This concentrates the filtrate as it moves down.

126. (c) The given figure is of *Paramoecium*, a ciliated protozoan. They are actively moving organisms because of the presence of thousands of cilia. Ciliated protozoans steer food - laden water into their gullet through the coordinated movement of rows of cilia.

127. (a) Fibres of the tracts, covered with the myelin sheath, constitute the inner part of cerebral hemisphere. They give an opaque white appearance and are called white matter.

128. (c) The correct match is A-1, B-2, C-3, D-4.
- Intrafascicular cambium is present between xylem and phloem.
- Interfascicular cambium refers to the parenchymatous cells of medullary rays.
- There are more than six (polyarch) xylem bundles in the monocot root.
- Heartwood is physiologically inactive.

129. (b) Cerebellum is involved in loss of control when a person consumes alcohol, as it maintains the equilibrium, posture and orientation of the body.

130. (b) Cortical layers are present below hypodermis that consist of rounded thin walled parenchymatous cells with conspicous intercellular spaces.

131. (a) The ring arrangement of vascular bundles is a characteristic of dicot stem. Each vascular bundle is conjoint, open and with endarch protoxylem.

132. (a) The ion gradients across the resting membrane are maintained by active transport of ions which transports $3Na^+$ outwards for $2K^+$ into the cell.

133. (a) The trachea is supported by C-shaped rings of cartilage, which hold them in place when there is less air inside it. This prevents their collapse.

134. (c) Both A and R true, but R is not the correct explanation of A. The bioresources are analysed for the identification of valuable biomolecules. Analysing bioresources for biomolecules is essential for disease diagnostics, food safety inspection, environmental monitoring and pharmaceutical development.

135. (a) In his experiment Mendel studied two contrasting traits, i.e. one dominant and another recessive.

	Characters	Dominant/ Recessive
1.	Stem height	Tall / Dwarf
2.	Flower colour	Violet / White
3.	Flower position	Axial / Terminal
4.	Pod shape	Inflated / Constricted
5.	Pod colour	Green / Yellow
6.	Seed shape	Round / Wrinkled
7.	Seed colour	Yellow / Green

136. (c) Statements I, III and V are correct, whereas statements II and IV are incorrect. These can be corrected as
- The cell wall provide shape to the cell, protects the cell from mechanical damage and infection. It also helps in cell to cell interaction.
- The middle lamella is a layer of calcium pectate, which holds or glues the different neighbouring cells together.

137. (d) Coenzyme/cofactors are organic substances which are loosely attached with apoenzymes. The factors which are tightly attached with apoenzymes are prosthetic groups. These are basically the category of cofactor.

138. (d) All the statements are correct, except statement in option (d) and it can be corrected as
In parasitic food chains, the size of parasites gradually decreases in successive trophic levels e.g, lice being eaten by microscopic bacteria and fungi.

139. (a) At the end of prophase, when cells are viewed under the microscope, the Golgi complexes, endoplasmic reticulum, nucleolus and the nuclear envelope are not seen.

140. (a) Statement I is incorrect, but statement II is correct. The incorrect statement can be corrected as In juxtamedullary nephrons, the blood first passes through the capillaries of glomerulus and then through the vasa recta.

141. (d) A is true, but R is false and it can be corrected as Decomposers produce inorganic raw materials for recycling.

142. (c) Green seed and constricted pod are the recessive characters used by the Mendel during his experiment.
Green seed and wrinkled seeds were recessive to yellow and round seeds. Whereas, yellow and constricted pods were recessive to green and inflated pods.

143. (d) In the presence of an inducer such as lactose or allolactose, the repressor is inactivated by interaction with inducer. This allows RNA polymerase access to the promoter and transcription proceeds.

144. (c) In the given figure of pectoral girdle and upper arm, *A* represents clavicle, *B* represents scapula, *C* represents radius, *D* represents ulna, *E* represents carpals, *F* represents metacarpals and *G* represents phalanges. The scapula (B) is a large triangular bone possessing slightly elevated ridge called the spine which projects as a flat, expanded process called acromion.

145. (d) Population of organisms evolves to maximise their reproductive fitness, i.e. Darwinian fitness in the habitat in which they live.
Under a particular set of selection pressures organisms evolve towards most efficient reproductive strategy. Life

history traits of organisms have evolved in relation to the constraints imposed by components of habitat in which they live.

However loss of energy does not relate to evolving populations.

146. (c) The correct matches are A-4, B-1, C-2, D-3.

Diseases	Symptoms
Typhoid	Sustained high fever (39°C - 40°C) stomach pain, headache, etc.
Pneumonia	Fever, chills, finger nails turn gray to bluish in colour, etc.
Ascariasis	Muscular pain, internal bleeding, blockage of intestinal passage, etc.
Filariasis	Genital organs are also affected resulting in gross deformities.

147. (a) If we use DNA polymerase, isolated from normal soil bacterium, in PCR, we cannot obtain even a single copy of DNA. This is because normal DNA polymerase cannot with stand high temperature of PCR and gets denatured.

148. (b) Most aerobic respiration takes place in the cell's mitochondria. So, the final product of glycolysis, pyruvate is transported to mitochondria.

149. (a) The correct matches are A-2, B-3, C-4, D-1.

- Pineal gland secretes a hormone called melatonin and is present on the dorsal side of forebrain.
- The thyroid gland is composed of follicles and stromal tissue.
- Parathyroid gland secretes parathyroid hormone that increases Ca^{2+} levels in blood.
- Thymus gland secretes the peptide hormone thymosin that plays a major role in differentiation of T-lymphocytes.

150. (c) Both statement I and statement II are incorrect and can be corrected as In urochordates like *Salpa*, *Ascidia*, etc. notochord is present only in larval tail, while in cephalochordates like *Branchiostoma* notochord extends from head to tail region and is persistent throughout their life.

151. (c) Statement in option (c) is incorrect and can be corrected as

In *Spirogyra* vegetative reproduction usually takes place by fragmentation or by formation of different types of spores.

152. (a) Statement I is incorrect, but statement II is correct. The incorrect statement can be corrected as

TSH stands for Thyroid Stimulating Hormone. It controls the secretion of thyroxine hormone.

153. (b) Electron micrographs of zygotene stage indicate that chromosome synapsis is accompanied by the formation of complex structure called synaptonemal complex.

154. (d) During protein formation, amino acid condense to produce protein and molecule of water is eliminated, i.e. dehydration takes place. Glycosidic bond is also formed by the removal of a molecule of water.

155. (b) Organisms like reptiles, birds and land snails, etc. excrete nitrogenous waste as uric acid in the form of pellet with a minimum loss of water, they are known as uricotelic animals.

156. (c) Oral contraceptive pill is a popular method of contraception used by females. They work by inhibiting ovulation and implantation. Saheli is a new oral contraceptive pill for females that contains a non-steroidal preparation. It is once a week pill with very few side effects and high contraceptive value.

157. (b) Statements I and IV are incorrect. These can be corrected as

- Columnar or cuboidal cells bearing cilia on their surface are called ciliated epithelium.
- The cuboidal epithelium lines salivary gland and pancreatic ducts.

Rest other statements are correct.

158. (d) Xenogamy is a type of cross-pollination in which pollens are transferred from anther of the different plants to the stigma of a different flower as seen in grasses.

159. (b) Calvin cycle requires 3 ATP, 2 NADPH molecules and one CO_2 for a single turn of the cycle.

160. (b) Beetles are coleopterans, which are killed by *Bacillus thuringiensis* (*Bt*). The bacterium is also toxic to nematodes.

161. (c) The set of organs having different structures, but evolving for the same function and hence have similarity are known as analogous organs, e.g. eye of mammals and octopus, flippers of penguins and dolphins, etc.

162. (b) Statement in option (b) is incorrect. It can be corrected as

The standing crop is measured as the mass of living organisms or the number in a unit area.

163. (c) In glomerulus, the afferent arteriole is shorter and wider than efferent arteriole, which is longer and narrower.

164. (a) Oxidative phosphorylation refers to the formation of ATP from ADP and Pi in the presence of O_2. The synthesis of ATP is driven by proton motive force developed during oxidation of reducing powers NADH and $FADH_2$ through electron transport chain. The use of proton motive force to drive transport of protons down the concentration gradient and simultaneous ADP phosphorylation represents chemiosmosis.

165. (b) Statements III, IV and V are correct. Statements I and II are incorrect and can be corrected as
- Western ghats have a greater amphibian species diversity than the Eastern ghats.
- India with its mangroves, coral reefs, wetlands and alpine meadows has a greater ecosystem diversity than a Scandinavian country like Norway.

166. (d) The correct match is A-3, B-1, C-4, D-2.
- Golden rice is a genetically modified variety of rice, which is enriched with vitamin - A.
- Alpha (α)- 1 - antitrypsin helps in the treatment of emphysema.
- *Flavr Savr* is a genetically modified variety of tomato, which is modified to increase the shelf life.
- First transgenic cow, Rosie produced human protein enriched milk (2.4 gms per litre).

167. (a) The correct matches are A-2, B-3, C-4, D-1.
- Golden rice is rich in vitamin-A. It is a genetically modified crop.
- Cry protein is a crystal protein that is poisonous to insects and is expressed by the *cry* gene of *B. thuringiensis*. Because of this, it is also known as *Bt* toxin.
- RNA interference is known as gene silencing. It involves silencing of a specific *m*RNA due to complementary *ds*RNA molecule that binds to *m*RNA and prevents its translation.
- Tobacco budworm and army worm are lepidopteran insects.

168. (a) The statement is option (a) is correct as the volume of blood pumped out by the right and left ventricles are same.

169. (b) Both A and R are true and R is the correct explanation of A. This can be explained as
The size of chromosome is measured best during metaphase as during this phase the chromosomes are in most condensed and coiled stage and are also aligned at the equator.

170. (a) Statements III and IV are incorrect and can be corrected as
- The centrosomes are surrounded by amorphous pericentriolar materials.
- The inclusion bodies like gas vacuoles, cyanophycean granules, etc. are not bound by any membrane system and lie free in the cytoplasm. Rest all statements are correct.

171. (b) Both A and R are true, and R is the correct explanation of A. The *Bt* toxin genes are isolated from *B. thuringiensis* and incorporated into several crop plants to kill the targeted pests or insect of that crop.

172. (b) Antrum is the fluid-filled cavity found in ovarian follicles, which is rich in hyaluronan and proteoglycans.

173. (b) In *Drosophila* the female has a pair of XX chromosome (homogametic) and the male has XY chromosomes (heterogametic) composition.

174. (a) The correct match is A-4, B-1, C-2, D-3. *Spirogyra* is an example of green algae. *Marchantia*, *Polytrichum*, *Dictyota* are the examples of liverworts, moss and brown algae, respectively.

175. (c) The vertebral column is differentiated into five groups. The first 7 are called cervical vertebrae, the next 12 are called thoracic vertebrae, the next 5 are lumbar vertebrae, the next 1 is sacral vertebrae and the next 1 is coccygeal vertebrae starting from the skull to the spine.

176. (c) *Salmonella typhi* causes typhoid fever. These pathogens generally enter the small intestine through food and water and migrate to other organs through blood.

177. (a) The side effects of anabolic steroids in females include masculinisation (features like males), excessive hairs on face, mood swings, enlargement of clitoris, abnormal menstrual cycles and deepening of voice.

178. (c) *C* represents coleoptile, which is a protective covering for plumule in the embryo.

179. (d) The option (d) is incorrectly matched pair. It can be corrected as

Dengue is a viral infection caused by the dengue virus transmitted to humans through the bite of infected *Aedes* mosquitoes.

180. (a) The correct matches are A-2, B-3, C-1, D-4.

Hormones	Functions
Human chorionic gonadotrophin	Maintains corpus luteum
Progesterone	Suppress uterine contractions
Oestrogen	Promotes growth of myometrium
Relaxin	Softens cervix to prepare for dilation

SECTION II
Mastery Builders

PRACTICE SET 6

Maximum Marks : 720 | Time : 3 hrs | No. of Questions : 180

Instructions

1. This question paper contains **180** multiple-choice questions (four options with a single correct answer) from **Physics, Chemistry** and **Biology**.
2. These questions are distributed as 45 questions, each from Physics and Chemistry and 90 questions in Biology. These are to be compulsorily attempted by the candidate.
3. Each question carries 4 marks. For each correct response, the candidate will get 4 marks. For each incorrect response, one mark will be deducted from the total scores.

PHYSICS

1. The respective speeds of five molecules are 1, 2, 3, 4 and 5 km/s. The ratio of their rms velocity and the average velocity will be

(a) $\sqrt{11}:3$ (b) $3:\sqrt{11}$ (c) $1:2$ (d) $3:4$

2. A coil in the shape of an equilateral triangle of side 0.02 m is suspended from its vertex, such that it is hanging in a vertical plane between the pole pieces of permanent magnet producing a uniform field of 5×10^{-2} T. If a current of 0.1 A is passed through the coil, what is the couple acting?

(a) $5\sqrt{3}\times10^{-7}$ N-m (b) $5\sqrt{3}\times10^{-10}$ N-m

(c) $\frac{\sqrt{3}}{5}\times10^{-7}$ N-m (d) None of these

3. A tuning fork of frequency 520 Hz is used in an experiment for measuring speed of sound (v) in air by resonance tube method. Resonance is observed to occur at two successive lengths of air column, $l_1=30$ cm and $l_2=70$ cm. Then, v is equal to

(a) 385 m/s (b) 395 m/s (c) 416 m/s (d) 428 m/s

4. The masses of neutron and proton are 1.0087 and 1.0073 amu, respectively. If neutrons and protons combine to form helium nucleus of mass 4.0015 amu, the binding energy of the helium nucleus will be

(a) 28.4 MeV (b) 20.8 MeV
(c) 27.3 MeV (d) 14.2 MeV

5. Calculate the work done by a gas as it is taken from 1 to 2, 2 to 3 and 3 to 1 as shown in the figure. The work done in cyclic process $1\rightarrow2\rightarrow3\rightarrow1$ is found to be $-np_0V_0$, the value of n is

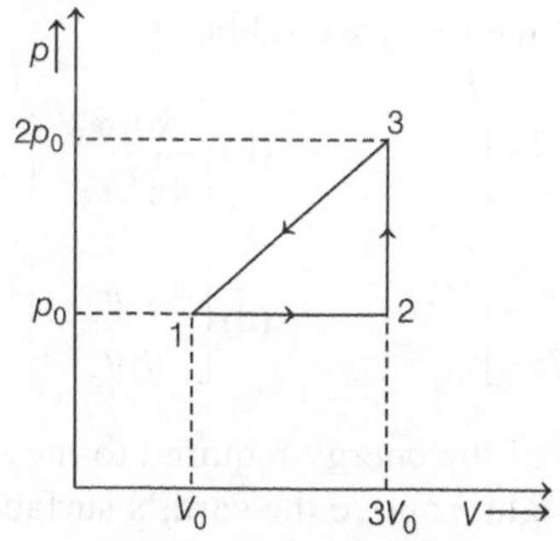

(a) 1 (b) 2
(c) 3 (d) 4

6. The two statements are given below

Statement I When unpolarised light is incident on the polariser, the intensity of the transmitted polarised light remains unchanged.

Statement II Polarisation is convincing proof of transverse nature of light wave.

In the light of above statements, choose the most appropriate answer from the options given below.
(a) Both Statement I and Statement II are correct.
(b) Both Statement I and Statement II are incorrect.
(c) Statement I is correct but Statement II is incorrect.
(d) Statement I is incorrect but Statement II is correct.

7. The stress *versus* strain graphs for wires of two materials A and B are as shown in figure. If Y_A and Y_B are the young's modulus of the materials, then

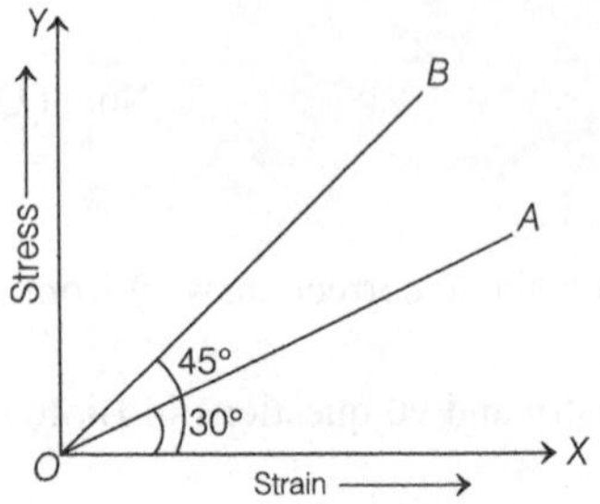

(a) $Y_A = 3Y_B$ (b) $Y_A = \sqrt{3}Y_B$
(c) $Y_B = 3Y_A$ (d) $Y_B = \sqrt{3}Y_A$

8. An α-particle is accelerated by V volt, experiences a force F, when it enters in a uniform magnetic field. When α-particle is accelerated by 3V, in same magnetic field, then force experienced by α-particle is
(a) $\sqrt{3}F$ (b) $\sqrt{2}F$ (c) $\frac{F}{3}$ (d) $\frac{F}{\sqrt{2}}$

9. Charge q_2 of mass m revolves around a stationary charge q_1 in a circular orbit of radius r. The orbital periodic time of q_2 would be
(a) $\left[\frac{4\pi^2 mr^2}{q_1 q_2}\right]^{\frac{1}{2}}$ (b) $\left[\frac{kq_1 q_2}{4\pi^2 mr^2}\right]^{\frac{1}{2}}$
(c) $\left[\frac{4\pi^2 mr^3}{kq_1 q_2}\right]^{\frac{1}{2}}$ (d) $\left[\frac{4\pi^2 mr^4}{q_1 q_2}\right]^{\frac{1}{2}}$

10. The ratio of the energy required to move a satellite upto a height h above the earth's surface of radius R to that the kinetic energy of satellite into that orbit is given by
(a) $R:2h$ (b) $R:h$ (c) $h:2R$ (d) $2h:R$

11. For an ideal gas of n moles, the temperature is increased from temperature T to $4T$ at pressure $p = aT^{-1}$, where a is a constant. What will be the work done by the gas ?
(a) $2nRT$ (b) nRT (c) $4nRT$ (d) $6nRT$

12. A pure inductor of 25 mH is connected to an AC source of 220 V and the frequency of the source is 50 Hz, the rms current in the circuit is
(a) 42 A (b) 28 A (c) 14 A (d) 7 A

13. A block of mass 10 kg is moving horizontally with a speed of 1.5 ms^{-1} on a smooth plane. If a constant vertical force of 10 N acts on it, then the displacement of the block from the point of application of the force at the end of 4s is
(a) 5 m (b) 20 m (c) 12 m (d) 10 m

14. A satellite is revolving around the earth, close to its surface with a kinetic energy E, then the energy required to be given to it, so that it escape from the earth is
(a) $2E$ (b) $\frac{E}{2}$ (c) E (d) $3E$

15. 22 g of CO_2 at 27°C is mixed with 16 g of O_2 at 37°C. The temperature of mixture is
[Assume degree of freedom of $CO_2 = 7$ and degree of freedom of $O_2 = 5$]
(a) 31.16°C (b) 27°C
(c) 37°C (d) 30°C

16. If $\frac{4}{3}$ and $\frac{3}{2}$ are the refractive indices of water and glass, respectively. A ray of light travelling in water is incident on the water-glass interface at 30°. The angle of refraction is given by
(a) $\sin^{-1}\left(\frac{4}{9}\right)$ (b) $\sin^{-1}\left(\frac{3}{2}\right)$
(c) $\sin^{-1}\left(\frac{18}{8}\right)$ (d) $\sin^{-1}\left(\frac{4}{3}\right)$

17. An α-particle after passing through a potential difference of V volts collides with a nucleus. If the atomic number of the nucleus is Z, then the distance of closest approach of α-particle to the nucleus will be
(a) $14.4\frac{Z}{V}$ Å (b) $14.4\frac{Z}{V}$ m
(c) $14.4\frac{Z}{V}$ cm (d) 1.44×10^{-15} m

18. The position x of a particle varies with time t as $x = 6 + 12t - 2t^2$, where x is in metres and t is in seconds. The distance travelled by the particle in first five seconds is
(a) 16 m (b) 26 m
(c) 10 m (d) 36 m

19. In a particular medium in an EM wave, if $E_0 = 9$ N/C and speed of light in free space is 3×10^8 ms^{-1}. The amplitude of magnetic field will be

(a) 1×10^{-8} T (b) 2×10^{-8} T
(c) 3×10^{-8} T (d) 2.5×10^{-8} T

20. The displacement of body along X-axis depends on time as $\sqrt{x} = t+1$, then the velocity of body

(a) increases with time (b) decreases with time
(c) independent of time (d) None of the above

21. Identify the logic gates marked X and Y in the following figure.

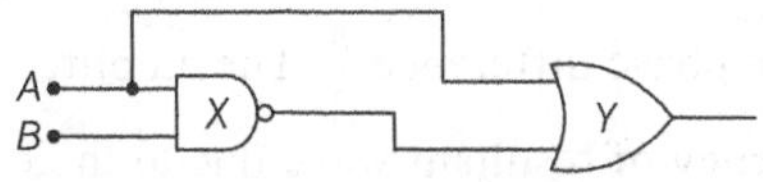

(a) OR, NAND (b) NAND, OR
(c) NOT, OR (d) AND, NOR

22. Match the column I (types of material) with column II (their properties).

	Column I		Column-II
A.	Diamagnetic	I.	$\mu_r >> 1$
B.	Paramagnetic	II.	$\mu_r > 1$
C.	Ferromagnetic	III.	$\mu_r = 0$
D.	Superconductor	IV.	$0 < \mu_r < 1$

Choose the correct answer from the given options.

	A	B	C	D		A	B	C	D
(a)	I	II	III	IV	(b)	IV	III	I	II
(c)	IV	II	III	I	(d)	IV	II	I	III

23. The velocity of electromagnetic wave is parallel to

(a) $\mathbf{B}\times\mathbf{E}$ (b) $\mathbf{E}$
(c) $\mathbf{E}\times\mathbf{B}$ (d) $\mathbf{B}$

24. In the relation, $p = \frac{\alpha}{\beta} e^{\frac{-\alpha z}{K\theta}}$, where p is pressure, z is distance, K is Boltzmann constant and θ is temperature. The dimensional formula of β will be

(a) $[M^0L^2T^0]$ (b) $[ML^2T]$
(c) $[ML^0T^{-1}]$ (d) $[M^0L^2T^{-1}]$

25. A. The n-type and p-type semiconductors are intrinsic semiconductors.

B. The number of free electrons in the conduction band is equal to the number of holes in the valence band in intrinsic semiconductors.

C. Electrical conductivity is high for extrinsic semiconductor.

Choose which of the above statements are correct from the given options.

(a) A and C only (b) B and C only
(c) A and B only (d) A, B and C

26. If number of turns per unit length of a coil of solenoid is doubled, then the self-inductance of the solenoid will

(a) be halved
(b) remain unchange
(c) be doubled
(d) become four times

27. If n equal resistors are used to produce a total resistance in circuit, then the ratio of maximum to the minimum resistance is

(a) $1:n^2$ (b) $n^2:1$
(c) $1:1$ (d) None of these

28. The bob A of simple pendulum is released, then the string makes an angle of 45° with the vertical. It hits another bob B of the same material and same mass kept at rest on the table. If the collision is elastic, then

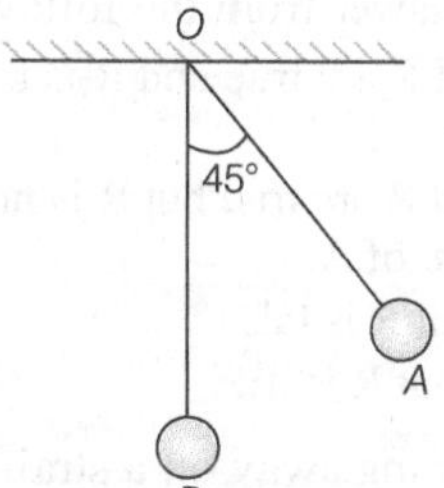

(a) Both A and B rise of the same height.
(b) Both A and B come to rest at B.
(c) Both A and B move with the same velocity of A.
(d) A comes to rest and B moves with the velocity of A.

29. For a coil having $L = 2$ mH, current flows through it is $i = t^2 e^{-t}$, then the time at which emf becomes zero.

(a) 1 s (b) 3 s
(c) 4 s (d) 2 s

30. Given below are two statements

Statement I In slide wire bridge, the value of known resistance is so selected that the null point is obtained at the middle of the wire.

Statement II The wire of meter bridge is made up of copper or aluminium.

In the above statement, choose the most appropriate answer from the option given below.
(a) Statement I is incorrect but Statement II is correct.
(b) Statement I is correct but Statement II is incorrect.
(c) Both Statement I and Statement II are correct.
(d) Both Statement I and Statement II are incorrect.

31. The ratio of the energies of the hydrogen atom in its first to second excited state is
(a) 9/4 (b) 4 (c) 1/4 (d) 4/9

32. Positive and negative charges of equal magnitude are kept at $A(0,0,\sqrt{a})$ and $B(0,0,-\sqrt{a})$ respectively. The work done by the electric field when another positive point charge is moved from $(-2a,0,0)$ to $(0,2a,0)$ is
(a) zero (b) positive
(c) negative
(d) charges are not given so data insufficient

33. **Assertion** (A) If an electron and proton enter a perpendicular magnetic field with equal momentum, then radius of curve for electron is more than that of proton.
Reason (R) Radius is directly proportional to momentum of the particle.
In the light of above statements, choose the most appropriate answer from the following.
(a) Both A and R are true and R is the correct explanation of A.
(b) Both A and R are true but R is not the correct explanation of A.
(c) A is true but R is false.
(d) A is false but R is true.

34. A thief is running away on a straight road with a speed of $9\ ms^{-1}$. A policeman chases him in a jeep moving at a speed of $10\ ms^{-1}$. If the instantaneous separation of the jeep from the thief is 100 m, how long will it take for the policeman to catch the thief?
(a) 100 s (b) 90 s
(c) 19 s (d) 1 s

35. In the circuit shown below, A is joined to B for a long time and then A is joined to C. The total heat produced in R is

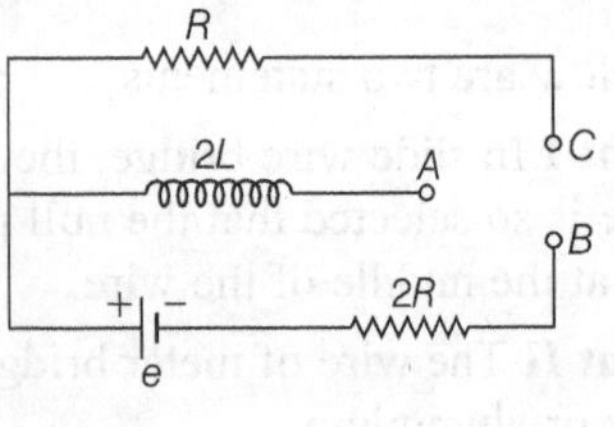

(a) $\frac{Le^2}{8R^2}$ (b) $\frac{Le^2}{2R^2}$
(c) $\frac{Le^2}{4R^2}$ (d) $\frac{Le^2}{R^2}$

36. From the top of a tower 19.6 m high, a ball is thrown horizontally. If the line joining the point of projection to the point where it hits the ground makes an angle of 45° with the horizontal, then the initial velocity of the ball is
(a) $2.8\ ms^{-1}$ (b) $9.8\ ms^{-1}$
(c) $4.9\ ms^{-1}$ (d) $14.7\ ms^{-1}$

37. Two waves each of amplitude a and frequency f have a phase difference $\frac{\pi}{2}$. The amplitude and frequency of resultant wave due to their superposition will be
(a) $\frac{a}{\sqrt{2}}, \frac{f}{2}$ (b) $\frac{a}{\sqrt{2}}, f$
(c) $2a, \frac{f}{2}$ (d) $\sqrt{2}a, f$

38. A block of mass 10 kg is pushed up on a smooth inclined plane of inclination 30°, so that it has acceleration $2\ m/s^2$. The applied force is
(a) 80 N (b) 50 N
(c) 60 N (d) 70 N

39. The work functions of three metals A, B and C are 1.92 eV, 2 eV and 5 eV, respectively. Which metals will emit photoelectrons for a radiation of wavelength 4100 Å?
(a) A only (b) B only
(c) Both A and B (d) C only

40. In the given figure, what will be the coefficient of mutual inductance?

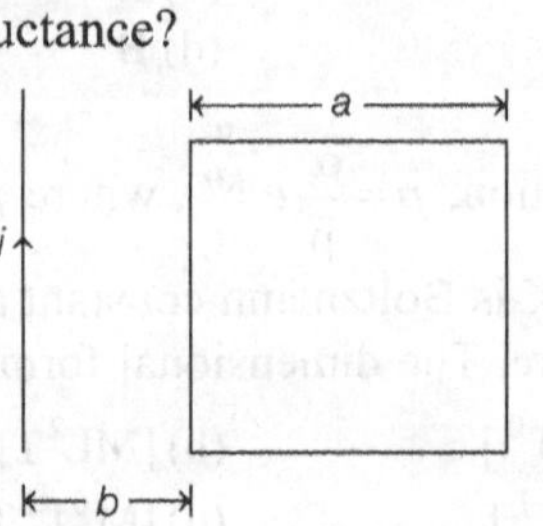

(a) $\frac{\mu_0 a}{2\pi} \ln\left(1+\frac{a}{2b}\right)$ (b) $\frac{\mu_0 a}{\pi} \ln\left(1+\frac{b}{2a}\right)$
(c) $\frac{\mu_0 a}{2\pi} \ln\left(1+\frac{a}{b}\right)$ (d) $\frac{\mu_0 a}{2\pi} \ln\left(1+\frac{b}{a}\right)$

41. In Young's double slit experiment, the distance between two slits is 0.8 mm and the fringes are observed 1m away. If it produces the second dark fringe at a distance of 1.5 mm from the middle position of central bright fringe, the wavelength of the monochromatic source of light used is

(a) 600 nm (b) 500 nm
(c) 450 nm (d) 480 nm

42. In an experiment, the measurement of diameter of a wire of length 5.0 cm with help of screw gauge, the main scale reads 1 mm and 48th division on circular scale coincides with the reference line. There are 100 divisions are on circular scale. If the pitch of the screw gauge is 1 mm, then volume of the wire is

(a) $0.019\,cm^3$ (b) $0.026\,cm^3$
(c) $0.086\,cm^3$ (d) $0.046\,cm^3$

43. Let the moment of inertia of a hollow cylinder of length 30 cm, inner radius 11 cm and outer radius 15 cm about its axis be I. The radius of a thin cylinder of the same mass such that its moment of inertia about its axis is also I, is found to be x cm, then the value of x is ....

(a) 14.5 (b) 10.5
(c) 13.1 (d) 18.5

44. In the following electric circuit, calculate the effective resistance between A and B.

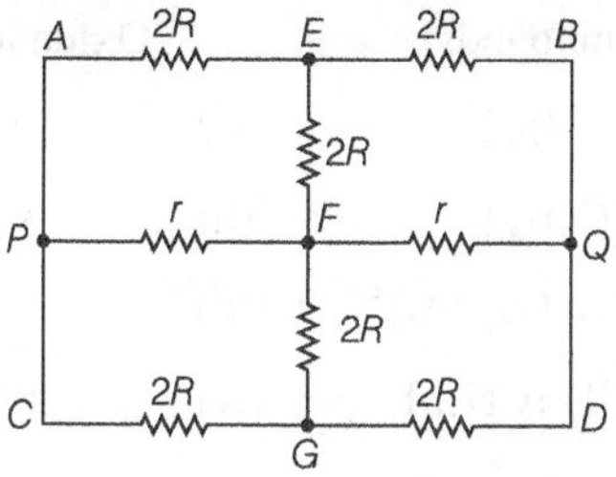

(a) $\frac{2Rr}{R+r}$ (b) $\frac{Rr}{2(R+r)}$
(c) $\frac{R^2}{r}+\frac{r^2}{R}$ (d) $\frac{2Rr}{3(R+r)}$

45. A solid conducting sphere having a charge Q is surrounded by an uncharged concentric conducting hollow spherical shell. Let the potential difference between the surface of solid sphere and that of the outer surface of hollow shell be V. What will be the new potential difference between the same two surfaces, if the shell is given a charge $-3Q$?

(a) $\frac{Q}{4\pi\varepsilon_0}\left(\frac{r_1}{r_2}-\frac{r_2}{r_1}\right)$ (b) $\frac{Q}{4\pi\varepsilon_0}\left(\frac{1}{r_1}-\frac{1}{r_2}\right)$
(c) $\frac{Q}{4\pi\varepsilon_0}\left(\frac{1}{r_2}-\frac{1}{r_1}\right)$ (d) $\frac{Q}{4\pi\varepsilon_0}\left(\frac{r}{r_1}-\frac{1}{r_2}\right)$

CHEMISTRY

46. The bond length of HCl is 3.40×10^{-10} m.

The percentage ionic character of HCl, if measured dipole moment is 6.28×10^{-30} Cm, is

(a) 12% (b) 8%
(c) 25% (d) 50%

47. For reaction $A\longrightarrow B$, rate constant $k_1=A_1e^{-\frac{E_{a1}}{RT}}$ and for the reaction $X\longrightarrow Y$, rate constant $k_2=A_2e^{-\frac{E_{a2}}{RT}}$. If $A_1=10^8$, $A_2=10^{10}$ and $E_{a_1}=600$ cal/mole, $E_{a_2}=1800$ cal/mole, then the temperature at which $k_1=k_2$ is

(Given : $R=2$ cal $K^{-1}mol^{-1}$)

(a) 1200 K (b) 1200×4.606 K
(c) $\frac{1200}{4.606}$ K (d) $\frac{600}{4.606}$ K

48. Hydrocarbon on reaction with steam produces hydrogen gas. Chemical reaction occurring in this process is given by

$$H_2O(g)+CH_4(g)\rightleftharpoons CO(g)+3H_2(g)$$

If $K_C=3.0\times10^{-4}$ at 1000 K, then the K_p would be

(a) 202 (b) 2.02 (c) 20.2 (d) 0.6740

49. Given below are two statements.

Statement I Surface tension is an intensive property.

Statement II Heat of neutralisation is always negative.

In the light of the above statements, choose the correct answer from the options given below:

(a) Both Statement I and Statement II are false.
(b) Statement I is true, but Statement II is false.
(c) Statement I is false, but Statement II is true.
(d) Both Statement I and Statement II are true.

50. Match the List-I with List-II.

List-I (Compounds)		List-II (Oxidation state)
A. $[Fe(CN)_6]^{3-}$	(i)	0
B. $[Ni(CO)_4]$	(ii)	+1
C. $[Fe(H_2O)_5NO]^{2+}$	(iii)	+3
D. $Fe_4[Fe(CN)_6]$	(iv)	+2

Choose the correct answer from the options given below.
(a) A-(iv), B-(iii), C-(i), D-(ii)
(b) A-(ii), B-(iv), C-(i), D-(iii)
(c) A-(iii), B-(i), C-(ii), D-(iv)
(d) A-(i), B-(ii), C-(iii), D-(iv)

51. Anisole $\xrightarrow[\text{Anhy. AlCl}_3]{(CH_3)_3CCl}$ $\xrightarrow{Cl_2/FeCl_3}$ $\xrightarrow[\text{Heat}]{HBr}$ '*A*'.

The product '*A*' in the above series of reaction is

(a) 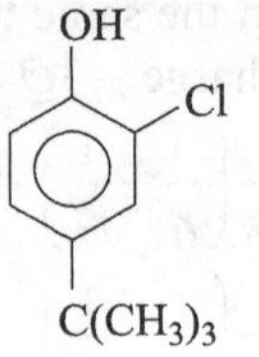

(b) 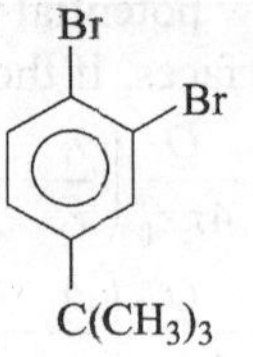

(c) 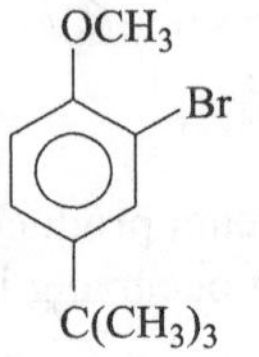

(d) 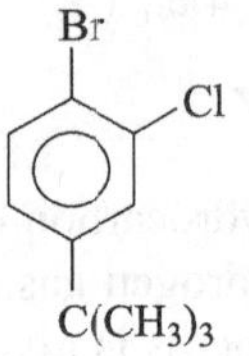

52. The reaction of propene with HOCl proceeds *via* the addition of
(a) OH^- in the first step
(b) H^+ in the first step
(c) Cl^+ in the first step
(d) Cl^+ and OH^- in a single step

53. K_a for HCN is 5×10^{-10} at 25°C. For maintaining a constant pH of 9, the volume of 5M KCN solution required to be added to 10 mL of 2M HCN solution is
(a) 4 mL (b) 2 mL (c) 8 mL (d) 10 mL

54. Given below are two statements, one is labelled as Assertion (A) and the other is labelled as Reason (R).

Assertion (A) Electron affinity of fluorine is less than that of chlorine.

Reason (R) Chlorine can accommodate an electron by utilising its vacant 3*d*-orbital.

In the light of the above statements, choose the most appropriate answer from the options given below.
(a) Both (A) and (R) are true but (R) is not the correct explanation of (A).
(b) (A) is true but (R) is false.
(c) (A) is false but (R) is true.
(d) Both (A) and (R) are true and (R) is the correct explanation of (A).

55. Select the incorrect statement for developing of an exposed camera film involving the reaction.

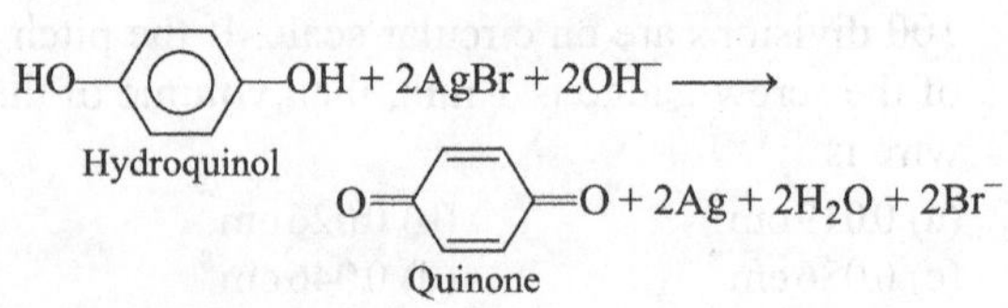

(a) Hydroquinol acts as reductant.
(b) Ag^+ acts as oxidant.
(c) Hydroquinol and AgBr undergoes redox change.
(d) It involves intramolecular change.

56. When acidified $K_2Cr_2O_7$ solution is added to Sn^{2+} salt then Sn^{2+} changes to
(a) Sn^+ (b) Sn^{3+}
(c) Sn (d) Sn^{4+}

57. Match List-I with List-II.

List-I		List-II	
A.	$TiCl_4$	I.	Adams catalyst in reduction.
B.	$PdCl_2$	II.	In preparation of $(CH_3)_2SiCl_2$
C.	Pt / PtO	III.	Used as the Natta catalyst
D.	Cu	IV.	Wacker process

Choose the correct answer from the options given below.
(a) A-I, B-IV, C-II, D-III
(b) A-II, B-III, C-I, D-IV
(c) A-III, B-IV, C-I, D-II
(d) A-IV, B-III, C-I, D-II

58. Which of the following is the strongest nucleophile?
(a) $CH_3—CH_2^-$ (b) $HC\equiv C^-$
(c) NH_2^- (d) $H_2C=CH^-$

59. Match the species in List-I with their structure in List-II.

List-I (Molecule)	List-II (Shape)
A. $XeOF_4$	I. *See-saw*
B. XeF_4	II. Trigonal bipyramidal
C. SF_2Cl_2	III. Square pyramidal
D. PCl_3F_2	IV. Square planar

Choose the correct answer from the options given below:
(a) A-III, B-I, C-IV, D-II
(b) A-III, B-IV, C-I, D-II
(c) A-II, B-IV, C-I, D-III
(d) A-II, B-I, C-IV, D-III

60. Given below are two statements, one is labelled as Assertion (A) and other is labelled as Reason (R).
Assertion (A) Both rhombic and monoclinic sulphur exist as S_8 but oxygen exists as O_2.
Reason (R) Oxygen forms $p\pi$-$p\pi$ multiple bond due to small size and small bond length but $p\pi$-$p\pi$ bonding is not possible in sulphur.
In the light of the above statements, choose the most appropriate answer from the options given below:
(a) Both (A) and (R) are true but (R) is not the correct explanation of (A).
(b) (A) is true but (R) is false.
(c) (A) is false but (R) are true.
(d) Both (A) and (R) are true and (R) is the correct explanation of (A).

61. Consider the graph given below and mark the correct option.

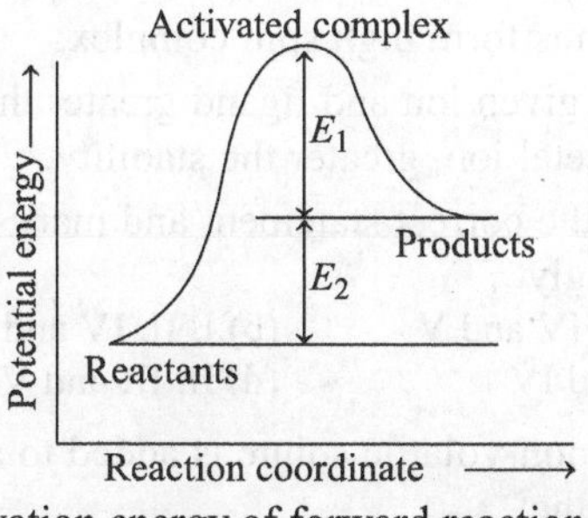

(a) Activation energy of forward reaction is $E_1 + E_2$ and product is less stable than reactant.
(b) Activation energy of forward reaction is $E_1 + E_2$ and product is more stable than reactant.
(c) Activation energy of forward and backward reaction is $E_1 + E_2$ and product is more stable than reactant.
(d) Activation energy of backward reaction is E_1 and product is less stable than reactant.

62. Which of the following conductometric titration represent the curve of HCl *vs* NaOH?
x-axis ⇒ Volume of alkali added
y-axis ⇒ Conductivity

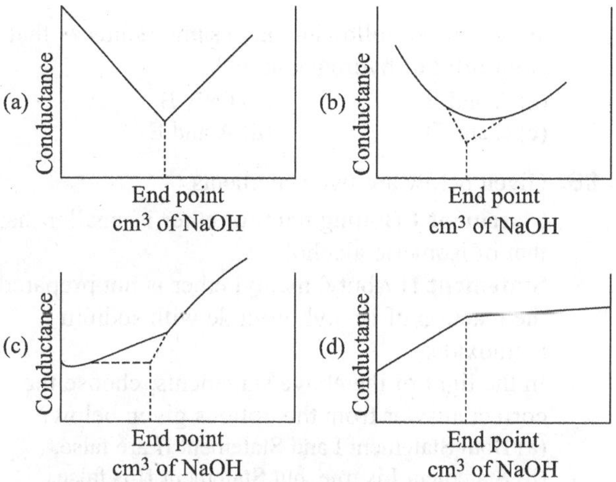

63. Given below are two statements.
Statement I A negative catalyst retards the rate of chemical reaction.
Statement II Presence of negative catalyst increases the energy of activation.
In the light of the above statements, choose the correct answer from the options given below.
(a) Both Statement I and Statement II are false.
(b) Statement I is true but Statement II is false.
(c) Statement I is false but Statement II is true.
(d) Both Statement I and Statement II are true.

64. Consider the following reaction sequence.

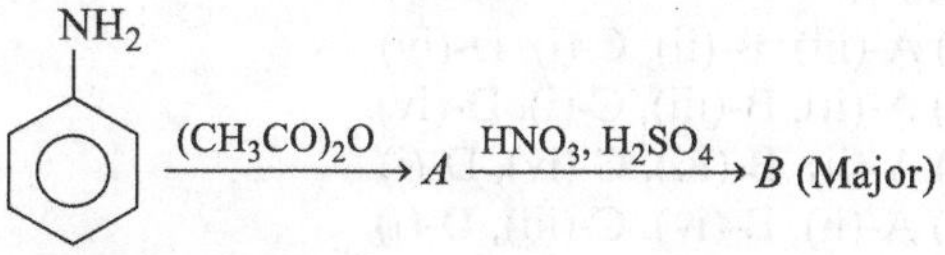

Major product B is

(a) 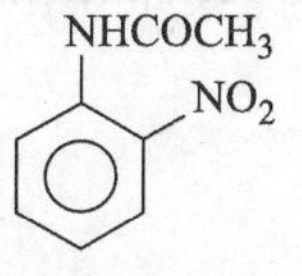

(b) 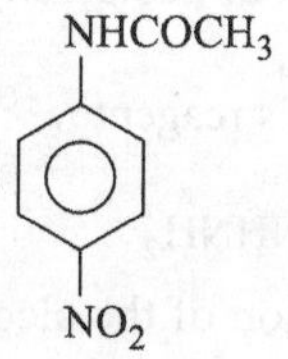

(c) 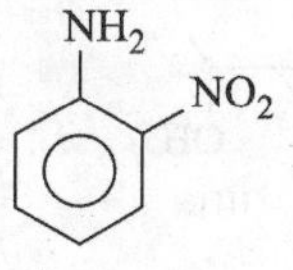

(d) 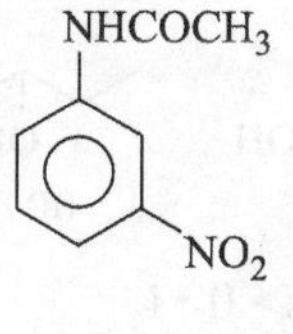

65. Consider the following hydrogen like species.

A. $n=2$, Li^{2+} B. $n=2$, Be^{3+}
C. $n=3$, He^{+} D. $n=3$, Na^{+}
E. $n=4$, Ca^{2+}

Which of the following have same radius as that of Bohr orbit of hydrogen atom?

(a) A and B (b) Only B
(c) C and D (d) A and E

66. Given below are two statements.

Statement I Boiling point of ether is smaller than that of isomeric alcohol.

Statement II *t*-butyl methyl ether is not prepared by the reaction of *t*-butyl bromide with sodium methoxide.

In the light of the above statements, choose the correct answer from the options given below:

(a) Both Statement I and Statement II are false.
(b) Statement I is true, but Statement II is false.
(c) Statement I is false, but Statement II is true.
(d) Both Statement I and Statement II are true.

67. Match the List-I with List-II.

List-I	List-II
A. Sucrose	(i) Glucose + fructose + galactose
B. Lactose	(ii) Glucose + fructose
C. Maltose	(iii) Glucose + galactose
D. Raffinose	(iv) Glucose + glucose

Choose the correct answer from the options given below.

(a) A-(iii), B-(ii), C-(i), D-(iv)
(b) A-(ii), B-(iii), C-(i), D-(iv)
(c) A-(ii), B-(iii), C-(iv), D-(i)
(d) A-(ii), B-(iv), C-(iii), D-(i)

68. Which of the following reagent is used for the separation of acetaldehyde from acetophenone?

(a) NH_2O_4
(b) Tollen's reagent
(c) NaOI
(d) $C_6H_5NHNH_2$

69. Dehydration of the alcohols will be in the order

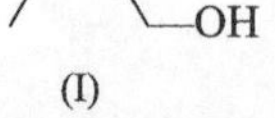
(I)

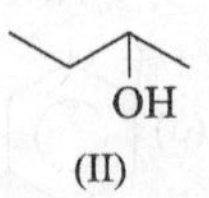
(II)

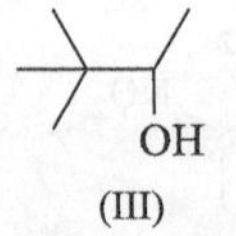
(III)

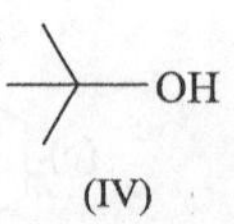
(IV)

(a) IV> III> II> I (b) I> II> III> IV
(c) IV> II> III> I (d) II> IV> I> III

70. The correct order of given compounds in decreasing order of their reactivity towards S_N1 reaction

I. 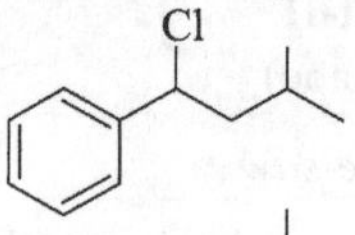

II. 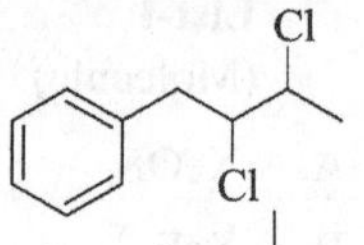

III. 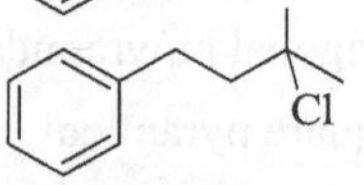

IV. 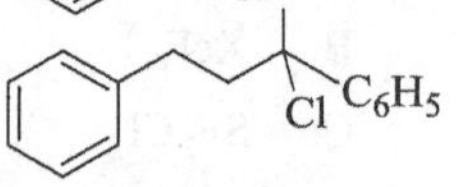

(a) IV> I> III> II (b) I> IV> III> II
(c) IV> I> II> III (d) I> II> III> IV

71. Which oxoacid of phosphorus contains highest number of oxygen atom in its chemical formula?

(a) Pyrophosphorus acid (b) Pyrophosphoric acid
(c) Hypophosphorus acid (d) Phosphoric acid

72. The actinoids exhibit more oxidation states in general than the lanthanoids. This is because

(a) the 5*f*-orbitals are more buried than the 4*f*-orbitals.
(b) there is a similarity between 4*f*-and 5*f*-orbitals in their angular part of the wave function.
(c) the actinoids are more reactive than the lanthanoids.
(d) the 5*f*-orbitals extend further from the nucleus than the 4*f*-orbitals.

73. Consider the following statements.

I. Chelate of higher denticity will give more stable complexes than chelate with lower denticity.
II. Macrocyclic ligands of appropriate size form more stable complexes than chelate ligands.
III. In $[Cu(NH_3)_4]SO_4$ the ligand has satisfied both primary and secondary valencies of ferric ion.
IV. For the complex, $[CoF_6]^{3-}$, F^- is a weak-field ligand, so that $\Delta_{oct} < P$ (electron-pairing energy) and thus form high spin complex.
V. For a given ion and ligand greater the charge on the metal ion, greater the stability.

Choose the correct statement and mark the option accordingly.

(a) I, III, IV and V (b) I, II, IV and V
(c) III and IV (d) II, III and V

74. When a non-volatile solute is added to a pure solvent, the

(a) vapour pressure of the solution becomes lower than that of the pure solvent.
(b) rate of evaporation of the pure solvent is increased.
(c) solute does not affect the boiling point of resulting solution.
(d) rate of the evaporation of the solution is equal to the rate of condensation of the solution at a lower vapour pressure than that in the case of the pure solvent.

75. Which of the following statements is not correct regarding $AlCl_3$?

(a) It achieves stability by forming a dimer.
(b) In acidified aqueous solution it forms octahedral $[Al(H_2O)_6]^{3+}$ ion.
(c) In complex with acidified water 3*d*-orbital is used
(d) Hybridisation involved in complex with acidified water is sp^3.

76. The formation of PH_4^+ is difficult compared to NH_4^+ because

(a) lone pair of phosphorus is optically inert.
(b) lone pair of phosphorus resides in almost pure *p*-orbital.
(c) lone pair of phosphorus resides at sp^3-orbital.
(d) lone pair of phosphorus resides in almost pure *s*-orbital.

77. The standard reduction potential for Zn^{2+}/Zn, Ni^{2+}/Ni and Fe^{2+}/Fe are -0.76, -0.23 and -0.44 V respectively. The reaction $X + Y^{2+} \longrightarrow X^{2+} + Y$ will be spontaneous when

(a) $X = Ni$, $Y = Zn$ (b) $X = Fe$, $Y = Zn$
(c) $X = Zn$, $Y = Ni$ (d) $X = Ni$, $Y = Fe$

78. The amount of bromine required to convert 3 g of phenol into 2, 4, 6-tribromophenol will be

(a) 15.32 g (b) 20.82 g
(c) 10.22 g (d) 4.89 g

79. A plot of $1/T$ *versus* $\ln k$ for a reaction gives the slope -2×10^4. The energy of activation for the reaction is (Given, $R = 8.314\ JK^{-1}\ mol^{-1}$)

(a) $166\ kJ\ mol^{-1}$ (b) $400\ kJ\ mol^{-1}$
(c) $67\ kJ\ mol^{-1}$ (d) $280\ kJ\ mol^{-1}$

80. The maximum work done in expanding 16 g of oxygen at 300 K and occupying a volume of 5 dm^3 isothermally until the volume becomes 25 dm^3 is

(a) 2.01×10^3 J (b) -4.03×10^4 J
(c) -2.01×10^3 J (d) 2.67×10^4 J

81. 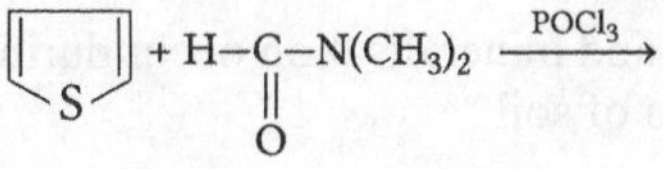

A; Product *A* will be

(a) 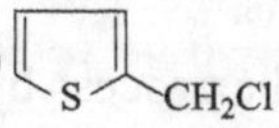

(b) 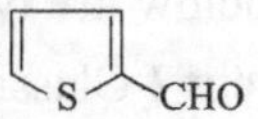

(c) 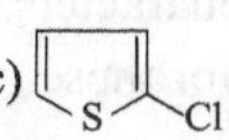

(d) 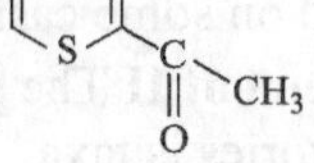

82. Benzoin condensation is the chemical properties of aromatic aldehydes only. The resultant product of this reaction is α-hydroxy ketones. Reagent used in benzoin condensation is

(a) KOH (b) KCN (c) H_2SO_4 (d) C_2H_5ONa

83. Cycloketone on reacting with NH_2OH gives *B* which further reacting with H_2SO_4 gives *C*. Find the product *C* and choose the correct option.

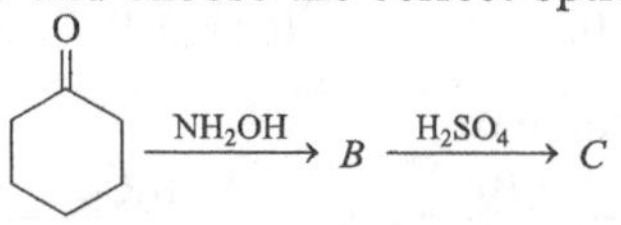

(a) Caprolactam (b) Cyclohexanone oxime
(c) Aniline (d) Anilide

84. Given below are two statements.

Statement I The molal elevation constant K_b is characteristic of a solvent and is independent of the solute added.

Statement II When a volatile solute is added to water, a depression in freezing point is observed.

In the light of the above statements, choose the correct answer from the options given below:

(a) Both Statement I and Statement II are false.
(b) Statement I is true, but Statement II is false.
(c) Statement I is false, but Statement II is true.
(d) Both Statement I and Statement II are true.

85. Given below are two statements.

Statement I Sublimation method is used to separate aniline from water.

Statement II Lassaigne's method is used to detect nitrogen, halogen, phosphorus and sulphur in organic compound.

In the light of the above statements, choose the correct answer from the options given below:

(a) Both Statement I and Statement II are false.
(b) Statement I is true, but Statement II is false.
(c) Statement I is false, but Statement II is true.
(d) Both Statement I and Statement II are true.

86. Match the List-I with List-II.

List-I	List-II
A. Al_2O_3	(i) Dimer
B. $AlCl_3$	(ii) Basic
C. MgO	(iii) Acidic
D. B_2O_3	(iv) Amphoteric

Choose the correct answer from the options given below.

(a) A-(iv), B-(iii), C-(ii), D-(i)
(b) A-(i), B-(iv), C-(iii), D-(ii)
(c) A-(ii), B-(iii), C-(iv), D-(i)
(d) A-(iv), B-(i), C-(ii), D-(iii)

87. The oxidation state of S-atoms in $S_4O_6^{2-}$ from left to right respectively are

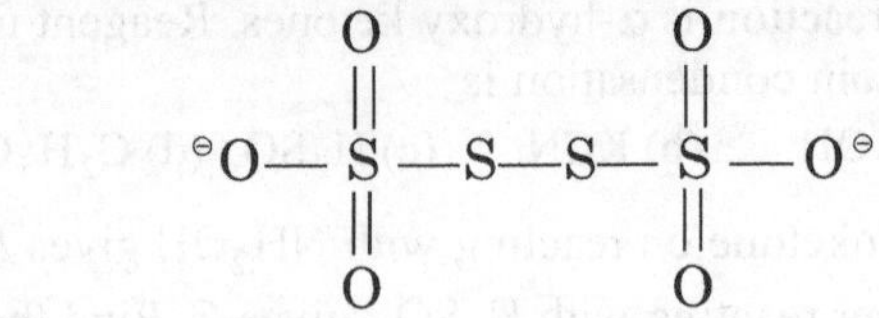

(a) +3, +1, +1, +3 (b) +4, +1, +1, +4
(c) +5, 0, 0, +5 (d) +6, 0, 0, +6

88. IUPAC name of

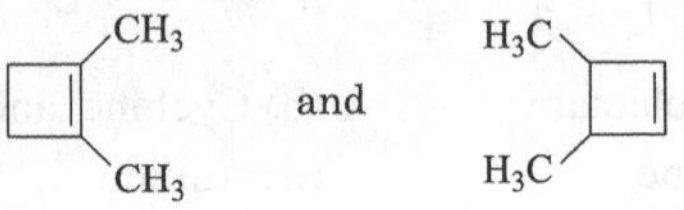

respectively are

(a) 1, 2-dimethylcyclobutane and 2, 3-dimethylbutene.
(b) 1, 2-dimethylcyclobut-1-ene and 3, 4-dimethyl cyclobut-1-ene.
(c) 2, 3-dimethylcyclobutene and 2, 3-dimethyl cyclobutane.
(d) 2, 3-dimethylbutene and 1, 2-dimethyl cyclobut-1-ene.

89. The observed osmotic pressure for a 0.10 M solution of $Fe(NH_4)_2(SO_4)_2$ at 25°C is 10.8 atm. The expected and experimental (observed) values of van't Hoff factor (i) will be respectively

$[R = 0.082 \text{ L atm K}^{-1}\text{mol}^{-1}]$

(a) 5 and 4.42 (b) 4 and 4.00
(c) 5 and 3.42 (d) 3 and 5.42

90. The correct order for N—O bond length in the given species is

I. NO II. NO^+ III. NO_2^- IV. NO_3^-

(a) I < II < III < IV (b) II < I < III < IV
(c) II < III < IV < I (d) I < III < IV < II

BIOLOGY

91. The relation between species richness and area is correctly depicted by

(a) $\log S = \log C - Z \log A$
(b) $\log S = Z \log A$
(c) $\log S = \log C$
(d) $\log S = \log C + Z \log A$

92. Which one of the following reaction represents photophosphorylation?

(a) ADP + AMP $\xrightarrow{\text{Light energy}}$ ATP
(b) ADP + inorganic phosphate $\xrightarrow{\text{Light energy}}$ ATP
(c) ADP + inorganic PO_4 $\longrightarrow$ ATP
(d) AMP + inorganic PO_4 $\xrightarrow[\text{energy}]{\text{light}}$ ATP

93. In which of the given plant groups, does gamete transfer occur by water?

1. Algae 2. Pteridophyte
3. Bryophyte 4. Gymnosperm

(a) Both 3 and 4 (d) Only 1
(c) Only 2 and 3 (d) 1, 2 and 3

94. During photorespiration, RuBP instead of being converted to two molecules of PGA, binds with O_2 to form

(a) one molecule of phosphoglycerate and phosphoenol pyruvate
(b) one molecule of phosphoglycolyte and one molecule of phosphoenol pyruvate
(c) one molecule of phosphoenol pyruvate and one molecule of oxaloacetic acid
(d) one molecule of phosphoglycolate and one molecule of phosphoglycerate

95. According to the fluid mosaic model the quasi fluid nature of lipid enables

(a) passive transport of molecules across the membrane
(b) lateral movement of proteins within the overall bilayer
(c) the neutral solutes may move across the membrane
(d) polar molecules can pass through the membrane

96. Which of the following statement is incorrect?

(a) Decomposition is a carbon dioxide requiring process
(b) Humus is colloidal in nature and serves as a reservoir of nutrient
(c) Warm and moist environment favours decomposition
(d) Humification and mineralisation occur during decomposition of soil

97. Given below are two statements.

Statement I Classification is the process by which anything is grouped into convenient categories based on some easily observable characters.

Statement II The scientific term for these categories is taxa.

In the light of above statements, choose the correct answer from the options given below.
(a) Statement I is incorrect, but statement II is correct
(b) Both statement I and statement II are correct
(c) Both statement I and statement II are incorrect
(d) Statement I is correct, but statement II is incorrect

98. What may be caused as a result of a marriage between close relatives?
(a) Erythroblastosis foetalis
(b) Mutations
(c) More recessive alleles will come together
(d) Incomplete dominance

99. Which of the following is incorrectly matched?

(a)	ICSI	Sperm directly injected into ovum
(b)	IUI	Sperm introduced artificially into uterus
(c)	GIFT	Embryo with more than 8 blastomeres transferred into Fallopian tube
(d)	IVF	Ferlitisation outside the body

100. Match List I with List II.

List-I	List-II
A. *Paramecium caudatum*	1. Obligate anaerobes
B. Fungi imperfect	2. Food supplement
C. Lichens	3. Binary fission
D. Archaebacteria	4. Molds
E. *Spirulina*	5. Phycobiont + Mycobiont

Choose the correct answer from the options given below.

	A	B	C	D	E		A	B	C	D	E
(a)	3	5	4	1	2	(b)	2	4	5	3	1
(c)	3	4	5	1	2	(d)	2	1	5	3	4

101. The transposons is a DNA sequence also known as ....
(a) silenced genes
(b) mobile genetic elements
(c) pleiotropic genes
(d) polymorphic genes

102. DNA fingerprinting relies on identifying minisatellite which are
(a) repetitive coding short DNA sequence
(b) repetitive non-coding short DNA sequences
(c) repetitive coding and non-coding short DNA sequences
(d) non-repetitive non-coding short DNA sequences

103. Read the following statements and choose the correct set of statements.
I. Cardiac muscle tissue is a contractile tissue present only in the heart.
II. Cartilage is solid and pliable and resists compression.
III. Osteocytes are present in spaces called bone matrix.
IV. Biceps are voluntary and striated muscles.
V. Columnar epithelium form walls of blood vessels.

Choose the correct answer from the options given below.
(a) I, II and IV (b) II, III and V
(c) III and V (d) III and IV

104. Read the following statements about tubular reabsorption.
I. It is absorption of water and useful solutes from the glomerular filtrate into blood.
II. It occurs mostly in PCT.
III. It takes place only by active transport.
IV. It occurs mostly in DCT.
V. About 50% of water is reabsorbed along with solutes.

Choose the correct set of statements from the options given below.
(a) I and II (b) II and III
(c) III and IV (d) II and IV

105. When a more complex structure form a simple structure for example, glucose becomes lactic acid in our skeletal muscle it is called
(a) amphibolic pathway (b) anabolic pathway
(c) catabolic pathway (d) endothermic pathway

106. Read the following statements regarding respiration.
I. Glycolysis occurs in the cytoplasm of the cell.
II. Aerobic respiration takes place within the mitochondria.
III. ETS is present in the outer mitochondrial membrane.
IV. $C_{51}H_{98}O_6$ is the chemical formula of tripalmitin fatty acid.

V. Respiratory quotient is defined as the ratio of volume of O_2 evolved to the volume of CO_2 consumed.

Choose the correct answer from the option given below.

(a) I, II and IV (b) II, III and IV
(c) III, IV and V (d) I, III and V

107. A couple has a haemophilic son, a normal son and a haemophilic daughter. What are the most likely genotypes of the mother and father, respectively in this case?

(a) XX^h, X^hY (b) XX, XY
(c) X^hX^h, X^hY^h (d) X^hY, XY^h

108. Match List I with List II.

List I	List II
A. Mollusca	1. Locomotion by comb plates
B. Ctenophora	2. Pseudocoelomate
C. Porifera	3. Presence of external skeleton of shell
D. Aschelminthes	4. Body with canals in walls

Choose the correct answer from the options given below.

	A	B	C	D
(a)	1	3	4	2
(b)	4	3	1	2
(c)	3	1	4	2
(d)	1	4	3	2

109. Mycelium is found to be coenocytic or aseptate in which of the given classes of fungi?

(a) Phycomycetes (b) Ascomycetes
(c) Basidiomycetes (d) Deuteromycetes

110. Given below are two statements.

Statement I In 1865, three scientists independently rediscovered Mendel's result on the inheritance of characters.

Statement II The two alleles of a gene pair are located on homologous sites on homologous chromosomes.

In the light of above statements, choose the correct answer from the options given below.

(a) Statement I is incorrect, but statement II is correct
(b) Both statement I and statement II are correct
(c) Both statement I and statement II are incorrect
(d) Statement I is correct, but statement II is incorrect

111. Match List I and List II.

List I	List II
A. Uremia	1. Presence of high ketone bodies in urine
B. Sweat gland	2. Lactic acid
C. Ketonuria	3. Presence of glucose in urine
D. Glycosuria	4. Presence of excess urea in blood

Choose the corect answer from the options given below.

	A	B	C	D
(a)	2	1	3	4
(b)	3	4	2	1
(c)	4	3	1	2
(d)	4	2	1	3

112. In Chondrichthyes, claspers are seen on

(a) pelvic fins of male
(b) pelvic fins of female
(c) operculum of both sexes
(d) around jaws

113. The anaphase of meiosis-II begins with the simultaneous splitting of the centromere of each chromosome allowing them to move towards the opposites poles of cell by

(a) shortening of microtubules attached to kinetochore
(b) shortening of microtubules attached to centromere
(c) cytokinesis followed by karyokinesis
(d) karyokinesis followed by cytokinesis

114. Given below are two statements.

Statement I The DNA molecule in eukaryotes is associated with histones and protamines.

Statement II The number of hydrogen bonds between adenine and thymine in DNA molecules is three.

In the light of the above statements, choose the correct answer from the options given below.

(a) Statement I is incorrect, but statement II is correct
(b) Both statement I and statement II are correct
(c) Both statement I and statement II are incorrect
(d) Statement I is correct, but statement II is incorrect

115. Find the incorrect match pair.

(a)	Cytoplasm	present between nucleus and plasma membrane
(b)	Nucleoplasm	Protoplasm of nucleus
(c)	Glycocalyx	Slime layer
(d)	Protoplasm	Cytoplasm excluding nucleus

116. In prophase-I of meiosis, during which substage can terminalisation of chiasmata be observed?

(a) Pachytene (b) Diplotene
(c) Diakinesis (d) Karyokinesis

117. Match List I with List II.

	List I		List II
A.	Monocot stem	1.	Vascular bundle closed
B.	Dicot stem	2.	Vascular bundle open
C.	Monocot root	3.	Polyarch xylem bundles
D.	Dicot root	4.	2-4 xylem bundles

Choose correct answer from the options given below.

	A	B	C	D		A	B	C	D
(a)	1	2	3	4	(b)	2	1	3	4
(c)	4	1	3	4	(d)	4	3	1	2

118. During the process of sexual reproduction in flowering plants, double fertilisation involves

(a) fertilisation of two egg cells by two male gametes brought by same pollen tube
(b) fertilisation of egg cell and a central cell by two male gametes brought by different pollen tubes
(c) fertilisation of egg cell by two male gametes
(d) fertilisation of egg cell and a central cell by two male gametes brought by same pollen tube

119. Identify the incorrect statement.

(a) Transformation is a procedure through which a piece of DNA is introduced in a bacterium
(b) Normally the genes encoding resistance to antibiotics like ampicillin, chloramphenicol, tetracycline, kanamycin, etc are considered useful selectable markers for *E. coli*
(c) The normal *E. coli* cells carry genes resistant against amplicillin, chloramphenicol, tetracycline and kanamycin.
(d) In order to link the alien DNA, the vector needs to have very few preferably single recognition site for the commonly used restriction enzymes

120. Select the correct pair of restriction enzymes, which produce blunt ends.

(a) *Bam* HI and *Hind* III (b) *Eco* RV and *Pst* I
(c) *Eco* RV and *Sma* I (d) *Eco* RI and *Sma* I

121. A transgenic plant containing *Bt* toxin gene, does not require

(a) irrigation (b) fertiliser
(c) insecticides (d) mineral

122. Identify the correct labelled part from the options given below.

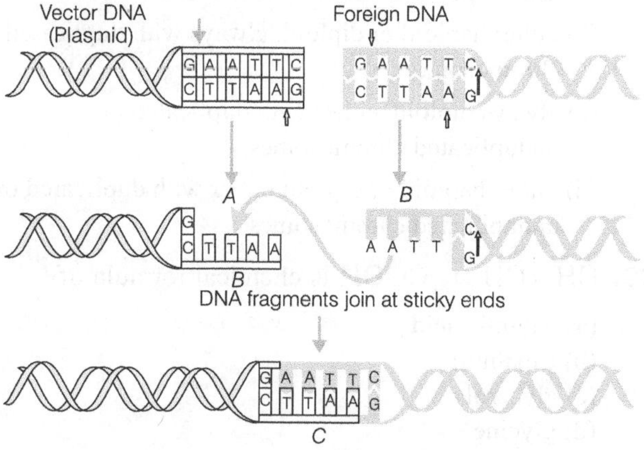

(a) *A*-*Hind* II, *B*-Blunt ends, *S*-Non-recombinant DNA
(b) *A*-*Bam* HI, *B*-Sticky ends, *C*-Recombinant DNA
(c) *A*-*Eco*RI, *B*-Sticky ends, *C*-Non-recombinant DNA
(d) A-*Eco*RI, *B*-Sticky ends, *C*-Recombinant DNA

123. Which of the given statements is correct in the context of observing DNA separated by agarose gel electrophoresis?

(a) DNA can be seen in visible light
(b) Ethidium bromide stained DNA can be seen orange in visible light
(c) DNA can be seen without staining in visible light
(d) Eithidium bromide stained DNA can be seen under exposure to UV light

124. Given below are two statements.

Statement I Slime moulds are characterised by the presence of a rigid cell wall and if motile, a flagellum is present.

Statement II Bacteria can live in extreme habitat such as hot springs, deserts, snow and deep oceans where very few other life forms can survive.

In the light of the above statements, choose the correct answer from the options given below.
(a) Statement I is incorrect, but statement II is correct
(b) Both statement I and statement II are correct
(c) Both statement I and statement II are incorrect
(d) Statement I is correct, but statement II is incorrect

125. A cell that is entering the M-phase of the cell cycle is
(a) always haploid with duplicated chromosomes
(b) either haploid or diploid, always with duplicated chromosome
(c) always diploid, either with duplicated or unduplicated chromosomes
(d) either haploid or diploid either with duplicated or unduplicated chromosomes

126. $CH_3(CH_2)_{14}COOH$ is chemical formula of
(a) palmitic acid
(b) tripalmitin
(c) glycerol
(d) glycine

127. Study the given pedigree chart and select the correct option regarding it.

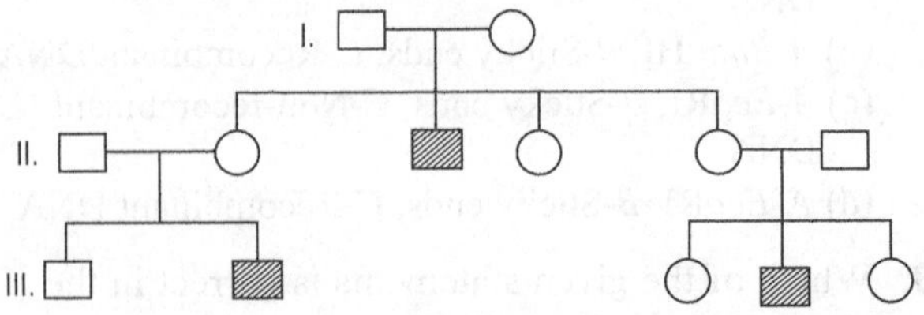

(a) The trait shown in above pedigree is a sex-linked recessive disease
(b) The genotype of affected female in II generation can be aa or Aa
(c) In first generation male cannot be carrier for the trait
(d) Gene for the above given trait is found in females only

128. Filamentous thalli, hyphae generally non-septate and multinucleate are vegetative features of
(a) Phycomycetes-*Rhizopus*
(b) Basidiomycetes-*Chlamydomonas*
(c) Ascomycetes-*Neurospora*
(d) Deuteromycetes-*Mycorrhiza*

129. Given below are two statements.
Statement I Selectable markers help in identifying and eliminating non-transformants and selectively permitting the growth of transformants.
Statement II If a recombinant DNA bearing gene for resistance of ampicillin is transferred into *E.coli* cells, the host cells become transformed into ampicillin resistant cells.
In the light of the above statements choose the correct answer from the options given below.
(a) Statement I is incorrect, but statement II is correct
(b) Both statement I and statement II are correct
(c) Both statement I and statement II are incorrect
(d) Statement I is correct, but statement II is incorrect

130. Which of the following organelle is involved in modification and routing of newly synthesised proteins to their destination?
(a) Mitochondria
(b) Endoplasmic reticulum
(c) Lysosome
(d) Chloroplast

131. The advantage of a DNA molecule having two complementary strands is that it
(a) promotes easy pairing between chromatids
(b) transcription and translation processes can occur simultaneously
(c) favours semiconservative replication
(d) replication takes less time

132. Read the following statements and choose the correct set of statements.
I. Some species of annelids exhibi metamerism, which is the segmentation of the body.
II. In arthropods, the exoskeleton is primarily composed of chitin.
III. Molluscs are the only phylum within the animal kingdom that lacks a true coelom.
IV. Echinoderms possess a primitive brain called a ganglion, which serves as their central nervous system.
V. Cephalisation is a characteristic feature of all animal phyla, ensuring the presence of a well-developed head region.

Choose the correct answer from the options given below.
(a) I, II and IV
(b) II and V
(c) I, II and III
(d) IV and V

133. Saheli a new oral contraceptive for females developed by Indian scientists is a
(a) steroidal preparation
(b) hormonal preparation
(c) non-steroidal preparation
(d) toxic preparation to kill sperm

134. In a polysaccharide the right end and left end are called
(a) N-terminal and C-terminal, respectively
(b) C-terminal and N-terminal, respectively
(c) Reducing end and non-reducing end, respectively
(d) Non-reducing end and reducing end, respectively

135. Which among the following statement is correct regarding dicot leaf ?
(a) Leaves are dorsiventral
(b) Bulliform cells are present
(c) Vascular bundle is not surrounded by parenchymatous bundle sheath
(d) Mesophyll is not differentiated into palisade and spongy parenchyma.

136. Read the following statements and choose the incorrect statement(s).
I. Yeast is a unicellular sac fungus that produces edible fruiting bodies.
II. Organism causing sleeping sickness has flagella for locomotion.
III. In *Agaricus,* karyogamy is delayed after plasmogamy.
IV. White spots seen on mustard leaves are due to a member of Phycomycetes.
V. *Saccharomyces cerevisiae* is widely used in baking industry.

Choose the correct answer from the options given below.
(a) I only (b) III and IV
(c) I and II (d) V only

137. The graph given below shows a relationship between population size and time. Under what conditions will the population growth rate of this graph be levelled up so as to give an S-shaped curve?

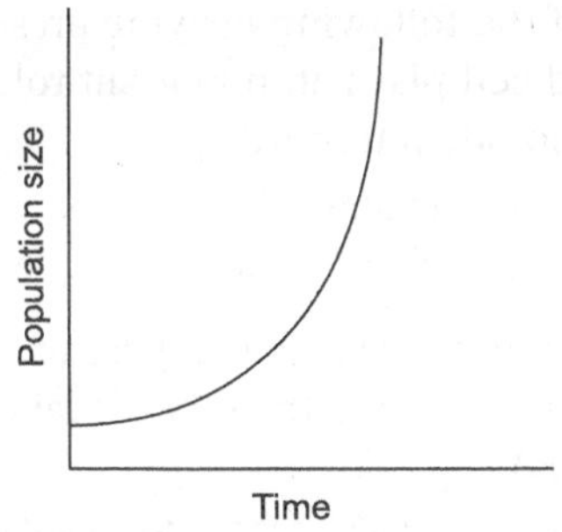

(a) When environmental conditions favour the growing population size.
(b) When the number of individuals increases upto an extent, resources start to be used up and population growth rate is slowed down
(c) When the predators are eliminated, thus, increasing the prey population
(d) When a hypothetical carrying capacity is considered as a limit for population size

138. Palm crease, short statured and furrowed tongue are the symptoms related to which disease?
(a) Klinefelter's syndrome
(b) Down's syndrome
(c) Turner's syndrome
(d) Patau syndrome

139. If the recombinant DNA is inserted within the coding sequence of *lac z* gene, then the host cells, which carry the recombinant DNA plasmid will form .... in the presence of X-gal.
(a) blue colonies
(b) white colonies
(c) orange colonies
(d) pink colonies

140. Given below are two statements; one is labelled as Assertion (A) and the other is labelled as Reason (R).
Assertion (A) The first evolved organic compounds required for origin of life were proteins and nucleic acid.
Reason (R) All early forms of life occurred in water only.
In the light of the above statements, choose the correct answer from the options given below.
(a) A is false, but R is true
(b) Both A and R are true and R is the correct explanation of A
(c) Both A and R are true, but R is not the correct explanation of A
(d) A is true, but R is false

141. Which of the following enzyme present in the red blood cell plays an important role in carbon dioxide transport?

(a) Carbonic anhydrase (b) Fibrinogen
(c) Carbonic acid (d) Carboxylase

142. Given below are two statements; one is labelled as Assertion (A) and the other is labelled as Reason (R).

Assertion (A) Hardy - Weinberg principle is applicable in a population having stable allelic frequency.

Reason (R) The sum total of the allelic frequency is more than one.

In the light of the above statements, choose the correct answer from the options given below.

(a) A is false, but R is true
(b) Both A and R are true and R is the correct explanation of A
(c) Both A and R are true, but R is not the correct explanation of A
(d) A is true, but R is false

143. Select the incorrect statement amongst the following.

(a) Eosinophils resist infection and are associated with allergic reactions.
(b) Leucocytes are nucleated and are relatively less in number.
(c) Lifespan of basophils are generally 2-3 days.
(d) Lymphocytes provide immunity by engulfing pathogens.

144. Read the following statements and choose the correct statements.

I. Amino acids are linked by peptide bond.
II. In a polysaccharide the individual monosaccharides are linked by phosphate group.
III. Peptide bond is formed when–COOH group of one amino acid reacts with —NH_2 group of next amino acid with elimination of water.
IV. Nucleic acid exhibit a wide variety of secondary structures.
V. The DNA backbone is formed by sugar phosphate nitrogenous base chain.

Choose the correct answer from the options given below.

(a) I, III and IV (b) II and V
(c) I, II and V (d) III, IV and V

145. Match List I with List II.

List I	List II
A. Simple leaf	1. In this leaf lamina is entire
B. Compound leaf	2. Leaflets are attached at common point
C. Pinnately compound leaf	3. If the incision of the lamina reach up to the midrib breaking it into a number of leaflets
D. Palmately compound leaf	4. Number of leaflets present on common axis, represents the mid rib of the leaf.

Choose correct answer from the options given below.

	A	B	C	D		A	B	C	D
(a)	1	3	4	2	(b)	2	1	3	4
(c)	2	3	1	4	(d)	1	3	2	4

146. Read the following statements and choose the correct set of statements.

I. The structural gene in the segment of DNA, exercise the control over transcription.
II. The regulator gene is responsible for the synthesis of repressor.
III. The terminator region is present upstream of structural gene at 5′ end of the coding strand.
IV. The promoter gene is the DNA segment at which RNA polymerase binds.
V. The operator gene carries code for the synthesis of protein.

Choose the correct answer from the options given below.

(a) II and V (b) I and III (c) II and IV (d) I and IV

147. Match List I with List II.

List I	List II
A. Cervical	1. 7
B. Thoracic	2. 1
C. Lumbar	3. 12
D. Sacral	4. 5

Choose the correct answer from the options given below.

	A	B	C	D		A	B	C	D
(a)	1	4	2	3	(b)	4	2	1	3
(c)	1	3	4	2	(d)	4	1	3	2

148. The cross-section of stem and root appears same when viewed by naked eye. But under microscope they can be differentiated by
(a) exarch condition of root and stem
(b) endarch condition of root and stem
(c) endarch condition of root and exarch condition of stem
(d) endarch conditions of stem and exarch condition of root.

149. Given below are two statements; one is labelled as Assertion (A) and other is labelled as Reason (R).

Assertion (A) In gel electrophoresis, DNA fragments are separated on the basis of their size.

Reason (R) DNA is negatively charged, so it moves towards anode under electric field.

In the light of the above statements, choose the correct answer from the options given below.
(a) A is false, but R is true
(b) Both A and R are true and R is the correct explanation of A
(c) Both A and R are true, but R is not the correct explanation of A
(d) A is true, but R is false

150. Given below are two staements; one is labelled as Assertion (A) and other is labelled Reason (R).

Assertion (A) *Streptococcus* sp. and *Haemophillus* sp. are responsible for pneumonia.

Reason (R) The alveoli getting filled with fluid leading to severe problems in respiration is the main symptom of pneumonia.

In the light of the above statements, choose the correct answer from the options given below.
(a) A is false, but R is true
(b) Both A and R are true and R is the correct explanation of A
(c) Both A and R are true, but R is not the correct explanation of A
(d) A is true, but R is false

151. Study the given diagram carefully and choose the correct option.

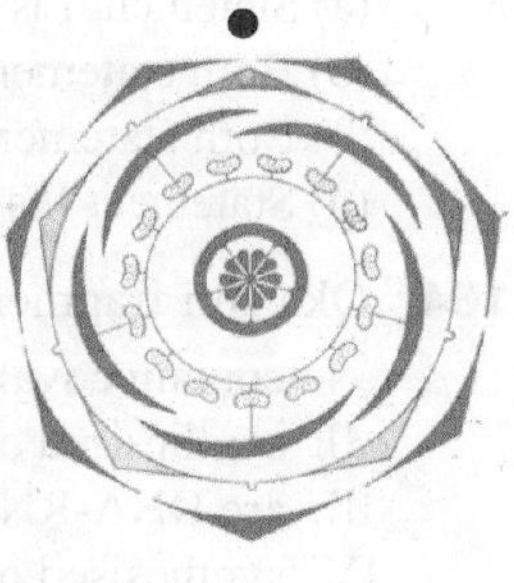

I. Small non-endospermic seed
II. Marginal placentation
III. Capsule or Schizocarp fruit
IV. Br. ⊕ ⚥ $Epi_{3\text{-}9}\ K_{5 \text{ or } (5)}\ \widehat{C_5\ A}_{(\infty)}\ \underline{G}_{(2\infty)}$

Choose the correct answer from the options given below.
(a) II and III (b) III and IV
(c) I and II (d) I and IV

152. Which of the following is incorrectly matched pair?
(a) Compositae → Absent or hairy pappus or scaly calyx
(b) Cruciferae → Six tepals arranged in two whorls (3 + 3).
(c) Leguminosae → Gamosepalous imbricate or valvate.
(d) Malvaceae → Epicalyx is formed by bracteoles.

153. Which of the following is one of the advantage of application of viruses as bioinsecticides?
(a) They are used in conventional farming
(b) They are effective for all insects
(c) They are species specific
(d) They have negative impact on humans

154. The steps in the life cycle of *Plasmodium* are given below. Arrange these steps in a correct sequence.
A. Gametocytes in human
B. Sporozoites reach the liver through blood
C. Gametocyte consumption with blood meal
D. Multiplication in female mosquito

Choose the correct answer from the options given below.
(a) B, A, C, D (b) A, B, C, D
(c) C, D, B, A (d) B, C, D, A

155. Which of the given events occur during S-phase of cell cycle?
1. DNA replication 2. Tubulin protein synthesis
3. Duplication of centrioles
4. Duplication of Golgi body
(a) Both 1 and 2 (b) Both 1 and 3
(c) Both 2 and 4 (d) Both 2 and 3

156. Match List I with List II.

List I	List II
A. Investment of oxygen during aerobic respiration	1. Pathway taking place in cytoplasm
B. Consumption of ATP	2. In matrix of mitochondria
C. α-ketoglutaric acid	3. F_1-particle
D. Oxidative phosphorylation	4. ETS

Codes

	A	B	C	D		A	B	C	D
(a)	1	3	2	4	(b)	3	1	4	2
(c)	4	1	2	3	(d)	2	1	3	4

157. Match List I with List II.

List I	List II
A. Centrioles	1. Basal body of cilia
B. Microtubules	2. Cytoskeleton
C. Chromatin net	3. Membrane bound minute vesicles
D. Microbodies	4. Interphase nucleus

Codes

	A	B	C	D		A	B	C	D
(a)	1	3	2	4	(b)	4	3	2	1
(c)	1	2	4	3	(d)	2	4	3	1

158. Given below are two statements.

Statement I MTP is essential where the continuation of the pregnancy could be harmful or even fatal either to the mother or to foetus or both.

Statement II MTP can also be used to get rid of pregnancy if the foetus is found to be female.

In the light of the above statements, choose the correct answer from the options given below.

(a) Statement I is incorrect, but statement II is correct
(b) Both statement I and statement II are correct
(c) Both statement I and statement II are incorrect
(d) Statement I is correct, but statement II is incorrect

159. Given below are two statements; one is labelled as Assertion (A) and others is labelled as Reason (R).

Assertion (A) Catecholamines increase the concentration of glucose in blood.

Reason (R) Catecholamines stimulate the glycogenolysis.

In the light of the above statements, choose the correct answer from the options given below.

(a) A is false, but R is true
(b) Both A and R are true and R is the correct explanation of A
(c) Both A and R are true, but R is not the correct explanation of A
(d) A is true, but R is false

160. Read the following statement and choose the set of correct statements.

I. Schleiden concluded that the presence of cell wall is a unique character of plant cell.
II. Rudolf Virchow first explained that cells divided and new cells are formed from pre-existing cells.
III. Centrosomes are special membranous structure which formed by the extension of plasma membrane.
IV. Several ribosomes form a chain called polysome by attaching to a single *m*RNA.
V. Fimbriae are small bristle like fibres, which are known to help attach the bacteria to the rocks in streams.

(a) I, III and V (b) II, IV and V
(c) I, III and IV (d) III, IV and V

161. In which of the following conversions does oxidative decarboxylation take place?

(a) Succinic acid → Fumaric acid
(b) Pyruvate → Acetyl Co-A
(c) Fumarate → Malate
(d) Isocitrate → Citrate

162. Bryophytes include the various mosses and liverworts that are found is moist shaded areas, they are

(a) non-vascular cryptogams
(b) first terrestrial plants
(c) vascular cryptogams
(d) homosporous

163. Given below are two statements.

Statement I First vertebrae is axis which articulates with occipital condyles.

Statement II Parietal bones and temporal bones of skull are joined together by fibrous joint.

In the light of the above statements, choose the correct answer from the options given below.

(a) Statement I is incorrect, but statement II is correct
(b) Both statement I and statement II are correct
(c) Both statement I and statement II are incorrect
(d) Statement I is correct, but statement II is incorrect

164. Okazaki fragments

I. contain covalently linked RNA and DNA.
II. synthesised on the template with polarity 5′-3′.
III. are DNA-RNA hybrids.
IV. synthesised on the template with polarity 3′-5′.

Choose the correct answer from the options given below.
(a) I and III only (b) I and II only
(c) II, III and IV (d) I, II and III

165. Which of the following works when the electron is circulated within the photosystem and the phosphorylation occurs due to cyclic flow of electrons?
(a) Photosystem-I only (b) Photosystems-I and II
(c) Photosystem-II only (d) Reaction centre P_{680}

166. Which of the given blood group(s) is/are not possible in progenies when parents have blood group AB and O?
1. A 2. AB
3. B 4. O
(a) 1 only (b) 2 only
(c) Both 2 and 4 (d) 4 only

167. Match List I with List II.

	List I		List II
A.	Osteoporosis	1.	Inflammation of joints due to accumulation of Uric acid
B.	Gout	2.	Decrease in bone mass, higher chance of fractures
C.	Myasthenia gravis	3.	Contraction in muscles due to low Ca^{++}
D.	Tetany	4.	Paralysis of skeletal muscle

Choose the correct answer from the options given below.

	A	B	C	D
(a)	1	3	4	2
(b)	1	2	4	3
(c)	4	1	2	3
(d)	2	1	4	3

168. Identify the incorrect match pair from the following.

(a)	Back cross	1. TT × tt
(b)	Monohybrid ratio	2. 3 : 1
(c)	Dihybrid ratio	3. 9 : 3 : 3 : 1
(d)	Test cross	4. Tt × tt

169. Which of the following is correctly matched?
(a) Auxin — Shoots
(b) Auxin and cytokinin — Callus
(c) Abscisic acid — Stem elongation
(d) Cytokinin — Somatic embryo

170. Given below are two statements; one is labelled as Assertion (A) and other is labelled as Reason (R).
Assertion (A) Origin of replication is a definite region in *E. coli* DNA, where the replication originates.
Reason (R) The vectors in *r*DNA procedures provide the origin of replication.
In the light of the above statements, choose the correct answer from the options given below.
(a) A is false, but R is true
(b) Both A and R are true and R is the correct explanation of A
(c) Both A and R are true, but R is not the correct explanation of A
(d) A is true, but R is false

171. The control of bacterial pathogens by sulpha drugs, is an example of
(a) competitive inhibition
(b) non-competitive inhibition
(c) protein denaturation
(d) increased activation energy

172. Given below are two statements; one is labelled as Assertion (A) and the other is labelled as Reason (R).
Assertion (A) The secondary spermatocytes are haploid.
Reason (R) Secondary spermatocytes are formed by Spermatogonia.
In the light of the above statements, choose the correct answer from the options given below.
(a) A is false, but R is true
(b) Both A and R are true and R is the correct explanation of A
(c) Both A and R are true, but R is not the correct explanation of A
(d) A is true, but R is false

173. Choose the incorrect match with respect to elements of phloem and their features.

(a)	Sieve tube element	Peripheral cytoplasm, large central vacuole, but lacks a nucleus
(b)	Companion cells	Maintain pressure gradient in sieve tubes
(c)	Phloem parenchyma	Storage of resins, latex mucilage and food materials
(d)	Phloem fibres	Generally absent in secondary phloem

174. The correct sequence of stages of prophase-I is
(a) zygotene, leptotene, pachytene, diakinesis and diplotene
(b) leptotene, zygotene, pachytene, diplotene and diakinesis
(c) leptotene, pachytene, zygotene, diakinesis and diplotene
(d) diplotene, diakinesis, pachytene, zygotene and leptotene

175. Which of the following statement is correct?
(a) The eyes of the frog are obligate unpaired structures situated in the orbit in skull
(b) The frog excretes urea and thus is a ureotelic animal
(c) The frogs do not constitute thymus and thyroid glands
(d) Frogs have underdeveloped male and female reproductive system

176. Match List I with List II.

List I	List II
A. Cerebrum	1. Controls pituitary
B. Cerebellum	2. Controls vision and hearing
C. Hypothalamus	3. Controls the rate of heartbeat
D. Mid brain	4. Seat of intelligence
	5. Maintains body posture

Choose the correct answer from the options given below.

	A	B	C	D
(a)	5	4	2	1
(b)	4	5	2	1
(c)	5	4	1	2
(d)	4	5	1	2

177. Which of the following statement is incorrect?
(a) The autosome linked recessive traits can be transmitted from parents to offspring when both the partners are carrier for the gene (or heterozygous)
(b) The mutation which arises due to substitution of Glu by Val, is referred to as point mutation
(c) Queen Victoria was a carrier of haemophilia with a number of haemophilic descendents in her family
(d) Accumulation of phenylalanine and phenyl pyruvic acid in brain results in neurodegeneration

178. Given below are two statements.

Statement I Nicotine, caffeine, quinine, strychnine and opium are produced by plants actually as defence against grazers and browsers.

Statement II Thorns of *Acacia* and cactus are most common physiological means of defence.

In the light of the above statements, choose the correct answer from the options gives below.
(a) Statement I is incorrect, but statement II is correct
(b) Both statement I and statement II are correct
(c) Both statement I and statement II are incorrect
(d) Statement I is correct, but statement II is incorrect

179. Read the following statements carefully and choose the options having correct statements.

I. Tilman found that plots with more species showed less year to year variation in total biomass.
II. Stable community should not show too much variation in year to year productivity.
III. Alien species invasions provide stability to the stable community.
IV. According to Tilman, biomass cannot be increased without increasing diversity.
V. The rivet popper hypothesis was given by Paul Ehrlich.

(a) I and III (b) I and IV
(c) I, II, IV and V (d) I, IV and V

180. Which statement regarding coenzyme is incorrect?
(a) Every coenzyme is a cofactor and every cofactor is a coenzyme
(b) Every coenzyme is a cofactor, but every cofactor is not a coenzyme
(c) Most of the coenzyme are nucleotides and are composed of vitamins
(d) Coenzymes are the active constituents of enzymes

Explanations

Physics

1. (a) $v_{rms} = \sqrt{\frac{v_1^2 + v_2^2 + v_3^2 + \ldots + v_n^2}{n}}$

$= \sqrt{\frac{1^2 + 2^2 + 3^2 + 4^2 + 5^2}{5}} = \sqrt{11}$ km/s

$v_{avg} = \frac{v_1 + v_2 + v_3 + \ldots + v_n}{n}$

$= \frac{1+2+3+4+5}{5} = 3$ km/s

$\therefore \quad \frac{v_{rms}}{v_{avg}} = \frac{\sqrt{11}}{3} = \sqrt{11} : 3$

2. (a) Given, $I = 0.1\,\text{A}, \theta = 90°$

$B = 5 \times 10^{-2}\,\text{T}$

$A = \frac{1}{2} \times \text{Base} \times \text{Height}$

or $\quad A = \frac{1}{2} a \times \frac{a\sqrt{3}}{2} = \frac{\sqrt{3}\,a^2}{4} = \frac{\sqrt{3} \times (0.02)^2}{4}$

$= \sqrt{3} \times 10^{-4}\,\text{m}^2$

$\therefore$ Torque, $\tau = IAB \sin\theta$

$\tau = 0.1 \times \sqrt{3} \times 10^{-4} \times 5 \times 10^{-2} \sin 90°$

$= 5\sqrt{3} \times 10^{-7}$ N-m

3. (c) Given, $f = 520\,\text{Hz}$,

Resonance lengths, $l_1 = 30\,\text{cm} = 0.3\,\text{m}$

$l_2 = 70\,\text{cm} = 0.7\,\text{m}$

$\therefore$ The speed of sound in air,

$v = 2f(l_2 - l_1)$

$= 2 \times 520 \times (0.7 - 0.3)$

$= 416\,\text{m/s}$

4. (a) Mass defect, $\Delta m = 2(m_n + m_p) - m_{He}$

(as helium nucleus has two protons and two neutrons)

$\Delta m = 2(1.0087 + 1.0073) - 4.0015$

$\Delta m = 4.032 - 4.0015 = 0.0305$ amu

binding energy, $E_b = \Delta m \times 931\,\text{MeV}$

$= 0.0305 \times 931 = 28.4$ MeV

5. (a) Work done in process $1 \rightarrow 2$,

$W_1 =$ Area under curve $1 \rightarrow 2$

$= (3V_0 - V_0)(p_0) = 2p_0V_0$

Work done in process $2 \rightarrow 3$,

$W_2 =$ Area under curve $2 \rightarrow 3$

$\because$ Volume is constant

$\therefore \quad W_2 = 0$

Work done in process $3 \rightarrow 1$,

$W_3 =$ Area under curve $3 \rightarrow 1$

$= -\left[2p_0V_0 + \frac{1}{2}(2p_0 - p_0)(3V_0 - V_0)\right]$

$= -2p_0V_0 - p_0V_0 = -3p_0V_0$

Now, the total work done in cyclic process $1 \rightarrow 2 \rightarrow 3 \rightarrow 1$,

$W = W_1 + W_2 + W_3$

$= 2p_0V_0 + 0 + (-3p_0V_0) = -p_0V_0$

$= -np_0V_0$ (Given)

$\therefore \quad n = 1$

6. (d) The wave nature of light is explained by polarisation. Since, only transverse wave can be polarsied. Thus, polarisation is convincing proof of transverse nature of light wave. When unpolarised light is incident on the polariser, the intensity of the transmitted polarised light remains half the intensity of unpolarised light.

7. (d) $\frac{Y_A}{Y_B} = \frac{\tan\theta_A}{\tan\theta_B} = \frac{\tan 30°}{\tan 45°} = \frac{\frac{1}{\sqrt{3}}}{1} = \frac{1}{\sqrt{3}}$

$\therefore \quad Y_B = \sqrt{3}\,Y_A$

8. (a) Work done = Kinetic energy

$qV = \frac{1}{2}mv^2 \Rightarrow v = \sqrt{\frac{2qV}{m}}$

Force experienced by α-particle,

$F = Bqv = Bq \cdot \sqrt{\frac{2qV}{m}}$

$F \propto \sqrt{V} \Rightarrow \frac{F_2}{F_1} = \sqrt{\frac{V_2}{V}} = \sqrt{3}$

$F_2 = \sqrt{3}\,F \qquad [\therefore F_1 = F, V_2 = 3V]$

9. (c) As we know, force

$F = \frac{1}{4\pi\varepsilon_0}\frac{q_1q_2}{r^2} \qquad \ldots\text{(i)}$

Also, $\quad F = mr\omega^2 = \frac{4\pi^2 mr}{T^2} \quad \left(\because \omega = \frac{2\pi}{T}\right) \qquad \ldots\text{(ii)}$

By Eqs (i) and (ii), we get

$T^2 = \frac{(4\pi\varepsilon_0)r^2(4\pi^2 mr)}{q_1q_2}$

So, $\quad T = \left[\frac{4\pi^2 mr^3}{kq_1q_2}\right]^{\frac{1}{2}}$

10. (d) Energy required to move the satellite to the height of h from earth's surface is given by

$$U = -\frac{GMm}{(R+h)} - \left(-\frac{GMm}{R}\right) = \frac{GMmh}{R(R+h)}$$

Now, the kinetic energy of the satellite is

$$KE = \frac{1}{2}mv_0^2$$

$$= \frac{1}{2}m\frac{GM}{(R+h)}$$

So, the ratio of energy required to the kinetic energy is given by

$$\frac{U}{KE} = \frac{\frac{GMmh}{R(R+h)}}{\frac{1}{2}m\frac{GM}{(R+h)}} = \frac{2h}{R}$$

$$\therefore \quad \frac{U}{KE} = \frac{2h}{R}$$

11. (d) From the ideal gas equation,

$$pV = nRT$$

$$\Rightarrow \quad V = \frac{nRT}{p}$$

$$\Rightarrow \quad V = \frac{nRT^2}{a} \qquad (\because p = aT^{-1})$$

$$\Rightarrow \quad dV = \frac{2nRT}{a}dT \qquad \ldots\text{(i)}$$

Now, the work done by the gas is given by

$$dW = pdV$$

$$W = \int_T^{4T} \frac{a}{T}\frac{2nRT}{a}dT$$

$$= [2nRT]_T^{4T}$$

$$W = 6nRT$$

12. (b) Here, $L = 25\,\text{mH} = 25\times10^{-3}\,\text{H}$

$f = 50\,\text{Hz}, V_{rms} = 220\,\text{V}$

The inductive reactance,

$$X_L = 2\pi fL$$

$$= 2\times\frac{22}{7}\times50\times25\times10^{-3}\,\Omega$$

The rms current in the circuit,

$$I_{rms} = \frac{V_{rms}}{X_L}$$

$$= \frac{220}{2\times\frac{22}{7}\times50\times25\times10^{-3}}$$

$$= \frac{7\times1000}{2\times5\times25}\,\text{A} = 28\,\text{A}$$

13. (d) $a_y = \frac{F}{m} = \frac{10}{10} = 1\,\text{ms}^{-2}$

Distance in vertical direction in 4 s,

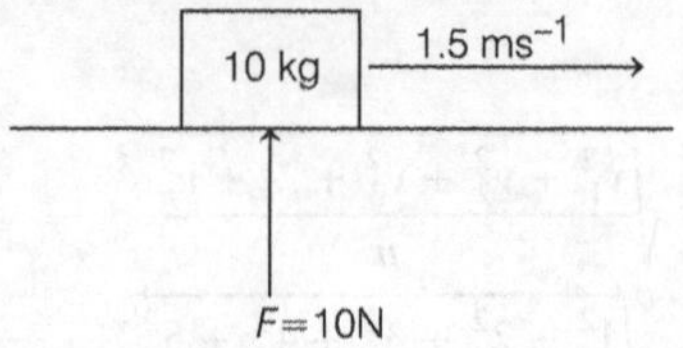

$$s_y = \frac{1}{2}a_yt^2 = \frac{1}{2}\times1\times16 = 8\,\text{m}$$

Distance in horizontal direction in 4 s,

$$s_x = 1.5\times4 = 6\,\text{m}$$

$$\therefore \text{ Displacement} = \sqrt{s_x^2+s_y^2} = \sqrt{8^2+6^2} = 10\,\text{m}$$

14. (c) The escape velocity and orbital velocity are related as $v_e = \sqrt{2}v_o$

Energy in a orbital velocity, $KE_o = \frac{1}{2}mv_o^2 = E$

Energy for escape velocity,

$$KE_e = \frac{1}{2}mv_e^2 = \frac{1}{2}m(\sqrt{2}v_o)^2 = 2E$$

Thus, energy required $= KE_e - KE_o = 2E - E = E$

15. (a) $n_{CO_2} = \frac{22}{44} = \frac{1}{2}, f_{CO_2} = 7, T_{CO_2} = 300\,\text{K}$

$$n_{O_2} = \frac{16}{32} = \frac{1}{2}, f_{O_2} = 5, T_{O_2} = 310\,\text{K}$$

where, n = number of moles,

f = degree of freedom

and T = initial temperature.

$$T_{mix} = \frac{[n_{CO_2}f_{CO_2}T_{CO_2} + n_{O_2}f_{O_2}T_{O_2}]}{n_{CO_2}f_{CO_2} + n_{O_2}f_{O_2}}$$

$$= \frac{\left[\frac{1}{2}\times7\times300\right] + \left[\frac{1}{2}\times5\times310\right]}{\left[7\times\frac{1}{2}\right] + \left[5\times\frac{1}{2}\right]}$$

$$= \frac{\frac{2100}{2} + \frac{1550}{2}}{\frac{7+5}{2}} = 304.16\,\text{K or } 31.16°\text{C}$$

16. (a) Given $\mu_w^a = \frac{4}{3}$

$$\mu_g^a = \frac{3}{2}$$

$$\mu_g^w = \frac{\mu_g^a}{\mu_w^a} = \frac{3/2}{4/3} = \frac{9}{8}$$

As, $\quad i = 30°$

$$\frac{\sin i}{\sin r} = \mu_g^w = \frac{9}{8}$$

$$\Rightarrow \quad \sin r = \frac{8}{9}\sin i = \frac{8}{9}\sin 30° = \frac{8}{9}\times\frac{1}{2} = \frac{4}{9}$$

$$\Rightarrow \quad r = \sin^{-1}\left(\frac{4}{9}\right)$$

17. (a) For closest approach,
Initial kinetic energy of α-particle = Potential energy of α-particle at closest approach

$$(2e)V = \frac{1}{4\pi\varepsilon_0}\frac{(2e)(Ze)}{d}$$

$$d = \frac{1}{4\pi\varepsilon_0}\frac{Ze}{V} = (9\times10^9)\frac{Z}{V}(1.6\times10^{-19}) = 14.4\frac{Z}{V}\,\text{Å}$$

18. (b) $x = 6 + 12t - 2t^2$

$$\frac{dx}{dt} = 12 - 4t$$

When particle stops travelling in forward direction, $v = 0$

$$12 - 4t = 0$$
$$t = 3\,\text{s}$$

Position at $t = 0$ s,
$$x = 6 + 12(0) - 2(0)^2$$
$$x = 6\,\text{m}$$

Position at $t = 3$ s,
$$x = 6 + 12(3) - 2(3)^2 = 24\,\text{m}$$

Position at $t = 5$ s,
$$x_3 = 6 + 12(5) - 2(5)^2 = 16\,\text{m}$$

Distance from 0s to 3s, $\Delta x = |24 - 6| = 18\,\text{m}$
Distance from 3s to 5s,
$$\Delta x' = |16 - 24| = 8\,\text{m}$$
Total distance travelled in first 5 s
$$= 18 + 8 = 26\,\text{m}$$

19. (c) Speed of light

$$= \frac{\text{Amplitude of electric field}}{\text{Amplitude of magnetic field}}$$

$$3\times10^8 = \frac{9}{B_0}$$

$$B_0 = \frac{9}{3}\times10^{-8}\,\text{T}$$

$$B_0 = 3\times10^{-8}\,\text{T}$$

20. (a) Given, $\sqrt{x} = t + 1$

$$\Rightarrow \quad x = (t+1)^2 \quad \Rightarrow \quad \frac{dx}{dt} = 2t + 2$$

$$\Rightarrow \quad v = 2t + 2 \quad \Rightarrow \quad v \propto t$$

21. (b) X is NAND gate and Y is OR gate.

22. (d) For diamagnetic, μ_r lies between 0 and 1
For paramegnetic, $\mu_r > 1$
For ferromagnetic, $\mu_r >> 1$
For superconductor, $\mu_r = 0$

23. (c) For electromagnetic wave

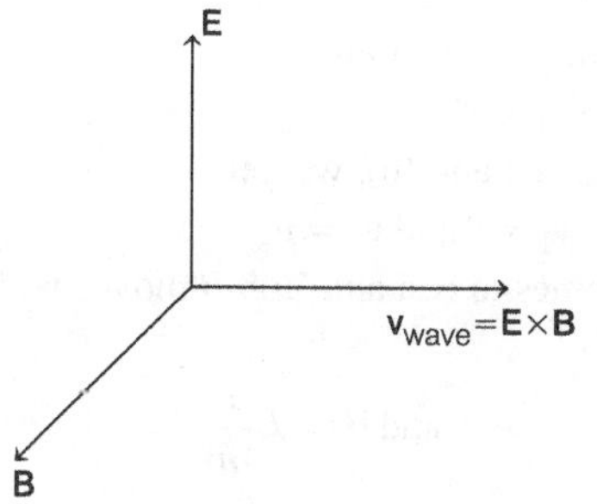

24. (a) Using the principle of homogeneity of dimensions, the quantity $\frac{\alpha z}{K\theta}$ is dimensionless.

$$\therefore \quad \alpha = \frac{K\theta}{z}$$

$$= \frac{[ML^2T^{-2}K^{-1}]\times[K]}{[L]} = [MLT^{-2}]$$

Also, $p = \frac{\alpha}{\beta}$

$$\Rightarrow \quad [\beta] = \left[\frac{\alpha}{p}\right] = \frac{[MLT^{-2}]}{[ML^{-1}T^{-2}]} = [M^0L^2T^0]$$

25. (b) Statement A is incorrect because the n-type and p-type semiconductors are extrinsic semiconductors.

26. (d) Self-inductance of solenoid = $\mu n^2 Al$
n = number of turns per unit length
∴ Self-induction $\propto n^2$
So, inductance becomes 4 times when n is doubled.

27. (b) Resistance will be maximum when connected in series,

$$\therefore \quad R_{series} = R + R + R\,.........\text{ upto } n$$
$$R_{series} = nR$$

Resistance will be minimum when connected in parallel,

$$\therefore \quad \frac{1}{R_{parallel}} = \frac{1}{R} + \frac{1}{R} + \ldots\ldots\text{upto } n$$

$$\Rightarrow \quad R_{parallel} = \frac{R}{n}$$

$$\therefore \quad \frac{R_{series}}{R_{parallel}} = \frac{nR}{\frac{R}{n}} = \frac{n^2}{1}$$

28. (d) As bob B is of same material and same mass as that of bob A, therefore on elastic collision, their velocities are exchanged.

By momentum conservation and $e = 1$, we have

$$e = \frac{\text{Speed of separation}}{\text{Speed of approach}} = \frac{v_2 - v_1}{u_1} = 1$$

$$\Rightarrow \quad v_2 - v_1 = u_1 \quad \ldots\text{(i)}$$

$$mu_1 = mv_1 + mv_2$$

$$\Rightarrow \quad v_2 + v_1 = u_1 \quad \ldots\text{(ii)}$$

Using Eqs. (i) and (ii), we get

$$v_1 = 0 \text{ and } v_2 = u_1$$

Bob A comes to rest and Bob B moves with the velocity of Bob A.

29. (d) As, $i = t^2 e^{-t}$ and $|\varepsilon| = L\frac{di}{dt}$

So, emf will be zero when $\frac{di}{dt} = 0$

Now, $\frac{di}{dt} = 2te^{-t} - t^2e^{-t} = 0$

$$\Rightarrow \quad 2te^{-t} - t^2e^{-t} = 0$$

$$\Rightarrow \quad te^{-t}(t-2) = 0$$

As, $t \neq \infty$ and $t \neq 0$

$\therefore \quad t = 2\text{ s}$

30. (b) In slide wire bridge (meter bridge), the balance point is obtained in the middle so as to increase its sensitivity and thereby no deflection in the galvanometer.

So, it minimizes error in measuring resistance with the help of slide wire bridge. The wire of slide wire bridge is made of manganin and constantan because it has low value of coefficient of thermal resistance.

31. (a) The energy of an electron in nth orbit of the hydrogen atom is given by

$$\therefore \quad E_n = \frac{-13.6}{n^2}\text{ eV}$$

For the first excited state, $n = 2$

$$\therefore \quad E_2 = \frac{-13.6}{2^2}\text{ eV}$$

For the second excited state, $n = 3$

$$\therefore \quad E_3 = \frac{-13.6}{3^2}\text{ eV}$$

$$\therefore \quad \frac{E_2}{E_3} = \frac{3^2}{2^2} = \frac{9}{4}$$

32. (a) Two equal and opposite charges make an electric dipole. P and Q points lie on the equatorial plane of the dipole.

Hence, potential at $P, V_P = 0$, potential at $Q, V_Q = 0$

Hence, work done,

$$W = q(V_P - V_Q) = q \times 0 = 0$$

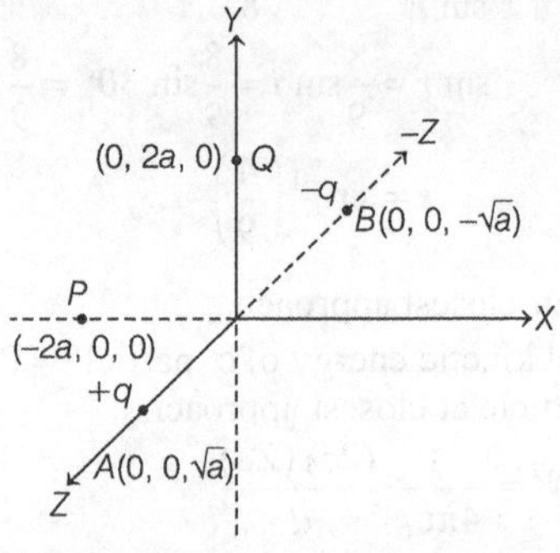

Problem Solving Tactics If potential difference between two points is zero, then the work done to bring a charge particle from one point to another point is also zero.

33. (d) $r = \frac{mv}{qB} = \frac{p}{qB}$

Both electron and proton have same p and q, so r is same for them. Hence, assertion is false but reason is true.

34. (a)

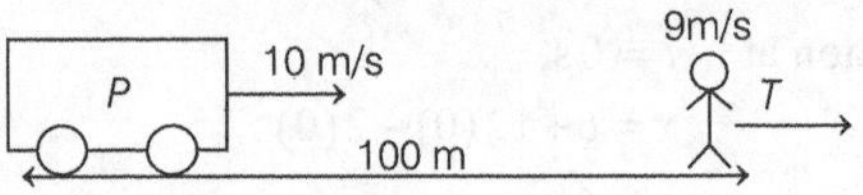

$$v_{PT} = v_P - v_T = 10 - 9 = 1\text{ m/s}$$

So time taken, $t = \frac{100}{v_{PT}} = \frac{100}{1} = 100\text{ s}$

35. (c) When A is joined to B, then peak value of current,

$$I_0 = \frac{e}{2R} \quad \ldots\text{(i)}$$

Now, when A is connected to C, then current flowing through R be I_0.

Hence, total heat produced across R is given by

$$H = \frac{1}{2}(L')I_0^2 = \frac{1}{2}(2L)\left(\frac{e}{2R}\right)^2 = \frac{Le^2}{4R^2}$$

36. (b) Since, angle with the horizontal is 45°, therefore vertical height = range

$$\tan 45° = \frac{H}{x} = 1$$

$$x = H = 19.6$$

Time of flight, $t = \sqrt{\frac{2H}{g}} = \sqrt{\frac{2 \times 19.6}{9.8}}$

$$t = 2\text{ s}$$

$$u = \frac{x}{t}$$

$$\Rightarrow \quad u = \frac{19.6}{2} = 9.8\text{ ms}^{-1}$$

37. (d) $y_1 = a\sin(2\pi ft)$

$$y_2 = a\sin\left(2\pi ft + \frac{\pi}{2}\right)$$

$$\therefore \quad y = y_1 + y_2$$

$$= 2a\sin\left(2\pi ft + \frac{\pi}{4}\right)\cos\frac{\pi}{4}$$

$$= \frac{2a}{\sqrt{2}}\sin\left(2\pi ft + \frac{\pi}{4}\right)$$

$$= \sqrt{2}\,a\sin\left(2\pi ft + \frac{\pi}{4}\right)$$

Thus, amplitude $= \sqrt{2}a$, frequency $= f$

38. (d)

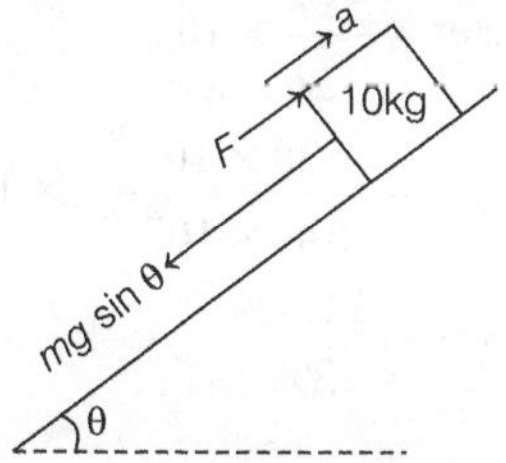

$$F - mg\sin\theta = ma$$

$$\Rightarrow \quad F - 10\times10\times\sin 30° = 10\times 2$$

$$\Rightarrow \quad F - 50 = 20 \Rightarrow F = 70\,\text{N}$$

39. (c) $W_0 = \frac{hc}{\lambda} = \frac{6.62\times10^{-34}\times3\times10^{8}}{4100\times10^{-10}}$

$$= 4.8\times10^{-19}\,\text{J} = 3\,\text{eV}$$

$W_A = 1.92\,\text{eV}$

$W_B = 2\,\text{eV}$

$W_C = 5\,\text{eV}$

Since, $W_A < W_0$

$W_B < W_0$

Hence, A and B will emit photoelectrons.

40. (c) Magnetic field due to wire,

$$B = \frac{\mu_0}{2\pi x}\cdot i$$

$$dA = a\,dx$$

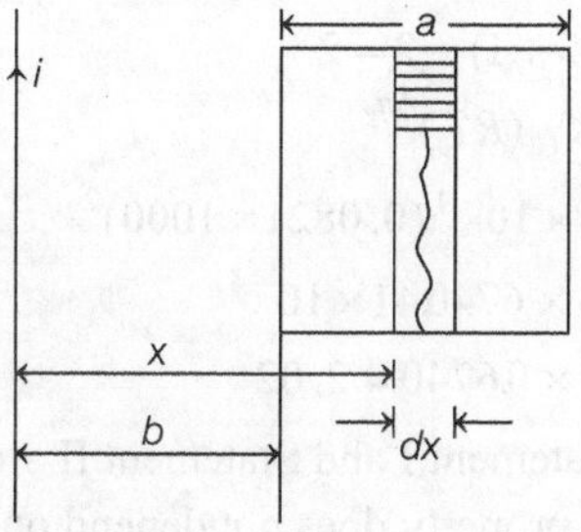

and $\quad d\phi = B\cdot dA$

On integrating both sides, we get

$$\int d\phi = \int B\,dA$$

$$\phi = \frac{\mu_0 i}{2\pi}\int_b^{a+b}\frac{a\cdot dx}{x}$$

$$\phi = \frac{\mu_0 i}{2\pi}a\ln[x]_b^{a+b} = \frac{\mu_0 i}{2\pi}a[\ln(a+b) - \ln b]$$

$$= \frac{\mu_0 i}{2\pi}a\left[\ln\left(1+\frac{a}{b}\right)\right] = Mi$$

where, M = coefficient of mutual inductance.

$$M = \frac{\mu_0 a}{2\pi}\ln\left(1+\frac{a}{b}\right)$$

41. (d) If β is fringe width, then spacing between second dark fringe and middle position of central bright fringe =

$$\frac{\beta}{2} + \beta + \beta = \frac{5\beta}{2}$$

Given, $\quad \frac{5\beta}{2} = 1.5\times10^{-3}$

$$\frac{5}{2}\times\frac{D\lambda}{d} = 1.5\times10^{-3} \Rightarrow \frac{5}{2}\times\frac{1\times\lambda}{0.8\times10^{-3}} = 1.5\times10^{-3}$$

$$\Rightarrow \quad \lambda = 480\,\text{nm}$$

42. (c) Given, length of the wire, $l = 5.0$ cm

Pitch = 1 mm

Least count of screw gauge,

$$\text{LC} = \frac{\text{pitch}}{\text{number of division on circular scale}}$$

$$= \frac{1\text{ mm}}{100} = 0.01\,\text{mm}$$

∴ Diameter of the wire, d

= Reading of main scale + Reading of circular scale

$= 1\,\text{mm} + 48\times\text{LC}$

$= 1\,\text{mm} + 48\times0.01 = 1.48\,\text{mm} = 1.48\times10^{-1}$ cm

∴ Volume of the wire $= \pi r^2 l$

$$= \pi\left(\frac{d}{2}\right)^2 l = \frac{\pi d^2 l}{4} \qquad \left(\because R = \frac{d}{2}\right)$$

$$= \frac{3.14\times(1.48\times10^{-1}\,\text{cm})^2\times5\,\text{cm}}{4}$$

$$= 0.0859732\,\text{cm}^3$$

$$= 0.086\,\text{cm}^3$$

43. (c) Given, moment of inertia of a hollow cylinder = I

Radius of hollow cylinder R_1 (inner radius), R_2 (outer radius) are 11cm, 15 cm, respectively.

Moment of inertia of hollow cylinder about its axis,

$$I_1 = \frac{M}{2}(R_1^2 + R_2^2)$$

Moment of inertia of thin hollow cylinder of radius R about its axis, $I_2 = MR^2$

Given, I_1 and I_2 is equal and both cylinders have same mass M, so

$$\frac{M}{2}(R_1^2 + R_2^2) = MR^2 \Rightarrow \frac{M}{2}(11^2 + 15^2) = MR^2$$

$$\frac{346}{2} = R^2$$

$$R = 13.15 \text{ cm}$$

44. (a) The equivalent circuit of the above figure can be written as

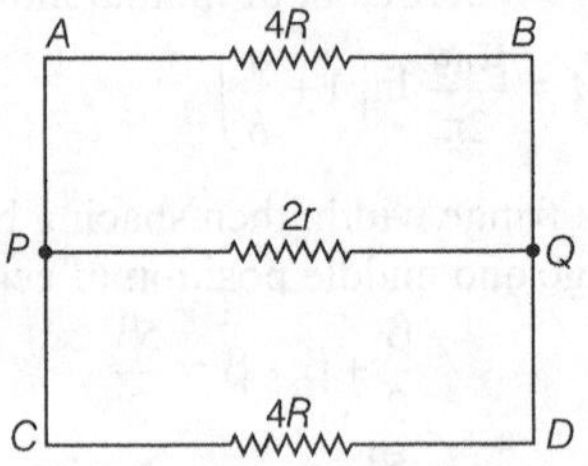

The branches AB, PQ and PQ, CD are a balanced Wheatstone bridge, therefore resistance between E and F and between F and G do not contribute and the circuit simplifies to the figure given above.

Hence, effective resistance R_e between P and Q will be

$$\frac{1}{R_e} = \frac{1}{4R} + \frac{1}{2r} + \frac{1}{4R}$$

$$R_e = \frac{2Rr}{(R+r)}$$

45. (b) In charged conducting sphere,

$$V_{in} = V_S = \frac{1}{4\pi\varepsilon_0} \cdot \frac{Q}{r_1}$$

In spherical shell, $V_{out} = \frac{1}{4\pi\varepsilon_0} \frac{Q}{r_2}$

where, r_1 and r_2 are the radii of sphere and spherical shell, respectively.

Potential at their surfaces,

$$V_{sphere} = \frac{1}{4\pi\varepsilon_0} \frac{Q}{r_1}$$

$$V_{shell} = \frac{1}{4\pi\varepsilon_0} \frac{Q}{r_2}$$

$$V = V_{sphere} - V_{shell} = \frac{Q}{4\pi\varepsilon_0}\left(\frac{1}{r_1} - \frac{1}{r_2}\right)$$

When the shell is given a charge $(-3Q)$ the potential at its surface and also inside will get charged by a potential V_0.

$$V_0 = \frac{1}{4\pi\varepsilon_0}\left(-\frac{3Q}{r_2}\right)$$

$$V'_{sphere} = \frac{1}{4\pi\varepsilon_0}\left(\frac{Q}{r_1}\right) + V_0$$

$$V'_{shell} = \frac{1}{4\pi\varepsilon_0}\left(\frac{Q}{r_2}\right) + V_0$$

$$V'_{sphere} - V'_{shell} = \frac{Q}{4\pi\varepsilon_0}\left(\frac{1}{r_1} - \frac{1}{r_2}\right) = V$$

Problem Solving Tactics	If any charge is given to an external shell, then voltage difference between external shell and internal sphere remain same.

Chemistry

46. (a) $\mu_{cal} = q \times d$

$$= 1.6 \times 10^{-19} \times 3.40 \times 10^{-10} \text{ Cm}$$

$$= 5.44 \times 10^{-29} \text{ Cm}$$

$$\% \text{ ionic character} = \frac{\mu_{exp}}{\mu_{cal}} \times 100$$

$$= \frac{6.28 \times 10^{-30}}{5.44 \times 10^{-29}} \times 100$$

$$= 11.5\%$$

$$\approx 12\%$$

47. (d) $k_1 = k_2$,

$$A_1 e^{-\frac{E_{a1}}{RT}} = A_2 e^{-\frac{E_{a2}}{RT}}$$

$$\Rightarrow \quad \frac{A_2}{A_1} = e^{\left(\frac{E_{a2}}{RT} - \frac{E_{a1}}{RT}\right)}$$

$$\Rightarrow \quad 10^2 = e^{\left(\frac{1200}{RT}\right)}$$

$$\ln(10)^2 = \ln e^{\left(\frac{1200}{RT}\right)}$$

$$\Rightarrow \quad 2 \ln 10 = \frac{1200}{RT} \ln e$$

$$\Rightarrow 2 \times 2.303 \times \log_{10} 10 = \frac{1200}{RT}$$

$$4.606 = \frac{1200}{RT}$$

$$T = \frac{600}{4.606} \text{ K}$$

48. (b) $\Delta n_g = (3+1) - 2 = 2$

$$K_p = K_C (RT)^{\Delta n_g}$$

$$= 3 \times 10^{-4} (0.0821 \times 1000)^2$$

$$= 3 \times 6740.41 \times 10^{-4}$$

$$= 3 \times 0.6740 = 2.02$$

49. (d) Both Statement I and Statement II are true.

I. Intensive property does not depend on mass.

II. Heat of neutralisation is always evolved.

50. (c) (A) $[Fe(CN)_6]^{3-}$

$$x+(-1)\times 6=-3$$
$$x-6=-3$$
$$x=-3+6$$
$$x=+3$$

(B) $[Ni(CO)_4]$

$$x+4(0)=0$$
$$x=0$$

(C) $[Fe(H_2O)_5NO]^{2+}$

$$x+5(0)+1=2$$
$$x=1$$

(D) $Fe_4[Fe(CN)_6]$

$$x+(-1)\times 6=-4$$
$$x-6=-4 \Rightarrow x=-4+6$$
$$x=+2$$

51. (a) Anisole reacts with *t*-butylchloride to give *p*-(*t*-butyl) anisole which further reacts with chlorine in dark to give 2-chloro-4-(*t*-butyl) anisole. This is then heated in HBr to give the desired product *A* (2-chloro-4-(*t*-butyl)-phenol).

The complete reaction sequence is as follows

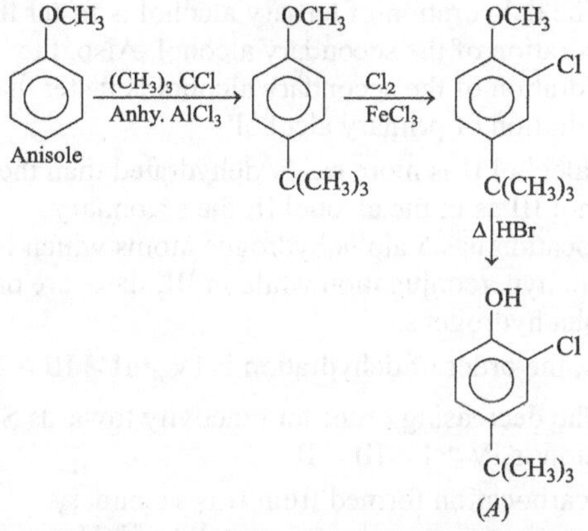

52. (c) The reaction of propene with HOCl proceeds *via* the addition of Cl^+ in the first step. HOCl has Cl^+ and OH^- ions.

The reaction takes place as follows

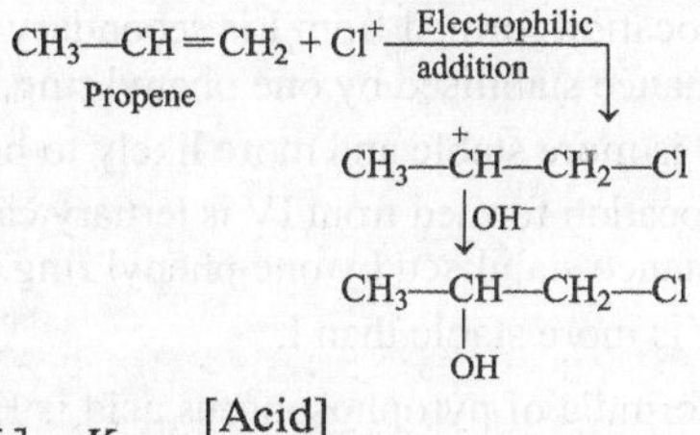

53. (b) $[H^+]=K_a\times\dfrac{[\text{Acid}]}{[\text{Salt}]}$

$$10^{-9}=5\times 10^{-10}\times\frac{10\times 2}{x\times 5}$$

$$x=\frac{5\times 10^{-10}\times 4}{10^{-9}}$$

$$x=\frac{20\times 10^{-10}}{10^{-9}}=20\times 10^{-1}=2\text{ mL}$$

54. (a) The electron affinity of fluorine is less than chlorine because fluorine is exceptionally small in size. Due to which energy has to be supplied to introduce an extra electron to overcome the electronic repulsions between the incoming electron and the electrons already present.

55. (d) Statement given is option (d) is false. It is an intermolecular redox change where AgBr reduces to Ag and hydroquinol oxidises to quinone.

56. (d) When acidified $K_2Cr_2O_7$ solution is added to Sn^{2+} salts then Sn^{2+} changes to Sn^{4+}. The balanced reaction is given below.

$$Cr_2O_7^{2-}+3Sn^{2+}+14H^+ \longrightarrow 3Sn^{4+}+2Cr^{3+}+7H_2O$$

57. (c) The correct match is A-III, B-IV, C-I, D-II.

58. (a) Among, $CH_3CH_2^-$, $HC\equiv C^-$ and $H_2C=CH^-$, $CH_3CH_2^-$ is the strongest nucleophile, as it is less electronegative (due to least *s*-character).

Problem Solving Tactics

In case of same nucleophilic site, nucleophilicity parallels the basicity while in case of different sites, nucleophilicity varies inversely with electronegativity.

The electronegativity of N > C so, the nucleophilicity of C > N.

59. (b) The correct match is A-III, B-IV, C-I, D-II.

The structure of the given species are as follows

(a) $\mathbf{XeOF_4}$ 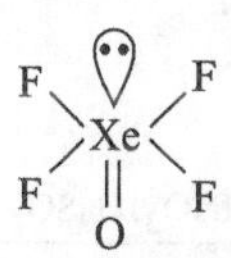 $\Rightarrow$ Square pyramidal

(b) $\mathbf{XeF_4}$ 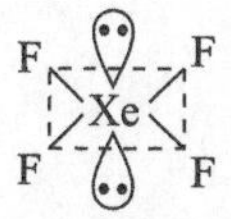 $\Rightarrow$ Square planar

(c) $\mathbf{SF_2Cl_2}$ 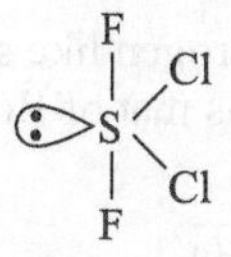 $\Rightarrow$ *See-saw*

(d) $\mathbf{PCl_3F_2}$ 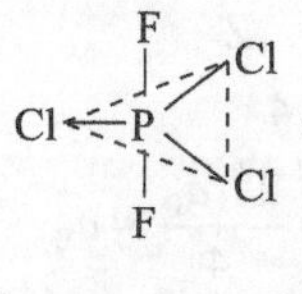 $\Rightarrow$ Trigonal bipyramidal

60. (d) Both A and R are true and R is the correct explanation of A.

61. (a) The product is less stable since energy of product is greater than the reactant and the activation energy is given by $E_1 + E_2$.

62. (a) The graph given in option (a) represents the curve of HCl *vs* NaOH, i.e. strong acid with a strong base.

Before the addition of NaOH, the conductance is high because of the presence of highly mobile hydrogen ions. While the base is added, the conductance falls due to the replacement of hydrogen ions through the added cation. As H^+ ions react along with OH^- ions to form undissociated water. Then decrease in the conductance continues till the equivalence point. At the equivalence point, a solution holds just NaCl. After the equivalence point, the conductance increases because of the huge conductivity of OH^- ions.

Problem Solving Tactics The electrical conductivity of a solution serves as a means of determining the end point in a chemical reaction, involved in the titration of acids, bases or precipitation.

63. (d) **Negative catalysts** (Inhibitors) A catalyst which decreases or retards the rate of reaction is called negative catalysts.

Presence of negative catalyst increase the energy of activation. Hence, Statement I and Statement II are true.

64. (b) The complete reaction is as follows

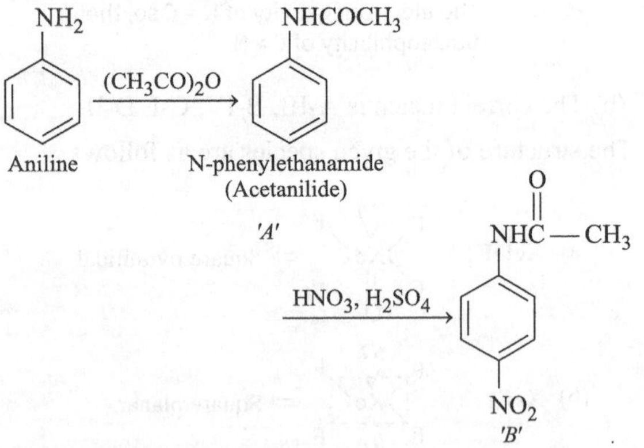

65. (b) Among the given hydrogen like species only one i.e. *B* will have same radius as that of Bohr orbit of hydrogen atom.

$$r_n = \frac{n^2 a_0}{Z}$$

In case of B, $n = 2$, $Z = 4$

$$r_n = \frac{2^2 \cdot a_0}{4} = a_0$$

66. (d) Both Statement I and Statement II are true.

67. (c)

(A) Sucrose is made up of glucose and fructose molecules. When sucrose is consumed, the enzyme separates sucrose into its individual sugar units of glucose and fructose.

(B) Lactose is a disaccharide, it is composed of two simple sugars, glucose and galactose.

(C) Maltose is made up of two molecules of glucose.

(D) Raffinose is a trisaccharide composed of galactose, glucose, and fructose.

Hence, the correct match is A-(ii), B-(iii), C-(iv), D-(i).

68. (b) Ammoniacal $AgNO_3$ is known as Tollen's reagent. It only gives positive test with aldehyde and not with ketone.

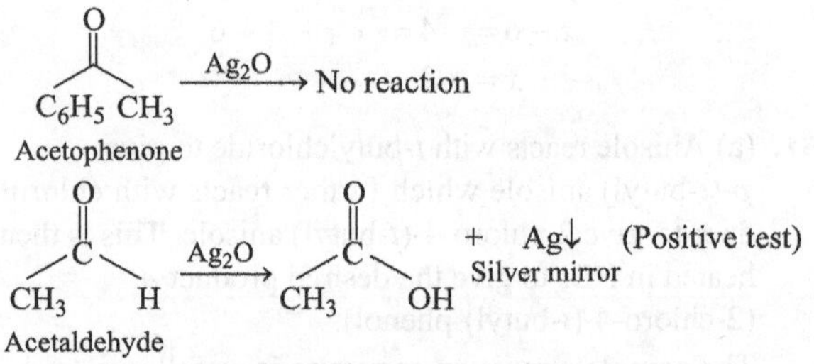

69. (c) The dehydration of tertiary alcohol is faster than the dehydration of the secondary alcohol. Also, the dehydration of the secondary alcohol is faster than the dehydration of primary alcohol.

The alcohol II is more easily dehydrated than the alcohol III as in the alcohol II, the secondary carbocation has 5 alpha hydrogen atoms which is taking part in hyperconjugation while in III, there are only 3 alpha hydrogens.

Thus, the order of dehydration is IV > II > III > I.

70. (a) The decreasing order for reactivity towards S_N1 reaction is IV > I > III > II.

The carbocation formed from II is secondary carbocation are not resonance stabilised. Hence, it is least stable and least likely to be formed.

The carbocation formed from III is tertiary carbocation and are not resonance stabilised. But, it is more stable then II and more likely to be formed.

The carbocation formed from I is secondary carbocation and resonance stabilised by one phenyl ring.

Hence, it is more stable and more likely to be formed.

The carbocation formed from IV is tertiary carbocation and resonance stabilised by one phenyl ring.

Hence, it is more stable than I.

71. (b) The formula of pyrophosphorus acid is $H_4P_2O_5$, Pyrophosphoric acid is $H_4P_2O_7$, Hypophosphorus acid is H_3PO_2 and phosphoric acid is H_3PO_3. Thus, pyrophosphoric acid contains highest number of oxygen atom in its chemical formula.

72. (d) In actinoids, the outermost 5*f*-orbitals are away from the nucleus and its energy is approximately similar in energies to 6*d* and 7*s*-orbitals.

Thus, transition of electron between these orbitals can take place easily and once they reach the valence orbital they can be ionised. This leads to the variability in oxidation states. In the case of lanthanoids, the outermost 4 *f*-orbitals are too close to the nucleus.

73. (b) Statements I, II, IV and V are correct but statement III is incorrect. It's correct form is

In $[Cu(NH_3)_4]SO_4$, the ligand has satisfied only secondary valencies of ferric ion.

74. (a) If we add a non-volatile solute to solvent such as water, it decrease the tendency for water molecules to evaporate into the gas phase. In essence, the solute particles obstruct the evaporation of water, as a result, finer molecules change from the liquid to the gas phase, thus reducing the vapour pressure and increases the boiling point of solution.

75. (d) $AlCl_3$ + aqueous acid $\longrightarrow [Al(H_2O)_6]^{3+}$

Al^{3+} ions give a complex ion in which Al^{3+} ion form six coordinate covalent bonds with six H_2O molecules. Hence, it shows sp^3d^2-hybridisation.

76. (d) The formation of PH_4^+ is difficult compared to NH_4^+ because lone pair of phosphorus resides in pure *s*-orbital. Due to this, phosphine lacks nucleophilicity and donation of lone pair to a proton becomes difficult.

77. (c) X should have high negative value of standard potential than Y so that it will be oxidised to X^{2+} by reducing Y^{2+} to Y. So, X = Zn, Y = Ni.

$$Zn + Ni^{2+} \longrightarrow Zn^{2+} + Ni$$

78. (a) The complete reaction is as follows

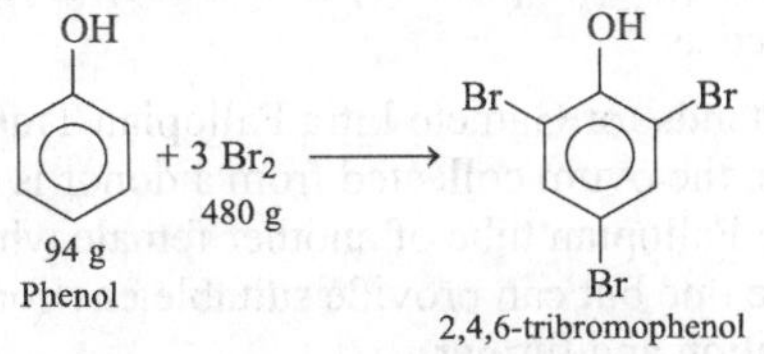

$\because$ 94 g of phenol requires = 480 g Br_2

$\therefore$ 3 g of phenol will require $= \frac{480}{94} \times 3 = 15.32$ g

79. (a) Arrhenius equation is given by

$$\ln k - \ln A = -\frac{E_a}{RT}$$

On comparing with equation of straight line, $y = mx + c$

$$\text{Slope} = -\frac{E_a}{R} \Rightarrow -2 \times 10^4 = -\frac{E_a}{8.314}$$

$$E_a = 166.28$$

$$E_a \approx 166 \text{ kJ/mol}$$

80. (c) Maximum work is always obtained in a reversible process.

$\therefore \quad W = -2.303\, nRT \log(V_2/V_1)$

$\because n_{O_2} = (w/M) = (16/32)$;

$R = 8.314 \text{ JK}^{-1}\text{mol}^{-1}$,

$T = 300 \text{ K}, V_1 = 5 \text{ dm}^3$,

$V_2 = 25 \text{ dm}^3$

$$\therefore \quad W = -2.303 \times (16/32)\, 8.314 \times 300 \times \log\left(\frac{25}{5}\right)$$

$$\simeq -2.01 \times 10^3 \text{ J}$$

81. (b) The formylation of thiophene α-position is carried out *via* the Vilsmeier-Haack reaction.

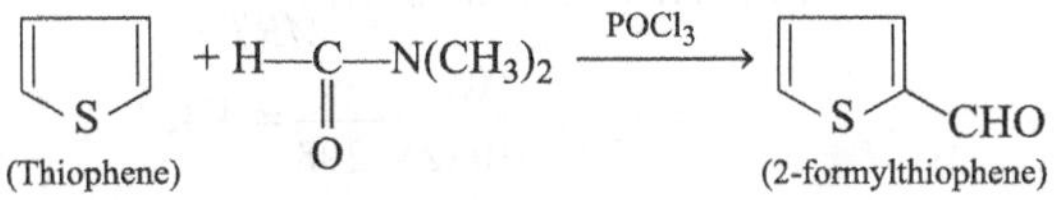

82. (b) Reagent used in benzoin condensation is KCN and reaction occurs as follows

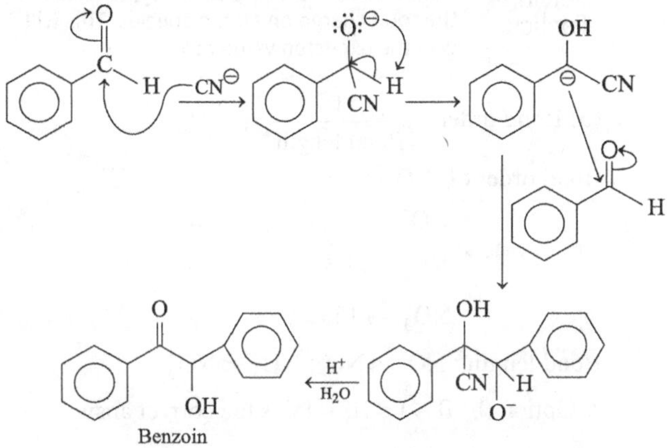

83. (a) Cycloketone reacts with hydroxylamine (NH_2OH) to give oxime (B) which further undergoes Beckmann's rearrangement to given caprolactam (C) as final product.

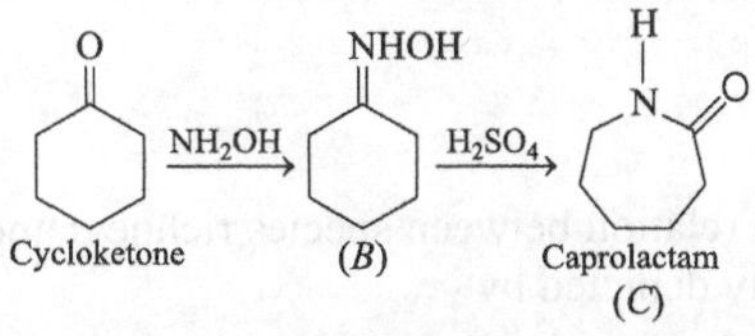

84. (d) Both Statement I and Statement II are true.

85. (c) Statement I is false but Statement II is true.

Aniline can be separated using the process of steam distillation because aniline is steam volatile and it is insoluble in water.

86. (d) Al_2O_3 is amphoteric and $AlCl_3$ forms a dimer. MgO is basic oxide while B_2O_3 is acidic in nature.

87. (c) For corner S-atom, + 2 from each (=O), + 1 from (O^-) and zero from sulphur atom present at centre. Therefore, its oxidation number is + 5. Middle S-atoms has zero oxidation number.

88. (b)

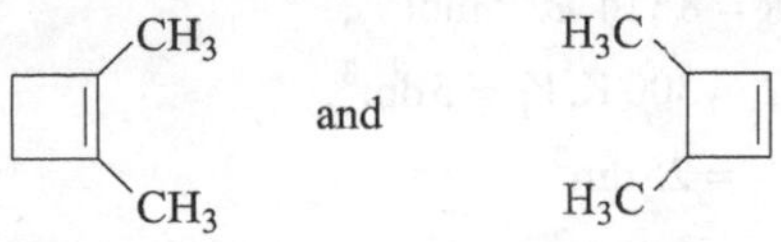

IUPAC name 1,2-dimethylcyclobut-1-ene

IUPAC name 3,4-dimethylcyclobut-1-ene

89. (a) $[Fe(NH_4)_2(SO_4)_2] \longrightarrow 2NH_4^+ + Fe^{2+} + 2SO_4^{2-}$

Expected value of $i = 5$

Now, observed van't Hoff factor $= \dfrac{\pi}{MRT}$

$$= \frac{10.8}{0.10 \times 0.082 \times 298} = 4.42$$

Problem Solving Tactics Write the balanced equation for the dissociation of $[Fe(NH_4)_2(SO_4)_2]$ and count the total charge on all the species. This will give the expected value of 'i'.

90. (b) Bond order $\propto \dfrac{1}{\text{Bond length}}$

Bond order of $NO \rightarrow 2.5$

$NO^+ \rightarrow 3$

$NO_2^- \rightarrow 1.5$

$NO_3^- \rightarrow 1.33$

Bond length : $NO^+ < NO < NO_2^- < NO_3^-$

$\therefore$ Option (b) II < I < III < IV is the correct answer

Problem Solving Tactics Remember the relation between bond order and bond length. So that by calculating the bond order you can predict the order of bond length.

Biology

91. (d) The relation between species richness and area is correctly depicted by

$$\log S = \log C + Z \log A$$

Where, S = Species richness

A = Area

Z = Slope of the line (regression coefficient)

C = Y-intercept

92. (b) Reaction in option (b) represents photo phosphorylation.

It is the process of utilising light energy from photosynthesis to convert ADP to ATP. It is of two types, i.e. cyclic photophosphorylation and non-cyclic photophosphorylation.

93. (d) Gamete transfer occurs by water in algae, bryophytes and pteriodophytes. This water-dependent gamete transfer is a primitive method of sexual reproduction. In contrast, gymnosperms have evolved more advance methods that are not dependent on water for fertilisation.

94. (d) During photorespiration, RuBP instead of being converted into two molecules of PGA, binds with O_2 to form one molecule of phosphoglycerate and one molecule of phosphoglycolate.

95. (b) Fluid mosaic model was proposed by Singer and Nicolson (1972). According to this the quasi fluid nature of lipids enables lateral movement of proteins within the overall bilayer.

96. (a) Statement in option (a) is incorrect and can be corrected as

Decomposition is an oxygen requiring process. In this process, the organic materials get decomposed in the presence of oxygen by bacteria and other microbes.

Rest statements are correct.

97. (b) Both statement I and statement II are correct. Classification is the process by which anything is grouped into convenient categories based on some easily observable characterstics.

The scientific term for these categories is taxa.

98. (c) Marriage between close family members can lead to genetic abnormalities in future offsprings. This is because certain recessive genes may get accumulated, which increases the chance of appearance of genetic abnormalities in their children.

99. (c) Match pair in option (c) is incorrect. It can be corrected as

GIFT stands for Gamete Intra Fallopian Transfer. In this process, the ovum collected from a donor is transferred into the Fallopian tube of another female who cannot produce one but can provide suitable environment for fertilisation and further development.

100. (c) The correct matches are A-3, B-4, C-5, D-1, E-2.

Paramecium caudatum reproduces by binary fission. Fungi (molds) belonging to class Deuteromycetes are known as fungi imperfect as only their asexual and vegetative phases are known.

Lichens are symbiotic association between algae and fungi, where the phycobiont is the algal componeent and mycobiont is the fungal component. Archaebacteria are obligate anaerobes. *Spirulina* is a source of protein and, thus is used as food supplement.

101. (b) The transposons are also known as mobile genetic elements or jumping genes. These are DNA sequences which move from one location to another.

102. (b) DNA fingerprinting relies on identifying minisatellite which are repetitive non-coding short DNA sequences.

103. (a) Statements I, II and IV are correct whereas statements III and V are incorrect and can be corrected as

Osteocytes are present in lacunae and are surrounded by matrix.
Columnar epithelium is found in the lining of stomach and intestine.

104. (a) Statements I and II are correct whereas other statements are incorrect and can be corrected as

The tubular reabsorption involves the absorption of water and useful solutes from the glomerular filtrate into the blood. About 90% of water is reabsorbed along with solute. It occurs by reverse diffusion and active transport. It occurs mostly in PCT. It does not occur in animals that lack glomerulus.

105. (c) When a more complex structure forms a simple structure for example, glucose becomes lactic acid in our skeletal muscle this pathway is called catabolic pathways.

106. (a) Statements I, II and IV are correct, but statements III and V are incorrect. These can be corrected as
Electron transport system is a chain of electron carrier, present in the inner mitochondrial membrane that carry the electron from NADH and $FADH_2$ produced in the mitochondrial matrix to the final acceptor, i.e. oxygen, resulting in the formation of H_2O. It is essential to release and utilise the energy stored in NADH and $FADH_2$.
Respiratory quotient is the ratio of volume of CO_2 evolved to the volume of O_2 consumed.

107. (a) Haemophilia is caused by a sex-linked recessive gene *h* located on the X-chromosome. A marriage between a carrier woman and a haemophilic man produces 50% normal and 50% haemophilic sons. Among the daughters, 50% will be carriers and remaining 50% will be affected by the disease.

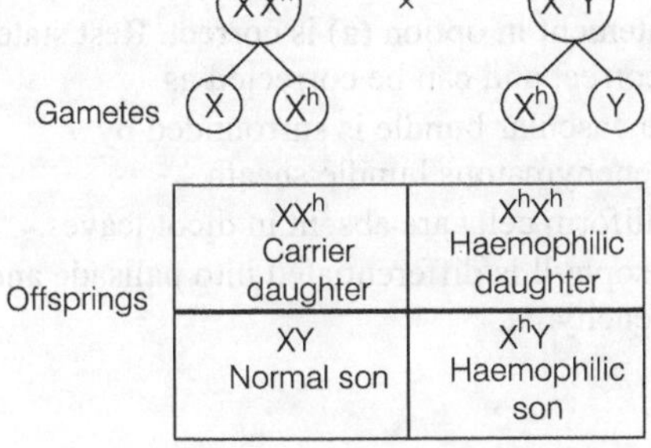

108. (c) The correct matches are A-3, B-1, C-4, D-2.
- The second largest phylum molluscs have their body covered by a calcareous shell.
- The body of ctenophores bear eight external rows of ciliated comb plates for locomotion.
- In poriferans, the body contains pores and canals in the walls.
- The body cavity is not lined by mesoderm in Aschelminthes, instead it is scattered as pouches in between the ectoderm and endoderm. Such animals possessing pseudocoelom are known as pseudocoelomates.

109. (a) Members of Phycomycetes have aseptate/coenocytic mycelium. They are found in aquatic habitats and on decaying wood in moist and damp places or as obligate parasites on plants. Some common examples are *Mucor, Rhizopus,* etc.

110. (a) Statement I is incorrect, but statement II is correct. Statement I can be corrected as

In 1900, three scientist (de Vries, Correns and von Tschermak) independently rediscovered Mendel's result on the inheritance of characters.

111. (d) The correct matches are A-4, B-2, C-1, D-3.
- Uremia–Presence of excess urea in blood
- Sweat produced by the sweat glands is a watery fluid containing NaCl, small amounts of urea, lactic acid, etc.
- Ketonuria–Presence of high ketone bodies in urine
- Glycosuria–Presence of glucose in urine

112. (a) In Chondrichthyes, Claspers are seen on the pelvic fins of male used for sperm transfer during copulation.

113. (a) The anaphase of meiosis-II begins with the simultaneous splitting of the centromere of each chromosome allowing them to move towards the opposite poles of cell by shortening of microtubules attached to kinetochores.

114. (d) Statement I is correct, but statement II is incorrect and it can be corrected as

The number of hydrogen bonds between adenine and thymine in DNA molecules is two.

115. (d) Match pair in option (d) is incorrect and it can be corrected as

Protoplasm is the living part of the cell, comprises of the cytoplasm, nucleus and other organelles. It can be denoted as

Protoplasm = Cytoplasm + Nucleoplasm

116. (c) In prophase-I of meiosis, during the susbtage diakinesis terminalisation of chiasmata can be observed. During this phase the chromosomes are fully condensed and the meiotic spindle is assembled to prepare the homologous chromosomes for separation.

117. (a) The correct matches are A-1, B-2, C-3, D-4.
Monocot stem has closed vascular bundle. Dicot stem has open vascular bundle due to the presence of cambium. In dicot root there are usually 2-4 xylem bundles and in monocot roots it has polyarch conditions, i.e. more than six xylem bundles.

118. (d) Double fertilisation involves fusion of the two male gametes brought by a pollen tube to two different cells, i.e. polar nuclei and egg cell, of the same female gametophyte.

119. (c) The incorrect statement is in option (c) and it can be corrected as,
The normal *E. coli* cells does not carry genes resistant against ampicillin, chloramphenicol, tetracyclins and kanamycin.

120. (c) *Eco* RV and *Sma* I is the correct pair of restriction enzymes, which produce blunt ends. They create a straight cut without overhangs on either sides.

121. (c) *Bt* toxin gene has been cloned from the bacteria and been expressed in plants to provide resistance to insects without the need of insecticides.

122. (d) *A-Eco*RI, *B*-Sticky ends, *C*-Recombinant DNA.
*Eco*RI cut off the sequence of GAATTC to generate sticky ends. These sticky ends are joined by complementary sequence to generate recombinant DNA.

123. (d) Statement in option (d) is correct.
Rest all other statements are incorrect and it can be corrected as
The separated DNA fragments can be visualised only after staining the DNA with a compound known as ethidium bromide followed by exposure to UV radiation. DNA cannot be seen without staining.

124. (a) Statement I is incorrect, but statement II is correct.
Incorrect statement can be corrected as
Slime moulds are unicellular saprophytic protists which form an aggregation called *Plasmodium*. They show amoeboid movement.

125. (b) A cell that is entering the M-phase of the cell cycle is either haploid or diploid and always with duplicated chromosomes.

126. (a) The chemical formula of palmitic acid is $CH_3(CH_2)_{14}COOH$. Rest can be explained as
Formula for Tripalmitin is $C_{51}H_{93}O_6$.
Formula for Glycerol is $C_3H_8O_3$.
Formula for Glycine is $CH-COOH-NH_2$.

127. (a) The given pedigree chart represents haemophilia. This is a sex-linked recessive disease, which shows its transmission from unaffected carrier female to the male progeny.
However, possibility of a female becoming a haemophilic is extremely rare.

128. (a) The features given are vegetative characteristics of fungi belonging to class Phycomycetes. e.g. *Rhizopus* (bread mould). Their hyphae are generally non-septate and multinucleate, i.e. coenocytic. The characteristic component of hyphal wall is chitin but cellulose may also be present along with it.

129. (b) Both statement I and statement II are correct.
Selectable markers helps in identifying and eliminating non-transformants and selectively permitting the growth of transformants. If a recombinant DNA bearing gene for resistance of ampicillin is transferred into *E.coli* cells, the host cells becomes transformed into ampicillin resistant cells. These genes are considered useful selectable marker for *E. coli*.

130. (b) Endoplasmic reticulum is involved in the modification and routing of newly synthesised proteins to their destinations.

131. (c) A DNA molecule is constituted by two complementary strands. This is advantageous because it promotes semiconservative mode of replication, where each parental strand gets paired with a newly formed daughter strand.

132. (a) Statements I, II and IV are correct, whereas statements III and V are incorrect. It can be corrected as
- Molluscs have a true coelom which is a fluid-filled body cavity between the body wall and the digestive tract.
- Cephalisation or the presence of a well-defined head region, is not a feature of all animal phyla. It is more prominent in bilaterally symmetrical animals, while animals with radial symmetry, like cnidarians, may lack a distinct head.

133. (c) Saheli a new oral contraceptive for female developed by Indian scientists is a non-steroidal preparation. It prevent unwanted pregnancy and has very low side effects.

134. (c) In polysaccharide like glycogen the right end contains the aldehyde group is called reducing end. The left end of the polysaccharide (glycogen) does not contain the aldehyde group and is called non-reducing end.

135. (a) Statement in option (a) is correct. Rest statements are incorrect and can be corrected as
- The vascular bundle is surrounded by parenchymatous bundle sheath.
- Bulliform cells are absent in dicot leaves.
- Mesophyll is differentiated into palisade and spongy parenchyma.

136. (a) The statement I is incorrect, whereas rest all the statements are correct.

Incorrect statement can be corrected as

Yeast is unicellular fungus, commonly used in baking and brewing. It does not produce edible fruiting bodies. Instead, it undergoes fermentation to produce CO_2 and alcohol.

137. (b) The given graph represents exponential growth curve where population size keeps on increasing with time since the resources are in abundance.

In order to level up this graph to a logistic or s-shaped curve, the population size should increase. This would permit the increased usage of resources and thereby, population growth rate is slowed down, giving an s-shaped curve.

138. (b) An additional copy of chromosome number 21 causes Down's syndrome. The affected individuals are short statured with furrowed tongue and partially open mouth.

139. (b) If the recombinant DNA is inserted within the coding sequence of *lac z* gene, then the host cells, which carry the recombinant DNA plasmid will form white colonies in the presence of *X*-gal.

140. (c) Both A and R are true but R is not the correct explanation of A.

Nucleic acids and proteins were the first evolved compounds (organic). They were required for origin of life. This explain the formation of life through chemical evolution.

All early forms of life occurred in water only.

141. (a) Carbonic anhydrase present in the red blood cell plays an important role in carbon dioxide transport. It is a zinc-containing enzyme which catalyses the hydration of carbon dioxide (CO_2), results in formation of carbonic acid (H_2CO_3)

142. (d) A is true, but R is false. R can be corrected as

Sum total of allelic frequency is 1. The Hardy-Weinberg principle says that the allele frequencies in a population are stable and is constant from generation to generation.

143. (d) Statement in option (d) is incorrect. It can be corrected as

Lymphocytes provide immunity by producing antibodies. Neutrophils and monocytes engulf pathogens.

144. (a) The statements I, III and IV are correct, while statements II and V are incorrect.

The incorrect statements can be corrected as

- In a polysaccharide the individval monosaccharides are linked by glycosidic bond.
- The DNA backbone is formed by the sugar phosphate-sugar chain. The nitrogenous bases are projected more or less perpendicular to backbone but face inside the strands.

145. (a) The correct matches are A-1, B-3, C-4, D-2.

- In simple leaf, lamina is entire.
- In compound leaves the incision of the lamina reach up to the midrib breaking it into a number of leaflets.
- In pinnately compound leaf a number of leaflets are present on common axis, the rachis which represent midrib of the leaf, e.g. neem.
- In palmately compound leaves, the leaflets are attached to common point, e.g. silk cotton.

146. (c) Statement II and IV are correct whereas rest of the statements are incorrect and it can be corrected as

The structural gene are the segments of DNA which carries codes for the synthesis of protein.

The terminator region is present down stream of structural gene at 3′ end of the coding strand.

The operator gene exercise the control over transcriptions.

147. (c) The correct matches are A-1, B-3, C-4, D-2.

Cervical vertebrae are seven in number and first cervical vertebra is called atlas.

Thoracic are present in the chest and are 12 in number.

Lumbar are five in number and present in the abdomen.

Sacral have five vertebrae and are fused in the adult forming one structure called sacrum.

148. (d) The cross-section of stem and root can be differentiated by endarch condition of stem and exarch condition of root, respectively. Endarch condition of xylem is found in the stem.

Here, the developement of protoxylem is directed towards the centre and meta xylem is directed towards the periphery. Whereas exarch condition of xylem is found in the root. Here, the protoxylem is directed towards the periphery and the metaxylem is directed towards the center.

149. (c) Both A and R are true, but R is not the correct explanation of A. It can be explained as

In gel electrophoresis DNA fragments are separated on the basis of their size, The smaller DNA molecules move more quickly through the gel matrix than the larger molecules through the sieving effect provided by the agarose gel.

150. (c) Both A and R are true and R is not the correct explanation of A.

Bacteria like *Streptococcus pneumoniae* and *Haemophilus influenzae* are responsible for the disease pneumonia.

As a result of the pneumonia, the alveoli get filled with fluid leading to severe problems in respiration. Some common symptoms include cough with phlegm, fever, chills, in severe case turning of finger nails bluish in colour is seen.

151. (b) The option (b) shows the correct description of the given floral diagram of family-Malvaceae.

It constitutes capsule or schizocarpous fruits. Its floral formula is

$$\text{Br} \; ⚥ \; \text{Epi}_{3\text{-}9} \, K_{5 \text{ or } (5)} \, \widehat{C_5 \, A_{(\infty)}} \, \underline{G}_{(2-\infty)} \cdot$$

152. (b) The pair in option (b) is incorrectly matched. It can be corrected as

In family-Cruciferae, the calyx is four polysepalous and arranged in two whorls. The calyx with six tepals in two whorls (3 + 3) is found in family-Liliaceae.

153. (c) *Nucleopolyhedrovirus* are excellent candidates for species-specific, narrow spectrum insecticidal application.

They are species specific. They have shown no negative impact on plants, mammals, birds, fishes, etc. These aid in integrated pest management programme.

154. (a) The correct sequence of the life cycle of *Plasmodium* is as follows —

Sporozoites are injected in human with mosquito bite → Sporozoties reach liver through blood→ Gametocytes develop in RBC→ Female mosquito takes up gametocytes with blood meal→ Fertilisation and development in mosquito's gut→ Mature infective sporozoite escape from gut and migrate to the salivary gland of mosquito.

155. (b) During S-phase, DNA replication begins in nucleus and centrioles duplicate in the cytoplasm.

156. (c) The correct matches are A-4, B-1, C-2, D-3.

- The investment of oxygen takes place under Electron Transport System (ETS) during aerobic respiration.
- The consumption of ATP occurs in various cytoplasmic pathways. One common example is glycolysis pathway.
- α-ketoglutaric acid is present in the matrix of mitochondria.
- F_1-particle are responsible for synthesising ATP and plays a crucial role in oxidative phosphorylation.

157. (c) The correct matches are A-1, B-2, C-4, D-3.

- The centrioles form the basal body of cilia or flagella.
- Microtubules are a structural component of the cytoskeleton in eukaryotic cells.
- The chromatin net represents the organisation of DNA and associated proteins in the nucleus, during interphase.
- Microbodies are membrane bound minute vesicles.

158. (d) Statement I is correct, but statement II is incorrect and can be corrected as

MTP is misused to get rid of pregnancy if the foetus is found to be female. It is illegal practice and dangerous for both the mother and the foetus.

159. (b) Both A and R are true and R is the correct explanation of A.

Catecholamines stimulate the breakdown of glycogen (glycogenolysis) which results in an increased concentrations of glucose in blood. In addition they also stimulate the breakdown of lipids and proteins.

160. (b) Statements II, IV and V are correct and rest of the statements are incorrect. These can be corrected as

- Schwann concluded that the presence of cell wall is a unique character of plant cell.
- Mesosomes in prokaryotic cell are special membranous structure, which are formed by the extensions of plasma membrane into the cell.

161. (b) In mitochondria, pyruvic acid formed by the glycolytic catabolism of carbohydrates in cytosol undergoes oxidative decarboxylation, i.e. removal of CO_2 in aerobic conditions, forming a key compound, i.e. acetyl Co-A by the action of pyruvic acid dehydrogenase (in mitochondrial matrix) through a series of reactions.

162. (a) Bryophytes are non-vascular cryptogams with thallus-like plant body. The sporophyte is attached to gametophyte. The gametophyte is the dominant phase in their life cycle.

163. (a) Statement I is incorrect, but statement II is correct. Incorrect statement can be corrected as

First vertebra is atlas which articulates with occipital condyles.

164. (d) Okazaki fragments contain covalently linked RNA and DNA. Okazaki fragments are short, newly synthesised DNA fragments that are formed on the template strand with polarity 5′–3′ during DNA replication.

165. (a) In the stroma lamellae, only PS-I is functional. The electron is circulated within the photosystem-I and the phosphorylation occurs due to cyclic flow of electrons. The process is known as cyclic photophosphorylation.

166. (c) The blood groups AB and O are not possible in this condition. Let us make a cross for the following.

$$I^A I^B \times I^O I^O$$

$$\downarrow$$

$$\underbrace{I^A I^O, \; I^A I^O}_{\text{Blood Group A}} \quad \underbrace{I^B I^O, \; I^B I^O}_{\text{Blood Group B}}$$

Hence, the progeny can only have either A or B blood group.

167. (d) The correct matches are A-2, B-1, C-4, D-3.

Osteoporosis is an age related disorder characterised by decreased bone mass and increased chances of fractures.
Gout is the inflammation of joints due to accumulation of uric acid crystals.
Myasthenia gravis is an autoimmune disorder affecting neuromuscular junction leading to fatigue and paralysis of skeletal muscle.
Tetany causes rapid contractions in muscle due to low Ca^{++} in body fluid.

168. (a) The incorrect match pair is in option (a).
It can be corrected as
Back cross is the process of crossing or mating a hybrid offspring with one of its parents.

169. (b) Match pair in option (b) is correct.
Auxin and cytokinin are plant growth promoters. When added in plant tissue culture media, they promote the formation of callus. Auxin promotes rooting and cytokinin accelerates shooting.
Rest options can be corrected as
Abscisic acid is a stress hormone. Auxin is used in the induction of somatic embryo.

170. (c) Both A and R are true, but R is not the correct explanation of A.
Origin of replication is a definite region in *E. coli* DNA, where the replication originates. This sequence is also responsible for controlling the copy number of the linked DNA.

Vectors are engineered in such a way that they must have origin of replication, selectable marker and cloning sites.

171. (a) The control of bacterial pathogens by sulpha drug, is an example of competitive inhibition. The sulpha drugs mimics a key substrate named Para Amino Benzoic Acid (PABA). These drugs compete with PABA for binding to the enzyme and disrupts the production of folic acid, in turn inhibits bacterial growth.

172. (d) A is true, but R is false and can be corrected as

The secondary spermatocytes are haploid formed by the meiotic division of the primary spermatocytes.

173. (d) The phloem fibres are generally present in secondary phloem of plants. These fibres provide structural support to the phloem tissue.

174. (b) The correct sequence of stages in prophase-I is

Leptotene, Zygotene, Pachytene, Diplotene and Diakinesis.

175. (b) Statement in option (b) is correct, whereas rest of the statements are incorrect. These can be corrected as

- The eyes of the frog are a pair of spherical structures situated in the orbit in skull.
- The frog constitutes prominent endocrine glands namely pituitary, thyroid, parathyroid, thymus, pineal, adrenals and gonads.
- Frogs have well organised male and female reproductive system.

176. (d) The correct matches are A-4, B-5, C-1, D-2.

- Cerebrum is the seat of intelligence.
- Cerebellum maintains body posture.
- Hypothalamus controls pituitary gland.
- Mid brain controls vision and hearing.

177. (b) Point mutations refer to those mutations which arises due to change in a single base pair of DNA.
This change may either be deletion or addition of one base pair or it may be due to substitution of one base pair by another.

178. (d) Statement I is correct, but statement II is incorrect and can be corrected as

Thorns of *Acacia* and cactus are most common morphological means of defence.

179. (c) Statements I, II, IV and V are correct, whereas statement III is incorrect and can be corrected as

Invasive alien species typically disrupt ecosystem rather than providing stability.

180. (a) Statement in option (a) is incorrect and can be corrected as

Coenzyme is an organic compound and their association with the apoenzyme is only transient .
Rest other statements are correct.

SECTION II

Mastery Builders

PRACTICE SET 7

Maximum Marks : 720	Time : 3 hrs	No. of Questions : 180

Instructions

1. This question paper contains **180** multiple-choice questions (four options with a single correct answer) from **Physics**, **Chemistry** and **Biology**.
2. These questions are distributed as 45 questions, each from Physics and Chemistry and 90 questions in Biology. These are to be compulsorily attempted by the candidate.
3. Each question carries 4 marks. For each correct response, the candidate will get 4 marks. For each incorrect response, one mark will be deducted from the total scores.

PHYSICS

1. Two balls of masses M_1 and M_2 are placed on a horizontal frictionless table connected by a spring as shown in figure. Now mass M_2 is pulled to the right with a force F. If the acceleration of mass M_1 is a, then acceleration of mass M_2 will be

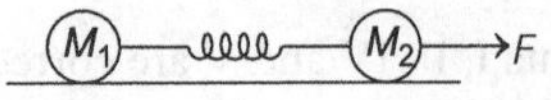

a) $\dfrac{F}{M_1}$ (b) $\dfrac{F - M_1 a}{M_2}$

(c) $\dfrac{F}{M_2}$ (d) None of these

2. The moment of inertia of a uniform rod about a perpendicular axis passing through one end is I_1. When it is bent into a ring, the moment of inertia about a diameter is I_2. Then, the ratio of $\dfrac{I_1}{I_2}$ is

(a) $\dfrac{4\pi^2}{3}$ (b) $\dfrac{2\pi^2}{3}$ (c) $\dfrac{\pi^2}{3}$ (d) $\dfrac{8\pi^2}{3}$

3. The total energy of a particle executing SHM of period 2π s is 10.24×10^{-3} J. The displacement of the particle at $\dfrac{\pi}{4}$ s is $0.08\sqrt{2}$ m. The mass of particle is

(a) 0.08 kg (b) 0.8 kg

(c) 0.16 kg (d) 1.6 kg

4. A piece of solid weighs 150 g in air, 120 g in water and 90g in liquid. The relative density of the solid and that of liquid are, respectively

(a) 5, 2 (b) 3, 2 (c) 4, 5 (d) 2, 5

5. At what point on the line joining two masses of 500 kg and 2000 kg, will the resultant gravitational field intensity is zero, if their separation is 2m ? (Take, $G = 6.67 \times 10^{-11}$ N-m^2 kg^{-2})

(a) 1 m from 500 kg (b) $\dfrac{2}{3}$ m from 2000 kg

(c) 1 m from 2000 kg (d) $\dfrac{2}{3}$ m from 500 kg

6. A body is projected vertically upward with speed of 40 m/s. The distance travelled by body in the last second of upward journey is [Take, $g = 10$ m/s^2 and neglect effect of air resistance]

(a) 10.0 m (b) 5.0 m (c) 12.5 m (d) 20.0 m

7. In Fraunhoffer's diffraction pattern, slit is illuminated by a light source of wavelength 4200 Å. If slit is illuminated by another monochromatic light source, then angular width is increased by 40%. Wavelength of new source is

(a) 5880 Å (b) 4200 Å

(c) 6000 Å (d) 5580 Å

8. A bar magnet has a magnetic moment 2.5 JT^{-1} and is placed in a magnetic field of 0.2 T. The work done in turning the magnet from parallel to anti-parallel position relative to field direction is
(a) 4J (b) 2 J (c) 3 J (d) 1 J

9. In the figure, a proton moves a distance d in a uniform electric field **E** as shown in the figure. Does the electric field do a positive or negative work on the proton ? Does the electric potential energy of the proton increase or decrease ?

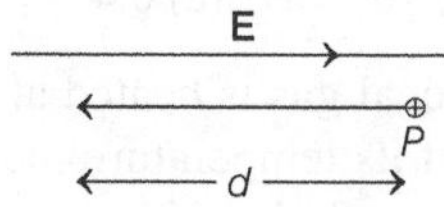

(a) Negative, increases (b) Positive, decreases
(c) Negative, decreases (d) Positive, increases

10. The average depth of Indian ocean is about 4 km. The fractional compression, $\frac{\Delta V}{V}$ of water at the bottom of ocean is (given that the Bulk modulus of the water $= 2.2 \times 10^9$ Nm^{-2} and $g = 10$ ms^{-2})
(a) 1.36% (b) 1.81% (c) 2.43% (d) 1.17%

11. A cyclic process is shown on the p-T diagram.

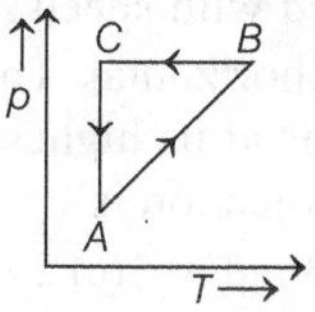

Which of the curve shows the same process on p-V diagram?

(a)
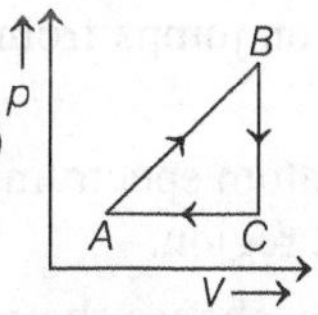

(b)
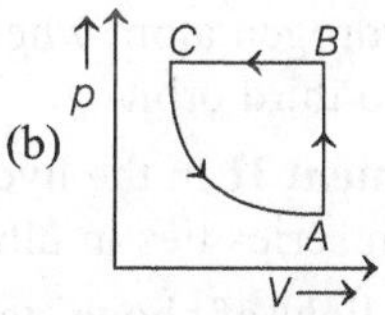

(c)
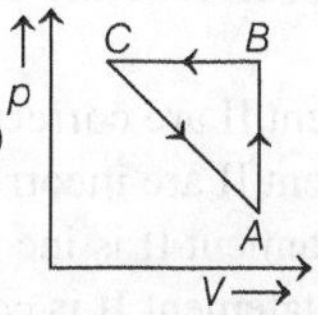

(d)
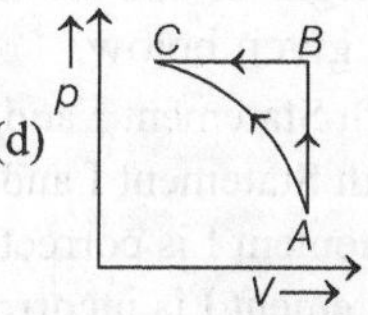

12. Two resistances are connected in two gaps of meter bridge. The balance point is 20 cm from the zero end. A resistance of 15Ω is connected in series with the smaller of the two. The null point shifts to 40 cm. The value of the smaller resistance (in ohm) is
(a) 12 (b) 9 (c) 3 (d) 6

13. In CGS system, density of a liquid is 0.625 g cm^{-3}. The magnitude of density in MKS system will be
(a) 0.625 (b) 0.0625 (c) 0.00625 (d) 625

14. A stone is dropped from the top of a fall cliff and after 3 s another stone is thrown vertically downwards with a speed of 8 ms^{-1}. Then, the second stone will overtake the first, below the top of cliff at a distance of

(a) $\frac{g}{2}\left[\frac{\left(24-\frac{9}{2}g\right)}{(8-3g)}\right]^2$ (b) $\frac{g}{2}\left[\frac{(8-3g)}{\left(24-\frac{9}{2}g\right)}\right]^2$

(c) $\frac{g}{2}\left[\frac{(8g-3)}{(24g-9)}\right]^2$ (d) $\frac{g}{2}\left[\frac{(24g-9)}{(3g-8)}\right]^2$

15. If the refractive index of water is $\frac{4}{3}$ and that of given slab of glass immersed in it is $\frac{5}{3}$, what is the critical angle for a ray of light tending to go from glass to water?
(a) $\sin^{-1}\left(\frac{3}{4}\right)$
(b) $\sin^{-1}\left(\frac{3}{5}\right)$
(c) $\sin^{-1}\left(\frac{4}{5}\right)$
(d) Data given are insufficient to make any calculation

16. The value of surface tension of water in SI unit is $7.2 \times 10^{-3} Nm^{-1}$. The value of surface tension in CGS unit is
(a) 72 dyne cm^{-1} (b) 7.2 dyne cm^{-1}
(c) 72×10^5 dyne cm^{-1} (d) 3.6 dyne cm^{-1}

17. In the given circuit, the reading of voltmeter V_L and V_C are 300 V each. The reading of the voltmeter V_R and ammeter A are respectively,

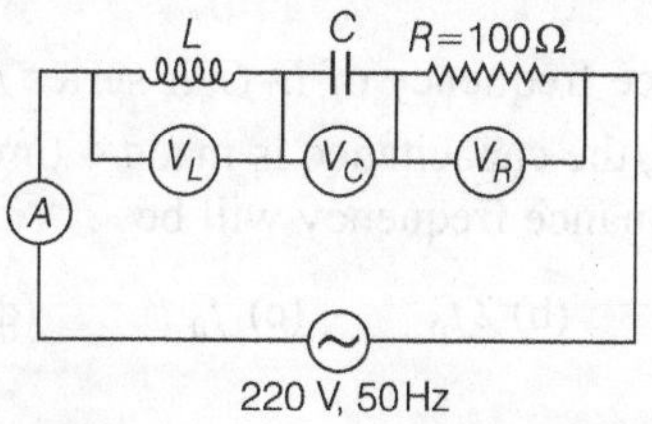

(a) 100 V, 2.0 A (b) 220 V, 2.2 A
(c) 150 V, 2.2 A (d) 220 V, 2.0 A

18. A resistance coil is made by joining in parallel two resistances each of 10 Ω. An emf of 1.0 V is applied between two ends of coil for 5 min. The heat produced (in cal) will be
(a) 10.3 (b) 14.3 (c) 16.3 (d) 18.3

19. The net force on an electric dipole placed parallel to the X-axis, where electric field is also parallel to X-axis, will be
(a) directed along, Y-axis (b) directed along X-axis
(c) directed along Z-axis (d) None of these

20. Three photodiodes D_1, D_2 and D_3 are made of semiconductors having band gaps of 2.6 eV, 1.9 eV and 3.2 eV, respectively. Which one will be able to detect light of wavelength of 6000Å?
(a) D_1 (b) D_2
(c) D_3 (d) D_1 and D_2

21. Given below are two statements.

Statement I Electromagnetic induction is a source of emf which based upon law of conservation of energy in which mechanical energy is converted into electrical energy.

Statement II If the coil is cut, then induced emf will be produced but the current will not flow.

In the light of above statements, choose the correct option given below.
(a) Both Statement I and Statement II are incorrect.
(b) Both Statement I and Statement II are correct.
(c) Statement I is correct but Statement II is incorrect.
(d) Statement I is incorrect but Statement II is correct.

22. If one main scale division of a vernier calliper is x cm and nth division of vernier scale coincides with $(n-1)$th division of main scale. The least count of the vernier calliper (in mm) is
(a) $\left(\frac{n-1}{10n}\right)x$ (b) $\left(\frac{10n}{n-1}\right)x$
(c) $\frac{10x}{n}$ (d) $\frac{10x}{n-1}$

23. Resonance frequency of L- C-R series AC circuit is f_0. Now, the capacitance is made 4 times, then the new resonance frequency will be
(a) $\frac{f_0}{4}$ (b) $2f_0$ (c) f_0 (d) $\frac{f_0}{2}$

24. The circuit shown below is working as 8 V DC regulated voltage source. When 12 V is used as input, the power dissipated (in mW) in each diode is (considering both Zener diode as identical)

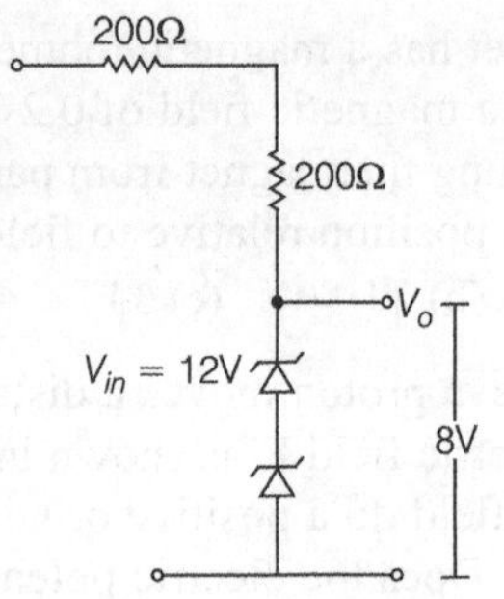

(a) 4 (b) 40 (c) 0.4 (d) 400

25. 3 moles of an ideal gas is heated at constant pressure, so that its temperature increases from 27°C to 177° C, then work done is
(a) 5732 J (b) 3735 J (c) 3243 J (d) 1775 J

26. A helium nucleus makes full rotation in a circle of radius 0.8 m in 2s. The value of the magnetic field B at the centre of the circle will be
(a) $\frac{10^{-19}}{\mu_0}$ (b) $10^{-19}\mu_0$
(c) $2\times 10^{-10}\mu_0$ (d) $\frac{2\times 10^{-10}}{\mu_0}$

27. A ball is projected with speed $20\sqrt{2}$ ms^{-1} at an angle of 45° above the horizontal. The angular velocity of the ball, when it is at its highest point of journey, about point of projection is
(a) 4 rad/s (b) 3 rad/s (c) 2 rad/s (d) 1 rad/s

28. Given below are two statements

Statement I Lines of Lyman series are emitted by the hydrogen atom when electron jumps from higher orbit to third orbit.

Statement II In the hydrogen atom spectrum, the Lyman series lies in ultraviolet region.

In the light of above statements, choose the correct option given below.
(a) Both Statement I and Statement II are correct.
(b) Both Statement I and Statement II are incorrect.
(c) Statement I is correct but Statement II is incorrect.
(d) Statement I is incorrect but Statement II is correct.

29. The earth is assumed to be a sphere of radius R. A platform is arranged at a height R from the surface of the earth. The escape velocity of a body from this platform is fv, where v is its escape velocity from the surface of the earth. The value of f is
(a) $\frac{1}{2}$ (b) $\sqrt{2}$ (c) $\frac{1}{\sqrt{2}}$ (d) $\frac{1}{3}$

30. Two batteries of emfs 3 V and 6 V with internal resistances 2Ω and 4Ω are connected in a circuit with resistance of 10Ω as shown in the figure. The current and potential difference between the points P and Q are

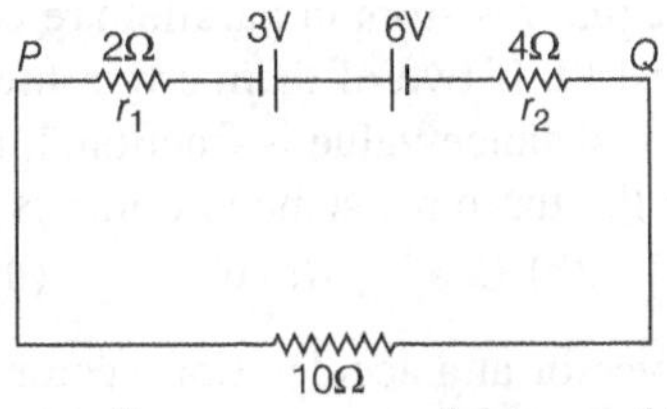

(a) $\frac{3}{16}$ A and $\frac{8}{15}$ V (b) $\frac{16}{3}$ A and $\frac{15}{8}$ V
(c) $\frac{3}{16}$ A and 8 V (d) $\frac{3}{16}$ A and $\frac{15}{8}$ V

31. The de-Broglie wavelength associated with an electron, accelerated through a potential difference of 400 V is

(a) 1.2×10^{-9} m (b) 0.06×10^{-9} m
(c) 3.6×10^{-9} m (d) 4.8×10^{-9} m

32. Two coherent sources of intensity ratio β interfere, then the value of $\frac{(I_{max}-I_{min})}{(I_{max}+I_{min})}$ is

(a) $\frac{1+\beta}{\sqrt{\beta}}$ (b) $\sqrt{\left(\frac{1+\beta}{\sqrt{\beta}}\right)}$
(c) $\frac{1+\beta}{2\sqrt{\beta}}$ (d) $\frac{2\sqrt{\beta}}{1+\beta}$

33. A parallel plate capacitor of area A, plate separation d and capacitance C is filled with three different dielectric materials having dielectric constants K_1, K_2 and K_3 are shown in following figure. If a single dielectric material is to be used to have the same capacitance C in this capacitor, then its dielectric constant K is given by

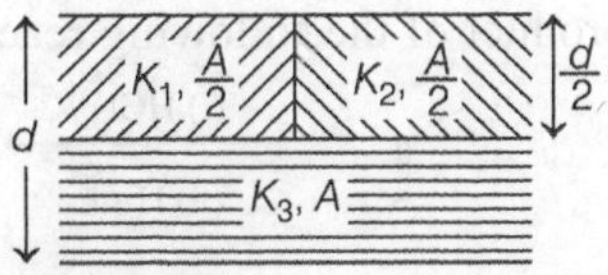

(a) $\frac{1}{K}=\frac{1}{K_1}+\frac{1}{K_2}+\frac{1}{2K_3}$
(b) $\frac{1}{K}=\frac{1}{K_1+K_2}+\frac{1}{2K_3}$
(c) $K=\frac{K_1K_2}{K_1+K_2}+2K_3$
(d) $K=K_1+K_2+K_3$

34. Infinite number of charges of magnitude $6\mu C$ each are lying at $y=2, 4, 8, 16 \ldots$ metre on Y-axis. The value of electric field intensity at point $y=0$ due to these charges will be

(a) 6.5×10^3 N/C (b) 4.05×10^4 N/C
(c) 7.2×10^3 N/C (d) 1.8×10^4 N/C

35. The correct statements about the EM waves among the following are

A. Like mechanical waves, EM waves require a material medium for propagation.
B. If an electromagnetic wave incident on a material surface is completely reflected, then it delivers momentum, $p=\frac{2U}{c}$ and U energy to the surface.
C. The velocity of electromagnetic waves in free space is equal to the velocity of light in free space.
D. EM waves of different radiations travel with the same speed in a medium.

Choose the correct answer from the options given below.

(a) C and D only (b) A and B only
(c) B and C only (d) A and D only

36. In which case, there is no current induced in the coil as shown in the figure?

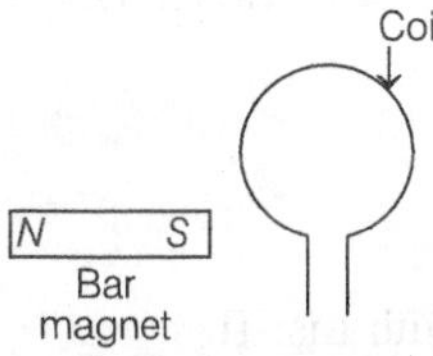

(a) When both moves towards each other.
(b) When magnet moves towards coil.
(c) When coil and magnet both move in same direction with same velocity.
(d) When both moves away from each other with same speed.

37. In Young's double slit experiment with sodium vapour lamp of wavelength 589 nm and the slits 0.589 mm apart, then the half angular width of the central maxima is

(a) $\sin^{-1}(0.01)$
(b) $\sin^{-1}(0.0001)$
(c) $\sin^{-1}(0.001)$
(d) $\sin^{-1}(0.1)$

38. A nucleus with mass number 240 breaks into two fragments of mass number 110 and 130 having binding energy per nucleon 7.8 MeV and 8.0 MeV, respectively. If binding energy per nucleon of unfragmented nuclei is 7.5 MeV, the energy released in the process is

(a) 216 MeV (b) 153 MeV
(c) 124 MeV (d) 98 MeV

39. Electromagnetic waves travel in a medium which has relative permeability 1.3 and relative permittivity 2.14, then the speed of electromagnetic waves in the medium will be

(a) 13.6×10^6 ms^{-1} (b) 1.8×10^8 ms^{-1}
(c) 3.6×10^8 ms^{-1} (d) 1.8×10^6 ms^{-1}

40. A 4m long ladder weighing 25 kg rests with its upper end against a smooth wall and lower end on rough ground. The minimum coefficient of friction between the ground and the ladder for it to be inclined at 60° with the horizontal without slipping (Take, $g = 10\text{ m/s}^2$) will be

(a) 0.3 (b) 0.289 (c) 0.25 (d) 0.298

41. The potential energy function for the force between two atoms in a diatomic molecule is approximately given by $U(x) = \frac{a}{x^{12}} - \frac{b}{x^6}$, where a and b are constants and x is the distance between the atoms. If the dissociation energy of the molecules is $D = [U(x=\infty) - U_{\text{at equlibrium}}]$, then D is equal to

(a) $\frac{b^2}{6a}$ (b) $\frac{b^2}{2a}$
(c) $\frac{b^2}{12a}$ (d) $\frac{b^2}{4a}$

42. Three unequal resistors in parallel are equivalent to a resistance 1 Ω. If two of them are in the ratio 1 : 2 and if no resistance value is fractional, then the largest of the three resistance in ohm is

(a) 5 (b) 12 (c) 6 (d) 4

43. Velocity vector and acceleration vector in a uniform circular motion are related as

(a) both in the same direction
(b) both in opposite direction
(c) perpendicular to each other
(d) not related to each other

44. Two identical wires A and B have the same length l and carry the same current I. Wire A is bent into a circle of radius R and wire B is bent to form a square of side a. If B_1 and B_2 are the values of magnetic induction at the centre of the circle and the centre of the square respectively, then the ratio B_1 / B_2 is

(a) $\pi^2/8$ (b) $\pi^2/8\sqrt{2}$ (c) $\pi^2/16$ (d) $\pi^2/16\sqrt{2}$

45. A wave has simple harmonic motion whose period is 5 s, while another wave which also possess simple harmonic motion has its period 4 s. If both are combined, the resultant wave will have the period equal to

(a) 12 s (b) 16 s (c) 20 s (d) 25 s

CHEMISTRY

46. Match List-I with List-II.

	List-I		List-II
A.	Number of sub-shells in a shell	I.	$2(2l+1)$
B.	Maximum number of electrons in a sub-shell	II.	$n-l-1$
C.	Number of spherical nodes	III.	n
D.	Number of spectral lines in Lyman series for a gas (for n to 1 transition)	IV.	$(n-1)$

Choose the correct answer from the options given below.

(a) A-III, B-I, C-IV, D-II (b) A-III, B-I, C-II, D-IV
(c) A-I, B-II, C-III, D-IV (d) A-I, B-IV, C-II, D-III

47. Major product of the following reaction is

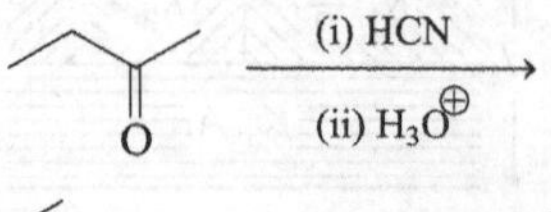

(a) 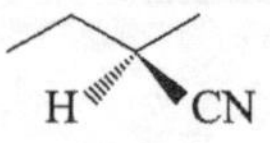

(b) 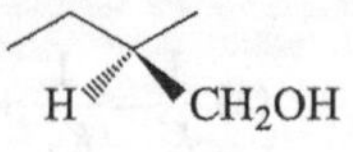

(c) 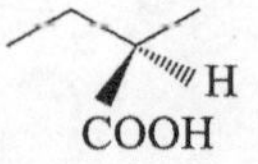

(d) 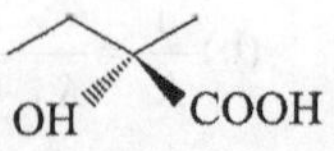

48. The correct order of decreasing second ionisation enthalpy of Ti, V, Cr and Mn is

(a) Cr > Mn > V > Ti (b) Ti > V > Cr > Mn
(c) V > Mn > Cr > Ti (d) Mn > Cr > Ti > V

49. Which of the following pair can be distinguish by Fehling's solution?

(a) CH_3CHO and C_6H_5CHO

(b) CH_3CHO and $CH_3\overset{\overset{\displaystyle O}{||}}{C}CH_2OH$

(c) $CH_3\overset{\overset{\displaystyle OH}{|}}{C}H—\overset{\overset{\displaystyle O}{||}}{C}CH_3$ and HCHO

(d) CH_3CHO and HCHO

50. For the first order reaction, the ratio of $t_{1/2}$ to $t_{1/3}$ for the amount of substance left will be [Given, log 2 = 0.3010; log 3 = 0.4771].

(a) 0.520 (b) 0.413
(c) 0.328 (d) 0.631

51. In molecule C_2, consider the following statements

I. Bond order is 2.
II. Both the bonds present in C_2 are π-bond.
III. The molecule is paramagnetic in nature.
IV. Double bond in C_2 consists of 1σ and 1π-bond.
V. Bond length of C_2 is greater than that of O_2 molecule.

Select the incorrect statements.

(a) III and IV (b) III and V
(c) I, II and III (d) I and V

52. During electrophilic substitution reaction of fullerene, the hybridisation of carbon atom

(a) remains sp^2 in reactant as well as product
(b) changes from sp^2 to sp^3 from reactant to product
(c) changes from sp^3 to sp^2 from reactant to product
(d) sp^2 to sp from reactant to product

53. Which of the following statement is correct?

(a) $[Co(en)_3]^{3+}$ is paramagnetic, inner orbital complex.
(b) $[Co(en)_3]^{3+}$ is diamagnetic, outer orbital complex.
(c) $[Co(en)_3]^{3+}$ is paramagnetic, outer orbital complex.
(d) $[Co(en)_3]^{3+}$ is diamagnetic, inner orbital complex.

54. Select the incorrect statement about cyclohexane from the following

(a) It exists in puckered chair and boat form conformation.
(b) Twist boat is less stable than chair conformation.
(c) Each carbon atom has an axial and equatorial hydrogen.
(d) Chair form is the least stable conformation.

55. Match the List-I with List-II.

List-I (Electronic configuration)		List-II (Electronegativity of element)	
A.	$1s^2, 2s^2, 2p^5$	(i)	3.04
B.	$1s^2, 2s^2, 2p^4$	(ii)	2.58
C.	$1s^2, 2s^2, 2p^3$	(iii)	3.98
D.	$1s^2, 2s^2, 2p^6, 3s^2, 3p^4$	(iv)	3.44

Choose the correct answer from the options given below.

(a) A-(iv), B-(iii), C-(i), D-(ii)
(b) A-(ii), B-(iv), C-(i), D-(iii)
(c) A-(iii), B-(iv), C-(i), D-(ii)
(d) A-(i), B-(ii), C-(iii), D-(iv)

56. Consider the following statements.

Statement I The solution of HCl and water, exhibits negative deviation from Raoult's law.

Statement II The mixture of $CHCl_3$ and acetone boils at a temperature higher than those of its either components.

In the light of the above statements, choose the correct answer from the options given below:

(a) Statement I is false but Statement II is true.
(b) Statement I is true but Statement II is false.
(c) Both Statement I and Statement II are true.
(b) Both Statement I and Statement II are false.

57. For a cell involving one electron $E^\circ_{cell} = 0.59$ V at 298K, the equilibrium constant for the cell reaction is

[Given that, $\frac{2.303RT}{F} = 0.059\text{V}$ at $T = 298$ K]

(a) 10^2
(b) 10^5
(c) 10^{10}
(d) 10^{30}

58. Consider the reaction,

$$Cl_2(g) + 2Br^-(aq) \longrightarrow 2Cl^-(aq) + Br_2(aq)$$

The emf of the cell when $[Cl^-] = [Br_2] = [Br^-] = 0.01$ M and Cl_2 gas at 1 atm pressure will be (E°_{cell} for the above reaction is = 0.29 volt).

(a) 0.65
(b) 0.35
(c) 0.85
(d) 1.35

59. Glucose $+ 3C_6H_5NH—NH_2 \xrightarrow{H^+/\Delta}$ Osazone $+ A + B$
A and B are

(a) 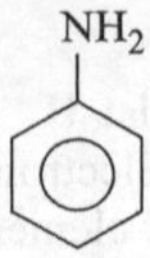 and NH_3 (b) 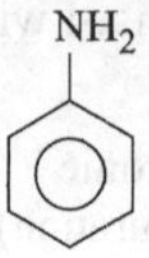 and NH_2OH

(c) 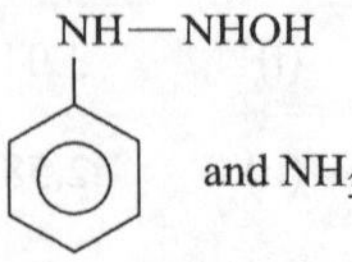 and NH_3 (d) NH_2OH and H_2O

60. Which of the following order is correct regarding acidic strength?

(a) $Cl_2O > Cl_2O_3 > Cl_2O_7$ (b) $Cl_2O > Cl_2O_7 > Cl_2O_3$
(c) $Cl_2O < Cl_2O_3 < Cl_2O_7$ (d) $Cl_2O < Cl_2O_7 < Cl_2O_3$

61. The reaction which is induced in the preparation of ethene from chloroethane is

(a) β-elimination (b) reduction
(c) α-elimination (d) dehalogenation

62. Given below are two statements.

Statement I Fluorine does not form polyhalide as it has low F—F bond energy.
Statement II Chlorine has most negative electron gain enthalpy.
In the light of the above statements, choose the correct answer from the options given below.

(a) Statement I is false but Statement II is true.
(b) Both Statement I and Statement II are true.
(c) Both Statement I and Statement II are false.
(d) Statement I is true but Statement II is false.

63. The nodal plane in the π-bond of ethene is located in

(a) the molecular plane.
(b) a plane parallel to the molecular plane.
(c) a plane perpendicular to the molecular plane which bisects the C—C σ-bond at right angle.
(d) a plane perpendicular to the molecular plane which contains the C—C σ-bond.

64. Which plot best represents the potential energy (E) of two hydrogen atoms as they approach one another to form a hydrogen molecule?

(a) 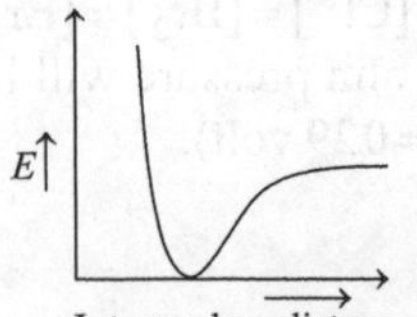

(b) 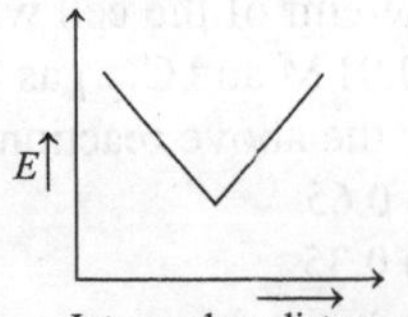

(c) 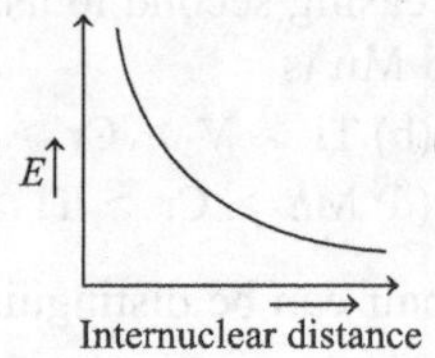

(d) 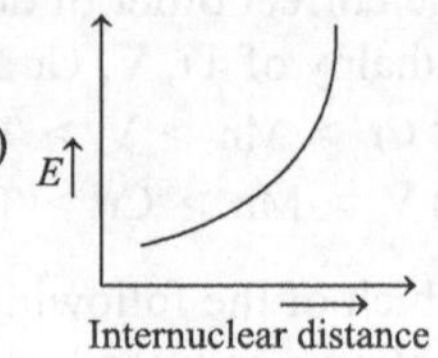

65. Consider the following compounds.

A. $C_6H_5COC_6H_5$
B. $C_6H_5COCH_3$
C. $C_6H_5COCH_2COCH_3$
D. $C_6H_5CH=CH—OH$
E. 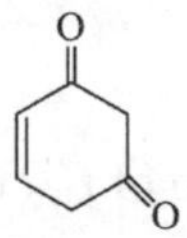

Which of the following compounds can exhibit keto-enol tautomerism?

(a) B and C (b) A and C
(c) B, C and E (d) A, B and C

66. Match the List-I with List-II.

	List-I		List-II
A.	Hess law is not applicable for	(i)	Not a state function
B.	All combustion reaction are	(ii)	Heat of dilution
C.	Work	(iii)	Exothermic
D.	Difference between two integral heats of solution	(iv)	Nuclear reaction

Choose the correct answer from the options given below.

(a) A-(i), B-(ii), C-(iii), D-(iv)
(b) A-(iv), B-(iii), C-(i), D-(ii)
(c) A-(ii), B-(i), C-(iii), D-(iv)
(d) A-(i), B-(ii), C-(iv), D-(iii)

67. Given below are two statements.

Statement I Blue chromate has two peroxide bonds.
Statement II Blue chromate reacts with H_2SO_4 to give oxygen.
In the light of the above statements, choose the correct answer from the options given below.

(a) Statement I is false but Statement II is true.
(b) Both Statement I and Statement II are true.
(c) Both Statement I and Statement II are false.
(d) Statement I is true but Statement II is false.

68. Given below are two statements, one is labelled as Assertion (A) and the other is labelled as Reason (R).

Assertion (A) Oxidation involves loss of electrons and reduction involves gain of electrons.

Reason (R) The overall reaction in which oxidation and reduction occurs simultaneously is called redox reaction.

In the light of the above statements, choose the most appropriate answer from the options given below.

(a) (A) is false but (R) is true.
(b) Both (A) and (R) are true and (R) is a correct explanation of (A).
(c) Both (A) and (R) are true but (R) is not a correct explanation of (A).
(d) (A) is true but (R) is false.

69. Find the value of ΔG° for the reaction having K_{eq} value 4×10^5 at 300 K temperature.

(a) 7.73 cal (b) 32.15 kcal
(c) 7.73 kJ (d) 32.18 kJ

70. Given below are two statements.

Statement I Be and Al form the amphoteric oxides.

Statement II Be and Al are metalloids.

In the light of the above statements, choose the correct answer from the options given below.

(a) Statement I is false but Statement II is true.
(b) Both Statement I and Statement II are true.
(c) Both Statement I and Statement II are false.
(d) Statement I is true but Statement II is false.

71. For a binary ideal liquid solution, the variation in total vapour pressure *versus* composition of the solution is given by which of the curves?

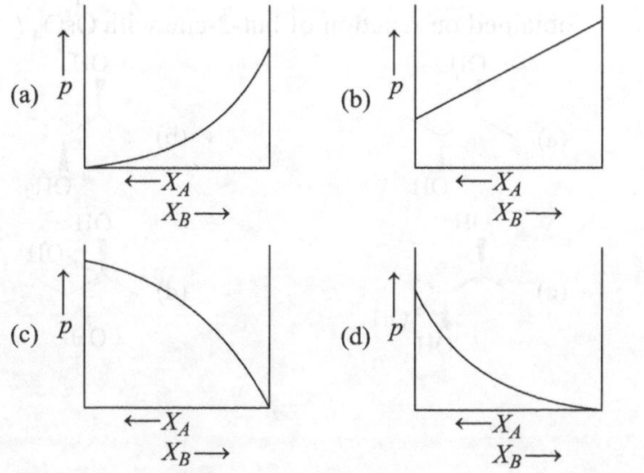

72. Given below are two statements.

Statement I For a solution of $AlCl_3$ in water, the van't Hoff factor (*i*) is greater than 1.

Statement II The solubility of gas is directly proportional to the pressure over the solutions at a given temperature.

In the light of the above statements, choose the correct answer from the options given below.

(a) Statement I is false but Statement II is true.
(b) Both Statement I and Statement II are true.
(c) Both Statement I and Statement II are false.
(d) Statement I is true but Statement II is false.

73.

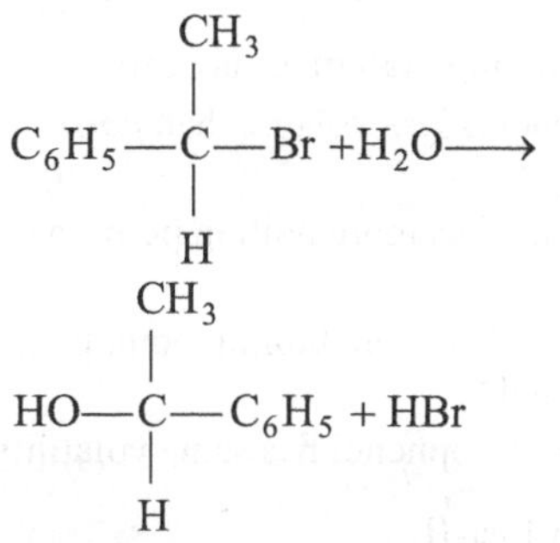

The above reaction results in 98% racemisation, the reaction mainly follows

(a) S_N1 mechanism
(b) S_N2 mechanism
(c) Can be both S_N1 and S_N2
(d) Neither S_N1 nor S_N2

74. Coordination compounds have great importance in biological systems. In this context which of the following statements is incorrect?

(a) Chlorophylls are green pigments in plants and contains calcium.
(b) Carboxypeptidase-A is an enzyme and contains zinc.
(c) Haemoglobin is the red pigment of blood and contains iron.
(d) Cyanocobalamin is B_{12} and contains cobalt.

75. Which of the following statements is incorrect?

(a) Silicon carbide has a three dimensional tetrahedral structure.
(b) Carbon can form C=S bond because C has the ability to form $d\pi$-$d\pi$ bond.
(c) Boron nitride has structure similar to that of graphite.
(d) Graphite conducts electricity because of the availability of delocalised π-electrons.

76. $CH_3MgX \xrightarrow[\text{Dry ether}]{CH_3COOCH_3} A \xrightarrow{Na} B \xrightarrow{C_2H_5Br} C$

Here, *C* is

(a) $C_2H_5OC_2H_5$ (b) $CH_3COOC_2H_5$
(c) CH_3COOCH_3 (d) $(CH_3)_3COC_2H_5$

77. Which one of the following is a wrong statement?
(a) ΔH_f° for $H^+ (aq)$ is taken as zero.
(b) Standard entropy of ethane is lower than that of methane.
(c) The final temperature of an ideal gas is less in adiabatic reversible expansion as compared to adiabatic irreversible expansion against a constant external pressure.
(d) For isothermal irreversible compression, $\Delta S_{sys} < 0$.

78. Which of the following statement is correct?
(a) *ortho*-nitrophenol is less volatile than *para* nitrophenol.
(b) *ortho*-nitrophenol has more boiling point than *para* nitrophenol.
(c) *para*-nitrophenol has more boiling point than *ortho*-nitrophenol.
(d) *ortho* and *para*-nitrophenol has same volatility.

79. Match List-I with List-II.

	List-I		List-II
A.	XeO_2F_2	(i)	Tetrahedral
B.	XeF_2	(ii)	Square planar
C.	XeF_4	(iii)	Linear
D.	XeO_3	(iv)	*See-saw*

Choose the correct answer from the options given below.
(a) A-(i), B-(ii), C-(iii), D-(iv)
(b) A-(i), B-(ii), C-(iv), D-(iii)
(c) A-(ii), B-(i), C-(iii), D-(iv)
(d) A-(iv), B-(iii), C-(ii), D-(i)

80. The product X in the reaction given below is

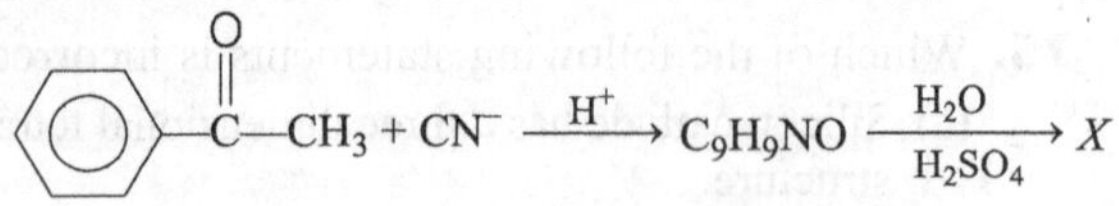

(a) 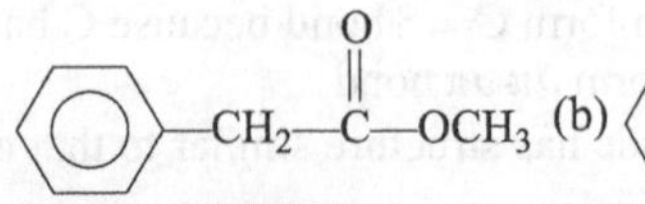

(b) 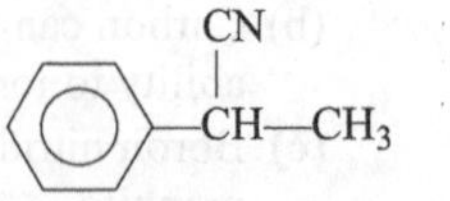

(c) 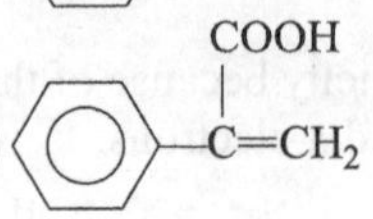

(d) 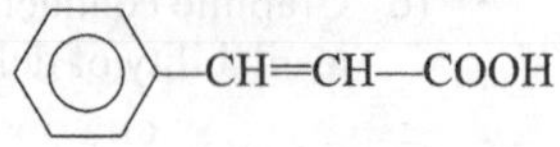

81. Match List-I with List-II.

	List-I		List-II
A.	Gabriel phthalimide synthesis	I.	Amine with a lesser number of carbon atoms.
B.	Carbylamine reaction	II.	Reaction of alkyl halides with NH_3
C.	Ammonolysis	III.	Reaction of phthalimide with KOH and $R—X$
D.	Hofmann Bromamide reaction	IV.	Detection test for primary amines.

Choose the correct answer from the options given below:
(a) A-I, B-II, C-III, D-IV
(b) A-III, B-IV, C-II, D-I
(c) A-II, B-IV, C-I, D-III
(d) A-IV, B-II, C-III, D-I

82. Acetophenone can be prepared by
I. oxidation of 1-phenyl ethanol.
II. reaction of benzaldehyde with methyl magnesium bromide.
III. Friedel-crafts reaction of benzene with acetyl chloride.
IV. distillation of calcium benzoate.
V. reaction of anisole with a mixture of conc. H_2SO_4 + conc. HNO_3.

Choose the correct answer from the options given below.
(a) I and III (b) V and IV (c) I and II (d) III and IV

83. What will be correct stereochemistry of product obtained on reaction of but-2-ene with OsO_4?

(a) 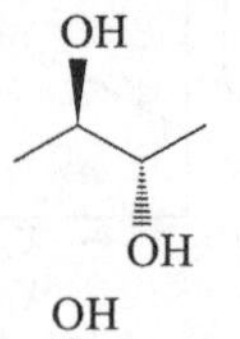

(b) 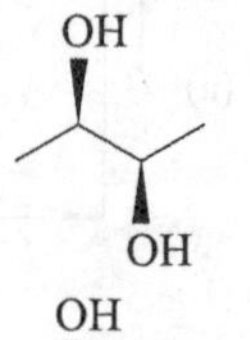

(c) 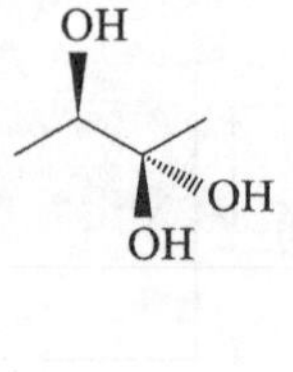

(d) 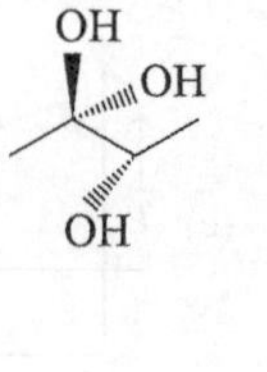

84. Suggest the suitable oxidising agent for the following conversions.

I. $CH_3CH_2CH{=}CHCH_2OH \longrightarrow CH_3CH_2CH{=}CHCHO$

II. 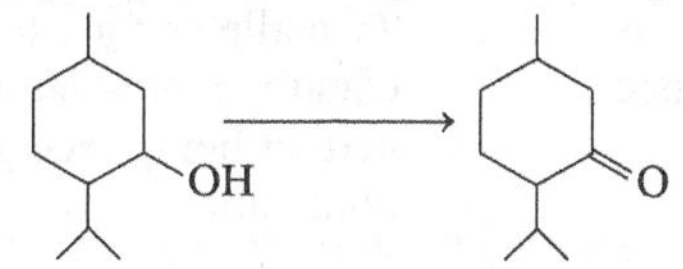

(a) MnO_2 in I and CrO_3 (in glacial acetic acid) in II
(b) CrO_3 in I and MnO_2 in II
(c) CrO_3 in both
(d) MnO_2 in both

85. 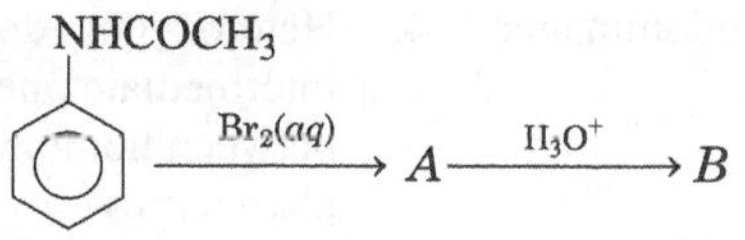

B may be
(a) *o*-bromoaniline
(b) *p*-bromoaniline
(c) mixture of (a) and (b)
(d) None of the above

86. Which of the following order is correct regarding the acidity of carboxylic group?
(a) $CH_3CH_2CH(Cl)COOH > CH_3CH(Cl)CH_2COOH > ClCH_2CH_2CH_2COOH$
(b) $CH_3CH_2CH(Cl)COOH < CH_3CH(Cl)CH_2COOH < ClCH_2CH_2CH_2COOH$
(c) $CH_3CH_2CH(Cl)COOH > CH_3CH(Cl)CH_2COOH < ClCH_2CH_2CH_2COOH$
(d) $CH_3CH_2CH(Cl)COOH < CH_3CH(Cl)CH_2COOH > ClCH_2CH_2CH_2COOH$

87. The radius of hydrogen atom in the ground state is 0.53 Å. The radius of Li^{2+} ion (atomic number = 3) in a similar state is
(a) 0.17 Å (b) 0.265 Å
(c) 0.53 Å (d) 1.06 Å

88. The half-life period of a first order chemical reaction is 6.93 minutes. The time required for the completion of 99% of chemical reaction will be ($\log 2 = 0.301$)
(a) 23.03 minutes (b) 46.06 minutes
(c) 460.6 minutes (d) 230.3 minutes

89. The solubility product of a salt having general formula MX_2 in water is 32×10^{-15}.
The concentration of M^{2+} ions in the aqueous solution of the salt is
(a) 2×10^{-5} M (b) 16×10^{-15} M
(c) 8×10^{-15} M (d) 0.8×10^{-6} M

90. 0.5 g of hydrocarbon gave 0.9 g water on combustion. The percentage of carbon in the hydrocarbon is
(a) 60.6 (b) 28.8 (c) 80.0 (d) 68.6

BIOLOGY

91. According to the operon concept, the regulatory gene regulates biochemical reaction in a cell by
(a) inhibiting transcription
(b) inactivating enzymes
(c) inactivating substrate
(d) inhibiting migration of *m*RNA

92. At certain region in bark, parenchymatous cells rupture the epidermis and form lens shaped openings which permit the
(a) transpiration (b) guttation
(c) gaseous exchange (d) photosynthesis

93. Given below are two statements.
Statement I Inability to conceive or produce children even after 2 years of unprotected sexual co-habitation is called infertility.
Statement II Female is responsible for the couple being childless.
In the light of the above statements, choose the most appropriate answer from the options given below.
(a) Statement I is incorrect, but statement II is correct
(b) Both statement I and statement II are correct
(c) Both statement I and statement II are incorrect
(d) Statement I is correct, but statement II is incorrect

94. Vasa efferentia is a male sex accessory duct that
(a) pulls down the testis during breeding season into the scrotal sac
(b) allows daily migration of the testis from the abdominal cavity into the scrotum
(c) facilitates ejaculation of spermatozoa from the testis
(d) opens into epididymis

95. Match List I with List II.

	List I		List II
A.	*Microsporum*	1.	Malaria
B.	*Wuchereria bancrofti*	2.	Amoebiasis
C.	*Trypanosoma gambiense*	3.	Ringworm
D.	*Entamoeba histolytica*	4.	Sleeping sickness
		5.	Filariasis

Choose the correct answer from the options given below.

	A	B	C	D
(a)	4	3	2	1
(b)	3	4	5	2
(c)	3	5	4	2
(d)	3	5	2	1

96. Gamosepalous calyx, imbricate aestivation and zygomorphic flowers are found in which of the following families of plants?

(a) Malvaceae
(b) Cruciferae
(c) Leguminosae
(d) Compositae

97. Inhibition of succinate dehydrogenase by malonate is an example of

(a) non-competitive inhibition
(b) competitive inhibition
(c) allosteric inhibition
(d) negative feedback

98. In a study on enzyme kinetics, a researcher introduces a molecule that closely resembles the enzyme's substrate and competes for the active site. This molecules is classified as which type of inhibitor?

(a) Non-competitive inhibitor
(b) Allosteric inhibitor
(c) Competitive inhibitor
(d) Irreversible inhibitor

99. ……… is a microbial product and is obtained by the bacterium *Acetobacter aceti*.

(a) Citric acid
(b) Vinegar
(c) Lactic acid
(d) Gluconic acid

100. Match List I with List II.

	List I		List II
A.	Incomplete dominance	1.	Two alleles for a trait are equally expressed with neither being recessive or dominant.
B.	Phenotype	2.	Expression of multiple traits by a single gene.
C.	Pleiotropy	3.	Physical characteristics of an individual
D.	Codominance	4.	Heterozygote displays intermediate phenotype between homozygous phenotypes

Choose the correct answer from the options given below.

	A	B	C	D
(a)	2	4	1	3
(b)	4	3	1	2
(c)	2	1	3	4
(d)	4	3	2	1

101. Which of the following steps of decomposition does not need action of microorganisms?

(a) fragmentation (b) humification
(c) mineralisation (d) leaching

102. Read the following statements.

I. Migration is the movement of individuals from a population to another population.
II. Emigration is the migration of individuals out of an area.
III. Immigration is the migration of individuals into an area.
IV. Gene flow cannot alter the genetic characteristics of populations.
V. Gene flow keeps separated populations genetically similar.

Choose the correct statements from the options given below.

(a) I, II, III and V (b) III and V
(c) I, II and IV (d) I, III and V

103. Biosphere reserves differ from national parks and wildlife sancturies because

(a) people are an integral part of the system
(b) human beings are not allowed to enter
(c) plants are paid greater attention than the animals
(d) living organisms are brought from all over the world and preserved for future

104. Given below are two statements; one is labelled as Assertion (A) and other is labelled as Reason (R).

Assertion (A) Most endonucleases optimally digest the target DNA at 37°C.

Reason (R) *Taq* I optimally digests the target DNA at temperature 65°C.

In the light of the above statements, choose the correct answer from the options given below.

(a) A is false, but R is true
(b) Both A and R are true and R is the correct explanation of A
(c) Both A and R are true, but R is not the correct explanation of A
(d) A is true, but R is false

105. Which of the following is not observed in telophase?

(a) Chromosome material condense to form compact mitotic chromosomes
(b) Nucleolus, Golgi complex and ER reform
(c) Nuclear envelop assembles around the chromosome clusters
(d) Chromosomes clusters at opposite spindle poles and their identity is lost as discrete elements

106. Which of the following statements is correct?

(a) The apical bud always suppresses the growth of axillary buds present beneath it, due to the presence of relatively higher quantities of auxin near the stem apex
(b) Gibberellins are strong acidic growth hormones having gibbane ring structure which cause cell elongation of intact plant
(c) The major sites of cytokinin production in plants are embryos, roots and young leaves near the shoot tip
(d) Some naturally occurring cytokinins are zeatin, ribosyl zeatin, etc. They are derivatives of pyrimidine-cytosine

107. The term used to refer the use of bioresources by multinational companies and other organisations without proper authorisation from the countries and people concerned without proper compensatory payment is known as

(a) biopatent
(b) biopiracy
(c) patent
(d) bioethics

108. Which of the following statements is incorrect with respect to 'human genome'?

(a) Human genome consist of 3×10^9 bp and about 30, 000 genes
(b) The average gene size is 3000 bp and dystrophin is the largest known human gene
(c) Chromosome 1 contains (2968) number of genes and Y-chromosome has 231 number of genes
(d) Repetitive sequences are not present

109. Match List I with List II.

	List I		List II
A.	Helper T-cell	1.	Cells that are active in production of antibodies.
B.	Plasma cells	2.	Activate B-lymphocytes to become plasma cells.
C.	Killer T-cell	3.	Protein produced by virus infected cell.
D.	Interferon	4.	Combine with antigen causing lysis

Choose the correct answer from the options given below.

	A	B	C	D
(a)	4	1	2	3
(b)	3	2	1	4
(c)	1	3	4	2
(d)	2	1	4	3

110. Krebs' cycle starts with the formation of a 6C atom compound by chemical reaction between

(a) succinic acid and acetyl Co-A
(b) fumaric acid and pyruvic acid
(c) oxaloacetic acid and acetyl Co-A
(d) malic acid and acetyl Co-A

111. Given below are two statements.

Statement I In directional selection more individuals acquire mean character value .

Statement II In disruption selection more individuals acquire peripheral character value at both ends of the distribution curve.

In the light of the above statements, choose the correct answer from the options given below.

(a) Statement I is incorrect, but statement II is correct
(b) Both statement I and statement II are correct
(c) Both statement I and statement II are incorrect
(d) Statement I is correct, but statement II is incorrect

112. The essential requirements for a gene amplification reaction are

I. 20 mg of DNA template
II. forward and reverse primer
III. *Taq* polymerase
IV. *cry* II Ab gene
V. Recombinant protein

Choose the correct option from the following.

(a) I and V (b) I, III and IV
(b) III and IV (d) I, II and III

113. Stratified squamous non-keratinised epithelium is present in the lining of

(a) buccal cavity, oesophagus, cornea of eye
(b) skin, hair, horn, nail
(c) small pancreatic ducts, thyroid follicles, ovary
(d) intestine, stomach, gall bladder

114. Given below are two statements.

Statement I The ATP molecules synthesised in the process of oxidative phosphorylation are utilised in dark reaction for CO_2 assimilation.
Statement II In oxidative phosphorylation, reduced NADH and $FADH_2$ are oxidised to form NAD^+ and FAD^+.

In the light of the above statements, choose the correct answer from the options given below.

(a) Statement I is incorrect, but statement II is correct
(b) Both statement I and statement II are correct
(c) Both statement I and statement II are incorrect
(d) Statement I is correct, but statement II is incorrect

115. Given below are the different geological periods. Arrange them in ascending order.

A. Permian - Extinction of *Pelycosaurs*
B. Tertiary - Extinction of dinosaurs
C. Triassic - Extinction of Therapsids
D. Jurassic - Age of dinosaurs

Choose the correct answer from the options given below.

(a) A, C, D, B (b) A, B, C, D
(c) B, A, C, D (d) D, A, B, C

116. At what stage of the cell cycle are histone proteins synthesised in a eukaryotic cell?

(a) During telophase
(b) During S-phase
(c) During G_2-stage of prophase
(d) During entire prophase

117. Match List I with List II.

	List I		List II
A.	Flying fox	1.	*Pterophyllum*
B.	Limbless amphibian	2.	*Exocoetus*
C.	Flying fish	3.	*Ichthyophis*
D.	Angel fish	4.	*Pteropus*

Choose the correct answer from the options given below.

	A	B	C	D		A	B	C	D
(a)	1	2	3	4	(b)	1	3	4	2
(c)	3	2	1	4	(d)	4	3	2	1

118. Read the following statements about the phytohormones and select the incorrect set of statements.

I. Auxin controls xylem differentiation and helps in cell division in plants.
II. Natural cytokinins are synthesised in regions where rapid cell division occurs.
III. Gibberellins promote nutrient mobilisation which helps in the delaying of leaf senescence.
IV. Ethephon is the most widely used compound as a source of cytokinins.
V. Application of minute quantity of ABA to the leaves can reduce transpiration.

Choose the correct answer from the options given below.

(a) I, III and V (b) III and IV
(c) III, IV and V (d) III and V

119. The technique in which a foreign DNA is coated on the surface of tungsten or gold particles and shot into the target cell is known as

(a) microinjection
(b) chemical-mediated genetic transformation
(c) electroporation
(d) biolistics

120. Match List I with List II.

	List I		List II
A.	Auxins	1.	Enhance respiration rate
B.	Gibberellins	2.	Antitranspirant
C.	Cytokinins	3.	Promote nutrient mobilisation
D.	Ethylene	4.	Increase yield in sugarcane
E.	Abscisic acid	5.	Initiates rooting in stem cuttings

Codes

	A	B	C	D	E
(a)	3	2	1	5	4
(b)	5	1	3	4	2
(c)	3	5	2	1	4
(d)	5	4	3	1	2

121. Identity the given tissue and its function from the options given below.

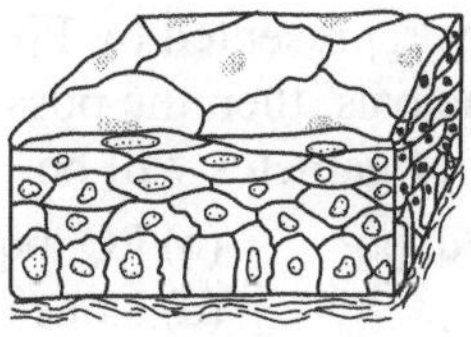

(a) Compound epithelium; provides protection against chemical and mechanical stresses
(b) Squamous epithelium; found in the walls of blood vessels
(c) Cuboidal epithelium; helps in secretion and absorption
(d) Column epithelium; found in the lining of stomac

122. A person is having problems with calcium and phosphorus metabolism in his body. Which one of the following glands may not be functioning properly?
(a) Parotid (b) Thyroid
(c) Pancreas (d) Parathyroid

123. Match List I with List II.

	List I		List II
A.	Formation of fruit without festilisation of ovary	1.	Apomixis
B.	The outermost proteinaceous layer of endosperm of maize grain.	2.	Anatropous ovule
C.	The body of the ovule is completely inverted	3.	Aleurone layer
D.	Production of seeds without fertilisation	4.	Parthenocarpic fruit

Choose the correct answer from the options given below.

	A	B	C	D		A	B	C	D
(a)	2	3	4	1	(b)	4	3	2	1
(c)	3	4	2	1	(d)	4	2	3	1

124. Given below are two statements; one is labelled as Assertion (A) and the other is labelled as Reason (R).

Assertion (A) In gymnosperms the male and female gametophytes do not have an independent free living existence.

Reason (R) They remain within the sporangia retained on the sporophytes.

In the light of the above statements, choose the correct answer from the options given below.
(a) A is false, but R is true
(b) Both A and R are true and R is the correct explanation of A
(c) Both A and R are true, but R is not the correct explanation of A
(d) A is true, but R is false

125. Polyembryo condition in citrus and mango varieties arises due to the
(a) synergids (b) nucellus cell
(c) antipodal cell (d) haploid egg

126. How *Ascidia* and *Pterophyllum* differs from *Echinus* and *Pila* ?
(a) Absence of post-anal tail
(b) Presence of ventral heart
(c) Presence of ventral central nervous system
(d) Absence of notochord

127. Which of the following statements is incorrect regarding the structure of proinsulin and mature insulin?
(a) C- polypeptide chain with 33 amino acids is removed prior to insulin formation
(b) Mature insulin is made up of 51 amino acids arranged in two polypeptide chains - A and B
(c) Pro-insulin and mature insulin are structurally similar
(d) Proinsulin is made up of three polypeptide chains

128. The lipids are arranged within the cell membrane with the polar head towards the outer sides and the hydrophobic tails towards the inner part, it ensures that the
(a) polar head of saturated hydrocarbons is protected from the aqueous environment.
(b) neutral molecules may move across the membrane
(c) non-polar tail of saturated hydrocarbons is protected from the aqueous environment.
(d) polar head of unsaturated hydrocarbons is protected from the aqueous environment

129. Consider the figure of a filamentous blue - green algae and identify the correct statement about part labelled as 'x'.

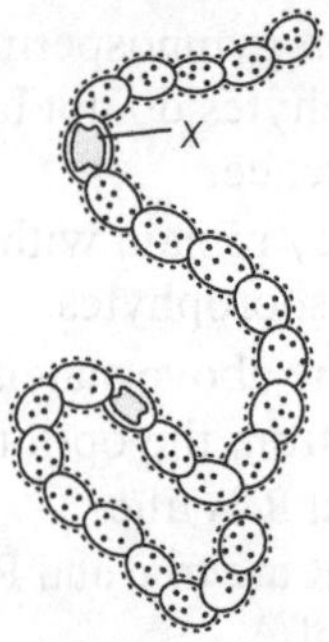

(a) Structure X is responsible for the sexual reproduction
(b) Structure X aids in fixing atmospheric nitrogen
(c) X is a specialised cell which is capable of recycling many nutrients
(d) X is harvested for the production of antibiotics

130. Given below are two statements; one is labelled as Assertion (A) and other is labelled as Reason (R).

Assertion (A) Axial skeleton comprises 80 bones distributed along the main axis of the body.

Reason (R) The skull, vertebral column, sternum and ribs constitute axial skeleton.

In the light of the above statements, choose the correct answer from the options given below.
(a) A is false, but R is true
(b) Both A and R are true and R is the correct explanation of A
(c) Both A and R are true, but R is not the correct explanation of A
(d) A is true, but R is false

131. Which one of the following palindromic bases sequences in DNA, can be easily cut at about the middle by some particular restriction enzymes?
(a) 5′ CACGTA 3′ and 3′ CTCAGT 5′
(b) 5′ CGTTCG 3′ and 3′ ATGGTA 5′
(c) 5′ GATATC 3′ and 3′ CTACTA 5′
(d) 5′ GAATTC 3′ and 3′ CTTAAG 5′

132. Given below are two statements.

Statement I The somatic neural system relays impulses from CNS to skeletal muscles.

Statement II The autonomic neural system transmits the impulse from involuntary organs to CNS.

In the light of the above statements, choose the correct answer from the options given below.
(a) Statement I is incorrect, but statement II is correct
(b) Both statement I and statement II are correct
(c) Both statement I and statement II are incorrect
(d) Statement I is correct, but statement II is incorrect

133. If a cell of an organism is heterozygous for two pairs of genes represented by Pp, Qq which undergoes meiosis, then the possible genotypic combination of gametes will be
(a) PQ, pQ, Pq, pq (b) PQ, pq
(c) Pp Qq (d) None of the above

134. Consider the following characteristics.
I. Twisted aestivation
II. Polypetalous cruciform
III. Actinomorphic
IV. Polyandrous tetradynamous dithecous
V. Axile placentation

Which of the following characters belongs to family-Cruciferae?
(a) I and V
(b) II, III and IV
(c) II, III and V
(d) I, II and III

135. Competition for food, light and space is most severe in
(a) closely related species growing in different habitat
(b) closely related species growing in the same area
(c) distantly related species growing in the different habitat
(d) distantly related species growing in the same

136. Given below are two statements.

Statement I Hardy-Weinberg equilibrium is not applicable for large population size.

Statement II Random mating is one of the necessary aspect for Hardy-Weinberg equilibrium.

In the light of above statements, choose the correct answer from the options given below.
(a) Statement I is incorrect, but statement II is correct
(b) Both statement I and statement II are correct
(c) Both statement I and statement II are incorrect
(d) Statement I is correct, but statement II is incorrect

137. Arrange the following skeletal bone according to the number of bones found in them, in increasing order.
Coxal bone, Cranial bone, Ribs, Facial bones
(a) Coxal bone, Cranial bone, Facial bones, Ribs
(b) Cranral bone, Coxal bone, Ribs, Facial bones
(c) Faceal bons, Cranial bone, Ribs, Coxal bone
(d) Coxal bone, Facial bones, Ribs, Cranial bone

138. Complete alimentary canal with a well developed muscular pharynx is observed in
(a) *Obelia* (b) *Ctenoplana*
(c) *Ascaris* (d) *Taenia*

139. Given below are two statements.
Statement I In meiosis, the daughter cells differ from parent cell as well as amongst themselves due to independent assortment and crossing over.
Statement II During complete meiosis DNA replication takes place once while cell division occurs twice.
In the light of the above statements, choose the correct answer from the options given below.
(a) Statement I is incorrect, but statement II is correct
(b) Both statement I and statement II are correct
(c) Both statement I and statement II are incorrect
(d) Statement I is correct, but statement II is incorrect

140. Match List I with List II.

	List I		List II
A.	C_4 plants	1.	Accessory photosynthetic pigment
B.	Chlorophyll-*b*	2.	Kranz anatomy
C.	PS-II	3.	Succulents
D.	CAM	4.	Photo-oxidation of H_2O

Choose the correct answer from the options given below.

	A	B	C	D		A	B	C	D
(a)	2	1	3	4	(b)	3	1	2	4
(c)	2	1	4	3	(d)	4	1	2	3

141. Select the incorrect match from the following.
(a) Terpenoids - Monoterpenes
(b) Lectins - Concanavalin-A
(c) Toxins - Anthocyanins
(d) Drugs - Vinblastin

142. Match the items given in List I with those in List II and choose the correct option.

List I	List II
A. Squamous epithelium	1. Pharynx and buccal cavity
B. Ciliated epithelium	2. PCT and intestine
C. Brush border epithelium	3. Endothelium and lung alveoli
D. Compound epithelium	4. Bronchi and Fallopian tube

Codes

	A	B	C	D		A	B	C	D
(a)	1	2	3	4	(b)	4	3	2	1
(c)	3	4	2	1	(d)	4	2	1	3

143. Cystic fibrosis is an autosomal recessive genetic disorder, what are the chances that the child would have the disease if any one of the parent is a carrier of the faulty cystic fibrosis gene?
(a) 100 per cent (b) 50 per cent
(c) 25 per cent (d) 0 per cent

144. Which of the following is true for endoplasmic reticulum?
I. It provides additional mechanical support to the cell by dividing the fluid content of the cell into compartment.
II. It is involved in secretion, storage and packaging of materials.
III. It is found to be greatly involved in glycoprotein and glycolipid metabolism.
IV. It is rich in almost all types of hydrolytic enzymes.
V. A modified form of SER is sarcoplasmic reticulum.
Choose the most appropriate answer from the options given below.
(a) I, II and IV (b) II, III and IV
(c) I and V (d) II, IV and V

145. Identify the incorrect set of statements.
I. In a dicot root, the vascular bundles are collateral and endarch.
II. The inner most layer of cortex in a dicot root is endodermis.
III. In a dicot root, the phloem masses are separated from the xylem by parenchymatous cells that are known as the conjunctive tissue.

IV. All tissues on the innerside of the endodermis such as phloem, xylem and pith constitute the pericycle.
V. Epiblema protrude in the form of unicellular root hairs.

Choose the correct answer from the options given below.

(a) II, III and V (b) I, II and IV
(c) III and IV (d) I and IV

146. Select the incorrectly matched pair.
(a) Mitosis - Cell repair
(b) Reductional division - Meiosis-I
(c) Equational division - Meiosis-II
(d) Crossing over - Non- homologous chromosome

147. Given below are two statements.
Statement I The majority of the members of Rhodophyceae are marine with greater concentrations found in warmer areas.
Statement II Members of Rhodophyceae occur only in well lighted regions close to the surface of water.
In the light of the above statements, choose the correct answer from the options given below.
(a) Statement I is incorrect, but statement II is correct
(b) Both statement I and statement II are correct
(c) Both statement I and statement II are incorrect
(d) Statement I is correct, but statement II is incorrect

148. Which part of nephron is involved in active reabsorption of sodium?
(a) Ascending limb of Henle's loop
(b) Descending limb of Henle's loop
(c) Collecting duct
(d) Proximal convoluted tubule

149. If you remove fimbriae from the bacterial cell, which of the following would you expect to happen?
(a) The bacteria could not longer swim
(b) Bacteria would not adhere to the host tissue
(c) Transportation of molecules across the membrane would stop
(d) The shape of bacteria would change

150. Who observed that the behaviours of chromosome at meiosis can serve as the cellular basis of both segregation and independent assortment ?
(a) Sutton and Boveri (b) Banden and Boveri
(c) W Flemming (d) Boveri and Braun

151. Read the following statements about the productivity.
I. Net primary productivity is the amount of biomass available for consumption of carnivores.
II. Secondary productivity is defined as the rate of energy storage at consumers level.
III. Primary productivity depends on the plants species inhabiting a particular area.
IV. The monthly net primary productivity of the whole biosphere is approximately 170 billion tons of organic matter.
V. Secondary productivity is equal to NPP minus the rate of respiration and other losses.

Choose the correct statements from the options given below.
(a) I, III and V (b) II and III
(c) I, IV and V (d) II and IV

152. In a garden, there are 4000 ants living in an ant hole. In a month there are 200 births and 100 ants died. What should be the growth rate of population of ants in that month?
(a) 100 ants/month
(b) 200 ants/month
(c) 300 ants/month
(d) 250 ants/month

153. Some features of frog are given below. Read them carefully and choose the feature which is incorrectly described.
(a) Parathyroid and pineal body are present
(b) There are ten cranial nerves only
(c) Optic lobes are situated in the midbrain
(d) The ventricle opens into the conus arteriosus

154. The disease causing chronic inflammation of the lower limbs and resulting in gross deformities is caused by
(a) *Ascaris lumbricoides*
(b) *Wuchereria bancrofti*
(c) *Ancylostoma duodenale*
(d) *Dracunculus medinensis*

155. Read the following statements on tobacco and find out the correct set of statements.
I. Tobacco contains nicotine which stimulates pituitary gland, resulting in high blood pressure and increased heart rate.
II. It is also used as a snuff.
III. Tobacco smoking increases the carbon dioxide content in the blood.

IV. Smoking also causes oxygen deficiency in the body by reducing the concentration of haem bound oxygen.
V. Tobacco chewing is associated with increased risk of lung cancer.

Choose the correct answer from the options given below.

(a) I, III and IV (b) III and V
(c) II and IV (d) II, IV and V

156. A gene locus has two alleles A and a. If the frequency of dominant allele A is 0.7, then what will be the frequency of homozygous dominant, heterozygous and homozygous recessive individuals in the population?

(a) 0.49 (AA); 0.21 (Aa); 0.09 (aa)
(b) 0.49 (AA); 0.42 (Aa); 0.09 (aa)
(c) 0.36 (AA); 0.48 (Aa); 0.16 (aa)
(d) 0.16 (AA); 0.36 (Aa); 0.48 (aa)

157. A flower having polypetalous, cruciform corolla, valvate aestivation, basifixed polyandrous stamens and superior ovary is found in

(a) mustard (b) cotton
(c) *Sesbania* (d) China rose

158. Which of the following is incorrectly matched ?

(a) Sap wood - Peripheral region of secondary xylem
(b) Bark - All tissues exterior to the vascular cambium
(c) Lenticels - Permit the exchange of gases
(d) Stele - All tissues on the outer side of the endodermis in dicot root

159. Read the following statements.

I. Cerebellum has very convoluted surface in order to provide space for more neurons.
II. The medulla is connected to the spinal cord.
III. Medulla contains controlling centers for respiration, cardiovascular reflexes and gastric secretion.
IV. Cerebral aqueduct forms the connections between the brain and spinal cord.
V. The two hemispheres of brain are connected by basal ganglia.

Choose the correct answer from the options given below.

(a) I, II and III (b) III, IV and V
(c) II and III (d) I, IV and V

160. The sequential event in the heart which is cyclically repeated is called the cardiac cycle and it consists of

(a) systole of both the atria and ventricles
(b) systole and diastole of both the atria and ventricles
(c) diastole of venticles only
(d) diastole of both the atria and ventricles

161. Read the following statements about chromosomal mapping and find out the incorrect set of statements.

I. Crossing-over is important in locating genes on chromosomes.
II. Recombination frequency depends on the distance between the genes.
III. Recombination frequency is inversely proportional to the distance between the genes.
IV. The sequences and the relative distance between various genes are graphically represented in terms of recombination frequencies.
V. First chromosomal map was given by Bateson and Morgan.

Choose the correct answer from the options given below.

(a) I, II and IV
(b) II, III and IV
(c) III and V
(d) III, IV and V

162. Which of the following is incorrect for hormonal contraceptive pills?

(a) They inhibits ovulation
(b) Alternation in uterine endometrium
(c) Change in cervical mucus, impairing its ability to allow the passage and transport of sperm
(d) Induction of implantation in Fallopian tube

163. Phellogen is made of narrow, thin walled and nearly rectangular cells which cuts off cells on both sides. In which

(a) outer cells differentiate into phelloderm and inner cells differentiate into phellem
(b) outer cells differentiate into secondary cortex and inner cells differentiate into cork
(c) outer cells differentiate into cork and inner cells differentiate into cortex
(d) outer cells differentiate into periderm and inner cells differentiate into sapwood

164. Match List I with List II.

	List I		List II
A.	14th day	1.	Formation of corpus luteum
B.	1st - 4th day	2.	Development of Graafian follicle
C.	15th - 28 th day	3.	Shedding of endometrial lining
D.	5th - 13th day	4.	Release of secondary oocyte

Choose the correct answer from the options givens below.

	A	B	C	D
(a)	1	2	3	4
(b)	4	3	1	2
(c)	2	1	4	3
(d)	1	2	4	3

165. Which of the following is incorrectly matched pair of taxonomic categories of wheat?

(a) Family - Poaceae
(b) Genus - *Triticum*
(c) Class - Monocotyledonae
(d) Order - Sapindales

166. At which stage the homologous chromosomes separate due to repulsion, but are yet held by chiasmata?

(a) Zygotene (b) Pachytene
(c) Diplotene (d) Diakinesis

167. Identify the correct set of statements. about the discovery of Stanley Cohen and Herbert Boyer.

I. They discovered recombinant DNA (*r*DNA) technology and this marks the birth of modern biotechnology.
II. The first instance of the construction of an artificial *r*DNA molecule was accomplished in 1982.
III. They isolated the antibiotic resistance gene by cutting out a piece of DNA from the plasmid which was responsible for conferring antibiotic resistance.
IV. They invented genetic engineering by combining a piece of foreign DNA containing a gene from a bacterium with a bacterium plasmid using the enzyme restriction endonuclease.
V. They used the plasmid of *Salmonella typhimurium*.

Choose the correct answer from the options given below.

(a) II, III and IV
(b) IV and V
(c) I, III, IV and V
(d) I, II, III, IV and V

168. Given below are two statements; one is labelled as Assertion (A) and other is labelled as Reason (R).

Assertion (A) Photosynthetically, C_4 plants are less efficient than C_3 plants.
Reason (R) The operation of C_4 pathway requires involvement of mesophyll and bundle sheath cells.

In the light of the above statements, choose the correct answer from the options given below.

(a) A is false, but R is true
(b) Both A and R are true and R is the correct explanation of A
(c) Both A and R are true, but R is not the correct explanation of A
(d) A is true, but R is false

169. The function of intracellular membrane is not to

(a) establish a number of compartments within the cell
(b) provides for the neat spatial organisation of enzymes and pigments
(c) keep the cell rigidity, so that it does not collapse
(d) provide a system of channel for the distribution of nutrients within the cell

170. Match List I with List II.

	List I		List II
A.	TCA cycle	1.	Inner mitochondrial membrane
B.	$F_0 - F_1$ particles	2.	Hans Krebs
C.	End product of glycolysis	3.	Oxidative decarboxylation
D.	Pyruvate dehydrogenase	4.	Pyruvic acid

Codes

	A	B	C	D
(a)	2	1	4	3
(b)	1	2	4	3
(c)	2	3	4	1
(d)	3	2	1	4

171. Given below are two statements.

Statement I All test cross are back cross.

Statement II In back cross, an individual is crossed with recessive parent.

In the light of the above statements, choose the correct answer from the options given below.

(a) Statement I is incorrect, but statement II is correct
(b) Both statement I and statement II are correct
(c) Both statement I and statement II are incorrect
(d) Statement I is correct, but statement II is incorrect

172. Which one of the following statements is not true regarding the secondary growth in the plants?

(a) Fusiform initials and ray initials are the constituents of cambium
(b) Amount of secondary xylem is more than secondary phloem because cambium is more active on the outer side
(c) The inner, darker and harder portion of secondary xylem that cannot conduct water in older dicot stem is called duramen
(d) Interfascicular cambium is found between two vascular bundles

173. Identify a characteristic that is not desirable in a cloning vector.

(a) Presence of two or more recognition sites
(b) An origin of replication site
(c) Selectable markers such as genes for antibiotic resistance
(d) One or more unique restriction endonuclease sites

174. Given below are two statements; one is labelled as Assertion (A) and the other is labelled as Reason (R).

Assertion (A) The longer polypeptide chains, which coiled to form specific structure are called secondary structure of proteins.

Reason (R) These structures of proteins are produced and maintained by disulphide bonds.

In the light of above statement, choose the correct answer from the option given below.

(a) A is false, but R is true
(b) Both A and R are true and R is the correct explanation of A
(c) Both A and R are true, but R is not the correct explanation of A
(d) A is true, but R is false

175. Approximately how many restriction enzymes have been isolated from the different strains of bacteria?

(a) 300 (b) 600 (c) 750 (d) 900

176. Given below are two statements.

Statement I About 97% of O_2 is transported by RBC in the blood.

Statement II Carbon dioxide cannot be transported by haemoglobin.

In the light of the above statements, choose the correct answer from the options given below.

(a) Statement I is incorrect, but statement II is correct
(b) Both statement I and statement II are correct
(c) Both statement I and statement II are incorrect
(d) Statement I is correct, but statement II is incorrect

177. Which of the following statements is incorrect for echinoderms?

(a) The most distinctive feature of echinoderms is the presence of water vascular system, which is a part of the coelom
(b) The main function of water vascular system is locomotion and the capture of food
(c) Echinoderms have no proper excretory system
(d) They have well-developed circulatory system

178. Which of the following is true for hormones released by temporary endocrine gland in ovary of a female?

(a) The first hormone to peak during luteal phase is progesterone
(b) The second hormone to peak during luteal phase is essential for maintenance of endometrium during pregnancy
(c) The hormones released by this temporary endocrine gland exerts positive feedback on hypothalamus
(d) These hormones appear in urine in menopausal phase

179. Read the following statements with respect to immunity.

I. The antibodies against smallpox pathogen are produced by B-lymphocytes.

II. Antibodies are proteins molecules, each of which has four light chains.

III. Preformed antibodies need to be injected to treat the bite by a viper snake.

IV. Rejection of a kidney graft is the function of T-lymphocytes.

V. The primary and secondary immune responses are carried out with the help of only B-lymphocytes.

Choose the incorrect statements from the options given below.

(a) I, II, III, IV and V (b) I, II, III and V
(c) II, III and IV (d) II and V

180. Gamete Intra Fallopian Transfer (GIFT) refers to

(a) Transfer of sperms of a healthy donor to a test tube containing ova.
(b) Transfer of an ovum from a donor to another female who cannot produce the ovum.
(c) Transfer of zygote upto 8 blastomeres into the Fallopian tube
(d) Transfer of sperms of a healthy person directly into the Fallopian tube

Explanations

Physics

1. (b) Force acting on mass M_1, $F_1 = M_1 a$.
Mass M_1 will pull mass M_2 towards left with a force f.
Net force acting on mass M_2, $F_2 = F - F_1$

$$= F - M_1 a$$

Acceleration of mass M_2, $a_2 = \frac{F - M_1 a}{M_2}$

2. (d) Moment of inertia of rod about one end is $I_1 = \frac{1}{3} ML^2$

Moment of inertia of this rod, when bent into a ring,

$$I_2 = \frac{MR^2}{2}$$

As, $R = \frac{L}{2\pi}$

$\therefore$ $I_2 = \frac{ML^2}{8\pi^2}$

Then, $\frac{I_1}{I_2} = \frac{(1/3) ML^2}{ML^2 / 8\pi^2} = \frac{8\pi^2}{3}$

3. (b) As, $y = A \sin \omega t = A \sin \frac{2\pi}{T} t$

$$0.08\sqrt{2} = A \sin \frac{2\pi}{2\pi} \times \frac{\pi}{4} = A \sin \frac{\pi}{4}$$

$\Rightarrow$ $A = 0.08 \times 2 = 0.16\,\text{m}$

Total energy $= \frac{1}{2} m\omega^2 A^2 = \frac{1}{2} m \left(\frac{2\pi}{T}\right)^2 A^2$

$$10.24 \times 10^{-3} = \frac{1}{2} \times m \times \left(\frac{2\pi}{2\pi}\right)^2 \times (0.16)^2$$

$\Rightarrow$ $m = \frac{10.24 \times 10^{-3} \times 2}{(0.16)^2} = 0.8\,\text{kg}$

4. (a) Relative density of solid

$$= \frac{\text{Weight in air}}{\text{Weight in air} - \text{Weight in water}}$$

$$= \frac{150}{150 - 120} = \frac{150}{30} = 5$$

Relative density of liquid

$$= \frac{\text{Weight in air} - \text{Weight in liquid}}{\text{Weight in air} - \text{Weight in water}}$$

$$= \frac{150 - 90}{150 - 120} = \frac{60}{30} = 2$$

5. (*d*) Let, x be the distance from 500 kg mass, then

$$\frac{G \times 500}{x^2} = \frac{G \times 2000}{(2-x)^2}$$

$\Rightarrow$ $(2-x)^2 = 4 \times x^2 \Rightarrow 2 - x = 2x$

$\Rightarrow$ $x = \frac{2}{3}$ m from 500 kg

6. (b) Let H be the distance covered vertically,

$\therefore$ $H = \frac{u^2}{2g} = \frac{1600}{2 \times 10} = 80\,\text{m}$

Now, the time taken by body to reach H distance,

$$t = \sqrt{\frac{2H}{g}} = 4\,\text{s}$$

$\because$ $s = ut + \frac{1}{2} gt^2$

$$H - d = (40)(t-1) - \frac{1}{2} g(t-1)^2$$

where, d = distance travelled in last second.

$$80 - d = 40(4-1) - \frac{1}{2} \times 10(4-1)^2$$

$$80 - d = 120 - 45$$

$$d = 5\,\text{m}$$

7. (*a*) Angular width, $\omega = 2\theta$

$$\omega = 2\frac{\lambda}{d}$$

$$\lambda = \frac{\omega d}{2}$$

$$\frac{\lambda_1}{\lambda_2} = \frac{\omega_1}{\omega_2} = \frac{\omega_1}{1.4\,\omega_1} \quad [\because \omega_2 = 1.4\omega_1]$$

$$\frac{\lambda_1}{\lambda_2} = \frac{1}{1.4}$$

$$\lambda_2 = 1.4\lambda_1 = 1.4 \times 4200 = 5880\,\text{Å}$$

8. (d) Work done in changing the orientation of a dipole of moment M in a magnetic field B from position θ_1 to θ_2 is given by

$$W = MB(\cos\theta_1 - \cos\theta_2)$$

$$(\because \theta_1 = 0° \text{ and } \theta_2 = 180°)$$

$$W = 2MB = 2 \times 2.5 \times 0.2 = 1\,\text{J}$$

9. (a) Since, the proton is moving against the direction of electric field, so work is done by the proton against electric field and hence, work done by the field is negative.
As, proton is moving in electric field from low potential region to high potential region. Hence, its potential energy increases.

10. (b) We know that, $B = \dfrac{p}{\Delta V / V}$

So, $\dfrac{\Delta V}{V} = \dfrac{p}{B} = \dfrac{\rho \times g \times h}{B}$

$$\frac{\Delta V}{V} \times 100 = \frac{1000 \times 10 \times 4000}{2.2 \times 10^9} \times 100$$

$$= 1.81\%$$

11. (b) We know, $\dfrac{pV}{T} =$ constant

AB = Isochoric process,
BC = Isobaric process and
CA = Isothermal process

So, option (b) is correct.

12. (b) $\dfrac{P}{Q} = \dfrac{20}{80} = \dfrac{1}{4}$ ... (i)

$$\frac{P + 15}{Q} = \frac{40}{60} = \frac{2}{3} \quad \text{...(ii)}$$

Dividing Eq. (i) by Eq. (ii), we get

$$\therefore \quad \frac{P}{P+15} = \frac{1/4}{2/3} = \frac{3}{8}$$

$$\Rightarrow \quad 8P = 3P + 45$$

$$\Rightarrow \quad 5P = 45$$

$$\Rightarrow \quad P = 9\Omega$$

13. (d) We know that,

$$n_1 u_1 = n_2 u_2$$

$$\Rightarrow \quad n_2 = n_1 \left[\frac{u_1}{u_2}\right]$$

$$= 0.625 \left[\frac{M_1}{M_2}\right]\left[\frac{L_1}{L_2}\right]^{-3}$$

$$= 0.625 \left[\frac{\text{g}}{\text{kg}}\right]\left[\frac{\text{m}}{\text{cm}}\right]^3$$

$$= 0.625 \left[\frac{\text{g}}{1000\text{g}}\right]\left[\frac{100\text{cm}}{\text{cm}}\right]^3$$

$$= 0.625 \left[\frac{1}{1000}\right][100]^3 = 625$$

14. (a) Let, two stones meet at time t.

The distance travelled by 1st stone,

$$s_1 = \frac{1}{2} g t^2 \quad [\because u = 0]$$

The distance travelled by 2nd stone,

$$s_2 = 8(t-3) + \frac{1}{2} g (t-3)^2$$

$$= 8t - 24 + \frac{1}{2} g t^2 + \frac{9}{2} g - 3gt$$

At time t, $s_1 = s_2$

$$\Rightarrow \frac{1}{2} g t^2 = 8t - 24 + \frac{1}{2} g t^2 + \frac{9}{2} g - 3gt$$

$$\Rightarrow \quad t = \frac{24 - \frac{9}{2} g}{8 - 3g}$$

Thus, distance after which second stone overtakes,

$$s_1 = \frac{g}{2}\left[\frac{\left(24 - \frac{9}{2} g\right)}{(8 - 3g)}\right]^2.$$

15. (c) Critical angle,

$$i_c = \sin^{-1}\left(\frac{\mu_w}{\mu_g}\right) = \sin^{-1}\left(\frac{\frac{4}{3}}{\frac{5}{3}}\right) = \sin^{-1}\left(\frac{4}{5}\right)$$

16. (b) We know that,

$$n_2 = n_1 \left[\frac{L_2}{L_1}\right]^a \left[\frac{M_2}{M_1}\right]^b \left[\frac{T_2}{T_1}\right]^c$$

But, surface tension = $[MT^{-2}]$

$$n_2 = n_1 \left[\frac{M_2}{M_1}\right]^1 \left[\frac{T_2}{T_1}\right]^{-2}$$

Here, $n_1 = 7.2 \times 10^{-3}$

$$\therefore \quad n_2 = 7.2 \times 10^{-3} \left[\frac{\text{kg}}{\text{g}}\right]\left[\frac{\text{s}}{\text{s}}\right]^{-2}$$

$$= 7.2 \times 10^{-3} \left[\frac{1000\text{g}}{\text{g}}\right]$$

$$= 7.2 \times 10^{-3} \times 10^3$$

$$= 7.2 \text{ dyne cm}^{-1}$$

17. (b) Given, $V_L = V_C = 300\text{ V}$

Given, L-C-R circuit in resonance

$$V = \sqrt{V_R^2 + (V_L - V_C)^2}$$

$$\therefore \quad V_R = V = 220\text{ V}$$

And circuit will be purely resistive, $Z = R = 100\ \Omega$

Current, $i = \dfrac{V}{Z} = \dfrac{220}{100} = 2.2\text{ A}$

18. (b) As two resistances are in parallel combination, so the effective resistance,

$$R' = \frac{10 \times 10}{10 + 10} = 5\ \Omega$$

Heat produced for 5 min $= \dfrac{V^2}{R'} \times t$

$$= \frac{1^2}{5} \times 5 \times 60\text{ J} = \frac{60}{4.2}\text{ cal} = 14.3\text{ cal}$$

19. (d) Resultant force on electric dipole can be equal to zero as **E** || **p**.

20. (b) Energy of incident light,

$$h\nu = \frac{hc}{\lambda} = \frac{6.6\times10^{-34}\times3\times10^{8}}{6\times10^{-7}\times1.6\times10^{-19}} = 2.06\,\text{eV}$$

2.06 is greater than the band gap of photodiode D_2.

21. (b) When the magnetic flux linked with coil varies continuously, the emf is induced across the coil and if circuit is closed, then induced current starts flowing. Thus, if coil is cut, then emf is produced but no current will flow. Electromagnetic induction is a source of emf which is based upon the law of conservation of energy in which mechanical energy is converted into electrical energy.

22. (c) Given, 1MSD = x cm

$$n\,\text{VSD} = (n-1)\,\text{MSD}$$

$$\therefore \quad 1\text{VSD} = \left(\frac{n-1}{n}\right)\text{MSD}$$

$\therefore$ Least count, LC = 1MSD − 1VSD

$$= \left(1-\frac{n-1}{n}\right)\text{MSD} = \frac{1}{n}\times x\,\text{cm}$$

$$= \frac{10x}{n}\,\text{mm}$$

23. (d) We know that, f_0 = resonance frequency

$$= \frac{1}{2\pi}\times\frac{1}{\sqrt{LC}}$$

$$\Rightarrow \quad f_0 \propto \frac{1}{\sqrt{C}}$$

When capacitance of the circuit is made 4 times, let new resonance frequency is f_0'.

$$\Rightarrow \quad \frac{f_0'}{f_0} = \frac{\sqrt{C}}{\sqrt{4C}} = \frac{1}{2}$$

$$\Rightarrow \quad f_0' = \frac{f_0}{2}$$

24. (b)

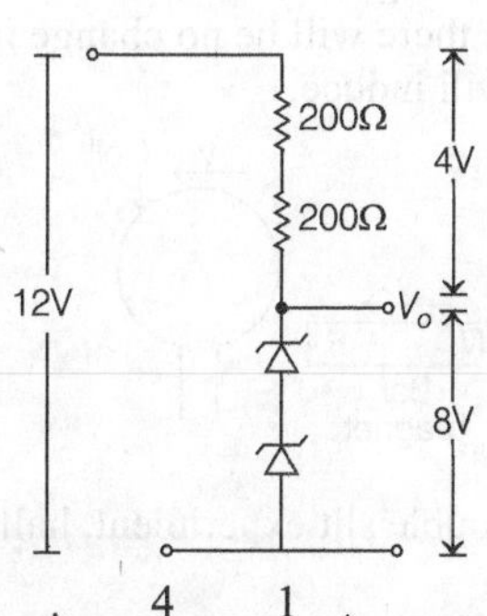

$$\text{Current in circuit} = \frac{4}{400} = \frac{1}{100}\,\text{A}$$

So, power dissipated in each diode = VI

$$= \left(4\times\frac{1}{100}\right)\text{W} = 40\times10^{-3}\,\text{W}$$

$$= 40\,\text{mW}$$

25. (b) $\Delta W = nR\Delta T$ $\quad [\because p\,\Delta V = nR\,\Delta T]$

$$= 3\times8.3\times(177-27) = 3735\,\text{J}$$

26. (b) Current, $i = \dfrac{q}{t} = \dfrac{2\times1.6\times10^{-19}}{2} = 1.6\times10^{-19}\,\text{A}$

$$\therefore \text{Magnetic field, } B = \frac{\mu_0 i}{2r} = \frac{\mu_0\times1.6\times10^{-19}}{2\times0.8}$$

$$= 10^{-19}\mu_0$$

27. (d) Given, $v = 20\sqrt{2}$ m/s

Resolving the component of velocity into horizontal and vertical.

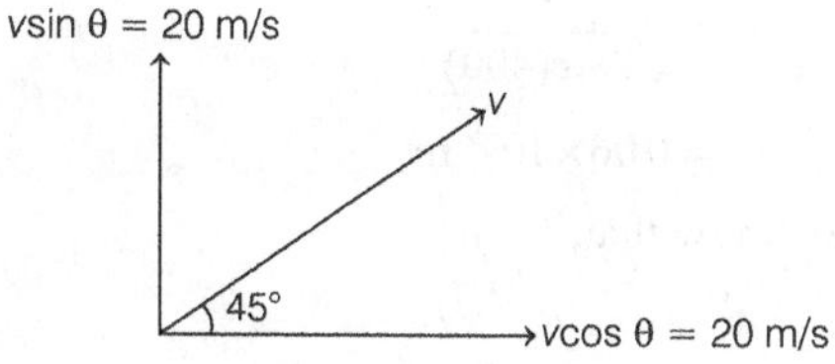

At maximum height, $v_x = 20\,\text{m/s}$

$$H_{\max} = \frac{v^2\sin2\theta}{2g} = \frac{(20)^2\times\sin90^\circ}{2\times10} = 20\,\text{m}$$

$\therefore$ Angular velocity, $\omega = v/H_{\max} = 20/20 = 1\,\text{rad/s}$

28. (*d*) Lines of Lyman series are emitted by the hydrogen atom when the electron jumps from higher orbit to first orbit, hence Statement I is incorrect. In the hydrogen atom spectrum, the Lyman series lies in ultraviolet region, hence Statement II is correct..

29. (c) According to the question and by using conservation of mechanical energy,

$$-\frac{GMm}{R+R} + \frac{1}{2}m(fv)^2 = 0$$

$$\Rightarrow \quad fv = \sqrt{\frac{GM}{R}} \text{ but } v = \sqrt{\frac{2GM}{R}}$$

$$\text{Therefore, } f\sqrt{\frac{2GM}{R}} = \sqrt{\frac{GM}{R}} \Rightarrow f = \frac{1}{\sqrt{2}}$$

30. (d) Applying Kirchhoff's voltage law in the given loop.

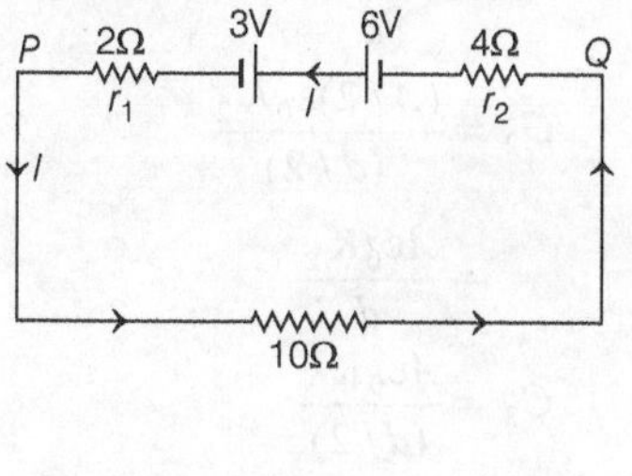

$$-4I + 6 - 3 - 2I - 10I = 0$$
$$-16I = -3$$
$$I = \frac{3}{16}\,\text{A}$$

$\because$ Potential difference across $PQ = \frac{3}{16} \times 10 = \frac{15}{8}$ V

31. (b) Here, potential difference = 400 V

$$\therefore \quad \frac{1}{2}mv^2 = e(400)$$
$$v = \sqrt{\frac{2e(400)}{m}}$$

Now, de-Broglie's wavelength,

$$\lambda = \frac{h}{mv} \Rightarrow \lambda = \frac{h}{m\sqrt{\frac{2e(400)}{m}}}$$
$$= \frac{h}{\sqrt{2me(400)}}$$
$$= 0.06 \times 10^{-9}\ \text{m}$$

32. (d) We know that, $I \propto a^2$

$$a \propto \sqrt{I}$$
$$\frac{I_1}{I_2} = \beta = \frac{a_1^2}{a_2^2}$$
$$\frac{I_{max}}{I_{min}} = \frac{(a_1 + a_2)^2}{(a_1 - a_2)^2} = \frac{(\sqrt{\beta}+1)^2}{(\sqrt{\beta}-1)^2}$$
$$\Rightarrow \quad \frac{I_{max} + I_{min}}{I_{max} - I_{min}} = \frac{(\sqrt{\beta}+1)^2 + (\sqrt{\beta}-1)^2}{(\sqrt{\beta}+1)^2 - (\sqrt{\beta}-1)^2}$$
$$= \frac{2(1+\beta)}{4\sqrt{\beta}}$$
$$\Rightarrow \quad \frac{I_{max} - I_{min}}{I_{max} + I_{min}} = \frac{2\sqrt{\beta}}{1+\beta}$$

33. (b) As we know, from the formula,

$$C = \frac{\varepsilon_0 AK}{d}$$

We have,
$$C_1 = \frac{(A/2)\varepsilon_0 K_1}{(d/2)}$$
$$= \frac{A\varepsilon_0 K_1}{d} \quad \ldots(\text{i})$$
$$C_2 = \frac{(A/2)\varepsilon_0 K_2}{(d/2)}$$
$$= \frac{A\varepsilon_0 K_2}{d} \quad \ldots(\text{ii})$$

and
$$C_3 = \frac{A\varepsilon_0 K_3}{(d/2)}$$
$$= \frac{2A\varepsilon_0 K_3}{d} \quad \ldots(\text{iii})$$

Two capacitors C_1 and C_2 are in parallel and their equivalent capacitance is,

$$C' = C_1 + C_2 = \frac{A\varepsilon_0}{d}(K_1 + K_2)$$

This combination is in series with capacitance C_3. Hence, the equivalent capacitance,

$$\frac{1}{C''} = \frac{1}{C'} + \frac{1}{C_3} = \frac{d}{A\varepsilon_0 (K_1 + K_2)} + \frac{d}{2A\varepsilon_0 K_3}$$
$$= \frac{d}{\varepsilon_0 A}\left[\frac{1}{K_1 + K_2} + \frac{1}{2K_3}\right]$$
$$C'' = \frac{A\varepsilon_0 K}{d}$$
$$\Rightarrow \quad \frac{1}{C''} = \frac{d}{A\varepsilon_0 K}$$
$$\therefore \quad \frac{1}{K} = \frac{1}{K_1 + K_2} + \frac{1}{2K_3}$$

34. (d) The value of resultant electric field at $y = 0$

$$E = \frac{q}{4\pi\varepsilon_0}\left[\frac{1}{2^2} + \frac{1}{4^2} + \frac{1}{8^2} + \ldots\infty\right]$$
$$= 6 \times 10^{-6} \times 9 \times 10^9 \left[\frac{\frac{1}{4}}{1 - \frac{1}{4}}\right]$$
$$= 54 \times 10^3 \times \frac{1}{3} = 1.8 \times 10^4\ \text{N/C}$$

35. (c) A. EM waves do not require a material medium for propagation.

D. EM waves of different radiations travel with the different speed in a medium and with the same speed in vacuum.

Statement B and statement C are correct.
Hence, option (c) is correct answer.

36. (c) When coil and magnet both move in same direction with same velocity, so there will be no change in flux and due to this, no current will induce.

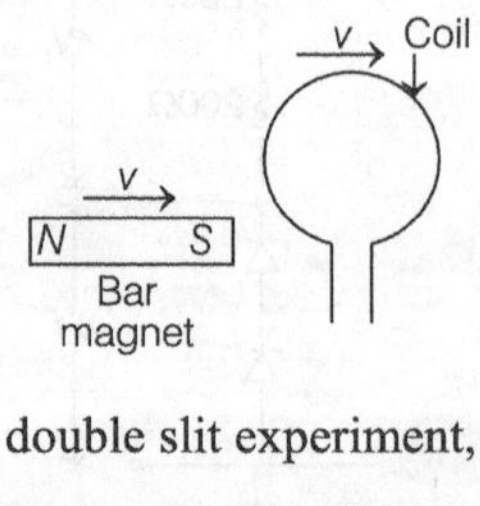

37. (c) In Young's double slit experiment, half angular width is given by

$$\sin\theta = \frac{\lambda}{d} = \frac{589 \times 10^{-9}}{0.589 \times 10^{-3}} = 10^{-3}$$
$$\Rightarrow \quad \theta = \sin^{-1}(0.001)$$

38. (d) The nuclear reaction is

$$X^{240} \rightarrow Y^{110} + Z^{130}$$

$$Q = (\text{BE})_{\text{product}} - (\text{BE})_{\text{reactant}}$$
$$= [(7.8 \times 110) + (8 \times 130)] - [240 \times 7.5]$$
$$= (858 + 1040) - 1800$$
$$= 1898 - 1800 = 98 \text{ MeV}$$

39. (b) The speed of electromagnetic waves in a medium of relative permittivity ε_r and relative permeability μ_r is given by

$$u = \frac{1}{\sqrt{\varepsilon_r \varepsilon_0 \mu_r \mu_0}} = \frac{c}{\sqrt{\mu_r \varepsilon_r}} \quad \left(\because c = \frac{1}{\sqrt{\mu_0 \varepsilon_0}} \right)$$

Given, $\varepsilon_r = 2.14$ and $\mu_r = 1.3$

$$\therefore \quad v = \frac{3 \times 10^8}{\sqrt{2.14 \times 1.3}} = 1.8 \times 10^8 \text{ ms}^{-1}$$

40. (b)

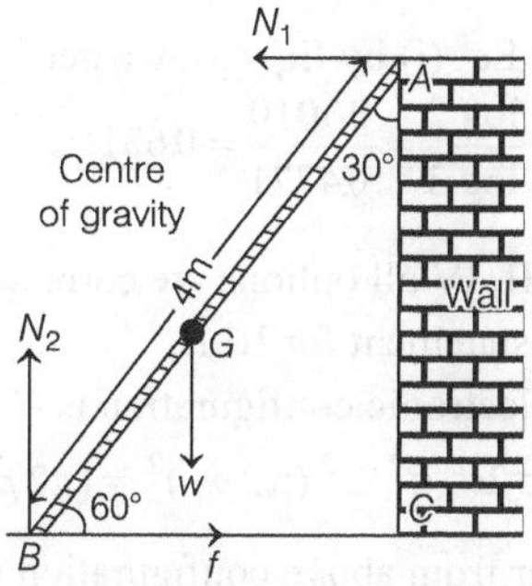

According to the question,
AB is the long ladder of weight w which acts at its centre of gravity G.
As given, $\angle ABC = 60° \therefore \angle BAC = 30°$
Let, N_1 be the reaction of the wall and N_2 be the reaction of the ground.
Force of friction f between the ladder and the ground acts along BC
For horizontal equilibrium, $f = N_1$
For vertical equilibrium, $N_2 = w$
Taking moments about B,
we get for equilibrium,

$$N_1 (4\cos 30°) - w(2\cos 60°) = 0$$

$$N_1 \times 4 \times \frac{\sqrt{3}}{2} - w \times 2 \times \frac{1}{2} = 0$$

$$w = N_1 \times 4 \times \frac{\sqrt{3}}{2} = 2\sqrt{3} N_1 = 2\sqrt{3} f$$

$$250 = 2\sqrt{3} f$$

$$\Rightarrow \quad f = \frac{250}{2 \times \sqrt{3}} = 72.16 \text{ N}$$

$$N_2 = 250 \text{N}$$

$$\therefore \quad f = \mu N_2$$

$$\mu = \frac{f}{N_2} = \frac{72.16}{250} = 0.289$$

41. (d) Given, potential energy function,

$$U(x) = \frac{a}{x^{12}} - \frac{b}{x^6} \quad \ldots \text{(i)}$$

$$\therefore \quad U(x = \infty) = 0$$

$$\text{Force, } F = -\frac{dU}{dx} = -\frac{d}{dx}\left(\frac{a}{x^{12}} - \frac{b}{x^6}\right)$$

$$F = -\left(-\frac{12a}{x^{13}} + \frac{6b}{x^7}\right) \quad \ldots \text{(ii)}$$

At equilibrium, $F = 0$.

Putting $F = 0$ in Eq. (ii), we get $x^6 = \frac{2a}{b}$

Now, substituting $x^6 = \frac{2a}{b}$ in Eq. (i), we get

$$U_{\text{at equilirbium}} = \frac{a}{\left(\frac{2a}{b}\right)^2} - \frac{b}{\left(\frac{2a}{b}\right)} = -\frac{b^2}{4a}$$

$$\therefore \quad D = [U \text{ at } (x = \infty) - U_{\text{at equilirbium}}]$$
$$= 0 - \left(-\frac{b^2}{4a}\right) = \frac{b^2}{4a}$$

42. (c) Given, $\frac{R_1}{R_2} = \frac{1}{2} \Rightarrow R_2 = 2R_1$

The equivalent resistance of parallel combination,

$$\frac{1}{R} = \frac{1}{R_1} + \frac{1}{R_2} + \frac{1}{R_3}$$
$$= \frac{1}{R_1} + \frac{1}{2R_1} + \frac{1}{R_3}$$
$$= \frac{3}{2R_1} + \frac{1}{R_3}$$

$$\Rightarrow \quad \frac{1}{R_3} = 1 - \frac{3}{2R_1}$$

$$\Rightarrow \quad 1 = R_3 - \frac{3}{2}\frac{R_3}{R_1}$$

$$\Rightarrow \quad R_3 = 1 + \frac{3}{2}\frac{R_3}{R_1}$$

Since, no resistance is in fraction, therefore minimum value of

$$\frac{R_3}{R_1} = \frac{2}{3}$$

$$\therefore \quad R_3 = 1 + \frac{3}{2} \times \frac{2}{3} = 2\Omega$$

and $R_1 = 3\Omega$

The maximum resistance value is

$$R_2 = 2R_1 = 2 \times 3 = 6\Omega$$

43. (c) In uniform circular motion, $a_t = 0$, so $\mathbf{a} = \mathbf{a}_c$

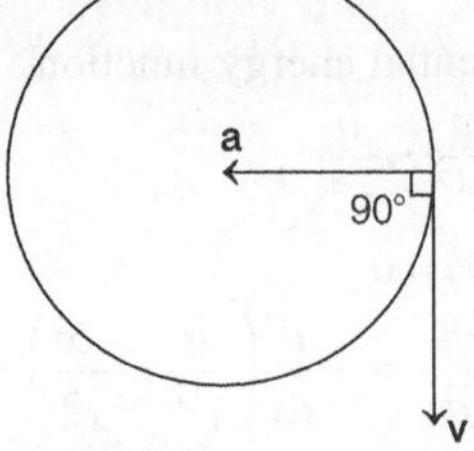

$\therefore$ **a** and **v** are perpendicular to each other.

44. (b) $\because B_1 = \frac{\mu_0}{4\pi} \times \frac{2\pi I}{R}$

$$= \frac{\mu_0}{4\pi} \times \frac{2\pi I \times 2\pi}{L} \quad \text{...(i)}$$

($\because L = 2\pi R$, for circular loop)

$$B_2 = \frac{\mu_0}{4\pi} \times \frac{I}{(a/2)} [\sin 45° + \sin 45°] \times 4$$

where, $a = L/4$ (for square)

$$\therefore \quad B_2 = \frac{\mu_0 I}{4\pi L} \times 8 \times 4 \times \left[\frac{1}{\sqrt{2}} + \frac{1}{\sqrt{2}}\right]$$

$$= \frac{\mu_0 I}{4\pi L} \times \frac{64}{\sqrt{2}}$$

$$\therefore \quad \frac{B_1}{B_2} = \left(\frac{\mu_0}{4\pi}\right) \frac{4\pi^2 I}{L} \Big/ \frac{\mu_0}{4\pi L} \times \frac{64 I}{\sqrt{2}}$$

or $$\frac{B_1}{B_2} = \frac{\pi^2}{8\sqrt{2}}$$

45. (c) Here, beats are produced.

So, frequency of beat will be

$$= \frac{1}{4} - \frac{1}{5} = \frac{5-4}{20} = \frac{1}{20} \text{ Hz}$$

$\therefore$ Time period = 20 s

Chemistry

46. (b) The correct answer is (b) A-III, B-I, C-II, D-IV.

n = Principal quantum number, l = Azimuthal quantum number

47. (d) Reaction takes place as follows

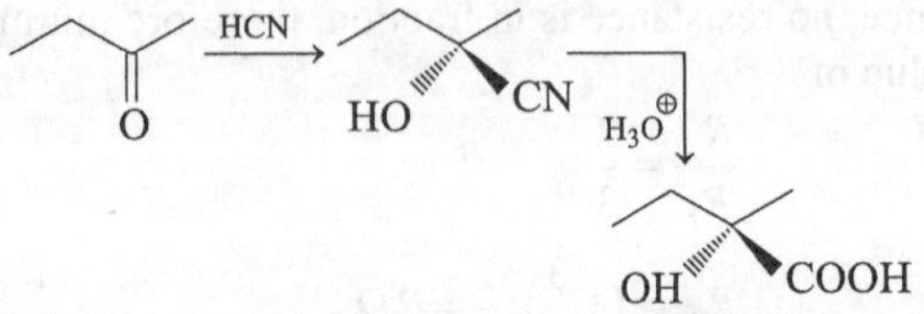

48. (a) Among Ti, V, Cr and Mn generally second ionisation energy increases with increase in atomic number but second ionisation energy of Cr ($3d^5\ 4s^1$) is greater than that of Mn because Cr attains exactly half-filled d-subshell after removal of one electron. Thus, the order of second ionisation enthalpy is Cr > Mn > V > Ti.

Problem Solving Tactics	To solve this question, focus on the electronic configuration and analyse which element need less or more energy to be just in its stable state.

49. (a) CH_3CHO gives positive Fehling's test whereas C_6H_5CHO gives negative Fehling's test. Hence, these aldehydes can be distinguish by using Fehling's solution.

50. (d) For first order reaction,

$$t_{\frac{1}{2}} = \frac{2.303}{k} \log\left(\frac{1}{1/2}\right) = \frac{2.303}{k} \log 2 \quad \text{...(i)}$$

$$t_{\frac{1}{3}} = \frac{2.303}{k} \log\left(\frac{1}{1/3}\right) = \frac{2.303}{k} \log 3 \quad \text{...(ii)}$$

On dividing Eq. (i) by Eq. (ii), we get

$$\frac{t_{1/2}}{t_{1/3}} = \frac{\log 2}{\log 3} = \frac{0.3010}{0.4771} = 0.631$$

51. (a) Except III, IV all options are correct.

The correct statement for III is,

Molecular electronic configuration is

$$\sigma 1s^2\ \sigma^* 1s^2\ \sigma 2s^2\ \sigma^* 2s^2\ (\pi 2p_x)^2 = (\pi 2p_y)^2$$

So, it is clear from above configuration that C_2 molecule has paired electrons both in π orbital and therefore it is diamagnetic in nature. The correct statement for IV is given in statement II.

52. (a) When fullerene undergoes electrophilic substitution, hybridisation of carbon atom remain sp^2 in reactant as well as product.

53. (d)

	3d	4s	4p
Co^{3+} =	⇅ ↑ ↑ ↑ ↑	☐	☐☐☐

In presence of ethylene diamine (strong field ligand), electrons get paired.

	3d	4s	4p
$[Co(en)_3]^{3+}$ =	⇅ ⇅ ⇅ ×× ××	××	×× ×× ××

(d^2sp^3)

$\therefore$ It is an inner orbital complex with no unpaired electrons.

54. (d) All the statements about cyclohexane are correct except (d).

The correct form of statement is

In chair conformation, the adjacent hydrogen atoms on all the neighbouring carbon atoms are staggered and the force of repulsion in them is the minimum. It also does not have any angle strain. So, it is most stable.

55. (c)

Configuration	Element	Electronegativity
$1s^2, 2s^2, 2p^5$	Fluorine (F)	3.98
$1s^2, 2s^2, 2p^4$	Oxygen (O)	3.44
$1s^2, 2s^2, 2p^3$	Nitrogen (N)	3.04
$1s^2, 2s^2, 2p^6, 3s^2, 3p^4$	Sulphur (S)	2.58

On moving down the group, atomic size increases and electronegativity decreases. While in period, electronegativity increases.

So, order will be $F > O > N > S$.

Hence, the correct match is A-(iii), B-(iv), C-(i), D-(ii).

56. (c) Both statements I and statement II are correct.

An azeotrope or a constant boiling mixture is a mixture of two or more liquids whose proportions can not be altered by simple distillation. It also deviated negatively from Raoult's Law and boils at higher temperature than those of either components.

57. (c) According to Nernst equation,

$$E_{cell} = E^\circ_{cell} - \frac{0.059}{n} \log Q \quad \ldots(i)$$

At equilibrium, $Q = K_{eq}$ and $E_{cell} = 0$

$$0 = E^\circ_{cell} - \frac{0.059}{n} \log K_{eq} \quad \text{[from (i)]}$$

$$\log K_{eq} = \frac{E^\circ_{cell} \times n}{0.059}$$

$$= \frac{E^\circ_{cell} \times 1}{0.059} = \frac{0.59}{0.059}$$

$$\log K_{eq} = 10$$

$$K_{eq} = \text{antilog } (10)$$

$$K_{eq} = 10^{10}$$

58. (b) $Cl_2(g) + 2Br^-(aq) \longrightarrow 2Cl^-(aq) + Br_2(aq)$;

$$E^\circ_{cell} = 0.29 \text{ V}$$

$$E_{cell} = E^\circ_{cell} - \frac{0.0591}{2} \log \frac{[Cl^-]^2[Br_2]}{[Br^-]^2[Cl_2]}$$

$$E_{cell} = 0.29 - \frac{0.0591}{2} \log \frac{(0.01)^2 \times 0.01}{(0.01)^2}$$

$$E_{cell} = 0.29 - \frac{0.0591}{2} \log 10^{-2}$$

$$E_{cell} = 0.29 + 2 \times \frac{0.0591}{2} \log 10$$

$$= 0.3491 \text{ V}$$

$$\approx 0.35 \text{ V}$$

59. (a)

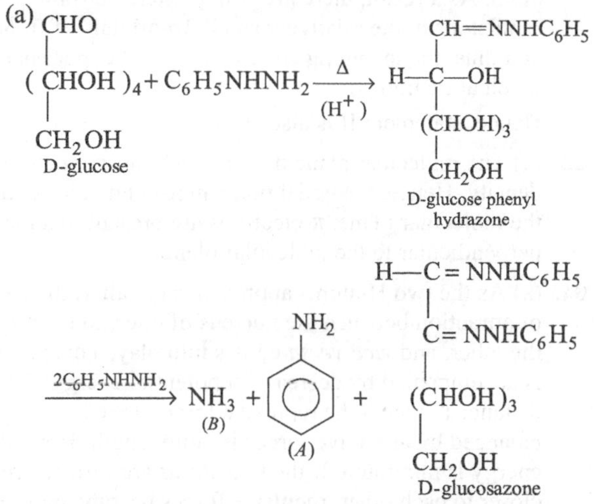

60. (c) As oxidation state of Cl increases, acidic strength of oxy acid of chlorine increases.

Oxidation state of Cl in $Cl_2O \Rightarrow 2 \times x - 2 = 0$

$$x = +1$$

Oxidation state of Cl in $Cl_2O_3 \Rightarrow 2x + 3 \times (-2) = 0$

$$x = +3$$

Oxidation state of Cl in $Cl_2O_7 \Rightarrow 2x + 7 \times (-2) = 0$

$$x = +7$$

∴ Correct order of acidic strength is

$$Cl_2O_7 > Cl_2O_3 > Cl_2O.$$

Problem Solving Tactics The chlorocompound that contains more number of oxygen will be more acidic.

61. (a) Alkyl halides on heating with alcoholic potash eliminate one molecule of halogen acid to form alkenes. This reaction is known as dehydrohalogenation reaction. This is an example of β-elimination reaction. The reaction is as follows

$$\overset{\beta}{H_3C}—\overset{\alpha}{CH_2}X \xrightarrow[-KX]{\text{Alc. KOH}} CH_2{=}CH_2 + H_2O$$

(Here, X=Cl, Br, I)

62. (b) Fluorine does not form any polyhalide as other halogens because

(i) it has maximum ionic character.

(ii) it has low F—F bond energy (38.5 kcal mol^{-1}).

(iii) of the absence of *d*-orbitals in the valence shell of fluorine.

(iv) It brings about maximum coordination number in other elements.

Hence, statement I is correct.

The negative electron gain enthalpy of fluorine is less than that of chlorine. It is due to small size of fluorine atom. As a result, there are strong interelectronic repulsions in the relatively small $2p$-orbitals of fluorine and thus, the incoming electron does not experience much attraction.

Hence, statement II is also correct.

63. (a) The molecular plane does not contain π-electron density. Hence, the nodal plane in π-bond is located in the molecular plane. π-electrons are present in a plane perpendicular to the molecular plane.

64. (a) As the two H-atoms approach each other, the force of attraction between the nucleus of one and electron of the other, and *vice-versa* comes into play. This process is accompanied by decrease in potential energy. The distance at which the repulsive forces are exactly balanced by attractive forces is bond length. Here, the energy is minimum. If the two atoms are further brought closer to each other, repulsive forces become more dominant and energy increases.

65. (c) Keto-enol tautomerism is shown by aldehydes and ketones that have a proton on the α-carbon.

Among the given compounds only three i.e. B, C and E can exhibit keto-enol tautomerism.

66. (b) Hess law is not applicable for nuclear reaction.

All combustion reactions are exothermic.

Work is a path function, not a state function.

Difference between two integral heats of solution is heat of dilution.

Hence, the correct match is A-(iv), B-(iii), C-(i), D-(ii).

67. (b) Blue chromate has two peroxide bonds. The structure is given below.

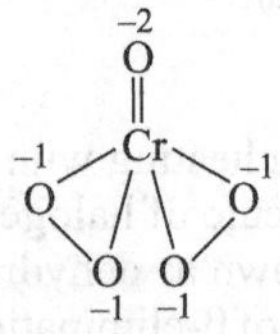

Blue chromate reacts with H_2SO_4 to give oxygen. The reaction is as follows

$$4CrO_5 + 6H_2SO_4 \longrightarrow 2Cr_2(SO_4)_3 + 7O_2 + 6H_2O$$

68. (c) As per the definition of oxidation and reduction. Oxidation involves loss of electrons while reduction involves gain of electrons.

The overall reaction in which oxidation and reduction occur simultaneously is called redox reaction.

Thus, both (A) and (R) are true but (R) is not the correct explanation for (A).

69. (d) $\Delta G^\circ = -2.303\,RT \log K_{eq}$

Given : $K_{eq} = 4 \times 10^5$

$R = 8.314\ JK^{-1}\ mol^{-1}$ and $T = 300\ K$

$$\Delta G^\circ = -2.303 \times 8.314 \times 300 \log (4 \times 10^5)$$
$$= 32179\ J/mol$$
$$\Delta G^\circ \approx 32.18\ kJ\ mol^{-1}$$

70. (d) Be and Al form amphoteric oxides, BeO and Al_2O_3 respectively. These oxides can behave both as base as well as acids.

Aluminium is a lightweight silvery-white metal and beryllium is also a steel-grey metal which is quite brittle at room temperature and resembles some of the properties of aluminium.

Hence, Statement I is true and Statement II is false.

71. (b) For a binary ideal liquid solution, the variation in total vapour pressure *versus* composition of the solution is given by graph (b) in which, total vapour pressure shows a linear composition of the solution. As the mole fraction of more volatile component increases, the total vapour pressure increases.

72. (b) For a solution of $AlCl_3$ in water, the van't Hoff factor (i) is greater than 1 due to hydrolysis.

$$AlCl_3 + 3H_2O \longrightarrow Al(OH)_3 + 3Cl^-$$

As the number of particles increases due to hydrolysis, the van't Hoff factor is more than 1. Hence, statement I is true. The solubility of gas in liquid is directly proportional to the pressure over the solutions at a given temperature. This is according to Henry's law. Hence, statement II is also true.

73. (a) An alkyl halide with chiral carbon forms a racemic mixture through S_N1 mechanism while S_N2 mechanism changes the configuration of a compound due to formation of the transition state.

S_N1 mechanism proceeds through carbocation formation. So, it's a two-step process and as stability of carbocation increases, reaction favours S_N1 mechanism.

3° carbocation are more stable than others and also polar solvent increases the stability of carbocation. So, they both favours S_N1 mechanism.

74. (a) Chlorophylls are green pigments in plants and contain magnesium.

They are useful during photosynthesis to store energy in the form of glucose from carbon dioxide and water in presence of sunlight.

75. (b) Carbon is not able to form $d\pi$-$d\pi$ bond due to absence of d-orbital.

76. (d) In first step

$$CH_3Mg{-}X + CH_3COOCH_3 \xrightarrow{\text{Dry ether}} \underset{(A)}{(CH_3)_3C{-}OH} + C_2H_5OMgX$$

Here, the tertiary butyl alcohol formed, which then reacts, with Na to give $(CH_3)_3CO^-Na^+$ (B).

So, when there is primary alkyl halide reacts with alkoxide then Williamson's ether synthesis takes place rather than elimination.

$$(CH_3)_3\overset{-}{C}ONa^+ \xrightarrow{C_2H_5Br} \underset{(C)}{(CH_3)_3COC_2H_5}$$

Williamson's ether synthesis goes through the S_N2 mechanism.

77. (b) The incorrect answer among all is (b).

The correct form of (b) is,

Standard entropy of ethane is higher than that of methane because it depends on the molar mass of the molecules.

More the mass of the molecules more will be the entropy of the molecule.

78. (c) The correct option is only (c).
The correct statements for rest options are

(a) *ortho*-nitrophenol is more volatile than *para*-nitrophenol due to presence of intramolecular H-bonding.

(b) *ortho*-nitrophenol has less boiling point than *para*-nitrophenol.

(d) They do not have same volatility, *ortho*-nitrophenol > *para*-nitrophenol

79. (d) XeO_3 has tetrahedral structure.

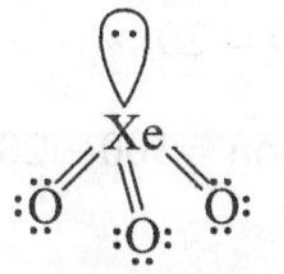

XeO_2F_2 has *see-saw* structure as shown below.

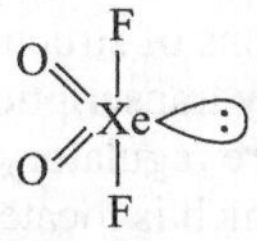

XeF_4 has square planar structure.

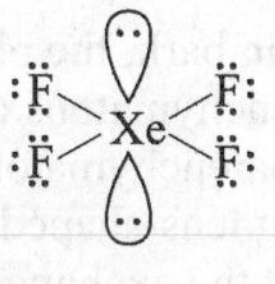

XeF_2 has linear structure.

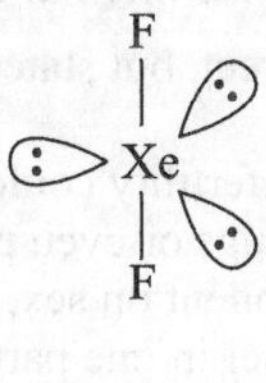

80. (c) The reaction proceeds as

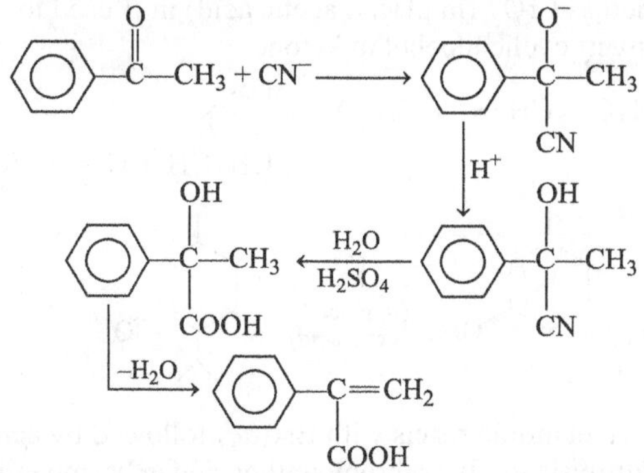

81. (b) The correct answer is (b) A-III, B-IV, C-II, D-I.

82. (a)

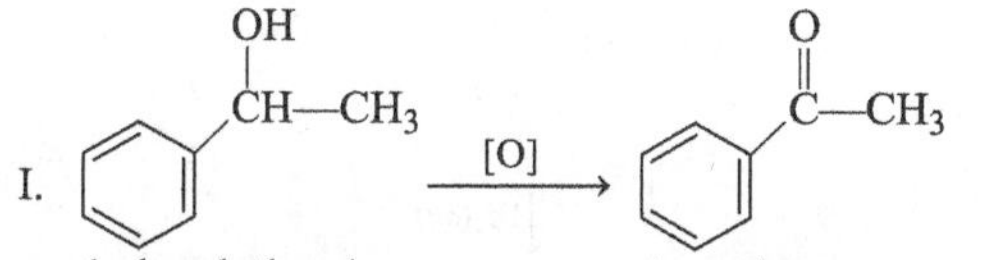

1-phenyl ethanol Acetophenone

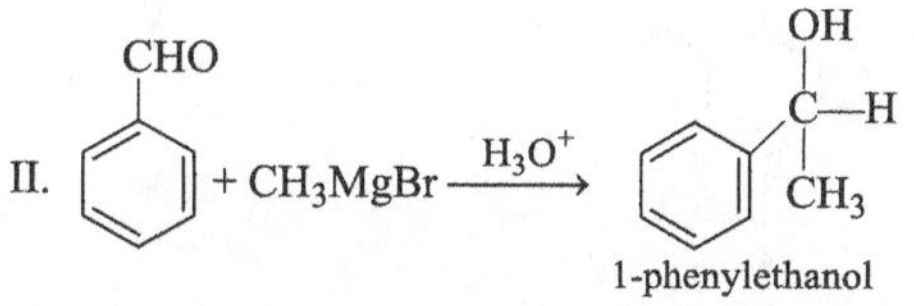

1-phenylethanol

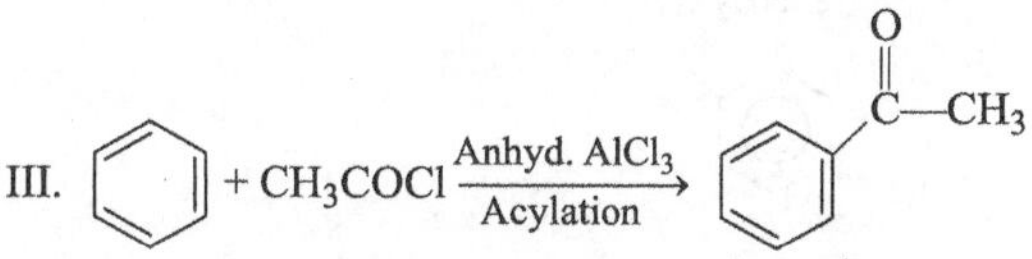

Acetophenone

IV. $(C_6H_5CO_2)_2Ca \xrightarrow{\text{Distillation}} C_6H_5{-}\underset{\overset{\|}{O}}{C}{-}C_6H_5 + CaCO_3$

Benzophenone

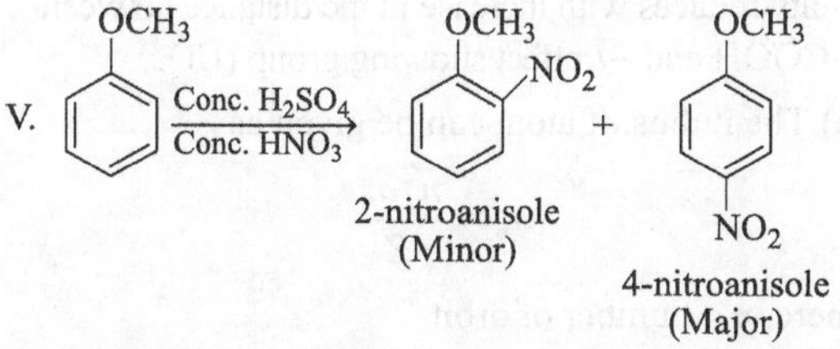

Hence, acetophenone is prepared by I and III reactions.

83. (b) OsO_4 causes *cis*-hydroxylation as shown below.

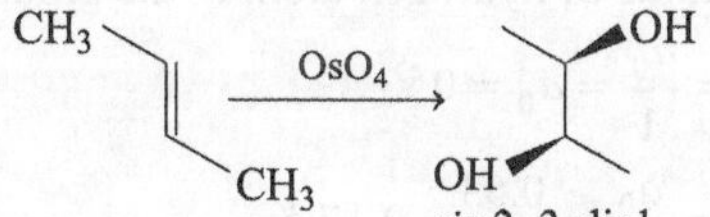

cis-2, 3-diol

84. (a) MnO_2 is used to convert alcohol into aldehyde whereas CrO_3 (in glacial acetic acid) in II used to convert cyclic alcohol to ketone.

$$CH_3CH_2CH{=}CHCH_2OH \xrightarrow{MnO_2} CH_3CH_2CH{=}CHCHO$$

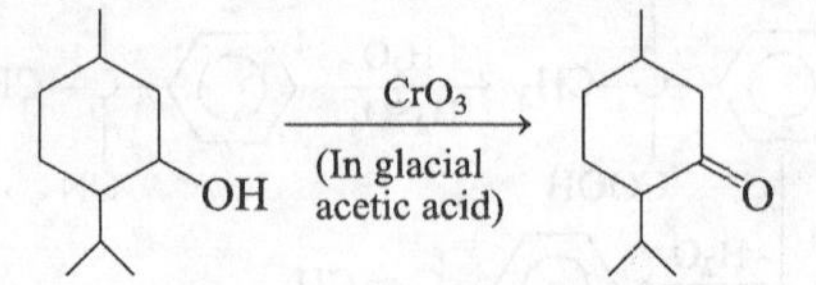

85. (c) Acetanilide reacts with $Br_2(aq)$ followed by acidic hydrolysis to give *o*-bromoaniline and *p*-bromoaniline as products.

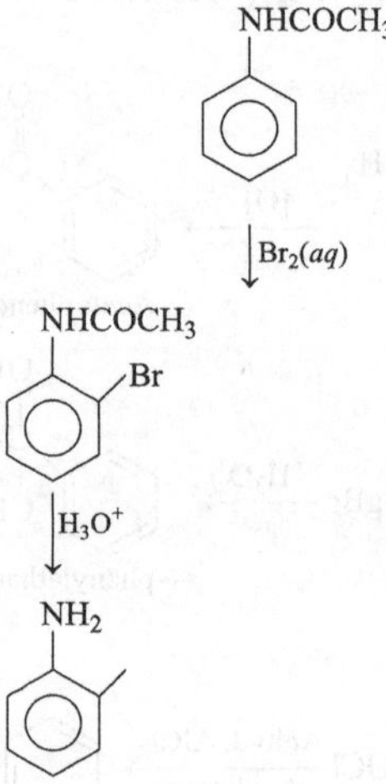

86. (a) Presence of $-I$ effect showing group like Cl increases the acidic character of carboxylic acids and the acidity reduces with increase in the distance between —COOH and $-I$ effect showing group (Cl).

87. (a) The radius of atom can be given as

$$r_n = \frac{n^2 a_0}{Z}$$

where, n = number of orbit

Z = atomic number

a_0 = constant value

So, the radius of hydrogen atom in the ground state.

$$r_1(\text{H}) = \frac{a_0}{1} = a_0 = 0.53\ \text{Å}$$

$$r_1(\text{Li}^{2+}) = \frac{a_0}{3} = \frac{0.53}{3} \approx 0.17\ \text{Å}$$

Hence, the radius of lithium ion in ground state = 0.17 Å.

88. (b) It is given that half-life, $t_{1/2} = \frac{0.693}{k} = 6.93$

$$k = 0.1$$

For a first order reaction,

$$k = \frac{2.303}{t}\log\frac{[A_0]}{[A_t]}$$

A_0 = initial concentration

A_t = concentration at time t

$$0.1 = \frac{2.303}{t}\log\frac{100}{1} = \frac{2.303}{t}\times 2$$

$$t = \frac{4.606}{0.1} = 46.06 \text{ minutes}$$

89. (a) $MX_2 \rightleftharpoons M^{2+} + 2X^-$

$$K_{sp} = [M^{2+}][X^-]^2$$

$$\therefore \quad K_{sp} = (S)(2S)^2 = 4S^3$$

$$4S^3 = 32\times 10^{-15}$$

Thus, $S = \sqrt[3]{8\times 10^{-15}}$

$$= 2\times 10^{-5}\ \text{M}$$

$$\Rightarrow \quad [M^{2+}] = 2\times 10^{-5}\ \text{M}$$

90. (c) Percentage of H

$$= \frac{2}{18}\times\frac{\text{Weight of } H_2O}{\text{Weight of organic compound}}\times 100$$

$$= \frac{2}{18}\times\frac{0.9}{0.5}\times 100 = 20\ \%$$

∴ Percentage of carbon = 100 – 20 = 80%

Biology

91. (a) According to *lac* operon concept, regulatory gene regulates the expressions of structural genes by its protein product that are mostly transcription factors. These transcription factors are regulatory proteins that, bind to the operator region which is located just upstream of the binding site of RNA polymerase and hence prevent the transcription.

92. (c) At certain region in bark, the phellogen cuts off closely arranged parenchymatous cells on the outer side of cork cells. These parenchymatous cells soon rupture the epidermis forming lens-shaped openings called lenticels. They permit the exchange of gases between the outer atmosphere and the internal tissue of the stem.

93. (d) Statement I is correct, but statement II is incorrect and it can be corrected as

The reasons for the infertility could be physical, congenital disease, drugs or even psychological. Infertility is not dependent on sex, the problem may lies in both partner or either in one partner.

94. (d) The male sex accessory ducts include rete testis, vasa efferentia, epididymis and vas deferens. The vasa efferentia leave the testis and open into epididymis located along the posterior surface of each testis.

95. (c) The correct matches are A-3, B-5, C-4, D-2.
- *Microsporum* is the causative agent of ringworm in humans.
- *Wuchereria bancrofti* is an aschelminthes which cause filariasis in humans.
- *Trypanosoma gambiense* is a protozoan which causes sleeping sickness.
- *Entamoeba histolytica* causes amoebiasis, i.e. amoebic dysentry in humans.

96. (c) Gamosepalous calyx, imbricate aestivation and zygomorphic flowers are found in Leguminosae (Fabaceae) family.

Many plants belonging to this family are gram, arhar, soybean plant, groundnut, etc.

97. (b) The inhibition of enzyme succinate dehydrogenase is a classical example of competitive inhibition with succinic acid as its substrate.

The compounds namely malonic acid, glutaric acid and oxalic acid, have structural similarities with succinic acid and compete with the substrate for binding at the active site of succinate dehydrogenase enzyme.

98. (c) A competitive inhibitor is a molecule that resembles the structure of the enzyme's substrate and can bind to the active site of the enzyme. Because of the similarity, it competes with the substrate for binding.

When the competitive inhibitor occupies the active site, the substrate cannot bind, which reduces the rate of the enzymatic reaction.

99. (b) Vinegar or acetic acid is a liquid substance consisting mainly of acetic acid and water. It is obtained by the bacterium *Acetobacter aceti*. Citric acid obtained from *Aspergillus* and lactic acid from *Lactobacillus*.

100. (d) The correct match is A-4, B-3, C-2, D-1.
- Incomplete dominance is the condition where heterozygote displays intermediate phenotype between homozygous phenotypes.
- The physical characteristics of an individual is known as phenotype.
- The phenomenon in which single gene affect multiple traits is known as pleiotropy.
- In codominance two alleles for a trait are equally expressed with neither being recessive or dominant.

101. (d) The important steps in the process of decomposition are fragmentation, leaching, catabolism, humification and mineralisation. All of these processes need microbial action except leaching. By the process of leaching, water soluble inorganic nutrients go down into the soil horizon and get precipitated as unavailable salts.

102. (a) Statements I, II, III and V are correct, whereas statement IV is incorrect and can be corrected as Gene flow can alter the genetic characteristics of population. For example, if the characteristic of newly arrived animal differs from those of the animals already living there, and if the newcomer is adapted well enough to the new area to survive and mate successfully, the genetic composition of the receiving population may alter.

103. (a) The biosphere reserves differ from national parks and wildlife sancturies because in national parks and wildlife sancturies species are protected from getting hunted, predated or poached. Here, the interaction of humans is banned.

Whereas biosphere is divided into different zones, i.e. core zone (no human activity is allowed), buffer zone (limited human activity is permitted) and the transition zone (participation of local people for cropping, recreation etc. is done). Thus, in biosphere people are an integral part of the system.

104. (c) Both A and R are true, but R is not the correct explanation of A.
Depending on the substrate DNA and the reaction conditions, restriction enzymes show a wide variation of cleavage. Most endonucleases optimally digest the target DNA at 37°C. However, there are some exceptions with lower or higher optimal temperature. For exampel, *Taq* I optimally digests at 65°C and *Apa* I digests at 25°C.

105. (a) Statement in option (a) is incorrect and can be corrected as
During telophase the chromosomes that have reached their respective poles decondense and lose their individualities.
The compact mitotic chromosomes are observed in prophase.
Rest of the statements are correct.

106. (a) Statement in option (a) is correct. Rest other statements are incorrect and can be corrected as
- Gibberellins are weak acidic growth hormones having gibbane ring structure, which cause cell elongation of intact plants and increased internodal length of genetically dwarfed plants.
- The major sites of gibberellin production in plants are embryos, roots and young leaves near the shoot tip.
- Some naturally occurring cytokinins are zeatin, ribosyl zeatin, etc. Cytokinins are derivates of purine–adenine.

107. (b) Biopiracy is the term used to refer to the use of bioresources by multinational companies and other organisation without proper authorisation from the countries and people concerned without proper compensatory payment.

Biopatents are intellectual property rights granted by the state for a limited period of time for inventions consisting of products made of biological material or processes with which biological material is produced.

108. (d) Statement in option (d) is incorrect and can be corrected as

Repetitive sequence are present in human genome. These sequences are nucleotide sequences that are repeated many times.They are thought to have no direct coding functions, but they shed light on chromosome structure , dynamics and evolution.

109. (d) The correct matches are A-2, B-1, C-4, D-3.

- Helper T-cells activate B-lymphocytes to become plasma cells.
- Plasma cells get active in production of antibodies.
- Killer T-cells combines with antigens causing lysis.
- Interferons are proteins produced by virus infected cells.

110. (c) Krebs' cycle starts with the formation of 6 C atom compound, i.e. citric acid by chemical reaction between 2 C compound, i.e. acetyl Co-A and 4 C compound, i.e. oxaloacetic acid. The reaction is catalysed by the enzyme citrate synthase and a molecule of Co-A is released.

111. (a) Statement I is incorrect, but statement II is correct. Incorrect statement can be corrected as

In directional selection more individuals acquire value other than the mean character value whereas in stabilisation selection more individuals acquire mean character value.

112. (d) The essential requirements for a gene amplification reaction are I, II and III. Other options are not associated with gene amplification.

- 20 mg of DNA template that contains the DNA region to be amplified.
- Two primers that are complementary to the 3′ ends of each of the sense and anti-sense strand of the target DNA.
- *Taq* polymerase with a temperature optimum at 70°C.

113. (a) Stratified squamous non-keratinised epithelium provides protection and serve as a lining or covering for moist internal cavity of the body such as buccal cavity, oesophagus and cornea of eye.

114. (a) Statement I is incorrect, but statement II is correct. Statement I can be corrected as

The ATP molecules synthesised in oxidative phosphorylation are used in metabolic process, whereas the ATP molecules synthesised in the process of photophosphorylation are used in dark reaction for CO_2 assimilation.

115. (a) The sequence in option (a) is correct.

The representation of evolutionary history of vertebrates through geological periods is as follows

Permian $\rightarrow$ Triassic $\rightarrow$ Jurassic $\rightarrow$ Cretaceous $\rightarrow$ Tertiary

The permian is a geological period that began nearly 300 mya. Therapsids are mammal-like reptiles that flourished in early permian and became extinct in Triassic period. *Pelycosaurs* are the earliest most primitive synapsids that become extinct before the origin of dinosaurs. Jurassic period is the golden time for dinosaurs. They become extinct in the tertiary period.

116. (b) During the S-phase of the cell cycle, the histone proteins are synthesised in a eukaryotic cell.

The major event in S-phase is DNA replication. The process create exactly two identical semi-conserved chromosomes.

117. (d) The correct matches are A-4, B-3, C-2, D-1.

- The scientific name of flying fox is *Pteropus.*
- The limbless amphibian is called *Ichthyophis*.
- The scientific name of flying fish is *Exocoetus obtusirostris.*
- The scientific name of angel fish is *Pterophyllum*.

118. (b) Statements III and IV are incorrect and can be corrected as

- Cytokinins promote nutrient mobilisation which helps in the delaying of leaf senescence.
- Ethephon is the most widely used compound as a source of ethylene. It hastens fruit ripening in tomatoes and apples and accelerates abscission in flowers and fruits.

119. (d) Biolistics or gene gun is a physical method used to introduce alien DNA into the host cells. In this method, a foreign DNA coated on the tungsten or gold particles is shot with high velocity on the target host cells.

120. (d) The correct matches are A-5, B-4, C-3, D-1, E-2.

- Auxin initiates rooting in stem cuttings, but inhibits the growth of roots at higher concentration.
- Gibberellins increases the length of sugarcane stem, thus increases the yield as much as 20 tonnes per acre.
- Cytokinins promote nutrient mobilisation.
- Ethylene enhances the rate of respiration during ripening of the fruits.
- Abscisic acid causes partial closure of stomata under drought, thus acts as antitranspirant.

121. (a) The given figure represents compound epithelium.

It is made up of more than one layer of cells and has limited role in secretion and absorption.

Their main function is to provide protection against chemical and mechanical stresses.

122. (d) If a person is having problem with calcium and phosphorus metabolism in his body, this indicates that his parathyroid gland may not be functioning properly. The parathyroid gland release parathyroid hormone. It takes part in the control of calcium and phosphorous homeostasis, as well as bone physiology.

123. (b) The correct matches are A-4, B-3, C-2, D-1.

- **Parthenocarpic fruit** These are fruits formed without fertilisation of ovary.
- **Aleurone layer** It is made up of parenchyma cells and forms the outer layer present in the periphery of an endosperm.
- **Anatropous ovule** The body of the ovule is completely inverted so that micropyle and hilum come to lie very close to each other.
- **Apomixis** Some species of Asteraceae and grasses have evolved special mechanism to produce seeds without fertilisation. This phenomenon is termed as apomixis.

124. (b) Both A and R are true and R is the correct explanation of A.

Unlike bryophytes and pteridophytes, in gymnosperms the male and female gametophytes do not have an independent free living existence. They remain within the sporangia retained on the sporophytes.

125. (b) In many citrus and mango varieties some of the nucellar cells surrounding the embryo sac start dividing protrude into the embryo sac and develop into the embryos. In such species, each ovule contains many embryos. Occurrence of more than one embryo in a seed is referred to as polyembryony .

126. (b) The chordates (*Ascidia* and *Pterophyllum*) differs from non-chordates (*Echinus* and *Pila*) by the presence of ventral heart, presence of notochord and post-anal tail.

127. (c) Statement in option (c) is incorrect and can be corrected as

Mature and proinsulin are structurally not similar because proinsulin contains an extra stretch called C-peptide. This C-peptide is not present in matrue insulin. Mature insulin is made up of two polypeptide chains.

Rest statements are true.

128. (c) The cell membrane is mainly composed of lipids and proteins. The major lipids are phospholipids that are arranged in a bilayer. Also the lipids are arranged within the membrane with the polar head towards the outside and the hydrophobic tails towards the inner parts. This ensures that the non-polar tail of saturated hydrocarbons is protected from the aqueous environment.

129. (b) Structure 'X' represents heterocyst which is specialised cell present in some organisms helping them in fixing atmospheric nitrogen.

130. (c) Both A and R are true, but R is not the correct explanation of A.

In human beings the skeletal system is made up of 206 bones and few cartilages. It is grouped into two principal divisions, i.e. the axial and the appendicular skeleton. Axial skeleton comprises 80 bones distributed along the main axis of the body. The bones of the limbs alongwith their girdles constitute the appendicular skeleton.

131. (d) A restriction enzymes is an enzyme that cuts DNA at or near specific recognition nucleotide sequences known as recognition sites.

The recognition sequences in DNA differ for each restriction enzyme producing different length, sequence and strand orientation of a sticky end of an enzymes.

For example, if the DNA is cut with *Eco*RI, it would be cut right from the middle. Hence, 5′ GAATTC 3′, 3′ CTTAAG 5′ palindrome sequence can be easily cut at about the middle by *Eco*R1 enzyme.

132. (d) Statement I is correct, but statement II is incorrect. The incorrect statement can be corrected as The autonomic neural system transmits the impulse from the CNS to involuntary organs and smooth muscles of the body. The autonomic neural system is further classified into sympathetic neural system and parasympathetic neural system.

133. (a) The cross between Pp and Qq is as follows

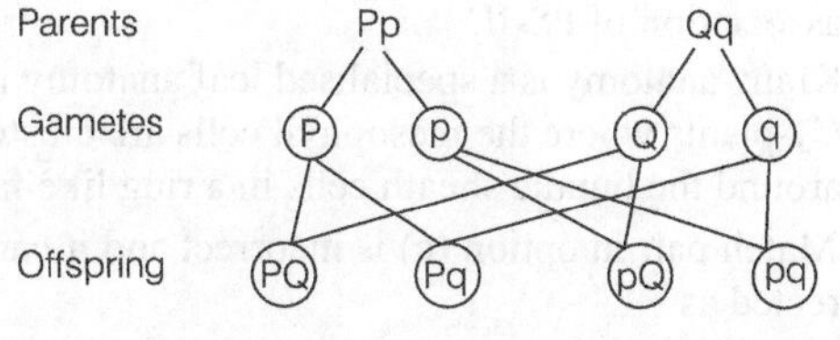

Thus, the possible genotype of the offspring will be PQ, Pq, pQ and pq.

134. (b) The characters in option (b) belong to family-Cruciferae. The members of this family are sources of food, e.g. *Brassica campestris* (mustard), etc.

135. (b) The competition mainly arises when the same species compete for the same niche, territory or resources. Hence, competition for food, light and space is most severe in closely related species growing in the same area.

136. (a) Statement I is incorrect, but statement II is correct. Incorrect statement can be corrected as

As per Hardy-Weinberg equilibrium, the frequency of dominant and recessive alleles in a population will remain constant from generation to generation, provided that certain condition exist, i.e. population should be large, mating should be random, no mutation occurs and no natural selection occur, etc.

137. (a) The correct order is as follows coxal bone, cranial bone, facial bones, ribs bone.

- Pelvic girdle consists of two coxal bones. Each coxal bones is formed by the fusion of 3 bones.
- Cranial bones are 8 in number.
- The facial region is made up of 14 skeletal elements.
- In human total 12 pairs of ribs are found.

138. (c) Aschelminthes are bilaterally symmetrical, triploblastic and pseudocoelomate animals. Alimentary canal is complete with a well-developed muscular pharynx, e.g. *Ascaris*.

139. (b) Both statement I and statement II are correct.

- In meiosis, the daughter cells differ from parent cell as well as amongst themselves due to segregation, independent assortment and crossing over. Meiosis leads to recombination of gene or characters. It involves two sequential cycles of cell division called meiosis-I and meiosis-II.
- The DNA replication, takes place only once in S-phase of cell cycle.

140. (c) The correct matches are A-2, B-1, C-4, D-3.

- CAM pathway is observed in succulents xerophytes these plants often grow in hot, dry climate and thus need to minimise water loss.
- Chlorophyll-*b* is an accessory photosynthetic pigment.
- Photo- oxidation or photolysis of water occurs in association of PS-II.
- Kranz anatomy is a specialised leaf anatomy in C_4-plants where the mesophyll cells are clustered around the bundle sheath cells in a ring like fashion.

141. (c) Match pair in option (c) is incorrect and it can be corrected as

Anthocyanins are pigments found in plants especially in flowers, fruits and tubers.

Abrin ricin are some examples of toxins.

142. (c) The correct matches are A-3, B-4, C-2, D-1.

- Squamous epithelium are found in the endothelium and lung alveoli.
- Ciliated epithelium are found in bronchi and Fallopian tube.
- Brush border epithelium are found in PCT and intestine.
- Compound epithelium are found in pharynx and buccal cavity.

143. (d) If only one of the parent is found to be a carrier then the chances that the offspring will have faulty cystic fibrosis gene is very low or zero.

Whereas if both the parents are carrier then, each pregnancy will have 25% chances of being affected with the disease.

144. (c) Statements I and V are correct. Rest other statements are incorrect and can be corrected as

- Golgi bodies are involved in the secretion, storage and packaging of materials.
- Golgi apparatus is the important site of formation of glycoproteins and glycolipids.
- The lysosomal vesicles have been found to be very rich in almost all types of hydrolytic enzymes optimally active at the acidic pH.

145. (d) Statements I and IV are incorrect and can be corrected as

- In dicot roots vascular bundles are radial and exarch.
- All tissues on the innerside of the endodermis such as pericycle, vascular bundles and pith constitute the stele.

Rest of the statements are correct.

146. (d) Match pair in option (d) is incorrect and can be corrected as

Crossing over is the exchange of genetic material between non-sister chromatids of homologous chromosome.

Rest other matched pairs are correct.

147. (d) Statement I is correct, but statement II is incorrect.

The incorrect statement can be corrected as

The members of Rhodophyceae also known as red algae occur in both well-lighted regions close to the surface of water and also at great depths in oceans where relatively little light penetrates.

148. (d) Proximal convoluted tubule is involved in active reabsorption of sodium as 70-80 percent of electrolytes and water are reabsorbed by this segment.

149. (b) Fimbriae are hair-like structures present in large number in bacteria. They help in attaching bacteria to solid surfaces or host tissues.

So, if fimbriae are removed from bacteria then it would not be able to adhere to the host tissue.

150. (a) Sutton and Boveri noted that the behaviour of chromosomes was nearly parallel to the behaviour of genes. They used chromosome movement to explain Mendel's law. According to them the pairing and segregation of a pair of chromosome lead to segregation of a pair of factors they carried.

151. (b) Statements II and III are correct and rest of the statements are incorrect and can be corrected as

- Net primary productivity is the available biomass for the consumption of heterotrophs.
- The annual net primary productivity of the whole biosphere is aproximately 170 billion tons of organic matter.
- Net primary productivity is equal to gross primary productivity minus respiration losses.

NPP = GPP $-R$

152. (a) Since, $\frac{dN}{dt} = rN$

and $r = b - d$

Per capita birth rate $(b) = \frac{200}{4000} = 0.05$

Per capita death rate $(d) = \frac{100}{4000} = 0.025$

$$r = b - d$$

$\Rightarrow$ $0.05 - 0.025 = 0.025$

Rate of population of ants, $\frac{dN}{dt} = rN$

$$= 0.025 \times 4000 = 100 \text{ ants/month}$$

153. (b) All the given features are correctly described except one in option (b). It can be corrected as

In frog 10 pairs of cranial nerves are present which arises from the brain.

154. (b) *Wuchereria bancrofti*, the filarial worm causes a slow developing chronic inflammation of the organs. This disease is known as elephantiasis or filariasis.

155. (c) Statements II and IV are correct and rest of the statements are incorrect. These can be corrected as

- Tobacco contains nicotine which stimulates adrenal gland to release adrenaline and nor-adrenaline into blood. Both of these hormones raise blood pressure and increase heart rate.
- Tobacco smoking increases carbon monoxide (CO) content in the blood and reduces the concentration of haem-bound oxygen.
- Tobacco chewing is associated with the increased risk of cancer of the oral cavity.

156. (b) Frequency of dominant allele (A) = 0.7

According to Hardy Weinberg $p + q = 1$

if the frequency of dominant allele $(A) = 0.7$

Then, $0.7 + q = 1$

$$q = 1 - 0.7$$

$$q = 0.3$$

and $p^2 + q^2 + 2pq = 1$

Here, $p^2 = (\text{AA})^2$

$$q^2 = (\text{aa})^2$$

$$2pq = (\text{Aa})^2$$

So, frequency of homozygous dominant allele

$$\text{AA} = (0.7)^2$$

$\Rightarrow$ 0.49

Frequency of homozygous recessive allele aa $= (0.3)^2$

$\Rightarrow$ 0.09

Frequency of heterozygous allele Aa $= 2 \times 0.7 \times 0.3$

$\Rightarrow$ 0.42

$\therefore$ AA = 0.49

Aa = 0.42

aa = 0.09

Hence, option (b) is correct.

157. (a) Mustard belongs to Cruciferae (Brassicaceae) family. Its flowers have polypetalous, cruciform corolla, valvate aestivation, basifixed polyandrous stamens and superior ovary. *Sesbania* flower shows vexillary aestivation whereas cotton and china rose shows twisted aestivation.

158. (d) Match pair in option (d) is incorrect and can be corrected as

All tissues on the innerside of endodermis such as pericycle, vascular bundles and pith constitute the stele.

159. (a) Statements I, II and III are correct whereas statements IV and V are incorrect and can be corrected as

- Brainstem forms the connections between the brain and spinal cord. Three major regions make up the brainstem, i.e. pons, midbrain and medulla oblongata. Cerebral aqueduct is a canal which passes through the midbrain.
- The two hemispheres of brain are connected by bundle of transverse fibres called corpus callosum.

160. (b) The sequential event in the heart which is cyclically repeated is called the cardiac cycle and it consists of systole and diastole of both the atria and ventricles. The contraction of the muscles of the heart is referred to as systole, while relaxation of the heart muscle is called diastole.

161. (c) Statements III and V are incorrect and can be corrected as

- Recombination frequency is directly proportional to the distance between the genes, while linkage is inversely proportional to it.
- The first chromosomal map was given by Sturevant and Morgan.

162. (d) Statement in option (d) is incorrect and can be corrected as

Hormonal pills inhibits ovulation and implantation as well as alter the quality of cervical mucus to prevent/retard entry of sperms.

163. (c) Phellogen is a couple of layers thick. It produces secondary cortex or phelloderm on innerside and cork or phellem on outerside.
The cells of phellem are dead, suberised and impervious to water. Cells of phelloderm are thin walled, living and store food.

164. (b) The correct matches are A-4, B-3, C-1, D-2.
- The cycle starts with menstrual phase, which last for 3-5 days, i.e. 1st-4th days of cycle. It results due to shedding of endometrial lining.
- Next phase is proliferative phase which last from 5th to 13th day. Here development of Graafian follicle takes place.
- At 14th day, due to rapid LH secretion, Graafian follicle ruptures resulting in ovulation.
- After ovulatory phase, the next phase is luteal phase which lasts from 15th to 28th day. Here, formation of corpus luteum occurs.
  This corpus luteum releases progesterone to maintain the endometrium lining. In the absence of fertilisation the lining sheds and the next cycle begins.

165. (d) Match pair in option (d) is incorrected. It can be corrected as
The order of wheat is Poales whereas Sapindales order belongs to Mango. The Poales is a large order of flowering plants in the monocotyledons.

166. (c) During diplotene stage, the homologous chromosomes separate due to repulsion, but yet held by chiasmata.These are X-shaped structures. In oocytes of some vertebrates, diplotene can last for months or years.

167. (c) Statements I, III, IV and V are correct for the discovery of Stanley Cohen and Herbert Boyer. Only statement II is incorrect and it can be corrected as
The first instance of the construction of an artificial rDNA molecule was accomplished in 1972 by Cohen and Boyer.

168. (a) A is false, but R is true. A can be corrected as
Photosynthetically, C_4 plants are more efficient than C_3 plants because these have Kranz anatomy (undifferentiated mesophyll around vascular bundles with chloroplast containing bundle sheath). Bundle sheath chloroplast are larger agranal and without PS-II activity and perform C_3 cycle.

169. (c) Intracellular membrane is involved in the establishing compartments in the cells and provides organisation of enzymes and pigments. It provides a channel for nutrient distribution. However, rigidity to the cell is provided by cell wall.

170. (a) The correct matches are A-2, B-1, C-4, D-3.
- TCA or Tri-Carboxylic Acid cycle commonly called as, Krebs' cycle was discovered by Hans Krebs.
- In the inner mitochondrial membrane ATP synthesis takes place with the help of ATP synthase (complex -V). This complex consists of two major components, F_1 and F_0. The F_1 contains the site for synthesis of ATP from ADP and inorganic phosphate. F_0 forms the channel through which protons cross the inner membrane.
- Pyruvic acid is the key/end product of glycolysis. Depending upon the cellular need there are three major ways in which cell utilise this. They are lactic acid fermentation, alcoholic fermentation and aerobic respiration.
- The oxidative decarboxylation reaction is catalysed by enzyme pyruvate dehydrogenase. This reaction require the participation of several co-enzymes, including NAD^+ and coenzyme-A.

171. (d) Statement I is correct, but statement II is incorrect and can be corrected as
In a back cross, an individual can be crossed with any of the parent, i.e. recessive or dominant. Whereas, in test cross an individual is crossed with only recessive parent.

172. (b) Statement in option (b) is not true and can be corrected as
The cambium cut off the cells towards pith mature into secondary xylem and the cells cut off towards periphery mature into secondary phloem. The amount of secondary xylem is more than secondary phloem because cambium is more active on the inner side.

173. (a) The presence of two or more recognition sites is not a desired characteristics in a cloning vector. The vector molecule should have a single recognition site. This help in easy ligation of the gene of interest at one specific location.

174. (d) A is true, but (R) is false. It can be corrected as
The secondary structure of protein is formed by the coiled long polypeptide chains. These structures of proteins are produced and maintained by hydrogen bond. Depending upon hydrogen bonding two main types of secondary structures are found, i.e. α-helix and the β-sheet.

175. (d) About 900 restriction enzymes have been isolated from over 230 strains of bacteria each of which recognise different recognition sequences.

176. (d) Statement I is correct but statement II is incorrect. It can be corrected as : Carbon dioxide can be transported by haemoglobin as carbaminohaemoglobin.

177. (d) Statement in option (d) is incorrect and can be corrected as

Echinoderms do not have well-developed circulatory system. Instead they have haemal or perihaemal system. There is no heart in them and the blood is often without a respiratory pigment.

Rest statements are correct.

178. (a) Statement in option (a) is true, while the rest of the statements are false and can be corrected as

- The progesterone is essential for maintenance of endometrium during pregnancy.
- Progesterone exerts negative feedback on hypothalamus.
- The FSH and LH are produced after menopause in large continuous quantities. Thus, these are excreted out in the urine.

179. (d) Statements II and V are incorrect and can be corrected as

- Antibodies are protein molecules. Each antibody molecule has four peptide chains which consist of two light chains and two heavy chains.
- The primary and secondary immune responses are carried out with the help of two special types of lymphocytes present in our blood, i.e. B-lymphocytes and T-lymphocytes.

180. (b) Gamete Intra Fallopian Transfer (GIFT) involves the transfer of an ovum collected from a donor into the Fallopian tube of another female who cannot produce one, but can provide suitable environment for development and fertilisation.

SECTION II
Mastery Builders

PRACTICE SET 8

Maximum Marks : 720	Time : 3 hrs	No. of Questions : 180

Instructions

1. This question paper contains **180** multiple-choice questions (four options with a single correct answer) from **Physics, Chemistry** and **Biology**.
2. These questions are distributed as 45 questions, each from Physics and Chemistry and 90 questions in Biology. These are to be compulsorily attempted by the candidate.
3. Each question carries 4 marks. For each correct response, the candidate will get 4 marks. For each incorrect response, one mark will be deducted from the total scores.

PHYSICS

1. In a vessel, the gas is at a pressure p. If the mass of all the molecules is halved and their speed is doubled, then the resultant pressure will be

(a) $4p$ (b) $2p$ (c) p (d) $p/2$

2. In an experiment with vernier callipers of least count 0.1 mm, when two jaws are joined together the zero of vernier scale lies right to the zero of the main scale and 6th division of vernier scale coincides with the main scale division. While measuring the diameter of a spherical bob, the zero of vernier scale lies in between 3.2 cm and 3.3 cm marks and 4th division of vernier scale coincides with the main scale division. The diameter of bob is measured as

(a) 3.26 cm (b) 3.22 cm (c) 3.25 cm (d) 3.18 cm

3. A galvanometer of resistance 35 Ω is shunted by a 3.5 Ω wire. The part of total current that flows through the galvanometer $\left(\frac{I_g}{I}\right)$ is given as

(a) $\frac{3}{11}$ (b) $\frac{2}{11}$ (c) $\frac{1}{11}$ (d) $\frac{4}{11}$

4. The power factor of the circuit shown in the figure is

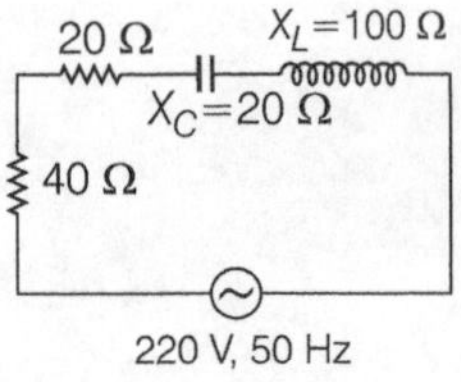

(a) 0.2 (b) 0.8
(c) 0.4 (d) 0.6

5. The equivalent resistance between A and B is

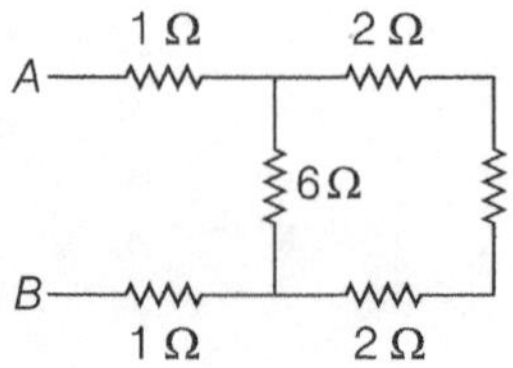

(a) 5Ω (b) 8Ω (c) 2.5Ω (d) 6.8Ω

6. A body is moving along X-axis with the speed of 5.00 ms^{-1}. If the mass of the body is 3.513 kg, then the magnitude of its momentum is recorded as

(a) 17.56 kg ms^{-1} (b) 15.56 kg ms^{-1}
(c) 16.65 kg ms^{-1} (d) 18.57 kg ms^{-1}

7. A coil of one turn is made of a wire of certain length and then from the same length, a coil of 4 turns is made. If the same current is passed in both the cases, then the ratio of magnetic field at their centres will be

(a) 4:1 (b) 1:4 (c) 16:1 (d) 1:16

8. A p-type semiconductor has acceptor level 50 meV above the valence band. Find the maximum wavelength of light that can create a hole.

(a) 1.24×10^{-3} m (b) 1.24×10^{-5} m
(c) 4.47×10^{-4} m (d) 2.47×10^{-5} m

9. A rectangular frame of copper wire enclosing a surface area A is covered with a soap film. If the area of the frame of copper wire is reduced 25%, the energy of the soap film will be changed by

(a) 25% (b) 50% (c) 75% (d) 35%

10. Suppose the speed of a planet at the perihelion P as in the figure be v_P and the sun-planet distance SP be r_P, then r_P, v_P are related to the corresponding quantities at the aphelion r_A, v_A as

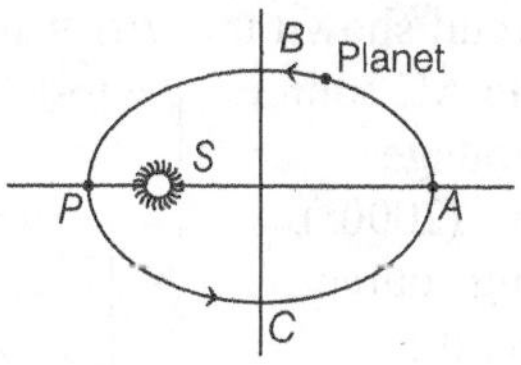

(a) $r_P > r_A, v_P > v_A$ (b) $r_P < r_A, v_P > v_A$
(c) $r_A > r_P, v_A > v_P$ (d) $r_A < v_P, v_A = v_P$

11. The interference pattern is obtained with two coherent light sources of intensity ratio n. In the interference pattern, the ratio $\frac{I_{max} - I_{min}}{I_{max} + I_{min}}$ will be

(a) $\frac{\sqrt{n}}{n+1}$ (b) $\frac{2\sqrt{n}}{n+1}$ (c) $\frac{\sqrt{n}}{(n+1)^2}$ (d) $\frac{2\sqrt{n}}{(n+1)^2}$

12. A scooter accelerates from rest for time t_1 at constant rate a_1 and then retards at constant rate a_2 for time t_2 and comes to rest. The correct value of $\frac{t_1}{t_2}$ will be

(a) $\frac{a_1 + a_2}{a_2}$ (b) $\frac{a_2}{a_1}$ (c) $\frac{a_1}{a_2}$ (d) $\frac{a_1 + a_2}{a_1}$

13. A brass rod of 1 m long is firmly clamped at the middle and one end is stroked by a resined cloth. What is the pitch of the note will be heard? (Young's modulus for brass $= 10^{12}$ dyne cm^{-2} and density $= 9$ g cm^{-3})

(a) 1652.5 Hz (b) 1600 Hz
(c) 1666.67 Hz (d) 1554.48 Hz

14. The time period of the electron orbiting in second orbit of hydrogen atom is 4×10^{-16} s. Hence, the time period in the third orbit will be

(a) 2.7×10^{-16} s (b) 1.35×10^{-16} s
(c) 2.7×10^{-15} s (d) 1.35×10^{-15} s

15. Treating the bulb of power 60W as a point source of electromagnetic radiation, i.e. about 5% efficient in converting electrical energy to visible light. The maximum magnitudes of the electric field of the light that is incident on a page, because of the visible light coming from a desk lamp is (distance between bulb and page is 30 cm)

(a) 40 V/m (b) 30 V/m
(c) 45 V/m (d) 25 V/m

16. A metal rod of length 2.5 m and negligible mass has two masses tied to its ends. If they have masses 0.5 kg and 1.5 kg respectively, then find the location of the point on this rod, where the rotational energy is minimum, when rod is rotated about that point.

(a) 1.875 m from 1.5 kg (b) 1.525 m from 1.5 kg
(c) 1.525 m from 0.5 kg (d) 1.875 m from 0.5 kg

17. A marble block of mass 2 kg lying on ice when given a velocity of 6 m/s is stopped by friction in 10 s. Then, the coefficient of friction is

(a) 0.06 (b) 0.01 (c) 0.03 (d) 0.02

18. Which of the following physical quantities do not have same dimensional formula ?

(a) Speed and $(\mu_0 \varepsilon_0)^{-1/2}$
(b) Torque and work
(c) Young's modulus and pressure
(d) Momentum and Planck's constant

19. The given below are two statements

Statement I If n identical capacitors of capacitance C each are connected in parallel, then their equivalent capacitance is equal to $\frac{C}{n}$.

Statement II Parallel combination of capacitors is used, when we require a large capacitance at a small potential.

(a) Both Statement I and Statement II are correct and Statement II is correct explanation of Statement I.
(b) Both Statement I and Statement II are correct but Statement II is not the correct explanation of Statement I.
(c) Statement I is correct but Statement II is incorrect
(d) Statement I is incorrect but Statement II is correct

20. The potential energy of a normal hydrogen atom in ground state is 27.2 eV, then its kinetic energy in the same state will be

(a) 9.07 eV (b) 13.6 eV
(c) −13.6 eV (d) 0

21. A block of mass M moving on the frictionless horizontal surface collides with a spring of spring constant k and compresses it by length L. The maximum momentum of the block is

(a) zero (b) $\frac{ML^2}{k}$ (c) $\sqrt{Mk} \cdot L$ (d) $\frac{kL^2}{2M}$

22. The diode used in the circuit shown in the figure has a constant voltage drop of 0.7 V at all currents and a maximum power rating of 140 mW. What should be the value of the resistance R, connected in series with diode, for obtaining maximum current?

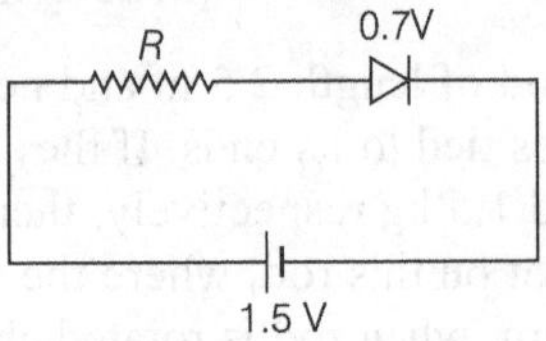

(a) 1.2Ω (b) 0.7Ω (c) 4Ω (d) 5Ω

23. The velocity of particle is $v = v_0 + gt + ft^2$. Its position is $x = 0$ at $t = 0$, then its displacement after time ($t = 1$s) is

(a) $v_0 + g + f$ (b) $v_0 + 2g + 3f$
(c) $v_0 + \frac{g}{2} + \frac{f}{3}$ (d) $v_0 + \frac{g}{2} + f$

24. The resultant resistance of the circuit between A and B is

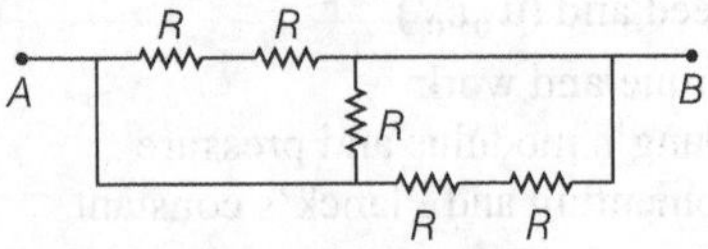

(a) R (b) $2R$ (c) $\frac{3R}{2}$ (d) $\frac{R}{2}$

25. For a satellite moving in an orbit around the earth, the ratio of magnitude of kinetic energy to potential energy is

(a) 2 (b) $\frac{1}{\sqrt{2}}$ (c) $\frac{1}{2}$ (d) $\sqrt{2}$

26. **Statement I** Resistivity of conductor increases with the increase of its temperature.

Statement II Relaxation time of electrons in conductor increase with the increase of its temperature.

(a) Both Statement I and Statement II are correct
(b) Statement I is correct and Statement II is incorrect
(c) Both Statement I and Statement II are incorrect
(d) Statement I is incorrect and Statement II is correct

27. The value of refractive index of a medium of polarising angle of 76° is (given, tan 76° = 4)

(a) 2 (b) 4 (c) 1.5 (d) None of these

28. The potential difference between X and Y in the following figure is

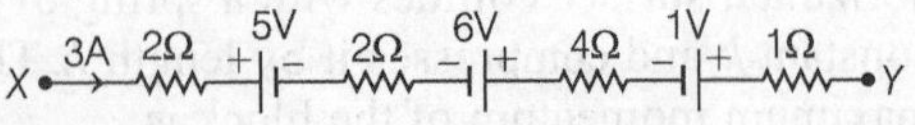

(a) 24 V (b) 25 V
(c) 18 V (d) 27 V

29. A body is projected with a velocity of 40 ms^{-1}. After 2 s, it crosses a vertical pole of height 20.4 m. The angle of projection be ($g = 9.8$ ms^{-2})

(a) 15° (b) 30° (c) 45° (d) 60°

30. A rope 1 cm in diameter breaks, if the tension in it exceeds 500 N. The maximum tension that may be given to a similar rope of diameter 2 cm is

(a) 250 N (b) 2000 N (c) 500 N (d) 1000 N

31. In the circuit shown in figure, the AC source gives a voltage $V = 20\cos(2000t)$. Neglecting source resistance, the voltmeter and ammeter readings will be

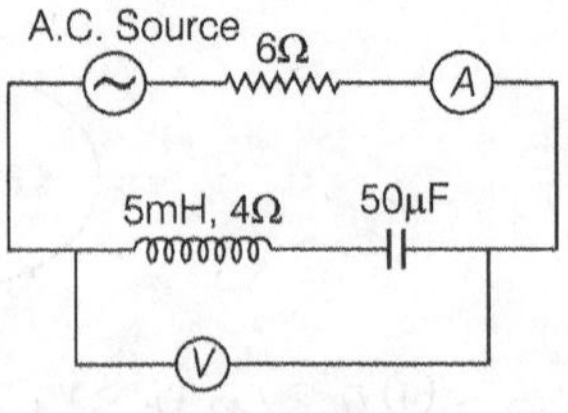

(a) 0 V, 2.0 A (b) 0 V, 1.4 A
(c) 5.6 V, 1.4 A (d) 8 V, 2.0 A

32 When a dielectric material is placed between the plate of capacitor, then its capacitance increases, because

(a) potential difference between the plates decreases
(b) electric field between the plates decreases
(c) Both (a) and (b)
(d) charges on plates decreases

33. An AC Voltage is applied to a resistance R and an inductor L in series. If R and the inductive reactance are both equal to 3Ω, the phase difference between the applied voltage and the current in the circuit is

(a) zero (b) $\pi/2$ (c) $\pi/4$ (d) $\pi/6$

34. A balloon with mass 16 kg is descending down with an acceleration 6.2 ms^{-2}. How much mass should be removed from it, so that it starts acceleration up with 6.2 ms^{-2}? (take, $g = 9.8$ ms^{-2})

(a) 12.4 kg (b) 12 kg (c) 11.5 kg (d) 13 kg

35. The energy level of the doubly ionised lithium (Li^{++}) has the same energy as the ground state energy of the hydrogen atom is

(a) 1 (b) 2 (c) 3 (d) 4

36. In a Young's double slit experiment performed with light of wavelength 8000 Å, the screen is placed 1 m from the slits. Fringes formed on the screen are observed by a student sitting close to the slits. The student's eye can distinguish two neighbouring fringes. If they subtend an angle more than 1 minute of arc, then the maximum distance between the slits, so that the fringes are clearly visible is

(a) 2.75 mm (b) 1.5 mm
(c) 4.25 mm (d) 3.36 mm

37. Three bricks each of length L and mass M are arranged as shown in figure. The distance of the centre of mass of the system from the wall is

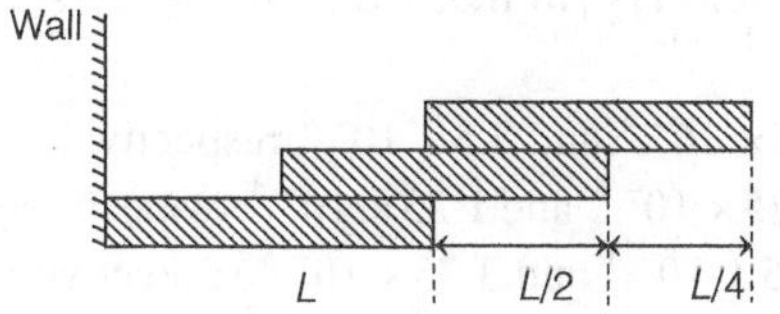

(a) $\frac{L}{2}$ (b) $\frac{L}{4}$ (c) $\frac{11}{12}L$ (d) $\frac{5}{6}L$

38. The power of a biconvex lens is 10 D and the radius of curvature of each surface is 10 cm, then the refractive index of the material of the lens is

(a) $\frac{3}{2}$ (b) $\frac{4}{3}$ (c) $\frac{9}{8}$ (d) $\frac{5}{3}$

39. Four points charges, each equal to $4\,\mu C$ are held at the corners of a square $ABCD$ of side $a = 10$ cm. The magnitude of a charge Q is placed at the centre of the square, so that the system of charges is in equilibrium, is

(a) $-(1+2\sqrt{2})\,\mu C$ (b) $2\sqrt{2}\,\mu C$
(c) $(1+2\sqrt{2})\,\mu C$ (d) $-2\sqrt{2}\,\mu C$

40. An electromagnetic wave is propagating along X-axis. At $x = 1$ m and $t = 10$ s, its electric vector $|\mathbf{E}| = 6$ V/m, then the magnitude of its magnetic vector is

(a) 5×10^{-7} T (b) 6×10^{-8} T
(c) 3×10^{-7} T (d) 2×10^{-8} T

41. An infinitely long straight conductor carries a current of 10 A as shown in figure. An electron is moving with a speed of v m/s parallel to the conductor. The perpendicular distance between the electron and the conductor is 20 cm at an instant. The magnitude of the force experienced by the electron at that instant is 8×10^{-20} N. Speed v of electron is

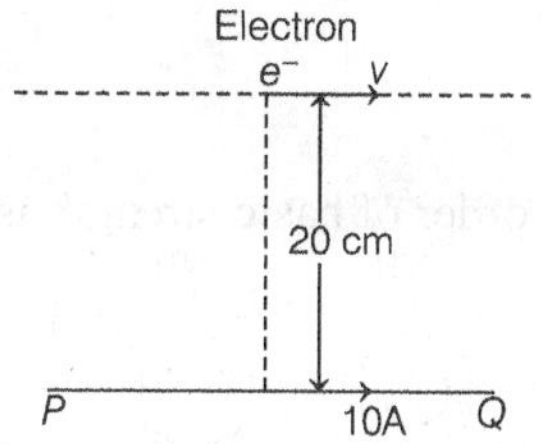

(a) 1.5×10^4 m/s (b) 15×10^4 m/s
(c) 0.5×10^4 m/s (d) 5×10^4 m/s

42. The velocity of a particle describing SHM is 16 cm s^{-1} at a distance of 8 cm from mean position and 8 cm s^{-1} at a distance of 12 cm from mean position. The amplitude of motion

(a) 15.5 cm (b) 18 cm
(c) 14.3 cm (d) 13.06 cm

43. The name of the following gate that the circuit shown in the figure

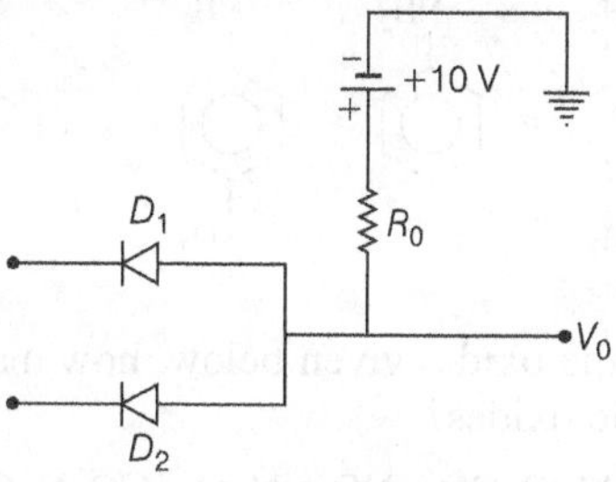

(a) AND gate (b) OR gate
(c) NOT gate (d) NOR gate

44. When a metal plate of negligible thickness is introduced between the two plates of a capacitor at middle position. Now, capacitance of capacitor will be

(a) half (b) double (c) same (d) infinite

45. The anode potential of a photocell is kept fixed. The wavelength λ of the light falling on the cathode is gradually increased. The photocurrent I of photocell varies with λ as

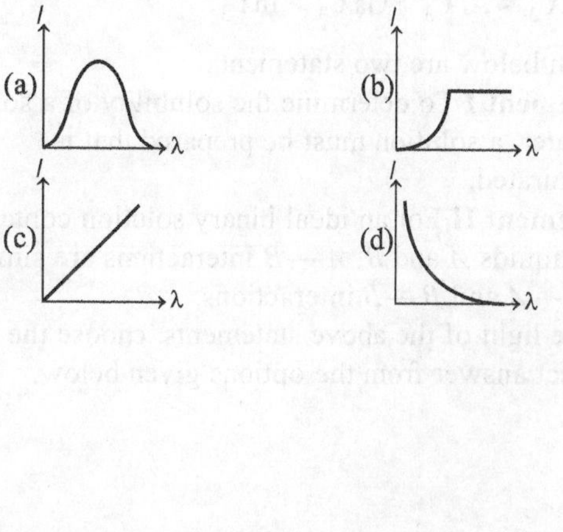

CHEMISTRY

46. The correct order of basic strength is

(a) 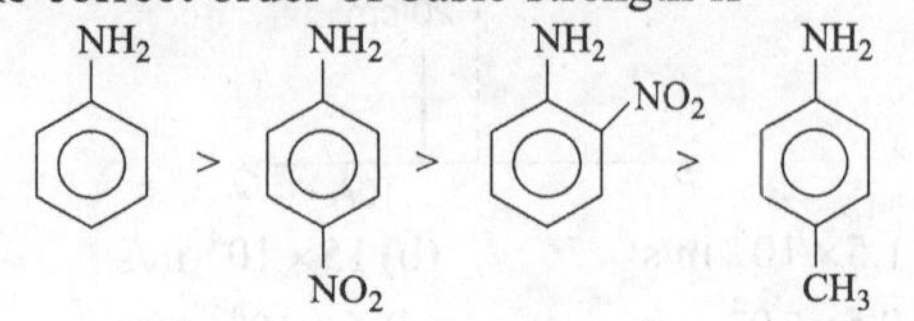

(b) 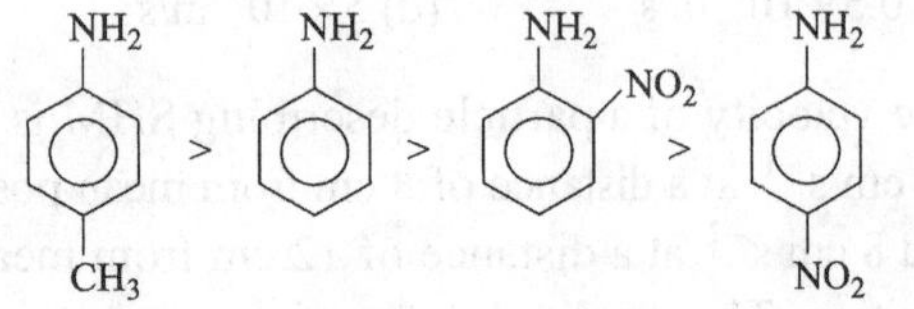

(c) 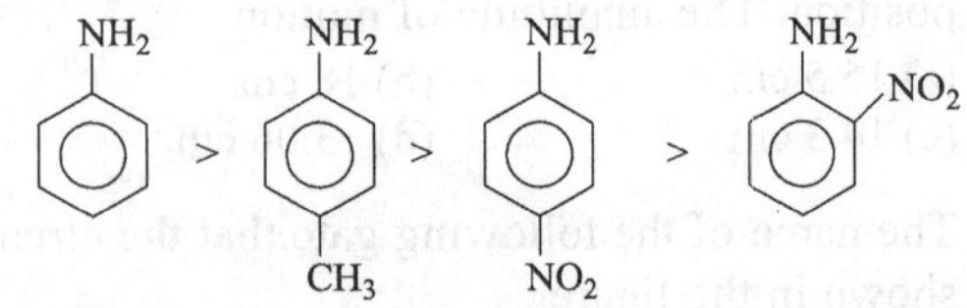

(d) 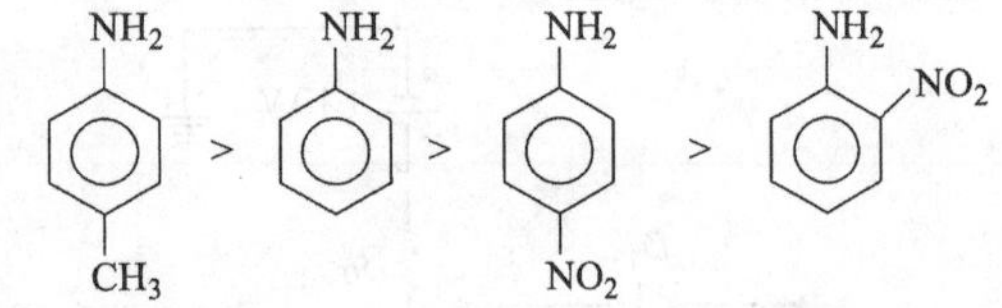

47. Among the oxides given below, how many of them are acidic oxides?

$MnO, CO_2, NO_2, N_2O_5, CO, N_2O$

(a) 2 (b) 3 (c) 4 (d) 5

48. In perchloric acid ($HClO_4$), the number of σ and π-bonds are

(a) 5σ and 4π-bonds (b) 6σ and 3π-bonds
(c) 5σ and 3π-bonds (d) 5σ and 2π-bonds

49. Arrange halides of group 13 elements in correct order of Lewis acidic strength. [where, X is a halogen]

(a) $BX_3 > AlX_3 > GaX_3 > InX_3$
(b) $BX_3 < AlX_3 < GaX_3 < InX_3$
(c) $BX_3 < AlX_3 > GaX_3 < InX_3$
(d) $BX_3 < AlX_3 > GaX_3 > InX_3$

50. Given below are two statements.

Statement I To determine the solubility of a solute in water, a solution must be prepared that is unsaturated.

Statement II For an ideal binary solution containing two liquids A and B, A—B interactions are similar to A—A and B—B interactions.

In the light of the above statements, choose the correct answer from the options given below.

(a) Statement I is false but Statement II is true.
(b) Both Statement I and Statement II are true.
(c) Both Statement I and Statement II are false.
(d) Statement I is true but Statement II is false.

51. The decomposition of NH_3 on Pt surface is zero order reaction. Calculate the rate of production of N_2 and H_2 [in $mol^{-1}L^{-1}$] if $k = 2.5\times 10^{-4}$ $mol\ L^{-1}s^{-1}$.

(a) 2.5×10^{-4} and 7.5×10^{-4} respectively.
(b) 3.75×10^{-4} and 1.25×10^{-4} respectively.
(c) 1.25×10^{-3} and 3.75×10^{-3} respectively.
(d) 3.75×10^{-3} and 1.25×10^{-3} respectively.

52. For the equilibrium in a closed vessel

$$PCl_5(g) \rightleftharpoons PCl_3(g) + Cl_2(g)$$

K_p is found to be double of K_C. This is at temperature attained when

(a) $T = 2K$ (b) $T = 12.18K$
(c) $T = 24.36K$ (d) $T = 27.3K$

53. The transition metal ion that has 'spin only' magnetic moment value of 5.92 BM is

(a) Mn^{2+} (b) Fe^{2+} (c) V^{2+} (d) Cu^{2+}

54. The radius of first Bohr orbit of hydrogen atom is 0.52 Å. The radius of the third orbit of H^+ will be

(a) 8.467 Å (b) 0.705 Å
(c) 1.590 Å (d) 4.761 Å

55. In reaction, $\underset{(A)}{C_5H_{10}Cl_2} + NaOH \longrightarrow \underset{(B)}{C_5H_{10}O}$

B is an aldehyde with no α-hydrogen. Thus, A is

(a) $(CH_3)_3CCHCl_2$
(b) $CH_3CH_2\underset{|}{C}HCHCl_2$ with CH_3 on the marked carbon
(c) $CH_3\underset{|}{C}HCH_2CHCl_2$ with CH_3 on the marked carbon
(d) $CH_3\underset{|}{\overset{|}{C}}CH_2CH_2CH_3$ with Cl above and Cl below the marked carbon

56. Given below are some compounds,

A. CH_3OH
B. CH_3CH_2OH
C. CH_3COCH_3
D. CH_3—$\underset{|}{CH}$—OH with CH_3 on CH
E. $CH_3CH_2CH_2CH_3$

Which of the above compounds on being warmed with iodine solution and NaOH will give iodoform?
(a) B, C and D
(b) A, B and D
(c) A and D
(d) Only C

57. Which of the following statement is incorrect?
(a) Boron shows only + 3 oxidation state while all other element of group 13 shows + 1 as well as + 3 oxidation state.
(b) Stability of + 1 oxidation state decreases from top to bottom along group 13.
(c) Compound of Tl(I) shows great resemblence with alkali metals.
(d) Aluminium trichloride occurs as dimeric structure.

58. Elimination of bromine from 2-bromobutane in presence of alc. (KOH) results in the formation of
(a) predominantly but-2-yne
(b) predominantly but-2-ene
(c) predominantly but-1-ene
(d) equimolar mixture of but-1-ene and but-2-ene

59. Consider a third order reaction which involves a single reactant. If the concentration of the reactant is doubled, the rate of the reaction will
(a) increases by a factor of two
(b) increases by a factor of four
(c) increases by a factor of eight
(d) increases by a factor of nine

60. Given below are two statements.
Statement I The highest oxidation state of osmium is + 7.
Statement II Osmium is a $5d$-block element.
In the light of the above statements, choose the correct answer from the options given below.
(a) Both Statement I and but Statement II are false.
(b) Statement I is true but Statement II is false.
(c) Statement I is false but Statement II is true.
(d) Both Statement I and Statement II are true.

61. Which of the following statement is incorrect?
(a) 3-ethylpentane is the lowest molecular mass alkane which has ethyl group as the substituent.
(b) Double bond is preferred over triple bond while naming the organic compound.
(c) Carbinol got its name from destructive distillation of wood.
(d) The IUPAC name of HOOC—CH(COOH)—COOH is propanetrioic acid.

62. Amount of work done when 2 mole of an ideal gas present in a vessel of 2 L capacity at 1 atm pressure is allowed to enter into an evacuated vessel of 10 L capacity
(a) 16 J
(b) 16×101.3 J
(c) 12×101.3 J
(d) Zero

63. Chlorination of toluene in presence of light and heat followed by treatment with aqueous NaOH gives
(a) *o*-cresol
(b) *p*-cresol
(c) 1, 3, 5-trihydroxytoluene
(d) benzoic acid

64. Major product of the following reaction is

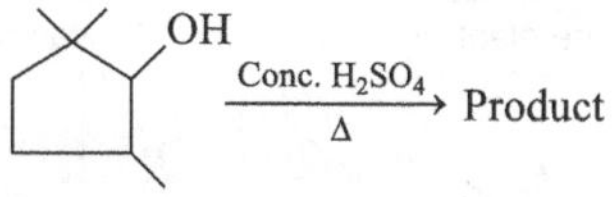

(a) 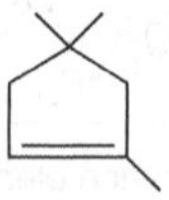
(b) 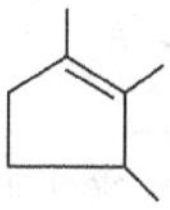
(c) 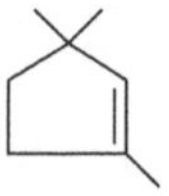
(d) 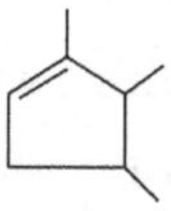

65. Which of the following is an incorrect statement?
(a) Electron withdrawing inductive effect of the carbonyl group in —COOH group weaken the O—H bond and favours ionisation of a carboxylic acid compared with an alcohol.
(b) Inductive effect of the chlorine destabilises the acid and stabilises the conjugate base.
(c) Aniline is weaker base than ammonia.
(d) Phenol is a weaker acid than water.

66. Given below are two statements.
Statement I D-glucose and D-mannose are epimers of each other.
Statement II The spatial arrangement of the two or more polypeptide chains with respect to each other is known as quaternary structure.
In the light of the above statements, choose the correct answer from the options given below.
(a) Statement I is false but Statement II is true.
(b) Both Statement I and Statement II are true.
(c) Both Statement I and Statement II are false.
(d) Statement I is true but Statement II is false.

67. The principle of column chromatography is
(a) differential adsorption of the substances on the solid phase
(b) capillary action
(c) differential absorption of the substances on the solid phase
(d) gravitational force

68. If P to T are second period p-block elements then which of the following graph show correct relation between valence electrons in P_2 to T_2 (corresponding molecules) and their bond order is

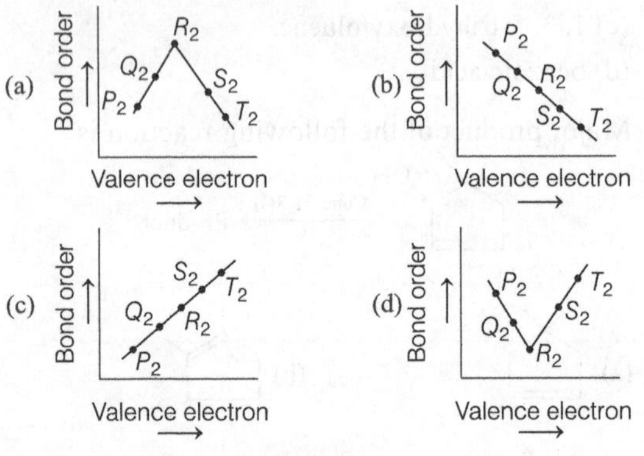

69. Match the List-I with List-II.

List-I	List-II
A. 105	(i) Uun
B. 107	(ii) Uns
C. 109	(iii) Unp
D. 110	(iv) Une

Choose the correct answer from the options given below.
(a) A-(iii), B-(ii), C-(i), D-(iv)
(b) A-(ii), B-(iii), C-(iv), D-(i)
(c) A-(ii), B-(iii), C-(i), D-(iv)
(d) A-(iii), B-(ii), C-(iv), D-(i)

70. The concentration of H_2O_2 in a solution containing 34 g in 500 mL is given in List-I and their corresponding values are given in List-II. Then match List-I with List-II.

List-I	List-II
A. Molarity (M)	(i) 68
B. Normality (N)	(ii) 22.4
C. % W/V	(iii) 4
D. Volume strength (g/L)	(iv) 2

Choose the correct answer from the options given below.
(a) A-(iv), B-(iii), C-(ii), D-(i)
(b) A-(iv), B-(iii), C-(i), D-(ii)
(c) A-(i), B-(ii), C-(iii), D-(iv)
(d) A-(iv), B-(ii), C-(iii), D-(i)

71. Match List-I with List-II.

List-I (Type of bond)	List-II (Method of formation)
A. σ-bond	(i) Sharing of electrons
B. Covalent bond	(ii) Axial overlapping
C. Ionic bond	(iii) Lateral overlapping
D. π-bond	(iv) Transfer of electrons

Choose the correct answer from the options given below.
(a) A-(ii), B-(i), C-(iv), D-(iii)
(b) A-(i), B-(ii), C-(iv), D-(iii)
(c) A-(ii), B-(i), C-(iii), D-(iv)
(d) A-(iv), B-(ii), C-(iii), D-(i)

72. Given below are two statements, one is labelled as Assertion (A) and the other is labelled as Reason (R).
Assertion (A) In dilute benzene solutions, equimolar addition of R_3N and HCl produce a substance with a dipole moment. In the same solvent, equimolar addition of R_3N and SO_3 produce a substance having an almost identical dipole moment.
Reason (R) SO_3 acts as a Lewis acids and can react with amine base to form polar substances.
In the light of the above statements, choose the most appropriate answer from the options given below.
(a) (A) is false but (R) is true.
(b) Both (A) and (R) are true and (R) is the correct explanation of (A).
(c) Both (A) and (R) are true but (R) is not the correct explanation of (A).
(d) (A) is true but (R) is false.

73. Match the List-I with List-II.

List-I (Compound)	List-II (Functional group)
A. Vinegar	(i) Ketone
B. C_2H_6	(ii) Alcohol
C. Ethanol	(iii) Alkane
D. Methanone	(iv) Carboxylic acid

Choose the correct answer from the options given below.

(a) A-(i), B-(iii), C-(ii), D-(iv)
(b) A-(i), B-(ii), C-(iii), D-(iv)
(c) A-(iv), B-(iii), C-(i), D-(ii)
(d) A-(iv), B-(iii), C-(ii), D-(i)

74. Diethyl ether is mostly used in solvent extraction due to all of the following reasons except.

(a) Its solvation capacity is very high.
(b) Being inert, it does not react with most organic compound.
(c) There are two lone pairs in it, therefore it acts as a strong nucleophile.
(d) Its boiling point is low, therefore, it can be easily separated by distillation.

75. Given below are two statements.

Statement I Toxic metal ions are removed by the chelating ligands.

Statement II Chelate complexes tend to be less stable.

In the light of the above statements, choose the correct answer from the options given below.

(a) Both Statement I and Statement II are false.
(b) Statement I is true Statement II is false.
(c) Statement I is false but Statement II is true.
(d) Both Statement I and Statement II are true.

76. The correct statement regarding a carbonyl compound with a hydrogen atom on its alpha carbon is

(a) a carbonyl compound with a hydrogen atom on its alpha-carbon never equilibrates with its corresponding enol.
(b) a carbonyl compound with a hydrogen atom on its alpha-carbon rapidly equilibrates with its corresponding enol and this process is known as aldehyde-ketone equilibration.
(c) a carbonyl compound with a hydrogen atom on its alpha-carbon rapidly equilibrates with its corresponding enol and this process is known as carbonylation.
(d) a carbonyl compound with a hydrogen atom on its alpha-carbon rapidly equilibrates with its corresponding enol and this process is known as keto-enol tautomerism.

77. The colour of $KMnO_4$ is purple due to

(a) *d-d* electronic transition
(b) ligand to metal charge transfer spectra
(c) metal to ligand charge transfer spectra
(d) transition of 4*s* electrons in Mn

78. The pH of ammonium phosphate solution, if pK_a of phosphoric acid and pK_b of ammonium hydroxide are 5.23 and 4.75 respectively is

(a) 7 (b) 6 (c) 5 (d) 4

79. In a first order reaction, the concentration of reactant decreases from 800 mol/dm^3 to 50 mol/dm^3 in 2×10^4 s. The rate constant (in s^{-1}) is

(a) 2×10^4 (b) 3.45×10^{-5}
(c) 1.386×10^{-4} (d) 2×10^{-4}

80. Consider the following reactions.

I. $Zn + \text{Dil. } H_2SO_4 \longrightarrow ZnSO_4 + H_2$
II. $Zn + \text{Conc. } H_2SO_4 \longrightarrow ZnSO_4 + SO_2 + H_2O$
III. $Zn + HNO_3 \longrightarrow Zn(NO_3)_2 + NH_4NO_3 + H_2O$
IV. $HCl(aq) + NaOH(aq) \longrightarrow NaCl(aq) + H_2O(l)$
V. $2HClO_4(aq) + CaCO_3(s) \longrightarrow Ca(ClO_4)_2 + H_2O(l) + CO_2(g)$

Oxidation number of hydrogen changes in

(a) I, II and III (b) I, II, III and IV
(c) I, II, III and IV (d) Only I

81. Cr^{3+} form four complexes with four different ligands which are $[Cr(Cl)_6]^{3-}$, $[Cr(H_2O)_6]^{3+}$, $[Cr(NH_3)_6]^{3+}$ and $[Cr(CN)_6]^{3-}$. The order of CFSE (Δ_o) in these complexes is

(a) $[Cr(Cl)_6]^{3-} = [Cr(H_2O)_6]^{3+} = [Cr(NH_3)_6]^{3+} = [Cr(CN)_6]^{3-}$
(b) $[Cr(Cl)_6]^{3-} < [Cr(H_2O)_6]^{3+} < [Cr(NH_3)_6]^{3+} < [Cr(CN)_6]^{3-}$
(c) $[Cr(Cl)_6]^{3-} > [Cr(H_2O)_6]^{3+} > [Cr(NH_3)_6]^{3+} < [Cr(CN)_6]^{3-}$
(d) $[Cr(Cl)_6]^{3-} < [Cr(H_2O)_6]^{3+} = [CrNH_3)_6]^{3+} < [Cr(CN)_6]^{3-}$

82. The values of standard electrode potentials of Zn^{2+}/Zn and Ag^+/Ag are -0.763 V and $+0.799$ V respectively. The standard potential of the cell is

(a) 1.56 V (b) -1.56 V (c) -0.036 V (d) $+0.036$ V

83. The specific conductance of a 0.1 N KCl solution at 23°C is 0.0112 ohm^{-1}cm^{-1}. The resistance of the cell containing the solution at the same temperature was found to be 55 ohm. The cell constant will be

(a) 0.142 cm^{-1} (b) 0.918 cm^{-1}
(c) 1.12 cm^{-1} (d) 0.616 cm^{-1}

84. What will be the product *B* in the following reaction?

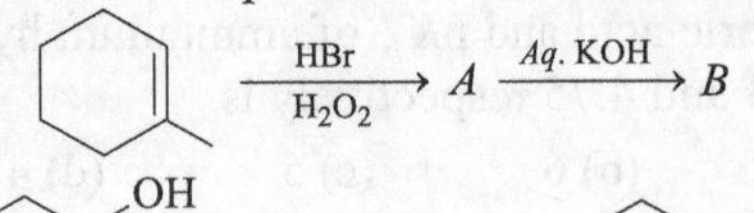

(a) 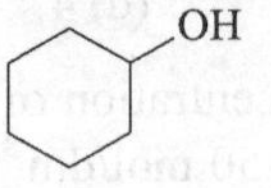 (b) 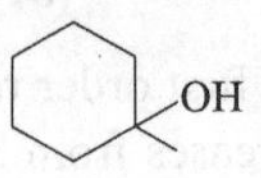

(c) 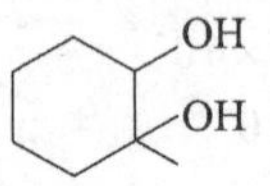 (d) 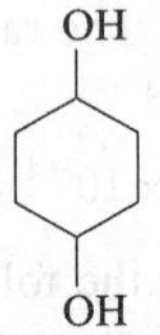

85. Which of the following compounds is square planar and does not have any unpaired electron?

(a) $[Ni(CO)_4]$ (b) $[Ni(H_2O)_6]^{2+}$
(c) $[NiCl_4]^{2-}$ (d) $[Ni(CN)_4]^{2-}$

86. Match List-I with List-II.

	List-I		List-II
A.	5.1 g of NH_3	(i)	5 N_A molecules
B.	100g H_2	(ii)	0.2 mole
C.	3.011×10^{24} molecules of CO_2	(iii)	6.72 L at STP
D.	11.2 L CH_4 gas at STP	(iv)	50 moles

Choose the correct option given below.

(a) A-(i) B-(ii) C-(iii) D-(iv)
(b) A-(iii) B-(iv) C-(i) D-(ii)
(c) A-(ii) B-(iv) C-(iii) D-(i)
(d) A-(iii) B-(iv) C-(ii) D-(i)

87. 1.2% NaCl solution is isotonic with 7.2% glucose solution. What will be the van't Hoff factor '*i*' for NaCl ?

(a) 0.5 (b) 1 (c) 2 (d) 6

88. Trichloroacetaldehyde CCl_3CHO reacts with chlorobenzene in presence of sulphuric acid to give

(a) 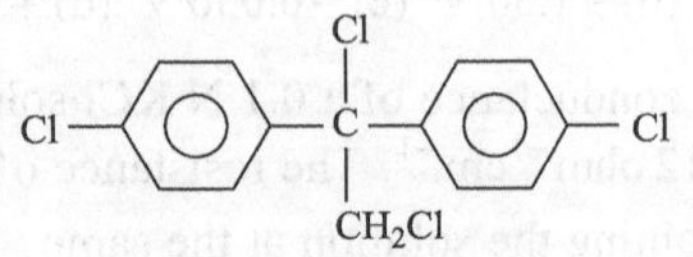

(b) 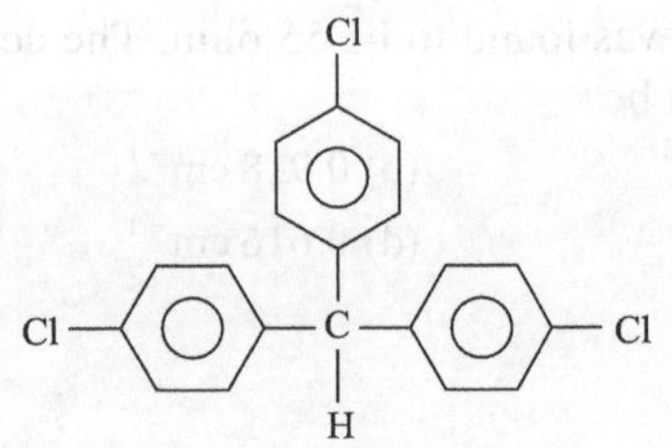

(c) 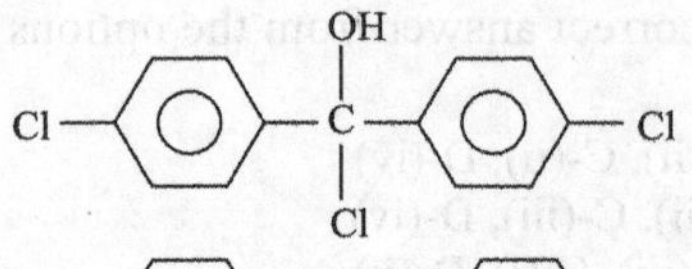

(d) 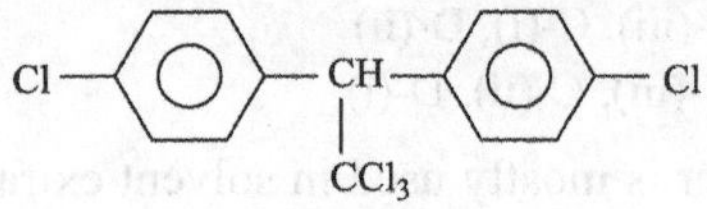

89. Given below are two statements.

Statement I Alkanes participate in substitution reaction.

Statement II Alkanes are unsaturated hydrocarbons.

In the light of the above statements, given below.

(a) Statement I is false but Statement II is true.
(b) Both Statement I and Statement II are true.
(c) Both Statement I and Statement II are false.
(d) Statement I is true but Statement II is false.

90. Match the List-I with List-II.

	List-I		List-II
A.	$CH_3-\overset{O}{\overset{\parallel}{C}}-Cl + H_2 \xrightarrow{Pd\text{-}C/BaSO_4} CH_3-\overset{O}{\overset{\parallel}{C}}-H$	(i)	HVZ reaction
B.	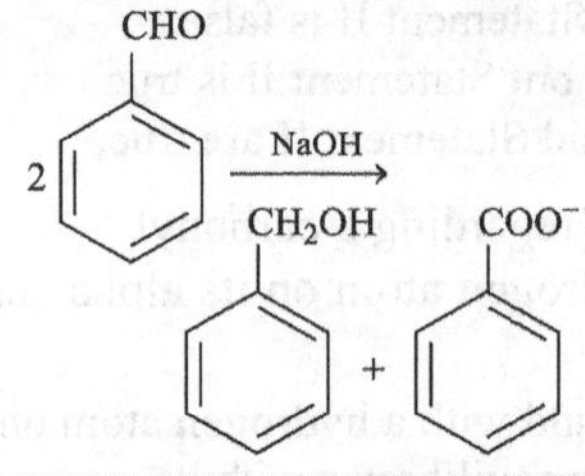	(ii)	Friedel-Crafts acylation
C.	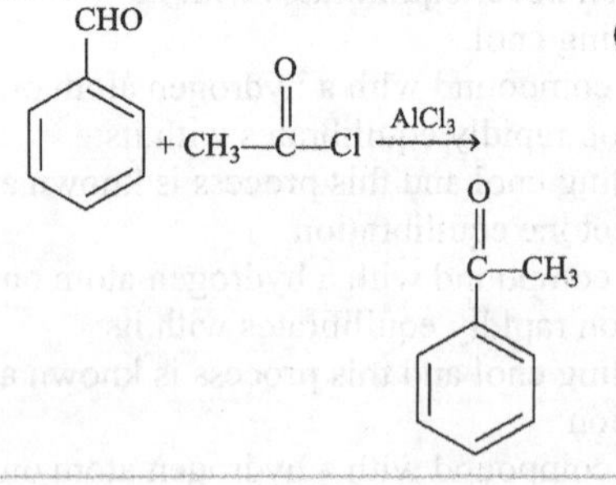	(iii)	Cannizzaro's reaction
D.	$R-CH_2-COOH \xrightarrow{Br_2/Red\ P} R-\underset{Br}{\underset{\mid}{CH}}-COOH$	(iv)	Rosenmund's reduction

Choose the correct answer from the options given below.

(a) A-(iv), B-(iii), C-(ii), D-(i)
(b) A-(i), B-(ii), C-(iii), D-(iv)
(c) A-(iv), B-(ii), C-(iii), D-(i)
(d) A-(iv), B-(iii), C-(i), D-(ii)

BIOLOGY

91. The protozoans that have a cavity (gullet) that opens to the outside of the cell surface are

(a) amoeboid (b) flagellated
(c) ciliated (d) sporozoans

92. A fatty acid has a carboxyl group attached to R group. The number of carbon atom in R group of a fatty acid may be

(a) 1 carbon to 19 carbon
(b) 2 carbon to 21 carbon
(c) 1 carbon to 20 carbon
(d) 2 carbon to 22 carbon

93. Match List I with List II.

	List I		List II
A.	pO_2 of alveoli	1.	159 mm Hg
B.	pO_2 of atmospheric air	2.	40 mm Hg
C.	pO_2 of blood (deoxygenated)	3.	95 mm Hg
D.	pO_2 of blood (oxygenated)	4.	104 mm Hg

Choose the correct answer from the options given below.

	A	B	C	D		A	B	C	D
(a)	4	2	1	3	(b)	1	2	3	4
(c)	4	1	3	2	(d)	4	1	2	3

94. The corpus callosum is a

(a) source of hypothalamic hormones
(b) neural pathway that connects the right and left hemispheres
(c) part of the neocortex
(d) structure in the cerebellum

95. Given below are, two statements.

Statement I Insulin promotes conversion of glucose to glycogen.

Statement II Insulin is secreted by α-(alpha) cells of islets of langerhans of pancreas.

In the light of the above statements, choose the correct answer from the options given below.

(a) Statement I is incorrect, but statement II is correct
(b) Both statement I and statement II are correct
(c) Both statement I and statement II are incorrect
(d) Statement I is correct, but statement II is incorrect

96. The relationship between species *X* and species *Y* is described as parasitism. This indicates that

(a) Both species derive mutual benefits like insect and pollinators
(b) Both species suffer as seen between *Plasmodium* and its vector
(c) *X* derives benefit while *Y* is harmed like lice living on human body
(d) Both *X* and *Y* compete for the same resources

97. In a flowering plant a tetraploid male plant is cross pollinated with a diploid female plant of the same angiospermic species. What would be the ploidy of endosperm and embryo developed, respectively?

(a) $5n$ and $2n$ (b) $4n$ and $3n$
(c) $3n$ and $3n$ (d) $3n$ and $2n$

98. Given below are two statements; one is labelled as Assertion (A) and the other is labelled as Reason (R).

Assertion (A) Bryophytes are also called amphibians of the plant kingdom.

Reason (R) These plants can live in soil, but are dependent on water for sexual reproduction.

In the light of the above statements, choose the correct answer from the options given below.

(a) A is false, but R is true
(b) Both A and R are true and R is the correct explanation of A
(c) Both A and R are true, but R is not the correct explanation of A
(d) A is true, but R is false

99. Given below are two statements; one is labelled as Assertion (A) and the other is labelled as Reason (R).

Assertion (A) Spermicides are effective when used along with condom or diaphragm.

Reason (R) They have high contraception efficiency even if used on their own.

In the light of the above statements, choose the correct answer form the options given below.

(a) A is false, but R is true
(b) Both A and R are true and R is the correct explanation of A.
(c) Both A and R are true, but R is not the correct explanation of A.
(d) A is true, but R is false.

100. A very low concentration of a pathogen, at a time when the symptoms of disease are not yet visible, can be detected by
(a) using enzyme linked immunosorbent assay
(b) serum and urine analysis
(c) amplification of their nucleic acid by PCR
(d) examining blood smear under microscope

101. Which of the following is incorrect for the activity of the cambium ring?
(a) The cambium is generally more active on inner side than on outer side
(b) The cells cut off towards pith, mature into secondary phloem and towards periphery mature into secondary xylem
(c) During secondary growth, amount of the secondary xylem produced is more than secondary phloem
(d) The secondary medullary rays are the narrow band of parenchyma passing through the secondary xylem and secondary phloem radially

102. Match List I with List II.

List I	List II
A. PCR	1. To make a gene
B. Antisense genes	2. To separate fragments of DNA
C. Gene synthesis	3. To stop the expression of a gene in a cell
D. Electrophoresis	4. Amplification of nucleic acid

Choose the correct answer from the options given below.

	A	B	C	D
(a)	1	2	3	4
(b)	4	2	1	3
(c)	4	3	1	2
(d)	3	2	1	4

103. The secretory granules originating from Golgi complex fuse with
(a) cell wall (b) plasmalemma
(c) vacuole (d) endoplasmic reticulum

104. Which among the following is not an application of DNA fingerprinting?
(a) It is a highly reliable method for identification of individuals involved in crime
(b) It is useful in guiding breeding programmes for endangered animals
(c) It provides information about human lineage and relationship with great apes
(d) Production of organisms which are genetically identical to their parents

105. Node of Ranvier occurs where
(a) nerve is covered with myelin sheath
(b) neurilemma is discontinuous
(c) neurilemma and myelin sheath are discontinuous
(d) myelin sheath is discontinuous

106. Proper development of the bone depends on ....
(a) thyroxine (b) epinephrine
(c) vasopressin (d) parathormone

107. A cell will not enter M-phase if
(a) cell is not sufficiently large
(b) there is lack of nutrients
(c) mitotic cyclin is overexpressed
(d) replication of DNA is not complete

108. Match List I with List II.

List I (Plant hormones)	List II (Action)
A. IAA	1. Stomatal closure
B. Gibberellins	2. Stem elongation
C. Cytokinins	3. Cell elongation
D. Abscisic acid	4. Cell division

Choose the correct answer from the options given below.

	A	B	C	D		A	B	C	D
(a)	3	2	4	1	(b)	1	2	3	4
(c)	4	3	2	1	(d)	2	4	1	3

109. Choose the incorrect statement.
(a) Tetany in muscle is due to low Ca^{2+} in body fluid
(b) Repeated stimulation of muscles leads to fatigue
(c) Muscular dystrophy is an autoimmune disorder
(d) Gout is an inherited disorder of purine metabolism

110. Identify the incorrect statement.
(a) Atrial natriuretic factor works opposite to RA mechanism
(b) The colour of urine is dependent upon the pigment urochrome
(c) Deamination is the removal of amine group from amino acids
(d) Nephritis is an inflammation of the urinary bladder

111. Match List I with List II.

List I		List II
A. Chasmogamous	1.	Transfer of pollen grains from anther to the stigma of a different plant.
B. Cleistogamous	2.	Transfer of pollen grains from anther to the stigma of another flower of the same plant.
C. Geitonogamy	3.	Flowers with exposed anthers and stigma.
D. Xenogamy	4.	Flowers in which anther stigma lie close to each other.

Choose the correct answer from the options given below.

	A	B	C	D
(a)	4	1	2	3
(b)	3	4	1	2
(c)	4	3	2	1
(d)	3	4	2	1

112. Which statement is incorrect for a food web?

(a) Network of food chains which interlink different trophic levels in an ecosystem is food web
(b) It provides stability to ecosystem
(c) It helps in the survival of top carnivores
(d) Energy flow is same to the organism sharing two trophic levels

113. In *lac* operon, the genes *a*, *i*, *y* and *z* code respectively for

(a) permease, transacetylase, repressor protein, β-galactosidase
(b) transacetylase, represssor protein, permease, β-galactosidase
(c) repressor protein, permease, β-galactosidase, transacetylase
(d) transacetylase, permease, β-galactosidase, repressor protein

114. Match List I with List II.

List I		List II
A. Man	1.	Sapindales
B. Housefly	2.	Poales
C. Mango	3.	Primata
D. Wheat	4.	Diptera

Choose the correct answer from the options given below.

	A	B	C	D		A	B	C	D
(a)	3	4	1	2	(b)	4	1	3	2
(c)	2	3	1	4	(d)	3	1	2	4

115. Read the following statements and choose the correct set of statements.

I. Apical meristems occur at the tips of roots and shoots and produce primary tissues.
II. Shoot apical meristem occupies closest region of the stem axis.
III. The meristem which occurs between mature tissues is known as intercalary meristem.
IV. Secondary meristem occurs in the mature regions of roots and shoots and produce woody axis.
V. Fascicular cambium, interfascicular cambium and cork cambium are the examples of intercalary meristem.

Choose the correct answer from the options given below.

(a) I, III and V
(b) I, II and IV
(c) III, IV and V
(d) I, III and IV

116. Identify the incorrectly matched pair.

(a) Dairy - *Lactobacillus*
(b) Vinegar industry - *Acetobacter aceti*
(c) Alcohol industry - *Clostridium acetobutylicum*
(d) Roquefort cheese - *Propionibacterium sharmanii*

117. Which of the following phytohormones is used for early maturity and seed production in juvenile conifers?

(a) Gibberellin
(b) Ethylene
(c) Auxin
(d) Cytokinin

118. Given below are two statements.

Statement I Selectable marker helps to select the host cells which contain the vector and eliminate the non-transformants.

Statement II For transformation with recombinant DNA, the bacterial cells must be first made competent to decrease their metabolic reaction.

In the light of the above statement, choose the correct answer from the options below.

(a) Statement I is incorrect, but statement II is correct
(b) Both statement I and statement II are correct
(c) Both statement I and statement II are incorrect
(d) Statement I is correct, but statement II is incorrect

119. In cell membrane peripheral proteins
(a) lie on the surface of membrane
(b) lie in the matrix of membrane
(c) buried in the membrane
(d) lie in between the membranes

120. Which one of the following is correct statement regarding the particular psychotropic drug specified?
(a) Barbiturates cause relaxation and temporary euphoria
(b) Hashish causes after thought perceptions and hallucinations
(c) Opium stimulates nervous system and causes hallucinations
(d) Morphine leads to delusions and disturbed emotions

121. Read the following statements.
I. ABO blood group types are an example of multiple alleles.
II. ABO blood group was discovered by Karl Landsteiner
III. Offspring with all four kinds of blood groups are possible in a cross between two parents homozygous for blood group A.
IV. Both I^A and I^B are dominant over i.
V. Person with genotype I^AI^B have both antibodies
Which of the above statements are incorrect ?
(a) I and III (b) III and V
(c) III and IV (d) II and III

122. Which of the following represents the correct sequence of human evolution?
(a) *Homo habilis* → *Homo neanderthalensis* → *Australopithecus* → *Homo erectus* → Cro-Magnon → *Homo sapiens*
(b) *Australopithecus* → *Homo neanderthalensis* → *Homo habilis* → *Homo erectus* → Cro-Magnon → *Homo sapiens*
(c) *Australopithecus* → *Homo habilis* → *Homo neanderthalensis* → *Homo erectus* → Cro-Magnon → *Homoapiens*
(d) *Australopithecus* → *Homo habilis* → *Homo erectus* → *Homo neanderthalensis* → Cro-Magnon

123. Given below are two statements.
Statement I In fermentation, there is a net gain of only two molecules of ATP for each molecule of glucose degraded into pyruvic acid.
Statement II If fatty acids are to be respired, they are first degraded into acetyl Co-A.
In the light of the above statement, choose the correct answer from the optins given below
(a) Statement I is incorrect, but statement II is correct
(b) Both statement I and statement II are correct
(c) Both statement I and statement II are incorrect
(d) Statement I is correct, but statement II is incorrect

124. Read the following statements and identify the incorrect statement.
I. In mustard plant, secondary roots and its branches constitute the tap root system.
II. In monocot plants, the primary root is short lived and replaced by the fibrous root system.
III. In *Monstera* and grasses, roots arise from parts of plant other than the radicle and are called stilt roots.
IV. The main functions of the root system are only absorption of water and minerals from the soil.
V. In sweet potato, adventitious roots get swollen and store the food material.
Choose the correct answer from the options given below.
(a) I and IV
(b) III and V
(c) I and III
(d) I, III and IV

125. Which of the following pairs is incorrectly matched ?
(a) Corpus luteum - Progesterone
(b) Morula - Transforms into blastocyst
(c) Acrosomal reaction - Zona pellucida
(d) Colostrum - Mammary gland

126. Which method is used when there are only a very few cells available, such as fertilised egg cells ?
(a) Heat shock
(b) Treatment with divalent cation
(c) Gene gun
(d) Microinjection

127. Given below are two statements.
Statement I Stroma lamellae membranes possess PS-I only, whereas grana lamellae membranes possess both PS-I and PS-II.
Statement II PS-II is involved in both cyclic and non-cyclic photophosphorylation.

In the light of the above statements, choose the correct answer from the options given below
(a) Statement I is incorrect, but statement II is correct
(b) Both statement I and statement II are correct
(c) Both statement I and statement II are incorrect
(d) Statement I is correct, but statement II is incorrect

128. Which of the following pair of plants prevent both autogamy and geitonogamy?
(a) Papaya and date palm
(b) Castor and maize
(c) Papaya and maize
(d) Date palm and castor

129. Given below are two statements; one is labelled as Assertion (A) and the other is labelled as Reason (R).
Assertion (A) Dinoflagellates have left behind large amount of cell wall deposits in their habitat.
Reason (R) Diatoms have cell walls that are indestructible.
In the light of the above statements, choose the correct answer from the options given below.
(a) A is false, but R is true
(b) Both A and R are true and R is the correct explanation of A
(c) Both A and R are true, but R is not the correct explanation of A
(d) A is true, but R is false

130. Read the following statements and choose the incorrect option.
(a) Grave's disease is due to hypersecretion of thyroxine
(b) Cretinism is due to hypersecretion of thyroxine.
(c) Acromegaly is due to hypersecretion of parathyroid
(d) Diabetes mellitus is caused due to hyposecretion of insulin

131. Study the given figure.

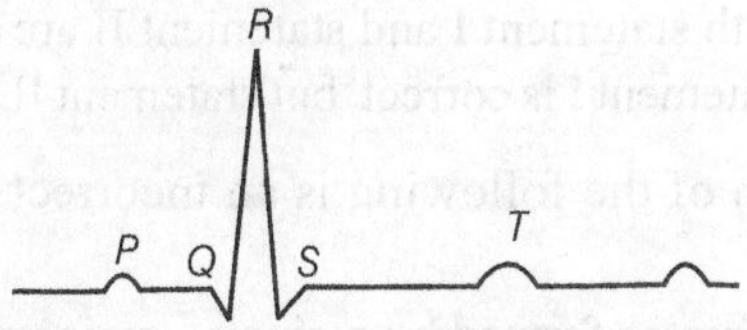

Which part of the figure can determine the heartbeat rate of the individual?
(a) P wave (b) T wave
(c) QRS complex (d) ST segment

132. Match List I with List II.

List I	List II
A. Grave's disease	1. β-cells (pancreas)
B. Irregular menstrual cycle	2. Hypothyroidism
C. Type I diabetes mellitus	3. Overactive thyroid
D. Addison's disease	4. Adrenal cortex

Choose the correct answer from the options given below.

	A	B	C	D
(a)	1	2	3	4
(b)	3	2	1	4
(c)	4	3	2	1
(d)	2	1	4	3

133. Which among the following does not come under the factors affecting primary productivity?
(a) Environmental factor
(b) Nutrients availability
(c) Photosynthetic efficiency of plants
(d) Leaching

134. Which of the following events does not take place during the mitotic prophase?
(a) Disappearance of nuclear envelope
(b) Nucleolar disaggregation
(c) DNA replication
(d) Coiling of chromosome

135. Consider the following statements.
I. During photosynthesis, the membrane system is responsible for the trapping the light energy and also for the synthesis of ATP and NADPH.
II. In stroma, enzymatic reactions synthesise starch, which in turn forms carbohydrates.
III. Chlorophyll *a* and *c* are the primary photosynthetic pigments present in plants
IV. In PS-I, the reaction centre chlorophyll *a* has an absorption peak at 700 nm.
V. The splitting of water is associated with the PSI, and water is split into $4H^+$, [O] and electrons
Choose the set of correct statements from the options given below.
(a) I, III, II
(b) II, III, V
(c) I, IV, V
(d) I, III, IV

136. High copy number in a vector
(a) provides more replicates of inserted DNA sequences in the cell
(b) aids in easy transformation to the host cells
(c) aids in easy isolation and purification
(d) has small size of low molecular weight for enhanced stability

137. Given below are two statements.
Statement I Genetic diversity comprises of different type of gene in same species as well as different type of species.
Statement II Amphibian species diversity is more in Eastern Ghats than the Western Ghats.
In the light of the above statement, choose the correct answer from the options given below.
(a) Statement I is incorrect, but statement II is correct
(b) Both statement I and statement II are correct
(c) Both statement I and statement II are incorrect
(d) Statement I is correct, but statement II is incorrect

138. Which statement is correct about passive immunity?
(a) Acquired through first exposure to the disease
(b) Achieved directly through readymade antibodies
(c) Inherited from parents
(d) Achieved through vaccination

139. Read the following statements with respect to Ti plasmid and identify the incorrect statement.
I. *Agrobacterium tumefaciens*, a pathogen of monocot plants is able to deliver T-DNA.
II. T-DNA transforms normal plant cells into a tumour and direct these cells to produce chemicals required by pathogens.
III. *A. tumefaciens* vectors are used for silencing nematode gene.
IV. *A. tumefaciens* has now been modified to a cloning vector which is still pathogenic to the plants.
V. Introduction of *Agrobacterium* vectors produces both antisense and sense RNA in the host cells.
Choose the correct answer from the option given below.
(a) I, II and III
(b) II and IV
(c) I and III
(d) I and IV

140. Families in plant kingdoms are characterised based on which of the following features ?
(a) Seasonal similarities and variations
(b) Anatomy of various parts
(c) External morphology
(d) Vegetative and reproductive parts

141. Match List I with List II.

List I	List II
(A) Terpenoides	1. Cotton
(B) Lectins	2. Concanavalin A
(C) Morphine	3. Alkaloid
(D) Cellulose	4. Diterpenes

Choose the correct answer from the options given below.

	A	B	C	D
(a)	2	4	3	1
(b)	2	3	4	1
(c)	4	2	3	1
(d)	1	3	4	2

142. A women with blood group 'A' marries a man with, blood group 'B'. The possibility of blood group AB in their children will be
(a) 0% (b) 50%
(c) 75% (d) 25%

143. Given below are two statements.
Statement I On reaching the Fallopian tube the spermatozoan undergoes some changes.
Statement II Fertilised ovum first divides into two cells by horizontal division.
In the light of the above statement, choose the correct statement from the options given below.
(a) Statement I is incorrect, but statement II is correct
(b) Both statement I and statement II are correct
(c) Both statement I and statement II are incorrect
(d) Statement I is correct, but statement II is incorrect

144. Which of the following is an incorrect match pair ?
(a) Gametes formed by meiosis - meiocytes
(b) Separation of chromatids and centromere - meiosis-II
(c) DNA duplication - S-phase
(d) Best stage to observe chromosome morphology and number - Interphase

145. Which one of the following shows the advantage of cleistogamy in flowers?
(a) Each visit of a pollinator results in transfer of hundreds of pollen grains
(b) Seed set is not dependent on pollinators
(c) Cleistogamy leads to greater genetic diversity
(d) Seed dispersal is more efficient and widespread

146. Read the following statements.
I. All the Ctenophores are exclusively fresh water.
II. Ctenophores are also known as comb jellies or sea walnuts.
III. They are Pseudocoelomate organisms.
IV. Digestion is both extracelluar and intracellular.
V. Nervous system is absent.
Which of the above statements with respect to ctenophores are correct ?
(a) II and IV (b) I and V
(c) III and IV (d) II and III

147. Which part of the brain controls the urge for eating and is important for enjoyment of life?
(a) Cerebrum (b) Hypothalamus
(c) Medulla (d) Pons

148. Main steps in the life cycle of HIV are given below. Arrange these steps in a correct sequence.
A. The progeny viruses released in the blood attack other helper T-lymphocytes.
B. RNA genome of virus replicates to form viral DNA with the help of reverse transcriptase.
C. The viral DNA gets incorporated into host cell's (macrophages and helper T-lymphocytes) DNA and directs the infected cells to produce virus DNA.
D. Progressive decrease in the number of helper T-lymphocytes in the body of infected person results in decline of cell mediated immunity.
Choose the correct answer from the options given below.
(a) B, A, C, D (b) B, C, A, D
(c) B, A, D, C (d) B, D, C, A

149. A graphic representation of energy flow from one trophic level to next is shaped like a pyramid because
(a) organisms at each level store most of the energy
(b) there are more producers than primary consumers
(c) eventually organisms die as they age
(d) most energy at each level is lost, leaving little for the next level

150. Which among the following statements is incorrect regarding gynoecium?
(a) It is made up of one or more carpels
(b) Stigma is the receptive surface for the pollen grains
(c) In lotus and rose, carpels are fused and are termed as syncarpous
(d) After fertilisation, the ovules develop into seeds and the ovary matures into fruit

151. The diagram given below is a schematic (Photosynthesis) representation of the Calvin cycle.

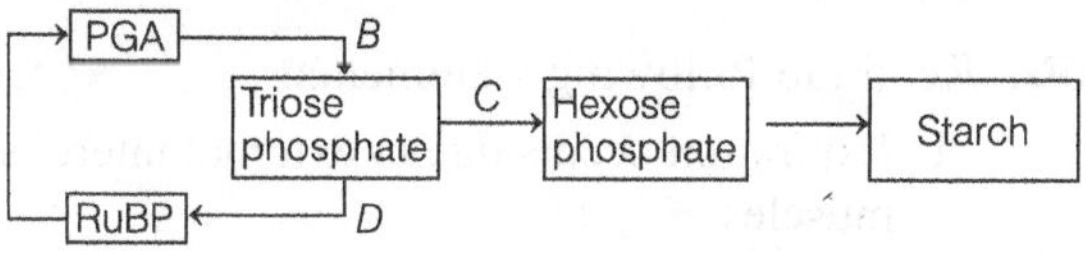

At which of the given stage, does CO_2 get incorporated?
(a) *B* (b) *A*
(c) *D* (d) *C*

152. Which of the following correctly defines amphibian heart?
(a) Two auricles and one ventricle
(b) Two auricles and two ventricles
(c) One auricle and two ventricles
(d) One auricle and one ventricle.

153. A group of compactly arranged homogenous cells called sporogenous tissue occupies the centre of each microsporangium. The cells of the sporogenous tissue undergo
(a) mitotic divisions to form microspores
(b) meiotic divisions to form microspore tetrads
(c) two mitotic divisions to form microspore tetrad
(d) karyokinesis to form many nuclei

154. Match List I with List II.

List I	List II
A. *Trichoderma polysporum*	1. Citric acid
B. *Aspergillus niger*	2. Ethanol
C. *Clostridium butylicium*	3. Cyclosporin-A
D. Yeast	4. Butyric acid

Choose the correct answer from the options given below.

	A	B	C	D
(a)	3	1	4	2
(b)	1	2	3	4
(c)	4	3	2	1
(d)	2	4	1	3

155. The lining of stomach is made up of
(a) ciliated epithelium
(b) simple columnar epithelium
(c) stratified squamous epithelium
(d) simple cuboidal epithelium

156. Read the following statements.
I. Expiration occurs due to external intercostal muscles.
II. Intrapulmonary pressure is higher than the atmospheric pressure during inspiration.
III. Inspiration occurs when atmospheric pressure is less than intrapulmonary pressure.
IV. Expiration is initiated due to contraction of diaphragm.
V. To increase the strength of inspiration, abdominal muscle relax, allowing further compression of abdominal organs by diaphragm.

Which of the above statements is /are correct?
(a) I, II and III (b) V only
(c) II and III (d) I, IV and V

157. Which of the following steps of krebs' cycle yield CO_2?
(a) Isocitric acid – Oxalosuccinic acid
(b) Isocitrate – α-ketoglutaric acid
(c) Succinic acid – Fumaric acid
(d) Malic acid – Oxalo acetic acid

158. The rate of decomposition is slower if
(a) detritus is rich in lignin
(b) detritus is rich in nitrogen
(c) detritus is rich in sugars
(d) detritus is rich in cellulose

159. Given below are two statements.

Statement I The opening between the right atrium and right ventricle is guarded by a valve formed of two muscular flaps/cusps, the bicuspid valve.

Statement II The valves in the heart allow the flow of blood only in one direction, i.e. from the atria to the ventricles and from the ventricles to the pulmonary artery or aorta.

In the light of the above statements, choose the correct answer from the options given below.
(a) Statement I is incorrect, but statement II is correct
(b) Both statement I and statement II are correct
(c) Both statement I and statement II are incorrect
(d) Statement I is correct, but statement II is incorrect

160. Consider the following statements regarding DNA fingerprinting.
I. VNTRs are also known as minisatellites.
II. The technique identifies a person on the basis of person's DNA specificity.
III. VNTRs are used as genetic markers.
IV. VNTRs are dissimilar in monozygotic twins.

The incorrect statement(s) is/are
(a) I and III (b) III and II
(c) Only III (d) Only IV

161. Match List I with List II.

	List I		List II
A.	Rivet popper hypothesis	1.	Paul Ehrlich
B.	Communities with more species	2.	Edward Wilson
C.	Communities with less species	3.	Less stable
D.	Term biodiversity	4.	More stable

Choose the correct answer from the options given below.

	A	B	C	D
(a)	1	4	3	2
(b)	2	4	3	1
(c)	1	3	4	2
(d)	1	4	2	3

162. Read the following statement and identify which is incorrect.
I. Back cross is the cross of the hybrids of F_1- generation with either of its parents.
II. Test cross is the cross of the individuals with its heterozygous dominant parent.
III. Law of segregation is based on the fact that the alleles do not show any blending and both the characters are recovered.
IV. Boveri coined the term linkage to describe physical association of genes on a chromosome.

V. Dominance is an autonomous feature of a gene.
Choose the correct answer from the options given below.
(a) I and IV (b) III and V
(c) II, IV and V (d) Only V

163. ________ has haploid number of chromosomes.
(a) Spermatogonium
(b) Primary oocyte
(c) Spermatozoa
(d) Primary spermatocytes

164. Immunity is a state of protection from foreign molecules. It is of two types, i.e. innate and adaptive immunity. Specificity, diversity, memory are characteristics of
(a) innate immunity (b) non-specific immunity
(c) acquired immunity (d) external defence

165. Find the odd one out in the given list.
I. Multiload 375 II. LNG-20
III. Lippes loop IV. Cervical cap
V. Progestasert
Choose the correct option.
(a) Only V (b) Only IV
(c) IV and V (d) III, IV and V

166. The occurrence of haemophilia is more likely in human males compared to females because
(a) females are heterogametic
(b) females can only be carriers
(c) the haemophilic allele is present only on X-chromosome
(d) the haemophilic allele is present only on Y-chromosome

167. Darwinism explained all the following, except that
(a) within each species, there are variations
(b) organism tend to produce more number of offspring that can survive
(c) offspring with better traits that over come competition are best suited for the environment
(d) variations are inherited from parents to offspring through genes

168. Which of the following organisms has been commercially utilised as blood cholesterol lowering agent?
(a) *Clostridium butylicum*
(b) *Saccharomyces cerevisiae*
(c) *Monascus purpureus*
(d) *Pseudomonas putida*

169. Match List I with List II.

List I (Reproductive organ)	List II (Characteristic)
A. Protonema	1. Vegetative propagation
B. Antheridium	2. Male sex organ
C. Archegonium	3. Female sex organ
D. Sporophyll	4. Bears sporangia

Choose the correct answer from the options given below.

	A	B	C	D		A	B	C	D
(a)	1	2	3	4	(b)	2	1	3	4
(c)	1	2	4	3	(d)	2	1	4	3

170. The most effective means of conserving biodiversity is
(a) getting rid of predators
(b) census species during breeding season
(c) preserving habitats
(d) shifting species to safer places

171. Given below are two statements.
Statement I Cardiac muscles taper at both ends and do not show striations.
Statement II Cardiac muscle tissues contract and relax throughout life and never get fatigued.
In the light of the above statements, choose the correct answer from the options given below
(a) Statement I is incorrect, but statement II is correct
(b) Both statement I and statement II are correct
(c) Both statement I and statement II are incorrect
(d) Statement I is correct, but statement II is incorrect

172. Which among the following is/are correctly matched regarding age pyramid ?
(a) Young population pyramid - Pyramid with broad base
(b) Stable population - Urn-shaped pyramid
(c) Declining population - Bell-shaped pyramid
(d) More post reproductive individuals - Inverted pyramid

173. Identify the correct statement w.r.t the blood vessels.

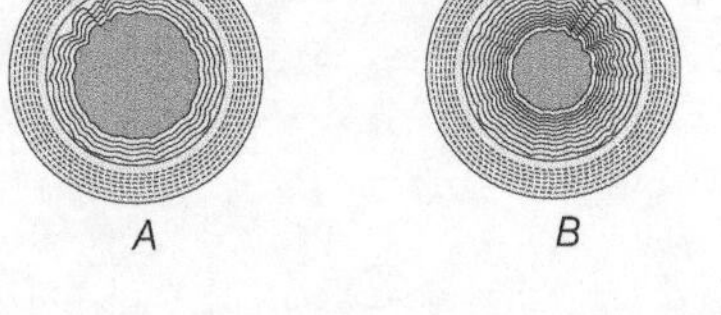

(a) *A* represents veins that carry deoxygenated blood from the body back to the heart.
(b) Blood flows with considerable pressure in *A* which has thick tunica media.
(c) *B* represents veins that allow fast and intermittent blood flow.
(d) *B* do not possess valves to prevent blood flow.

174. Identify the incorrect statement.
(a) In Arthropoda, jointed appendages help in locomotion
(b) Radula for feeding are present in mollusca
(c) Water vascular system is present in Echinodermata
(d) Roundworm is an example of Platyhelminthes

175. Match List I with List II.

	List I		List II
A.	DNA ligase	1.	Adenylate residues
B.	Tailing	2.	*r*RNA
C.	RNA polymerase-I	3.	Removal of introns
D.	Splicing	4.	To join the cuts in DNA.

Choose the correct answer from the options given below.

	A	B	C	D		A	B	C	D
(a)	4	1	2	3	(b)	4	1	3	2
(c)	1	2	4	3	(d)	2	4	3	1

176. Convolvulaceae and Solanaceae are kept under order–Polymoniales because they have similar
(a) vegetative characters
(b) natural distribution
(c) floral characters
(d) leaf characters

177. The only living element of the xylem tissue is
(a) vessels (b) tracheids
(c) xylem fibre (d) xylem parenchyma

178. Read the following statements carefully and identify the correct statements.
I. Whales, bats, cheetah share similarities in the pattern of bones of forelimbs.
II. Analogous structures are a result of divergent evolution.
III. Karl Ernst von Baer noted that embryos never pass through the adult stages of other animals.
IV. Homology indicates common ancestry.
V. Sweet potato and potato is an example of homology.

Choose the correct answer from the options given below.
(a) I, II and IV (b) I, II and V
(c) I, II, IV and V (d) I, III and IV

179. Given below are two statements.
Statement I The individual suffering from Klinefelter syndrome has masculine development and gynaecomastia.
Statement II Teenagers who suffer from klinefelter's are shorter than average stature, have weak bones and short legs.
In the light of the above statements, choose the correct answer from the options given below.
(a) Statement I is incorrect, but statement II is correct
(b) Both statement I and statement II are correct
(c) Both statement I and statement II are incorrect
(d) Statement I is correct, but statement II is incorrect

180. Given below are two statements; one is labelled as Assertion (A) and the other is labelled as Reason (R).
Assertion (A) Cilia facilitates the passage of ova through the female reproductive tract.
Reason (R) Ciliary movement helps us in removing waste substances inhaled.
In the light of the above statements, choose the correct answer form the options given below.
(a) A is false, but R is true
(b) Both A and R are true and R is the correct explanation of A
(c) Both A and R are true, but R is not the correct explanation of A
(d) A is true, but R is false

Explanations

Physics

1. (b) According to kinetic theory of gases, the pressure exerted by the gas,

$$p = \frac{1}{3} \times \frac{mn}{V} v^2$$

$$\Rightarrow \quad p \propto mv^2 \text{ and } p' \propto \left(\frac{m}{2}\right)(2v)^2$$

$$\therefore \quad \frac{p'}{p} = 2 \Rightarrow p' = 2p$$

2. (d) Given, Least Count,

$$(\text{LC}) = 0.1\,\text{mm} = 10^{-4}\,\text{m}$$

$$\text{Zero error} = 6 \times \text{LC} = 0.6\,\text{mm}$$
$$= 6 \times 10^{-4}\,\text{m}$$

Reading

$$= \text{MSR} + \text{VSR} \times \text{LC} - \text{zero error}$$
$$= [32\,\text{mm} + (0.1) \times 4\,\text{mm}] - 0.6\,\text{mm}$$
$$= 31.8\,\text{mm} = 3.18\,\text{cm}$$

3. (c) Shunt resistance,

$$S = \frac{I_g G}{I - I_g} \Rightarrow I - I_g = \frac{I_g G}{S}$$

$$\frac{I}{I_g} - 1 = \frac{G}{S} = \frac{35}{3.5} = 10$$

$$\frac{I}{I_g} = 11 \Rightarrow \frac{I_g}{I} = \frac{1}{11}$$

4. (d) $R = 40 + 20 = 60\,\Omega$

$$\text{Power factor} = \frac{R}{\sqrt{R^2 + (X_L - X_C)^2}}$$

$$= \frac{60}{\sqrt{60^2 + (100 - 20)^2}} = 0.6$$

5. (a) Equivalent circuit is shown below

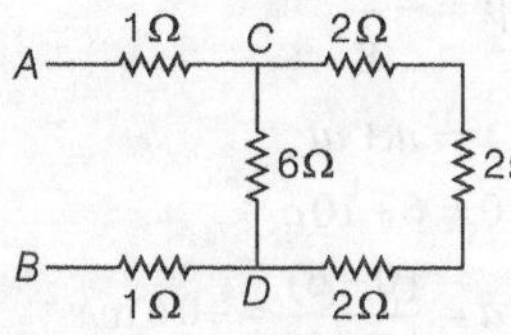

Here, $2\,\Omega$ resistors are in series combination.

$$\therefore \quad R = 2 + 2 + 2 = 6\,\Omega$$

R and $6\,\Omega$ are in parallel combination.

$$\therefore \quad R_{CD} = \frac{6 \times 6}{6 + 6}\,\Omega$$

$$\text{So,} \quad R_{AB} = 1 + 1 + \left(\frac{6 \times 6}{6 + 6}\right)$$
$$= 5\,\Omega$$

6. (a) Given, $m = 3.513$ kg

$$v = 5.00\,\text{ms}^{-1}$$

$\therefore$ Momentum of moving body,

$$p = mv$$
$$= 3.513 \times 5.00$$
$$= 17.565\,\text{kg ms}^{-1}$$

7. (c) Suppose the length of wire is l.

Ist case $\quad l = 2\pi r \Rightarrow r = \frac{l}{2\pi}$

$$\therefore \quad B = \frac{n\mu_0 I}{2r} = \frac{\mu_0 \pi I}{l} \qquad [\because n = 1] \ldots \text{(i)}$$

IInd case

$$l = 4(2\pi r') \Rightarrow r' = \frac{l}{8\pi}$$

$$\therefore \quad B' = \frac{n\mu_0 I}{2r'} = \frac{4\mu_0 I}{2(l/8\pi)} \qquad [\because n = 4]$$

$$= \frac{16\mu_0 \pi I}{l}$$

$$B' = 16B \Rightarrow \frac{B'}{B} = 16:1 \qquad \text{[using Eq. (i)]}$$

Problem Solving Tactics

If a current carrying circular loop is turned into a coil having n turns, then magnetic field at the centre of loop becomes $(B)_{n\,\text{turn}} = n^2 B_{(\text{circular loop})}$

8. (d) To create a hole, an electron of valence band has to be excited into one of the acceptor levels which are 50 meV above the valence band. Hence, a minimum of 50 meV energy is needed to create a hole.

$$\text{As} \quad E_{\min} = \frac{hc}{\lambda_{\max}}$$

$$\therefore \quad \lambda_{\max} = \frac{hc}{E_{\min}}$$

$$= \frac{6.6 \times 10^{-34} \times 3 \times 10^8}{50 \times 10^{-3} \times 1.6 \times 10^{-19}}$$

$$= 2.47 \times 10^{-5}\,\text{m}$$

9. (a) Surface energy, $E = T\times 2A$

New surface energy,

$$E' = T\times 2\left(\frac{3}{4}A\right) = \frac{3}{2}TA$$

Percentage decrease in $E = \frac{E-E'}{E}\times 100 = 25\%$

10. (b) The radius and velocity vectors of the planet are mutually perpendicular at any point, then the angular momentum at point P is $L_P = m_P r_P v_P$

Similarly, at point A is $L_A = m_P r_A v_A$

By conservation of angular momentum,

$$L_P = L_A \Rightarrow r_P v_P = r_A v_A$$

or $\quad \frac{v_P}{v_A} = \frac{r_A}{r_P}$

As, $\quad r_A > r_P$

So, $\quad v_P > v_A$

11. (b) It is given that,

$$\frac{I_2}{I_1} = n \Rightarrow I_2 = nI_1$$

$\therefore$ Ratio of intensities is given by

$$\frac{I_{\max}-I_{\min}}{I_{\max}+I_{\min}} = \frac{(\sqrt{I_2}+\sqrt{I_1})^2-(\sqrt{I_2}-\sqrt{I_1})^2}{(\sqrt{I_1}+\sqrt{I_2})^2+(\sqrt{I_2}-\sqrt{I_1})^2}$$

$$= \frac{\left(\sqrt{\frac{I_2}{I_1}}+1\right)^2-\left(\sqrt{\frac{I_2}{I_1}}-1\right)^2}{\left(\sqrt{\frac{I_2}{I_1}}+1\right)^2+\left(\sqrt{\frac{I_2}{I_1}}-1\right)^2}$$

$$= \frac{(\sqrt{n}+1)^2-(\sqrt{n}-1)^2}{(\sqrt{n}+1)^2+(\sqrt{n}-1)^2} = \frac{2\sqrt{n}}{n+1}$$

12. (b) Draw v-t curve

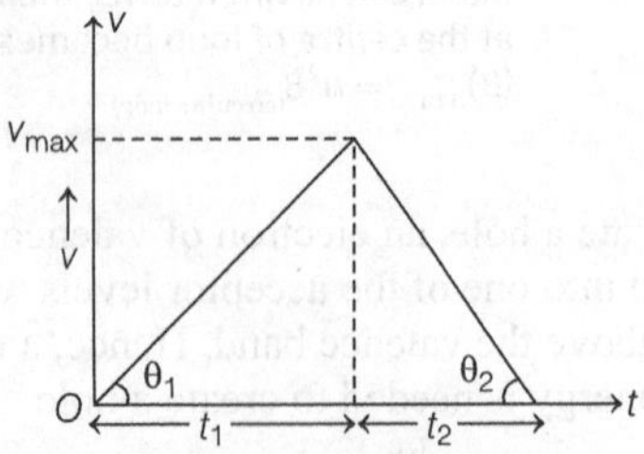

$$\tan\theta_1 = a_1 = \frac{v_{\max}}{t_1} \quad \dots\text{(i)}$$

and $$\tan\theta_2 = a_2 = \frac{v_{\max}}{t_2} \quad \dots\text{(ii)}$$

Dividing Eq. (ii) by Eq. (i), we get $\frac{t_1}{t_2} = \frac{a_2}{a_1}$

13. (c) Speed of sound in brass rod,

$$v = \sqrt{\frac{Y}{\rho}} = \sqrt{\frac{10^{12}}{9}} = \frac{10^6}{3}\text{ cm s}^{-1}$$

Length of rod, $L = 1\text{ m} = 100\text{ cm}$

Frequency of note, $\nu = \frac{v}{\lambda} = \frac{v}{2L}$

$$= \frac{10^6}{3\times 2\times 100} = 1666.67\text{ Hz}$$

14. (d) Time period, $T \propto n^3$

$$\therefore \quad \frac{T_2}{T_3} = \frac{(2)^3}{(3)^3}$$

$$T_3 = \frac{27T_2}{8}$$

$$= \frac{27}{8}\times 4\times 10^{-16}$$

$$= 1.35\times 10^{-15}\text{ s}$$

15. (c) As, wave intensity,

$$I = \frac{P_{av}}{4\pi r^2} = \frac{E^2_{\max}}{2\mu_0 c}$$

$$\Rightarrow \quad E_{\max} = \sqrt{\frac{\mu_0 c P_{av}}{2\pi r^2}}$$

$$= \sqrt{\frac{(4\pi\times 10^{-7})(3\times 10^8)(3)}{2\pi(0.30)^2}}$$

$$= 44.7\text{ V/m}$$

$$\simeq 45\text{ V/m}$$

16. (d) Rotational energy is minimum when moment of inertia is minimum. If the distance of point is x from mass 0.5 kg, then

$$I = 0.5x^2 + 1.5(2.5-x)^2$$

Now, for minimum value of I, $\frac{dI}{dx} = 0$

$$\Rightarrow \quad x + 3(2.5-x)(-1) = 0$$

$$\Rightarrow \quad x = 1.875\text{ m}$$

17. (a) $\quad F = ma$

$$\therefore \quad -\mu mg = ma$$

$$\Rightarrow \quad \mu = -\frac{a}{g}$$

$$\because \quad v = u + at$$

$$\Rightarrow \quad 0 = 6 + 10a$$

$$\Rightarrow \quad a = \frac{(0-6)}{10} = -0.6\text{ m/s}^2$$

$$\therefore \quad \mu = \frac{0.6}{10} = 0.06$$

18. (d) We know that,

$$E = h\nu$$

$$\Rightarrow \quad h = \frac{E}{\nu} = ET \qquad \left[\because \nu = \frac{1}{T}\right]$$

$$\therefore \quad [h] = [E][T] = [ML^2T^{-2}][T] = [ML^2T^{-1}]$$

Momentum, $p = mv$

$$\therefore \quad [p] = [m][v] = [M][LT^{-1}] = [MLT^{-1}] \qquad \left[\because v = \frac{L}{T}\right]$$

Thus, momentum and Planck's constant do not have same dimensions.

19. (d) Parallel combination of capacitors is used when we require a large capacitance at a small potential.

In this combination.

$$C_{eq} = C_1 + C_2 + C_3 + \ldots.. C_n$$

Here, $C_1 = C_2 = C_3 = \ldots.. C_n = C$

$$\therefore \quad C_{eq} = C + C + C + \ldots\ldots + C = nC$$

20. (b) We know that, PE = − 2KE

$$\Rightarrow \quad -27.2 = -2KE$$

$$\Rightarrow \quad KE = 13.6\,eV$$

21. (c) From law of conservation of energy,

$$\frac{1}{2}Mv^2 = \frac{1}{2}kL^2 \Rightarrow v = \sqrt{\frac{k}{M}} \cdot L$$

Maximum momentum,

$$p = Mv = M\sqrt{\frac{k}{M}} \cdot L = \sqrt{Mk} \cdot L$$

22. (c) Resistance, $R = \dfrac{\text{Voltage drop } (V)}{\text{Current } (I)}$

Current, $I = \dfrac{P}{V} = \dfrac{140 \times 10^{-3}}{0.7} = 0.2\,A$

$$R = \frac{1.5 - 0.7}{0.2} = \frac{0.8}{0.2} = 4\,\Omega$$

23. (c) $v = v_0 + gt + ft^2$

$$\Rightarrow \quad \frac{ds}{dt} = v_0 + gt + ft^2$$

$$\Rightarrow \quad \int ds = \int_0^1 (v_0 + gt + ft^2)\,dt$$

$$\Rightarrow \quad s = \left[v_0 t + \frac{gt^2}{2} + \frac{ft^3}{3}\right]_0^1$$

$$\Rightarrow \quad s = v_0 + \frac{g}{2} + \frac{f}{3}$$

24. (d) The equivalent circuit is as shown in figure

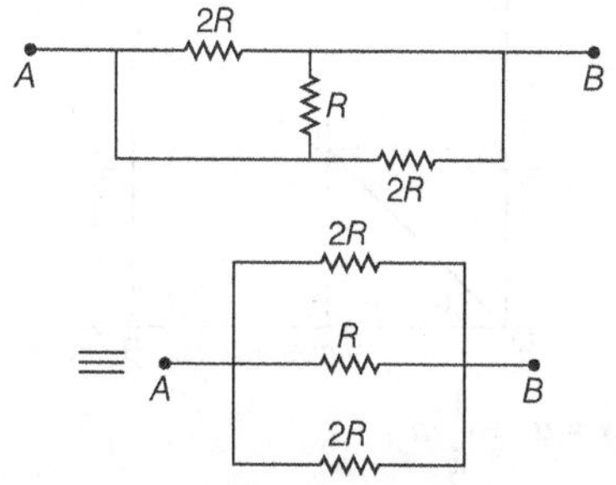

The resultant resistance between A and B,

$$\frac{1}{R_{AB}} = \frac{1}{2R} + \frac{1}{R} + \frac{1}{2R} = \frac{4}{2R}$$

$$\Rightarrow \quad R_{AB} = \frac{R}{2}$$

25. (c) Since we know, KE and PE of a satellite,

$$KE = \frac{GMm}{2R}$$

and $\quad PE = -\dfrac{GMm}{R}$

$$\therefore \quad |KE| = \frac{|PE|}{2}$$

$$\therefore \quad \frac{|KE|}{|PE|} = \frac{1}{2}$$

26. (b) Resistivity of conductor increases with increase of its temperature.

We know that, resistivity of a conductor,

$$\rho = \frac{m}{ne^2\tau}$$

$$\Rightarrow \quad \rho \propto \frac{1}{\tau} \qquad \ldots(i)$$

where, τ is relaxation time.

With the increase of temperature of conductor, mean free path for the electrons decreases. Hence, relaxation time (τ) also decreases with the increase of temperature.

27. (b) Refractive index, $\mu = \tan i_p = \tan 76° \simeq 4$

28. (b) If V_{XY} be the potential difference between X and Y, then applying Kirchhoff's voltage law,

$$V_X - 6 - 5 - 6 + 6 - 12 + 1 - 3 - V_Y = 0$$

$$\Rightarrow \quad V_X - V_Y = 25\,V$$

or $\quad V_{XY} = 25\,V$

29. (b) Taking vertical motion of projectile from O to A,
$u_y = u\sin\theta = 40\sin\theta$

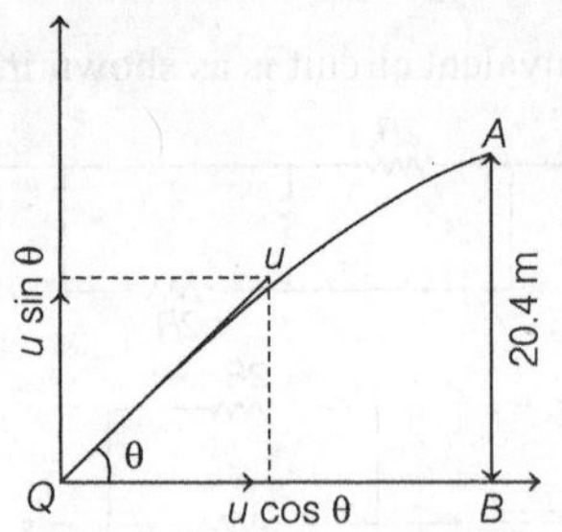

As, $s = ut + \frac{1}{2}at^2$

$\Rightarrow\ 20.4 = (40\sin\theta)(2) + \frac{1}{2}(-9.8)(2)^2$

$\Rightarrow\ 20.4 = 80\sin\theta - 19.6$

$\Rightarrow\ \sin\theta = \frac{40}{80} = \frac{1}{2} = \sin 30^\circ$

$\Rightarrow\ \theta = 30^\circ$

30. (b) The fracture point for a given material happens at a breaking stress.

Breaking stress $= \frac{500\text{N}}{\pi\,(1\text{cm})^2} = \frac{T_{max}}{\pi\,(2\text{cm})^2}$

$\Rightarrow\ T_{max} = 500\text{N} \times 4 = 2000\,\text{N}$

31. (c) $X_L = \omega L = 2000 \times 5 \times 10^{-3} = 10\,\Omega$

$X_C = \frac{1}{\omega C} = \frac{1}{2000 \times 50 \times 10^{-6}} = 10\,\Omega$

$X_L = X_C$. It is the case of resonance

$i = \frac{V}{R} = \frac{\frac{20}{\sqrt{2}}}{10} = \sqrt{2}\,\text{A} = 1.4\,\text{A}$

$V = iR = 1.4 \times 4 = 5.6\,\text{V}$

32. (c) $\because C_K = C_0 K$

Here, K is always greater than 1.
Since, due to polarisation of dielectric material, net electric field decreases.
Hence, potential difference also decreases. i.e. $V \propto E$

33. (c) Here, $R = 3\,\Omega$

Inductive reactance, $X_L = 3\,\Omega$
The phase difference between the applied voltage and the current in the circuit is

$\tan\phi = \frac{X_L}{R} = \frac{3\,\Omega}{3\Omega} = 1$

or $\phi = \tan^{-1}(1)$

or $\phi = \frac{\pi}{4}$

34. (a) In first case,

$mg - F_b = ma$ ...(i)

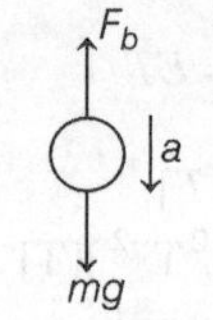

Let m_0 mass is removed, then

$F_b - (m - m_0)g = (m - m_0)a$ ...(ii)

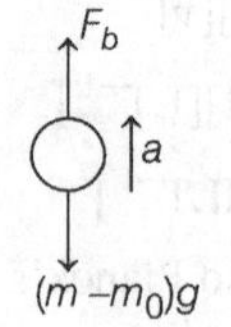

From Eqs. (i) and (ii), we get

$m_0 = \frac{2ma}{g + a} = \frac{2 \times 16 \times 6.2}{9.8 + 6.2} = 12.4\,\text{kg}$

35. (c) $E_n \propto \frac{Z^2}{n^2}$

$\therefore\ E_{n[\text{Li}^{++}]} = E_{1[\text{H}]}$

$\left[\frac{Z^2}{n^2}\right]_{\text{Li}^{++}} = \left[\frac{Z^2}{1^2}\right]_{\text{H}} \Rightarrow \frac{3^2}{n^2} = \frac{1^2}{1^2}$

$\Rightarrow\ n = 3$

36. (a) Given, wavelength, $\lambda = 8000\,\text{Å} = 8 \times 10^{-7}$ m

Distance of screen, $D = 1\,\text{m}$
Subtended angle, $\beta_\theta = 1'$
Now, The angular fringe width, i.e, the angle subtended by a fringe at the centre of slits is given by

$\beta_\theta = \frac{\beta}{D} = \frac{\lambda}{d}$

From the given condition,

$\beta_\theta = \frac{\lambda}{d} \geq \frac{\pi}{180 \times 60}$

As, $1' = \frac{\pi}{180 \times 60}$ rad

So, $\frac{\lambda}{d} \geq \frac{\pi}{180 \times 60}$

$\frac{8 \times 10^{-7}}{d} \geq \frac{\pi}{180 \times 60}$

So, $d \leq \frac{8 \times 10^{-7} \times 180 \times 60}{\pi}$

$d \leq 2.75 \times 10^{-3}$ m

Thus, $d_{max} = 2.75 \times 10^{-3}$ m

$= 2.75\,\text{mm}$

37. (c) $x_1 = \frac{L}{2}, x_2 = \frac{L}{2} + \frac{L}{2} = L,$

$$x_3 = L + \frac{L}{2} - \frac{L}{4} = \frac{5L}{4}$$

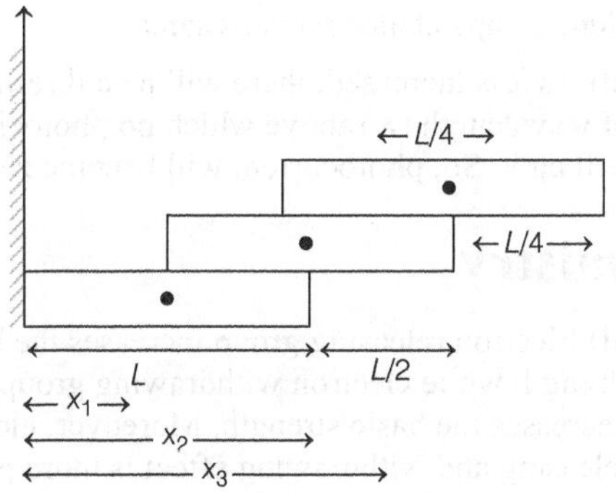

Centre of mass of system,

$$X_{CM} = \frac{m_1 x_1 + m_2 x_2 + m_3 x_3}{m_1 + m_2 + m_3}$$

$$= \frac{M\frac{L}{2} + ML + M\frac{5L}{4}}{M + M + M} = \frac{11ML/4}{3M} = \frac{11}{12}L$$

38. (a) Power of lens,

$$P \text{ (in D)} = \frac{100}{\text{Focal length } f \text{(in cm)}}$$

$$f = \frac{100}{10} = 10 \text{ cm}$$

According to lens Maker's formula,

$$\frac{1}{f} = (\mu - 1)\left(\frac{1}{R_1} - \frac{1}{R_2}\right)$$

For biconvex lens, $R_1 = +R, R_2 = -R$

$$\frac{1}{f} = (\mu - 1)\left(\frac{1}{R} + \frac{1}{R}\right)$$

$$\Rightarrow \frac{1}{f} = (\mu - 1)\left(\frac{2}{R}\right) \Rightarrow \frac{1}{10} = (\mu - 1)\left(\frac{2}{10}\right)$$

$$(\mu - 1) = \frac{1}{2} \text{ or } \mu = \frac{3}{2}$$

39. (a)

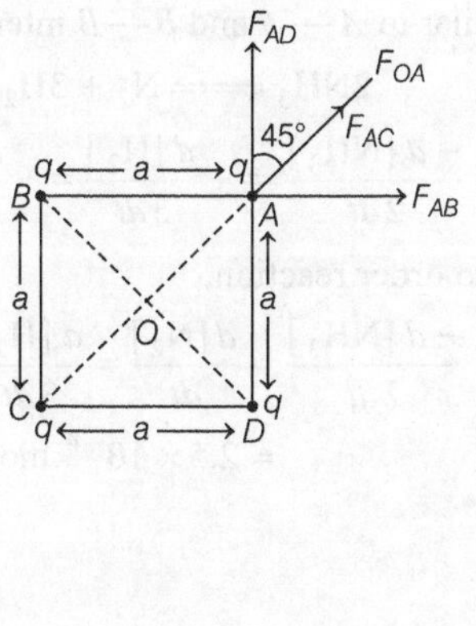

As diagonal, $AC = \sqrt{a^2 + a^2}$
$= \sqrt{2}a$

Let us consider the equilibrium of charge q at A.
Force exerted on charge at A by charge at B,

$$F_{AB} = \frac{kq^2}{a^2}\hat{\mathbf{i}}, \text{ where } k = \frac{1}{4\pi\varepsilon_0}$$

Similarly, $F_{AD} = \frac{kq^2}{a^2}\hat{\mathbf{j}}$

$$F_{AC} = \frac{kq^2}{(a\sqrt{2})^2}(\cos 45° \hat{\mathbf{i}} + \sin 45° \hat{\mathbf{j}})$$

$$= \frac{kq^2}{a^2 2\sqrt{2}}(\hat{\mathbf{i}} + \hat{\mathbf{j}})$$

and $$F_{OA} = \frac{kqQ}{\left(\frac{a}{\sqrt{2}}\right)^2}(\cos 45° \hat{\mathbf{i}} + \sin 45° \hat{\mathbf{j}})$$

$$= \sqrt{2}\frac{kqQ}{a^2}(\hat{\mathbf{i}} + \hat{\mathbf{j}})$$

Net force on charge q at A in the x-direction,

$$F_x = \left(\frac{kq^2}{a^2} + \frac{kq^2}{a^2 2\sqrt{2}} + \frac{\sqrt{2}kqQ}{a^2}\right)\hat{\mathbf{i}}$$

$$= \frac{kq}{a^2}\left(q + \frac{q}{2\sqrt{2}} + \sqrt{2}Q\right)\hat{\mathbf{i}} = \alpha\hat{\mathbf{i}}$$

$$\alpha = \frac{kq}{a^2}\left(q + \frac{q}{2\sqrt{2}} + \sqrt{2}Q\right)$$

Similarly, net force on charge q at A in the y-direction is

$$F_y = \alpha\,\hat{\mathbf{j}}$$

∴ Resultant force on charge q at A,

$$F = \sqrt{F_x^2 + F_y^2} = \sqrt{\alpha^2 + \alpha^2}$$

$$= \sqrt{2}\alpha$$

Charge q will be in equilibrium, if

i.e. if $F = 0 \Rightarrow \sqrt{2}\alpha = 0,\ \alpha = 0$

i.e., if $\frac{kq}{a^2}\left(q + \frac{q}{2\sqrt{2}} + \sqrt{2}Q\right) = 0$

$$\Rightarrow Q = -\frac{q}{4}(1 + 2\sqrt{2}) = -\frac{4}{4}(1 + 2\sqrt{2})$$

$$= -(1 + 2\sqrt{2})\ \mu\text{C}$$

40. (d) Here, $|\mathbf{E}| = 6$ V/m

The magnitude of magnetic vector,

$$|\mathbf{B}| = \frac{|\mathbf{E}|}{c} = \frac{6}{3 \times 10^8} = 2 \times 10^{-8} \text{ T}$$

41. (d)

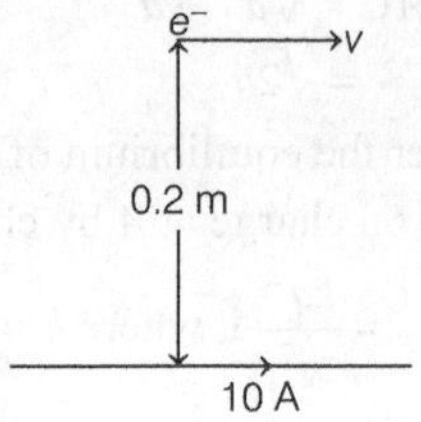

$$F = qvB$$

$$\Rightarrow \quad F = ev\left(\frac{\mu_0 i}{2\pi r}\right)$$

$$\Rightarrow \quad v = \frac{F(2\pi r)}{\mu_0 ie} = \frac{8\times 10^{-20}\times 2\pi \times 0.2}{4\pi \times 10^{-7}\times 10\times 1.6\times 10^{-19}}$$

$$\Rightarrow \quad v = 5\times 10^4 \text{ m/s}$$

42. (d) $v = \omega(A^2 - y^2)$

For 1st case

$$16 = \omega\sqrt{A^2 - 8^2} \quad \ldots\text{(i)}$$

For 2nd case

$$8 = \omega\sqrt{A^2 - 12^2} \quad \ldots\text{(ii)}$$

On dividing Eq. (i) by Eq. (ii), we get

$$\Rightarrow \quad \frac{16}{8} = \frac{\sqrt{A^2-8^2}}{\sqrt{A^2-12^2}} \Rightarrow 2^2 = \frac{A^2-64}{A^2-144}$$

$$\Rightarrow \quad 4A^2 - 576 = A^2 - 64$$

$$\Rightarrow \quad A^2 = 170.6$$

$$\Rightarrow \quad A = 13.06 \text{ cm}$$

43. (a) (i) If $D_1 = D_2 = 0$, then $V_0 = 0$.

Because there is no voltage drop across an ideal diode.

(ii) If D_1 or D_2 any one is high and other is grounded, then also $V_0 = 0$.

(iii) If both D_1 and D_2 are +10 V, then output is 10 V which mean high.

So, it performs like an AND gate.

44. (c) At initial condition,

Capacitance of a capacitor,

$$C = \frac{\varepsilon_0 A}{d} \quad \ldots\text{(i)}$$

When a metal plate of negligible thickness is introduced between the plates of capacitor, then it is equivalent to two capacitor connected in series. The distance between the plates of new capacitor is $\frac{d}{2}$ and area of plates remains same.

$$\therefore \quad C_1 = C_2 = \frac{\varepsilon_0 A}{d/2} = \frac{2\varepsilon_0 A}{d}$$

Using Eq. (i), we get

$$C_1 = C_2 = 2C$$

Now, the effective capacitance C_{eff} in series is

$$\frac{1}{C_{\text{eff}}} = \frac{1}{C_1} + \frac{1}{C_2} = \frac{1}{2C} + \frac{1}{2C}$$

$$\Rightarrow \quad C_{\text{eff}} = C$$

Hence, capacitance remains same.

45. (d) As λ is increased, there will be a threshold value of wavelength (λ) above which no photoelectron will emit. So, photocurrent will become zero.

Chemistry

46. (d) Electron releasing group increases the basic strength while electron withdrawing group decreases the basic strength. Moreover, electron releasing and withdrawing effect is more prominent at *ortho*-position. Thus, the correct sequence is as follows

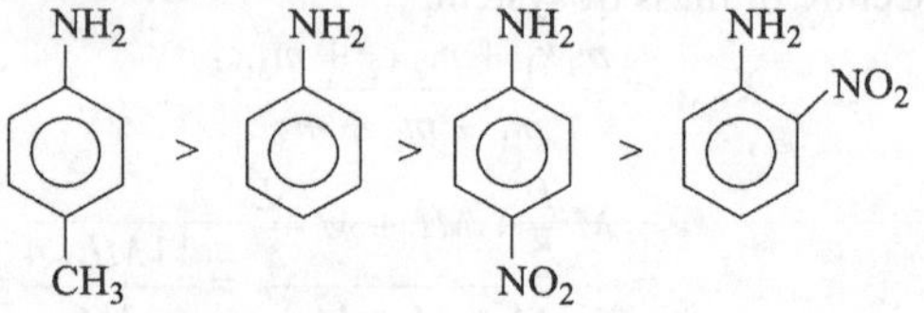

47. (b) Among the given oxides CO_2, NO_2 and N_2O_5 are acidic oxides.

48. (c) The structure of perchloric acid ($HClO_4$) has 5σ and 3π-bonds.

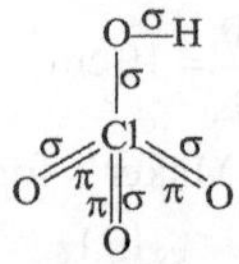

49. (a) The tendency to behave as Lewis acid decreases with increase in the size of central ion. Thus, the correct order of Lewis acid strength is

$$BX_3 > AlX_3 > GaX_3 > InX_3.$$

50. (a) Statement I is false as solution with the maximum possible amount of solute is saturated. Hence, a saturated solution must be prepared to determine the solubility of a solute in water.

Statement II is true as for an ideal binary solution containing two liquids *A* and *B*, *A*—*B* interactions are similar to *A*—*A* and *B*—*B* interactions.

51. (a)

$$2NH_3 \rightleftharpoons N_2 + 3H_2$$

$$\text{Rate} = \frac{-d[NH_3]}{2dt} = +\frac{d[H_2]}{3dt} = +\frac{d[N_2]}{dt}$$

For zero order reaction,

$$\text{So,} \quad \frac{-d[NH_3]}{2dt} = \frac{d[N_2]}{dt} = \frac{d[H_2]}{3dt} = k$$

$$= 2.5\times 10^{-4} \text{ mol L}^{-1}\text{s}^{-1}$$

$\therefore$ Rate of production of $N_2 = \dfrac{d[N_2]}{dt}$

$= 2.5 \times 10^{-4}$ mol $L^{-1}s^{-1}$

$\therefore$ Rate of production of H_2

$= 3 \times (2.5 \times 10^{-4}$ mol $L^{-1}s^{-1})$

$= 7.5 \times 10^{-4}$ mol $L^{-1}s^{-1}$

Problem Solving Tactics To solve this problem, the balanced chemical equation should be written first. For the zero order reaction, rate is equal to k.

52. (c) $PCl_5(g) \rightleftharpoons PCl_3(g) + Cl_2(g);\ \Delta n_g = 1$

$$K_p = K_C (RT)^{\Delta n_g}$$

$$\Rightarrow K_p = K_C RT \quad (\because \Delta n_g = 1)$$

$$\Rightarrow 2K_C = K_C RT \quad (\because K_p = 2K_C)$$

$$RT = 2$$

$$T = \frac{2}{R} = \frac{2}{0.0821} = 24.36\text{K}$$

53. (a) The electronic configuration of Mn^{2+} is $[Ar]: 3d^5 4s^0$ (5 unpaired electrons)

Spin only magnetic moment $(\mu_s) = \sqrt{n(n+2)}$

For $Mn^{2+}: \mu_s = \sqrt{5(5+2)} = 5.92$ B.M

While for other options the value of spin only magnetic moment are as follows

$Fe^{2+} = 4.90$ BM

$V^{2+} = 3.87$ BM

$Cu^{2+} = 1.73$ BM

54. (d) According to Bohr model, radius of hydrogen atom

$$r_n = \frac{0.529 \times n^2}{Z} \text{Å}$$

where, n = number of orbit

Z = atomic number ($Z = 1$ for hydrogen)

$$r_3 = \frac{0.529 \times (3)^2}{1} = 0.529 \times 9$$

$$= 4.761 \text{Å}$$

55. (a) Compound given in option (a), i.e. 1, 1-dichloro-2, 2-dimethylpropane (A) reacts with sodium hydroxide to give 2, 2-dimethylpropanal (B) with no α-hydrogen. The reaction involved is as follows

$$\underset{(A)}{(CH_3)_3CCHCl_2} + NaOH \longrightarrow (CH_3)_3CCH(OH)_2 \xrightarrow{-H_2O} \underset{(B)\uparrow}{(CH_3)_3CCHO}$$

α-C with no H

56. (a) Compounds with $CH_3-CH(OH)-$ or $CH_3-C(=O)-$ gives positive iodoform test.

Hence, compounds given in B, C and D will give positive iodoform test.

57. (b) Stability of +1 oxidation state increases from top to bottom due to inert pair effect, because of reluctance in the participation of inner s-electrons to participate in bond formation.

58. (b) The reaction of 2-bromobutane in presence of (alc.) KOH is as follows

$$\underset{\text{2-bromobutane}}{CH_3CH_2CH(Br)CH_3} + KOH\ (\text{alc.})$$

$$\downarrow -Br^-$$

$$CH_3CH_2\overset{\oplus}{C}HCH_3$$

$$\downarrow -H^+$$

$$\underset{\text{But-1-ene, (less substituted) I}}{CH_3CH_2CH{=}CH_2} + \underset{\text{But-2-ene, (more substituted) II}}{CH_3CH{=}CHCH_3}$$

Stability of II > I, hence II (i.e. but-2-ene) is the predominant product.

Problem Solving Tactics This problem is based on Saytzeff rule. This rule predicts the major product for elimination reactions of haloalkanes and alcohols. According to this rule, the most stable product is the one that is the most substituted.

59. (c) For third order reaction, Rate$_1 = k[A]^3$

On increasing the concentration of A by 2 times, new rate will be

$$\text{Rate}_2 = k[2A]^3$$

$$\therefore \frac{\text{Rate}_2}{\text{Rate}_1} = \frac{8}{1}$$

Thus, rate will increase by a factor of 8.

60. (c) Statement I false white II is true. The highest oxidation state of osmium is + 8.

61. (d) The IUPAC name of the compound $HOOC-CH(COOH)-COOH$ is methane tricarboxylic acid.

62. (d) As work done is given as, $W = -p_{ext} \times \Delta V$

Since, gas enters the vacuum bulb and pressure in vacuum is zero, And expression against vacuum i.e. $p_{ext} = 0$.

$\therefore$ Work done is zero.

63. (d) The complete reaction can be written as

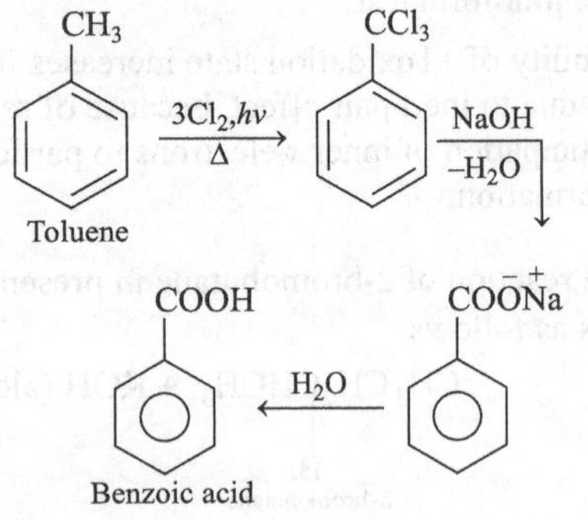

64. (c)

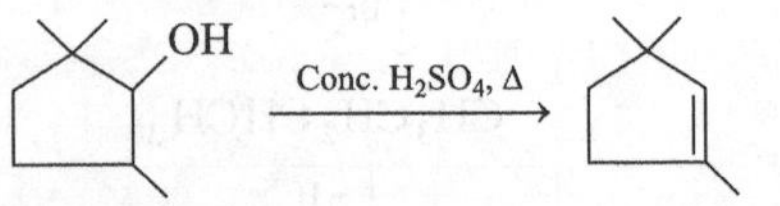

65. (d) Statement (d) is false.

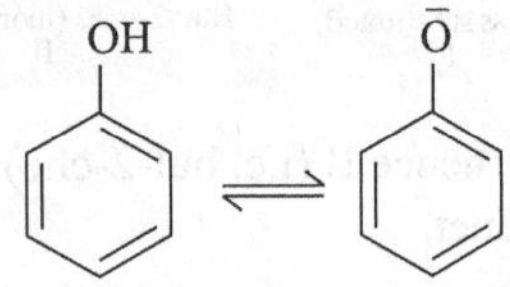

Resonance stabilised phenoxide ion

The resonance stabilised phenoxide ion makes phenol more acidic than water.

66. (b) Statement-I is true as D-mannose and D-glucose differ at configuration at C-2 only. Hence, they are epimers. The structure of D-mannose and D-glucose are as follows

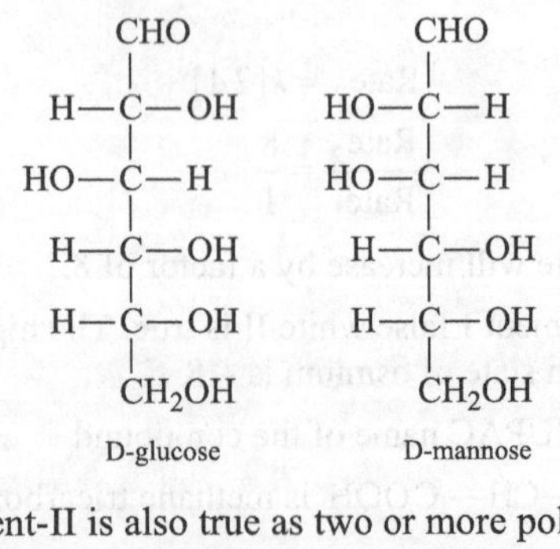

D-glucose D-mannose

Statement-II is also true as two or more polypeptide chains may associate to give rise to the quaternary structure.

These are held together by non-covalent forces such as hydrogen bonds, electrostatic interactions and van der Waals' interactions.

Problem Solving Tactics	In stereochemistry, an epimer is one of a pair of diastereomers. However, epimers are carbohydrates that differ in the position of —OH group.

67. (a) The principle of column chromatography is differential adsorption of the substances on the solid phase.

68. (a)

Species	$P_2:(B_2)$	$Q_2:(C_2)$	$R_2:(N_2)$	$S_2:(O_2)$	$T_2:(F_2)$
Bond order	1.0	2.0	3.0	2.0	1.0
Total no. of valence e^-s	6	8	10	12	14

69. (d) 105-Unnilpentium-Unp
107-Unnilseptium-Uns
109-Unnilennium-Une
110-Ununnilium-Uun

The elements with atomic number greater than 100 are named according to IUPAC nomenclature. For its nomenclature first letter of each number is taken. For example: 105 is named as Unp .U for un, n for nil and *p* for pent.

Hence, the correct match is A-(iii), B-(ii), C-(iv), D-(i).

70. (b)

(A) The molar mass of hydrogen peroxide is 34 g/mol, The molarity of 34 g of hydrogen peroxide in 500 mL is $\frac{34}{34} \times \frac{1000}{500} = 2\text{ M}$

(B) The normality of hydrogen peroxide is twice its molarity. It is $2 \times 2 = 4\text{ N}$

(C) Percent w/V of hydrogen peroxide solution is $\frac{34\text{g} \times 1000\text{ mL/L}}{500\text{mL}} = 68\%$.

(D) Volume strength $= 11.2 \times$ molarity
$= 11.2 \times 2$
$= 22.4$ g/L

Hence, the correct match is A-(iv), B-(iii), C-(i), D-(ii).

71. (a) σ-bond undergoes axial overlapping, covalent bond is formed by sharing of electrons, ionic bond is formed by transfer of electrons and π-bond undergoes lateral overlapping.

72. (b) In dilute benzene solutions, equimolar addition of R_3N and HCl produce a substance with a dipole moment. In the same solvent, equimolar addition of R_3N and SO_3 produce a substance having an almost identical dipole moment.

This is because, SO_3 acts as a Lewis acids and can react with the amine base to form polar substances which undergo ionic dissociation in a solvent sufficiently more

polar than benzene. Moreover, (N—S) bond is a more polar bond.
Thus, both (A) and (R) are true and (R) is the correct explanation of (A).

73. (d)(A) Vinegar is acetic acid belongs to carboxylic acid and has a functional group —COOH.
(B) C_2H_6 is belongs to the family of alkane as it follows general formula C_nH_{2n+2}.
(C) Ethanol belongs to the alcohol family; it has a functional group —OH.
(D) Methanone belongs to ketone family.
Hence, the correct match is A-(iv), B-(iii), C-(ii), D-(i).

74. (c) In diethylether ($C_2H_5OC_2H_5$), there are two lone pairs in it but being inert,it does not react with most organic compound.

75. (b) Statement I is true but Statement II is false. Chelate complexes tend to be more stable.

76. (d) "A carbonyl compound with a hydrogen atom on its alpha-carbon rapidly equilibrates with its corresponding enol and this process is known as keto-enol tautomerism."
For example, the keto enol tautomerism for acetaldehyde is as shown.

$$CH_3CHO \rightleftharpoons CH_2{=}CHOH$$

The inter conversion of the two forms (keto and enol) involves the movement of an alpha hydrogen and the shifting of bonding electrons.

77. (b) The colour of $KMnO_4$ is purple due to ligand to metal charge transfer.

78. (a) For a salt of weak acid and weak base;

$$pH = 7 + \frac{1}{2}(pK_a - pK_b)$$

$$= 7 + \frac{1}{2}(5.23 - 4.75)$$

$$= 7.24 \approx 7$$

79. (c) As for first order reaction,

$$k = \frac{2.303}{t}\log\frac{a}{a-x}$$

$$= \frac{2.303}{2\times10^4}\log\frac{800}{50} = \frac{2.303}{2\times10^4}\log 16$$

$$= 1.386\times10^{-4}\ s^{-1}$$

80. (d) I. $\overset{0}{Zn} + 2\overset{+1}{H^+} + SO_4^{2-} \longrightarrow Zn^{2+} + SO_4^{2-} + \overset{0}{H_2}$
(Change in oxidation number of hydrogen takes place)

II. $Zn + 2\underset{+1}{H^+} + SO_4^{2-} \longrightarrow Zn^{2+} + SO_4^{2-} + SO_2 + \underset{+1}{H_2O}$
(No change in oxidation number of hydrogen takes place)

III. $Zn + \underset{+1}{H^+} + NO_3^- \longrightarrow Zn^{2+} + NH_4^+ + \underset{+1}{H_2O}$
(No change in oxidation number of hydrogen takes place)

IV. $\overset{+1}{HCl}(aq) + NaOH \longrightarrow NaCl(aq) + \overset{+1}{H_2O}$
(No change in oxidation number of hydrogen takes place)

V. $2\overset{+1}{HClO_4}(aq) + CaCO_3(s) \longrightarrow Ca(ClO_4)_2(aq) + \overset{+1}{H_2O}(l) + CO_2(g)$
(No change in oxidation number of hydrogen takes place)

Thus, in (I) only oxidation number of hydrogen changes.

81. (b) The order of CFSE (Δ_o) in these complexes is $[CrCl_6]^{3-} < [Cr(H_2O)_6]^{3+} < [Cr(NH_3)_6]^{3+} < [Cr(CN)_6]^{3-}$. It is because more is the strength of ligand field higher is the CFSE.
The order of ligand is as follows

$$Cl^- < H_2O < NH_3 < CN^-$$

Problem Solving Tactics Strong field ligands are those which produce larger splittings between *d*-orbitals and form low spin complexes, While, weak field ligands are those which produce small splittings between *d*-orbitals and form high spin complexes.

82. (a) Half-cell reactions are
(i) $Zn \longrightarrow Zn^{2+} + 2e^-$; $E^\circ = +0.763$ V
(ii) $Ag^+ + e \longrightarrow Ag$; $E^\circ = 0.799$ V
From Eqs. (i) and (ii), we get

$$Zn + Ag^+ \longrightarrow Zn^{2+} + Ag;\ E^\circ = 0.763 + 0.799 = 1.56\ V$$

83. (d) $k = GG^*$
where, k = specific conductance = $0.0112\ ohm^{-1}cm^{-1}$

G = conductance

$$= \frac{1}{55} = 0.01818\ ohm^{-1}$$

G^* = cell constant

$$0.0112 = 0.01818 \times G^*$$

$$G^* = 0.616\ cm^{-1}$$

84. (b) In presence of H_2O_2, reaction undergoes through free radical pathways.

$$H—Br + H_2O_2 \longrightarrow \dot{H} + \dot{Br}$$

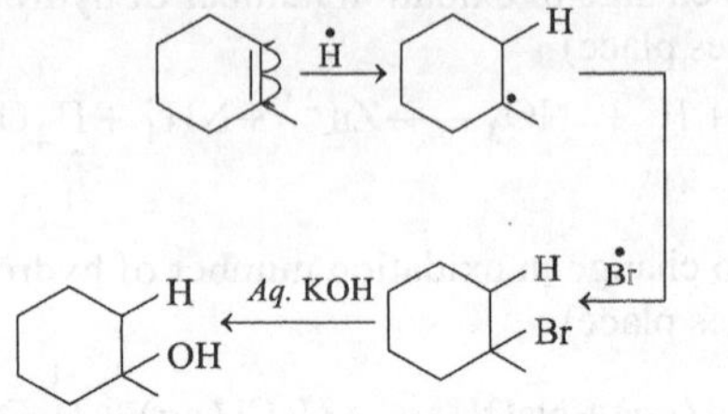

85. (d) In $[Ni(CN)_4]^{2-}$, Ni is in +2 oxidation state $Ni^{2+} \longrightarrow [Ar]\,3d^8$.

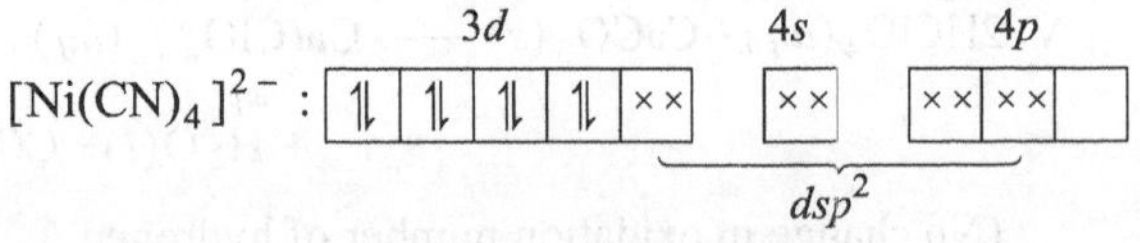

dsp^2-hybridisation results in square planar geometry, with no unpaired electron.

86. (b) The correct match is A-(iii), B-(iv), C-(i), D-(ii).

A. 5.1 g of $NH_3 = \frac{5.1}{17}$ mol = 0.3 mol
$= 0.3 \times 22.4$ L at STP
$= 6.72$ L

B. 100 g of $H_2 = \frac{100}{2} = 50$ mol

C. 3.011×10^{24} molecules of $CO_2 = \frac{3.011 \times 10^{24}}{6.022 \times 10^{23}}$
$= 5$ mol
$= 5N_A$ molecules

D. 11.2 L CH_4 gas at STP $= \frac{11.2}{22.4}$ mol = 0.2 mol

87. (c) For NaCl, $\pi_1 V_1 = i \times n_1 RT$

$$\pi_1 \times \frac{100}{1000} = \frac{1.2}{58.5} \times 0.0821 \times T \times i \quad ...(i)$$

For glucose, $\pi_2 V_2 = n_2 RT$

$$\pi_2 \times \frac{100}{1000} = \frac{7.2}{180} \times 0.0821 \times T \times 1 \quad ...(ii)$$

($\because$ For glucose, $i = 1$)

$\because$ NaCl and glucose solutions are isotonic.

$\therefore \quad \pi_1 = \pi_2$

$\Rightarrow \quad i = \frac{7.2}{180} \times \frac{58.5}{1.2}$

$= 1.95 \approx 2$

88. (d) When trichloroacetaldehyde CCl_3CHO reacts with chlorobenzene in the presence of sulphuric acid produces DDT (dichloro-diphenyl-trichloroethane). The reaction is as shown below.

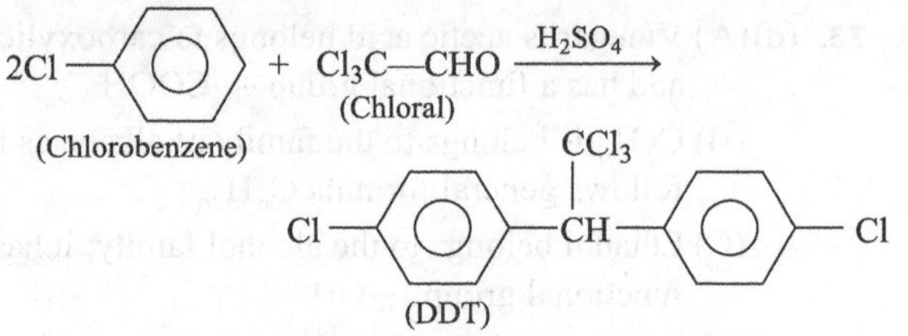

89. (d) Alkanes participate in substitution reactions. Hence, Statement I is true.

The example includes free radical halogenation reaction in which H-atom of an alkane is replaced with a halogen atom.

$$CH_3—CH_3 + Cl_2 + \text{Light} \longrightarrow CH_3CH_2Cl$$

Statement II is false as alkanes are saturated hydrocarbons. Saturated hydrocarbons are hydrocarbons that contain only single bonds between carbon atoms.

90. (a) The Rosenmund reduction is a hydrogenation process in which an acyl chloride is selectively reduced to an aldehyde.

$$CH_3—\overset{O}{\overset{\|}{C}}—Cl + H_2 \xrightarrow{Pd\text{-}C/BaSO_4} CH_3—\overset{O}{\overset{\|}{C}}—H$$

Cannizzaro reaction is an organic reaction of an aldehyde without active hydrogen that undergoes a redox reaction under the action of a strong base.

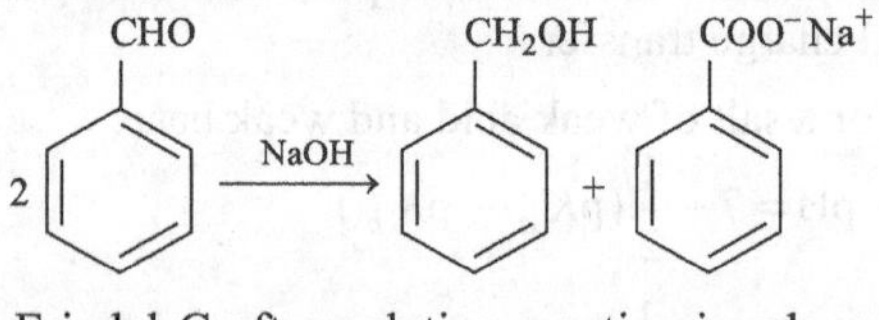

The Friedel-Crafts acylation reaction involves the addition of an acyl-group to an aromatic ring.

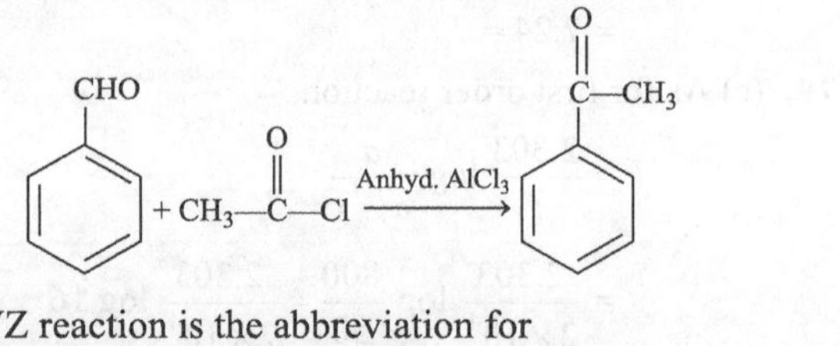

HVZ reaction is the abbreviation for Hell-Volhard-Zelinsky reaction. It is a halogenation reaction, i.e. addition reaction which adds one or more halogen to the compound. It halogenates carboxylic acids at the alpha carbon position.

$$R—CH_2—COOH \xrightarrow{Br_2/\text{Red P}} R—\underset{Br}{\underset{|}{C}H}—COOH$$

Hence, the correct match is A-(iv), B-(iii), C-(ii), D-(i).

Biology

91. (c) The cilliated protozoans have a cavity (gullet) that open to the outside of the cell surface. The coordinated movement of rows of cilia causes the water laden with food to be stered into the gullet.

92. (a) A fatty acid has a carboxyl group attached to an R group. The number of carbon atom in R group of a fatty acid may be 1 carbon to 19 carbon.

93. (d) The correct matches are A-4, B-1, C-2, D-3.
The partial pressure of oxygen (in mm Hg) at different parts involved in diffusion in comparison to those in atmosphere is as follows

- pO_2 of alveoli is 104 mm Hg.
- pO_2 of atmospheric air is 159 mm Hg.
- pO_2 of blood (deoxygenated) is 40 mm Hg.
- pO_2 of blood (oxygenated) is 95 mm Hg.

94. (b) The corpus callosum is a neural pathway that connects the right and the left hemispheres.

95. (d) Statement I is correct, but statement II is incorrect.

Incorrect statement can be corrected as

- α - cells of islets of Langerhans of pancreas secrete glycogen which increases blood sugar whereas β-cells of islets of langerhans secrete insulin.
- The insulin lowers the blood glucose level by promoting the uptake of glucose by cell and it conversion of glucose into glycogen by liver and skeletal muscle.

96. (c) In parasitism, one species (called parasite) derives benefit while the other species (called host) is harmed like lice living on human body.

97. (*b*) The ploidy of endosperm and embryo developed will be 4*n* and 3*n*, respectively.

- When the male plant is tetraploid then the gamete formed after meiotic division is diploid.
- Female plant is diploid, then the gamete formed after division will be haploid.
- Endosperm is formed by the fusion of two polar nuclei and one male gamete.
- Therefore, ploidy of endosperm will be $= n + n + 2n = 4n$
- Similarly embryo is formed by the fusion of male and female gametes $= 2n + n = 3n$.

98. (b) Both A and R are true and R is the correct explanation of A.

Bryophytes include the various mosses and liverworts that are found commonly growing in moist shaded areas in the hills. They are also called as amphibians of plant kingdom because they can live in soil, but are dependent on water for sexual reproduction.

99. (d) A is true, but R is false. R can be corrected as

The spermicides which kill sperms are in the form of creams. They have high contraception efficiency if used along with other barrier methods.

Otherwise, spermicide alone is only 70% effective in preventing pregnancy.

100. (c) Presence of a pathogen is normally suspected only when the pathogen has produced disease symptoms. However, very low concentration of a bacteria or virus, at a time when the symptoms of the diseases are not visible yet, can be detected by amplification of their nucleic acid by PCR.

101. (b) Statement in option (b) is incorrect and can be corrected as

The cambium ring becomes active and begins to cutoff new cells, both towards the inner and the outer side.

The cells cutoff towards pith, mature into secondary xylem and the cells cut off towards periphery mature into secondary phloem.
Rest of the statements are correct.

102. (c) The correct matches are A-4, B-3, C-1, D-2.

- PCR involves amplification of nucleic acids.
- Antisense genes are used to turn off the expression of a gene in a cell.
- Gene synthesis is to synthesise gene.
- Electrophoresis method is used to separate fragments of DNA on agarose gel.

103. (b) The secretory granules originating from Golgi complex fuse with plasmalemma.

Thus, they contribute to the renewal of membrane constituents.

104. (d) Cloning is the production of living structures or organisms, which are genetically identical to their parents, and is not an application of DNA fingerprinting.

105. (d) Node of Ranvier occurs where myelin sheath is discontinuous. The myelinated nerve fibres are enveloped with Schwann cells, which form a myelin sheath around the axon.

106. (d) The parathyroid hormone increases the Ca^{2+} levels in the blood. It acts on bones and stimulates the process of bone resorption (dissolution/demineralisation). Thus, helping in proper development of bones.

107. (d) A cell will not enter M-phase if replication of DNA is not complete. DNA replication takes place in the S-phase.

Doubling of chromosomes is necessary before the cell division takes place.

108. (a) The correct matches are A-3, B-2, C-4, D-1.
- IAA (Indole-Acetic Acid) is an auxin which helps to stimulate cell elongation.
- Gibberellin helps to promote stem elongation.
- Cytokinins promote cell division or cytokinesis.
- Abscisic Acid (ABA) inhibits stomatal opening and induces stomatal closure.

109. (c) Statement in option (c) is incorrect and can be corrected as
Muscular dystrophy is a genetic disease that weakens the muscular skeletal system and hamper locomotion.

The disease is characterised by progressive skeletal muscle weakness, defects in muscle proteins and the death of muscle cells and tissues.

110. (d) The statement (d) is incorrect statement.

It can be corrected as

Nephritis is the inflammation of renal pelvis, calyces and interstitial tissue due to local bacterial infection.

111. (d) The correct matches are A-3, B-4, C-2, D-1.
- Chasmogamous flowers are flowers with exposed anthers and stigma.
- Cleistogamous flowers do not open at all. In such flowers, the anthers and stigma lie close to each other.
- Geitonogamy is the transfer of pollen grains from the anther to the stigma of another flower of the same plant.
- Xenogamy is the transfer of pollen grains from anther to the stigma of a different plant.

112. (d) Statement in option (d) is incorrect. It can be corrected as

The transfer of energy follows 10 per cent law, i.e. only 10% of the energy is transferred to each trophic level from the lower trophic level.

A particular organism may occupy different trophic levels in two different individual food chains. Thus, energy flow will be different.

113. (b) *Lac* operon consists of one regulatory (i-gene) and three structural genes *a,y* and *z*. In *lac*operon, the genes *a, i, y*, and *z* code for transacetylase, repressor protein, permease, β-galactosidase, respectively.

114. (a) The correct matches are A-3, B-4, C-1, D-2.
Homo sapiens (Human) belongs to the order Primata. Housefly belongs to the order diptera of the class insecta. The order of mango (*Mangifera indica*) is sapindales and that of wheat (*T. aestivum*) is poales.

115. (d) Statements I, III and IV are correct. Rest of the statements are incorrect and can be corrected as

Shoot apical meristem occupies the distant most region of the stem axis.

Fascicular vascular cambium, interfascicular cambium and cork cambium are the examples of lateral meristems. These are responsible for producing the secondary tissues.

116. (d) option (d) is incorrectly matched pair. It can be corrected as *Propionibacterium sharmanii* is used for production of swiss cheese.

117. (a) Spraying juvenile conifers with GAs hastens the maturity period, thus leading to early seed production.

118. (d) Statement I is correct but statement II is incorrect. It can be corrected as

For transformation with recombinant DNA, the bacterial cells must first made competent to increase efficiency with which DNA enters the bacterium.

119. (a) In cell membrane, peripheral proteins lie on the surface of membrane. These proteins do not cross the membrane and aid in transportation of substances.

120. (b) Hashish causes after thought perceptions and hallucinations is the correct statement regarding the particular psychotropic drug specified in the given question.

121. (b) Statements I, II and IV are correct whereas statements III and V are incorrect and can be corrected as :

Offspring with all four kinds of blood groups are possible in a cross between two parents heterozygous for blood group A and B.

♀ \ ♂	I^A	i
I^B	I^AI^B (AB)	I^B (B)
i	I^Ai (A)	ii (O)

Person with genotype $I^A I^B$ have both antigens but no antibodies.

122. (d) The correct sequence of human evolution is
Australopithecus → *Homo habilis* → *Homo erectus*→ *Homo neanderthalensis* → Cro-Magnon

123. (b) Both statement I and statement II are correct.

In fermentation, there is a net gain of 2 molecules of ATP for each molecule of glucose degraded into pyruvic acid.
If fatty acids and glycerol are to be respired, they are first degraded into acetyl Co-A.

124. (d) Statements I, III and IV are incorrect and can be corrected as
- In mustard plant, primary roots and its branches constitute the tap root system.
- In some plants, like grasses, *Monstera* and banyan tree, roots arise from parts of the plant other than the radicle and are called adventitious roots.

- The main functions of the root system are absorption of water and minerals from the soil, providing a proper anchorage to the plants parts, storing reserve food materials and synthesis of plant growth regulators.

125. (c) Match pair in option (c) is incorrect and it can be corrected as
Acrosomal reaction involves hyaluronidase (hydrolysis enzyme), present in the head of sperm. This enzyme dissolves the zona pellucida and helps in penetration of sperm into the ova (egg).

126. (d) Microinjection method is used when there are only a very few cells available, such as fertilised animal egg cells. In this method, a cell is held on a glass pipette, under a microscope and the foreign DNA is injected directly into the nucleus using an incredibly fine micro injection needle.

127. (d) Statement I is correct, but statement II is incorrect and it can be corrected as

PS-II is involved only in non-cyclic photophosphorylation.

128. (a) Papaya and date palm are dioecious plants in which male and female flowers are present on different plants, i.e. each plant is either male or female. This condition prevents both autogamy and geitonogamy.
Whereas, castor and maize are monoecious plants, This condition prevents autogamy, but not geitonogamy.

129. (a) A is false, but R is true. A can be corrected as

The cell walls of diatoms are embedded with silica that makes them indestructible. Thus, they left behind large amount of cell wall deposits in their habitat. This accumulation over billions of years is referred to as diatomaceous earth'.

130. (c) All statements are correct except, statement given in option (c) which can be corrected as
Acromegaly is due to hypersecretion of growth hormone

131. (c) The QRS complex represents the depolarisation of the ventricle, which initiates the ventricular contraction. By counting the number of QRS complex that occur in a given time period, one can determine the heartbeat rate of an individual.

132. (b) The correct matches are A-3, B-2, C-1, D-4.
Grave's disease is an autoimmune disease that causes hyperthyroidism, or overactive thyroid. In this disease immune system attacks the thyroid causing it to produce more thyroid hormone than the body needs.
In adult women, hypothyroidism may cause menstrual cycle to become irregular.

In type I diabetes mellitus, pancreatic beta cells are destroyed by T-cells of patient's own immune system. This results in hyposecretion of insulin

Addison's disease is an autoimmune disease caused due to undersecretion of adrenal (cortex) hormones.

133. (d) Leaching is not a factor affecting primary productivity. It is the process, by which water soluble inorganic nutrients go down into the soil horizon and get precipitated as unavailable salts.

134. (c) DNA replication does not take place during the M-phase. It takes place during the S-Phase of the cell cycle. Other events are associated with mitotic prophase

135. (d) Statements I, III, IV are correct and rest of the statements are incorrect. These can be corrected as
- In stroma, enzymatic reactions synthesise sugar, which in turn forms starch.
- The splitting of water is associated with PS II, and water is split into $2H^+$,[O] and electrons.

136. (a) High copy number aims to provide more replicates of inserted DNA sequences in the cell. It refers to the average or reported number of copies per host cell. Plasmids have either low, medium or high copy number.

137. (d) Statement I is correct, but statement II is incorrect and can be corrected as

Amphibian species diversity is more in Western ghats than in the Eastern ghats.

138. (b) Passive immunity can occur when antibodies formed within other organisms are introduced into the patient's body through injection and it can naturally pass from mother to foetus *via* placenta.

139. (d) Statement I and IV are incorrect. These can be corrected as
Agrobacterium tumefaciens is a pathogen of dicot plants and is able to deliver T-DNA. It is modified into a cloning vector which is no more pathogenic to plant, but is still able to use the mechanism to deliver genes of interest into a variety of plants.

140. (d) Family is a subdivision of an order consisting of a group of related genera and species. The families in plant kingdom are classified based on the vegetative and reproductive parts of the plant species.

141. (c) The correct matches are A-4, B-2, C-3, D-1.
Diterpenes are example of terpenoides and concanavalin-A is a lectin. Morphine is constituted under alkaloid and cotton is a cellulose. All these are secondary metabolites.

142. (d) The genotype of the partner with 'A' blood group (female) will be either $I^A I^A$ or $I^A i$. Whereas, the genotype of the partner with B blood group will be either $I^B I^B$ or $I^B i$.

If parents were heterozygous, genotype of mother will be $I^A i$ and that of father will be $I^B i$.

Representing the condition by a Punnett square.

♀ \ ♂	I^B	i
I^A	I^AI^B (AB)	I^Ai (A)
i	I^Bi (B)	ii (O)

Thus, the progeny will have all the four types of blood groups 25% O, 25% A, 25% B, and 25% AB.
If mother and father were homozygous then the probability of AB blood group in their children will be 100%.

143. (d) Statement I is correct, but statement II is incorrect. It can be corrected as
Fertilised ovum first divides into two cells by a vertical division that takes place about 30 hours after fertilisation.

144. (d) Match pair in option (d) is incorrect and can be corrected as
The best stage to observe chromosome morphology and number is metaphase.
In this stage chromosomes are clearly visible, each chromosome having two chromatids.

145. (b) In cleistogamy seed is not dependent on pollinators. Such flowers never expose their sex organs to environment. Thus, assuring seed set due to self pollination or autogamy.

146. (a) Statements II and IV are correct. Statements I, III and V are incorrect. They can be corrected as
All the Ctenophores are exclusively marine. They are acoelomate organisms.
The nervous system in Ctenophores is in the form of a nerve net or plexus, formed by nerve cells.

147. (b) Hypothalamus is the important part of brain and contain centres for controlling body temperature, urge for drinking and eating.

148. (b) The correct sequence is B, C, A, D.
- RNA genome of virus replicates to form viral DNA with the help of reverse transcriptase.
- The viral DNA gets incorporated into host cell's DNA and directs the infected cells to produce virus DNA.
- The progeny viruses released in the blood attack other helper T-lymphocytes.
- Progressive decrease in the number of helper T-lymphocytes is observed in the body of infected person. This results in a decline of cell mediated immunity.

149. (d) At each trophic level, most of the energy, gets lost as heat in metabolic reactions. As a result, there occurs a progressive decrease in energy at each trophic level.
This results in a pyramid shaped structure.

150. (c) Statement in option (c) is incorrect and can be corrected as,
In lotus and rose more than one carpel is present, which may be free this condition is called apocarpous.

151. (b) Stage *A* represents carboxylation step wherein CO_2 is utilised for carboxylation of RuBP.

152. (a) The heart of amphibians is 3 chambered, i.e. two auricles and one ventricle. This is due to the requirement of less oxygen and hence a lower metabolic rate.

153. (b) The cells of the sporogenous tissue undergo meiotic divisions to form microspore tetrads.
As the anthers mature and dehydrate, the microspores dissociate from each other and develop into pollen grains.

154. (a) The correct matches are A-3, B-1, C-4, D-2.
- *Trichoderma polysporum* yields cyclosporin - A.
- *Aspergillus niger* yields citric acid.
- Butyric acid is sourced form *Clostridium butylicum.*
- Yeast is used for commercial production of ethanol.

155. (b) The columnar epithelium is composed of a single layer of tall and slender cells. Their nuclei are located at the base. They are found in the lining of stomach and intestine and help in the secretion and absorption.

156. (b) Only statement V is correct. Other statements can be corrected as
Expiration occurs when atmospheric pressure is lower than the intrapulmonary pressure. Internal intercostal muscles are active during this process.
Inspiration occurs when intrapulmonary pressure is less than atmospheric pressure.
The relaxation of diaphragm causes expiration.

157. (b) During complete krebs' cycle, decarboxylation reaction occurs twice resulting in CO_2 evolution. First, when isocitrate is converted to α-ketoglutaric acid, a 5C compound.
The other CO_2 molecule is evolved when formation of succinyl CO-A takes place from α-ketoglutaric acid.

158. (a) The rate of decomposition is slow, if detritus is rich in lignin and chitin. While, it is quicker if it is composed of nitrogen and water soluble substances like sugars.

159. (a) Statement I is incorrect, but statement II is correct. Statement I can be corrected as
The opening between the right atrium and right ventricle is guarded by a valve formed of three muscular flaps/cusps, the tricuspid valve.

160. (d) The statement IV is incorrect. It can be corrected as
VNTRs(Variable Number Tandem Repeats) are similar in monozygotic (identical) twins only.
Rest of the statements are correct.

161. (a) The correct matches are A-1, B-4, C-3, D-2.
- Rivet popper hypothesis was given by Stanford ecologist Paul Ehrlich.
- Communities with more species are more stable.
- Communities with less species are less stable.
- Term biodiversity was popularised by the sociobiologist Edward Wilson to describe the combined diversity at all levels of biological organisation.

162. (c) Statement II, IV and V are incorrect and can be corrected as
- Test cross is the cross of the individuals with its homozygous recessive parent. In other words, it is a specialised back cross of F_1 hybrid with its homozygous recessive parent.
- Morgan coined the term linkage to describe the physical association of genes on a chromosome.
- Dominance is not an autonomous feature of a gene or the product that it has information for.
- Rest of the statements are correct.

163. (c) The spermatozoa is formed by the process of spermiogenesis by the transformation of spermatids. It contains haploid (n) chromosome, while spermatogonium, primary oocyte, primary spermatocytes have diploid (2n) chromosomes.

164. (c) Specificity diversity, memory are characteristics of acquired immunity. Adaptive immune system is also known as acquired immune system.

Specificity is able to distinguish among various kinds of foreign molecules/particles. It has the ability to recognise a vast variety of foreign molecules. It retains the memory of the antigen which has encountered earlier.

165. (b) Cervical cap is the odd one out among the list. All the others are Intra Uterine Device (IUDs). These devices are inserted by doctors or expert nurses.

However, the cervical cap is one of the barrier methods to prevent unwanted pregnancy. It is made up of rubber and may be self inserted into the female reproductive tract.

166. (c) Statement in option (c) is correct.

Haemophilia is sex-linked recessive disease whose (recessive) allele is present on X-chromosomes. Females are homogametic, i.e. have XX-chromosomes, whereas males are heterogametic, i.e. XY.

Males only require one recessive allele for expressing haemophilic trait. However, females need two copies of recessive alleles for the diseased condition, which is very rare.

167. (d) Darwinism was unable to explain that variations are inherited from parents to offspring through genes.

168. (c) *Monascus purpureus* is a species of mold belonging to division *Ascomycetes*. It is commercially important as it produces number of statins, which are used to lower blood cholesterol.

169. (a) The correct matches are A-1, B-2, C-3, D-4.
Protonema is involved in vegetative propagation in mosses like *Funaria*. Antheridium is the male sex organ. Archegonium is the female sex organ. Sporophyll bears sporangia.

170. (c) The best and the most effective means of conserving biodiversity is to preserve species in their natural habitat. This strategy is called *in situ* conservation and involves setting up of national parks, hotspots, etc.

171. (a) Statement I is incorrect, but statement II is correct. The incorrect statement can be corrected as

Smooth muscles taper at both ends and do not show striation. Also, cardiac muscles do not taper at ends and show striation.

172. (a) In young population pyramid, the birth rate is high and population growth may be exponential. Hence, age pyramid with broad base is observed.

The stable population has moderate proportion of young to old. Hence, a bell-shaped age pyramid is observed. In declining population, young individuals are in low percentage as compared to post reproductive ones. Hence, an urn-shaped age pyramid is observed.

173. (b) *A* represents arteries and *B* represents veins, arteries carry blood from heart to be distributed in the body. The arteries have thick tunica media, narrow lumen and possess no valves.

Veins carry deoxygenated blood from parts to the heart except pulmonary veins. The flow of blood is slow and steady.

174. (d) Statement in option (d) is incorrect. It can be corrected as

Roundworm is an example of Aschelminthes. The Platyhelminthes also called flatworm includes *Taenia* (Tapeworm), *Fasciola* (Liver fluke), etc.

175. (a) The correct matches are A-4, B-1, C-2, D-3.
- DNA ligase is used to join the cuts in DNA. The 5′ and 3′ ends of okazaki fragments are joined by them.
- In tailing, adenylate residues (200-300) are added at 3′-end in a template independent manner.

- In splicing, introns are removed and exons are joined in a defined order.
- The RNA polymerase-I transcribes *r*RNAs (28S, 18S and 5.8S)

176. (c) Convolvulaceae and Solanaceae are kept under order Polymoniales because they have similar floral characters. Such as the structure and arrangement of flowers.

177. (d) Xylem parenchyma is the only living component of xylem, that helps in conduction of water and minerals and also in the storage of food.

178. (d) Statements I, III and IV are correct whereas statements II and V are incorrect and can be corrected as

- Analogous structures are a result of convergent evolution.
- Sweet potato (root modification) and potato (stem modification) are example of analogy.

179. (d) Statement I is correct, but statement II is incorrect. It can be corrected as

Teenagers suffering from Klinefelter's syndrome are taller than average stature, have weak bones but longer legs.

180. (c) Both A and R are true, but R is not the correct explanation of A.

As cilia are hair-like structures seen in the cells of Fallopian tube, they facilitate the movement of ovum to uterus. Thus, allowing passage of ova through the female reproductive tract.

SECTION II
Mastery Builders

PRACTICE SET 9

Maximum Marks : 720	Time : 3 hrs	No. of Questions : 180

Instructions

1. This question paper contains **180** multiple-choice questions (four options with a single correct answer) from **Physics, Chemistry** and **Biology**.
2. These questions are distributed as 45 questions, each from Physics and Chemistry and 90 questions in Biology. These are to be compulsorily attempted by the candidate.
3. Each question carries 4 marks. For each correct response, the candidate will get 4 marks. For each incorrect response, one mark will be deducted from the total scores.

PHYSICS

1. The kinetic energy of electron in the first Bohr orbit of the hydrogen atom is

(a) -13.6 eV (b) 13.6 eV (c) -6.5 eV (d) -27.2 eV

2. An electromagnetic wave passing through vacuum is described by $E = E_0 \sin(kx - \omega t)$, $B = B_0 \sin(kx - \omega t)$. The correct equation is

(a) $E_0 B_0 = \omega k$ (b) $E_0 k = B_0 \omega$

(c) $E_0 \omega = B_0 k$ (d) $\frac{k}{\omega} = \sqrt{\frac{E_0}{B_0}}$

3. In a series LCR circuit, $R = 200\,\Omega$ and the voltage and frequency of the main supply is 220 V and 50 Hz, respectively. On taking out the capacitance from the circuit, the current lags behind the voltage by 30°. On taking out the inductor from the circuit, the current leads the voltage by 30°. The power dissipated in the LCR circuit is

(a) 242 W (b) 305 W (c) 210 W (d) zero

4. The dependence of binding energy per nucleon (ΔE_{bn}) on the mass number A is represented by

(a) ΔE_{bn}
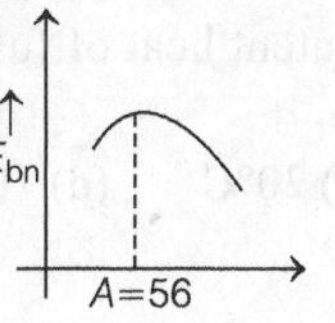

(b) ΔE_{bn}
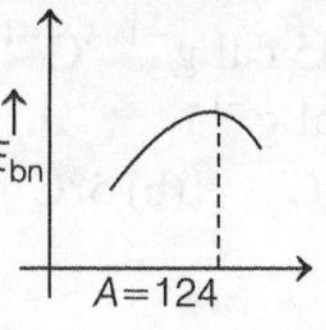

(c) ΔE_{bn}
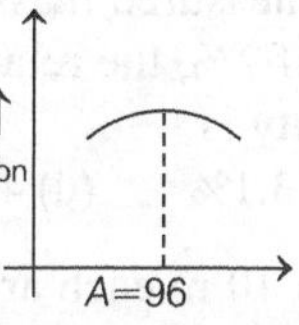

(d) ΔE_{bn}
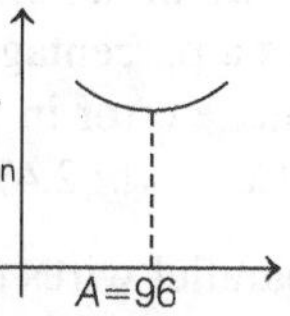

5. A man sits on a chair which is supported by a rope passing over a frictionless fixed pulley. The man of weight 1000 N exerts a force of 450 N on the chair downwards, while pulling the rope on the other side. If the chair's weight is 250 N and g is 10 ms^{-2}, then the acceleration of the chair is

(a) 0.45 ms^{-2}
(b) zero
(c) $\frac{9}{25}$ ms^{-2}
(d) 2 ms^{-2}

6. A player kicks a football with an initial speed of 25 ms^{-1} at an angle of 45° from the ground. What are the maximum height and the time taken by the football to reach at the highest point during motion? (Take, $g = 10$ ms^{-2})

(a) $h_{max} = 3.54$ m, $T = 0.125$ s
(b) $h_{max} = 15.625$ m, $T = 1.77$ s
(c) $h_{max} = 10$ m, $T = 2.5$ s
(d) $h_{max} = 15.625$ m, $T = 3.54$ s

7. The electrostatic potential V at a distance r from the centre of a charged metallic sphere of radius R for $r< R$ will vary according to relation

(a) $V \propto \frac{1}{r}$ (b) $V \propto r$ (c) $V \propto \frac{1}{r^2}$ (d) $V \propto r^0$

8. Two cells of emf E are connected in series through an external resistance R. The internal resistance of the cells are r_1 and r_2 $(r_1 > r_2)$. When the circuit is closed, the potential difference across the first cell is zero. The value of R is

(a) $r_1 + r_2$ (b) $\frac{r_1 + r_2}{2}$ (c) $\frac{r_1 + r_2}{2}$ (d) $r_1 - r_2$

9. In a capillary tube, water rises to 4 mm. The height of water that will rise in another capillary tube having one-fourth radius of the first tube is

(a) 16 mm (b) 14 mm
(c) 12 mm (d) 9 mm

10. The density of a solid ball is to be determined in an experiment. The diameter of the ball is measured with a screw gauge, whose pitch is 0.5 mm and there are 50 divisions on the circular scale. The reading on the main scale is 2.5 mm and that on the circular scale is 20 divisions. If the measured mass of the ball has a percentage error of 2%, the relative percentage error in the density is

(a) 0.9% (b) 2.4% (c) 3.1% (d) 4.2%

11. Two parallel wires of length 10 m each are separated by a distance of 0.1 m. If they carry equal currents in the same direction and exerts a total force of 2×10^{-7} N on each other, then the value of current must be

(a) 0.5 A (b) 0.4 A
(c) 0.3 A (d) 0.1 A

12. A carpet of mass m, made of inextensible material is rolled along its length in the form of a cylinder of radius r and kept on a rough floor. If it is unrolled to radius $\frac{r}{2}$ without sliding, the decrease in potential energy is

(a) $\frac{3}{4}mgr$ (b) $\frac{7}{8}mgr$ (c) $\frac{1}{2}mgr$ (d) $\frac{1}{8}mgr$

13. The binding energy of deuteron is 2.2 MeV and that of ${}_2^4He$ is 28 MeV. If two deuterons are fused to form one ${}_2^4He$, then the energy released is

(a) 25.8 MeV (b) 23.6 MeV
(c) 19.2 MeV (d) 30.2 MeV

14. In the following circuit diagram, current through 5Ω resistor is

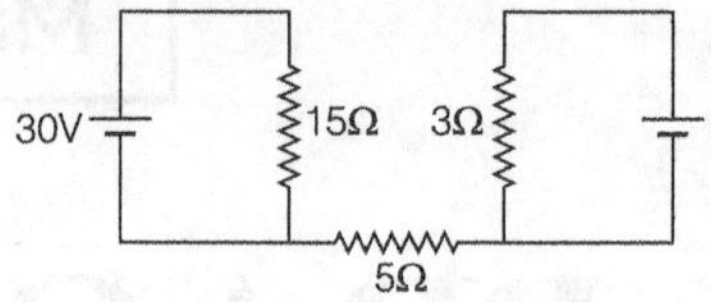

(a) 4A (b) 2.5A (c) zero (d) 3A

15. A transformer is used to light a 100 W, 110 V lamp. If the mains current and voltage are 0.5A and 220 V respectively, then the efficiency of the transformer is approximately

(a) 30% (b) 50% (c) 90% (d) 10%

16. Given below are two statements.

Statement I If the width of the slit is increased in Young's double slit experiment, then fringe width remains unchanged.

Statement II If the slit is sufficiently wide, then each part gives a pattern which overlaps and the fringes gets obliterated.

In the light of above statements. Choose the correct one.

(a) Both Statement I and Statement II are correct.
(b) Both Statement I and Statement II are incorrect.
(c) Statement I is correct but Statement II is incorrect.
(d) Statement I is incorrect but Statement II is correct.

17. If the width of one slit is doubled to the another slit in Young's double slit experiment, then the ratio of maximum intensities to minimum intensities in the interference pattern is

(a) 9 : 1 (b) 1 : 9 (c) 3 : 1 (d) 1 : 3

18. A pure Si wafer is doped with Al. The number density of acceptor atoms is approximately 10^{22} m^{-3}, if density of the hole in an intrinsic semiconductor is approximately $10^{20} m^{-3}$.

The number density of electron in the wafer is

(a) 10^4 m^{-3} (b) 10^{12} m^{-3}
(c) 10^{18} m^{-3} (d) 10^{24} m^{-3}

19. 20 g of water at 50°C and 8 g of ice at −20°C are mixed together in a calorimetry. What is the final temperature of the mixture? (Given, specific heat of ice = 0.5 cal g^{-1} °C^{-1} and latent heat of fusion of ice = 80 cal g^{-1})

(a) −5°C (b) 5°C (c) 20°C (d) 10°C

20. The output of the given circuit in the figure

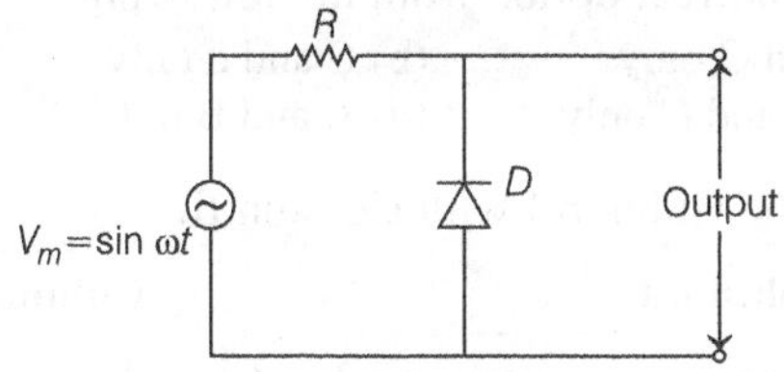

(a) would be zero at all times
(b) would be like that of a full wave rectifier
(c) would be like a half-wave rectifier with positive cycle in output
(d) would be like a half-wave rectifier with negative cycle in output

21. A raw egg and a hard boiled egg are made to spin on a table with the same angular speed about the same axis. The ratio of time taken by the two eggs to stop is
(a) equal to 1 (b) less than 1
(c) greater than 1 (d) zero

22. The wavelength of the first line of Balmer series of hydrogen atom is λ Å. The wavelength of this line of a double ionised lithium atom ($Z = 3$) is
(a) $\frac{\lambda}{3}$ Å (b) $\frac{\lambda}{9}$ Å
(c) $\frac{\lambda}{8}$ Å (d) $\frac{\lambda}{27}$ Å

23. A ray of light strikes a material slab at an angle of incidence 30°. If the reflected and refracted rays are perpendicular to each other, the refractive index of the material is
(a) $\sqrt{3}$ (b) $\sqrt{2}$
(c) $\frac{1}{\sqrt{2}}$ (d) $\frac{1}{\sqrt{3}}$

24. An ideal gas undergoes a thermodynamic process a to b as shown on pressure-volume (p-V) diagram. The work done by the gas during this process is

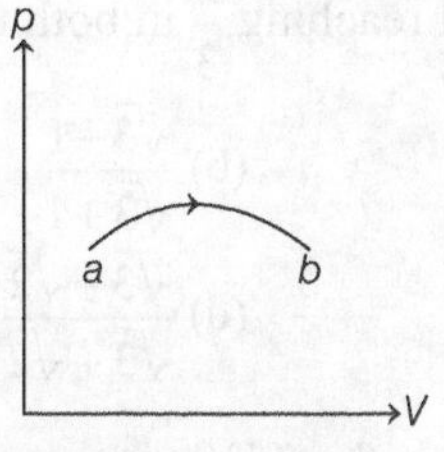

(a) first decreases then increases
(b) first increases then decreases
(c) continuously increases
(d) continuously decreases

25. A simple harmonic wave train of amplitude 1 cm and frequency 100 vibrations is travelling in positive x-direction with velocity 15 ms^{-1}. The displacement y, at $x = 180$ cm from the origin at $t = 5$ s, is
(a) zero (b) 2400 cm (c) 1200 cm (d) 900 cm

26. Assuming earth to be a perfect sphere of radius 6400 km. The value of acceleration due to gravity changes by what value from poles to equator for a period of 1 day?
(a) 3.5×10^{-2} ms^{-2} (b) 3.38×10^{-2} ms^{-2}
(c) 3×10^{-2} ms^{-2} (d) 225×10^{-2} ms^{-2}

27. At what temperature is the root mean square velocity of gaseous hydrogen molecules equal to that of oxygen molecules at 47°C ?
(a) 3K (b) −73 K (c) 80 K (d) 20 K

28. The level of water in a tank is 5 m high. A hole of area 10 cm^2 is made in the bottom of the tank. The rate of leakage of water from the hole is
(take, $g = 10$ m/s^2)
(a) 10^3 m^3s^{-1} (b) 10^{-4} m^3s^{-1}
(c) 10^{-3} m^3s^{-1} (d) 10^{-2} m^3s^{-1}

29. An equation is given as

$$\left(p + \frac{a}{V^2}\right)(V - b) = RT$$

where all the symbols have their usual meaning. If a and b are constants, then the dimensions of a can be written as
(a) $[ML^5T^{-2}]$ (b) $[ML^5T^1]$
(c) $[M^{-1}L^5T^2]$ (d) $[ML^{-5}T^{-1}]$

30. In hydrogen spectrum, the ratio of the longest wavelength of Lyman series to the longest wavelength in the Balmer series is given by
(a) $\frac{4}{9}$ (b) $\frac{9}{4}$
(c) $\frac{5}{27}$ (d) $\frac{27}{5}$

31. The equivalent resistance between A and B in the given circuit is

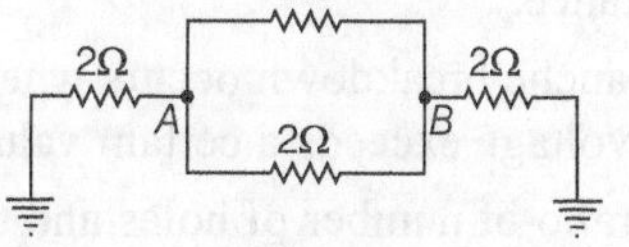

(a) 0.8 Ω (b) 1 Ω
(c) 5 Ω (d) 10 Ω

32. Parallel plate capacitor is constructed using three different dielectric materials as shown in the figure. The parallel plates, across which potential difference is applied of area 200 cm^2 and separated by a distance 10 cm, then the capacitance across P and Q is

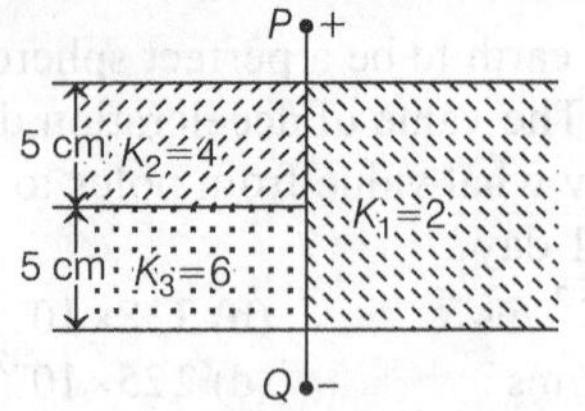

(a) 6pF (b) 6μF (c) 12pF (d) 12μF

33. Two concentric metallic spheres kept in air have radii r_1 and r_2 ($r_1 > r_2$). They have similar charge and equal surface density σ, the electric potential at their common centre is

(a) $\frac{\sigma}{\varepsilon_0}(r_1 + r_2)$ (b) $\frac{\sigma}{\varepsilon_0}(r_2 - r_1)$

(c) $\frac{\sigma}{\varepsilon_0}(r_1 - r_2)$ (d) $\frac{\sigma}{\varepsilon_0(r_2 - r_1)}$

34. A man is 45 m behind the bus, when the bus starts accelerating from rest with acceleration 2.5 ms^{-2}. With what minimum velocity should the man start running to catch the bus?

(a) 15 ms^{-1} (b) 10 ms^{-1}

(c) 7.5ms^{-1} (d) 5 ms^{-1}

35. Two circular coils 1 and 2 are made from the same wire, but the radius of the 1st coil is twice that of the 2nd coil. What is the ratio of potential difference applied across them, so that the magnetic field at their centres is the same?

(a) 3 (b) 4 (c) 6 (d) 2

36. How many NOR gates are required to form an AND gate?

(a) 1 (b) 2

(c) 3 (d) 4

37. A. An ideal current source is one which has infinite internal resistance.

B. An ideal voltage source has zero internal resistance.

C. Avalanche breakdown occurs when the forward bias voltage exceeds a certain value.

D. The ratio of number of holes and the number of conduction electrons in an n-type extrinsic semiconductor is more than 1.

Choose which of the above statements are true and tick the correct option from the following.

(a) A and C only (b) C and d only

(c) A, B and C only (d) A and B only

38. Match the Column I with Column II.

	Column I		Column II
A.	Root means square speed of gas molecules.	I.	$\frac{1}{3}nm\bar{v}^2$
B.	Pressure exerted by ideal gas.	II.	$\sqrt{\frac{3RT}{M}}$
C.	Average kinetic energy of a molecule	III.	$\frac{5}{2}RT$
D.	Total internal energy of 1 mole of a diatomic gas.	IV.	$\frac{3}{2}k_BT$

Choose the correct answer from the options given below.

	A	B	C	D
(a)	I	II	III	IV
(b)	III	II	I	IV
(c)	II	I	IV	III
(d)	IV	III	II	I

39. The drive shaft of an automobile rotates at 3600 rpm and transmits 80 HP up from the engine to the rear wheels. The torque developed by the engine is

(a) 16.58 N-m (b) 0.022 N-m

(c) 158.38 N-m (d) 141.6 N-m

40. Two electric bulbs, rated at 25 W, 220 V and 100 W, 220V are connected in series across a 220 V voltage source. If the 25 W and 100 W bulbs draw powers P_1 and P_2 respectively, then

(a) $P_1 = 9\,W, P_2 = 16\,W$ (b) $P_1 = 16\,W, P_2 = 9\,W$

(c) $P_1 = 4\,W, P_2 = 16\,W$ (d) $P_1 = 16\,W, P_2 = 4\,W$

41. A ball is thrown up with a certain velocity, so that it reaches a height h. Find the ratio of the two different times of the ball reaching $\frac{h}{3}$ in both the directions.

(a) $\frac{1}{3}$ (b) $\frac{\sqrt{3}-1}{\sqrt{3}+1}$

(c) $\frac{\sqrt{2}-1}{\sqrt{2}+1}$ (d) $\frac{\sqrt{3}-\sqrt{2}}{\sqrt{3}+\sqrt{2}}$

42. If the earth shrinks by 25% of its present radius and mass remaining the same, the value of acceleration due to gravity increases by

(a) 50% (b) 75% (c) 25% (d) 60%

43. Two springs are joined and connected to a mass m as shown in the figure. If the force constants of the two springs are k_1 and k_2, then the frequency of oscillation of mass m is

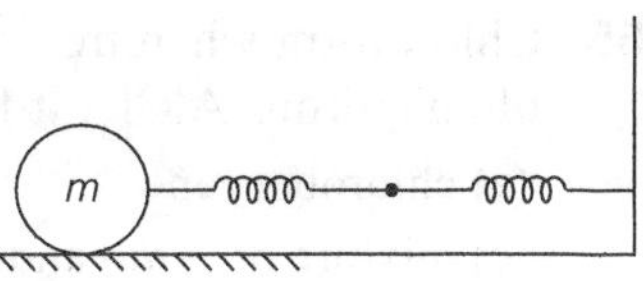

(a) $\nu = \frac{1}{2\pi}\sqrt{\frac{k_1 k_2}{(k_1 + k_2)m}}$ (b) $\nu = \frac{1}{2\pi}\sqrt{\frac{(k_1 + k_2)}{(k_1 k_2)m}}$

(c) $\nu = \frac{1}{2\pi}\sqrt{\frac{(k_1 k_2)m}{k_1 + k_2}}$ (d) $\nu = \frac{1}{2\pi}\sqrt{\frac{(k_1 + k_2)m}{k_1 k_2}}$

44. In the following figure, the capacitance is

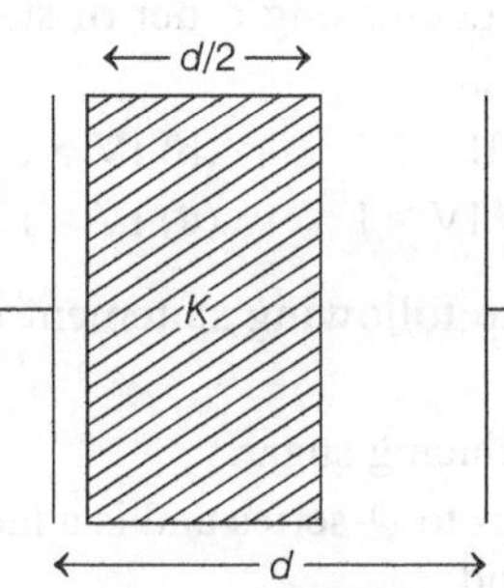

(a) $\frac{2KA\varepsilon_0}{(K+1)d}$ (b) $\frac{2KA\varepsilon_0}{d}$

(c) $\frac{(K+1)A\varepsilon_0}{2d}$ (d) $\frac{2KA\varepsilon_0}{(K^2+1)d}$

45. Two substances P and Q of equal masses m are heated at uniform rate of 6 cal/sec under the similar conditions. A graph between temperature and time is shown in the figure. Ratio of heat absorbed H_P/H_Q by them for complete fusion is

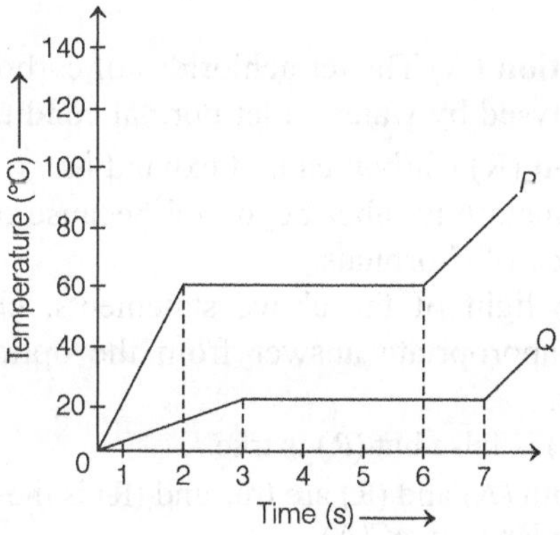

(a) 2 : 3 (b) 2 : 1 (c) 1 : 1 (d) 1 : 2

CHEMISTRY

46. Consider the following groups,

—OAc; —OMe; —OSO_2Me; —OSO_2CF_3
I II III IV

The correct order of leaving group ability is

(a) I > II > III > IV
(b) IV > III > I > II
(c) III > II > I > IV
(d) II > III > IV > I

47. Ethanal reacts with HCN and the addition product so obtained is hydrolysed to form a new compound. This compound shows

(a) optical isomerism (b) geometrical isomerism
(c) tautomerism (d) metamerism

48. For the following reaction,

$$H_2(g) + I_2(g) \rightleftharpoons 2HI(g).$$

If value of equilibrium constant is 50 at 25°C, then the value of ΔG will be

(a) – 6.964 kJ (b) – 4.964 kJ
(c) – 9.694 kJ (d) – 6.496 kJ

49. Given below are two statements.

Statement I The transition metals and their compounds are studied for their catalytic activity due to their capability to adopt multiple oxidation states and complexes.

Statement II Cr^{2+} (d^4) is a stronger reducing agent than Fe^{2+} (d^6) in water.

In the light of the above statements, choose the correct answer from the options given below.

(a) Both Statement I and Statement II are false.
(b) Statement I is true but Statement II is false.
(c) Statement I is false but Statement II is true.
(d) Both Statement I and Statement II are true.

50. For the equilibrium, $CO(g) + \frac{1}{2}O_2(g) \rightleftharpoons CO_2(g)$.

The correct relationship is

(a) $K_p = K_C(RT)^{-1}$ (b) $K_p = K_C(RT)^{-\frac{1}{2}}$

(c) $K_p = K_C(RT)$ (d) $K_p = K_C(RT)^{\frac{1}{2}}$

51. Number of oxygen atom in 0.2 mole of $Na_2S_2O_3$ is

(a) 0.2
(b) 0.4
(c) 0.4 N_A
(d) 0.6 N_A

52. Given below are two statements, one is labelled as Assertion (A) and the other is labelled as Reason (R).

Assertion (A) The tetrachlorides of carbon are not hydrolysed by water under normal conditions.
Reason (R) Carbon cannot expand its coordination number beyond 4 because of the absence of *d*-orbitals.
In the light of the above statements, choose the most appropriate answer from the options given below.

(a) (A) is false but (R) is true.
(b) Both (A) and (R) are true and (R) is the correct explanation of (A).
(c) Both (A) and (R) are true but (R) is not the correct explanation of (A).
(d) (A) is true but (R) is false.

53. Given below are two statements, one is labelled as Assertion (A) and the other is labelled as Reason (R).

Assertion (A) The O—O bond length in H_2O_2 is shorter than that of O_2F_2.
Reason (R) H_2O_2 is a covalent compound.
In the light of the above statements, choose the most appropriate answer from the options given below.

(a) (A) is false but (R) is true.
(b) Both (A) and (R) are true and (R) is the correct explanation of (A).
(c) Both (A) and (R) are true but (R) is not the correct explanation of (A).
(d) (A) is true but (R) is false.

54. Identify *Z* in the sequence of reactions,

$$CH_3CH_2CH=CH_2 \xrightarrow{HBr/H_2O_2} Y \xrightarrow{C_2H_5ONa} Z$$

(a) $CH_3—(CH_2)_3—O—CH_2CH_3$
(b) $(CH_3)_2CH_2—O—CH_2CH_3$
(c) $CH_3(CH_2)_4—O—CH_3$
(d) $CH_3CH_2—CH(CH_3)—O—CH_2CH_3$

55. Chloroform when treated with benzene in presence of anhydrous $AlCl_3$, it forms

(a) chlorobenzene (b) toluene
(c) mixture of *ortho* and *para*-chlorotoluene
(d) triphenyl methane

56. Consider the following compounds,

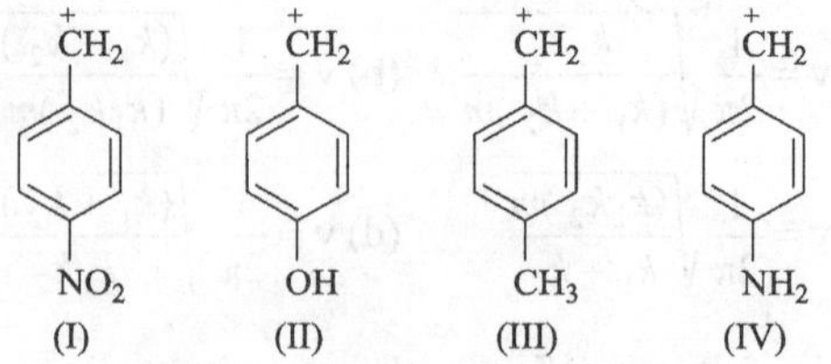

The correct decreasing order of stability of compounds is

(a) I > III > II > IV (b) IV > II > III > I
(c) III > II > IV > I (d) IV > I > III > II

57. Which of the following statement is not true about fructose?

(a) It is a reducing sugar.
(b) It belongs to D-series and is a laevorotatory compound.
(c) It is an aldohexose.
(d) It contains five hydroxyl groups.

58. The hybridisation state of Co in *cis*- $[Co(NH_3)_4Cl_2]^+$ is

(a) d^2sp^3 (b) dsp^2 (c) sp^3 (d) sp^3d^2

59. Given below are two statements.

Statement I Lead storage battery is a secondary cell.
Statement II Faraday's law of electrolysis is related to equivalent weight of electrolyte.
In the light of the above statements, choose the correct answer from the options given below.

(a) Statement I is false but Statement II is true.
(b) Both Statement I and Statement II are true.
(c) Both Statement I and Statement II are false.
(d) Statement I is true but Statement II is false.

60. Which of the following method is correct for the formation of benzene?

(a) Mixture of calcium benzoate and calcium acetate is heated.
(b) Calcium benzoate is heated.
(c) Sodium benzoate is heated with sodalime.
(d) All of the above

61. In reversible isothermal expansion of an ideal gas.

A. $w = 0$ B. $U_1 = U_2$

C. $H_1 = H_2$ D. $q = nRT \ln \frac{V_2}{V_1}$ E. $w = q$

Choose the correct answer from the options given below.

(a) A, B and D (b) A and E
(c) B, C and D (d) Only B

62. Minimum amount of work required to compress 5.00 moles of an ideal gas isothermally from 200 L to 40 L is [Given : log 0.2 = −0.7]

(a) +20.1 kJ (b) −20.1 kJ
(c) −20.1 J (d) +20.1 J

63. Molarity of a solution obtained by mixing 800 mL of 0.6 M HCl with 200 mL of 1 M HCl will be

(a) 0.4 M (b) 1.6 M
(c) 0.68 M (d) 1.68 M

64. Consider the reaction, $M^{3+} + 3e^- \longrightarrow M$; If 0.415 g of metal M is deposited at the cathode due to passage of 2A of current for 965 s, then the atomic weight of the metal M is

(a) 124.5 g (b) 62.25 g (c) 18.75 g (d) 27.5 g

65. Match the following columns.

Oxide	Nature
A. Cr_2O_3	I. Basic
B. V_2O_3	II. Neutral
C. CO	III. Acidic
D. Cl_2O_7	IV. Amphoteric

Which of the following is correct option?

(a) A-IV, B-I, C-II, D-III
(b) A-III, B-II, C-I, D-IV
(c) A-IV, B-III, C-II, D-I
(d) A-I, B-II, C-IV, D-III

66. Assuming 100% dissociation, maximum van't Hoff factor is of

(a) $CaCl_2$
(b) $K_4[Fe(CN)_6]$
(c) $AlCl_3$
(d) NH_2CONH_2

67. Match the List-I with List-II.

List-I	List-II
A. KCl	(i) Polar covalent compound
B. NH_3	(ii) *sp*-hybridisation in carbon atoms
C. Acetylene	(iii) Trigonal pyramidal shape
D. H_2O	(iv) Ionic compound

Choose the correct answer from the options given below.

(a) A-(iv), B-(iii), C-(ii), D-(i)
(b) A-(iii), B-(iv), C-(i), D-(ii)
(c) A-(iv), B-(iii), C-(i), D-(ii)
(d) A-(i), B-(iv), C-(ii), D-(iii)

68. Given below are two statements.

Statement I π-bond is formed by sidewise overlapping of $d_{x^2-y^2}$ and p_y orbital along x-axis.

Statement II An increase in s-character give rise to a decrease in size of orbitals.

In the light of the above statements, choose the correct answer from the options given below.

(a) Statement I is false but Statement II is true.
(b) Both Statement I and Statement II are true.
(c) Both Statement I and Statement II are false.
(d) Statement I is true but Statement II is false.

69. Match the List-I with List-II.

List-I	List-II
A. H_3O^+	(i) Tetrahedral
B. $HC \equiv CH$	(ii) Angular
C. ClO_2^-	(iii) Linear
D. NH_4^+	(iv) Pyramidal

Choose the correct answer from the options given below.

(a) A-(iv), B-(iii), C-(ii), D-(i)
(b) A-(i), B-(ii), C-(iii), D-(iv)
(c) A-(iv), B-(iii), C-(i), D-(ii)
(d) A-(iii), B-(ii), C-(i), D-(iv)

70. According to Moseley, a straight line graph is obtained on plotting.
(a) The frequencies of characteristics of X-rays of elements against their atomic numbers.
(b) The square of the frequencies of characteristics of X-rays of elements against their atomic numbers.
(c) The square root of the frequencies of characteristics of X-rays of elements against their atomic numbers.
(d) The reciprocal of frequencies of characteristics of X-rays of elements against their atomic numbers.

71. Match the complexes in List-I with their informations in List-II.

	List-I	List-II
A.	$[Cu(NH_3)_4]SO_4$	(i) dsp^3
B.	$[Fe(CO)_5]$	(ii) d^2sp^3
C.	$K_4[Fe(CN)_6]$	(iii) sp^3d^2
D.	$[Fe(H_2O)_6]Cl_3$	(iv) dsp^2

Choose the correct answer from the options given below.
(a) A-(iv), B-(i), C-(ii), D-(iii)
(b) A-(iv), B-(i), C-(iii), D-(ii)
(c) A-(iii), B-(i), C-(ii), D-(iv)
(d) A-(iii), B-(ii), C-(i), D-(iv)

72. A solution contains Fe^{2+}, Fe^{3+} and I^- ions. This solution was treated with iodine at 35°C. E_0 for Fe^{3+}/Fe^{2+} is + 0.77 V and $E°$ for $I_2/2I^- = 0.536$ V. The favourable redox reaction is
(a) I_2 will be reduced to I^-
(b) there will be no redox reaction
(c) I^- will be oxidised to I_2
(d) Fe^{2+} will be oxidised to Fe^{3+}

73. What is observed when excess of dilute NaOH solution added to an aqueous solution of aluminium chloride?
(a) A white precipitate which dissolves in excess NaOH.
(b) A permanent white precipitate is formed immediately.
(c) A green precipitate forms which turns red on standing in air.
(d) No change is noted at first; a white precipitate is formed on standing.

74. Which of the given amino acids are classified as basic amino acids?
I. Lysine II. Arginine
III. Histidine IV. Glycine
V. Aspartic acid
Choose the most appropriate answer from the options given below.
(a) I, II, III (b) II, III, IV
(c) I, II, III, IV, V (d) I, II, V

75. Among the following species,
(i) XeO_3 (ii) $XeOF_4$
(iii) XeF_6 (iv) XeF_2
(v) SO_4^{2-} (vi) XeO_2
(vii) XeO_2F_2
The number of species having same number of lone pairs are
(a) 5 (b) 2 (c) 1 (d) 4

76. Decomposition of $NH_4NO_2(aq)$ into $N_2(g)$ and $2H_2O(l)$ is first order reaction. Which of the following graph is correct?

(a) 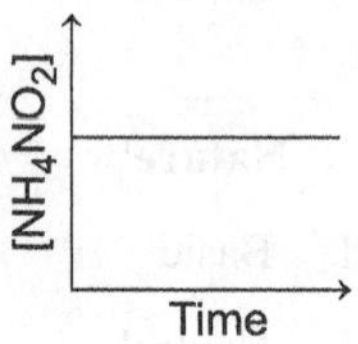

(b) 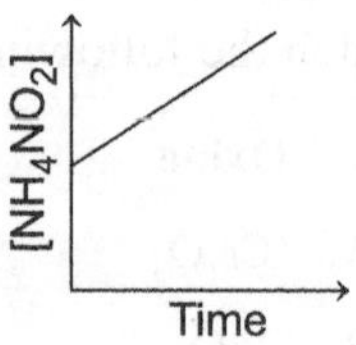

(c) 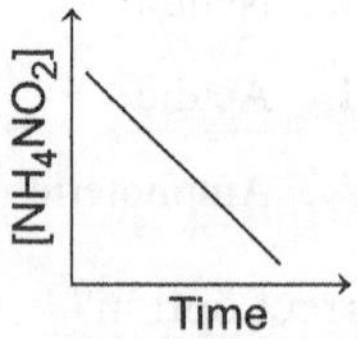

(d) 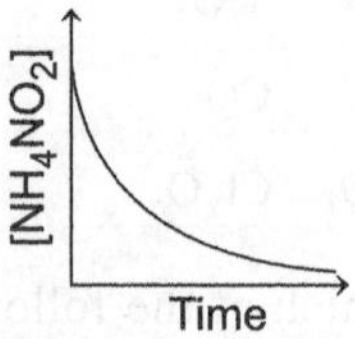

77. Which of the following compounds gives orange precipitate when treated with 2, 4-dinitrophenyl hydrazine?

(a) 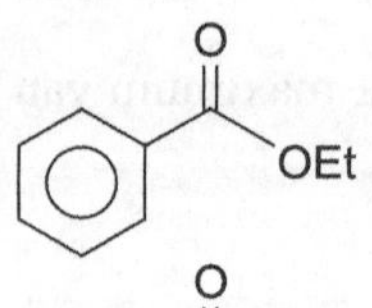

(b) 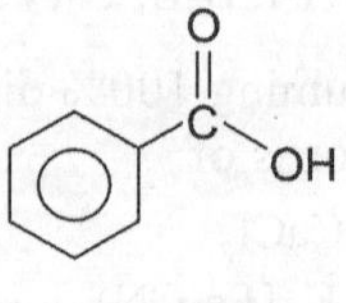

(c) 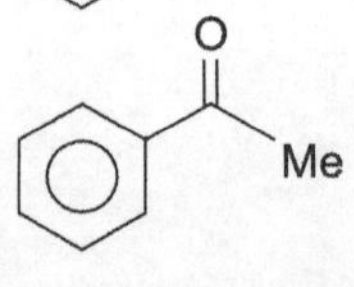

(d) 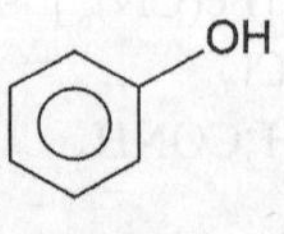

78. Which of the following complex ion is not expected to absorb visible light?

(a) $[NiCl_4]^{-2}$ (b) $[Ni(CN)_4]^{-2}$

(c) $[Cr(NH_3)_6]^{+3}$ (d) $[FeF_6]^{-3}$

79. Methyl amine reacts with $NaNO_2$ in the presence of HCl to form

I. N_2 II. HCl

III. CH_3OH IV. CH_3CHO

V. CH_3Cl

Choose the correct option.

(a) I, II and V (b) I and III

(c) I, IV and V (d) I, II and III

80. Choose the correct order of acidic strength of the following compounds.

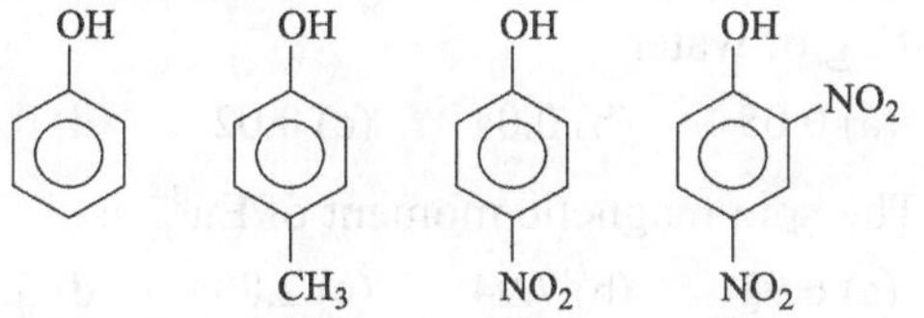

(I) (II) (III) (IV)

(a) I < II < III < IV (b) I < II < IV < III

(c) II < I < III < IV (d) III < I > II < IV

81. Match the List-I and List-II.

List-I (Reaction name)	List- II (Product)
A. Etard reaction	(i) Cinnamic acid
B. Reformatsky reaction	(ii) Benzaldehyde
C. Friedel-Craft's acylation	(iii) Dibenzoketone
D. Perkin reaction	(iv) α , β-unsaturated ester

Choose the correct answer from the options given below.

(a) A-(ii), B-(iv), C-(iii), D-(i)

(b) A-(ii), B-(iv), C-(i), D-(iii)

(c) A-(iv), B-(ii), C-(iii), D-(i)

(d) A-(i), B-(iv), C-(ii), D-(iii)

82. Given below are two statements.

Statement I Actinoids have magnetic moments less than theoretically predicted value.

Statement II Actinoids have larger number of oxidation states than lanthanoids.

In the light of the above statements, choose the correct answer from the options given below.

(a) Statement I is false but Statement II is true.

(b) Both Statement I and Statement II are true.

(c) Both Statement I and Statement II are false.

(d) Statement I is true but Statement II is false.

83.

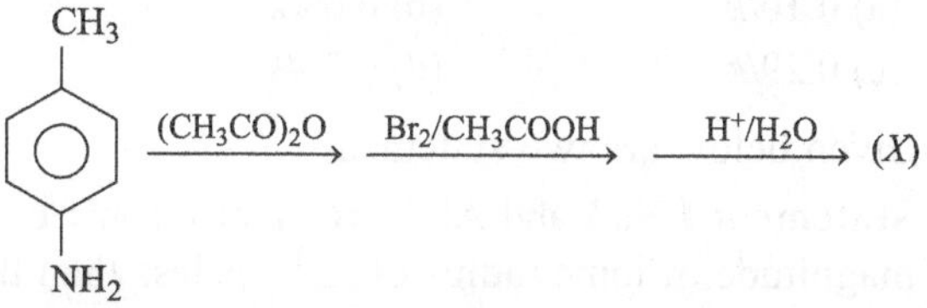

X is

(a)

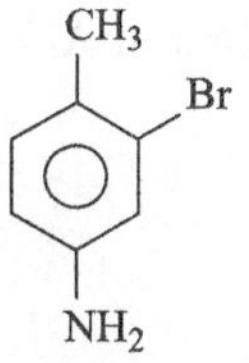

(b)

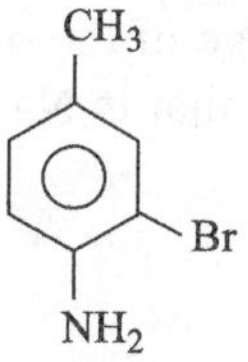

(c)

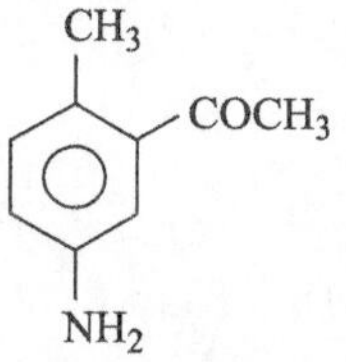

(d)

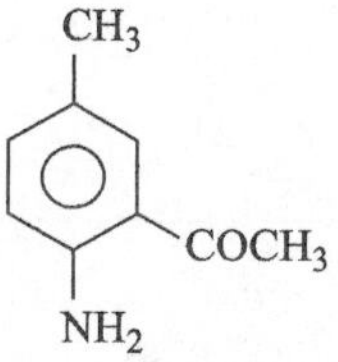

84. OsO_4 is highly toxic volatile substance. It is 518 times more soluble in CCl_4 than in water. Product obtained on reaction of cyclopentene with osmium tetraoxide at 25°C followed by reaction with Na_2SO_3 is

(a) *cis*-cyclopentan-1, 3-diol

(b) *trans*-cyclopentan-1, 3-diol

(c) *trans*-cyclopentan-1, 2-diol

(d) *cis*-cyclopentan-1, 2-diol

85. In base *vs* acid titration, at the end point methyl orange is present as
(a) quinonoid form
(b) benzenoid form
(c) heterocyclic form
(d) phenolic form

86. $t_{1/4}$ can be defined as the time taken for the concentration of a reactant to drop to 3/4th of its initial value. If the rate constant for a first order reaction is k, then $t_{1/4}$ can be given as $[\log 1.33 = 0.124]$
(a) $0.10/k$ (b) $0.69/k$
(c) $0.29/k$ (d) $0.75/k$

87. Given below are two statements.
Statement I Na^+ and Al^{3+} are isoelectronic but the magnitude of ionic radius of Al^{3+} is less than that of Na^+.
Statement II The magnitude of effective nuclear charge of the outer shell electrons in Al^{3+} is lesser than that in Na^+.
In the light of the above statements, choose the correct answer from the options given below.
(a) Statement I is false but Statement II is true.
(b) Both Statement I and Statement II are true.
(c) Both Statement I and Statement II are false.
(d) Statement I is true but Statement II is false.

88. What is the lowest energy of the spectral line emitted by the hydrogen atom in the Lyman series?
(a) $\frac{5hcR_H}{36}$ (b) $\frac{4hcR_H}{3}$
(c) $\frac{3hcR_H}{4}$ (d) $\frac{7hcR_H}{144}$

89. What will be the value of relative lowering of vapour pressure when 3 g urea is dissolved in 45 g of water?
(a) 0.05 (b) 0.04 (c) 0.02 (d) 0.01

90. The spin magnetic moment of Eu^{3+} is
(a) 6.93 (b) 7.94 (c) 2.83 (d) 3.87

BIOLOGY

91. A stilt root system is best adapted to perform which one of the following functions?

(a) Storage of food
(b) Absorption of water and minerals from the soil
(c) Transport of water and organic food
(d) Anchorage of the plant into the soil

92. Given below are two statements; one is labelled as Assertion (A) and other is labelled as Reason (R).

Assertion (A) Members of Sphenopsida are commonly called horsetails.

Reason (R) The present day Sphenopsida includes only one living genus–*Equisetum*.

In the light of the above statements, choose the correct answer from the options given below.

(a) A is false, but R is true
(b) Both A and R are true and R is the correct explanation of A
(c) Both A and R are true, but R is not the correct explanation of A
(d) A is true, but R is false

93. Match List I with List II.

	List I		List II
A.	Afferent neurons	1.	Carry sensory impulses from receptors to CNS
B.	Efferent neurons	2.	Carry motor impulses from CNS to effectors
C.	Unipolar neurons	3.	Found in the cerebral cortex
D.	Multipolar neurons	4.	Usually found in embryonic stage

Choose the correct answer from the options given below.

	A	B	C	D
(a)	1	2	3	4
(b)	4	3	1	2
(c)	1	2	4	3
(d)	2	1	3	4

94. Consider the given statements and choose the correct set of statements. .

I. Increase in mass and increase in number of individuals are twin characteristics of growth.
II. All organism can sense and respond to environmental cues except prokaryotes.
III. Unicellular organisms show growth by cell division.
IV. As new areas are explored, biodiversity tends to decrease.
V. Biological names are generally written in Latin.

Choose the correct answer from the options given below.

(a) II and IV
(b) II, III and V
(c) I, III and V
(d) II and IV only

95. Choose the incorrect matched pair.

(a) Amyloplasts – Store proteins granules
(b) Elaioplasts – Store oils or fats
(c) Chlorophlasts – Contain chlorophyll pigments
(d) Chromoplasts – Contain pigments other than chlorophyll

96. Which of the following statements correctly characterise ribosomes?

(a) They are the only site of RNA replication
(b) They are composed of two equal subunits
(c) They contain fewer identical components in prokaryotes and eukaryotes
(d) They are the site of protein synthesis

97. Which of the following statements is incorrect?

(a) Xeromorphic characters are inherited
(b) Autoecology deals with the study of a group of organisms
(c) Key stone species are low in abundance than the dominant species
(d) A major adaptation of tropical plants is the presence of mycorrhizae

98. Which of the following option gives the correct sequences of events during mitosis?

(a) Condensation → Nuclear membrane disassembly → Crossing over → Segregation → Telophase.
(b) Condensation → Nuclear membrane disassembly→ Arrangement at equator→ Centromere division → Seggregation → Telophase.

(c) Condensation → Crossing over → Nuclear membrane disassembly → Seggregation → Telophase.
(d) Condensation → Arrangement at equator → Centromere division→ Seggregation → Telophase.

99. Match List I with List II.

	List I		List II
A.	Brassicaceae	1.	Br ⊕ ⚥ Epi_{3-9} $K_{5 \text{ or } (5)}$ $\widehat{C_5 A_{(\infty)}}$ $\underline{G}_{(2-\infty)}$
B.	Fabaceae	2.	Br % ⚥ $P_2 A_3 G_1$
C.	Malvaceae	3.	% ⚥ $K_{(5)} C_{1+2+(2)} A_{(9)+1} \underline{G_1}$
D.	Gramineae	4.	⊕ ⚥ $K_{2+2} C_4 A_{2+4} \underline{G}_{(2)}$

Choose the correct answer from the options given below.

	A	B	C	D		A	B	C	D
(a)	3	1	2	4	(b)	4	3	1	2
(c)	4	1	2	3	(d)	2	3	1	4

100. Given below are two statements; one is labelled as Assertion (A) and other is labelled as Reason (R).
Assertion (A) A decrease in species diversity occurs as we ascend a high mountain.
Reason (R) Drop in temperature and lower seasonal variability at higher altitude increases diversity.
In the light of the above statements, choose the correct answer from the options given below.
(a) A is false, but R is true
(b) Both A and R are true and R is the correct explanation of A
(c) Both A and R are true, but R is not the correct explanation of A
(d) A is true, but R is false

101. The actin and myosin filaments can be best explained as
(a) when myofilament slide pass each other myosin filaments shorten, while action filaments do not shorten
(b) the light band contains actin, whereas the dark band contains myosin
(c) the light band contains myosin, whereas the dark band contains actin
(d) myosin filaments are thinner as compared to actin filaments

102. How many meiotic divisions will be necessary to produce 280 pollen grains?
(a) 100 (b) 70
(c) 99 (d) 140

103. Given below are two statements.
Statement I Grasshopper shows female heterogamety at earlier stage of development.
Statement II Genetic map is one that establishes various stages in gene evolution.
In the light of the above statements, choose the correct answer from the options given below.
(a) Statement I is incorrect, but Statement II is correct
(b) Both statement I and Statement II are correct
(c) Both statement I and Statement II are incorrect
(d) Statement I is correct, but Statement II is incorrect

104. Identify the incorrect statement.
(a) Henking discovered an X-body, while Y-body was discovered by Stevens
(b) Gynaecomastia is associated with Turner's syndrome
(c) Accumulation of phenylalanine acid in the brain results in mental retardation
(d) Only 8 per cent of males and 0.4 per cent of females suffer from colour blindness

105. Identify the incorrect statement.
(a) Members of Basidiomycetes have branched and septate mycelium
(b) Members of Deuteromycetes include *Alternaria, Trichoderma* and *Puccinia*
(c) Ciliated protozoans are actively moving organisms
(d) *Euglena* has a protein rich layer called pellicle

106. Consider the following statements.
I. In an aquatic ecosystem, DFC is the major conduit for energy flow.
II. In ecosystem, the trophic level represents a functional level, not a species as such.
III. Species cannot occupy more than one trophic level in the same ecosystem at the same time.
IV. In most ecosystem, the pyramids of number, energy and biomass are upright.
V. The pyramid of biomass in sea is also upright.

Choose the correct answer from the options given below.

(a) I, III and IV (b) I, IV and V
(c) II, III and IV (d) II and IV only

107. Match List I with List II.

	List I		List II
A.	Sex-linked trait	1.	Furrowed tongue with broad palm
B.	Autosomal recessive traits	2.	Non-stop bleeding
C.	$Hb^S Hb^S$	3.	Abnormal haemoglobin
D.	Chromosomal disorder	4.	Genotype of disease sickle-cell anaemia

Choose the correct answer from the options given below.

	A	B	C	D		A	B	C	D
(a)	2	3	4	1	(b)	2	3	1	4
(c)	1	4	3	2	(d)	2	4	1	3

108. In addition to *ori*, the vector requires a ...., which helps in identifying non-transformants and selectively permitting the growth of transformants.

(a) cloning site (b) selectable marker
(c) recognition site (d) restriction enzyme

109. Which of the following statements is incorrect about decomposition?

(a) Detritivores like earthworm breakdown the detritus
(b) In leaching the soluble inorganic nutrients go down into the soil horizon.
(c) The bacterial and fungal enzymes degrades detritus into simple inorganic salts by the process of fragmentation
(d) It is an aerobic process

110. Match List I with List II.

	List I		List II
A.	Storage of urine	1.	Proximal convoluted tubule
B.	Reabsorption	2.	Ureter
C.	Ultrafiltration	3.	Malpighian corpuscle
D.	Transport of urine	4.	Urinary bladder

Choose the correct answer from the options given below.

	A	B	C	D		A	B	C	D
(a)	4	1	3	2	(b)	4	1	2	3
(c)	4	2	3	1	(d)	2	3	4	1

111. Given below are two statements, one is labelled as Assertion (A) and other is labelled as Reason (R).

Assertion (A) Restriction endonuclease recognise short palindromic sequence and cut at specific sites.

Reason (R) When a restriction endonuclease acts on palindrome site, it cleaves both the strands of DNA molecule.

In the light of the above statements, choose the correct answer from the options given below.

(a) A is false, but R is true
(b) Both A and R are true and R is the correct explanation of A
(c) Both A and R are true, but R is not the correct explanation of A
(d) A is true, but R is false

112. Which of the following has circular smooth muscles and elastic fibres?

(a) Tunica interna (b) Tunica externa
(c) Tunica media (d) None of these

113. In lungs there is definite exchange of ions between RBC and plasma. Removal of CO_2 from blood involves

(a) influx of Cl^- into RBC
(b) efflux of Cl^- from RBC
(c) infflux of HCO_3^- ion in RBC
(d) efflux of HCO_3^- ions from RBC

114. Thyroid hormones support .... and control metabolism of ....

(a) WBC formation, carbohydrate
(b) Platelet formation, calcium
(c) Water-electrolyte balance, vitamins
(d) RBC formation, protein

115. Which enzyme catalyses the separation of DNA strands during DNA replication?

(a) DNA polymerase (b) Helicase
(c) Ligase (d) Primase

116. In a certain taxon of insects some have 32 chromosomes and the others have 31 chromosomes. The 32 and 31 chromosomes-bearing organisms are
(a) Males and females, respectively
(b) Females and males, respectively
(c) Drones and males, respectively
(d) Females and drones, respectively

117. Given below are two statements; one is labelled as Assertion (A) and other is labelled as Reason (R).

Assertion (A) Whisky and brandy are the products of fermentation.

Reason (R) Wine and beer are alcoholic beverages produced by the distillation of fermented broth.

In the light of the above statements, choose the correct answer from the options given below.
(a) A is false, but R is true
(b) Both A and R are true and R is the correct explanation of A
(c) Both A and R are true, but R is not the correct explanation of A
(d) A is true, but R is false

118. Match the List I with List II.

	List I		List II
A.	Parenchyma	1.	Absent in monocots
B.	Collenchyma	2.	Aerenchyma
C.	Sclerenchyma	3.	Complex permanent tissue
D.	Xylem	4.	Leaves of tea

	A	B	C	D		A	B	C	D
(a)	2	1	4	3	(b)	2	1	3	4
(c)	1	2	4	3	(d)	2	4	3	1

119. The minimum number of meiotic divisions required to produce 70 seeds in *Cyperus* are
(a) 125
(b) 250
(c) 140
(d) 40

120. Given below are two statements.

Statement I *Plasmodium malariae* is the most serious type of *Plasmodium* species which affects the brain.

Statement II The sporozoites of *Plasmodium* are injected into the human blood *via* vector, i.e. *Anopheles* mosquito.

In the light of the above statements, choose the correct answer from the options given below.
(a) Statement I is incorrect, but Statement II is correct
(b) Both statement I and Statement II are correct
(c) Both statement I and Statement II are incorrect
(d) Statement I is correct, but Statement II is incorrect

121. Read the following statements.
I. On an average, human kidneys filter about 1/5th of the blood pumped out by each ventricle of the heart in a minute.
II. The P-wave in ECG represents the repolarisation of atria.
III. Reduction in pH of blood will reduce the rate of heartbeat.
IV. During inspiration the lungs act as suction pump.
V. Muscles containing high content of myoglobin has plenty of mitochondria.

Choose the correct answer from the options given below.
(a) I, II and IV
(b) I, IV and V
(c) I, III and V
(d) I, II and III

122. Select the correct sequence of electron transfer from the options given below.
(a) $P_{680} \rightarrow P_{700} \rightarrow$ Cytochrome $\rightarrow$ PQ
(b) $P_{680} \rightarrow$ PQ $\rightarrow$ Q $\rightarrow$ Cytochrome
(c) $P_{680} \rightarrow$ PQ $\rightarrow$ Cytochrome $\rightarrow$ PC
(d) $P_{680} \rightarrow$ PQ $\rightarrow$ Cytochrome $\rightarrow$ PS-II

123. Alternation of asexual and sexual phases is observed in the phylum ....
(a) *Meandrina* and *Gorgonia*
(b) *Ctenoplana* and *Adamsia*
(c) *Taenia* and *Ancylostoma*
(d) *Antedon* and *Pennatula*

124. Given below are two statements; one is labelled as Assertion (A) and the other is labelled as Reason (R).

Assertion (A) Claspers are a distinguishing feature of males in class– Chondrichthyes.

Reason (R) Claspers help in copulation.

In the light of the above statements, choose the correct answer from the options given below.
(a) A is false, but R is true
(b) Both A and R are true and R is the correct explanation of A
(c) Both A and R are true, but R is not the correct explanation of A
(d) A is true, but R is false

125. Indole acetic acid promotes the cell elongation by
(a) decrease in osmotic solutes
(b) decrease in wall pressure
(c) decrease in permeability of cytoplasm to water
(d) decrease in wall synthesis

126. Match List I with List II.

	List I		List II
A.	Bilateral symmetry	1.	Porifera
B.	Radial symmetry	2.	Echinoderm larvae
C.	Asymmetry	3.	Ctenophora
D.	Radial symmetry	4.	Cnidaria

Choose the correct answer from the options given below.

	A	B	C	D
(a)	2	3	1	4
(b)	2	3	4	1
(c)	3	2	1	4
(d)	1	2	3	4

127. During mid-1960s three independent researchers reported the purification and chemical characterisation of three different kinds of inhibitors, i.e. Inhibitor – B, abscission II and dormin. Later all the three were proven to be chemically identical. It is named as
(a) Indole acetic acid
(b) Indole butylic acid
(c) Naphthalene acetic acid
(d) Abscisic acid

128. Given below are two statements.
Statement I In brinjal, stamens are attached to the petals and are called as epipetalous.
Statement II In China rosa, diadelphous types of stamens are present.
In the light of the above statements, choose the correct answer from the options given below.
(a) Statement I is incorrect, but Statement II is correct
(b) Both Statement I and Statement II are correct
(c) Both Statement I and Statement II are incorrect
(d) Statement I is correct, but Statement II is incorrect

129. Given below are two statements.
Statement I Oral contraceptives prevent the entry of sperms into female reproductive tract.
Statement II Emergency contraceptives have been proved effective to prevent pregnancy by the use of progestogen within 24 hours.
In the light of the above statements, choose the correct answer from the options given below.
(a) Statement I is incorrect, but Statement II is correct
(b) Both Statement I and Statement II are correct
(c) Both Statement I and Statement II are incorrect
(d) Statement I is correct, but Statement II is incorrect

130. Given below are two statements.
Statement I In plant kingdom, families are characterised on the basis of vegetative and reproductive features.
Statement II From species to kingdom, the number of common characteristics goes on increasing.
In the light of the above statements, choose the correct answer from the options given below.
(a) Statement I is incorrect, but Statement II is correct
(b) Both Statement I and Statement II are correct
(c) Both Statement I and Statement II are incorrect
(d) Statement I is correct, but Statement II is incorrect

131. Given below are two statements.
Statement I *Bt* plants are resistant to the attack of insect pests.
Statement II The scientists have introduced *B. thuringiensis* toxin genes into the animals.
In the light of the above statements, choose the correct answer from the options given below.
(a) Statement I is incorrect, but Statement II is correct
(b) Both Statement I and Statement II are correct
(c) Both Statement I and Statement II are incorrect
(d) Statement I is correct, but Statement II is incorrect

132. The 24 hrs rhythm of our body such as the sleep-wake cycle is regulated by ...*A*... hormone secreted by ...*B*... .

	A	*B*
(a)	glucocorticoids	pituitary gland
(b)	calcitonin	parathyroid gland
(c)	melatonin	pineal gland
(d)	thymosin	thymus

133. In a prokaryotic cell, the inclusion bodies
(a) are bounded by membrane system
(b) lie freely in the cytoplasm
(c) Both (a) and (b)
(d) they do not store reserve food material

134. Consider the following statements.
I. Lysosomes are membrane bound vesicular structures formed by the process of packaging in the Golgi apparatus.
II. Mitochondria divide by the fragmentation process.
III. 70S ribosomes are composed of two subunits whereas 50S ribosomes are composed of three subunits.
IV. ER helps in the transport of substances, synthesis of proteins, lipoproteins and glycogen.
V. Mitochondria help in oxidative phosphorylation and generation of ATP.

Choose the correct answer from the options given below.
(a) I, II and III (b) II, IV and V
(c) I, III and IV (d) I, IV and V

135. .... is famous for hosting thousands of migratory birds coming from Siberia every winter.
(a) Keoladeo National Park, Rajasthan
(b) Kanha National park, Balaghat
(c) Corbett National Park, Uttarakhand
(d) Kaziranga National Park, Assam

136. Which of the following statements is correct?
(a) Arteries carry blood away from the heart to different organs
(b) Pulmonary artery carries the oxygenated blood
(c) In mammals, the arteries differs from veins in having internal valves
(d) Maximum surface area is observed in veins

137. Which of the following is expected to have the highest value ($gm/m^2/yr$) in a grassland ecosystem?
(a) Secondary Production (SP)
(b) Tertiary Production (TP)
(c) Gross Production (GP)
(d) Net Production (NP)

138. Which of the following is the correct recognition site of *Eco*RI restriction endonuclease?

(a) 5′ – A – G ↓ C – T – 3′
3′ – T – C ↑ G – A – 5′

(b) 5′ – G ↓ A – A – T – T – C – 3′
3′ – C – T – T – A – A ↑ G – 5′

(c) 5′ – G – G ↓ C – C – 3′
3′ – C – C ↑ G – G – 5′

(d) 5′ – G ↓ G – A – T – C – C – 3′
3′ – C – C – T – A – G ↑ G – 5′

139. Given below are two statements.
Statement I Syphilis can pass from the mother to the developing foetus.
Statement II Placenta is impermeable to the pathogens.
In the light of the above statements, choose the correct answer from the options given below.
(a) Statement I is incorrect, but statement II is correct
(b) Both Statement I and Statement II are correct
(c) Both Statement I and Statement II are incorrect
(d) Statement I is correct, but Statement II is incorrect

140. Identify the incorrect statement.
(a) Evolution is a stochastic process based on chance events in nature and chance mutation in organisms
(b) In a mixed population the better adapted ones often survive and grow in population size and the variants are wiped out
(c) First cellular form of life did not possibly originate till about 2000 mya
(d) Whales, bats, cheetah share similarities in patterns of bones of forelimbs.

141. Match List I with List II.

	List I		List II
A.	UUU	1.	Serine
B.	GGG	2.	Phenylalanine
C.	UCU	3.	Glycine
D.	CCC	4.	Proline

Choose the correct answer from the options given below.

	A	B	C	D
(a)	2	3	1	4
(b)	4	1	2	3
(c)	3	4	1	2
(d)	2	1	3	4

142. 'Mummies' of Egypt still have their arteries preserved due to the presence of

(a) yellow elastic connective tissue fibres
(b) white fibrous connective tissue fibres
(c) cartilages
(d) valves

143. Identify the correct set of statements.

I. During gel electrophoresis the smallest DNA fragment will move to the farthest point towards cathode.
II. The restriction endonuclease enzyme binds to the DNA and cuts each of the two strands at specific points in their base sugar bonds.
III. The high sensitivity of PCR permits virus detection soon after infection and even before the onset of disease.
IV. pBR322 has genes for resistance against tetracycline or amipicillin.
V. Polyethylene glycol method is used for gene transfer without a vector.

Choose the correct answer from the options given below.

(a) II, III and V
(b) I, II and IV
(c) I, III and V
(d) III, IV and V

144. Consider the given section of a particular plant part.

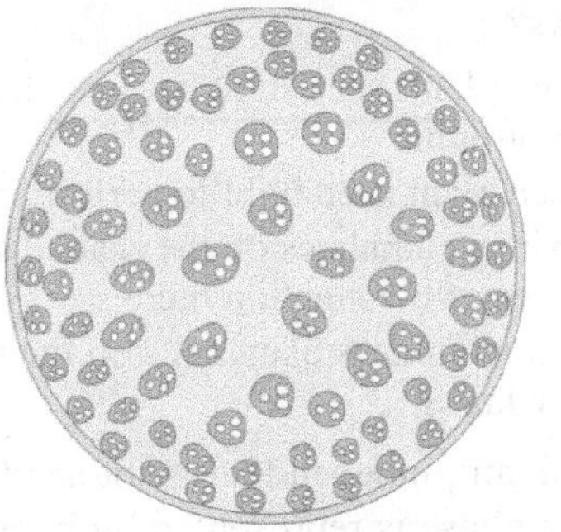

Choose the incorrect statement w.r.t. the given figure.

(a) Peripheral vascular bundles are generally smaller than the centrally located ones.
(b) Primary xylem shows endarch arrangement.
(c) Lysigenos cavity is present within each vascular bundle.
(d) Each vascular bundle is surrounded by parenchymatous bundle sheath.

145. Which of the following hormones stimulates corpus luteum to produce progesterone?

(a) FSH
(b) Oestrogen
(c) Chorionic corticotropin
(d) hCG

146. In addition to the prolactin which hormone has lactogenic properties?

(a) hPL
(b) Chorionic thyrotropin
(c) Oestrogen
(d) Progesterone

147. YACs are constructed artificially in the laboratory by joining segments of

(a) original DNA bacteria and linear plasmid from yeast
(b) original DNA of yeast and linear RNA from virus
(c) original DNA of yeast and linear plasmid from bacteria
(d) protein of virus and linear plasmid from bacteria

148. What causes a green plant exposed to the light, on only one side, to bend towards the source of light as it grows?

(a) Green plants seek light because they are phototrophic
(b) Green plant need light to perform photosynthesis
(c) Auxin accumulates on the shaded side, stimulating greater cell elongation there
(d) Light stimulates plant cells on the well-lit side to grow faster

149. A dominant, independent, photosynthetic, thalloid or erect phase is represented by haploid gametophytes and it alternates with the short lived multicellular sporophyte totally or partially dependent on the gametophytes for this anchorage and nutrition. This type of pattern is present in

(a) Mosses and liverworts (b) Ferns and horsetails
(c) *Cycas* and *Pinus* (d) *Ulothrix* and *Spirogyra*

150. Which property among these listed below is not a criterion for a molecule to act as a genetic material?

(a) It should be able to generate its replica
(b) It should be stable chemically and structurally.
(c) It should be degraded at high temperature
(d) It should mutate slowly to facilitate the evolution

151. Competitive inhibition of enzyme is affected by

(a) end product of reaction
(b) substrate concentration
(c) intermediate products formed
(d) Non-availability of activation energy

152. A phase that is common in anaerobic and aerobic respiration is

(a) TCA cycle (b) glycolysis
(c) glycogenolysis (d) ETS

153. The carrying capacity of an area is 500 and the population density is 400. If the intrinsic rate of natural increase is 0.01 then what will be the value of $\frac{dN}{dt}$ for this population?

(a) 0.01 (b) 0.8 (c) 80 (d) 40

154. Which of the following pairs should be chosen in order to perform critical study of secondary growth in plants?

(a) Deodar and fern
(b) Teak and pine
(c) Wheat and maiden hair fern
(d) Sugarcane and sunflower

155. Given below are two statements.

Statement I The haemoglobin of the foetus has a higher affinity for oxygen than that of adult haemoglobin.

Statement II Oxygen-haemoglobin dissociation curve for foetal haemoglobin will appear on the right side.

In the light of the above statements, choose the correct answer from the options given below.

(a) Statement I is incorrect, but Statement II is correct
(b) Both Statement I and Statement II are correct
(c) Both Statement I and Statement II are incorrect
(d) Statement I is correct, but Statement II is incorrect

156. Match List I with List II.

	List I		List II
A.	Epicotyl	1.	Place where pollen grain land
B.	Hypocotyl	2.	Site for seed development
C.	Stigma	3.	Portion of embryonal axis above the level of cotyledons
D.	Ovary	4.	Portion below the level of cotyledons

Choose the correct answer from the options given below.

	A	B	C	D		A	B	C	D
(a)	3	4	1	2	(b)	4	3	2	1
(c)	3	4	2	1	(d)	2	1	3	4

157. Consider the following figure and choose the parts (labelled A-D) that degenerate after fertilisation in flowering plants.

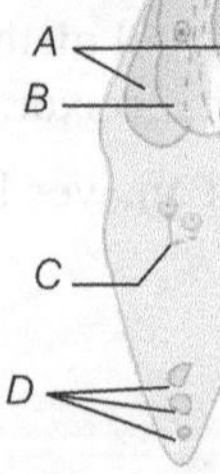

(a) *A*, *B* and *D* (b) *B* and *D*
(c) *A* and *C* (d) *A* and *D*

158. Identify the correct set of infectious disease.

I. Cancer II. Influenza
III. Allergy IV. Smallpox
V. Common cold

Choose the correct answer from the options given below.

(a) I and II (b) II, IV and V
(c) I, II, IV and V (d) II and IV

159. Given below are two statements; one is labelled as Assertion (A) and other is labelled as Reason (R).

Assertion (A) LSD and charas are hallucinogenic drugs.

Reason (R) These drugs alter thought, feelings and perceptions.

In the light of the above statements, choose the correct answer from the options given below.

(a) A is false, but R is true
(b) Both A and R are true and R is the correct explanation of A
(c) Both A and R are true, but R is not the correct explanation of A
(d) A is true, but R is false

160. If chromosome number of diploid cell is 20 at the G_1, how many chromosomes will be present during G_2-phase ?

(a) 20 (b) 40 (c) 60 (d) 10

161. Given below are two statements; one is labelled as Assertion (A) and other is labelled as Reason (R).

Assertion (A) Diakinesis is the final stage of meiotic prophase-I.

Reason (R) It is marked by terminalisation of chiasmata.

In the light of the above statements, choose the correct answer from the options given below.

(a) A is false, but R is true
(b) Both A and R are true and R is the correct explanation of A
(c) Both A and R are true, but R is not the correct explanation of A
(d) A is true, but R is false

162. Which of the following is used as vector for cloning genes in higher organisms?

(a) Aderoviruses (b) Lambda phage
(c) Retrovirus (d) Baculoviruses

163. The conus arteriosus is located on

(a) ventral surface of the heart of frog
(b) dorsal surface of the heart of frog
(c) dorsal surface of the kidney of frog
(d) ventral surface of the kidney of frog

164. Which of the following statements is not true regarding bioreactor?

(a) A bioreactor can process large volume of culture
(b) They are vessels in which raw materials are biologically converted into specific products
(c) It cannot be possible to maintain optimal growth conditions in a bioreactor because it is a closed system
(d) The curved base of stirred tank reactor facilitates the mixing of its contents

165. Identify the correct statement about the structure labelled as A in the given diagram.

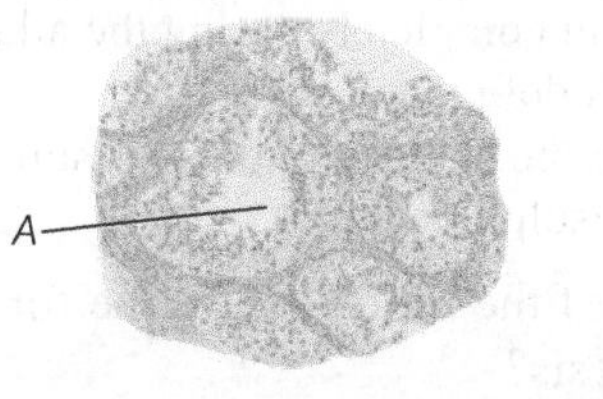

(a) It helps in the production of testosterone hormone.
(b) It is responsible for the production of sperm cells.
(c) It provide nutrition to the germ cell.
(d) It is located in the epididymis.

166. Match List I with List II.

	List I		List II
A.	First line of defence	1.	Cell-mediated immune response
B.	T-lymphocytes	2.	Antibody mediated immunity
C.	Active natural immunity	3.	Direct contact with pathogens
D.	B-lymphocytes	4.	Surface barriers

Choose the correct answer from the options given below.

	A	B	C	D
(a)	4	1	3	2
(b)	1	2	3	4
(c)	4	2	3	1
(d)	4	2	1	3

167. Calculate the sum total of phenotypes in F_2-generation if a character is controlled by five pairs of polygene.

(a) 11 (b) 7
(c) 34 (d) 27

168. What does the test cross ratio 7 : 1 : 1 : 7 indicate?
(a) A tendency of the recessive alleles to remain together
(b) The tendency of all genes to inherit together
(c) The extreme phenotypes are rare
(d) A tendency of the dominant alleles to remain together

169. Identify the incorrect statement.
(a) Genetically modified organisms have reduced reliance on chemical pesticides
(b) Non-human insulin caused some patients to develop allergy
(c) Enzyme replacement therapy has played a major role in completely curing the adult patients with ADA deficiency
(d) Both the chains of human insulin are combined by disulphide bonds

170. Which of the following is true for chemiosmotic hypothesis?
(a) Electron transfer leads to release of protons in the stroma
(b) Within the chloroplast, protons in the thylakoid lumen decreases in number
(c) Proton gradient is established across the thylakoid membrane
(d) It increases the pH in the lumen

171. Which among the following is the incorrect statement regarding exponential growth?
(a) The intrinsic rate of natural increase is different for different species
(b) *r* value of Norway rat lies exactly same as that of flour beetle
(c) Resources are unlimited
(d) Species growing under exponential growth can reach to large population densities in a short time

172. Which of the following is incorrect with respect to placenta?
(a) It is formed by association of both foetal and maternal tissue
(b) Vigrous contraction of the uterus at the end of pregnancy causes expulsion of the foetus
(c) Placenta and umbilical cord are rich sources of stem cells
(d) Placenta secretes relaxin hormone which induces parturition

173. Select the incorrect statement regarding carcinogen.
(a) Radiations like X-rays and UV-rays can cause DNA damage which leads to neoplastic transformation
(b) Tobacco smoke contains chemical carcinogens which can cause lung cancer
(c) Proto-oncogenes gets inactivated in normal conditions which leads to the oncogenic transformation of the cells
(d) They are physical, chemical and biological agents

174. The first dehydrogenation reaction in Krebs' cycle take place in the presence of which enzyme?
(a) α - ketoglutaric dehydrogenase
(b) Isocitric dehydrogenase
(c) Succinic thiokinase
(d) Succinic dehydrogenase

175. Read the following statements.
I. In bacteria translation begins much before *m*RNA is fully transcribed.
II. The regulatory gene regulates biochemical reaction in cell by inactivating enzymes.
III. The Human Genome Project was coordinated by the US Department of Energy and the National Institute of Health.
IV. AUG codon has dual functions. It codes for methionine and also act as stop codon.
V. Less than 2% of the human genome code for proteins.

Choose the correct set of statements answer from the options given below.
(a) I, III and V
(b) II, III and V
(c) I, IV and V
(d) II, IV and V

176. Given below are two statements.
Statement I The convex disc of RBC permits it to squeeze through small capillaries.
Statement II The surface remain moist and cells are living with distinct nuclei in non-keratinised stratified squamous epithelium.

In the light of the above statements, choose the correct answer from the options given below.
(a) Statement I is incorrect, but Statement II is correct
(b) Both Statement I and Statement II are correct
(c) Both Statement I and Statement II are incorrect
(d) Statement I is correct, but Statement II is incorrect

177. During light dependent reactions, light energy is converted to chemical potential energy through the process of chemiosmosis in the chloroplasts. Which of the following statements about this process is false ?

I. The electron carriers of phosphorylation are located in the thylakoid.
II. During phosphorylation, the chloroplast stroma becomes more acidic than the interior of thylakoid membrane.
III. Protons diffuse through the protein channels which are ATP synthetase molecules.
IV. ATP is formed from ADP + Pi on the stroma side of the thylakoid in the chloroplast.
V. During phosphorylation, water ionises to form $H^+ + 2OH^-$, yielding an e^- to PS-II.

(a) I, II and IV (b) Only II
(c) III and IV (d) Only IV

178. Given below are two statements; one is labelled as Assertion (A) and other is labelled as Reason (R).

Assertion (A) Interferons protect non-infected cells.
Reason (R) Interferons are the cellular barrier which protect the body.

In the light of the above statements, choose the correct answer from the options given below.
(a) A is false, but R is true
(b) Both A and R are true and R is the correct explanation of A
(c) Both A and R are true, but R is not the correct explanation of A
(d) A is true, but R is false

179. Read the following statements and identify the incorrect statements.

I. Mammary glands under normal state are also concerned with the secretion of hormone.
II. Progesterone is active during the follicular phase of menstrual cycle.
III. Oxytocin stimulates the contraction of mammary glands.
IV. Progesterone decline can trigger the menstruation.
V. Oestrogen is active during the proliferative phase of menstrual cycle.

Choose the correct answer from the options given below.
(a) I, II, III and V (b) I, IV and V
(c) I and II (d) I and V

180. Which one of the following is not characteristic feature of poriferans?
(a) Presence of ostia
(b) Cellular level of organisation
(c) Collar cells
(d) Body supported by chitin

Explanations

Physics

1. (b) KE = – Total energy $= -(-13.6 \text{ eV}) = +13.6 \text{ eV}$

2. (b) As, $\frac{E_0}{B_0} = c$ (where, c is velocity of light)

$$\frac{E_0}{B_0} = \nu\lambda \qquad (\because c = \nu\lambda) \quad ...(i)$$

Also, $$k = \frac{2\pi}{\lambda}$$

$$\Rightarrow \lambda = \frac{2\pi}{k} \quad ...(ii)$$

$$\Rightarrow \omega = 2\pi\nu$$

$$\Rightarrow \nu = \frac{\omega}{2\pi} \quad ...(iii)$$

So, combining Eqs. (i), (ii) and (iii), we have

$$\frac{E_0}{B_0} = \frac{\omega}{2\pi} \times \frac{2\pi}{k}$$

$$\Rightarrow E_0 k = B_0 \omega$$

3. (a) We know, $\tan\phi = \frac{X_L - X_C}{R}$

$$\tan 30° = \frac{X_C}{R}$$

$$\Rightarrow X_C = \frac{R}{\sqrt{3}}$$

$$\tan 30° = \frac{X_L}{R}$$

$$\Rightarrow X_L = \frac{R}{\sqrt{3}}$$

$$X_L = X_C \text{ (Condition for resonance)}$$

So $$\phi = 0°$$

$$P = VI\cos 0°$$

$$P = \frac{V^2}{R} = \frac{(220)^2}{200} = 242 \text{ W}$$

4. (a) The binding energy per nucleon increases to maximum of about 8.7 meV per nucleon for $A = 56(_{26}Fe^{56})$.

5. (d) According to Newton's law of motion of man-chair system,

$$2T - 1000 - 250 = \left(\frac{1000}{10} + \frac{250}{10}\right)a$$

$$\Rightarrow T = \frac{125a + 1250}{2} \quad ...(i)$$

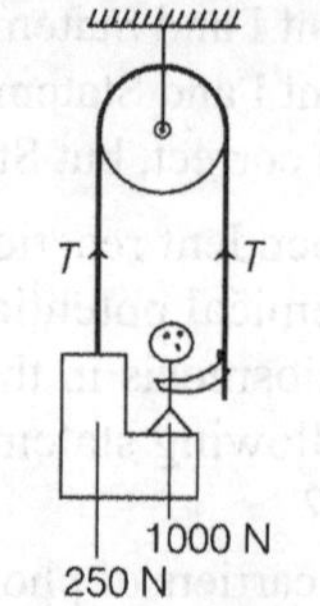

For upward motion of the chair,

$$T - 450 - 250 = \left(\frac{250}{10}\right)a$$

$$\Rightarrow T = 700 + 25a \quad ...(ii)$$

From Eqs. (i) and (ii), we get

$$\frac{125a + 1250}{2} = 700 + 25a$$

$$\Rightarrow a = \frac{150}{75} = 2 \text{ ms}^{-2}$$

6. (b) $$h_{max} = \frac{u^2 \sin^2\theta}{2g}$$

$$= \frac{(25)^2 \cdot (\sin 45°)^2}{2 \times 10} = 15.625 \text{ m}$$

$$T = \frac{u\sin\theta}{g} = \frac{25 \times \sin 45°}{10}$$

$$T = 2.5 \times 0.7 = 1.77 \text{ s}$$

7. (d) For an internal point $(r < R)$ in a charged conducting sphere,

$$V_{in} = V_{surface}$$

$$= \frac{q}{4\pi\varepsilon_0 R} = \text{constant}$$

$$V \propto r^0$$

8. (d) Current in the circuit is given by Ohm's law.
Net resistance of the circuit $= r_1 + r_2 + R$

$$\text{Net emf} = E + E = 2E$$

$\therefore$ Current in the circuit is given by

$$I = \frac{2E}{r_1 + r_2 + R} \quad ...(i)$$

As the circuit is closed, potential difference across the first cell is zero.

$$V = E - Ir_1 = 0$$

$$I = \frac{E}{r_1} \quad ...(ii)$$

From Eqs. (i) and (ii),

$$\frac{E}{r_1} = \frac{2E}{r_1 + r_2 + R}$$

$$\Rightarrow \quad 2r_1 = r_1 + r_2 + R$$

$\therefore$ External resistance, $R = r_1 - r_2$

9. (a) We know that, $h = \dfrac{2T\cos\theta}{r\rho g}$

$$\Rightarrow \quad h \propto \frac{1}{r}$$

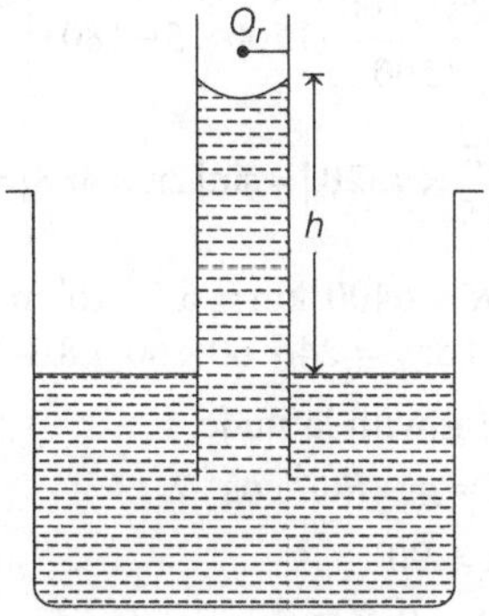

So, $\dfrac{h_1}{h_2} = \dfrac{r_2}{r_1} \Rightarrow \dfrac{4}{h_2} = \dfrac{1}{4}$

$$h_2 = 16\,\text{mm}$$

10. (c) Least count of screw gauge

$$= \frac{0.5}{50} = 0.01\,\text{mm} = \Delta r$$

Diameter, $r = 2.5\,\text{mm} + 20 \times 0.01 = 2.70\,\text{mm}$

$$\frac{\Delta r}{r} = \frac{0.01}{2.70} \text{ or } \frac{\Delta r}{r} \times 100 = \frac{1}{2.7}$$

Now, density, $d = \dfrac{m}{V} = \dfrac{m}{\dfrac{4}{3}\pi\left(\dfrac{r}{2}\right)^3}$

Here, r is the diameter.

$$\therefore \frac{\Delta d}{d} \times 100 = \left\{\frac{\Delta m}{m} + 3\left(\frac{\Delta r}{r}\right)\right\} \times 100$$

$$= \frac{\Delta m}{m} \times 100 + 3 \times \left(\frac{\Delta r}{r}\right) \times 100$$

$$= 2\% + 3 \times \frac{1}{2.7}\% = 3.1\%$$

11. (d) $F = \dfrac{\mu_0}{4\pi} \cdot \dfrac{2 \cdot I \cdot I \cdot L}{r}$

$$I^2 = \frac{2 \times 10^{-7} \times 0.1}{10^{-7} \times 2 \times 10}$$

$$= 0.01$$

$$I = 0.1\,\text{A}$$

12. (b) When carpet is unrolled to radius $\dfrac{r}{2}$, the centre of mass is at a height of $\dfrac{r}{2}$.

The mass left unrolled, $M = \dfrac{m\pi\left(\dfrac{r}{2}\right)^2}{\pi r^2} = \dfrac{m}{4}$

So, the decrease in potential energy

$$= mgr - \left(\frac{m}{4}\right)g\left(\frac{r}{2}\right) = \frac{7}{8}mgr$$

13. (b) The reaction can be written as

$${}_1H^2 + {}_1H^2 \longrightarrow {}_2He^4 + \text{energy}$$

The energy released in the reaction, is difference of binding energies of daughter and parent nuclei.

Hence, energy released = binding energy of ${}_2He^4 - 2 \times$ binding energy of ${}_1H^2$

$$= 28 - 2 \times 2.2 = 23.6\,\text{MeV}$$

14. (c)

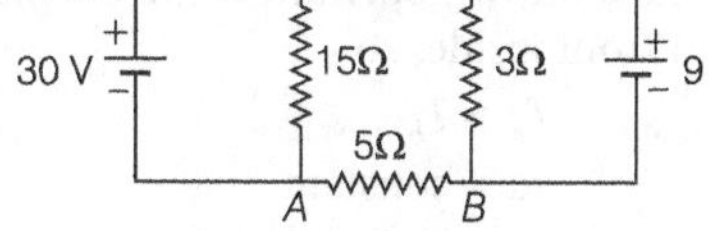

As, $V_A = V_B = 0$

$\therefore$ $V_{AB} = 0$, so no current flows in branch AB.

15. (c) The efficiency of transformer,

$$\eta = \frac{\text{Energy obtained from the secondary coil}}{\text{Energy given to the primary coil}}$$

or $\eta = \dfrac{\text{Output power}}{\text{Input power}}$ or $\eta = \dfrac{V_s I_s}{V_p I_p}$

Given, $V_s I_s = 100\,\text{W}, V_p = 220\,\text{V}$

$$I_p = 0.5\,\text{A}$$

Hence, $\eta = \dfrac{100}{220 \times 0.5} = 0.91 = 91\% \simeq 90\%$

16. (d) If the width of the slit in YDSE is increased, then distance between slits increases and hence, fringe width decreases. If the slit is sufficiently wide, then each part gives a pattern which overlaps and the fringes gets obliterated. In order to avoid this, the slit width must be smaller than fringe width.

17. (a) Let the amplitudes of light waves are a_1 and a_2.
Given, $a_1 = 2a$ and $a_2 = a$

$$a_{\max} = a_1 + a_2 = 3a$$

$$a_{\min} = a_1 - a_2 = a$$

$$\therefore \frac{I_{\max}}{I_{\min}} = \frac{a^2_{\max}}{a^2_{\min}} = \frac{(3a)^2}{(a)^2} = \frac{9}{1}$$

$$I_{\max} : I_{\min} = 9:1$$

18. (d) For intrinsic semiconductor, $n_i = 10^{22}\text{ m}^{-3}$

Density of holes, $n_h = 10^{20}\text{ m}^{-3}$

As, $n_h \cdot n_e = n_i^2$

$$\Rightarrow \quad n_e = \frac{(10^{22})^2}{10^{20}} = 10^{24}\text{ m}^{-3}$$

19. (d) Let final temperature of mixture be t°C.
Heat lost by water in calories,

$$H_1 = 20\times 1\times(50-t) = 1000-20t$$

Heat taken by ice, $H_2 = ms_{\text{ice}}\Delta t + mL + ms_w t$

$$= 8\times 0.5\times 20 + 8\times 80 + 8\times 1\times t$$

$$H_2 = 720 + 8t$$

$$\Rightarrow \quad 720 + 8t = 1000 - 20t \quad [\because H_1 = H_2]$$

$$t = 10°\text{C}$$

20. (d) The diode become reverse bias in positive half cycle, so only negative half cycles appear across the output.

21. (c) The raw egg has some fluid in it and thus on spinning the egg fluid is thrown outward while the hard boiled egg is solid from inside, so

$$I_r > I_b$$

As, $I\omega = \text{constant}$

$\therefore \quad \omega_r < \omega_b$

or $\quad \dfrac{\omega_r}{\omega_b} < 1$

or $\quad \dfrac{T_r}{T_b} > 1 \quad \left[\therefore \omega = \dfrac{2\pi}{T}\right]$

22. (b) Wavelength, $\dfrac{1}{\lambda} = RZ^2\left(\dfrac{1}{n_1^2} - \dfrac{1}{n_2^2}\right)$

Here, transition is same.

So, $\lambda \propto \dfrac{1}{Z^2}$

$$\frac{\lambda_H}{\lambda_{Li}} = \frac{(Z_{Li})^2}{(Z_H)^2} = \frac{(3)^2}{(1)^2} = 9$$

$$\lambda_{Li} = \frac{\lambda_H}{9} = \frac{\lambda}{9}\text{ Å}$$

23. (d) By Brewster's law,

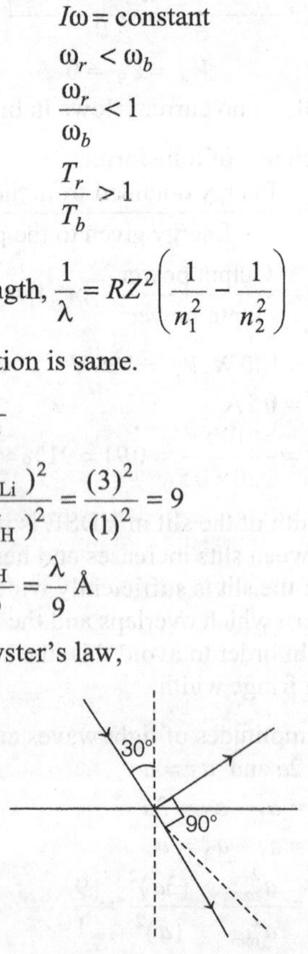

$$\mu = \tan i_p = \tan 30° = \frac{1}{\sqrt{3}}$$

24. (c) As seen from p-V diagram, the volume of gas is increasing continuously. Therefore, work done will increase continuously.

25. (a) Given, $A = 1\text{ cm}$, $\nu = 100\text{ Hz}$,

$v = 15\text{ ms}^{-1} = 1500\text{ cms}^{-1}$, $x = 180\text{ cm}$, $t = 5\text{ s}$

The displacement of wave is given by

$$y = A\sin\frac{2\pi}{\lambda}(vt - x) = A\sin\frac{2\pi\nu_{(\text{frequency})}}{v}(vt - x)$$

$$y = 1\sin\left[\frac{2\pi\times 100}{1500}(1500\times 5 - 180)\right]$$

$$= \sin\left[\frac{2\pi}{15}\times 7320\right] = \sin[2\pi\times 488] = 0$$

26. (b) Given, $R = 6400\text{ km} = 6.4\times 10^6\text{ m}$

$T = 1\text{ day} = 24\times 60\times 60 = 8.64\times 10^4\text{ s}$

The value of g with latitude,

$$g' = g - R\omega^2\cos^2\lambda$$

At poles, $\lambda = 90°$

$\Rightarrow \quad \cos\lambda = 0$, then

$$g_p = g - R\omega^2(0) = g \quad \text{...(i)}$$

At equator, $\lambda = 0°$

$\Rightarrow \quad \cos\lambda = 1$, then

$$g_e = g - R\omega^2 \quad \text{...(ii)}$$

The change in value of g is

$$g_p - g_e = R\omega^2 = 6.4\times 10^6\times\left(\frac{2\pi}{T}\right)^2$$

$$= 6.4\times 10^6\times\left(\frac{2\times 3.14}{8.64\times 10^4}\right)^2$$

$$= 3.38\times 10^{-2}\text{ ms}^{-2}$$

27. (d) $(v_{\text{rms}})_{H_2} = (v_{\text{rms}})_{O_2}$

$$\sqrt{\frac{3RT_{H_2}}{(M_0)_{H_2}}} = \sqrt{\frac{3RT_{O_2}}{(M_0)_{O_2}}}$$

$$\Rightarrow \quad \sqrt{\frac{T_{H_2}}{2}} = \sqrt{\frac{(273+47)}{32}} \Rightarrow T_{H_2} = 20\text{ K}$$

28. (d) Velocity of leakage of water, $v = \sqrt{2gh}$

Volume of liquid flowing out per second

$$= v\times A = \sqrt{2gh}\times A$$

$$= \sqrt{2\times 10\times 5}\times(10\times 10^{-4}) = 10^{-2}\text{ m}^3\text{s}^{-1}$$

29. (a) From the principle of homogeneity,

$$[p] = \left[\frac{a}{V^2}\right] \Rightarrow \frac{[F]}{[A]} = \frac{[a]}{[V^2]}$$

$$\Rightarrow \quad \frac{[\text{MLT}^{-2}]}{[\text{L}^2]} = \frac{a}{[\text{L}^3]^2} \Rightarrow a = [\text{ML}^5\text{T}^{-2}]$$

30. (c) For Lyman series,

$$\frac{1}{\lambda_L} = R\left[\frac{1}{1^2} - \frac{1}{2^2}\right] = \frac{3R}{4}$$

For Balmer series,

$$\frac{1}{\lambda_B} = R\left[\frac{1}{4} - \frac{1}{9}\right] = \frac{5R}{36}$$

$$\Rightarrow \quad \frac{\lambda_L}{\lambda_B} = \frac{4/3R}{36/5R} = \frac{5}{27}$$

Problem Solving Tactics For longest wavelength of lyman series, $n_1 = 1$ and $n_2 = 2$ and for longest wavelength of balmer series, $n_1 = 2$ and $n_2 = 3$. Use above in the formula $\frac{1}{\lambda} = R\left(\frac{1}{n_1^2} - \frac{1}{n_2^2}\right)$ to get required result.

31. (a) Redraw the circuit,

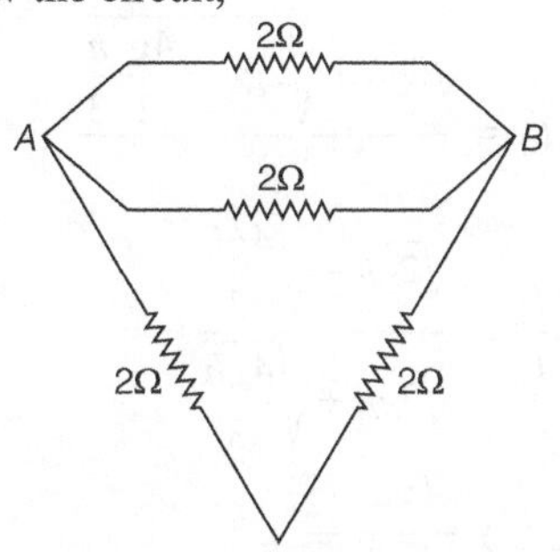

Let R_{AB} is equivalent resistance between A and B

$$\therefore \quad \frac{1}{R_{AB}} = \frac{1}{2} + \frac{1}{2} + \frac{1}{4} = \frac{5}{4} \quad \text{or} \quad R_{AB} = \frac{4}{5}\Omega = 0.8\Omega$$

32. (a) Given, $A = 200 \text{ cm}^2 = 2\times10^{-2}\text{m}^2$

If capacitance of capacitors having dielectric constants K_1, K_2 and K_3 are C_1, C_2 and C_3, respectively then

$$C_1 = \frac{K_1\varepsilon_0 A/2}{d}$$

$$= \frac{2\times8.86\times10^{-12}\times10^{-2}}{10\times10^{-2}} = 1.77\times10^{-12}\text{F}$$

$$C_2 = \frac{K_2\varepsilon_0 A/2}{d/2}$$

$$= \frac{4\times8.86\times10^{-12}\times10^{-2}}{5\times10^{-2}} = 7.1\times10^{-12}\text{F}$$

$$C_3 = \frac{K_3\varepsilon_0 A/2}{d/2} = \frac{6\times8.86\times10^{-12}\times10^{-2}}{5\times10^{-2}}$$

$$= 10.6\times10^{-12}\text{F}$$

C_2 and C_3 are in series and C_1 is parallel to both.

$$\therefore \quad C_{eq} = \frac{C_2C_3}{C_2 + C_3} + C_1$$

$$= \left(\frac{7.1\times10.6}{7.1+10.6}\right)\times10^{-12} + 1.77\times10^{-12}$$

$$= 4.25\times10^{-12} + 1.77\times10^{-12}$$

$$\simeq 6\times10^{-12} = 6\text{pF}$$

33. (a) If q be the charge on each sphere, then $q = \sigma\cdot4\pi r_1^2 = \sigma\cdot4\pi r_2^2$

$\therefore$ The potential on the surface and at any point inside the surface for inner sphere (radius r_2) is same.

$$\therefore \quad V_2 = \frac{1}{4\pi\varepsilon_0}\cdot\frac{q}{r_2}$$

$$= \frac{1}{4\pi\varepsilon_0}\cdot\frac{\sigma\cdot4\pi r_2^2}{r_2} = \frac{\sigma r_2}{\varepsilon_0}$$

Similarly, $V_1 = \frac{\sigma r_1}{\varepsilon_0}$

$\therefore$ Resultant potential, $V = V_1 + V_2 = \frac{\sigma}{\varepsilon_0}(r_1 + r_2)$

34. (a) Let t be the time, then distance covered by man is ut, similarly distance covered by bus will be $\frac{1}{2}at^2$.

According to given situation,

$$ut = 45 + \frac{1}{2}at^2 = 45 + \frac{1}{2}\times2.5\times t^2$$

$$= 45 + 1.25t^2 \text{ or } u = \frac{45}{t} + 1.25t$$

For the minimum velocity, $\frac{du}{dt} = 0$

$$\Rightarrow \quad \frac{-45}{t^2} + 1.25 = 0 \Rightarrow t = \sqrt{\frac{4500}{125}} = 6\text{ s}$$

$$\therefore \quad u = \frac{45}{6} + 1.25(6) = 15\text{ ms}^{-1}$$

35. (b) Magnetic field at the centre of circular coil is

$$B = \frac{\mu_0}{4\pi}\times\frac{2\pi I}{r}$$

where, I is current flowing in the coil and r is radius of coil.

At the centre of coil 1,

$$B_1 = \frac{\mu_0}{4\pi}\times\frac{2\pi I_1}{r_1} \quad \ldots\text{(i)}$$

At the centre of coil 2, $B_2 = \frac{\mu_0}{4\pi}\times\frac{2\pi I_2}{r_2}$ ...(ii)

But $B_1 = B_2$

$$\therefore \quad \frac{\mu_0}{4\pi}\frac{2\pi I_1}{r_1} = \frac{\mu_0}{4\pi}\frac{2\pi I_2}{r_2} \text{ or } \frac{I_1}{r_1} = \frac{I_2}{r_2}$$

As, $r_1 = 2r_2$

$\therefore \quad \frac{I_1}{2r_2} = \frac{I_2}{r_2}$ or $I_1 = 2I_2$ ...(iii)

Now, ratio of potential differences,

$$\frac{V_2}{V_1} = \frac{I_2 \times r_2}{I_1 \times r_1} = \frac{I_2 \times r_2}{2I_2 \times 2r_2} = \frac{1}{4}$$

$$\therefore \quad \frac{V_1}{V_2} = \frac{4}{1}$$

36. (c) AND gate using NOR gates

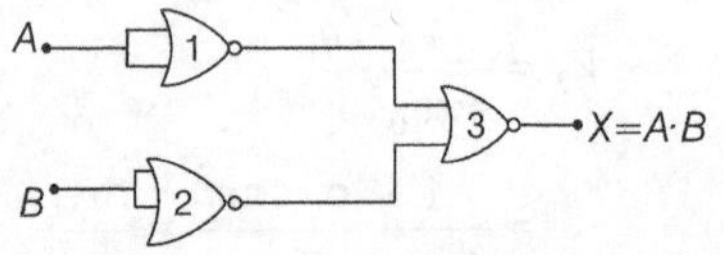

$\therefore$ 3 NOR gates are required to form an AND gate.

37. (d) Both statements A and B are correct.

Statement C is incorrect because avalanche breakdown occurs when the reversed bias voltage exceeds a certain value.

Statement D is incorrect because the ratio of number of holes and the number of conduction electrons in an *n*-type extrinsic semiconductor is less than 1.

38. (c) (A) Root mean square speed of gas molecules is $\sqrt{\frac{3RT}{M}}$

(B) Pressure exerted by ideal gas is $\frac{1}{3}nmv^2$

(C) Average kinetic energy of a molecule is $\frac{3}{2}k_BT$

(D) Total internal energy of 1 mole of a diatomic gas is $\frac{5}{2}RT$.

39. (c) From $P = \tau\omega \Rightarrow \tau = \frac{P}{\omega}$

It is given, $P = 80\text{HP} = 80 \times 746\text{ W} = 59680\text{ N-ms}^{-1}$

$$\omega = 3600\text{ rpm} = \frac{3600}{60} \times 2\pi\text{ rad s}^{-1}$$

$$= 120\pi\text{ rad s}^{-1}$$

So, $\tau = 158.38\text{ Nm}$

40. (d) $R_1 = \frac{(220)^2}{25} = 1936\,\Omega$

$$R_2 = \frac{(220)^2}{100} = 484\,\Omega$$

$$i = \frac{220}{R_1 + R_2} = 0.09\text{ A}$$

Power in 25 W bulb,

$$P_1 = i^2 R_1$$

$$P_1 = (0.09)^2 \times (1936) = 15.68 \simeq 16\text{ W}$$

Power in 100 W bulb,

$$P_2 = i^2 R_2$$

$$= (0.09)^2 (484) = 3.92 \approx 4\text{ W}$$

41. (d) $u = \sqrt{2gh}$

Now, $s = \frac{h}{3}$

$$s = ut + \frac{1}{2}at^2$$

$$\frac{h}{3} = (\sqrt{2gh})t + \frac{1}{2}(-g)t^2 \quad (a = -g)$$

$$t^2\left(\frac{g}{2}\right) - (\sqrt{2gh})t + \frac{h}{3} = 0$$

From quadratic equation,

$$t_1, t_2 = \frac{\sqrt{2gh} \pm \sqrt{2gh - \frac{4g}{2}\frac{h}{3}}}{g}$$

$$\frac{t_1}{t_2} = \frac{\sqrt{2gh} - \sqrt{\frac{4gh}{3}}}{\sqrt{2gh} + \sqrt{\frac{4gh}{3}}}$$

$$= \frac{\sqrt{3} - \sqrt{2}}{\sqrt{3} + \sqrt{2}}$$

42. (a) The acceleration due to gravity on the earth's surface,

$$g = \frac{GM}{R^2}$$

Differentiating it w.r.t. radius R, we get

$$\frac{dg}{dR} = \frac{-2GM}{R^3}$$

Then, $\frac{dg}{g} = -\frac{2dR}{R}$

When the earth shrinks by 25%, then

$$\frac{dR}{R} = \frac{-25}{100} = -\frac{1}{4}$$

$$\therefore \quad \frac{dg}{g} \times 100 = -\frac{2dR}{R} \times 100$$

$$= -2\left(-\frac{1}{4}\right) \times 100 = 50\%$$

43. (a) Let x_1, x_2 be the displacements in two springs for force F, then

$$F = -k_1x_1 = -k_2x_2$$

Total extension,

$$x = x_1 + x_2 = -F\left(\frac{1}{k_1} + \frac{1}{k_2}\right)$$

$$= -F\left(\frac{k_1 + k_2}{k_1 k_2}\right)$$

$$\Rightarrow \quad F = -\left(\frac{k_1 k_2}{k_1 + k_2}\right)x$$

Thus, $k = \dfrac{k_1 k_2}{k_1 + k_2}$

$\therefore$ Frequency $= \dfrac{1}{2\pi}\sqrt{\dfrac{k}{m}} = \dfrac{1}{2\pi}\sqrt{\dfrac{k_1 k_2}{(k_1 + k_2)m}}$

44. (a) This combination is same as the two capacitors are connected in series and distance between plates of each capacitor is $\frac{d}{2}$.

So, $C_1 = \dfrac{K\varepsilon_0 A}{\frac{d}{2}}$ and $C_2 = \dfrac{\varepsilon_0 A}{\frac{d}{2}}$

Hence, $C_{\text{net}} = \dfrac{C_1 C_2}{C_1 + C_2}$

$$= \frac{\left(\frac{2K\varepsilon_0 A}{d}\right)\left(\frac{2\varepsilon_0 A}{d}\right)}{\left(\frac{2K\varepsilon_0 A}{d} + \frac{2\varepsilon_0 A}{d}\right)}$$

$$= \frac{2KA\varepsilon_0}{(K+1)d}$$

45. (c) $H_P = (6\,\text{cal/sec}) \times (6-2)\,\text{s} = 24\,\text{s}$

$H_Q = (6\,\text{cal/sec}) \times (7-3)\,\text{s} = 24\,\text{s}$

$\therefore \quad \dfrac{H_P}{H_Q} = \dfrac{24}{24} = 1:1$

Chemistry

46. (b) Leaving group ability depends upon basicity of group. The weaker is base, the greater is its leaving group ability. Alternatively, the stronger is conjugate acid, the greater the leaving group ability of the base. The strength of conjugate acid is

$$HOSO_2CF_3 > HOSO_2Me > HOAc > HOMe.$$

Hence, correct order of leaving group ability is

$$IV > III > I > II.$$

47. (a) Ethanal reacts with HCN and the addition product so obtained is hydrolysed to form an optically active compound. Hence, it shows optical isomerism.

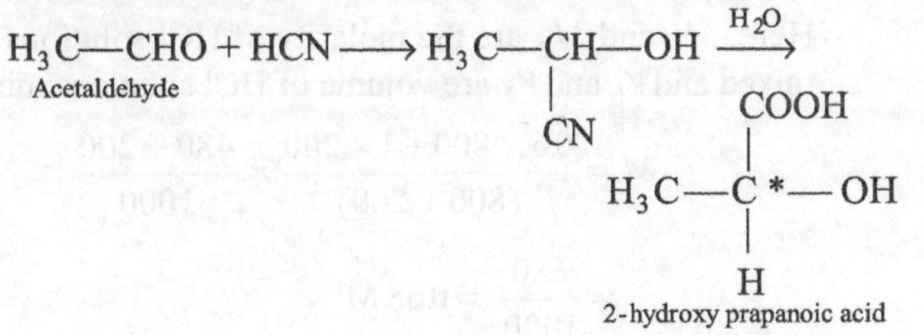

2-hydroxy prapanoic acid (Optically active)

Problem Solving Tactics	Optical isomerism occurs mainly in those compounds in which there is asymmetric carbon atom, i.e. has four different substituents attached to it.

48. (c) We know that,

$$\Delta G = -2.303RT \log K$$
$$= -2.303 \times 8.314 \times 298 \log 50$$
$$= -9694\ \text{J} = -9.694\ \text{kJ}$$

49. (d) Statement I is true as the transition metal ions can change their oxidation states, they become more effective as catalysts. Therefore, the catalytic activity of the transition metals and their compounds is due to their ability to adopt multiple oxidation states and their complexing ability.

Also, statement II is true, i.e. Cr^{2+} (d^4) is a stronger reducing agent than Fe^{2+} (d^6). This can be explained on the basis of the standard electrode potential values.

$E°(Cr^{3+}/Cr^{2+} = -0.41\ \text{V})$ and

$E°(Fe^{3+}/Fe^{2+} = +0.77\ \text{V})$.

The larger the value of the standard potential the easier it is for the element to be reduced (gain electrons) or act as a better oxidising agent. Hence, it is easy for Cr^{2+} to oxidise Cr^{3+} as compare to Fe^{2+} to Fe^{3+}.

50. (b) The relation between $K_p = K_C(RT)^{\Delta n_g}$

$$\Delta n_g = 1 - \left(1 + \frac{1}{2}\right) = 1 - \frac{3}{2} = -\frac{1}{2}$$

So, $K_p = K_C(RT)^{-\frac{1}{2}}$

51. (d) 1 mole of $Na_2S_2O_3$ contains 3 atoms of oxygen.
0.2 mole will contain $= 0.2 \times 3 = 0.6$
Hence, number of oxygen atoms $= 0.6 \times N_A$.

52. (b) Both (A) and (R) are true and (R) is the correct explanation of (A). Tetrachlorides of group 14 elements are easily hydrolysed except CCl_4 because all other elements have vacant *d*-orbital which can accommodate the lone pair of electrons from oxygen atom of water molecules but carbon does not have vacant *d*-orbitals.

53. (a) (A) is false but (R) is true. H_2O_2 is a covalent compound.

In O_2F_2, O—O bond is shorter than in H_2O_2 due to higher electronegativity of F.

54. (a) When HBr is added to unsymmetrical alkenes in the presence of peroxide, 1-bromobutane is formed. This reaction is known as Kharasch effect or peroxide effect.

$$\underset{\text{Butene}}{CH_3CH_2CH{=}CH_2} + HBr \xrightarrow{\text{Peroxide}} \underset{\substack{(Y)\\ \text{Bromobutane}}}{CH_3CH_2CH_2CH_2Br}$$

Williamson's ether synthesis involve an alkoxide that reacts with a primary haloalkane to produce ether. It is used for the preparation of symmetrical as well as unsymmetrical ethers.

$$\underset{\substack{(Y)\\ \text{Bromobutane}}}{CH_3CH_2CH_2CH_2Br} + C_2H_5\overset{-}{O}\overset{+}{Na} \longrightarrow \underset{\substack{(Z)\\ \text{Ethyl butyl ether}}}{CH_3CH_2CH_2CH_2OC_2H_5}$$

Thus, Z is ethyl butyl ether.

55. (d) The given reaction can be written as

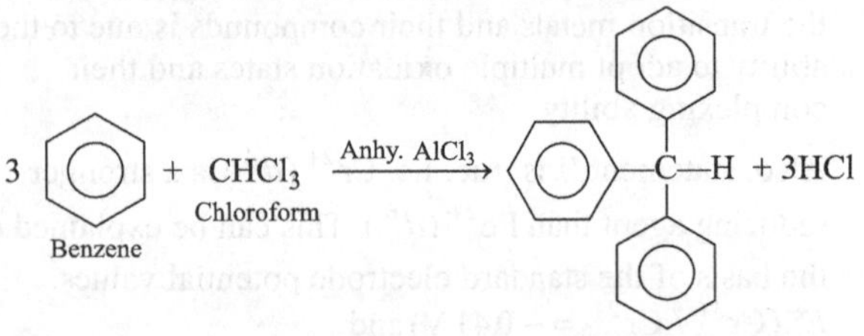

Triphenyl methane

56. (b) $+M$ effect of —NH_2 > $+M$ effect of —OH group that disperse the charge of carbocation and —CH_3 group shows $+I$ effect, so it will disperse the charge less than —NH_2, —OH group.

Hence, increases the stability whereas —NO_2 group shows $-M/-I$ effect due to which the positive charge on the carbocation increases. Hence, stability decreases.

$\therefore$ The correct order of stability is IV > II > III > I.

Problem Solving Tactics Carbocation is an electron deficient species. So, anything which can donate electron will stabilise the carbocation like electron donating group (CH_3). Conversely carbocation will be destabilised by an electron withdrawing group (F, Cl).

57. (c) Fructose is not an aldohexose sugar. It's structure can be represented as

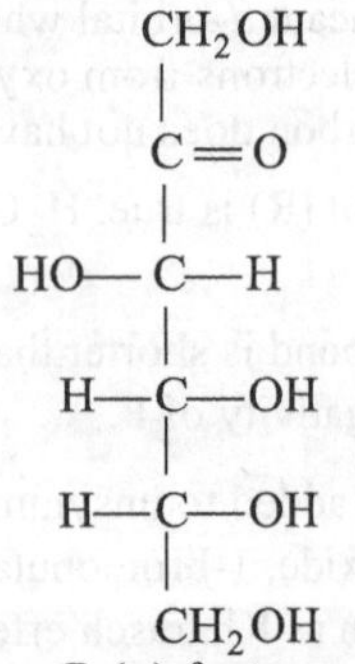

D-(−)-fructose

58. (a) In *cis*- $[Co(NH_3)_4Cl_2]^+$, Co is d^2sp^3-hybridised because NH_3 is a strong field ligand thus, pair up the $3d^6$ electrons of Co.

$$Co^{3+} = [Ar]\,3d^6\,4s^0$$

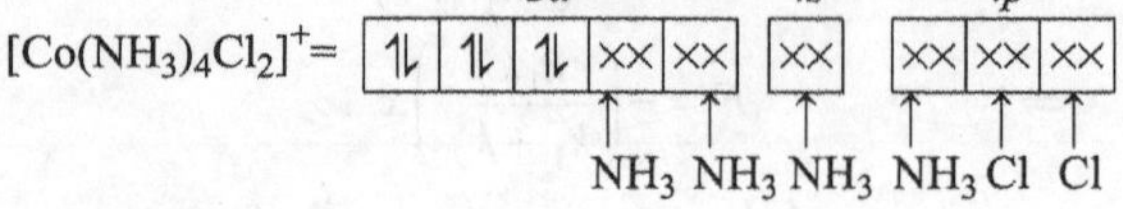

It is d^2sp^3-hybridised.

59. (b) Both statements I and II are true.

60. (c)

- Mixture of calcium benzoate and calcium acetate is heated to give methyl phenyl ether.
- Calcium benzoate is heated to form diphenyl ether.
- Sodium benzoate is heated with sodalime to form benzene.

$$\underset{\substack{\text{Calcium}\\ \text{benzoate}}}{(C_6H_5COO)_2\,Ca} + \underset{\substack{\text{Calcium}\\ \text{acetate}}}{(CH_3COO)_2\,Ca} \xrightarrow{\Delta} \underset{\text{Methyl phenyl ether}}{2C_6H_5OCH_3} + CaCO_3$$

$$\underset{\text{Calcium benzoate}}{(C_6H_5COO)_2\,Ca} \xrightarrow{\Delta} \underset{\substack{\text{Diphenyl}\\ \text{ether}}}{C_6H_5OC_6H_5} + CaCO_3$$

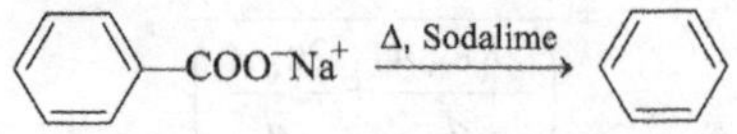

Sodium benzoate Benzene

61. (c) Among the given options (B), (C) and (D) are correct.

$\Delta U = 0 \quad \therefore \quad U_2 - U_1 = 0$

or $\quad U_2 = U_1$

Similarly, $\Delta\mu = 0$

$$q = -w = nRT\ln\frac{V_2}{V_1}$$

62. (a) Work done in an isothermal compression can be calculated as follows

$$W = -nRT\ln\frac{V_2}{V_1}$$

$$= -5\times 8.314\times 300\times 2.303\log\frac{40}{200}$$

$$= -1500\times 8.314\times 2.303\times(\log 0.2) = +20.1\,\text{kJ}$$

63. (c) Let M be the molarity of solution obtained by mixing HCl solutions.

$$\therefore \quad M = \frac{M_1V_1 + M_2V_2}{V_1+V_2}$$

Here, M_1 and M_2 are the molarity of HCl solutions mixed and V_1 and V_2 are volume of HCl solutions mixed.

$$M = \frac{0.6\times 800 + 1\times 200}{(800+200)} = \frac{480+200}{1000}$$

$$= \frac{680}{1000} = 0.68\,\text{M}$$

64. (b) According to first law of electrolysis,
Mass of metal deposited (w)

$$= \frac{\text{atomic weight}}{\text{electrons exchanged} \times 96500} \times i \times t$$

$$\therefore \quad 0.415 = \frac{\text{atomic weight}}{3 \times 96500} \times 2 \times 965$$

Thus, atomic weight $= \frac{0.415 \times 3 \times 96500}{2 \times 965}$

$= 62.25 \text{ g}$

65. (a) The correct match is A-IV, B-I, C-II, D-III.

66. (b) The dissociation of the given compounds are as follows

$$CaCl_2 \longrightarrow Ca^{2+} + 2Cl^-; i = 3$$

$$K_4[Fe(CN)_6] \longrightarrow 4K^+ + [Fe(CN)_6]^{4-}; i = 5$$

$$AlCl_3 \longrightarrow Al^{3+} + 3Cl^-; i = 4$$

$$NH_2CONH_2 \longrightarrow \text{does not dissociate}, i = 1$$

Since, $K_4[Fe(CN)_6]$ give 5 ions in the solution. Hence, has maximum van't Hoff factor.

67. (a) KCl $\rightarrow$ There is more electronegative difference between both the atoms. Hence, KCl is an ionic compound.

$NH_3 \rightarrow$ It has 3 bond pairs and 1 lone pair. Hence, its shape is trigonal pyramidal.

Acetylene $\rightarrow HC \equiv CH$ has triple bond and *sp*-hybridisation in carbon atoms.

$H_2O \rightarrow$ More electronegativity difference but it's a covalent compound. It has polar covalent bond.

Hence, the correct match is A-(iv), B-(iii), C-(ii), D-(i).

68. (a) Statement I is false but Statement II is true.

Non-bonding *MO* is formed by sideways overlapping of $d_{x^2-y^2}$ and p_y orbital along *x*-axis.

69. (a)

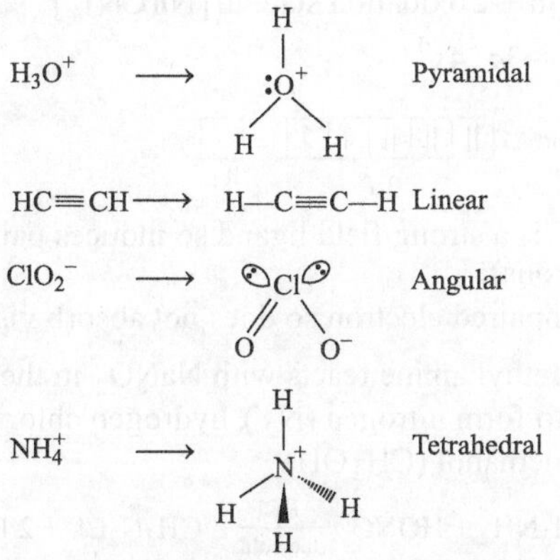

$\therefore$ The correct match is A-(iv), B-(iii), C-(ii), D-(i).

70. (c) According to Moseley, a straight line graph is obtained on plotting the square root of the frequencies of characteristics of X-rays of elements ($\sqrt{v}$) against their atomic numbers (Z).

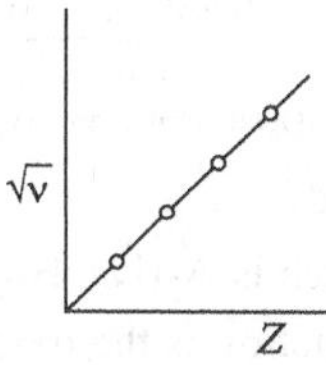

71. (a) Cu in $[Cu(NH_3)_4]SO_4$ has + 2 oxidation state.

$Cu^{2+} = [Ar]\,3d^9$

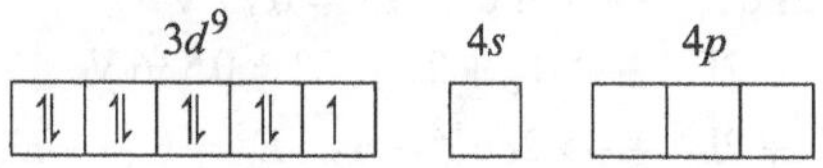

$[Cu(NH_3)_4]^{2+}$

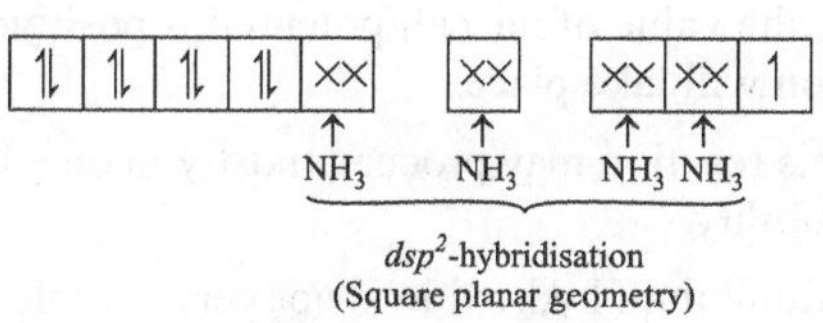

($\because$ NH_3 is strong ligand)

Fe has zero oxidation state in $[Fe(CO)_5]$

$Fe = [Ar]3d^6 4s^2$

$[Fe(CO)_5]$

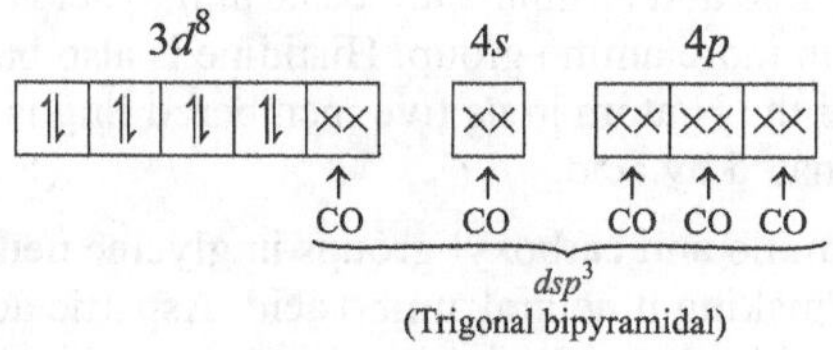

($\because$ CO is strong field ligand)

Fe in $K_4[Fe(CN)_6]$ has + 2 oxidation state.

$Fe^{2+} = [Ar]\,3d^6$

$[Fe(CN)_6]^{4-}$

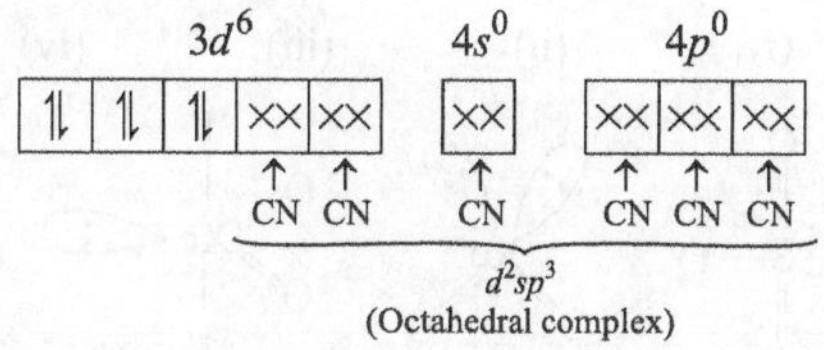

($\because$ CN is strong ligand)

$[Fe(H_2O)_6]Cl_3 \Rightarrow$ Fe has + 3 oxidation state

$Fe^{3+} = [Ar]3d^5$

$[Fe(H_2O)_6]^{3+}$

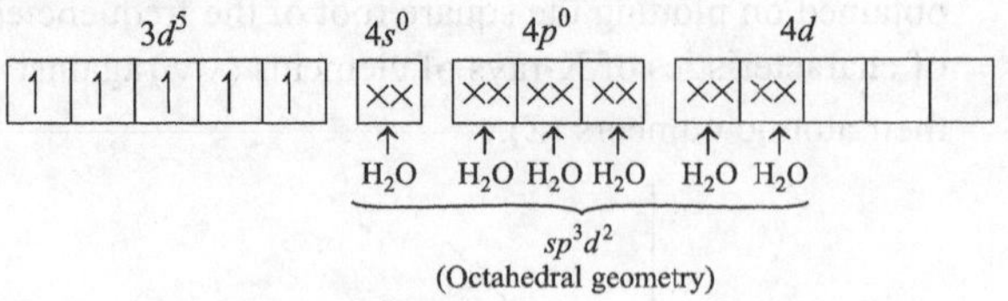

∵ (H_2O is weak ligand)

Hence, the correct match is A-(iv), B-(i), C-(ii), D-(iii).

72. (c) The favourable reaction is the oxidation of iodide ion to iodine.

I^- will be oxidised to I_2.

$$2e^- + 2Fe^{+3} \longrightarrow 2Fe^{2+};\ E° = 0.77\text{ V}$$

$$2I^- \longrightarrow I_2 + 2e^-;\ E° = 0.536\text{ V}$$

$$2Fe^{+3} + 2I^- \longrightarrow 2Fe^{+2} + I_2;\ E° = E°_{ox} + E°_{red}$$

$$= 0.77 - 0.536 = 0.234\text{ V}$$

Since, the value of the cell potential is positive, the reaction will take place.

73. (a) This reaction may proceed mostly in one direction due to solubility.

e.g. Aluminium hydroxide is not very soluble (0.0001 g/100 mL at 20°C). So, the overall reaction will be

$$AlCl_3 + 3NaOH \longrightarrow Al(OH)_3 + 3NaCl$$

$$Al(OH)_3 + 3NaOH \longrightarrow \underset{\substack{\text{Soluble} \\ \text{(white ppt.)}}}{Na_3[Al(OH)_6]}$$

74. (a) Lysine and Arginine are basic amino acids as they contain more amino group. Histidine is also basic as its one of the N atom in its five membered ring is readily protonated by acid.

The amino and carboxyl groups in glycine neutralise each other making it neutral amino acid. Aspartic acid has an acidic side chain. So, it is acidic amino acid.

75. (d)

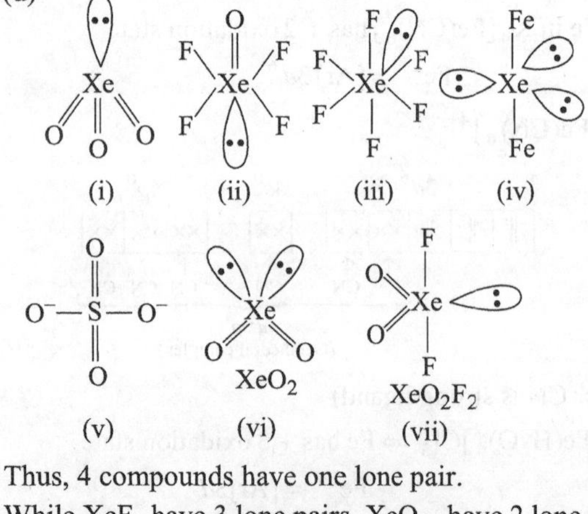

Thus, 4 compounds have one lone pair.

While XeF_2 have 3 lone pairs, XeO_2 have 2 lone pairs and SO_4^{2-} does not have any lone pair

Problem Solving Tactics To solve this problem, determine the valence electrons involved in the molecules and then substract the total number of bonding electrons from the valence electrons to calculate the number of lone pairs.

Lone pairs = (Valence electrons in the molecule − Bonding electrons in the molecule)

76. (d) The decomposition of NH_4NO_2 is as follows

$$NH_4NO_2(aq) \longrightarrow N_2(g) + 2H_2O(l)$$

Rate of reaction= $k[NH_4NO_2]^1$

For first order reaction $[A]_t = [A]_0 e^{-kt}$

So, the concentration of the reactant exponentially decreases with increasing time.

Hence, (d) is correct.

77. (c) 2, 4-dinitrophenyl hydrazine test is used to identify the aldehyde and ketone group. It gives yellow/orange precipitate with carbonyl containing compounds.

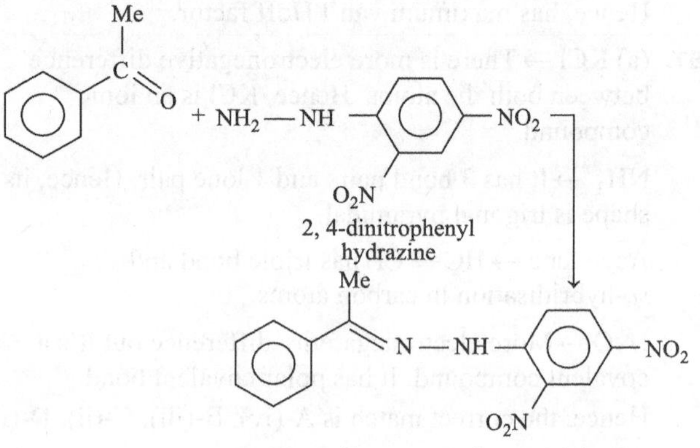

(Orange or yellow precipitate)

78. (b) A transition metal complex absorbs visible light if it has unpaired electrons.

Ni is in + 2 oxidation state in $[Ni(CN)_4]^{2-}$

$Ni^{2+} \rightarrow 3d^8 4s^0$

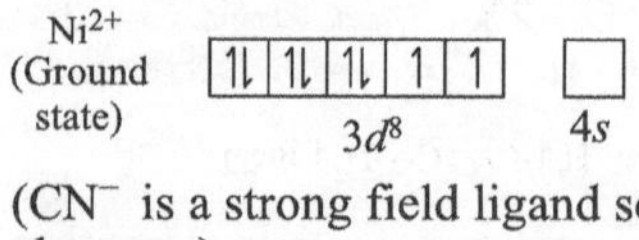

(CN^- is a strong field ligand so induces pairing of electrons).

No unpaired electron so does not absorb visible light.

79. (d) Methyl amine reacts with $NaNO_2$ in the presence of HCl to form nitrogen (N_2), hydrogen chloride (HCl) and methanol (CH_3OH).

$$CH_3NH_2 + HONO \xrightarrow[\text{Ice cold}]{\text{HCl}} CH_3\overset{\oplus}{N_2}\overset{\ominus}{Cl} + 2H_2O$$

$$\xrightarrow{\text{Unstable}} CH_3OH + N_2 + HCl$$

80. (c) Presence of electron withdrawing group on ring or aromatic nucleus such as NO_2 group increases its acidic strength by decreasing electron density of phenol.

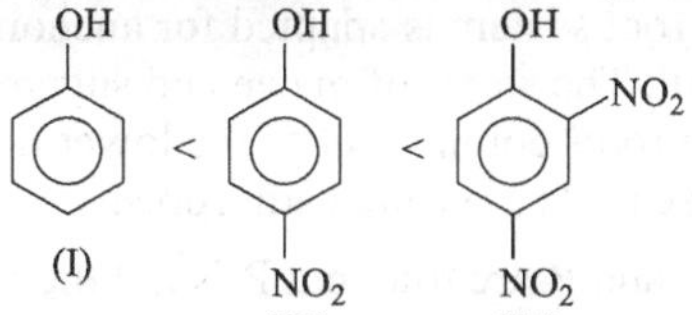

(I) (III) (IV)

On the other hand, electron donating group present on aromatic nucleus (here) decreases acidic strength due to increase in electron density around nucleus.

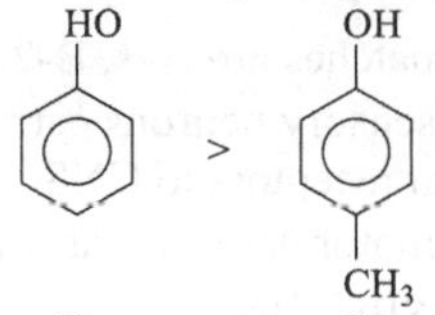

(I) (II)

Thus, the correct order of acidic strength of the given compounds is II < I < III < IV.

81. (a) **Etard reaction** is used to oxidise an aromatic methyl group or heterocyclic bound methyl group to an aldehyde using chromyl chloride.

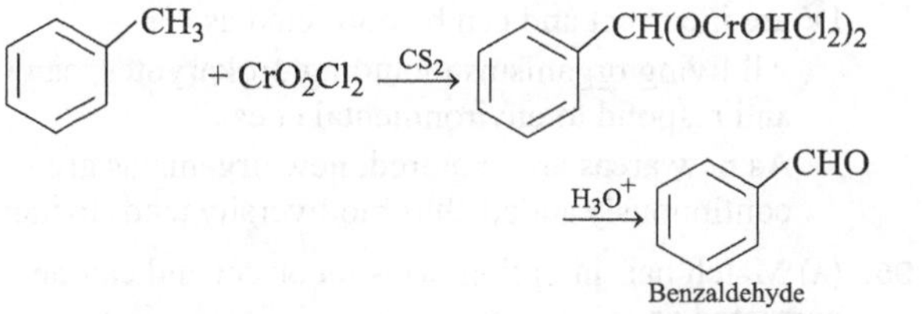

Benzaldehyde

Reformatsky reaction is an organic reaction which condenses aldehydes or ketones, with α-halo esters, using a metallic zinc to form α, β-unsaturated ester.

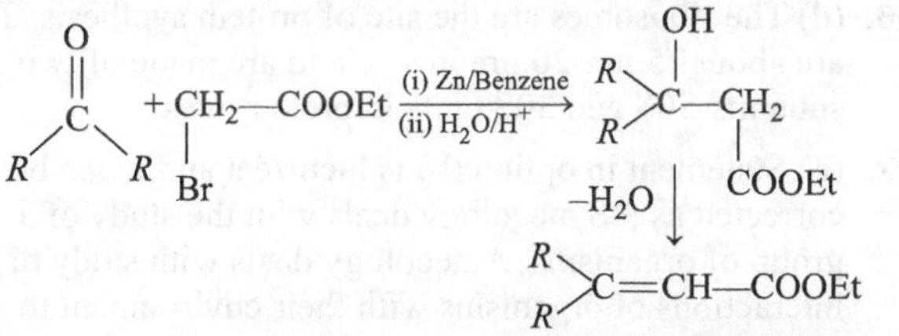

α, β-unsaturated ester

Friedel-Craft's acylation reaction involves formation of a complex between the Lewis acid and the chlorine atom of the acid chloride.

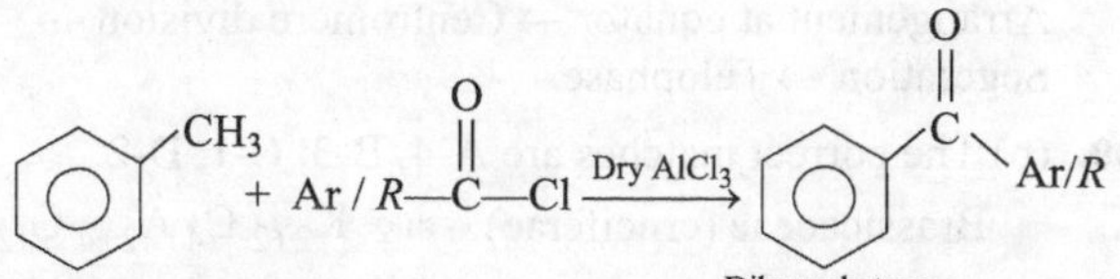

Dibenzoketone

Perkin's reaction mechanism includes the reaction between aromatic aldehydes, the aliphatic acid anhydride and the alkali salt of the acid to give cinnamic acid.

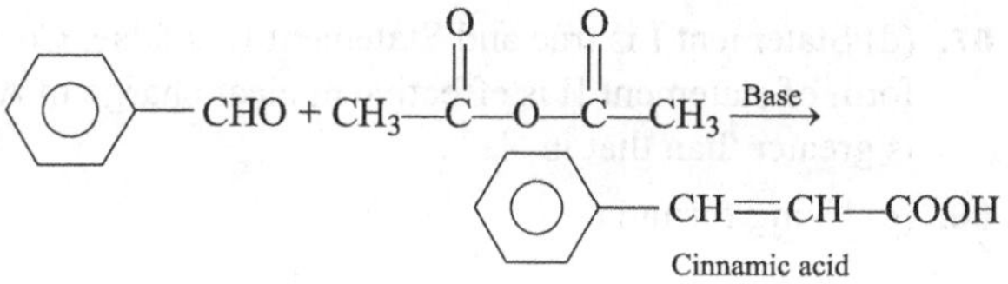

Cinnamic acid

Hence, the correct match is A-(ii), B-(iv), C-(iii), D-(i).

82. (b) Both Statement I and Statement II are true.

Actinoids exhibit a larger number of oxidation states than lanthanoids because, there is a very small energy gap between $5f$, $6d$ and $7s$ orbitals.

Also, $5f$ electron in actinoids are less effectively shielded resulting in quenching of orbital magnetic moment. So, their magnetic moment are less than theoretically predicted value.

83. (b)

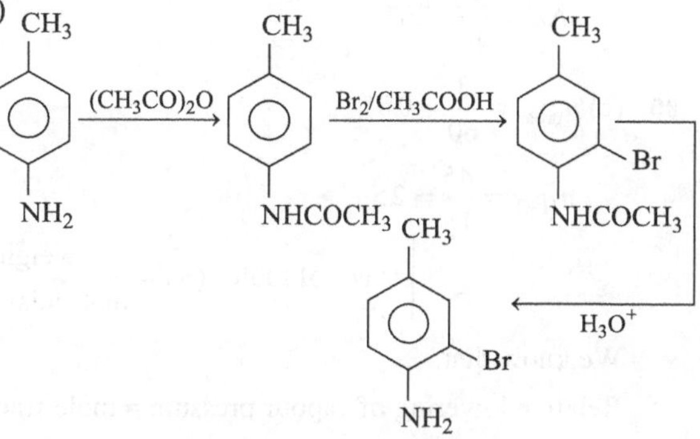

(X)

84. (d) The reaction involved is

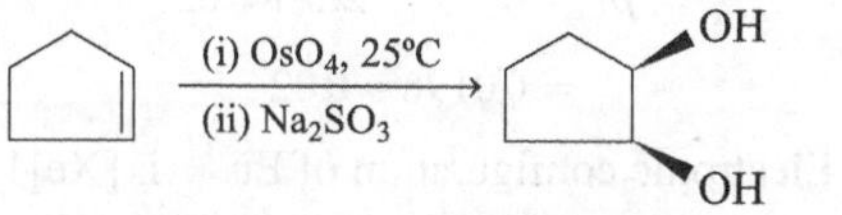

cis-cyclopentan-1, 2-diol

85. (a) In base *vs* acid titration, at the end point methyl orange is present as quinonoid form.

86. (c)

	$A \longrightarrow P$	
Initially	a	0
After time, t	$a-x$	x
After $t_{1/4}$	$a-\frac{a}{4}$	$\frac{a}{4}$

For first order reaction,

$$k=\frac{2.303}{t}\log\left(\frac{a}{a-x}\right)$$

$$k=\frac{2.303}{t_{1/4}}\log\frac{a}{\frac{3a}{4}}$$

$$\Rightarrow \quad t_{1/4}=\frac{2.303}{k}\log\frac{4}{3}$$

$$\therefore \quad t_{1/4}=\frac{0.29}{k}$$

87. (d) Statement I is true and Statement II is false. Correct form of statement II is effective nuclear charge in Al^{3+} is greater than that in Na^{+}.

88. (c) Using formula

$$\Delta E = hcR_H\left[\frac{1}{n_1^2}-\frac{1}{n_2^2}\right]$$

For lowest energy of spectral lines in Lyman series,

$n_1 = 1, n_2 = 2$

$$\text{So, } \Delta E = hcR_H\left[\frac{1}{(1)^2}-\frac{1}{(2)^2}\right]$$

$$= hcR_H \times \frac{3}{4}$$

$$\Delta E = \frac{3}{4}hcR_H$$

89. (c) $n_{urea} = \frac{3}{60} = 0.05,$

$$n_{H_2O} = \frac{45}{18} = 2.5$$

$$\left[\because \text{no. of moles } (n) = \frac{\text{weight}}{\text{molecular mass}}\right]$$

We know that,

Relative lowering of vapour pressure = mole fraction of urea.

$$\frac{\Delta p}{p^\circ} = \chi_{urea} = \frac{0.05}{2.5+0.05}$$

$$= 0.0196 \approx 0.02$$

90. (a) Electronic configuration of Eu^{3+} is $[Xe]4f^6 5d^0 6s^0$.

= | 1 | 1 | 1 | 1 | 1 | 1 | |
|---|---|---|---|---|---|---|

4f

$$\therefore \quad \mu_{cal} = \sqrt{n(n+2)}$$

$$\because \quad n = 6 \Rightarrow \mu_{cal} = \sqrt{48} = 6.93$$

where, n = no. of unpaired electrons.

Problem Solving Tactics

Spin only magnetic moment can be predicted (approximately) simply by knowing the number of unpaired electrons. For n number of unpaired electrons, the magnetic moment lies in the range of n to $n+1$.

No of unpaired electrons	Spin magnetic moment
1	1.73
2	2.82
3	3.87

Biology

91. (d) A stilt root system is adapted for anchorage of plant into the soil. The stems of maize and sugarcane have supporting roots coming out of the lower nodes of the stem. These roots are called stilt roots.

92. (c) Both A and R are true, but R is not the correct explanation of A.

Members of Sphenopsida are commonly called horsetails. The present day Sphenopsida includes only one living genus–*Equisetum*.

93. (c) The correct matches are A-1, B-2, C-4, D-3.

- The afferent/sensory neurons carry the sensory impulses from receptors to CNS.
- The efferent/motor neurons carry motor impulses from CNS to effectors.
- The unipolar neurons emerge from one pole of the cell body and are usually found in embryonic stage.
- The multipolar neurons have their cell body composed with one axon and two or more dendrites. They are usually found in the cerebral cortex.

94. (c) Statements I, III and V are correct. Statements II and IV are incorrect and can be corrected as

- All living organisms including prokaryotes, can sense and respond to environmental cues.
- As new areas are explored, new organisms are continuously added, thus biodiversity tends to increase.

95. (a) Match pair in option (a) is incorrect and can be corrected as

Amyloplasts store starch granules.
Rest match pairs are correct.

96. (d) The ribosomes are the site of protein synthesis. They are about 15 nm-20 nm in size and are made of two subunits-50S and 30S units in prokaryotes.

97. (b) Statement in option (b) is incorrect and it can be corrected as ; Synecology deals with the study of a group of organisms. Autecology deals with study of interactions of organisms with their environment to explain their distribution and abundance.

98. (b) The correct sequence of events during mitosis is as follows

Condensation → Nuclear membrane disassembly → Arrangement at equator → Centromere division → Segeration → Telophase.

99. (b) The correct matches are A-4, B-3, C-1, D-2.

- Brassicaceae (cruciferae) – ⊕ ⚥ $K_{2+2}\ C_4\ A_{2+4}\ \underline{G}_{(2)}$
- Fabaceae – % ⚥ $K_{(5)}\ C_{1+2+(2)}\ A_{(9)+1}\ \underline{G_1}$
- Malvaceae – Br ⊕ ⚥ $Epi_{3\text{-}9}\ K_{5 \text{ or } (5)}\ \widehat{C_5\ A_{(\infty)}}\ \underline{G}_{(2\text{-}\infty)}$
- Gramineae – Br % ⚥ $P_2\ A_3\ G_1$

100. (d) A is true, but R is false, it can be corrected as

Drop in temperature and greater seasonal variability at higher altitudes are the major factors that reduce diversity.

101. (b) Each myofibril has alternate dark and light bands on it. The light band contain actin and is called isotropic band, whereas the dark band contain myosin and is called anisotropic band. The actin filaments are thinner as compared to myosin filaments.

102. (b) Formation of number of pollen grains $= \frac{n}{4}$

$n = 280$ pollen grains $= \frac{280}{4} = 70$

Thus, 70 meiotic divisions are necessary to produce 280 pollen grains.

103. (c) Both Statement I and Statement II are incorrect. These can be corrected as

- Grasshopper shows male heterogamety and is the example of XO type of sex-determination. The males have only one X-chromosome besides the autosomes whereas, females have a pair of X- chromosome.
- Genetic map is one that establishes sites of gene on a chromosome.

104. (b) Statement in option (b) is incorrect and can be corrected as

Gynaecomastia, i.e. development of breast is observed in the individual suffering from Klinefelter's syndrome. It is caused due to the presence of an additional copy of X-chromosome.

105. (b) Statement in option (b) is incorrect and can be corrected as

Deuteromycetes is a class of fungi, commonly known as imperfect fungi. These include members like *Alternaria, Trichoderma, Colletotrichum* whereas *Puccinia* belongs to Basidiomycetes.

106. (d) Statements II and IV are correct and rest of the statements are incorrect. These can be corrected as

- In an aquatic ecosystem, GFC is the major conduit for energy flow.
- In an ecosystem, any given species may occupy more than one trophic level in the same ecosystem at the same time.
- The pyramid of biomass in sea is generally inverted because the biomass of fishes far exceeds that of phytoplankton.

107. (a) The correct matches are A-2, B-3, C-4, D-1.

- The trait linked with sex-chromosome is called sex-linked trait. Haemophilia is the example of sex-linked recessive trait. In this disease, a single protein that is a part of the cascade of proteins involved in the clotting of blood is affected. Due to which a simple cut results in non-stop bleeding in affected individual.
- Autosomal linked recessive trait includes sickle-cell anaemia, phenylketonuria, thalassemia, etc. Thalassemia which occurs due to mutation or deletion results into anaemia.
- Out of the three possible genotypes for sickle cell anaemia ($Hb^A Hb^A$, $Hb^A Hb^S$, $Hb^S Hb^S$), the individuals homozygous for Hb^S, i.e. $Hb^S Hb^S$ show diseased phenotype.
- Chromosomal disorder includes the Down's syndrome, Klinefelter's syndrome, Turner's syndrome, etc. In Down's syndrome the affected individual is short statured with furrowed tongue and broad palm.

108. (b) In addition to *ori*, the vector requires a selectable marker, which helps in identifying non-transformants and selectively permitting the growth of transformants, e.g. The ampicillin resistance gene acts a selectable marker when ampicillin is transferred into *E. coli* cells.

109. (c) Statement in option (c) is incorrect and can be corected as

Bacterial and fungal enzymes degrade detritus into simple inorganic salts by the process known as catabolism.

110. (a) The correct matches are A-4, B-1, C-3, D-2.

- Urine is formed by the nephron, but is stored in the urinary bladder till a voluntary signal is received.
- About 70-80% of the electrolytes and water are reabsorbed in the proximal convoluted tubule.
- Ultrafiltration occurs in the Malpighian corpuscle, where blood is filtered finely through the membrane of Malpighian corpuscle.
- On an average 1 to 1.5 litres of urine is produced per day, which is transported through the ureter.

111. (c) Both A and R are true, but R is not the correct explanation of A.

The restriction endonuclease cut the DNA sequences at a specific site and produce DNA strands with the sticky ends. It cuts both the strands of DNA at the palindrome sites.

112. (c) Tunica media has circular smooth muscles and elastic fibres.

Tunica interna has an inner endothelium of long, thin cells of squamous epithelium.

Tunica externa is rich in collagen fibres, but has less elastin fibres.

113. (a) Chloride shift is the movement of chloride ions from the plasma into red blood cells as a result of the transfer of carbon dioxide from tissues to the plasma, a process that serves to maintain blood pH. Bicarbonate and chloride ions are transported across the RBCs membrane in opposite directions by the bicarbonate chloride carrier proteins. Thus, removal of CO_2 from blood involves influx of Cl^- into RBCs.

114. (d) Thyroid hormones play an important role in regulating basal metabolic rate. These hormones control metabolism of carbohydrates, fats, proteins and also support the process of RBC formation.

115. (b) The enzyme helicase is responsible for breaking of hydrogen bonds between two strands of DNA molecules.

Other can be explained as

- Primase is responsible for synthesis of RNA primer.
- Ligase ligate okazaki segments with each other.
- DNA polymerase adds deoxyribonucleotides to the 3′–OH end of the polynucleotide chain.

116. (b) Some insects like grasshoppers have XO type of sex determination. In this the males have only one X-chromosome besides the autosomes, whereas females have a pair of X-chromosomes. Therefore, in such insects females have 32 chromosomes and males have 31 chromosomes.

117. (d) A is true, but R is false. It can be corrected as

Wine and beer are produced without distillation whereas, whisky and rum are prepared by distillation of the fermented broth.

118. (a) The correct matches are A-2, B-1, C-4, D-3.

- Aerenchyma are specialised modified parenchymatous tissues containing air chambers between cells. They provide buoyancy to aquatic plants.
- Collenchyma are simple tissues which are absent in monocotyledonous plant, but are present below the epidermis in dicotyledonous plants.
- Sclerenchyma provide mechanical support to plant organ. These consist of long narrow cells with thick and lignified cell walls having a few or numerous pits. These are commonly found in leaves of tea.
- Xylem is a complex permanent tissue which helps in conduction of water and minerals from roots to the stem and leaves.

119. (c) Seed (Ovule) is formed by the fusion of one male gamete and one egg cell.

In *Cyperus*, one microspore mother cell ($2n$) upon meiosis produce only one functional pollen grain as in case of megasporogenesis. Therefore, 70 meiotic divisions are required to produce 70 male gametes or pollen grains. Similarly one megaspore mother cell ($2n$), upon meiosis, produce one functional egg cell. Therefore, 70 meiotic divisions required to produce 70 egg cells.

Total meiotic division for producing 70 seeds in *Cyperus* = 70 meiotic divisions for male gamete + 70 meiotic division for egg cell. = 140 meiotic divisions.

Thus, 140 meiotic divisions are required to produce 70 seeds in *Cyperus*.

120. (a) Statement I is incorrect but Statement II is correct. The incorrect statement can be corrected as

There are four species of *Plasmodium* among them *P. falciparum* causes the most serious type of malaria as it affects the brain.

121. (b) Statements I, IV and V are correct, whereas statements II and III are incorrect and can be corrected as

- The P-wave in the ECG represents the electrical excitation (or depolarisation) of the atria.
- Reduction in pH of blood will reduce the blood supply to the brain.

122. (c) In the excited state of chlorophyll molecule an electron is expelled from P_{680} and is donated to PQ then the electron from PQ passes into cytochrome ($b_6 f$). The reduced form of cytochrome donates the electron to PC system which further donates electrons to PS - I.

123. (a) The members of phylum–Coelenterata exhibit alternation of generation known as metagenesis. The polyps produce medusae asexually, while the medusae produce polyps sexually. Both *Meandrina* and *Gorgonia* belongs to phylum–Coelenterata and exhibits the property of alternation of generation.

124. (c) Both A and R are true, but R is not the correct explanation of A.

In Chondrichthyes, males can be distinguished from the female, as the former has a pair of hard elongated claspers attached to the pelvic fins. The claspers help in the copulation.

125. (b) Indole acetic acid promotes the cell elongation by decrease in wall pressure. Rest options are incorrect and can be corrected as

Indole acetic acid promotes the cell elongation by increase in osmotic solutes, increase in permeability of cytoplasm to water and increase in wall synthesis.

126. (a) The correct matches are A-2, B-3, C-1, D-4.

- The adult echinoderm are radially symmetrical while the larval forms are bilaterally symmetrical.
- Members of phylum–Ctenophora exhibit radial symmetry. Bioluminescence is well marked in ctenophores.
- Members of phylum–Porifera exhibit asymmetry. They are generally marine.
- Members of phylum–Cnidaria are free-swimming and exhibit biradial symmetry.

127. (d) During mid-1960s three independent researches reports the purification and chemical characterisation of three different kinds of inhibitors, i.e. inhibitor $-B_1$ abscission- II and dormin. Later all the three were proven to be chemically identical and named as abscisic acid.

128. (d) Statement I is correct but Statement II is incorrect. The incorrect statement can be corrected as

In China rose, the stamens are united into one bunch or one bundle and are known as monoadelphous.

129. (d) Statement I is correct but Statement II is incorrect. It can be corrected as
The emergency contraceptives have been proved effective to prevent pregnancy if used within 72 hours of coitus.

130. (d) Statement I is correct but Statement II is incorrect. The incorrect statement can be corrected as
As we go higher from species to kingdom, the number of common characteristics goes on decreasing.

131. (d) Statement I is correct but Statement II is incorrect, it can be corrected as

The development of methods of genetic engineering in the last decade have improved the quality of crops. The scientists have introduced *B. thuringiensis* toxin genes into the plants. This has made crops such as *Bt* cotton resistant to insect pests.

132. (c) The 24 hrs rhythm of our body such as the sleep-wake cycle is regulated by melatonin hormone secreted by pineal gland. Its production increases with evening darkness, promoting healthy sleep and helping to orient our circadian rhythm.

133. (b) Reserve material in prokaryotes is stored in the form of inclusion bodies and they are not bound by any membrane system and lie free in the cytoplasm.

134. (d) Statements I, IV and V are correct and rest of the statements are incorrect. These can be corrected as
- Mitochondria divide by the fission. Since, mitochondria were created by bacterial endosymbiosis, they divide by using a method similar to prokaryotic binary fission.
- Both 70S and 80S ribosomes are composed of two subunits.

135. (a) Every winter the famous Keoladeo National Park (Bharatpur) in Rajasthan hots thousands of migratory birds coming from Siberia and other extremely cold Northern regions.

136. (a) Only statement in option (a) is correct. Rest all statements are incorrect and can be corrected as
- Pulmonary artery carries the deoxygenated blood.
- In mammals, veins differ from arteries in having internal valves.
- Maximum surface area of circulating system is observed in capillaries.

137. (c) The gross production has highest value in grassland ecosystem. The rate of total capture of energy or the rate of total production of organic material is Gross Production or Gross Primary Productivity (GPP), while the balance or biomass remaining after meeting the cost of respiration of producers is Net Primary Productivity (NPP).

138. (b) *Eco*RI is an endonuclease enzyme which recognises and cuts the strand at specific restriction sites and produces sticky ends. The recognition sequence and site is GAATTC.

139. (d) Statement I is correct, but statement II is incorrect. It can be corrected as
At the time of parturition, the parasite of syphilis enters the newborn baby through the placental blood as it become permeable to some pathogens.

140. (b) Statement is option (b) is incorrect. It can be corrected as
In a mixed population the better adapted ones often survive and grow in population size. No variants are wiped out.

141. (a) The correct matches are A-2, B-3, C-1, D-4.
- RNA sequence UUU is coded for the amino acid phenylalanine.
- GGG codes for glycine.
- UCU codes for serine.
- CCC codes for amino acid proline.

142. (a) The yellow elastic connective tissue fibres have considerable strengths and exceptional elasticity that allows stretching of various organs.

Consequently, Egyptian 'mummies' still have intact arteries due to well-preserved yellow elastic fibres.

143. (d) Statements III, IV and V are correct. Only statements I and II are incorrect and can be corrected as
- During gel electrophoresis the smallest fragment moves to the farthest point towards anode.
- The restriction endonuclease enzyme binds to the DNA and cut each of the two strands at specific points in their sugar-phosphate backbones.

144. (d) The given figure represents the transverse section of monocot stem. The incorrect statement w.r.t. it can be corrected as:

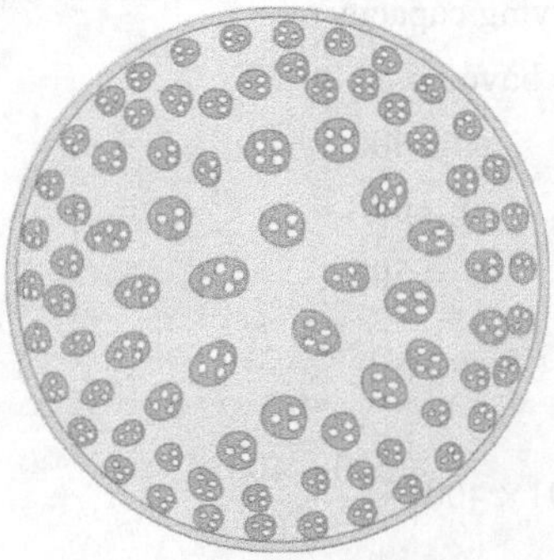

Each vascular bundle is surrounded by sclerenchymatous bundle sheath.

145. (d) hCG stimulates corpus luteum to produce progesterone in order to maintain pregnancy.

146. (a) Chorionic somatomammotropin also called hPL is secreted by placenta probably also has lactogenic properties, thus supporting the prolactin from the mother's pituitary during pregnancy.

147. (c) YACs are constructed artificially in the laboratory by joining segments of original DNA of yeast and linear plasmid from bacteria. YACs are prepared for gene transfer in eukaryotes and are found to be much more efficient than plasmids.

148. (c) Auxin is responsible for the bending of plant towards the source of light. Auxin accumulate on the shaded side, stimulating greater cell elongation there.

This means that the shaded side grows longer, causing the shoot to bend towards the light.

149. (a) A dominant independent photosynthetic, thalloid or erect phase is represented by haploid gametophyte and it alternater with the short lived multicellular sporophyte totally or partially dependent on the gametophytes for this anchorage and nutrition. This type of pattern is present in mosses and liverworts.

150. (c) Degradation at high temperature is not an criteria for a molecule to act as a genetic material. At high temperature DNA become fully separated but does not degrade.

151. (b) Competitive inhibition is affected by substrate concentration. It can be overcome by increasing the substrate concentration.

152. (b) Glycolysis is an essential phase and is the first path of respiration. It is common in both aerobic and anaerobic respiration.

153. (b) The logistic population growth model is represented by

$$\Rightarrow \frac{dN}{dt} = rN\left(\frac{K-N}{K}\right)$$

where, N = Population density at time 't'

r = Intrinsic rate of natural increase

K = Carrying capacity

Now, we have given

$$N = 400$$
$$r = 0.01$$
$$K = 500$$

if, $\frac{dN}{dt} = rN\left(\frac{K-N}{K}\right)$

then, $0.01 \times 400\left(\frac{500-400}{500}\right)$

$$\Rightarrow 0.01 \times 400\left(\frac{100}{500}\right)$$
$$\Rightarrow 0.01 \times 400 \times 0.2$$
$$\Rightarrow 0.8$$

154. (b) Secondary growth results in increase in the girth or diameter of the stem by the formation of secondary tissue by the activity of lateral meristem. It is clearly observed in dicots and gymnosperm. It is rarely observed in monocots and cannot be seen in pteridophytes.

Thus, for the study of secondary growth teak and pine are best suited.

155. (d) Statement I is correct, but statement II is incorrect. Statement II can be corrected as Oxygen-haemoglobin dissociation curve for foetal haemoglobin will appear on the left side. Foetal haemoglobin has two alpha and two gamma subunits. It carries 30% more oxygen than maternal haemoglobin.

156. (a) The correct matches are A-3, B-4, C-1, D-2.
- Epicotyl is the portion of embryonal axis above the level of cotyledons. It pushes the plant above the soil in early growth.
- Cylindrical portion below the level of cotyledons is hypocotyl. It lifts the growing tip above the ground bearing embryonic leaves.
- Stigma is the place where pollen grains land. It is present in the center of flower.
- Ovary is the site where seeds develop.

157. (d) The given figure is of a mature embryo sac.

After fertilisation, its different parts face different fates.
- Synergids (A) - degenerate
- Egg (B) - form zygote and then embryo (after fusion with male gamete)
- Polar nuclei (C) - form PEN and then endosperm
- Antipodals (D) - degenerate

158. (b) The infectious (communicable) diseases are the diseases which spread from person to person *via* several agents.

Some of the infectious diseases are influenza, smallpox, common cold, dengue, typhoid, etc.

159. (d) Both A and R are true and R is the correct explanation of A.

Hallucinogens are the drugs, which can alter a person's thought, feelings and perceptions. The sensations may be pleasant or more usually unpleasant, e.g, LSD, charas, hashish, etc.

160. (a) If chromosome number of diploid cell is 20 at the G_1-phase, even in G_2-phase the number of chromosomes remains the same, i.e. 20.

161. (c) Both A and R are true, but R is not the correct explanation of A

Final stage of meiotic prophase-I is diakinesis. During this phase the chromosomes are fully condensed and meiotic spindle prepares the separation of homologous chromosomes.
This stage marks the terminalisation of chiasmata.

162. (c) Retrovirus is used as a vector for cloning genes into higher organisms. They have the ability to transform their single-stranded RNA genome into a double-stranded DNA molecule that stably integrates into the target cell genome.

163. (a) In frog, the ventricle opens into a sac like conus arteriosus present on the ventral side of the heart.

164. (c) Statement in option (c) is incorrect and can be corrected as

Bioreactor provides optimal conditions for achieving the desired product by providing optimal growth conditions.

165. (c) The given diagram refers to the sectional view of seminiferous tubule in which 'A' represent sertoli cells.

Sertoli cells are located in the seminiferous tubules and provide nutrition to the germ cells.

166. (a) The correct matches are A-4, B-1, C-3, D-2.
- The surface barriers act as the first line of defence.
- The T-lymphocytes mediate the Cell-Mediated Immunity (CMI).
- Naturally acquired active immunity is the natural infection generated by a pathogen.
- The B-lymphocytes mediate antibody mediated immunity.

167. (a) Number of phenotypes for polygene $= 2n+1$ where n is number of heterozygotes in one polygene, $= (2\times 5+1) = 11$

168. (d) The test cross ratio of 7 : 1 : 1 : 7 indicates that there is a tendency of the dominant alleles to remain together.

169. (c) The statement in option (c) is incorrect. It can be corrected as

The therapies like bone marrow transplantation and enzyme replacement therapy cannot completely cure the patients with ADA deficiency. Gene isolation from bone marrow cells introduced at early embryonic stage can be a permanent cure.

Rest all the statements are correct.

170. (c) Only statement in option (c) is true. Rest other statements are incorrect and can be corrected as
- Electron transfer leads to release of protons in the thylakoid lumen.
- Within the chloroplast, protons in the stroma decreases in number.
- It decreases the pH in lumen.

171. (b) Statement in option (b) is incorrect and can be corrected as

The intrinsic rate of natural increase, i.e. r is different for different species.

The r value of Norway rat (0.015) is lesser compared to flour beetle (0.12).

172. (d) All the statements are correct except the statement in option (d). The incorrect statement can be corrected as

Relaxin is secreted by ovary and placenta at the end of gestation period because it aids in parturition.

173. (c) Statement in option (c) is incorrect and can be corrected as

The cellular oncogenes or proto-oncogenes gets activated in certain conditions that leads to oncogenic transformation of the cells.

174. (b) Dehydrogenation-I is the first oxidation step of the Krebs' cycle. Here, two hydrogen ions are removed from isocitric acid and oxalosuccinic acid are formed in the presence of the enzyme isocitric dehydrogenase.

175. (a) Statements I, III and V are correct, but statements II and IV are incorrect and can be corrected as
- The regulatory gene regulates biochemical reaction in a cell by inhibiting transcription.
- AUG codon has dual function. It codes for methionine and also acts as initiation codon.

176. (a) Statement I is incorrect, but statement II is correct. Incorrect statement can be corrected as

The biconcave discs of RBC permits it to squeeze through small capillaries.

177. (b) Only Statement II is incorrect and can be corrected as

During phosphorylation, the chloroplast stroma becomes less acidic than the interior of thylakoid membrane.
Rest other statements are correct.

178. (d) A is true, but R is false. It can be corrected as Interferons are group of signalling proteins released by host cells. These are the cytokine barriers, which protect the non-infected cells.

179. (c) Statements I and II are incorrect. These can be corrected as
- Mammary glands are not concerned with the secretion of hormone, but during pregnancy period progesterone and prolactin are released by mammary gland.
- Progesterone is active during the secretory phase of menstrual cycle.

Rest all the statements are correct.

180. (d) The body of the poriferans is supported by a skeleton made of spicules or spongin fibres, e.g. *Sycon*, *Spongilla*, etc.

SECTION II

Mastery Builders

PRACTICE SET 10

Maximum Marks : 720	Time : 3 hrs	No. of Questions : 180

Instructions

1. This question paper contains **180** multiple-choice questions (four options with a single correct answer) from **Physics, Chemistry** and **Biology**.
2. These questions are distributed as 45 questions, each from Physics and Chemistry and 90 questions in Biology. These are to be compulsorily attempted by the candidate.
3. Each question carries 4 marks. For each correct response, the candidate will get 4 marks. For each incorrect response, one mark will be deducted from the total scores.

PHYSICS

1. A uniform cylinder has a radius R and length L. If the moment of inertia of this cylinder about an axis passing through its centre and normal to its circular face is equal to the moment of inertia of the same cylinder about an axis passing through its centre and perpendicular to its length, then

(a) $L=\sqrt{3}R$ (b) $L=R$

(c) $L=R/\sqrt{3}$ (d) $L=2R$

2. In Young's double slit experiment, the intensity at centre of screen is I. If one of the slit is closed, the intensity at centre now will be

(a) I (b) $\frac{I}{3}$ (c) $\frac{I}{4}$ (d) $\frac{I}{2}$

3. The angular momentum of an electron orbiting in the third orbit of an atom is [given, $h=6.6\times10^{-34}$ J-s]

(a) 8.25×10^{-34} J-s (b) 6.55×10^{-34} J-s

(c) 3.15×10^{-34} J-s (d) 4×10^{-34} J-s

4. Consider the junction diode is ideal. The value of current in the figure is

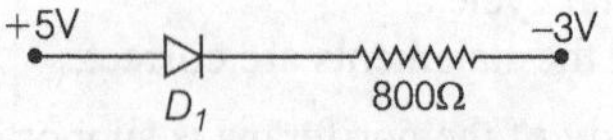

(a) zero (b) 10×10^{-2} A

(c) 10^{-1} A (d) 10 mA

5. The horizontal range and the maximum height of a projectile are equal. The angle of projection of the projectile is

(a) $\theta=\tan^{-1}(4)$ (b) $\theta=\tan^{-1}\left(\frac{1}{4}\right)$

(c) $\theta=45°$ (d) $\theta=60°$

6. For a p-type semiconductor, which of the following statements is false?

(a) Electrons are majority carriers and pentavalent atoms are the dopants.

(b) Holes are majority carriers and trivalent atoms are the dopants.

(c) Electrons are minority carriers and doping are of trivalent impurities.

(d) Impurities of third group (B, Al, Ga, In) are added.

7. When a proton is accelerated through 2V, then its kinetic energy will be

(a) 4.8×10^{-19} J

(b) 3.2×10^{-19} J

(c) 6.4×10^{-19} J

(d) 1.6×10^{-19} J

8. Statement I Non-polar molecules do not have permanent dipole moment.

Statement II In non-polar molecules, the centres of positive and negative charges are coincides.

In the light of above statements, choose the most appropriate answer from the option given below.
(a) Both Statement I and Statement II are correct.
(b) Both Statement I and Statement II are incorrect.
(c) Statement I is correct but Statement II is incorrect.
(d) Statement I is incorrect but Statement II is correct.

9. The current (i) in the inductance is varying with time according to the plot shown in the figure. Which one of the following is the correct variation of voltage with time in the coil ?

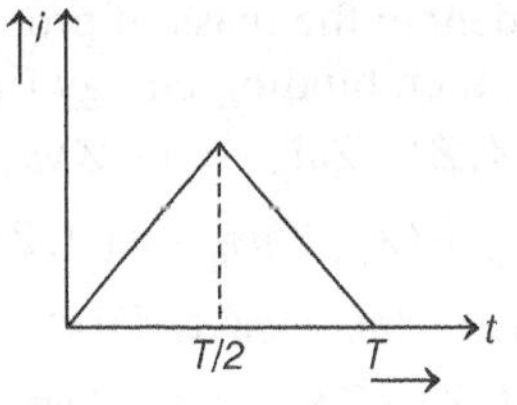

(a)
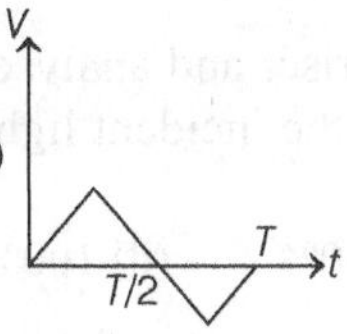

(b)
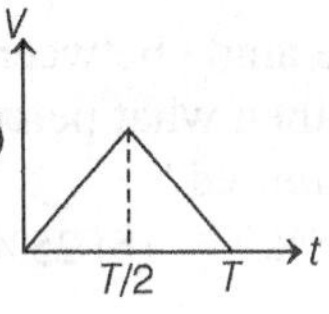

(c)
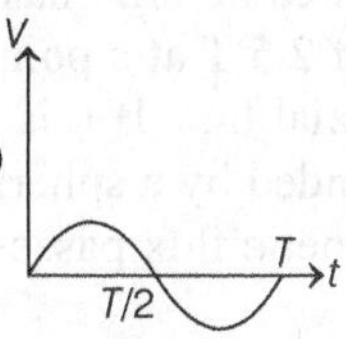

(d)
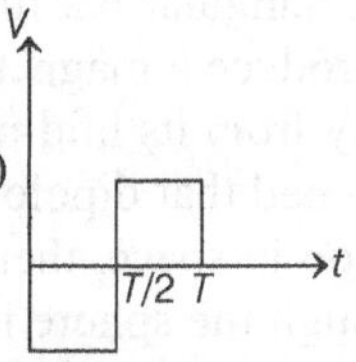

10. The Young's modulus of the material of a wire is 5×10^{10} N/m^2. If the elongation strain is 2%, then the energy stored in the wire per unit volume (in Jm^{-3}) is
(a) 10^7 (b) 2×10^7
(c) 0.5×10^7 (d) 10^8

11. An electromagnetic radiation has an energy of 13.2 keV, then the radiation belongs to the region of
(a) X-ray (b) infrared
(c) ultraviolet (d) visible light

12. A brass sphere of mass 5 kg is heated in a furnance to a temperature 500°C and then placed on a large ice block. The mass of ice that will melt in this process will be (specific heat of brass $= 500\text{ J kg}^{-1}\,°\text{C}^{-1}$ and heat of fusion of ice $= 336\text{ kJ kg}^{-1}$)
(a) 5.25 kg (b) 3.86 kg
(c) 2.56 kg (d) 3.72 kg

13. A 6 μF capacitor is charged to 360V. If its plates are joined through a resistance, then heat produced in the resistor is
(a) 0.78 J (b) 0.68 J
(c) 1.2 J (d) 0.39 J

14. In case of free expansion,
(a) no work to be required to do
(b) no heat exchange takes place
(c) change in internal energy is zero
(d) All of the above

15. If R is the radius of the earth and g is the acceleration due to gravity on the earth's surface, the mean density of the earth is
(a) $4\pi G / 3gR$ (b) $3\pi R / 4g G$
(c) $3g / 4\pi RG$ (d) $\pi RG / 12G$

16. The magnetic flux through a circuit of resistance R changes by an amount $\Delta\phi$ in a time Δt, then the total quantity of electric charge Q that passes at any point in the circuit during the time Δt is represented by
(a) $\frac{\Delta\phi}{R}$ (b) $\frac{1}{R}\frac{\Delta\phi}{\Delta t}$ (c) $R\frac{\Delta\phi}{\Delta t}$ (d) $\frac{\Delta\phi}{\Delta t}$

17. The average drift velocity of electrons inside a conducting rod of length 1 m when a potential difference of 100 V is applied across its ends, will be (Take, $\sigma = 5.81\times10^7\,\Omega^{-1}$ and $n = 8.5\times10^{28}\text{ m}^{-3}$)
(a) 0.63 m/s (b) 0.82 m/s
(c) 0.43 m/s (d) 0.92 m/s

18. Preeti reached the metro station and found that the escalator was not working. She walked up the stationary escalator in time t_1. On other days, if she remains stationary on the moving escalator, then the escalator takes her up in time t_2. The time taken by her to walk up on the moving escalator will be
(a) $\frac{t_1+t_2}{2}$ (b) $\frac{t_1t_2}{t_2-t_1}$ (c) $\frac{t_1t_2}{t_2+t_1}$ (d) t_1-t_2

19. A ball is released from the top of a tower of height h metre. It takes T second to reach the ground. What is the position of the ball in (T / 3) second ?
(a) $\left(\frac{h}{9}\right)$ m from the ground
(b) $\left(\frac{17h}{18}\right)$ m from the ground
(c) $\left(\frac{7h}{9}\right)$ m from the ground
(d) $\left(\frac{8h}{9}\right)$ m from the ground

20. A wire of resistance 10Ω is bent to from a complete circle. Find its resistance between two diametrically opposite points.

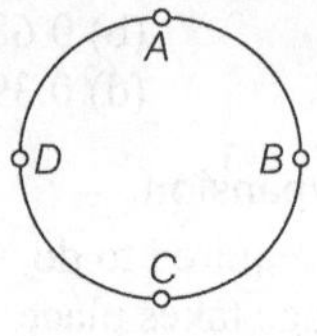

(a) 5Ω (b) 2.5Ω (c) 1.25Ω (d) $\frac{10}{3}\Omega$

21. When a charged particle moving with velocity **v** is subjected to a magnetic field of induction **B**, the force on it is non-zero. This implies that

(a) angle between them is either zero or 180°
(b) angle between them can have any value other than zero or 180°
(c) angle between them is necessary 90°
(d) angle between them can have any value other than 90°

22. If μ_0 and ε_0 represent the permeability and permittivity of free space respectively, then dimensional formula of $\mu_0\varepsilon_0$ will be

(a) $[LT^{-1}]$ (b) $[L^2T^{-2}]$ (c) $[L^{-1}T]$ (d) $[L^{-2}T^2]$

23. The current in the resistance of 2Ω in the following circuit is (diodes are ideal)

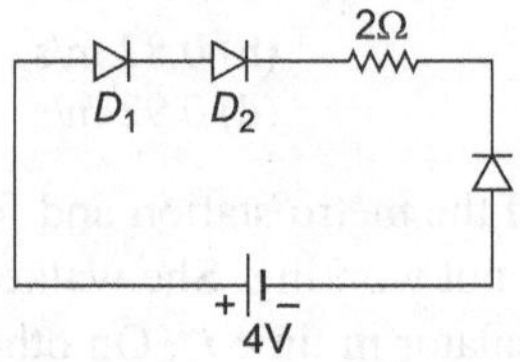

(a) 2 A (b) 1 A (c) 4 A (d) 0 A

24. Two blocks A and B of masses 4 kg and 8 kg respectively are placed on a smooth plane surface. A force F of 12 N is applied on A as shown. Find the force of contact (in N) between A and B.

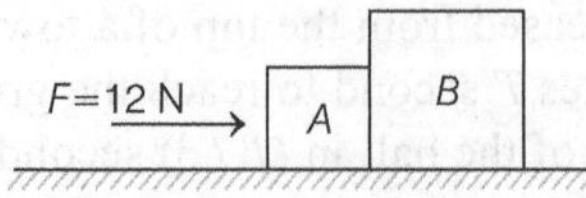

(a) 5 (b) 6
(c) 7 (d) 8

25. A given sample of an ideal gas occupies a volume V at a pressure p and absolute temperature T. The mass of each molecule of the gas is m. Which of the following gives the density of the gas ?

(a) mKT (b) p/KT
(c) pm/KT (d) p/KTV

26. Three electric dipoles are enclosed with in Gaussian spherical surface of radius 2 cm. If electric dipole moment of each dipole is 20 μC, then total electric flux passing through the surface is

(a) $\frac{10\times10^{-8}}{\varepsilon_0}$ (b) 0
(c) $\frac{5\times10^{-8}}{\varepsilon_0}$ (d) $\frac{20\times10^{-8}}{\varepsilon_0}$

27. A nucleus ${}^A_Z X$ has mass represented by $m(A, Z)$. If m_p and m_n denote the mass of proton and neutron, respectively, then binding energy (in MeV) is

(a) $BE = [m(A, Z) - Zm_p - (A - Z)m_n]c^2$
(b) $BE = [Zm_p + (A - Z)m_n - m(A, Z)]c^2$
(c) $BE = [Zm_p - Am_n - m(A, Z)]c^2$
(d) $BE = m(A, Z) - Zm_p - (A - Z)m_n$

28. If the angle between the polariser and analyser is 30°, then what percentage of the incident light is transmitted?

(a) 75% (b) 25% (c) 50% (d) 100%

29. A rectangular bar magnet of area 20 cm^2 has ability to produce a magnetic field of 2.5 T at a point 30 cm away from its mid-point on axial line. If it is assumed that dipole is surrounded by a spherical region in space, then net magnetic flux passes through the sphere is

(a) 0 (b) 0.005 Wb
(c) 0.15 Wb (d) 0.05 Wb

30. Two stones were projected simultaneously in the same vertical plane from same point obliquely, with different speeds and angles with the horizontal. The trajectory of path followed by one, as seen by the other, is

(a) parabola (b) straight line
(c) circle (d) hyperbola

31. A body weight 30 N in air and 26 N when fully immersed in water. Its relative density is

(a) 7.5 (b) 6.5
(c) 6 (d) 7

32. An experiment is performed to determine the I-V characteristics of a zener diode, which has a protective resistance of $R = 100\,\Omega$ and a maximum power of dissipation rating of 1 W. The minimum voltage range of the DC source in the circuit is

(a) 0-5 V (b) 0-24 V
(c) 0-12 V (d) 0-8 V

33. The vertical motion of a huge piston in a machine is approximately simple harmonic with a frequency of $0.5\,s^{-1}$. A block of 20 kg is placed on the piston. The maximum amplitude of the piston's SHM, for the block and the piston to remains together is

(a) 0.99 m (b) 1.5 m
(c) 1.99 m (d) 2.8 m

34. An open pipe is suddenly closed at one end. As a result of which, the frequency of the third harmonic of the closed pipe is found to be higher by 100 Hz than the fundamental frequency of the open pipe. The fundamental frequency of the open pipe is

(a) 200 Hz (b) 300 Hz
(c) 240 Hz (d) 480 Hz

35. If minimum deviation $=30°$, then speed of light in shown prism will be

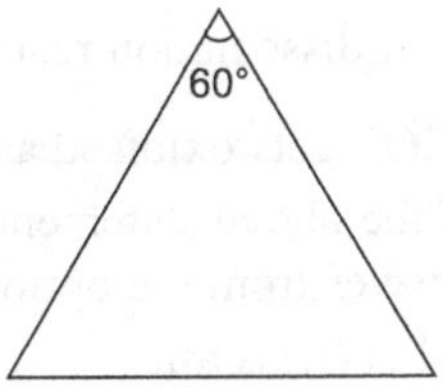

(a) $\frac{3}{\sqrt{2}}\times 10^8$ m/s (b) $\frac{1}{\sqrt{2}}\times 10^8$ m/s
(c) $\frac{2}{\sqrt{3}}\times 10^8$ m/s (d) $\frac{2}{3}\times 10^8$ m/s

36. The amount of energy released in the fusion of $_1H^2$ to form $_2He^4$ nucleus will be [BE per nucleon of $_1H^2 = 1.1$ MeV and $_2He^4 = 7$ MeV]

(a) 8.1 MeV (b) 5.9 MeV
(c) 23.6 MeV (d) 2 MeV

37. A square wire of side 2.0 cm is placed 20 cm in front of a concave mirror of focal length 10 cm with its centre on the axis of the mirror and its plane normal to the axis. The area enclosed by the image of wire is

(a) $7.5\,cm^2$ (b) $6\,cm^2$ (c) $2\,cm^2$ (d) $4\,cm^2$

38. A. The maximum kinetic energy of emitted electrons decreases as the work function of metal increases.
B. Stopping potential increases as the intensity of incident radiation in a photocell is increased.
C. The kinetic energy of photoelectrons increases as intensity of incident light increase.

Choose which of the above statements are correct and tick the correct option from the following.

(a) Only A (b) Only B and C
(c) Only C and A (d) Only A and B

39. **Statement I** Eddy currents heat up the core of a transformer and dissipate electrical energy in the form of heat.
Statement II Eddy currents are produce in any metallic conductor when magnetic flux is changed around it.
In the light of above statements, choose the most appropriate answer from the option given below.

(a) Both Statement I and Statement II are incorrect.
(b) Both Statement I and Statement II are correct.
(c) Statement I is correct but Statement II is incorrect.
(d) Statement I is incorrect but Statement II is correct.

40. A current of 2 mA was passed through an unknown resistor which dissipated a power of 4.4 W, then the dissipated power when an ideal power supply of 11 V is connected across it is

(a) 11×10^{-5} W (b) 11×10^{-4} W
(c) 11×10^{-3} W (d) 11×10^{5} W

41. If the percentage error in measuring the mass and the diameter are found to be 6.0% and 1.5% respectively, then maximum error in the measurement of density of solid metal sphere is found to be $\frac{x}{100}$ %, then the value of x is

(a) 950 (b) 850 (c) 1050 (d) 1250

42. Infinite number of masses, each of 1 kg are placed along the X-axis at $x = \pm 1$ m, ± 2m, ± 4m, ± 8m, ± 16m, ... The magnitude of the resultant gravitational potential in terms of gravitational constant G at the origin $(x=0)$ is

(a) G (b) $2G$ (c) $3\,G$ (d) $4G$

43. An EM wave which is passing by a vacuum is shown by the equations $E = E_0 \sin(kx - \omega t)$ and $B = B_0 \sin(kx - \omega t)$, then

(a) $E_0 \omega k B_0$ (b) $E_0 k = B_0 \omega$
(c) $E_0 \omega = B_0 k$ (d) $E_0 = B_0$

44. Assuming Bohr model of hydrogen atom. If an electron jumps from first excited state to the ground state of hydrogen atom, then the percentage change in the speed of electron will be

(a) 25% (b) 50%
(c) 100% (d) 200%

45. The work function of a given material is 6.1 eV. The wavelength of the incident radiation for which the stopping potential is 5V lies in the

(a) ultraviolet region (b) visible region
(c) X-ray region (d) infrared region

CHEMISTRY

46. Which of the following is correct graph regarding photoelectric effect?

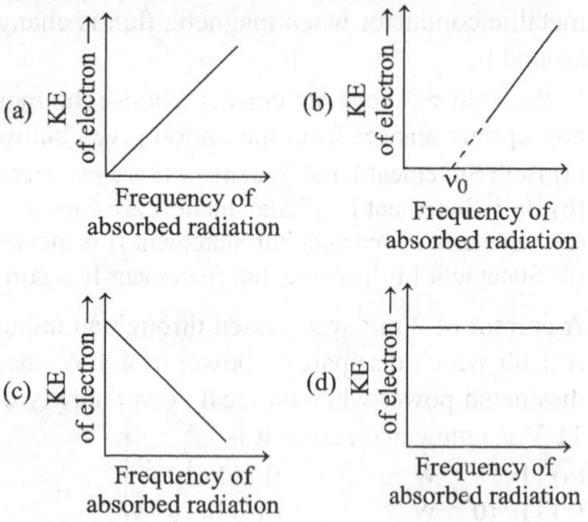

47. Introduction of inert gas (at same temperature) will affect the equilibrium if

(a) volume is constant and $\Delta n_g = 0$
(b) volume is constant and $\Delta n_g \neq 0$
(c) pressure is constant and $\Delta n_g \neq 0$
(d) pressure is constant and $\Delta n_g = 0$

48. Which of the following statements about the composition of vapour over an ideal 1 : 1 molar mixture of benzene and toluene is correct?
[Assume temperature is constant at 25°C and vapour pressure of benzene and toluene at 25°C are 12.8 kPa and 3.85 kPa respectively]

(a) The vapour will contain a higher % of benzene.
(b) The vapour will contain a higher % of toluene.
(c) The vapour will contain equal amount of benzene and toluene.
(d) Not enough information is given to make predictions.

49. Given below are two statements, one is labelled as Assertion (A) and the other is labelled as Reason (R).

Assertion (A) Na^+ ions are discharged in preference to H^+ ions at a mercury electrode.

Reason (R) The nature of cathode can affect the order of discharge of ions.

In the light of the above statements, choose the most appropriate answer from the options given below.

(a) (A) is false but (R) is true.
(b) Both (A) and (R) are true and (R) is the correct explanation of (A).
(c) Both (A) and (R) are true but (R) is not the correct explanation of (A).
(d) (A) is true but (R) is false.

50.

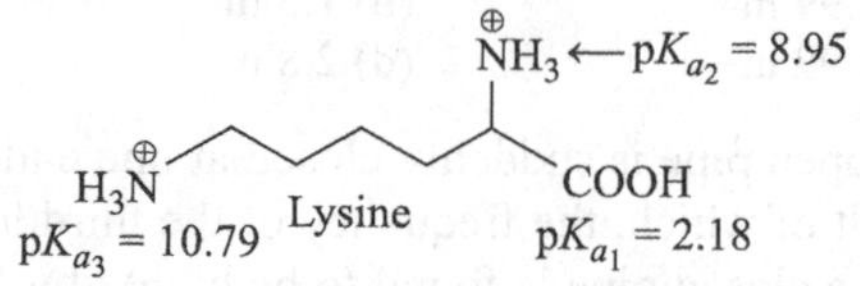

The isoelectric point for lysine will be

(a) 9.87 (b) 10.96 (c) 5.56 (d) 6.48

51. Given below are two statements, one is labelled as Assertion (A) and the other is labelled as Reason (R).

Assertion (A) $3ClO^-(aq) \longrightarrow ClO_3^-(aq) + 2Cl^-(aq)$ is an example of dissociation reaction.

Reason (R) ClO^- gets oxidised as well as reduced.

In the light of the above statements, choose the most appropriate answer from the options given below.

(a) (A) is false but (R) is true.
(b) Both (A) and (R) are true and (R) is the correct explanation of (A).
(c) Both (A) and (R) are true but (R) is not the correct explanation of (A).
(d) (A) is true but (R) is false.

52.

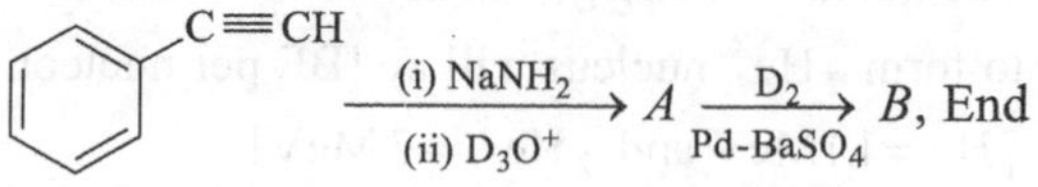

product '*B*' is

(a) 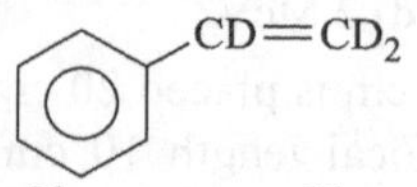

(b) 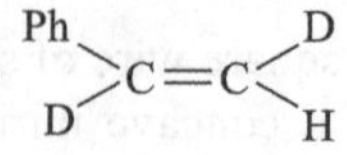

(c) 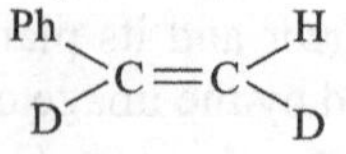

(d) Ph—C≡CD

53. The dark purple colour of $KMnO_4$ disappears in the titration with oxalic acid in acidic medium. The overall change in the oxidation number of manganese in the reaction is

(a) 5 (b) 1 (c) 3 (d) 2

54. Which of the following is correct statement?

(a) Starch is a polymer of α-glucose.
(b) All carbohydrates break down into glucose.
(c) Proteins are composed of only one type of amino acid.
(d) In cyclic structure of fructose, there are four carbons and one oxygen atom.

55. Consider the following tests;

A. Ferric chloride test B. Carbylamine test
C. Litmus test D. Liebermann's nitroso test
E. Phthalein test

Which of the following test is not given by phenols?

(a) B and E (b) Only B
(c) B and D (d) A and C

56. Select the option that has correct order of greater extent of overlapping of pure orbitals.

(a) $2s$-$2s > 2s$-$2p > 2p$-$2p$
(b) $2p$-$2p > 2s$-$2p > 2s$-$2s$
(c) $2s$-$2s > 2p$-$2p > 2s$-$2p$
(d) All have same extent of overlapping since all have same orbital

57. The ebullioscopic constant for a solvent is 0.5 K molal^{-1}. The boiling point of a solution containing 0.05 mole of a non-volatile, non-electrolytic solute in 0.25 kg solvent will increase by

(a) 10 K (b) 1 K (c) 0.1 K (d) 100 K

58. Which of the following is the correct order of boiling point?

(a) $HF > H_2O > NH_3 > CH_4$
(b) $H_2O > HF > NH_3 > CH_4$
(c) $HF > H_2O > CH_4 > NH_3$
(d) $CrO > VO > FeO > TiO$

59. Given below are two statements.

Statement I Tertiary amine shows carbylamine test.

Statement II Primary amines boil at higher temperature than tertiary amine.

In the light of the above statement choose the correct answer from the options given below.

(a) Statement I is false but Statement II is true.
(b) Both Statement I and Statement II are true.
(c) Both Statement I and Statement II are false.
(d) Statement I is true but Statement II is false.

60. The basic character of the transition metal monoxides follows the order.

(a) $TiO > FeO > VO > CrO$
(b) $TiO > VO > CrO > FeO$
(c) $VO > CrO > TiO > FeO$
(d) $CrO > VO > FeO > TiO$

61. de-Broglie wavelength of electron accelerated through V volt is given by

(a) $\sqrt{\frac{150}{V}}$ Å (b) $\frac{150}{V}$ Å
(c) $\left(\frac{150}{V}\right)^2$ Å (d) $\sqrt[3/2]{\frac{150}{V}}$ Å

62. XeF_6 on complete hydrolysis yields 'X'. The molecular formula of X and its shape respectively are

(a) XeO_4 and tetrahedral
(b) XeO_3 and trigonal planar
(c) XeO_3 and pyramidal
(d) XeO_2 and linear

63. The combustion of glucose takes place as

$$C_6H_{12}O_6 + 6O_2 \longrightarrow 6CO_2 + 6H_2O,$$
$$\Delta H = x \text{ kcal mol}^{-1}$$

The energy released by the combustion of 1.6g of glucose is – 0.64 kcal. What is the value of x ?

(a) -80 kcal mol^{-1} (b) -72 kcal mol^{-1}
(c) $+72$ kcal mol^{-1} (d) -108 kcal mol^{-1}

64. Ether in contact with air for a long time form peroxides. The presence of peroxide in ether can be tested by adding Fe^{2+} ions and then further adding

(a) KCN (b) $SnCl_2$
(c) $HgCl_2$ (d) KCNS

65. An exothermic chemical reaction occurs in two steps as follows

I. $A + B \longrightarrow X$ (Fast) II. $X \longrightarrow AB$ (Slow)

The progress of the reaction can be best represented by

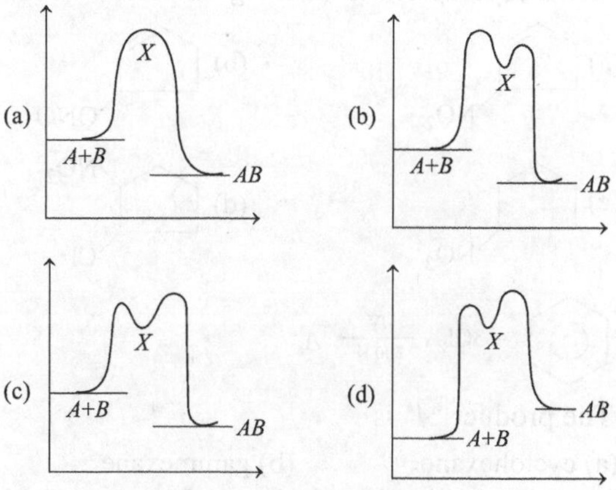

66. Which of the following are Newman projections of *meso*-2, 3-butanediol?

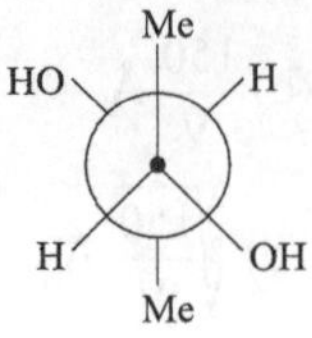

(I)

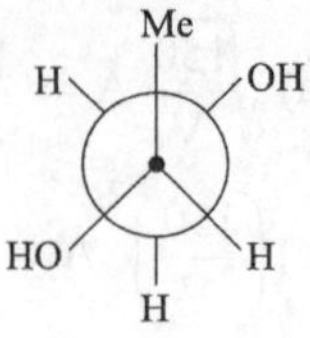

(II)

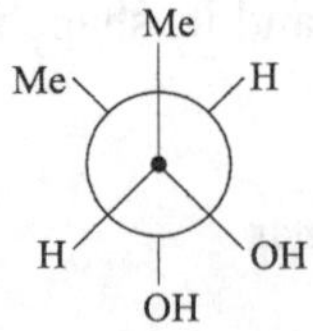

(III)

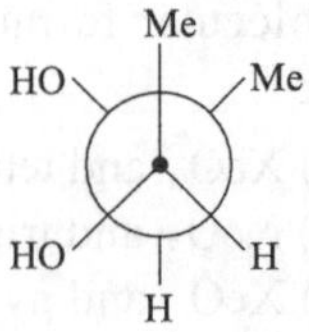

(IV)

Choose the correct answer from the options given below.

(a) I, IV (b) I, II (c) III, IV (d) II, III

67. Which one of the following pairs of compound can be used as starting material in the synthesis of 2-phenylbutan-2-ol?

(a) C_6H_5Br and $(CH_3)_3CCH=O$

(b) $C_6H_5-\overset{\overset{O}{\|}}{C}-CH_2CH_3$ and CH_3Br

(c) $C_6H_5-\overset{\overset{Br}{|}}{C}HCH_3$ and CH_3CHO

(d) $C_6H_5-\overset{\overset{O}{\|}}{C}-H$ and $CH_3-\underset{\underset{CH_3}{|}}{\overset{\overset{CH_3}{|}}{C}}-CH_3$

68. Product obtained on reaction of 3-chlorocyclopentene with $AgNO_2$ is

(a) 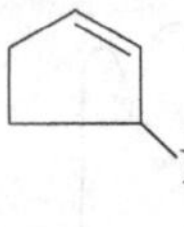

(b) 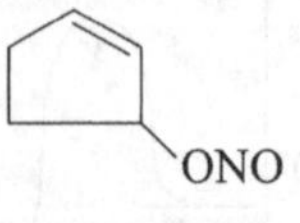

(c) 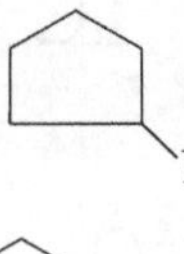

(d) 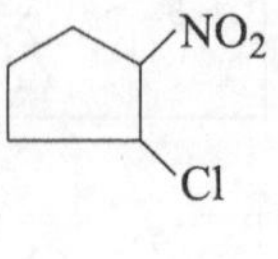

69. 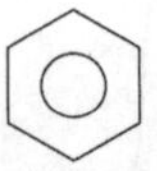 $+ 3Cl_2 \xrightarrow[500\text{ K}]{UV} A,$

The product '*A*' is

(a) cyclohexane (b) gammexane

(c) benzene chloride (d) cyclohexane chloride

70. Match List-I with List-II.

List-I (Coordination compounds)	List-II (Magnetic moment)
A. $[Fe(CN)_6]^{3-}$	(i) 5.92 BM
B. $[Fe(H_2O)_6]^{3+}$	(ii) 0 BM
C. $[Fe(CN)_6]^{4-}$	(iii) 4.90 BM
D. $[Fe(H_2O)_6]^{2+}$	(iv) 1.73 BM

Choose the correct answer from the options given below.

(a) A-(iv), B-(ii), C-(i), D-(iii)
(b) A-(ii), B-(iv), C-(iii), D-(i)
(c) A-(i), B-(iii), C-(iv), D-(ii)
(d) A-(iv), B-(i), C-(ii), D-(iii)

71. Given below are two statements.

Statement I In Lucas test, primary, secondary and tertiary alcohols are distinguished on the basis of their reactivity with conc. $HCl + ZnCl_2$, known as Lucas reagent.

Statement II Primary alcohols are most reactive and immediately produce turbidity at room temperature on reaction with Lucas reagent.

In the light of the above statements, choose the correct answer from the options given below.

(a) Statement I is false but Statement II is true.
(b) Both Statement I and Statement II are true.
(c) Both Statement I and Statement II are false.
(d) Statement I is true but Statement II is false.

72. 29.5 mg of an organic compound containing nitrogen was digested according to Kjeldahl method and the evolved ammonia was absorbed in 20 mL of 0.1 N HCl solution The excess of the acid required 15 mL of 0.1 N NaOH solution for complete neutralisation.

The percentage of nitrogen in the compound is

(a) 29.5% (b) 59.0% (c) 47.4% (d) 23.7%

73. Match List-I with List-II.

List-I	List-II
A. Diamond	(i) sp^2
B. Graphite	(ii) $CO + H_2$
C. Producer gas	(iii) sp^3
D. Water gas	(iv) $CO + N_2$

Choose the correct answer from the options given below.

(a) A-(ii), B-(i), C-(iv), D-(iii)
(b) A-(ii), B-(iv), C-(i), D-(iii)
(c) A-(iii), B-(i), C-(iv), D-(ii)
(d) A-(iii), B-(iv), C-(i), D-(ii)

74. Match List-I with List-II.

	List-I		List-II
A.	$CH_3(CH_2)_3OH \xrightarrow[H_2SO_4(\Delta)]{NaBr}$	I.	$CH_3CH(Br)CH_2CH_3$
B.	$(CH_3)_3COH \xrightarrow[\text{Room temp}]{\text{Conc. HCl}}$	II.	$CH_3—CH_2—CH_2Cl$
C.	$CH_3CH(OH)CH_2CH_3 \xrightarrow{PBr_3}$	III.	$(CH_3)_3C—Cl$
D.	$CH_3CH_2CH_2OH \xrightarrow{SOCl_2}$	IV.	$CH_3(CH_2)_3Br$

Choose the correct answer from the options given below:

(a) A-IV, B-III, C-I, D-II
(b) A-IV, B-II, C-I, D-III
(c) A-I, B-II, C-III, D-IV
(d) A-III, B-IV, C-II, D-I

75. Which of the following statement is correct for S_N1 mechanism?

(a) The first step is dissociation into an intimate ion pair.
(b) In second step, the leaving group attacks from back side.
(c) There is inversion of configuration.
(d) An external nucleophile attacks the substrate comparable molecular masses.

76. Given below are two statements.

Statement I The boiling points of aldehydes and ketones are higher than those of hydrocarbons and ethers of comparable molecular masses.

Statement II Aldehydes and ketones undergo intermolecular association due to dipole-dipole interactions.

In the light of the above statements, choose the correct answer from the options given below.

(a) Statement I is false but Statement II is true.
(b) Both Statement I and Statement II are true.
(c) Both Statement I and Statement II are false.
(d) Statement I is true but Statement II is false.

77. Consider the following species.

I. 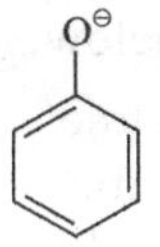

II. CH_3OH

III. $CH_3\overset{\ominus}{S}$

IV. $CH_3\overset{O}{\overset{\|}{C}}\overset{\ominus}{O}$

Which of the following is correct decreasing order of nucleophilicity in an aqueous solution?

(a) IV > II > I > III
(b) III > I > IV > II
(c) I > III > II > IV
(d) III > I > II > IV

78. Which of the following statement is incorrect regarding allotropes of carbon?

I. Carbon exists in more than one allotropic form.
II. Diamond is semiconductor while graphite is conductor.
III. Diamond has layered structure while graphite has tetrahedral structure.
IV. Diamond is a non-conductor of electricity.
V. Graphite and diamond both have giant structures.

Choose the correct answer from the options given below.

(a) I and II
(b) II and III
(c) I and IV
(d) I and V

79. Match List-I with List-II.

	List-I (Elements)		List-II (Outer electronic configuration)
A.	Thorium	(i)	$4f^0, 5d^1, 6s^2$
B.	Americium	(ii)	$3d^5, 4s^1$
C.	Lanthanum	(iii)	$5f^0, 6d^2, 7s^2$
D.	Chromium	(iv)	$5f^7, 6d^0, 7s^2$

Choose the correct answer from the options given below.

(a) A-(iii), B-(iv), C-(i), D-(ii)
(b) A-(ii), B-(i), C-(iii), D-(iv)
(c) A-(i), B-(ii), C(iii), D-(iv)
(d) A-(iv), B-(i), C-(ii), D-(iii)

80. Given below are two statements.

Statement I E_{cell} should have a positive value for the cell to function.

Statement II E_{cell} is an intensive property while Δ_rG of cell reaction is an extensive property.

In the light of the above statements, choose the correct answer from the options given below:

(a) Statement I is false but statement II is true.
(b) Both Statement I and Statement II are true.
(c) Both Statement I and Statement II are false.
(d) Statement I is true, but Statement II is false.

81. The rate constant for the reaction, $2N_2O_5 \longrightarrow 4NO_2 + O_2$ is $3.0\times 10^{-5}s^{-1}$. If the rate is 2.40×10^{-5} mol $L^{-1}s^{-1}$, then the concentration of N_2O_5 (in mol L^{-1}) is

(a) 0.04 (b) 1.2
(c) 1.4 (d) 0.8

82. Calculate the value of E°_{cell} if standard reduction potential of Fe^{2+} / Fe and Sn^{2+} / Sn electrodes are − 0.44 V and − 0.14 V respectively. The cell reaction is $Fe^{2+} + Sn \longrightarrow Fe + Sn^{2+}$

(a) 0.42 V (b) − 0.42 V
(c) − 0.30 V (d) − 1.10 V

83. Which of the following statements regarding chemical properties of acetophenone are incorrect?

I. It is reduced to methyl phenyl carbinol by sodium and ethanol.
II. It is oxidised to benzoic acid with acidified $KMnO_4$.
III. It does not undergo electrophilic substitution like nitration at *meta*-position.
IV. It does not undergo iodoform reaction with iodine and alkali.
V. Benzoic acid reacts with $Br_2/FeBr_3$ to give acetophenone.

Choose the correct answer from the options given below.

(a) I and II (b) II and IV
(c) III, IV and V (d) II and III

84. 0.7 g of $Na_2CO_3 \cdot xH_2O$ were dissolved in water and the volume was made upto 100 mL. 20 mL of this solution required 19.8 mL of *N*/10 HCl for complete neutralisation. The value of *x* is

(a) 7 (b) 3
(c) 2 (d) 5

85. Value of equilibrium constant for following reaction, $N_2(g) + 3H_2(g) \longrightarrow 2NH_3, (g)$ is 0.50 at 400°C. What is the value of K_p at 400°C?

(a) 1.64×10^{-3}
(b) 1.64×10^{4}
(c) 1.64×10^{-4}
(d) 164×10^{4}

86. Which of the following product is formed when cyclohexanone reacts with OH^- ions followed by heating?

(a) 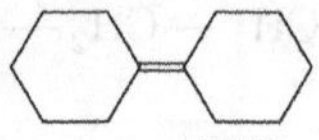
(b) 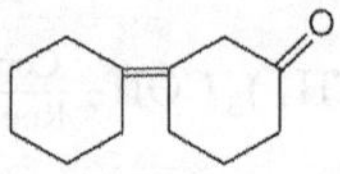
(c) 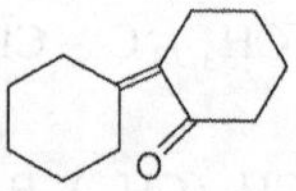

(d) 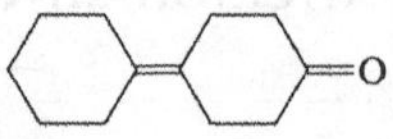

87. Which of the following statements is incorrect about the given reaction?

$[(CH_3)_3N^{\oplus}CH_2CH_3]OH^{\ominus} \xrightarrow{\Delta}$

(a) Less substituted alkene is the predominant alkene.
(b) OH^- ion function as a base in E2 elimination.
(c) The above reaction is known as Hofmann elimination.
(d) Primary amine is formed as one of the product.

88. Match List-I with List-II.

	List-I		List-II
A.	Ionisation energy comparable to O_2	I.	Helium
B.	Provides inert atmosphere in metallurgy	II.	Argon
C.	Cryogenic	III.	Neon
D.	Advertising sign	IV.	Xenon

Choose the correct answer from the options given below:

(a) A-I, B-II, C-III, D-IV
(b) A-IV, B-II, C-I, D-III
(c) A-II, B-I, C-III, D-IV
(d) A-IV, B-I, C-II, D-III

89. Given below are two statements.

Statement I For an element with an atomic number of 17, the most probable oxidation number is +1.

Statement II The outer energy level of the halogen family has a tendency to add one electron to itself.

In the light of the above statements, choose the correct answer from the options given below.

(a) Statement I is false but Statement II is true.
(b) Both Statement I and Statement II are true.
(c) Both Statement I and Statement II are false.
(d) Statement I is true but Statement II is false.

90. Arrange the following in increasing order of stability, O_2, N_2, Li_2, H_2.

(a) $Li_2 < H_2 < O_2 < N_2$ (b) $H_2 < Li_2 < O_2 < N_2$
(c) $N_2 < O_2 < Li_2 < H_2$ (d) $H_2 < Li_2 < N_2 < O_2$

BIOLOGY

91. A cell has 16 chromosomes. It undergoes mitotic division. Choose the correct option with respect to its chromosome number (N) during metaphase and DNA content (C) after mitotic metaphase?

	N	C		N	C
(a)	32	2C	(b)	16	4C
(c)	16	2C	(d)	32	4C

92. The liquid endosperm of *Cocos nucifera* is the product of

(a) mitosis without involving cytokinesis
(b) mitosis involving cytokinesis
(c) amitosis without involving cytokinesis
(d) amitosis involving cytokinesis.

93. Crown gall disease in plants is caused by

(a) Ti-plasmid (b) Pi-plasmid
(c) bacteria (d) virus

94. The separated bands of DNA are cut out from the agarose gel and extracted from the gel piece. This step is called

(a) electrophoresis (b) resolutions
(c) spooling (d) elution

95. During PCR, primers are paired to *ss*DNA segment. This step is

(a) denaturation (b) isolation
(c) annealing (d) polymerisation

96. .... is a popular method of contraception that increases phagocytosis of sperm within the uterus.

(a) Cervical caps
(b) Vaults
(c) Lippes loop
(d) Diaphragms

97. The Golgi complex plays a major role

(a) as energy transferring organelles
(b) in trapping the light and transforming it into chemical energy
(c) in digesting proteins and carbohydrates
(d) in post translational modification of proteins and glycosylations of lipids.

98. Given below are two statements; one is labeled as Assertion (A) and the other one is Reason (R)

Assertion (A) The three steps in the process of decomposition operate on the detritus simultaneously.

Reason (R) Humification and mineralisation occur during decomposition in the soil.

In the light of the above statements, choose the correct answer from the options given below.

(a) A is false, but R is true
(b) Both A and R are true and R is the correct explanation of A.
(c) Both A and R are true, but R is not the correct explanation of A
(d) A is true, but R is false

99. Consider the following matches and identify the incorrect match.

(a) Ectoparasites—Human body lice
(b) Endoparasites–Rat flea
(c) Parasitism—*Cuscuta*
(d) Brood parasitism—Cuckoo

100. Given below are two statements.

Statement I The seminal plasma along with the sperms constitute the semen.

Statement II The secondary oocyte forms a new membrane called Graafian follicle.

In the light of the above statements, choose the correct answer from the options givens below.

(a) Statement I is incorrect, but statement II is correct.
(b) Both statement I and statement II are correct.
(c) Both statement I and statement II are incorrect.
(d) Statement I is correct, but statement II is incorrect.

101. ELISA is the technique that serves the purpose of early diagnosis and is based on the principle of

(a) antigen-antigen interaction
(b) antigen-antibody interaction
(c) antibody-antibody interaction
(d) antigen-immune cells interaction

102. Match List-I with List-II.

	List-I		List-II
A.	Chlamydospores	1.	Formed in lower group of fungi of Phycomycetes
B.	Zoospores	2.	Non-motile structures
C.	Aplanospores	3.	Exogenous spores
D.	Conidia	4.	Resistant spores formed under unfavourable conditions

	A	B	C	D		A	B	C	D
(a)	1	2	3	4	(b)	4	3	2	1
(c)	1	2	4	3	(d)	4	1	2	3

103. Given below are two statements; one is labelled as Assertion (A) and the other one is labelled as Reason (R).

Assertion (A) Deoxyribonucleoside triphosphates serve dual purpose in replication process.

Reason (R) Deoxyribonucleoside triphosphates act as substrates and also provide energy for polymerisation

In the light of the above statements, choose the correct answer from the options given below.

(a) A is false, but R is true.
(b) Both A and R are true and R is the correct explanation of A.
(c) Both A and R are true, but R is not the correct explanation of A.
(d) A is true, but R is false.

104. Which of the following statements is incorrect about menopause?

(a) It is a phase in woman's life when ovulation comes to a halt
(b) Usually, menopause occurs at an age of 45-50 years
(c) Being physically active and exercising causes severe post menopause symptoms
(d) Menophase marks the end of a womans fertility

105. A plant hormone which allows the seeds to ignore environmental conditions and germinate is

(a) abscisic acid (b) ethylene
(c) cytokinin (d) gibberellins

106. Consider the following features.

I. Presence of pappus
II. Five fused petals
III. Showy flowering plants
IV. Monocarpellary ovary
V. Five fused sepals

How many of the above features describe (s) family-Compositae?

(a) 4 (b) 3
(c) 1 (d) 5

107. Which among the following statement(s) is/are correct regarding detritus food chain?

I. It begins from dead organic matter.
II. Energy comes from the primary producers.
III. It begins from the primary producers.
IV. Energy comes from sun.
V. This food chain helps in releasing inorganic nutrients.

Choose the correct answer from the options given below.

(a) I and V (b) only I
(c) only II (d) I, III and IV

108. Which part of the plant is best to study meiosis?

(a) Root apex (b) Shoot apex
(c) Growing embryo (d) Anther

109. The following hormones are released from the adenohypophysis, except

(a) adrenocorticotropic hormone
(b) growth hormone
(c) somatotropin hormone
(d) prolactin release inhibiting hormone

110. Match List I with List II.

List I		List II	
A.	Corticoids	1.	Glucagon
B.	Aldosterone	2.	Adrenal cortex
C.	α-cells	3.	Mineralocorticoid
D.	β-cells	4.	Insulin

Codes

	A	B	C	D
(a)	2	3	4	1
(b)	2	3	1	4
(c)	1	3	2	4
(d)	2	1	3	2

111. Given below are two statements.

Statement I Tracheid cells have more lignified and thick walls with wide lumen as compared to vessels.

Statement II Vessels are absent in pteridophytes and gymnosperms that's why these groups of plant have non-porous wood.

In the light of the above statements, choose the correct answer from the options below.

(a) Statement I is incorrect, but statement II is correct
(b) Both statement I and statement II are correct
(c) Both statement I and statement II are incorrect
(d) Statement I is correct, but statement II is incorrect

112. *Parthenium hysterophorus* and *Lantana camara* are examples of

(a) overexploitation
(b) alien species invasion
(c) coextinction
(d) habitat fragmentation

113. Name the leucocytes which are the largest in all types of leucocytes and constitute 2-10% of blood leucocytes.

(a) Neutrophils (b) N-K cells
(c) Monocytes (d) Lymphocyte

114. Which one of the following statements is true?

(a) In certain cases, multiple copies code for *r*RNA such a DNA is called *r*DNA
(b) Duplication of chromosomal segments has the potential to amplify the number of copies of individual genes
(c) Inheritance of a characters is affected by promoter and regulatory sequences of a structural gene
(d) All are true

115. Which of the following statements is incorrect with respect to the plant photosynthesis?

(a) Despite the presence of all other factors, the plant may not photosynthesise if the temperature is very low
(b) When the intensity of light is high, the rate of photosynthesis does not increase further
(c) In high temperature, C_4 plants show lower rate of photosynthesis
(d) Tropical plants have a higher temperature optimum than the plants adapted to temperate climates

116. A few epidermal cells in the vicinity of the guard cells become specialised in their shape and size. These enhance certain morphologies that affect gas exchange and are known as

(a) bulliform cells
(b) subsidiary cells
(c) epidermal cells
(d) stomatal pore

117. Given below are two statements.

Statement I The intercalated discs in cardiac muscles are meant for the transport of K^+ which maintain the rhythmicity in contraction.

Statement II Bones of old persons are brittle and undergo fracture more readily because they contain more organic matter.

In the light of the above statements, choose the correct answer from the options givens below.

(a) Statement I is incorrect, but statement II is correct
(b) Both statement I and statement II are correct
(c) Both statement I and statement II are incorrect
(d) Statement I is correct, but statement II is incorrect

118. The centre present in the pons region of the brain, which can moderate the functions of the respiratory rhythm centre is called

(a) chemosensitive area
(b) regulatory centre
(c) respiratory rhythm centre
(d) pneumotaxic centre

119. Given below are two statements.

Statement I *Pila* have amphibious type of respiration.
Statement II They have 8-shaped nervous system.
In the light of the above statements, choose the most appropriate answer form the options given below

(a) Statement I is incorrect, but statement II is correct
(b) Both statement I and statements II are correct
(c) Both statement I and statements II are incorrect
(d) Statement I is correct, but statement II is incorrect

120. Read the following statements with respect to the structure of collenchyma. Identify the incorrect statement.

I. Cell wall is made up of cellulose with localised thickenings of pectin and hemicellulose, lignin is absent.
II. Primary pits are present in those collenchyma cells where the walls are irregular/non uniform.
III. Protoplasm includes a very large central vacuole surrounded by a thin layer of cytoplasm.
IV. Nucleus is prominent, cell organelles are in functional state.
V. Cells are isodiametric, with intercellular spaces.

Choose the correct answer from the options given below.

(a) I, III and V (b) II and V
(c) III and IV (d) II, III and IV

121. The genotypes of a husband and wife are I^AI^B and I^Ai. Among the blood types of their children, how many different genotypes and phenotypes are possible?

(a) 3 genotypes; 3 phenotypes
(b) 3 genotypes; 4 phenotypes
(c) 4 genotypes; 3 phenotypes
(d) 4 genotypes; 4 phenotypes

122. The figure given below is a representation of member of a group of bacteria. Consider the figure and identify the incorrect statement w.r.t it.

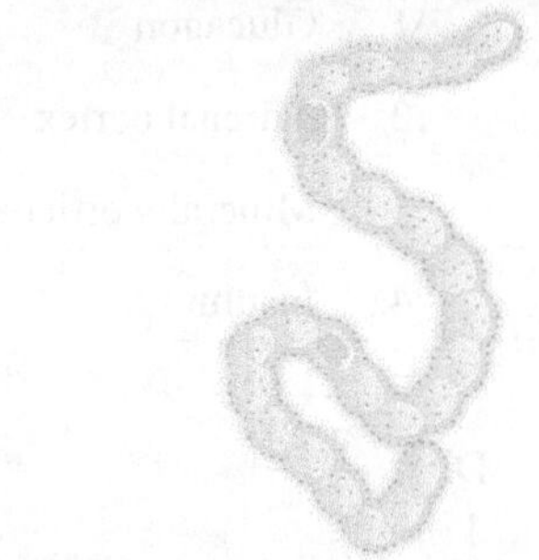

(a) Members of the group are called myxophyceae and perform oxygenic photosynthesis.
(b) These are predominantly freshwater forms with exception of few marine forms.
(c) They possess specialised, thick walled cells called heterocysts that aid in N_2 fixation.
(d) Photosynthetic pigments include chlorophyll-*a* carotenoids and C-phycocyanin

123. Which of the following is not true about transport of CO_2?

(a) CO_2 is carried by haemoglobin as carbaminohaemoglobin
(b) pCO_2 is high and pO_2 is low in the tissues
(c) In the tissues, pCO_2 is high and it diffuses into blood and forms CO_2 and H_2O
(d) Every 100 mL of deoxygenated blood delivers approximately 4 mL of CO_2 to the alveoli

124. Which of the following match pair is incorrect regarding the anatomy of frog?

(a) Brain box—cranium
(b) Forebrain—cerebellum
(c) Midbrain—optic lobes
(d) Hindbrain—medulla oblongata

125. Read the following statements about human evolution and identify the incorrect statements.

I. *Dryopithecus africanus* was discovered from Miocene rocks of Africa and Europe.
II. The fossils of *Ramapithecus* and *Homo habilis* were discovered in the pilocene rocks of Shivalik hills.
III. *Homo erectus* was 1.5 to 1.8 metre tall with brain size 900 cm^3 and had erect posture.

IV. Cro-Magnon man were the first to use skin clothing and practice of burning dead.

V. The fossil of *Homo erectus* was discovered in Java in 1891.

Choose the correct answer from the option.

(a) I and V (b) II and IV
(c) III and V (d) I and III

126. Consider the given floral formula.

$$\% \, ⚥ K_{(5)} C_{1+2+(2)} A_{(9)} +_{1} \underline{G}_{1}$$

Identify the correct feature of the family associated with the given formula.

(a) Monocarpellary ovary
(b) Monoadephous stamens
(c) Polysepalous condition
(d) Radial symmetry

127. Given below are two statements.

Statement I Respiratory roots help in the exchange of gases with the help of pneumatophores or lenticels.

Statement II Respiratory roots do not possess any definite organ for the exchange of gases.

In the light of the above statements, choose the correct answer from the options givens below.

(a) Statement I is incorrect, but statement II is correct
(b) Both statement I and statement II are correct
(c) Both statement I and statement II are incorrect
(d) Statement I is correct, but statement II is incorrect

128. Which of the following statements is incorrect?

(a) The Amazon rainforest is being cut and cleared for cultivating soybeans
(b) The degradation of many habitats by pollution also threatens the survival of many species
(c) Species extinctions like Stellar's sea cow and passenger pigeon were due to habitat loss
(d) Many marine fish populations are over harvested, endangering the continued existence of some commercially important species

129. High myoglobin content and intermediate glycolytic enzyme activity are the characteristics of which of the following?

(a) White fibres type of muscles
(b) Fast oxidative or aerobic muscles
(c) Cross-bridge structure
(d) None of the above

130. Given below are two statements; one is labelled as Assertion (A) and the other is labelled as Reason (R).

Assertion (A) Ion concentration is higher in the vacuole than in the cytoplasm of a plant cell.

Reason (R) Vacuole is important for osmoregulation and excretion.

In the light of the above statements, choose the correct answer from the options given below.

(a) A is false, but R is true
(b) Both A and R are true and R is the correct explanation of A.
(c) Both A and R are true, but R is not the correct explanation of A
(d) A is true, but R is false

131. Carboxylation is the most crucial step of the Calvin cycle, where CO_2 is utilised for the carboxylation of

(a) 3-PGA (b) RuBP
(c) Oxaloacetic acid (d) C_3 acid

132. Read the following statements about Anemophily.

I. Pollen grains are light, small and non-sticky.
II. Stamens are short and hidden inside the flowers.
III. Stigma are large and feathery to easily trap air borne pollen grains.
IV. These flowers often have a single ovule in each ovary and numerous flowers packed into an inflorescence.
V. It is a regular mode of gametes transport for the lower plant group such as algae, bryophytes and pteridophytes.

Choose the correct set of statements from the options given below.

(a) I, III and V (b) II, III and IV
(c) I, III and IV (d) II, III and V

133. One molecule of an enzyme is able to catalyse conversion of two molecules of substrate into products in 5 minutes. Ten molecules of enzymes and 25 molecules of substrate are mixed in a test tube. At the end of 10 min the test tube will have

(a) products only
(b) products and enzyme molecules
(c) products and 5 unreacted substrate molecules
(d) products, enzymes molecules and 5 molecules of substrate

134. Match List I with List II.

List I	List II
A. Haemopoiesis	1. Formation of RBCs
B. Cardiac output	2. Production of blood cells and platelets
C. Erythropoiesis	3. Ventricular depolarisation
D. QRS complex	4. Stroke volume × heart rate

Choose the correct answer form the options given below.

	A	B	C	D
(a)	2	4	1	3
(b)	1	3	2	4
(c)	3	2	4	1
(d)	4	1	3	2

135. Select the correct combination of the respiratory substrates and their respective RQs.

(a) Proteins-1. Fatty acid-0.9, Carbohydrates-0
(b) Proteins-0.7, Fatty acid-0, Carbohydrates-1
(c) Proteins-0.9, Fatty acid-0.7, Carbohydrates-1
(d) Proteins-0.7, Fatty acid-1, Carbohydrates-0.9

136. Read the following statements.

I. Habitat is the place or set of environmental conditions, in which a particular organism lives.
II. Habitat can have number of niches.
III. Niche have many species.
IV. Niche is profession of an organism.
V. Microhabitat is a small part of the habitats with its own characteristic and environmental features.

The incorrect statement is

(a) Only I
(b) Only II
(c) Only III
(d) Only IV

137. Fimbriae are membranous extensions present on the overall surface of a bacterium and more concentrated towards the poles.
If these extensions are removed which of the following is likely to happen?

(a) Bacteria could no longer swim
(b) Bacteria would change its shape
(c) Transport of material will be stopped
(d) Adherence to host tissue inhibited

138. Match List I with List II.

List I	List II
A. Spicules	1. Cnidaria
B. Hypostome	2. Ctenophora
C. Comb plates	3. Platyhelminthes
D. Hooks	4. Porifera

Codes

	A	B	C	D
(a)	2	3	1	4
(b)	2	1	4	3
(c)	1	3	2	4
(d)	4	1	2	3

139. In Hershey Chase experiment DNA as genetic material was concluded based on

(a) the presence of radioactivity in the bacteria when ^{35}S was used
(b) the presence of radicactivity in supernatant when $^{35}S$was used
(c) the presence of radioactivity in bacteria when ^{32}P was used
(d) the presence of radioactivity in supernatant when ^{32}P was used

140. After how many days the foetus develops the limbs and digits ?

(a) 30 days (b) 60 days
(c) 72 days (d) 25 days

141. Disruptive selection favors

(a) one extreme form of a trait
(b) intermediate form of a trait
(c) two extreme forms of trait
(d) no form of a trait

142. Identify the incorrect characteristic about TCA

(a) Consumption of ATP
(b) Cyclic pathway
(c) Occurs in mitochondrial matrix
(d) Complcte oxidation of acetyl Co-A

143. Given below are two statements.

Statement I Complex-IV refers to cytochrome-bc_1 complex.

Statement II Ubiquinone also receives reducing equivalents *via* $FADH_2$.

In the light of the above statements, choose the correct answer from the options given below.

(a) Statement I is incorrect, but statement II is correct
(b) Both statement I and statement II are correct
(c) Both statement I and statement II are incorrect
(d) Statement I is correct, but statement II is incorrect

144. The function of glycocalyx in bacteria is all, except

(a) protection from phagocytosis
(b) prevention of desiccation
(c) enable them to adhere to the surfaces
(d) facilitating cell movement

145. Given below are two statements; one is labelled as Assertion (A) and the other is labelled as Reason (R).

Assertion (A) Selectable markers can differentiate between the recombinant and non-recombinants by insertional inactivation.

Reason (R) Blue colour indicates the absence of chromogenic substrate.

In the light of the above statements, choose the correct answer from the options given below.

(a) A is false, but R is true
(b) Both A and R are true and R is the correct explanation of A.
(c) Both A and R are true, but R is not the correct explanation of A
(d) A is true, but R is false

146. Which one of the following is true for pest resistant plants ?

(a) *Bt* toxins are thousands of times more powerful
(b) These crops increase the use of chemical pesticides
(c) These plants contain *ds*RNA that initiate RNAi and silence the specific *m*RNA of pest
(d) These plants are more resistant to viral infection than bacterial

147. A zoologist studied the population of pigs in an abundant yard. He found that the average natality was 270, average mortality 240, immigration 20 and emigration 30. The net increase in population is

(a) 0 (b) 10
(c) 15 (d) 20

148. Which bacterium was the first to be used as biopesticide on the commercial scale in the world?

(a) *Bacillus thuringiensis*
(b) *Escherichia coli*
(c) *Pseudomonas aeruginosa*
(d) *Agrobacterium tumefaciens*

149. The given diagram shows mode of action of steroid hormone wherein the hormone receptor complex binds to specific regions on DNA called HRE to allow expression of certain genes.

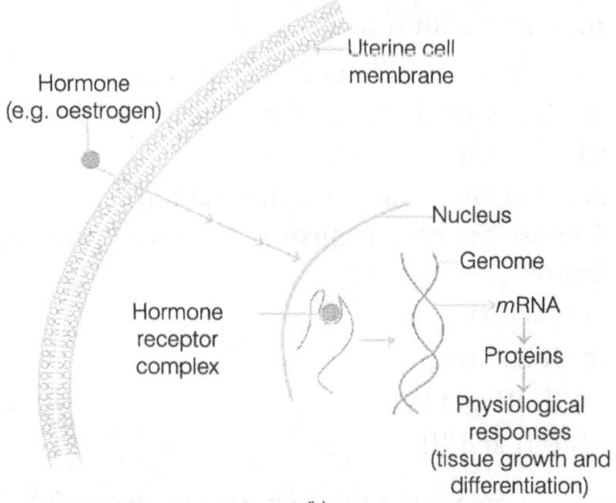

(b)

Failure of this binding will lead to

(a) easy diffusion of hormone
(b) normal synthesis of the protein
(c) no effect on metabolism
(d) failure of transcription

150. Which of the following organelles serves as a major packaging region for molecules distributed all over the cell?

(a) Vacuole
(b) Chloroplast
(c) Golgi complex
(d) Ribosome

151. Stem cuttings of grapes, sugarcane, etc. are dipped in which solution prior to being sowed?

(a) IBA
(b) GA_3
(c) ABA
(d) Ethylene

152. Anterior lobe of pituitary is concerned with production of ...*A*... and ...*B*....

Identify *A* and *B*.

	A	*B*
(a)	LH	Melatonin
(b)	FSH	LH
(c)	Oxytocin	MSH
(d)	MSH	FSH

153. Which of the following statement(s) is/are incorrect with respect to urine?

I. It is amber coloured watery fluid.
II. It is slightly basic with pH around 8.0.
III. It consists of 96% of urea.
IV. It is faintly aromatic in fresh form.

Choose the correct answer from the options given below.

(a) I and IV
(b) II and III
(c) II, III and IV
(d) I, II and III

154. Given below are two statements; one is labelled as Assertion (A) and the other is labelled as Reason (R).

Assertion (A) Amphibian have a common chamber called cloaca.

Reason (R) Alimentary canal, urinary and reproductive tracts open into the cloaca.

In the light of the above statements, choose the correct answer from the options given below.

(a) A is false, but R is true
(b) Both A and R are true and R is the correct explanation of A.
(c) Both A and R are true, but R is not the correct explanation of A
(d) A is true, but R is false

155. The two important types of secondary structures of proteins are

(a) motifs and domains
(b) α-helix, β-pleated sheet
(c) peptide bond, hydrogen bond
(d) *R* group, amino group

156. An otherwise tall plant when grown in a nutrient deficient soil, remained dwarf.

When this plant is made to cross with a dwarf variety. The resultant expected can be

(a) all hybrid dwarf plants
(b) all hybrid tall plants
(c) 50% tall and 50% dwarf progeny
(d) 75% tall and 25% dwarf progeny

157. Match List I with List II.

	List I		List II
A.	Family	1.	Poaceae
B.	Order	2.	Poales
C.	Class	3.	Monocotyledonae
D.	Division	4.	Angiospermae

	A	B	C	D
(a)	1	2	3	4
(b)	2	1	4	3
(c)	4	3	2	1
(d)	4	2	3	1

158. Given below are two statements.

Statement I Platelets also called thrombocytes, are cell fragments produced from megakaryocytes.

Statement II Platelets can release a variety of substances most of which are involved in the coagulation of blood.

In the light of the above statements, choose the correct answer from the options givens below.

(a) Statement I is incorrect, but statement II is correct
(b) Both statement I and statement II are correct
(c) Both statement I and statement II are incorrect
(d) Statement I is correct, but statement II is incorrect

159. Which of the following statement is not correct with respect to Down syndrome?

(a) It caused due to non-disjunction of chromosome number 21 during meiosis
(b) It is a monosomic condition
(c) Children with this syndrome have affectionate and loving nature.
(d) Individuals with this syndrome have a characteristic prominent epicanthic fold in each eye

160. Which of the following statements is incorrect?
(a) Non-albuminous seeds have no residual endosperm
(b) Groundnut is example of ex-albuminous seed
(c) Albuminous seeds retain a part of endosperm
(d) Pea is an example of albuminous seed

161. The common feature shared by guard cells and mesophyll cells is
(a) the presence of chloroplast
(b) dumb-bell shaped structure
(c) differentially thick cell wall
(d) Uniformly thick cell wall

162. An organism having cytoplasm, DNA and RNA, but no cell wall is
(a) Cyanobacterium
(b) Mycoplasma
(c) Bacterium
(d) Virus

163. Given below are two statements; one is labelled as Assertion (A) and other one is labelled Reason (R).
Assertion (A) Crossing over between the genes is directly proportional to distance
Reason (R) Greater distance between the genes reduces the possibility of linkage.
In the light of the above statements, choose the correct answer from the options given below.
(a) A is false, but R is true
(b) Both A and R are true and R is the correct explanation of A
(c) Both A and R are true, but R is not the correct explanation of A
(d) A is true, but R is false

164. Match List I with List II.

List I	List II
A. Cirrhosis	1. CNS stimulant
B. Cocaine	2. binds to receptors present on CNS
C. Opioids	3. α – interferons
D. Cancer	4. Liver disease

Choose the correct answers the options given below.

	A	B	C	D
(a)	4	2	3	1
(b)	4	1	3	2
(c)	3	4	1	2
(d)	4	1	2	3

165. Which of the following is incorrect in relation with the Human Genome Project (HGP)?
(a) Its aim was to map the whole human genome at the level of nucleotide sequences
(b) It was started in 1988 and completed in 2002
(c) Its aim included storing the information gathered from the project in databases and develop tools for data analysis
(d) Its aim was to solve any ethical, legal or social problems which may arise from the project

166. Match List I with List II.

List I	List II
A. RH Whittaker	1. Prions
B. MW Beijerinck	2. Viroids
C. TO Diener	3. *Contagium vivum fluidum*
D. Cr Jacob disease	4. Five kingdom classification

	A	B	C	D
(a)	4	3	2	1
(b)	2	1	4	3
(c)	3	4	2	1
(d)	4	3	1	2

167. Intron transcripts in heterogenous nuclear RNA (*hn*-RNA) are removed and exon transcripts are joined together under the direction of protein complexes. These complexes are
(a) Polysomes (b) Cdk complex
(c) Endopeptidases (d) Spliceosomes

168. Most of the members of .... have one or more storage bodies called pyrenoids that contain protein besides starch.
(a) Phaeophyceae (b) Liverworts
(c) Moss (d) Chlorophyceae

169. Read the following statements.
I. Secretions of epididymis, vas deferens and seminal vesicle are essential for sperm motility.
II. Spermatogonia present on the inside wall of semniferous tubule multiply mitotically.
III. A human male ejaculates about 50-100 million sperms during coitus.

IV. Androgens maintain or regulate the functioning of male sex accessory glands.
V. Sperm head contains haploid nucleus.

The incorrect statement is
(a) only I (b) only II
(c) only III (d) only IV

170. Control of gene expression in eukaryotes includes all of following given below, except
(a) methylation of DNA
(b) feedback inhibition of enzyme activity via allosteric modification
(c) transcription factors activity
(d) alternative splicing of RNA transcripts

171. The organism that are photosynthetic in the presence of sunlight, but behave like heterotrophs when deprived of sunlight is
(a) *Gonyaulax* (b) *Nostoc*
(c) *Euglena* (d) *Anabaena*

172. Identify the type of pistil in the diagram.

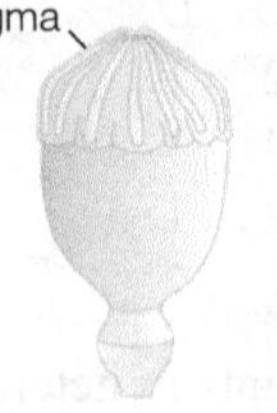

(a) Multicarpellary, apocarpous; *Papaver*
(b) Multicarpellary, syncarpous; *Papaver*
(c) Multicarpellary, pistillate, Brinjal
(d) Monocarpellary, apocarpous; Papaya

173. Which of the following statement is incorrect?
(a) Stem tendrils, which develop from axillary buds are slender
(b) Tendrils help plants to climb
(c) Thorns are found in plants like grapevine
(d) Thorns protect plants from browsing animals

174. Read the following statements and choose the correct ones about the mechanism of hormonal control.
I. Protein hormones like epinephrine require membrane bound receptors to bind to specific receptor sites.
II. Thyroid hormone does not require any receptor for binding with its target site.
III. The hormones behave as a second messenger in the cytoplasm.
IV. Steroid hormones such as testosterone enter the cytoplasm of target cell to produce effect.
V. Histamine is synthesised by the mast cell and basophils.

Choose the correct answer from the options given below.
(a) Only I (b) Only II
(c) I, IV and V (d) Only III

175. Restriction endonuclease binds to DNA and cuts two strands of double helix at specific points in their
(a) sugar-phosphate backbone
(b) hydrogen bond
(c) glycosidic bonds
(d) phosphodiester bond

176. Read the following statements.
I. The rate of biomass production is called productivity.
II. Catabolism leads to accumulation of a dark coloured amorphous substance.
III. Humification and mineralisation occur during decomposition in the soil.
IV. Primary productivity depends on the plant species inhabiting a particular area.
V. The consumers are represented by the fungi, bacteria and flagellates.

Choose the correct set of statement from the options given below.
(a) I and IV (b) I, III and IV
(c) III and V (d) II, IV and V

177. Match List I with List II.

	List I		List II
A.	Pigments	1.	Anthocyanins
B.	Terpenoids	2.	Diterpenes
C.	Alkaloids	3.	Codeine
D.	Lectins	4.	Concanavalin-A

Choose the correct answer from the options given below.

	A	B	C	D		A	B	C	D
(a)	1	2	3	4	(b)	2	3	4	1
(c)	3	1	2	4	(d)	4	1	2	3

178. Which of the following pairs of organisms got extinct due to over-exploitation?

(a) *Lantana* and *Eicchornia*
(b) Steller's sea cow and Passenger pigeon
(c) Bengal tiger and Dodo
(d) Red panda and Stellar sea cow

179. Which statement correctly defines the unipolar neuron ?

(a) Cell body with one dendrite
(b) Cell body with one axon
(c) Cell body with one axon and one dendrite
(d) Cell body with two axon

180. The outer layer of nuclear membrane is a part of

(a) mitochondrial membrane
(b) plasma membrane
(c) endoplasmic reticulum
(d) nucleoplasm

Explanations

Physics

1. (a) Moment of inertia of a cylinder about an axis passing through its centre and parallel to its length $= \dfrac{MR^2}{2}$.

Moment of inertia about its centre and perpendicular to its length

$$= M\left(\frac{L^2}{12} + \frac{R^2}{4}\right)$$

Equating both values, we get

$$\frac{MR^2}{2} = \frac{ML^2}{12} + \frac{MR^2}{4}$$

$$\Rightarrow \quad \frac{1}{4}R^2 = \frac{1}{12}L^2$$

$$\Rightarrow \quad \sqrt{3}R = L$$

$$\text{or} \quad L = \sqrt{3}R$$

2. (c) If I_0 is the intensity after closing one slit, then it satisfies

$$I_0 \propto a^2 \Rightarrow I_0 = ka^2$$

(where, a = amplitude of light wave)

When both slits open, then intensity

$$\therefore \quad I \propto (2a)^2 \propto 4a^2 \Rightarrow I = 4ka^2 \Rightarrow I = 4I_0$$

$$\therefore \quad I_0 = I/4$$

3. (c) Angular momentum,

$$L = \frac{nh}{2\pi} = \frac{3 \times 6.6 \times 10^{-34}}{2 \times 3.14}$$

$$= 3.15 \times 10^{-34} \text{ J-s}$$

4. (d) As, $I_f = \dfrac{\Delta V}{R} = \dfrac{5-(-3)}{800} = 10^{-2}\text{ A} = 10 \text{ mA}$

5. (a) Horizontal range, $R = \dfrac{u^2 \sin 2\theta}{g}$

where u is the velocity of projection and θ is the angle of projection.

Maximum height, $H = \dfrac{u^2 \sin^2\theta}{2g}$

According to question $R = H$

$$\frac{u^2 \sin 2\theta}{g} = \frac{u^2 \sin^2\theta}{2g}$$

$$\therefore \quad \tan\theta = 4$$

$$\Rightarrow \quad \theta = \tan^{-1}(4)$$

6. (a) Holes are majority carriers in p-type semiconductor and trivalent atoms are dopants. So, statement given in (a) is false.

7. (b) Kinetic energy,

$$K = eV = 1.6 \times 10^{-19} \times 2 = 3.2 \times 10^{-19} \text{ J}$$

8. (a) In a non-polar molecule, the centers of positive and negative charges coincide. So, net dipole moment comes to zero. Hence, non-polar molecules do not have permanent dipole moment.

9. (d) Since, $V = -L\left(\dfrac{di}{dt}\right)$

i.e., V is proportional to the slope of the i-t graph. The slope is constant and positive for the first half (0 to $T/2$) and negative for the second half ($T/2$ to T).

Thus, for the first half, V is negative and for the second half, it is positive.

10. (a) Energy stored per unit volume

$$= \frac{1}{2}Y\,(\text{strain})^2 = \frac{1}{2}Y\left(\frac{\Delta L}{L}\right)^2$$

Given, elongation strain = 2%

$$\Rightarrow \quad Y = \frac{1}{2} \times 5 \times 10^{10} \times \left(\frac{2L}{100\,L}\right)^2$$

$$= 10^7 \text{ Jm}^{-3}$$

11. (a) Given $E = 13.2$ keV

$$\lambda\,(\text{in Å}) = \frac{hc}{E\,(\text{eV})}$$

$$= \frac{12400}{13.2 \times 10^3} = 0.939\text{Å} \approx 1\text{Å}$$

X-rays covers wavelengths ranging from about 10^{-8} m (10 nm) to 10^{-13} m (10^{-4} nm).

An electromagnetic radiation of energy 13.2 keV belongs to X-ray region of electromagnetic spectrum.

12. (d) Fall in temperature of brass sphere,

$$\Delta T = 500 - 0 = 500^\circ \text{C}$$

Heat loss by sphere, $Q = ms\Delta T = 5 \times 500 \times 500$

$$= 1250 \text{ kJ}$$

Heat for melting m_2 kg of ice,

$$Q_2 = m_2 L = m_2 \times 336$$

From principle of calorimetry,

$$1250 = m_2 \times 336$$

$$m_2 = \frac{1250}{336} \text{ kg} = 3.72 \text{ kg}$$

13. (d) Heat produced in the resistor

$$= \text{Energy of capacitor} = \frac{1}{2}CV^2$$

$$= \frac{1}{2} \times 6 \times 10^{-6} \times 360 \times 360$$

$$= 0.39 \text{ J}$$

14. (d) All thermodynamic changes are zero.

15. (c) We know the relation of gravity, $g = \frac{GM}{R^2}$

$$\therefore \quad M = \frac{gR^2}{G} \quad \ldots\text{(i)}$$

Volume of the earth, $V = \frac{4}{3}\pi R^3$

Let, mean density of earth is d.

$$\Rightarrow \quad M = d \times V \quad \ldots\text{(ii)}$$

Solving Eqs. (i) and (ii), we get

$$\Rightarrow \quad d = \frac{3g}{4\pi RG}$$

16. (a) Induced emf is given by

$$E_{\text{ind}} = \frac{\Delta\phi}{\Delta t}$$

$$I = \frac{E}{R}$$

$$I = \frac{\Delta\phi}{R\,\Delta t}$$

Current, $I = \frac{Q}{\Delta t}$

$$\Rightarrow \quad Q = \frac{\Delta\phi}{R}$$

17. (c) We know that,

$$E = \frac{\Delta V}{l} = \frac{100}{1} = 100\,\text{Vm}^{-1}$$

$$\therefore \quad n = 8.5 \times 10^{28}\,\text{m}^{-3}$$

$$\therefore \quad v_d = \frac{I}{neA} = \frac{J}{en} = \frac{\sigma E}{en} \quad \left[\because J = \sigma E \text{ and } J = \frac{I}{A}\right]$$

$$= \frac{5.81 \times 10^7 \times 100}{1.6 \times 10^{-19} \times 8.5 \times 10^{28}}$$

$$\simeq 0.43\,\text{ms}^{-1}$$

18. (c) Speed of walking $= \frac{h}{t_1} = v_1$

Speed of escalator $= \frac{h}{t_2} = v_2$

Time taken when she walks over running escalator,

$$t = \frac{h}{v_1 + v_2}$$

$$\Rightarrow \quad \frac{1}{t} = \frac{v_1}{h} + \frac{v_2}{h}$$

$$= \frac{1}{t_1} + \frac{1}{t_2}$$

$$\Rightarrow \quad t = \frac{t_1 t_2}{t_1 + t_2}$$

19. (d) Using equation of motion,

$$s = ut + \frac{1}{2}gt^2$$

$$h = 0 + \frac{1}{2}gT^2$$

$$\Rightarrow \quad 2h = gT^2 \quad \ldots\text{(i)}$$

After $(T/3)$ s,

$$s = 0 + \frac{1}{2} \times g(T/3)^2 = \frac{gT^2}{18}$$

$$18s = gT^2 \quad \ldots\text{(ii)}$$

From Eqs. (i) and (ii), we get

$$18s = 2h$$

$$s = \left(\frac{h}{9}\right) \text{m from top}$$

Height from ground $= h - h/9 = \left(\frac{8h}{9}\right)$ m

20. (b) The wires ADC and ABC will have resistance 5 Ω each. These two are joined in parallel between A and C. The equivalent resistance R between A and C is given by

$$R = \frac{5\,\Omega \times 5\,\Omega}{5\,\Omega + 5\,\Omega} = 2.5\,\Omega$$

21. (b) As $\mathbf{F} = q(\mathbf{v} \times \mathbf{B}) \Rightarrow F = qvB\sin\theta$

At $\theta = 0°$, $F = 0$

At $\theta = 90°$, $F = qvB$

At $\theta = 180°$, $F = 0$

So, for non-zero force angle between **v** and **B** can have any value other than zero or 180°.

22. (d) We know that, velocity of EM wave is equal to $\frac{1}{\sqrt{\mu_0 \varepsilon_0}}$.

i.e., $c = \frac{1}{\sqrt{\mu_0 \varepsilon_0}}$

$$\Rightarrow \quad c^2 = \frac{1}{\mu_0 \varepsilon_0}$$

$$\Rightarrow \quad \mu_0 \varepsilon_0 = \frac{1}{c^2}$$

$$\Rightarrow \quad [\mu_0 \varepsilon_0] = \frac{1}{[c^2]}$$

$$= \frac{1}{[LT^{-1}]^2}$$

$$= [L^{-2}T^2]$$

23. (d) Here, diode D_3 is in reverse bias, so current flow is 0 A.

24. (d)

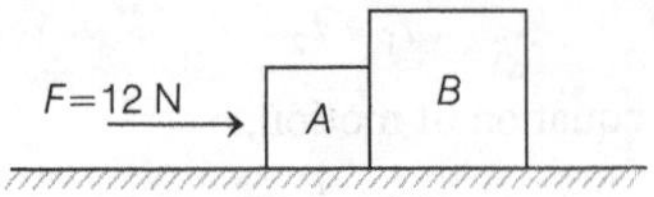

$$a = \frac{F}{M} = \frac{12}{8+4} = 1\,m/s^2$$

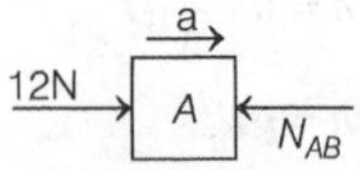

$\Rightarrow \quad 12 - N_{AB} = 4(1)$

$\Rightarrow \quad N_{AB} = 8N$

25. (c) Number of moles of the gas,

$$\mu = \frac{pV}{RT} = \frac{\text{Mass }(m)}{\text{Molar mass }(M_0)}$$

$$\therefore \quad \text{Density} = \frac{\text{mass }(m)}{\text{volume }(V)}$$

$$= \frac{(M_0)p}{RT} \quad \text{...(i)}$$

Since, number of moles, $\mu = \frac{m}{M_0} = \frac{N}{N_A}$ ... (ii)

where, $N =$ number of molecules

and $N_A =$ Avogadro's number.

Molar mass, $M_0 = N_A m$, for $N = 1$ [From Eq. (i)]

$$\therefore \text{ Density} = \frac{(mN_A)p}{RT} \quad \text{[from Eq. (i)]}$$

$$= \frac{pm}{KT} \quad [\because R = KN_A]$$

26. (b) Since, electric dipole has equal amount of positive and negative charges, therefore total outward flux is equal to total inward flux. Hence, net electric flux will be zero.

27. (b) Mass defect is given by

$$\Delta m = Zm_p + Nm_n - m(A, Z)$$

where, $m(A, Z)$ is the mass of the atom of mass number A and atomic number Z. Hence, the binding energy of nucleus is

$$BE = [Zm_p + Nm_n - m(A, Z)]c^2$$

$$BE = [Zm_p + (A - Z)m_n - m(A, Z)]c^2$$

28. (a) From the law of Malus, $I = I_0 \cos^2 30° = \frac{3}{4} I_0$

$\therefore$ Percentage of incident light transmitted

$$= \frac{I}{I_0} \times 100 = \frac{3}{4} \times 100 = 75\%$$

29. (a) Net magnetic flux through a closed surface enclosing a bar magnet is always zero.

30. (b) Velocities of the stones at some instant t can be given as

$$\mathbf{v}_1 = u_1 \cos\theta_1 \hat{\mathbf{i}} + (u_1 \sin\theta_1 - gt)\hat{\mathbf{j}}$$

and $\quad \mathbf{v}_2 = u_2 \cos\theta_2 \hat{\mathbf{i}} + (u_2 \sin\theta_2 - gt)\hat{\mathbf{j}}$

$\Rightarrow$ Relative velocity,

$$\mathbf{v}_1 - \mathbf{v}_2 = (u_1 \cos\theta_1 - u_2 \cos\theta_2)\hat{\mathbf{i}} + (u_1 \sin\theta_1 - u_2 \sin\theta_2)\hat{\mathbf{j}}$$

$$= \text{constant}$$

Since, their relative velocity is constant.

So, the trajectory of path followed by one as seen by other will be straight line, making a constant angle with horizontal.

31. (a) Weight of body in air = 30 N

Weight of body in water = 26 N

Loss in weigh of body = 30 − 26 = 4 N

$$\text{Relative density} = \frac{\text{Weight of body in air}}{\text{Loss in weight of body}}$$

$$= \frac{30}{4} = 7.5$$

32. (b) Given power, $P = 1\,W$

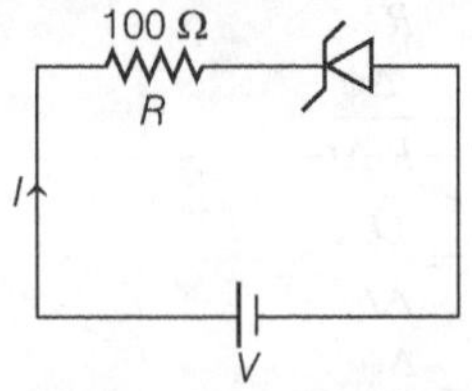

Potential drop across zener diode,

$$V_Z = V - IR = V - 100I$$

Power, $P = V_Z I_Z = (V - 100I)I$

$\therefore (V - 100I)I = 1$

or $100I^2 - VI + 1 = 0$

For I to be real, $V^2 - 4 \times 100 \times 1 \geq 0$ or $V \geq 20\,V$

33. (a) The maximum acceleration for SHM is given by

$$a_{max} = \omega^2 A = (2\pi\nu)^2 A = 4\pi^2\nu^2 A$$

The block will remain in contact with the piston, if

$$a_{max} \leq g \text{ or } 4\pi^2\nu^2 A \leq g$$

$\therefore$ Maximum amplitude of piston will be

$$A_{max} = \frac{g}{4\pi^2\nu^2} = \frac{9.8}{4\pi^2(0.5)^2}$$

$$= 0.99\,m$$

34. (a) Given, frequency of third harmonic = 100 Hz

Fundamental frequency of the open pipe

$$\therefore \quad \frac{3v}{4l} = 100 + \frac{v}{2l}$$

$\Rightarrow \quad \frac{v}{4l} = 100$

Fundamental frequency of the open pipe,

$$f = \frac{v}{2l} = 200\,\text{Hz}$$

35. (a) Given, $A = 60°, \delta_m = 30°$
According to prism formula,

$$\mu = \frac{\sin\left(\frac{A + \delta_m}{2}\right)}{\sin\left(\frac{A}{2}\right)}$$

$$\mu = \frac{\sin\left(\frac{60° + 30°}{2}\right)}{\sin \frac{60°}{2}} = \frac{\sin 45°}{\sin 30°}$$

or $\quad \mu = \sqrt{2}$

$\therefore \quad \mu = \frac{\text{Speed of light in air } (c)}{\text{Speed of light in prism } (v)}$

$$v = \frac{c}{\mu} = \frac{3\times10^8}{\sqrt{2}} = \frac{3}{\sqrt{2}}\times10^8\,\text{m/s}$$

36. (c) The nuclear reaction is $2\,{}_1H^2 \rightarrow {}_2He^4$

As we know that,
Energy released = Binding energy of products − Binding energy of reactants
and total binding energy = number of nucleons × binding energy per nucleon

$\therefore$ Energy released $= 4\times7 - 2\times2\times1.1 = 28 - 4.4 = 23.6\,\text{MeV}$

37. (d) Given, square wire of side = 2 cm,
$u = -20\,\text{cm}, f = -10\,\text{cm}$

$\therefore \quad \frac{1}{v} + \frac{1}{u} = \frac{1}{f}$

$\Rightarrow \quad \frac{1}{v} + \frac{1}{(-20)} = \frac{1}{-10}$

$\Rightarrow \quad \frac{1}{v} = -\frac{1}{10} + \frac{1}{20}$

$\Rightarrow \quad v = -20\,\text{cm}$

We know that, $m = -\frac{v}{u} = \frac{-(-20)}{-20} = -1$

$\because \quad \frac{\text{Area of image}}{\text{Area of object}} = m^2$

$\Rightarrow \quad \frac{A_i}{A_o} = (-1)^2$

$$A_o = a^2 = 2\times2 = 4\,\text{cm}^2$$

$$\frac{A_i}{4} = 1$$

$\Rightarrow \quad A_i = 4\,\text{cm}^2$

Problem Solving Tactics The magnification of a concave mirror is mainly negative because it forms real and inverted image except one case (i.e between F and P) and according to sign convention rule, the distance of object and image always measured from pole.

38. (a) Statement B is incorrect because there is no effect of intensity on stopping potential.

Statement C is incorrect because the kinetic energy of photoelectrons does not depend upon intensity of incident light.

39. (b) Eddy currents are produced in any metallic conductor when magnetic flux around it is changed. Eddy currents are undesirable which heat up the core of a transformer and dissipate electrical energy in the form of heat.

40. (a) We know that, $P = I^2R$

$\Rightarrow \quad 4.4 = (2\times10^{-3})^2 R$

$\Rightarrow \quad 4.4 = 4\times10^{-6} R$

$\Rightarrow \quad R = 1.1\times10^{6}\,\Omega$

$\therefore \quad P' = \frac{V^2}{R}$

$$P' = \frac{11^2}{R} = \frac{11^2}{11}\times10^{-6}$$

$$= 11\times10^{-5}\,\text{W}$$

41. (c) Given, relative error in mass,

$$\frac{\Delta m}{m}\times100 = 6\%$$

Percentage error in diameter,

$$\frac{\Delta d}{d}\times100 = 1.5\%$$

Density of sphere, $\rho = \frac{\text{Mass}}{\text{Volume}}$

$$= \frac{m}{\frac{4}{3}\pi r^3} = \frac{m}{\frac{4}{3}\pi\left(\frac{d}{2}\right)^3}$$

$\Rightarrow \quad \rho = \frac{6}{\pi} md^{-3}$

$\Rightarrow \quad \rho \propto md^{-3}$

For maximum error in density,

$$\frac{\Delta\rho}{\rho}\times100 = \left(\frac{\Delta m}{m} + 3\times\frac{\Delta d}{d}\right)\times100$$

$$= 6\% + 3\times1.5\% = 10.5\%$$

$$= \frac{1050}{100}\%$$

$$= \frac{x}{100}\% \quad \text{(given)}$$

$$\therefore \quad x = 1050$$

42. (d) Total gravitational potential at point O due to each of mass 1 kg,

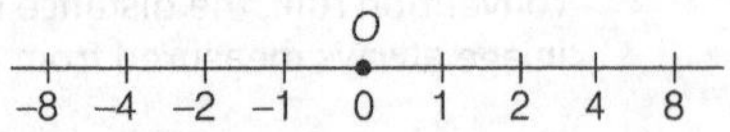

$$V = 2\left[-\frac{G\times 1}{1} - \frac{G\times 1}{2} - \frac{G\times 1}{4} - \frac{G\times 1}{8} \cdots\right]$$

$$= -2G\left[1 + \frac{1}{2} + \frac{1}{2^2} + \frac{1}{2^3} + \ldots\right]$$

$$= -2G\left[\frac{1}{\left(1-\frac{1}{2}\right)}\right] = -4G$$

Magnitude of $V = 4G$

43. (b) Given, $E = E_0 \sin(kx - \omega t)$ and
$B = B_0 \sin(kx - \omega t)$

Relation between E_0 and B_0 is

$$E_0 = cB_0 \quad \ldots\text{(i)}$$

Velocity of light $(c) = \nu\lambda = \frac{\omega}{2\pi}\lambda = \frac{\omega}{k}$ (where $k = \frac{2\pi}{\lambda}$)

Substituting this value of c in Eq. (i), we get

$$E_0 = \frac{\omega}{k}B_0 \text{ or } E_0 k = B_0 \omega$$

44. (b) Velocity of electron in nth orbit, $v_n \propto \frac{1}{n}$

First excited state corresponds to $n = 2$ and ground state corresponds to $n = 1$,

$$\frac{v_2}{v_1} = \frac{1}{2} \Rightarrow v_2 = \frac{v_1}{2}$$

$\therefore$ Change in velocity, $\Delta v = v_1 - v_2 = \frac{v_1}{2}$ i.e. 50%.

45. (c) According to Einstein's photoelectric equation, kinetic energy of photoelectron,

$$KE = h\nu - W_0 = eV_0$$
$$h\nu = eV_0 + W_0$$
$$= 5\text{eV} + 6.1\text{ eV} = 11.1\text{eV}$$

So, $$\lambda = \frac{1250 \text{ eV-nm}}{11.1\text{eV}} = 112.6\text{nm}$$

X-rays covers wavelengths ranging from about 10^{-8} m to 10^{-13} m.

$\therefore$ Wavelength lies in X-ray region.

Chemistry

46. (b) The correct graph regarding photoelectric effect is

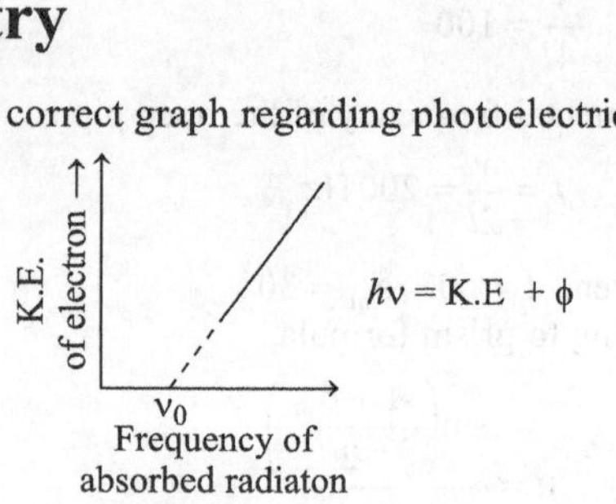

47. (c) The equilibrium is affected when the pressure is constant and the value of $\Delta n_g \neq 0$.

48. (a) Let A denotes benzene and B denotes toluene
In 1 : 1 molar mixture of A and B,
Mole fraction of A and B are

$$x_A = \frac{1}{2}, x_B = \frac{1}{2}$$

Vapour pressure of $A = p^{\circ}_A x_A = 12.8 \times \frac{1}{2} = 6.4$ kPa

Vapour pressure of $B = p^{\circ}_B x_B = 3.85 \times \frac{1}{2} = 1.925$ kPa

Thus, vapour will contain high percentage of benzene than toluene.

49. (b) Both (A) and (R) are true and (R) is correct explanation of (A). Although H^+ ions are discharged in preference to Na^+ ions normally but at mercury electrode, sodium ions are discharged first due to formation of amalgam. Hence, nature of cathode can affect the order of discharge of ions.

50. (a) For basic amino acids

$$\text{P.I} = \frac{pK_{a_2} + pK_{a_3}}{2}$$

$$= \frac{8.95 + 10.79}{2}$$

$$= \frac{19.74}{2} = 9.87$$

So, option (a) is correct.

51. (a) The given reaction is an example of disproportionation reaction. In this reaction, chlorine is oxidised as well as reduced.

The oxidation states of chlorine in $ClO^-(aq)$, $ClO_3^-(aq)$ and Cl^- are + 1, + 5 and – 1 respectively.

Hence, (A) is false but (R) is true.

Problem Solving Tactics	Disproportionation reaction is a redox reaction in which an element is oxidised as well as reduced in the same reaction.

52. (a)

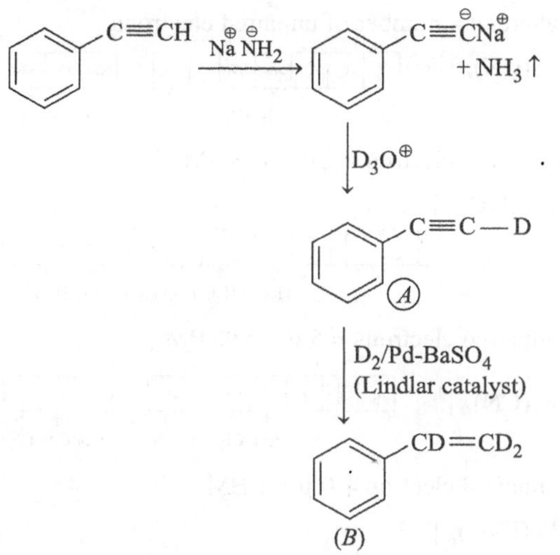

53. (a) In acidic medium the reaction for $KMnO_4$ is

$$\underset{+7}{Mn}O_4^- + 8H^+ + 5e^- \longrightarrow \underset{+2}{Mn}^{2+} + 4H_2O$$

Change in oxidation state = 7 − 2 = 5

54. (a) Starch is also known as amylum which occurs in all green plants. A molecule of starch $(C_6H_{10}O_5)_n$ is built of a large number of α-glucose ring joined through oxygen-atom.

55. (b) Among the given test only one i.e (B) carbylamine test is not given by phenols because carbylamine test is given by primary amines.

56. (b) On the basis of extent of overlapping, greater the area of overlapping greater is the strength of bond. Since, the area of overlapping is greatest in case of *p*-*p*-bond due to its dumb bell shape followed by *s*-*p* and then *s*-*s*. Hence, bond strength decreases in the order

$p—p > s—p > s—s$. So, the correct option is (b) $2p—2p > 2s—2p > 2s—2s$.

57. (c) $\Delta T_b = K_b \times m$

$$= 0.5 \times \left[\frac{n_A}{W_A}\right] = 0.5 \times \frac{0.05}{0.25}$$

$$\Delta T_b = 0.1\text{K}$$

58. (b) The correct order of boiling point is

$$H_2O > HF > NH_3 > CH_4.$$

59. (a) Only primary amines show carbylamine test whereas secondary and tertiary amines fail to undergo the carbylamine test. Since, primary amines need more amount of heat to break these hydrogen bonds, it have higher boiling points.

Therefore, primary amines have a higher boiling point than tertiary amines.

60. (b) Basic character of oxides decreases with increase in atomic number. So, the correct basicity order will be TiO > VO > CrO > FeO.

61. (a) de-Broglie wavelength of electron,

$$\lambda = \frac{h}{mv} = \frac{h}{\sqrt{2eVm}} \qquad \left(\because eV = \frac{1}{2}mv^2\right)$$

$$= \frac{6.626 \times 10^{-34}}{\sqrt{2 \times 1.6 \times 10^{-19} \times V \times 9.1 \times 10^{-31}}}$$

$$= \frac{6.626 \times 10^{-34}}{5.396 \times 10^{-25}\,[V]^{1/2}}$$

$$= \frac{1.227 \times 10^{-9}}{[V]^{1/2}}\text{ m}$$

$$= \frac{12.27 \times 10^{-10}}{[V]^{1/2}}\text{ m}$$

$$= \frac{12.27}{[V]^{1/2}}\text{Å} \approx \left[\frac{150}{V}\right]^{1/2}\text{Å}$$

62. (c) $XeF_6 + 3H_2O \longrightarrow \underset{(X)}{XeO_3} + 6HF$

XeO_3 is a colourless explosive solid and has a pyramidal molecular structure.

63. (b) For production of 180 g of glucose; heat energy is required = x kcal mol^{-1}

Number of moles of glucose to be produced $= \dfrac{1.6}{180}$

$$-0.64 = \frac{x}{180} \times 1.6$$

$$x = \frac{-0.64 \times 180}{1.60} \Rightarrow -72\text{ kcal mol}^{-1}$$

64. (d) Peroxide will oxidise Fe^{2+} to Fe^{3+} which gives a blood red colour with KCNS.

$$O_2^{2-} + 2Fe^{2+} + 4H^+ \longrightarrow 2Fe^{3+} + 2H_2O$$

$$Fe^{3+} + 3CNS^- \longrightarrow \underset{\text{(Blood red colour)}}{Fe(CNS)_3}$$

65. (c) The reaction occurring in two steps has two activation energy peaks.

The first step being fast needs less activation energy. The second step being slow, needs more activation energy.

Therefore, second peak will be higher than the first. Hence, graph (c) is correct.

66. (a) The structure of *meso*-2, 3-butanediol is

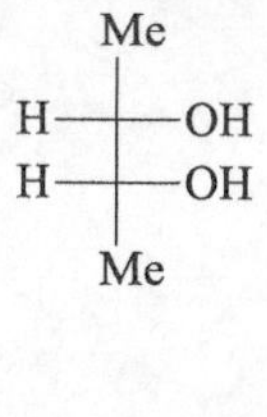

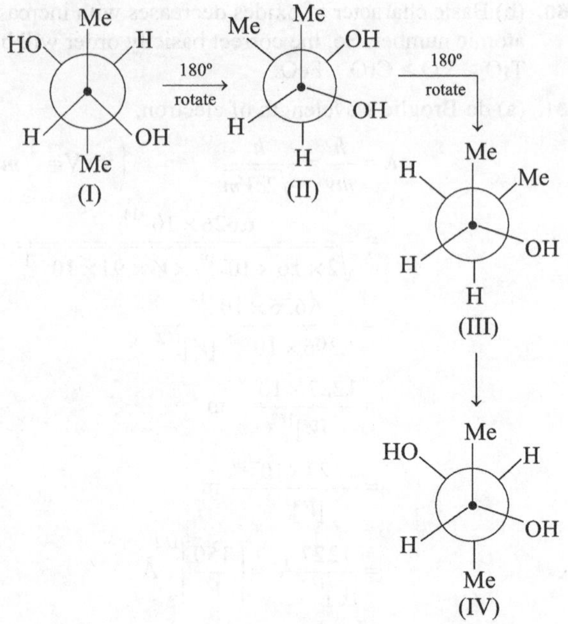

Hence, among the given structures only I and IV are Newmann projections of meso-2, 3-butanedial.

67. (b) First methyl bromide reacts with magnesium in the presence of dry ether to form Grignard reagent which further reacts with ethyl phenyl ketone to give 2-phenyl butan-2-ol.

$$CH_3Br + Mg \xrightarrow{Et_2O} CH_3MgBr \xrightarrow[H^+]{C_6H_5COCH_2CH_3} C_6H_5-\underset{CH_3}{\overset{OH}{C}}-CH_2CH_3$$

2-phenyl-butan-2-ol

68. (a) 3-chlorocyclopentene reacts with $AgNO_2$ to form 3-nitrocyclopentene.

69. (b)Benzene reacts with chlorine molecules in presence of ultraviolet light and give a compound gammexane (benzene hexachloride) which acts as an insecticide.

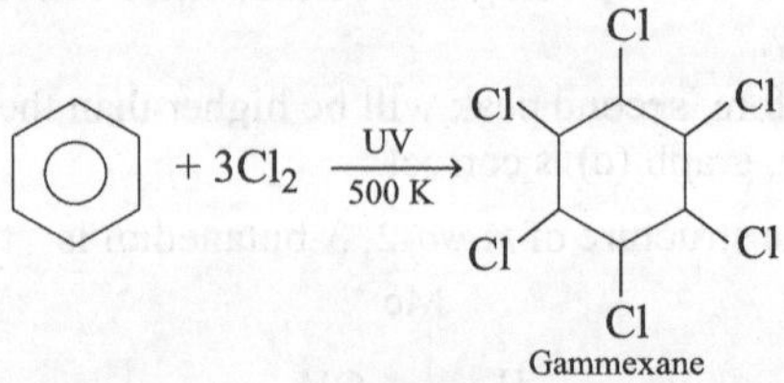

Gammexane
(*A*)

70. (d) Magnetic moment, $\mu = \sqrt{n(n+2)}$

where, n = number of unpaired electrons.

$[Fe(CN)_6]^{3-}$;

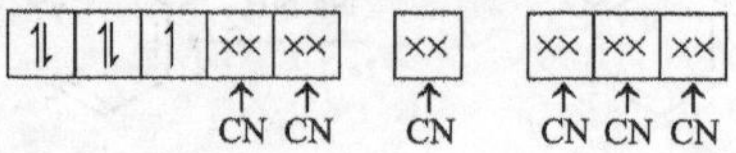

Unpaired electron = 1, μ = 1.73 BM

$[Fe(H_2O)_6]^{3+}$;

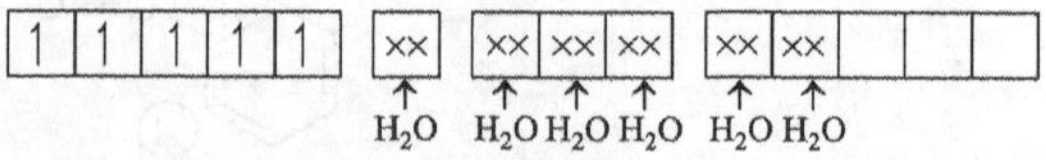

Unpaired electrons = 5, μ = 5.92 BM

$[Fe(CN)_6]^{4-}$;

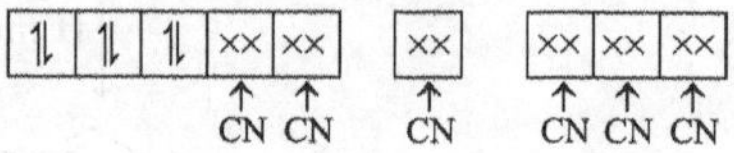

Unpaired electron = 0, μ = 0 BM

$[Fe(H_2O)_6]^{2+}$,

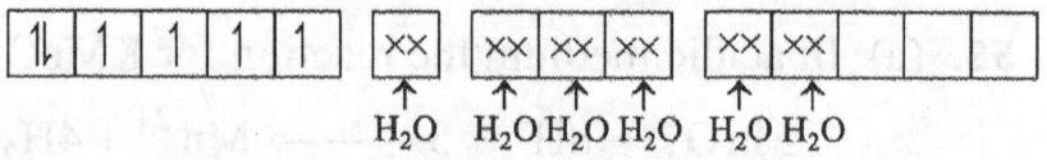

Unpaired electrons = 4, μ = 4.90 BM

71. (d) Primary, secondary and tertiary alcohols can be differentiated by their reaction with (HCl + anhy. $ZnCl_2$) Lucas reagent.

In the presence of Lucas reagent 3° alcohol produces immediate turbidity at room temperature 2° alcohol produces turbidity after 5 minutes at room temperature while 1° alcohol do not gives turbidity at room temperature. Hence, Statement I is true while Statement II is false.

72. (d) Moles of HCl reacting with ammonia

= (moles of HCl absorbed) − (moles of NaOH solution required)

$= (20 \times 0.1 \times 10^{-3}) - (15 \times 0.1 \times 10^{-3})$

$= 0.5 \times 10^{-3}$ = Moles of NH_3 released.

∴ Weight of nitrogen in organic compound

$= 0.5 \times 10^{-3} \times 14 = 7 \times 10^{-3}$ g

$$\% \text{ of } N = \frac{7 \times 10^{-3}}{29.5 \times 10^{-3}} \times 100 = 23.7\%$$

73. (c) The correct match is A-(iii), B-(i), C-(iv), D-(ii).

Diamond $\rightarrow sp^3$

Graphite $\rightarrow sp^2$

Producer gas $\rightarrow CO + N_2$

Water gas $\rightarrow CO + H_2$

74. (a) A. $CH_3(CH_2)_3OH \xrightarrow[H_2SO_4(\Delta)]{NaBr} CH_3(CH_2)_3Br$

B. $(CH_3)_3C{-}OH \xrightarrow[\text{Room temp.}]{\text{Conc. HCl}} (CH_3)_3C{-}Cl$

C. $CH_3CH(OH)(CH_2)CH_3 \xrightarrow{PBr_3} H_3CCH(Br)CH_2CH_3$

D. $CH_3—CH_2—CH_2—OH \xrightarrow{SOCl_2} CH_3—CH_2—CH_2—Cl$

75. (a) S_N1 = Unimolecular nucleophilic substitution reaction.

In S_N1 mechanism, retention of configuration will be observed.

The first step is dissociation into an intimate ion pair.

Mechanism

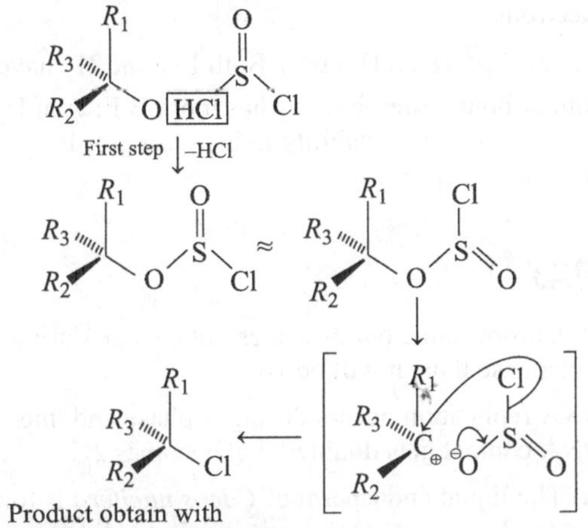

Product obtain with retention in configuration

76. (b) The boiling points of aldehydes and ketones are higher than hydrocarbons and ethers of comparable molecular masses. It is due to weak molecular association in aldehydes and ketones arising out of the dipole-dipole interactions.

Hence, Statements I and II both are true.

77. (b) Among the given species, CH_3OH being neutral will have least nucleophilicity. In species I and IV the (– ve) charge is involved in delocalisation hence, the nucleophilicity would be less than III.

The correct order is : III > I > IV > II.

78. (b) Diamond is a non-conductor while graphite is a conductor. Both have giant structure. Diamond has tetrahedral structure while graphite has layered structure.

79. (a) A. Thorium (90) = $5f^0\,6d^2\,7s^2$

B. Americium (95) = $5f^7\,6d^0\,7s^2$

C. Lanthanum (57) = $4f^0\,5d^1\,6s^2$

D. Chromium (24) = $3d^5\,4s^1$

Hence, the correct match is A-(iii), B-(iv), C-(i), D-(ii).

80. (b) Both Statement I and Statement II are true.

81. (d) For first order reaction,

$$\text{rate} = k[N_2O_5]$$

$$2.40\times10^{-5} = 3.0\times10^{-5}[N_2O_5]$$

$$\therefore\quad [N_2O_5] = 0.8$$

82. (c) Half-cell reactions are

(i) At cathode,

$$Fe^{2+} + 2e^- \longrightarrow Fe;\ E^\circ_{Fe^{2+}/Fe} = -0.44\ V$$

(ii) At anode,

$$Sn \longrightarrow Sn^{2+} + 2e^-;\ E^\circ_{Sn^{2+}/Sn} = -0.14\ V$$

$$E^\circ_{cell} = E^\circ_{Fe^{2+}/Fe} - E^\circ_{Sn^{2+}/Sn}$$

$$= -0.44 + 0.14$$

$$= -0.30\ V$$

83. (c) Acetophenone 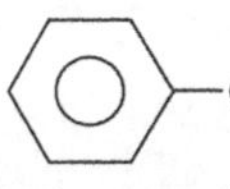 $—COCH_3$ undergoes usual electrophilic substitution reaction and also gives positive iodoform test with iodine and alkali.

Also benzoic acid reacts with $Br_2/FeBr_3$ to give *m*-bromobenzoic acids.

84. (c) For reaction,

$$Na_2CO_3\cdot xH_2O + 2HCl \longrightarrow 2NaCl + CO_2 + (x+1)H_2O$$

$$N_1V_1 = N_2V_2$$

$$n_1M_1V_1 = n_2M_2V_2$$

where, M_1 = molarity of $NaCO_3\cdot xH_2O$

V_1 = volume of $Na_2CO_3\cdot xH_2O$ solution

M_2 = molarity of HCl

V_2 = volume of HCl

n_1 and n_2 are acidity and basicity of Na_2CO_3 and HCl respectively.

$$2\times M_1\times 20 = 1\times\frac{1}{10}\times 19.8$$

$$M_1 = \frac{1}{10}\times 19.8\times\frac{1}{2}\times\frac{1}{20}$$

$$M_1 = 0.0495\ M$$

Now, strength = molar mass × molarity

$$7 = \text{Molar mass of } Na_2CO_3\cdot xH_2O \times 0.0495$$

Molar mass of $Na_2CO_3\cdot xH_2O$

$$= \frac{7}{0.0495} = 141.4\ g/mol$$

But molar mass of $Na_2CO_3\cdot xH_2O$

= Mass of anhydrous Na_2CO_3 + Mass of xH_2O

= 106 + 18*x* molecule

Therefore, $106 + 18x = 141.4$ g/mol

So, $x = 1.966$

Hence, $x \approx 2.0$

85. (c) We know that, $K_p = K_C (RT)^{\Delta n_g}$

$\Delta n_g = 2 - 4 = -2$

$K_p = 0.50(RT)^{-2} = 0.50\,(0.082 \times 673)^{-2} = 1.64 \times 10^{-4}$

86. (c) Cyclohexanone undergoes aldol condensation on reaction with OH^- followed by heating.

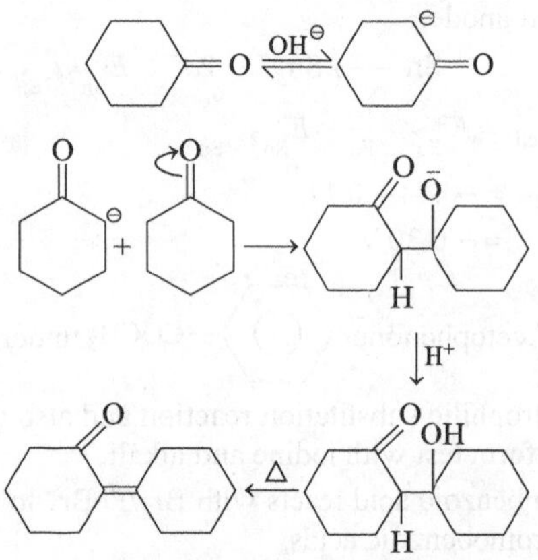

Problem Solving Tactics Condensation between two molecules of an aldehyde or ketone to form a β-hydroxy aldehyde or β-hydroxy ketone is called aldol condensation. The requirement for this reaction is atleast one α-H atom present in carbonyl compound.

87. (d) All the given statements are correct except (d). Quaternary ammonium hydroxide on heating strongly decomposes to yield water, a tertiary amine and alkene.

$$[(CH_3)_3N^{\oplus}CH_2CH_3]OH^{\ominus} \xrightarrow{\Delta} (CH_3)_3N + CH_2{=}CH_2 + H_2O$$

This method proceeds *via* E2-elimination in which the hydroxide ion functions as the base.

Elimination in alkyl-trimethyl ammonium hydroxide proceeds in the direction that gives the less substituted alkene.

88. (b) A-IV, B-II, C-I, D-III

- Xenon has a comparable I.E. as O_2.
- Argon provides inert atmosphere in metallurgy.
- Helium is utilised in the field of cryogenics.
- Neon gas produces red-orange colour so, it can glow in dark situation too. Hence, used is advertising sign.

89. (a) Statement I is false as with atomic number 17 the element has tendency to gain one electron to complete its octet. So, the most probable oxidation number is −1.
Statement II is true. Since, halogen elements are short of one electron in their valence shell, so they have the tendency to gain electron.

90. (b) In N_2, there is a triple bond while in O_2, there is a double bond and the atoms of Li_2 and H_2 are connected by a single bond. The bond energy will increase as the number of bonds between atoms increases.
So, bond energy of N_2 and O_2 will be more than Li_2 and H_2. Between Li_2 and H_2, Li_2 has more bonding electrons $(1s^2 2s^2 2p^2)$ than H_2 $(1s^2)$. Both Li_2 and H_2 have similar bond order, but Li_2 has more B.E. than H_2.
Thus, the order of stability in increasing order is $H_2 < Li_2 < O_2 < N_2$.

Biology

91. (c) Chromosome number does not change during metaphase thus, it will be 16.

DNA replication occurs during S-phase and thus the DNA content gets doubled, i.e. becomes 2C.

92. (a) The liquid endosperm of *Cocos nucifera* is formed due to absence of cytokinesis in mitotic division.

93. (a) Crown gall disease in plants is caused by (Ti) tumour inducing plasmid. Crown gall bacterium, *Agrobacterium tumefaciens* enters the plant through a wound.

It then inserts a portion of its own DNA into the DNA of the plant.

Crown gall is especially interesting because it results from nature's own genetic engineering.

94. (d) The separated bands of DNA are cut out from the agarose gel and extracted from the gel piece. This step is called elution.

The purified DNA fragments are then used in construction of *r*DNA.

95. (c) PCR, involves three steps namely denaturation annealing and polymerisation.

During annealing primers are paired to *ss*DNA. These primers are extended into complete DNA strand during polymerisation or extension.

96. (c) Lippes loop is an Intra Uterine Device (IUD). It increases the phagocytosis of the sperm within the uterus. It is made of plastic in a double S-shape and can be inserted for long periods.

97. (d) The Golgi apparatus plays a major role in post translational modification of proteins and glycosylation, of lipids. It was first reported by Camillo Golgi in 1898.

98. (c) Both A and R are true, but R is not the correct explanation of A.

The three steps in the decomposition, i.e. fragmentation, leaching and catabolism operate on the detritus simultaneously.

Humification and mineralisation occur during decomposition in the soil.

99. (b) Match pair in option (b) is incorrect and can be corrected as

Endoparasites are parasites, which live within the host's body as in the digestive tract, body cavities, various organs, or blood or other tissues of the host. e.g., *Plasmodium malariae*.

Rat flea is an ectoparasite. These are the parasites, which live on the outside of host body.

100. (d) Statement I is correct, but statement II is incorrect. It can be corrected as

The secondary oocyte forms a new membrane called zona pellucida surrounding it.

101. (b) ELISA is based on the principle of antigen-antibody interaction. In this, infection by a pathogen can be detected by the presence of antigens or by detecting antibodies synthesised against pathogen.

102. (d) The correct matches are A-4, B-1, C-2, D-3.

- Chlamydospores are resistant spores formed under unfavourable conditions.
- Zoospores are motile, flagellated formed in lower group of fungi of Phycomycetes.
- Aplanospores are non-motile structures formed in certain fungi.
- Conidia are exogenous spores.

103. (b) Both A and R are true and R is the correct explanation of A. Deoxyribonucleoside triphosphates serve dual purpose in replication process. In addition to acting as substrates they provide energy for polymerisation reaction.

104. (c) The incorrect statement is represented by option (c) Menopause is a phase in woman's life wherein ovulation and menstruation stop. It generally occurs between 45-50 years of age, thus marking the end of fertility period. However, physical exercise tend to relieve from post menopause symptoms.

105. (d) Gibberellins break the dormancy of seeds due to environmental conditions and promote germination. Seed dormancy arises in the seeds to overcome the unfavourable conditions for seedling and germination.

106. (b) Members of the family-Asteraceae or compositae are plants with showy flowers.
Instead of sepals these have thread like hairy structures called pappus. Petals are 5 in number in fused condition.

107. (a) The statements I and V are correct regarding detritus food chain.

The series of organisms eating one and being eaten by the other is called the food chain.

The detritus food chain begins from dead organic matter. It is made up of decomposers.

It helps in releasing inorganic nutrients.

108. (d) Anther is the best part of the plant to study meiosis since pollen grains are produced by meiotic division. Rest show mitosis.

109. (d) Prolactin release inhibiting hormone is a polypeptide hormone produced in the hypothalamus.

Growth or somatotropin hormone and adrenocorticotropic hormone are secreted by adenohypophysis.

110. (b) The correct matches are A-2, B-3, C-1, D-4.

- The adrenal cortex secretes many hormones commonly called as corticoids.
- Aldosterone is the main mineralocorticoid in our body.
- The two main types of cells in the islets of Langerhans are called α-cells and β-cells. The α-cells, secrete a hormone called glucagon, while the β-cells secrete insulin.

111. (a) Statement I is incorrect, but statement II is correct. Incorrect statements can be corrected as

Tracheid cells have less lignified walls. Thus, lumen is wide.

More lignified and thick walls are found in the cells of vessels.

112. (b) *Parthenium hysterophorus* and *Lantana camara* are examples of alien species invasion.

The alien species are introduced, unintentionally or deliberately for a specific purpose. Some of them turn invasive and cause decline or extinction of indigenous species.

114. (d) All the given statements are true. When multiple copies code for *r*RNA, such a DNA is called *r*DNA and its main source is gene duplication process.

Inheritance of a characters is affected by promoter and regulatory sequences of a structural gene.

113. (c) Monocytes are the largest of all types of leucocytes and are amoeboid in shape.

Monocytes constitute 2-10% of blood leucocytes. They generally change into macrophages after entering tissue spaces.

Neutrophils constitute about 65% of blood leucocytes. NK cells are natural killer cells.

115. (c) Statement in option (c) is incorrect and can be corrected as

The C_4 plants respond to higher temperatures and show higher rate of photosynthesis while C_3 plants have a much lower temperature optimum.

116. (b) Subsidiary cells are the accessory cells to guard cells in the epidermis of plants.

117. (d) Statement I is correct but statement II is incorrect and can be corrected as

Bones of old person are brittle and fracture more readily occur because they contain more inorganic matter.

118. (d) Pneumotaxic centre is present in the pons region which can moderate the functions of the respiratory rhythm centre.

119. (b) Both statement I and statement II are correct.

Pila are herbivorous animals, they lead an amphibious life as gaseous exchange occurs by means of gills and by lungs. They bear 8-shaped nervous system.

120. (b) Statement II and V are incorrect and can be corrected as

In the cells of collenchyma primary pits are present where the walls are uniform in thickness.

Collenchyma cells may be oval, polygonal or spherical and lack intercellular spaces.

Rest of the statements about collenchyma are correct.

121. (c) A cross between a husband and wife one with AB blood group and other with A blood group will produce four genotypes and three phenotypes. It has been depicted by the cross given below

Husband

Wife ♀ \ ♂	I^A	I^B
I^A	I^AI^A	I^AI^B
i	I^Ai	I^Bi

Thus, the genotypes and the phenotypes of the offspring would be

Genotypes : 4(I^AI^A, I^AI^B, I^Ai, I^Bi)

Phenotypes : 3(A, B, AB)

122. (d) The given figure is of *Nostoc*, a member of the group cyanobacteria or blue green algae. These perform oxygenic photosynthesis. Photosynthetic pigments include chlorophyll-*a*, carotenoids, C-phycocyanin, C-phycoerythrin which impart *Nostoc* its colour.

123. (c) At the tissue site, pCO_2 is high due to catabolism, CO_2 diffuses into blood and forms HCO_3^- and H^+.

At the alveolar site, pCO_2 is low. This results in formation of CO_2 and H_2O.

124. (b) The incorrect match is in option (b). It can be corrected as

Forebrain includes olfactory lobes, paired cerebral hemisphere and unpaired diencephalon.

125. (b) Statements II and IV are incorrect and it can be corrected as

The fossils of *Ramapithecus* and *Sivapithecus* were discovered in the Pilocene rocks of shivalik hills.

Neanderthal man were the first to use skin clothing and practice of burning the dead.

126. (a) The given formula belongs to family-Fabaceae or Leguminosae. The calyx shows gamosepalous condition, diadelphous stamens. These are zygomorphic and thus show bilateral symmetry. Ovary is monocarpellary and superior.

127. (b) Both Statement I and Statement II are correct

Respiratory roots help in the exchange of gases with the help of pneumatophores or lenticels.

These roots do not posses any definite organ for the exchange of gases.

128. (c) Statement in option (c) is incorrect and can be corrected as

Species extinctions in the last 500 years like Stellar's sea cow and passenger pigeon were due to over exploitation by humans.

129. (b) The above mentioned are characteristics of aerobic muscles.

Myoglobin content and number of mitochondria are high in some muscles. They are called red muscle fibres. The high myoglobin content in them facilitates production of ATP by oxidative phosphorylation. They also have a moderate ability to generate ATP through glycolytic pathway.

In white muscle fibres, there is accumulation of low or no myoglobin.

130. (c) Both A and R are true, but R is not the correct explanation of A.

In plant cells, vacuole occupy upto 90 per cent of the volume of the cell. The tonoplast facilitates the transport of a number of ions and other materials against concentration gradients into the vacuole. Hence, their concentration is significantly higher in the vacuole than in the cytoplasm.

131. (b) CO_2 is utilised for the carboxylation of Ribulose Bisphosphate (RuBP) in the first step of Calvin cycle. This reaction is catalysed by the enzyme RuBisCO.

132. (c) Statement I, III and IV are correct and rest of the statements are incorrect. These can be corrected as

- In wind pollinated plants, stamens are large and well exposed to the air currents.
- Wind pollination is quite common in grasses whereas water is a regular mode of transport for the male gametes among the lower plant groups such as Algae, Bryophytes and Pteridophytes.

133. (b) An enzyme reacts and binds with substrate to yield product. At the end of 10 minutes there will be presence of both products and enzyme in the test tube since enzymes are catalysts in the reaction and do not get consumed in it.

134. (a) The correct matches are A-2, B-4, C-1, D-3.
- Haemopoiesis is the process of formation of blood cells. It continues throughout the life of an individual.
- Cardiac output is defined as the volume of blood pumped out by each ventricle per minute. It can be calculated as stroke volume × heart rate.
- Erythropoiesis is the process that produces RBCs. QRS complex represents depolarisation of ventricles.

135. (c) When carbohydrates are used as substrate and are completely oxidised the RQ will be 1.

When fats are used in respiration the RQ is less than 1.

When Proteins are respiratory substrates the ratio would be about 0.9.

136. (c) The statement III is incorrect. It is corrected as follows

Niche have only one species. It is a functional description of the role, a species plays in a community.

137. (d) Fimbriae are long extensions arising from cell membrane of a bacterial cell. These aid the bacteria in adhering to the host tissue. Thus, if these extensions are removed, the adherence of bacteria to the host tissue is inhibited.

138. (d) The correct matches are A-4, B-1, C-2, D-3.
- The body of Porifera is supported by a skeleton made up of spicules or spongin fibres.
- Cnidarians have a central gastro-vascular cavity with a single opening, mouth on hypostome.
- The body of Ctenophora bears eight external rows of ciliated comb plates.
- Hooks and suckers are present in parasitic forms in Platyhelminthes.

139. (c) In Hershey Chase experiment DNA as genetic material was concluded, based on the presence of radioactivity in bacteria when 32P was used.

Hershey and Chase, during experiment observed that the set of viruses cultured in medium having radioactive phosphorous 32P consisted of radioactive DNA, but not proteins as DNA contains phosphorous, but protein does not.

Similarly viruses grown on radioactive sulphur contained radioactive protein, but not radioactive DNA. It was later concluded that the set of viruses having radioactive DNA transfered their DNA to the bacteria, but nothing was transfered in the latter case. This led to the conclusion that DNA is the genetic material.

140. (b) By the end of second month (60 days) of pregnancy the foetus develops limbs and digits.

By the end of first trimester the extenal genital organs are well developed.

141. (c) Disruptive or diversifying selection describes changes in poplulation genetics wherein two extreme values for a trait are preferred over intermediate values..

142. (a) TCA or Krebs' cycle is a cyclic pathway that does not consume ATP. It takes place in aerobic respiration only.

143. (a) Statement I is incorrect, but statement II is correct. Incorrect statement can be corrected as

Complex-IV refers to cytochrome-*c* oxidase complex containing cytochromes-*a* and a_3 and two copper centres.

144. (d) The function of glycocalyx in bacteria is protection from phagocytosis and prevention of desiccation. It also enables them to adhere to the surfaces.

Glycocalyx is made up of gelatinous polysaccharide or polypeptide.
However, it does not facilitate cell movement.

145. (d) A is true, but R is false. It can be corrected as

To differentiate between recombinant and non-recombinant insertional inactivation is used in which the presence of chromogenic substrate gives blue coloured colonies.

146. (c) Option (c) is true for pest-resistant plants. RNA interference is a gene silencing mechanism triggered by providing double-stranded RNA (dsRNA), that when ingested into insects can lead to death or affect the viability of the target pest.

147. (d) Net increase in population

(Natality + Immigration) − (Mortality + Emigration)

$= (270 + 20) - (240 + 30)$

$= 290 - 270 = 20$

148. (a) *Bacillus thuringiensis* spores were first used as biopesticides on a commercial scale in the world. *Bt* toxin gene has been cloned from the bacteria and has been expressed in plants to provide resistance to insects without the need of insecticides.

149. (d) Binding of hormone of intracellular receptor results in a hormone-receptor complex which further binds to Hormone Responsive Elements (HRE) in order to activate and transcribe a particular gene. In case of failure of this binding, transcription will be inhibited and therefore, specific proteins are not synthesised.

150. (c) Golgi bodies or golgi apparatus or complex are organelles present in eukaryotic cells. These aid in packaging, processing and distributing molecules within the cell.

151. (a) IBA or Indole-3 butyric acid, is a plant hormone in auxin family. It is an ingredient in many commercial horticulture plant rooting products because stem cuttings of some plants like grapes and sugarcane do not produce roots readily and have to be treated with a root promoting hormone such as IAA, IBA, etc.

152. (b) Anterior lobe of pituitary is concerned with the production of FSH and LH.

Both of these hormones play an important role in males by stimulating sperm production and testosterone (male).

In females, FSH stimulates growth of follicles in ovary whereas LH causes ovulation.

153. (b) The statements II and III are incorrect.

They can be corrected as

Urine is acidic with pH around 6.0 and it consists of 96% of water.

154. (c) Both A and R is true, but R is not the correct explanation of A.

In amphibians the alimentary canal, urinary and reproductive tracts open into the a common chamber called cloaca.

It common chamber for urine, sperm and faeces release.

155. (b) The two important types of secondary structures of proteins are α-helix and β-pleated sheet, β-sheets consist of β-strands connected laterally by atleast two or three backbone H-bonds, forming a generally twisted, pleated sheet. A β-strand is a stretch of polypeptide chain, 3-10 amino acids long with backbone in an extended conformation.

In α-helix, the chain is spirally coiled, generally in a right-handed manner.

This structure is formed through H-bonding in single amino acid chain only.

156. (b) A tall plant has a constitution of tall plant even though it was grown in nutrient deficient soil. Thus, a cross between such a plant and a dwarf plant will result in f_2 progeny with all tall plants.

157. (a) The correct matches are A-1, B-2, C-3, D-4.

- Poaceae is the family of monocotyledonous flowering plants commoly known as grasses (wheat).
- Poales are a large order of flowering plants in the monocotyledonous such as grasses (wheat).
- Monocotyledonous is the class of grasses (wheat).
- Wheat belongs to the division-Angiospermae.

158. (b) Both statement I and statement II are correct.

Platelets also called thrombocytes, are cell fragments produced from megakaryocytes. Blood normally contains 1,500,00-3,500,00 platelets mm^{-3}. Platelets can release many substances most of which are involved in the coagulation of blood.

159. (b) The statement in option (b) is incorrect regarding Down syndrome.

Down syndrome results due to trisomy $(2n + 1)$ of chromosome 21, caused due to non-disjunction of chromosome 21.

Down syndrome, also known as 21 trisomy, is not a monosomic condition.

Childern with Down syndrome have affectionate and loving nature and individuals have a characteristic prominent epicanthic fold in each eye.

160. (d) Statement in option (d) is incorrect. It can be corrected as

Wheat, maize, castor are examples of albuminous seed. The endosperm is not completely used up during embryo development.

Pea does not retain endosperm and is non-endospermic or ex-albuminous.

161. (a) The presence of chloroplast is a common feature shared by guard cells and mesophyll cells.

Guard cells, mesophyll cells and chloroplast are present in leaves of the plant. The chloroplasts are present in guard cells and mesophyll cells and are the site for photosynthesis.

162. (b) Mycoplasma lacks cells wall, but show multiplication like bacteria, so that they are termed as wall less bacteria.

163. (c) Both A and R are true, but R is not the correct explanation of A.

Frequency of crossing over is directly proportional to the distance between the genes. As distance between the genes increases the possibility of crossing over will also increases while it will reduce the possibility of linkage.

164. (d) The correct matches are A-4, B-1, C-2, D-3.

Cirrhosis is the severe scarring of liver. This can be caused due to several conditions and can lead to liver failure.

Cocaine is a powerful addictive drug made from leaves of *Erythroxylem coca*. It acts as CNS stimulant.

Opioids are drugs that bind to specific opioid receptors present in our CNS.

Patients suffering from cancer are usually given α-interferons to activated their immune system. Thus, help in fighting cancer.

165. (b) The statement in option (b) is incorrect. It can be corrected as follows

An International Human Genome Project was started in 1990 with the triple aim of mapping the whole human genone at the level of nucleotide sequences, to store the information from project in databases and develop tools for data analysis, to solve ethical, legal or social problems which may arise from the project. The project was completed on June 26, 2000.

166. (a) The correct matches are A-4, B-3, C-2, D-1.
- RH Whittaker proposed five kingdom classification.
- MW Beijerinck demonstrated that the extract of the infected plant of tobacco could cause infection in healthy plants and called the fluid *Contagium vivum fluidum*.
- In 1971, TO Diener discovered a new infectious agent called viroids.
- Cr. Jacob disease in humans is the most notable disease caused by prions.

167. (d) Intron transcripts in heterogenous nuclear RNA (*hn*RNA) are removed and exon transcripts are joined together under the direction of protein complexes. These complexes are spliceosomes. They are primarily found in nucleus of eukaryotes.

168. (d) Most of the members of Chlorophyceae have one or more storage bodies called pyrenoids located in the chloroplasts. Pyrenoids contain protein besides starch.

169. (c) Statement III is incorrect and can be corrected as

An adult human male ejaculates about 200 to 300 million sperms during a coitus of this 60% must have normal shape and size and 40% of these must be vigorously motile to perform successful fertilisation.

170. (b) Except option (b), all other strategies are used for controlling the expression of genes in eukaryotes. feedback inhibition via allosteric modification controls the enzyme activity.

171. (c) Euglenoids are photosynthetic in the presence of sunlight, but they behave like heterotrophs by predating on other smaller organisms, e.g. *Euglena.*

172. (b) The diagram represents the multicarpellary, syncarpous pistil of *Papaver*. The gynoecium of this plant consists of more than one pistil showing multicarpellary condition. These pistils are fused together and hence are called syncarpous.

173. (c) Statement in option (c) is incorrect. It can be corrected as

Thorns are found in many plants such as *Citrus* and *Bougainvillea.*

174. (c) Statements I, IV and V are correct, while statements II and III are incorrect and these can be corrected as

Hormones are first messengers and thyroid hormone needs receptors to bind target sites. Hormones that are too large like epinephrine, to pass cell membranes, require specific receptors to reach their target sites. Steroid hormones like testosterone are lipid soluble and can enter cytoplasm of target cells.

175. (a) Restriction endonucleases recognise their specific sequence and bind to the DNA and cuts each of the two strands of the double helix at specific points in their sugar-phosphate back bone.

176. (b) Statements I, III and IV are correct, while statements II and V are incorrect and can be corrected as
- Humification leads to accumulation of a dark coloured amorphous substance called humus that is highly resistant to microbial action.
- The consumers are represented by the zooplankton, which are the free swimming and bottom dewelling forms.

177. (a) The correct matches are A–1, B–2, C–3, D–4.

Secondary metabolites are the intermediate products produced during metabolism, catalysed by various enzymes that occur naturally within cells, e.g.

Pigments – Anthocyanins
Terpenoids – Diterpenes
Alkaloids – Codeine
Lectins – Concanavalin-A

178. (b) Steller's sea cow and Passenger pigeon are the organisms that have become extinct due to over-exploitation by humans.

Both of these were hunted for their skin and meat.

179. (b) Based on the number of axon and dendites neurons can be multi, bi or unipolar.

The unipolar neurons found in the embryonic stage have the cell body with one axon only.

180. (c) The nuclear envelope consists of two lipid bilayer membranes, i.e. an inner nuclear membrane and an outer nuclear membrane. The outer nuclear membrane is continuous with the endoplasmic reticulum membrane.

The space between the membranes is called the perinuclear space.

SECTION II

Mastery Builders

PRACTICE SET 11

Maximum Marks : 720	Time : 3 hrs	No. of Questions : 180

Instructions

1. This question paper contains **180** multiple-choice questions (four options with a single correct answer) from **Physics, Chemistry and Biology.**
2. These questions are distributed as 45 questions, each from Physics and Chemistry and 90 questions in Biology. These are to be compulsorily attempted by the candidate.
3. Each question carries 4 marks. For each correct response, the candidate will get 4 marks. For each incorrect response, one mark will be deducted from the total scores.

PHYSICS

1. The graph shows the variation of acceleration with position of a 3 kg particle, initially at rest, the acceleration results due to an applied force. The work done by the force on the particle by the time it reaches $x = 6$ m is

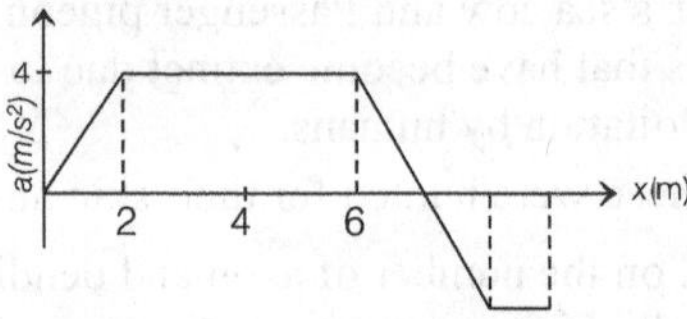

(a) 20 J (b) 30 J
(c) 40 J (d) 60 J

2. An apple of mass 0.25 kg falls from a tree. The ratio of acceleration of the apple towards the earth and of the earth towards the apple is (mass of earth $= 6 \times 10^{24}$ kg, radius of earth $= 6.4 \times 10^{6}$ m and $G = 6.67 \times 10^{-11}$ N-m^{2}kg^{-2})

(a) $\frac{1}{24 \times 10^{-24}}$ (b) 24×10^{24}
(c) 24×10^{-24} (d) $\frac{1}{24 \times 10^{24}}$

3. The refractive index of glass is 1.5. The speed of light in glass is

(a) 3×10^{8} m/s (b) 2×10^{8} m/s
(c) 1×10^{8} m/s (d) 4×10^{8} m/s

4. The co-ordinates of a particle in xy-plane are given as $x = 2t^2 + t$ and $y = 16t^2 + 8t$
The motion of the particle is

(a) along a straight line with uniform acceleration
(b) along a circular path with uniform acceleration
(c) along a parabolic path with uniform velocity
(d) along a hyperbolic path with uniform velocity

5. Two discs of moment of inertia I_1 and I_2 and angular speeds ω_1 and ω_2 are rotating along collinear axis passing through their centre of mass and perpendicular to their plane. If both discs are pressed face to face to rotate combinedly along same axis, then rotational KE of system is

(a) $\frac{I_1\omega_1 + I_2\omega_2}{2(I_1 + I_2)}$ (b) $\frac{(I_1 + I_2)(\omega_1 + \omega_2)^2}{2}$
(c) $\frac{(I_1\omega_1 + I_2\omega_2)^2}{2(I_1 + I_2)}$ (d) None of these

6. A portion of a meteor moving at a constant rate of 50 kmh^{-1} gets separated from its surface, when it enter earth's atmosphere. Find the velocity of the portion of meteor at the instant after it gets separated.

(a) 100 kmh^{-1} (b) 50 kmh^{-1}
(c) 0 kmh^{-1} (d) 200 kmh^{-1}

7. Two wires of same material and same diameters have lengths in the ratio 2 : 9. They are stretched by same force. The ratio of work done in stretching them is

(a) 9:2 (b) 4:8 (c) $\sqrt{9}:\sqrt{2}$ (d) 2:9

8. A pole PQ is held vertically with its one end P on the floor and is then allowed to fall. The speed of the other end Q, when it strikes the floor is

(a) $\sqrt{2gL}$ (b) $\sqrt{3gL}$ (c) $\sqrt{\frac{2g}{L}}$ (d) $\sqrt{\frac{3g}{L}}$

9. A man stands on a weighing machine placed on a horizontal platform. The machine reads 50 kg. By means of a suitable mechanism, the platform is made to execute harmonic vibrations of frequency 2 vibration per second. The change in the reading of the weighing machine observed due to oscillatory motion is (take, amplitude = 5 cm and $g = 10\ \text{ms}^{-2}$)

(a) 79 kg-f (b) 89.5 kg-f
(c) 10.5 kg-f (d) 100 kg-f

10. A double convex thin lens made of glass (refractive index, $\mu = 1.83$) has both radii of curvature of magnitude 30 cm. Incident light rays parallel to the axis of the lens will converge at a distance L, such that

(a) 30 m (b) 25 cm
(c) 18 cm (d) 13 cm

11. A 20 μF capacitor charged to 50V is connected in parallel to another 10 μF capacitor to 20V. Find the resulting potential across the combination.

(a) 40 V (b) 45 V
(c) 50 V (d) 55 V

12. In an AC circuit, $I = 10\sin\left(100\pi t - \frac{\pi}{3}\right)$ A and $E = 220\sin 100\pi t$ V. Calculate average power consumed in the circuit.

(a) 550 W (b) 410 W
(c) 350 W (d) 610 W

13. Match the thermodynamic process in column I with their respective slopes in column II for the p-V graph shown below.

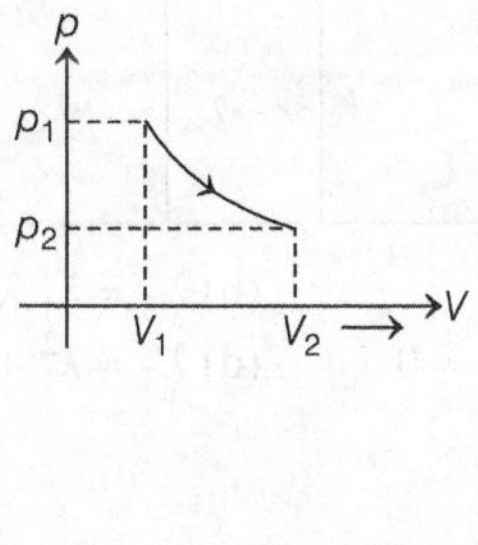

	Column I		Column II
A.	Isochoric Process	I.	$\frac{nR}{p}$
B.	Isobaric Process	II.	$\frac{nR}{V}$
C.	Isothermal Process	III.	$-\frac{\gamma p}{V}$
D.	Adiabatic Process	IV.	$-\frac{p}{V}$

Choose the correct answer from the given options.

	A	B	C	D		A	B	C	D
(a)	II	I	IV	III	(b)	IV	III	II	I
(c)	I	III	IV	II	(d)	III	II	I	IV

14. The typical I-V characteristic graph for photodiode is

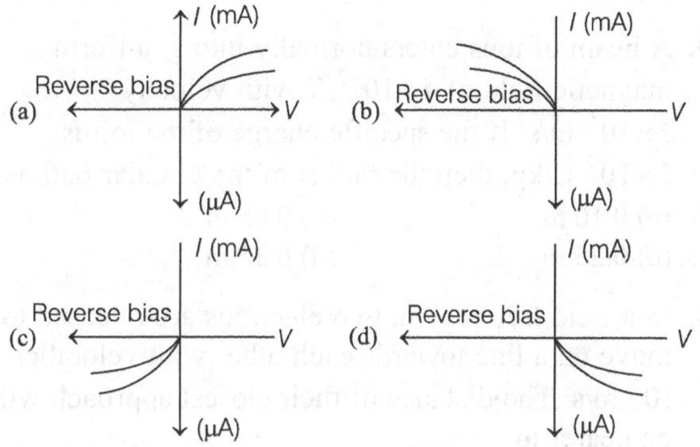

15. The variation of resistance with temperature as shown in the graph.

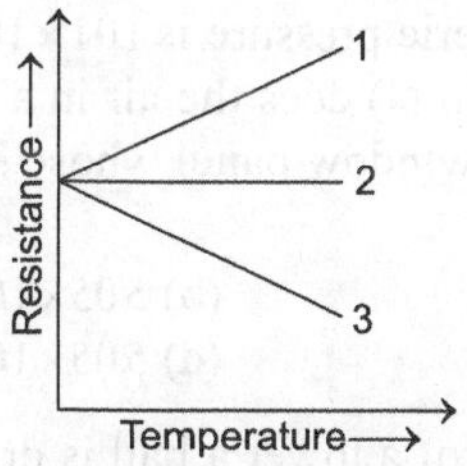

Graphs 1, 2 and 3 are drawn respectively for
(a) copper, constantan, germanium
(b) constantan, copper, germanium
(c) copper, germanium, constantan
(d) germanium, constantan, copper

16. A reverse bias in a junction diode is changed from 4V to 12 V, then the value of the current changes from 20 μA to 60 μA. The resistance of junction diode will be

(a) $2\times10^5\,\Omega$ (b) $2.5\times10^5\,\Omega$
(c) $3\times10^5\,\Omega$ (d) $4\times10^5\,\Omega$

17. If the density of oxygen is 8 times the density of hydrogen, then at what temperature the velocity of sound in hydrogen is same as in oxygen at 87° C ?

(a) 230°C (b) −230° C
(c) −228° C (d) 228° C

18. **Statement I** The drift velocity of electrons in a metallic wire increases with the increase of temperature of wire.
Statement II On increasing the temperature, conductivity of metallic wire decreases.
In the light of above statement, choose the correct option given below.

(a) Both Statement I and Statement II are correct.
(b) Both Statement I and Statement II are incorrect.
(c) Statement I is correct but Statement II is incorrect.
(d) Statement I is incorrect but Statement II is correct.

19. A beam of ions enters normally into a uniform magnetic field of 4×10^{-2} T with velocity 2×10^{5} m/s. If the specific charge of the ion is 5×10^{7} C/kg, then the radius of the circular path is

(a) 0.10 m (b) 0.08 m
(c) 0.25 m (d) 0.35 m

20. In a field free region, two electrons are released to move on a line towards each other with velocities 10^{7} m/s. The distance of their closest approach will be nearer to

(a) 1.28×10^{-10} m (b) 1.92×10^{-10} m
(c) 2.56×10^{-12} m (d) 3.84×10^{-10} m

21. The atmospheric pressure is 1.01×10^{5} Pa. How much force (in N) does the air in a room exert on the side of a window panel whose size is 50 cm × 10 cm ?

(a) 5.05×10^{3} (b) 5.05×10^{6}
(c) 5.05×10^{4} (d) 5.05×10^{5}

22. From the top of a tower a ball is dropped. If the total distance covered by it in last second of its motion is equal to the distance covered by it in its first 5 s, then the time for which it remains in air is

(a) 5 s (b) 10 s
(c) 13 s (d) 9 s

23. The ratio of electric field and electric potential due to electric dipole at a distance r from its mean position is

(a) r (b) $\frac{1}{r^2}$
(c) $\frac{1}{r}$ (d) r^2

24. If a cell of emf 12 V is connected with load of 5Ω provides a current of 2 A, then internal resistance of the cell is

(a) 1.5Ω (b) 2Ω (c) 2.5Ω (d) 1Ω

25. **Statement I** A dimensionally incorrect equation must be incorrect.
Statement II A dimensionally correct equation may or may not be correct.
In the light of above statements, choose the most appropriate answer from the options given below

(a) Both Statement I and Statement II are correct.
(b) Both Statement I and Statement II are incorrect.
(c) Statement I is correct but Statement II is incorrect.
(d) Statement I is incorrect but Statement II is correct.

26. A. Velocity of photon is different in different media.
B. Photons are deflected by electric fields but remains undeflected in magnetic fields.
C. In a photon-electron collision, the total energy remains conserved.
D. If intensity of light of a given wavelength increases, then photon energy increases.

Choose which of the above statements are true and tick the correct option from the following

(a) A and B only (b) A and C only
(c) B and D only (d) B and C only

27. A cube of side l is placed in a uniform electric field $\mathbf{E} = E\,\hat{\mathbf{i}}$. The net electric flux through the cube is

(a) zero (b) $4l^2E$
(c) l^2E (d) $6l^2Er$

28. If e/m of electron is 1.76×10^{12} C kg^{-1} and the stopping potential is 0.81 V, then maximum velocity of the photoelectron is

(a) 1.69×10^{6} m/s (b) 2.71×10^{7} m/s
(c) 3.1×10^{6} m/s (d) 4.1×10^{2} m/s

29. Energy levels A, B and C of a certain atom correspond to increasing values of energy, i.e., $E_A < E_B < E_C$. If λ_1, λ_2 and λ_3 are wavelengths of photon corresponding to transitions shown, then

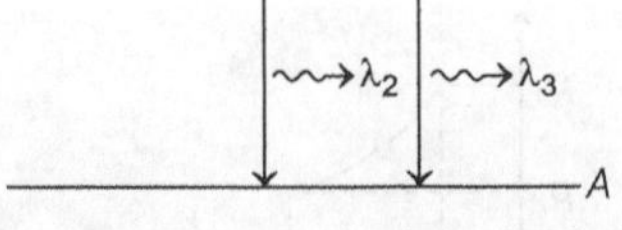

(a) $\lambda_3 = \lambda_1 + \lambda_2$ (b) $\lambda_3 = \lambda_1\lambda_2/\lambda_1 + \lambda_2$
(c) $\lambda_1 + \lambda_2 + \lambda_3 = 0$ (d) $\lambda_3^2 = \lambda_1^2 + \lambda_2^2$

30. If the reading of voltmeter V_1 and V_2 in the given circuit.diagram are 300 V each, then reading of voltmeter V_3 and ammeter A are, respectively

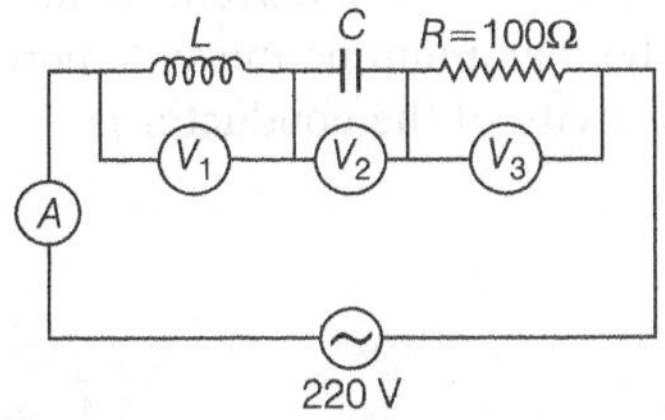

(a) 100 V, 2.0 A (b) 150 V, 2.2 A
(c) 220 V, 2.2 A (d) 220 V, 2.0 A

31. If the electric amplitude of the electromagnetic wave is 5 V m^{-1}, then its magnetic amplitude will be
(a) 5×10^{-10} T (b) 1.67×10^{-10} T
(c) 5×10^{-8} T (d) 1.67×10^{-8} T

32. A sphere has bulk modulus B. It is placed inside a pressure chamber, if a constant pressure p is maintained inside chamber. The fractional decrement in diameter is
(a) $\frac{p}{2B}$ (b) $\frac{3p}{B}$ (c) $\frac{p}{3B}$ (d) $\frac{p}{B}$

33. If binding energy of electron in a hydrogen atom is 13.6 eV, then energy required to remove the electron from the first excited state of Li^{++} is
(a) 13.6 eV (b) 3.4 eV (c) 30.6 eV (d) 122.4 eV

34. Choose the graph for an ideal gas that best represents the behaviour of the molecules mean free path time t between two successive collisions as a function of temperature T.

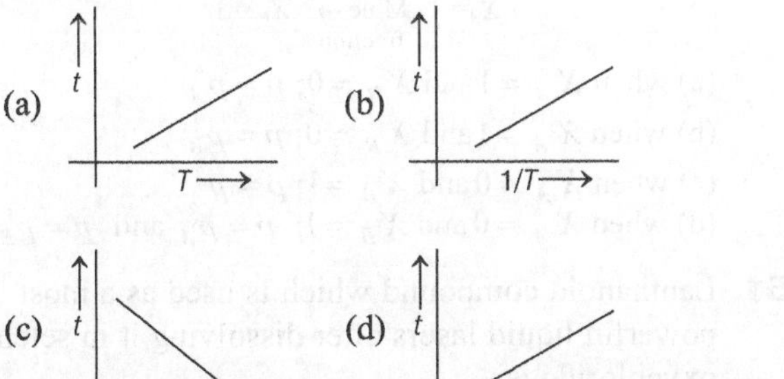

35. The driver of a train A moving with a uniform speed of 30 ms^{-1} sees another train B moving with uniform speed 10 ms^{-1} on the same track in the same direction. He immediately applies brakes and achieves a uniform retardation of 2ms^{-1} and finally stops. To avoid collision, the minimum distance between the trains must be
(a) 140 m (b) 75 m
(c) 80 m (d) 120 m

36. A positively charged particle enters a magnetic field of value $B\,\hat{\mathbf{i}}$ with a velocity $v\,\hat{\mathbf{j}}$, then the instantaneous direction of particle will be along
(a) Z-axis (b) $-Z$-axis
(c) $-X$-axis (d) $-Y$-axis

37. The plane face of a plano-convex lens is silvered. If μ be the refractive index and R be the radius of curvature of curved surface, then system will behave like a concave mirror of radius of curvature
(a) μR (b) R^2/μ
(c) $R/(\mu-1)$ (d) $[(\mu+1)/(\mu-1)]R$

38. **Assertion** (A) The fringe width decreases for the apparatus immersed in water.

Reason (R) The wavelength of light in water is less than that in air.

In the light of above statements, choose the most appropriate answer from the options given below.
(a) Both assertion and reason are true and reason is the correct explanation of assertion.
(b) Both assertion and reason are true but reason is not the correct explanation of assertion.
(c) Assertion is true but reason is false.
(d) Assertion is false but reason is true.

39. A body is released from 1600 km above the surface of earth. The velocity with which it strikes the surface of earth is (take, radius of earth = 6400 km and $g = 10\ ms^{-2}$)
(a) 18.2×10^3 kmh^{-1} (b) $3.5\times10^2 kmh^{-1}$
(c) 4×10^2 kmh^{-1} (d) 2.25×10^2 kmh^{-1}

40. A particle executes SHM with a time period of 2s and amplitude 5 cm. Starting from the mean position, its displacement and velocity after $\frac{1}{3}$ s are
(a) 4.33 cm, 7.85 cms^{-1}
(b) 4.5 cm, 6.75 cms^{-1}
(c) 7.85 cm, 4.33 cms^{-1}
(d) 6.75 cm, 4.5 cms^{-1}

41. In a single slit diffraction pattern, distance between screen and slit is 2.5 m and slit width is 0.25 mm. The separation of second dark band from central maxima is 1.5 cm, then the wavelength of light is
(a) 7000 Å (b) 6000 Å
(c) 6500 Å (d) 7500 Å

42. A transformer is used to light a 100 W and 110 V lamp from a 220 V mains. If the main current is 0.5 A, the efficiency of the transformer is approximately

(a) 50% (b) 91% (c) 10% (d) 30%

43. In the following electrical network, the equivalent resistance between point B and C is

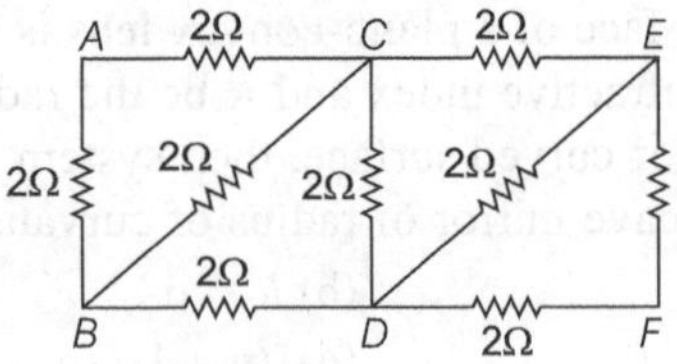

(a) $\frac{26}{27}\Omega$ (b) $\frac{29}{31}\Omega$ (c) $\frac{52}{55}\Omega$ (d) $\frac{58}{57}\Omega$

44. In the experiment of Ohm's law, a potential difference of 5.0 V is applied across the end of a conductor of length 10.0 cm and diameter of 5.00 mm. The measured current in the conductor is 2.00 A. The maximum permissible percentage error in the resistivity of the conductor is

(a) 3.9
(b) 8.4
(c) 7.5
(d) 3.0

45. The equations of motion of a projectile are given by $x = 18t$ and $2y = 54t - 9.8t^2$. The angle θ of projection is

(a) $\tan^{-1}(3)$ (b) $\tan^{-1}(1.5)$
(c) $\sin^{-1}\frac{2}{3}$ (d) $\cos^{-1}\frac{2}{3}$

CHEMISTRY

46. Glucose is a monosaccharide, aldohexose and reducing sugar. In the combined state, it occur in glucosides, dissaccharides and polysaccharides. Glucose on reaction with Br_2/H_2O produces

(a) gluconic acid (b) levulinic acid
(c) glucaric acid (d) n-hexane

47. If a particle of mass 500 mg is moving with a velocity of 100 m/s then the de-Broglie wavelength of the particle will be ($h = 6.625 \times 10^{-34}$ Js)

(a) 1.32×10^{-35} m (b) 1.32×10^{-32} m
(c) 1.32×10^{-34} m (d) 1.32×10^{-31} m

48. Which of the following ions shows paramagnetic property?

I. Fe^{3+} II. Mn^{2+} III. Zn^{2+}
IV. V^{2+} V. Cu^{2+}

Choose the most appropriate answer from the options given below.

(a) I, II, III (b) I, II, IV, V
(c) I, II, III, IV (d) II, III, IV

49. Which of the following statements are correct?

I. Decarboxylation of isobutyric acid leads to propane.
II. 1-pentene with HCl gives 3-chloropentane.
III. Propyne and propene can be distinguished by $AgNO_3$ in ammonia.
IV. Chloroethane on reacting with zinc and dil. HCl give ethane.
V. 2-butene shows geometrical isomerism due to restricted rotation about double bond.

Choose the correct answer the from the options given below.

(a) I, III, IV and V
(b) II and IV
(c) I and III
(d) II, III and V

50. The following is a graph plotted between two volatile liquids against their respective mole fractions. Which of the following statement is correct?

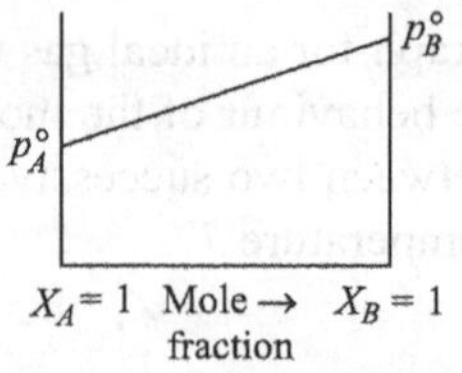

(a) when $X_A = 1$ and $X_B = 0$; $p = p_A^\circ$
(b) when $X_A = 1$ and $X_B = 0$; $p = p_B^\circ$
(c) when $X_A = 0$ and $X_B = 1$; $p = p_A^\circ$
(d) when $X_A = 0$ and $X_B = 1$; $p = p_A^\circ$ and $p = p_B^\circ$

51. Lanthanoid compound which is used as a most powerful liquid lasers after dissolving it in selenium oxychloride is

(a) ceric sulphate (b) promethium sulphate
(c) cerium oxide (d) neodymium oxide

52. 200 mL of an aqueous solution contains 0.01 mole of the solute AB. If its specific conductance is x S cm^{-1}, its molar conductance in Sm^2 mol^{-1} will be

(a) x (b) $2x$
(c) $200x$ (d) $40x$

53. Equilibrium constant of a chemical reaction is 1.5 and rate constant of backward reaction is 7.5×10^{-4}. Then, rate constant of forward reaction will be
(a) 1.125×10^{-3} (b) 2.225×10^{-3}
(c) 3.335×10^{-5} (d) 1.125×10^{-1}

54. The pH of the solution is defined as the negative logarithm of the concentration of hydrogen ions which it contains. pH of 0.365 g L^{-1} HCl solution will be
(a) 1 (b) 2 (c) 3 (d) 0.1

55. Consider the compounds (I) and (II):

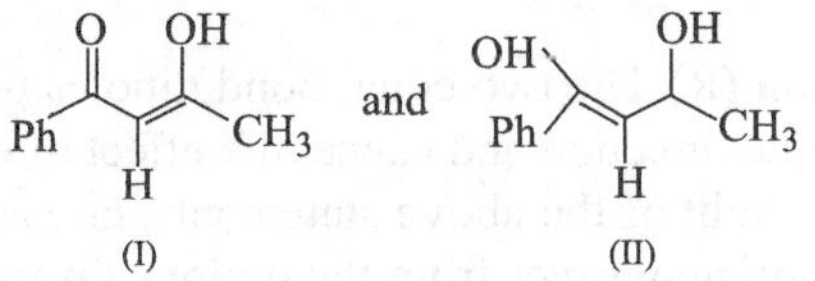

Which of the following statement is true for the above two compounds?
(a) Above pairs are resonance contributors.
(b) They are chain isomers.
(c) They are group isomers.
(d) They are tautomers.

56. What will be the product obtained when *A* reacts with heavy water?

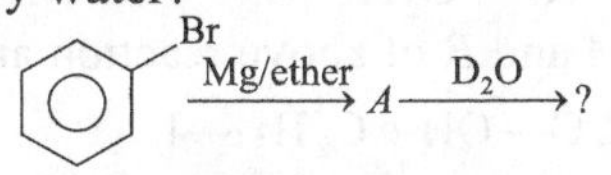

Choose the correct option regarding product.

(a) 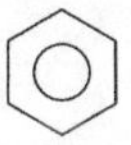 (b) 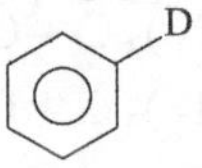

(c) 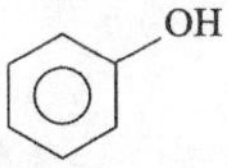

(d) 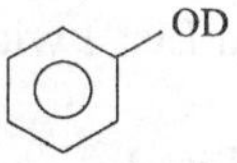

57. When propionic acid is treated with aqueous sodium bicarbonate, CO_2 is liberated. The C from CO_2 comes from
(a) methyl group (b) carboxylic acid group
(c) methylene group (d) bicarbonate

58. Which of the following order of electron gain enthalpy is correct?
(a) F < Cl < Br < I (b) F < Cl > Br < I
(c) I > Br > F < Cl (d) I < Cl < Br > F

59. Which of the following is a disproportionation reaction?
(a) $CaCO_3 + 2H^- \longrightarrow Ca^{2+} + H_2O + CO_2$
(b) $CuS + O_2 \longrightarrow Cu + SO_2$
(c) $2HCuCl_2 \longrightarrow 2Cu + Cu^{2+} + 4Cl^- + 2H^+$
(d) $3ClO^- + 2Cr(OH)_4^- \longrightarrow 2CrO_4^{2-} + 3Cl^-$

60. Which of the following will not undergo S_N2 reaction?
(a) $CH_2=CH—CH_2—Cl$
(b) 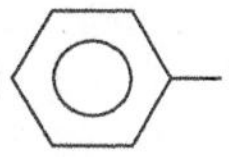 $—CH_2—Cl$
(c) $CH_2=CH—Cl$
(d) $CH_3—CH_2—CH_2—Cl$

61. In which of the options, order of arrangement does not agree with the variation of property indicated against it?
(a) C < N < O < F (Electronegativity)
(b) C < B < Be < Li (Atomic radius)
(c) F < N < Be < Ne (First ionisation enthalpy)
(d) He < Xe < Ar < Ne (Positive electron gain enthalpy)

62. 2 moles of an ideal gas expands reversibly and isothermally from 1 L to 10 L at 27°C. The entropy change during the process is
(a) 690 R (b) 600 R
(c) 2.3 R (d) 4.6 R

63. Match the List-I with List-II.

List-I (Products)	List-II (Reactions)
A. Ethane	(i) Sabatier-Senderens reaction of propylene
B. Propane	(ii) Wurtz reaction of methyl iodide
C. Methane	(iii) Sodium propanoate by Kolbe's electrolysis
D. Butane	(iv) Decarboxylation of sodium acetate

Choose the correct answer from the options given below.
(a) A-(ii), B-(i), C-(iv), D-(iii)
(b) A-(ii), B-(i), C-(iii), D-(iv)
(c) A-(i), B-(ii), C-(iv), D-(iii)
(d) A-(i), B-(iii), C-(iv), D-(ii)

64. The major product obtained in the reaction is expected to

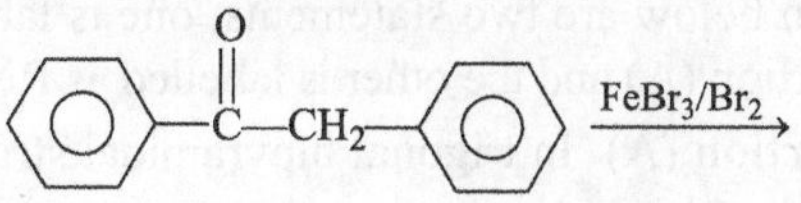

(a) 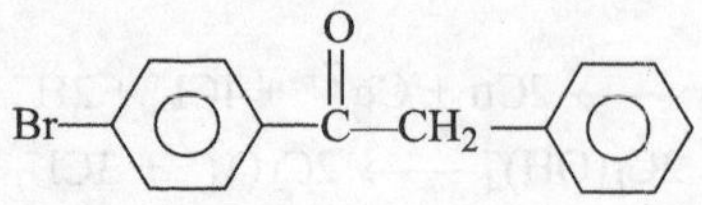

(b) 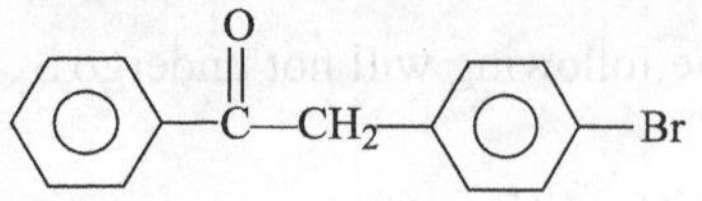

(c) 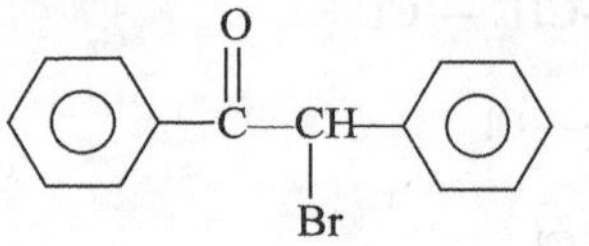

(d) 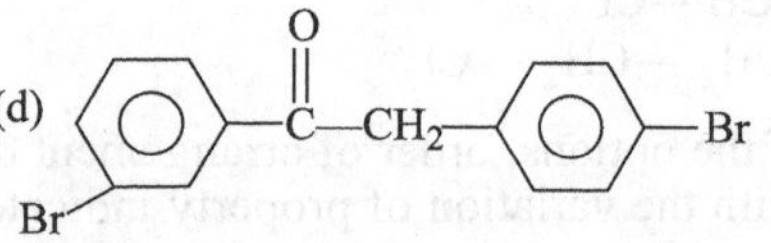

65. Arrange the following in increasing order of their acidic strength.

I. 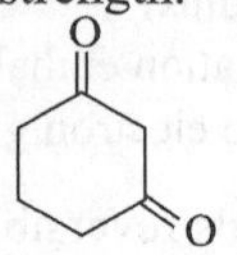

II. 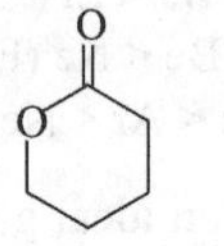

III. 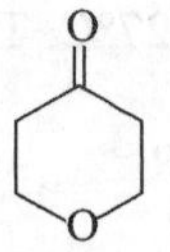

IV. 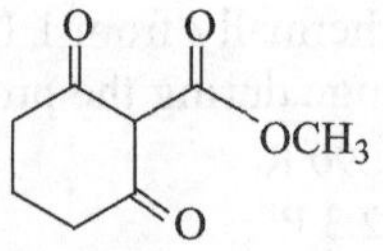

(a) I < II < III < IV
(b) II < III < IV < I
(c) III < II < I < IV
(d) II < III < I < IV

66. Given below are two statements.

Statement I CCl_4 acts as Lewis acid.

Statement II Silanes are strong reducing agents.

In the light of the above statements, choose the correct answer from the options given below.

(a) Statement I is false but Statement II is true.
(b) Both Statement I and Statement II are true.
(c) Both Statement I and Statement II are false.
(d) Statement I is true but Statement II is false.

67. Which among the following combinations illustrates the law of reciprocal proportions?

A. N_2O_3, N_2O_4, N_2O_5
B. NaCl, NaBr, NaI
C. H_2O, H_2S, SO_2
D. PH_3, P_2O_3, P_2O_5
E. CS_2, CO_2, SO_2

Choose the most appropriate answer from the options given below.

(a) A and D only
(b) C and E only
(c) B and C only
(d) D and E only

68. Given below are two statements, one is labelled as Assertion (A) and the other is labelled as Reason (R).

Assertion (A) In trigonal bipyramidal structure two axial bonds are longer than the equatorial bonds.

Reason (R) Axial bonds suffer more repulsion as compared to equatorial bonds.

In the light of the above statements, choose the most appropriate answer from the options given below.

(a) (A) is false but (R) is true.
(b) Both (A) and (R) are true and (R) is the correct explanation of (A).
(c) Both (A) and (R) are true but (R) is not the correct explanation of (A).
(d) (A) is true but (R) is false.

69. Given below are two statements, one is labelled as Assertion (A) and the other is labelled as Reason (R).

Assertion (A) The dipole moment in case of BeF_2 is zero.

Reason (R) The two equal bond dipoles point in opposite direction and cancel the effect of each other.

In the light of the above statements, choose the must appropriate answer from the options given below.

(a) (A) is false but (R) is true.
(b) Both (A) and (R) are true and (R) is the correct explanation of (A).
(c) Both (A) and (R) are true but (R) is not the correct explanation of (A).
(d) (A) is true but (R) is false.

70. Consider the following reaction

$(CH_3)_3C—O—C_2H_5 \xrightarrow{\text{HI (1 eq)}} A + B$

Products A and B of above reaction are

(a) $(CH_3)_3C—OH + C_2H_5—I$
(b) $(CH_3)_3C—I + C_2H_5I$
(c) $(CH_3)_3C—OH + C_2H_5—OH$
(d) $(CH_3)_3C—I + C_2H_5—OH$

71. Match List-I with List-II.

List-I (Metal ion)		List-II (Group in qualitative analysis)	
A.	Mn^{2+}	I.	Group-III
B.	As^{3+}	II.	Group-IIA
C.	Cu^{2+}	III.	Group-IV
D.	Fe^{3+}	IV.	Group-IIB

Choose the correct answer from the options given below:

(a) A-I, B-II, C-III, D-IV
(b) A-III, B-IV, C-II, D-I
(c) A-I, B-IV, C-II, D-III
(d) A-IV, B-II, C-III, D-I

72. The conversion of vinyl allyl ether to pent-4-enol follows first-order kinetics. The following plot is obtained for such a reaction. The rate constant for the reaction is

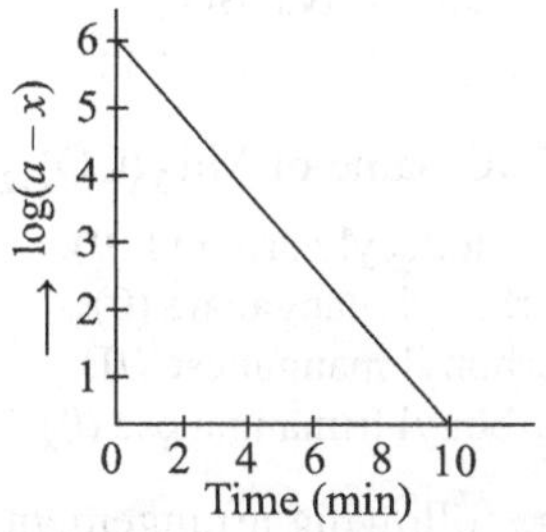

(a) $4.6 \times 10^{-2} s^{-1}$ (b) $1.2 \times 10^{-2} s^{-1}$
(c) $2.3 \times 10^{-2} s^{-1}$ (d) $8.4 \times 10^{-2} s^{-1}$

73. If rate constant of a chemical reaction is $4.606 \times 10^{-3} s^{-1}$ then the time required for the completion of 50% of the reaction is

(a) 150.5 s (b) 300 s (c) 200.5 s (d) 400 s

74. Ammonia gas is not prepared by

(a) reduction of sodium nitrite or sodium nitrate by the reaction of zinc dust and sodium hydroxide.
(b) hydrolysis of calcium cyanamide.
(c) heating ammonium chloride with slaked lime.
(d) heating of $(NH_4)_2Cr_2O_7$.

75. Given below are two statements.

Statement I ClO^- is isoelectronic with ClF.
Statement II HClO is stronger acid than HBrO.
In the light of the above statements, choose the correct answer from the options given below.

(a) Statement I is false but Statement II is true.
(b) Both Statement I and Statement II are true.
(c) Both Statement I and Statement II are false.
(d) Statement I is true but Statement II is false.

76. Match List-I with List-II.

List-I		List-II
A.	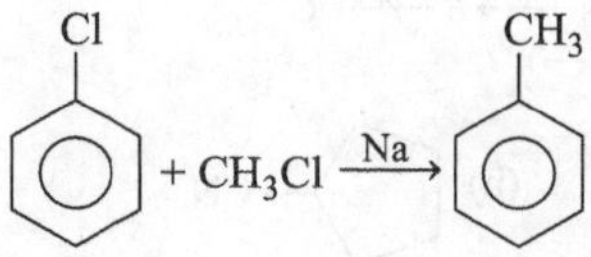	I. Fitting reaction
B.	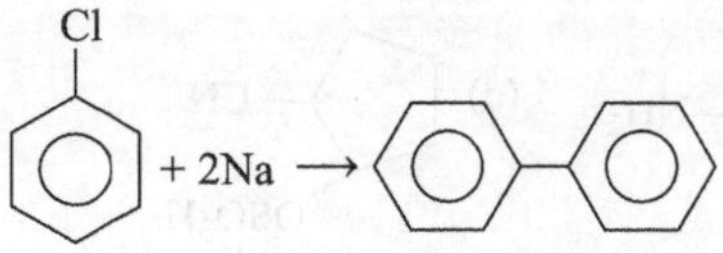	II. Wurtz Fittig reaction
C.	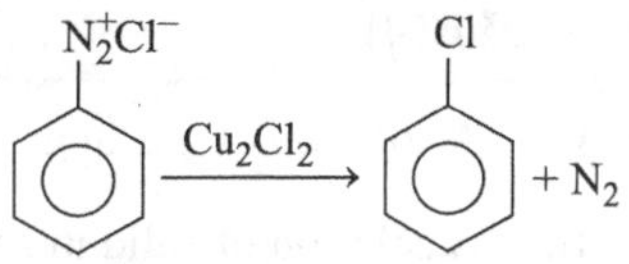	III. Finkelstein reaction
D.	$C_2H_5Cl + NaI \longrightarrow C_2H_5I + NaCl$	IV. Sandmeyer reaction

Choose the correct answer from the options given below:

(a) A-II, B-I, C-III, D-IV (b) A-II, B-I, C-IV, D-III
(c) A-IV, B-II, C-III, D-I (d) A-III, B-II, C-IV, D-I

77. In the preparation of *p*-nitro acctanilidc from anilinc, nitration is not done by nitrating mixture (a mixture of conc. H_2SO_4 and conc. HNO_3) because

(a) on nitration it gives *o*-nitroacetanilide.
(b) it gives a mixture of *o* and *p*-nitroaniline.
(c) —NH_2 group gets oxidised.
(d) it forms a mixture of *o* and *p*-nitro acetanilide.

78. Given below are two statements.

Statement I Dimethylglyoximato nickel (II) can show geometrical isomerism.
Statement II Tetrahedral complexes with chiral structures exhibit optical isomerism.
In the light of the above statements, choose the correct answer from the options given below.

(a) Statement I is false but Statement II is true.
(b) Both Statement I and Statement II are true.
(c) Both Statement I and Statement II are false.
(d) Statement I is true but Statement II is false.

79. If 10 moles of an ideal gas expands reversibly and isothermally from 10 L to 100 L at 300 K, then entropy change will be

(a) $191.47 JK^{-1} mol^{-1}$ (b) $191.24 JK^{-1}$
(c) $83.03 JK^{-1}$ (d) $83.03 JK^{-1} mol^{-1}$

80. Which is a possible set of quantum numbers for a valence electron in ground state atom of phosphorus ($Z = 15$)?

	n	l	m_l	m_s
(a)	2	1	0	+1/2
(b)	3	0	0	0
(c)	3	1	−1	+1/2
(d)	3	2	0	−1/2

81. Match List-I with List-II.

List-I		List-II	
A.	German silver	I.	A solution of gas in gas
B.	Soda water	II.	A solution of solid in solid
C.	Hydrogen gas in palladium	III.	A solution of gas in liquid
D.	Air	IV.	A solution of gas in solid

Choose the correct answer from the options given below:
(a) A-I, B-II, C-III, D-IV
(b) A-II, B-III, C-IV, D-I
(c) A-III, B-II, C-I, D-IV
(d) A-IV, B-III, C-II, D-I

82. Arrange the following elements in the order of their decreasing metallic character: Na, Si, Cl, Mg, Al.
(a) Cl > Si > Al > Mg > Na
(b) Na > Al > Mg > Cl > Si
(c) Na > Mg > Al > Si > Cl
(d) Al > Na > Si > Ca > Mg

83. What is/are advantage(s) of thin layer chromatography over column chromatography?
I. TLC is smaller and hence requires lesser amount of material.
II. More distinct individual spots which make determination easy.
III. R_f can be easily measured.
IV. TLC is slower and requires time.
V. TLC generally use silica gel as the stationary phase.
(a) I, II, IV
(b) IV only
(c) I, II, III, IV and V
(d) I, II, III and IV

84. Given below are two statements.
Statement I Phenol reacts with CCl_4 and NaOH followed by hydrolysis to give salicylic acid.
Statement II *Tert*-butyl methylether on heating with HI gives a mixture of *tert*-butyl iodide and methanol.
In the light of the above statements, choose the correct answer from the options given below.
(a) Statement I is false but Statement II is true.
(b) Both Statement I and Statement II are true.
(c) Both Statement I and Statement II are false.
(d) Statement I is true but Statement II is false.

85. The freezing point depression constant for water is 1.86°C m^{-1}. If 5g Na_2SO_4 is dissolved in 45g H_2O the freezing point is changed by 3.82°C. Calculate van't Hoff factor for Na_2SO_4.
(a) 2.05 (b) 2.62 (c) 3.11 (d) 0.381

80. Correct IUPAC name of $Mn_3(CO)_{12}$ is
(a) manganesedodecyl carbonyl (0)
(b) dodecacarbonyl manganate (0)
(c) dodecacarbonyl manganese (II)
(d) dodecacarbonyl trimanganese (0)

87. Which of the following arrangement of bond dissociation enthalpy of halogens is correct?
(a) F—F > Cl—Cl > Br—Br
(b) F—F < Cl—Cl < Br—Br
(c) F—> Cl—Cl < Br—Br
(d) F—F < Cl—Cl > Br—Br

88. Match the List-I with List-II.

List-I (Amine)		List-II (pK_a values)	
A.	*p*-toluidine	(i)	4.69
B.	*m*-toluidine	(ii)	5.12
C.	*o*-toluidine	(iii)	4.58
D.	Aniline	(iv)	4.39

Choose the correct answer from the options given below.
(a) A-(ii), B-(i), C-(iv), D-(iii)
(b) A-(iii), B-(iv), C-(i), D-(ii)
(c) A-(iv), B-(i), C-(ii), D-(iii)
(d) A-(i), B-(ii), C-(iii), D-(iv)

89. $C_2H_5Cl \xrightarrow{KCN} A \xrightarrow{H_3O^+} B$
Compound (*B*) in below reaction is
(a) ethylene chloride (b) acetic acid
(c) propionic aicd (d) ethyl cyanide

90. The major product obtained in reaction is

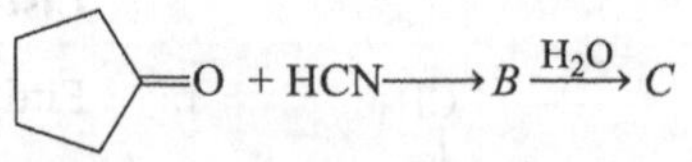

(a) 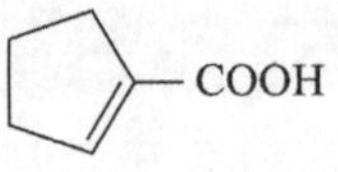

(b) 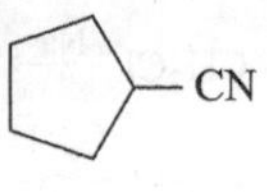

(c) 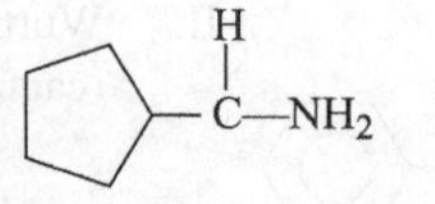

(d) 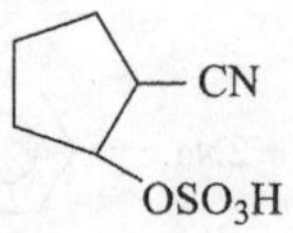

BIOLOGY

91. A species of fungus which can be used as a biocontrol agent is
(a) *Ashbya gossypii*
(b) *Trichoderma*
(c) *Aspergillus giganteus*
(d) *Penicillium chrysogenum*

92. Where is the major amount of cytokinin produced in vascular plants?
(a) Flowers (b) Leaves (c) Shoots (d) Roots

93. Given below are two statements.
Statement I In basal placentation, the placenta develops at the base of ovary and multiple ovules are attached to it.
Statement II In mustard, ovary is one chambered, but it becomes two chambered due to the formation of false septum.
In the light of the above statements, choose the correct answer from the options given below.
(a) Statement I is incorrect, but statement II is correct
(b) Both statement I and statement II are correct
(c) Both statement I and statement II are incorrect
(d) Statement I is correct, but statement II is incorrect

94. What will happen to the structure labelled as '*A*' in the diagram during contraction?

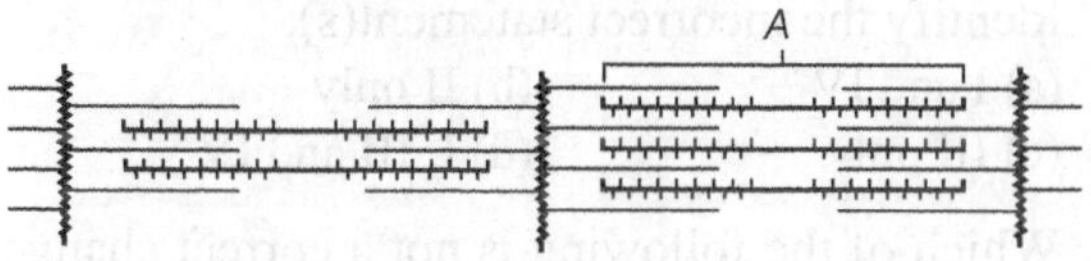

(a) Increases in length
(b) Decreases in length
(c) Remains same
(d) Disappear entirely

95. Consider the following set of statements.
I. Ctenophores are commonly known as sea walnuts or cnidocytes.
II. *Physalia* (Portuguese man of war) belongs to Coelenterata.
III. Platyhelminthes have specialised cells called flame cells for excretion.
IV. Digestion is both extracellular and intracellular in Ctenophora.
V. *Sycon* (Scypha) belongs to Ctenophora.

Choose the correct statements from the options given below.
(a) I, II and III
(b) III and V
(c) II, III and IV
(d) IV and V

96. Which of the following pair of alga is employed as food for human being?
(a) *Ulothrix; Volvox*
(b) *Chlorella* ; *Spirullina*
(c) *Polysiphonia ; Volvox*
(d) *Spirogyra* ; *Spirullina*

97. Given below are two statements.
Statement I The content of nucleolus is separated from nucleoplasm as it is a membrane bound structure.
Statement II Cells which are actively carrying out protein synthesis contain large and more numerous nucleoli.
In the light of the above statements, choose the correct answer from the options given below.
(a) Statement I is incorrect, but statement II is correct
(b) Both statement I and statement II are correct
(c) Both statement I and statement II are incorrect
(d) Statement I is correct, but statement II is incorrect

98. Which of the following statements is not correct with respect to Mendelian disorders?
(a) These disorders are determined by mutation in a single gene
(b) Phenylketonuria is an example of Mendelian disorder
(c) These disorders are mainly recessive
(d) Pattern of inheritance of such disorders can be made by pedigree analysis

99. Match List I with List II.

List I	List II
A. Psilopsida	1. *Adiantum*
B. Lycopsida	2. *Selaginella*
C. Sphenopsida	3. *Psilotum*
D. Pteropsida	4. *Equisetum*

Choose the correct answer from the options given below.

	A	B	C	D		A	B	C	D
(a)	3	1	2	4	(b)	3	2	4	1
(c)	2	4	3	1	(d)	3	1	4	2

100. Which of the following statements is incorrect regarding Assisted Reproductive Technologies (ART)?

(a) Artificial introduction of sperms of a healthy donor into the vagina
(b) Transfer of embryo upto 8 blastomere into the Fallopian tube
(c) Introduction of semen from donor into the clitoris
(d) Transfer of ovum from a donor into the Fallopian tube

101. Given below are two statements; one is labelled as Assertion (A) and the other is labelled as Reason (R).

Assertion (A) Nematode parasites cannot survive in a transgenic host expressing specific interfering RNA.

Reason (R) These RNAs initiate the RNAi process which silence the specific *m*RNA of parasite.

In the light of the above statements, choose the correct answer from the options given below.

(a) A is false, but R is true
(b) Both A and R are true and R is the correct explanation of A
(c) Both A and R are true, but R is not the correct explanation of A
(d) A is true, but R is false

102. Which one of the following statement is incorrect about the gross primary productivity?

(a) It is the rate of production of organic matter during photosynthesis
(b) A considerable amount of GPP is utilised by plants in respiration
(c) Gross primary productivity plus respiration loss (R), is the Net Primary Productivity (NPP)
(d) Gross primary productivity is always more than net primary productivity

103. The tertiary structure of a protein molecule results from all of the given, except

(a) electrostatic bonding (b) hydrophobic bonding
(c) hydrogen bonding (d) glycosidic bonding

104. Match List I with List II.

	List I		List II
A.	Gestation	1.	Delivery of baby from uterus
B.	Conception	2.	Rupture of Graafian follicle
C.	Parturition	3.	Process of fusion of a sperm with an ovum
D.	Ovulation	4.	Duration between pregnancy and birth

Choose the correct answer from the options given below.

	A	B	C	D
(a)	4	2	1	3
(b)	1	2	3	4
(c)	4	3	1	2
(d)	3	2	4	1

105. Consider the following statements.

I. Chloroplasts may be spherical, ovoid or disc shaped.
II. Mitochondria can be easily found in wings of an insect.
III. The ER membrane is thicker than the plasma membrane.
IV. Plant and fungal cells have a single stack of Golgi apparatus called dictyosomes.
V. Peroxisomes are also involved in photorespiration.

Identify the incorrect statement(s).

(a) I and IV (b) II only
(c) III only (d) I, III and IV

106. Which of the following is not a correct change about the seed development?

(a) As the seed matures, its water content is reduced
(b) Integuments of ovules harden to form a tough protective seed coat
(c) The general metabolic activity of embryo increase
(d) The micropyle remains as a small pore in the seed coat

107. Identify the incorrectly matched pair.

(a) Marginal placentation—Pea
(b) Axile placentation—Lemon
(c) Parietal placentation—Tomato
(d) Basal placentation—Sunflower

108. Graafian follicle contains large central follicular cavity called .... which ....
(a) stroma ; provides suitable environment for oocyte
(b) antrum; provides suitable environment for oocyte
(c) infundibulum ; aids in fertilisation
(d) ostium ; aids in fertilisation

109. Given below are two statements; one is labelled as Assertion (A) and the other is labelled as Reason (R).
Assertion (A) All factors in our body are favourable for diffusion of O_2 from tissue to alveoli and that of CO_2 from alveoli to tissues.
Reason (R) The thickness of diffusion membrane is much less than a millimeter.
In the light of the above statements, choose the correct answer from the options given below
(a) A is false, but R is true
(b) Both A and R are true and R is the correct explanation of A
(c) Both A and R are true, but R is not the correct explanation of A
(d) A is true, but R is false

110. What is the main function of the protein GLUT-4?
(a) Enables glucose transports into cells
(b) Fights against infectious organisms
(c) Serves as an enzyme as reaction booster
(d) Acts as a catalyst

111. Given below are two statements.
Statement I In banana the embryo develops parthenogenetically from the haploid egg.
Statement II Karyokinesis may occur after each meiotic division leading to the formation of isobilateral tetrad of microspore.
In the light of the above statements, choose the correct answer from the options given below.
(a) Statement I is incorrect, but statement II is correct
(b) Both statement I and statement II are correct
(c) Both statement I and statement II are incorrect
(d) Statement I is correct, but statement II is incorrect

112. Match List I with List II.

List I	List II
A. Bryophytes	1. Non-vascular, lacking seeds
B. Pteridophytes	2. Vascular, lacking seeds
C. Gymnosperms	3. Vascular, naked seeded plants
D. Algae	4. Flagellated zoospores

Choose the correct answer from the options given below.

	A	B	C	D		A	B	C	D
(a)	1	2	4	3	(b)	2	1	4	3
(c)	1	2	3	4	(d)	2	1	3	4

113. Which one of the following pairs of bacteria has been found to have extensive use in genetic engineering work in plants?
(a) *Bacillus coagulens ; Bacillus thuringiensis*
(b) *E. coli* ; *A. tumefaciens*
(c) *Salmonella typhi ; M. incognita*
(d) *Agrobacterium tumefaciens* ; *B. thuringiensis*

114. Name the enzyme used in dissolving blood clots in heart patients.
(a) Cyclosporin-A (b) Statins
(c) Amylase (d) Streptokinase

115. Match List I with List II.

List I	List II
A. Muscular pharynx	1. *Bombyx*
B. Metameres	2. *Ascaris*
C. Jointed appendages	3. *Pila*
D. Muscular foot	4. *Hirudinaria*

Codes

	A	B	C	D
(a)	1	3	2	4
(b)	2	4	1	3
(c)	3	2	4	1
(d)	3	1	4	2

116. Cryopreservation is an example of
(a) *ex situ* conservation strategies
(b) *in situ* conservation strategies
(c) tissue culture
(d) totipotent culture

117. Which among the following is the consumable form of marine fish?
(a) *Catla* (b) Mackerel
(c) Rohu (d) Common carp

118. The organism that is found in decaying wood in moist and damp places and reproduce asexually by aplanospores is
(a) *Mucor* and *Penicillium*
(b) *Neurospora* and *Alternaria*
(c) *Mucor* and *Albugo*
(d) *Neurospora* and *Penicillin*

119. Consider the following statements and select the correct set of statements.
I. On either side of frog's eyes a membrane tympanum receives sound signals.
II. Ears of frog are covered by a nictitating membrane.
III. Frog has only one pair of lymph hearts.
IV. Frog has 10 pairs of cranial nerves.
V. The midbrain of frog is characterised by a pair of optic lobes.

Choose the correct answer from the options given below.
(a) III and IV (b) I, IV and V
(c) II, III and V (d) I, II and IV

120. Given below are steps related to RNA processing in eukaryotes.
I. Cleavage of 3′ end and addition of adenylate residue.
II. Removal of phosphate group from terminal nucleotide.
III. Removal of introns and re-attachment of exons.
IV. Addition of methyl guanosine triphosphate to 5′ end of *hn*RNA.

Arrange the above steps in proper sequence and choose the correct option.
(a) II→I→III→IV
(b) III→I→II→IV
(c) IV→I→II→III
(d) II→IV→I→III

121. The core of a cilium called ...*A*... possess a number of microtubules running in direction ...*B*... to long axis.

	A	B
(a)	Linker	Tilled
(b)	Axoneme	Parallel
(c)	Linker	Perpendicular
(d)	Axoneme	Right angle

122. Which of the following set of RNAs are transcribed by the RNA polymerase I?
(a) 28S *r*RNA, 5S *r*RNA, 5.8S *r*RNA
(b) 28S *r*RNA, 18S *r*RNA, 5.8S *r*RNA
(c) *t*RNA, 5S *r*RNA, *sn*RNA
(d) *t*RNA, 5S *r*RNA, *hn*RNA

123. Match List I with List II.

List I		List II	
A.	Family	1.	Angiospermae
B.	Order	2.	Dicotyledonae
C.	Class	3.	Anacardiaceae
D.	Division	4.	Sapindales

Choose the correct answer from the options given below.

	A	B	C	D		A	B	C	D
(a)	1	2	3	4	(b)	4	3	2	1
(c)	3	4	2	1	(d)	2	3	4	1

124. The variations in chromosome structure is due to
I. deletion II. duplication
III. translocation IV. inversion

The correct option is
(a) I and II (b) III and IV
(c) II, III and IV (d) I, II, III and IV

125. A tetrad consists of
(a) four chromatids and four centromeres
(b) four chromatids and two centromeres
(c) two chromatids and four centromeres
(d) two chromatids and five centromeres

126. Given below are two statements.

Statement I The tunica intima is a middle layer of smooth muscle and elastic fibres.

Statement II Tunica externa is the external layer of fibrous connective tissue.

In the light of the above statements, choose the correct answer from the options given below.
(a) Statement I is incorrect, but statement II is correct
(b) Both statement I and statement II are correct
(c) Both statement I and statement II are incorrect
(d) Statement I is correct, but statement II is incorrect

127. Which of the following is true about prions?
(a) They have RNA with protein coat
(b) They consist of abnormally folded proteins only
(c) They are smaller in size than viruses
(d) They have free RNA without protein coat

128. Given below are two statements; one is labelled as Assertion (A) and the other is labelled as Reason (R).

Assertion Coronary Artery Disease affects the heart's major blood vessels.
Reason It is caused when no enough oxygen reaches the heart muscles.
In the light of the above statements, choose the correct answer from the options given below.
(a) A is false, but R is true
(b) Both A and R are true and R is the correct explanation of A
(c) Both A and R are true, but R is not the correct explanation of A
(d) A is true, but R is false

129. Given below are two statements.
Statement I Interkinesis is generally long lived.
Statement II Interkinesis is necessary for bringing true haploid DNA in daughter cells.
In the light of the above statement, choose the correct answer from the options given below.
(a) Statement I is incorrect, but statement II is correct
(b) Both statement I and statement II are correct
(c) Both statement I and statement II are incorrect
(d) Statement I is correct, but statement II is incorrect

130. Consider the following statements and choose the incorrect statements among them.
I. Typhoid is named after a cook Mary Mallon.
II. *Plasmodium falciparum* is the most serious type of malarial species.
III. *Ascarias* is the filarial worm that causes slowly developing chronic inflammation.
IV. B-lymphocytes mediate the cell mediated immunity.
V. Ringworms are acquired from the soil.
Choose the correct answer from the options given below.
(a) III and V (b) I, II and III
(c) III and IV (d) I, III and IV

131. Given below are two statements; one is labelled as Assertion (A) and the other is labelled as Reason (R).

Assertion (A) All aquatic plants are not hydrophilous.
Reason (R) Some hydrophytes like water hyacinth and water lily are entomophilous.
In the light of the above statements, choose the correct answer from the options given below.
(a) A is false, but R is true
(b) Both A and R are true and R is the correct explanation of A
(c) Both A and R are true, but R is not the correct explanation of A
(d) A is true, but R is false

132. Given below are two statements
Statement I The genetic information is available in monomeric units within the polymer.
Statement II In a nucleotide, the phosphate molecule is attached to third carbon atom of the deoxyribose molecules.
In the light of the above statements, choose the correct answer from the options given below.
(a) Statement I is incorrect, but statement II is correct
(b) Both statement I and statement II are correct
(c) Both statement I and statement II are incorrect
(d) Statement I is correct, but statement II is incorrect

133. In plant species like *Tamarindus* and *Orchid*, the endosperm is utilised by embryo and no endosperm is left at maturity. Such seeds are called
(a) ex-albuminous (b) albuminous
(c) xenia (d) metaxenia

134. Which of the following is correctly matched pair?
(a) HIV—Humoral immune virus
(b) AIDS—Acute immune deficiency syndrome
(c) ELISA—Enzyme linked immuno syndrome assay
(d) MALT—Mucosal Associated Lymphoid Tissue

135. Consider the following statements.

I. Only PS-I is functional in cyclic phosphorylation.
II. Cyclic phosphorylation results into synthesis of ATP and $NADPH_2$.
III. Z scheme of light reaction takes place in presence of PS-I only.
IV. Stroma lamellae lack PS-II as well as NADP.
V. Cyclic phosphorylation also occurs when only light of wavelengths beyond 680 nm are available for excitation.

Choose the correct set of statements from the options given below.
(a) I, III and IV (b) II, IV and V
(c) I, II and III (d) I, IV and V

136. Given below are two statements.
Statement I Gene therapy allows correction of a gene defect that has been diagnosed in a child/embryo.
Statement II In 1983, Eli lilly prepared three DNA sequence corresponding to chains of human insulin.
In the light of the above statements, choose the correct answer from the options given below.
(a) Statement I is incorrect, but statement II is correct
(b) Both statement I and statement II are correct
(c) Both statement I and statement II are incorrect
(d) Statement I is correct, but statement II is incorrect

137. How many molecules of CO_2 are evolved in glycolysis?
(a) 1 (b) 2 (c) 3 (d) 0

138. Which among the following statements is not correct regarding secondary growth in dicot stem?
(a) The vascular cambial ring develops as a circular ring since beginning
(b) The vascular rays are narrow since beginning
(c) Annual rings occur quite commonly
(d) Cambial ring formed is circular in the beginning and later becomes wavy

139. The muscle contraction requires energy which comes from ATP hydrolysis. The enzyme ATPase for this is present in
(a) globular head of meromyosin
(b) tropomyosin
(c) light meromyosin
(d) cisternae of sarcoplasmic reticulum

140. Identify the correct match with respect to dicot stem.
(a) Ground tissue – Lacks differentiation
(b) Secondary growth – Cambium present
(c) Hypodermis – Sclerenchymatous
(d) Vascular bundle – Conjoint and closed

141. The peripheral region of the secondary xylem which is lighter in colour is known as
(a) late wood (b) spring wood
(c) heart wood (d) sapwood

142. Mineralocorticoids are steroid hormones produced from
(a) zona fasciculata
(b) zona glomerulosa
(c) zona reticularis
(d) zona pellucida

143. The function of companion cell is to
(a) help the sieve tube members in translocation of food material
(b) provide mechanical support
(c) store food material
(d) accumulate tannins

144. The primary CO_2 acceptor which is present in the mesophyll cells is called
(a) PEP (b) RuBisCO
(c) RuBP (d) PEPcase

145. Which of the following statements are incorrect regarding mitochondria?

I. Mitochondrial matrix contains single circular DNA molecule and ribosome.
II. Outer membrane is permeable to monomers of carbohydrates, fats and proteins.
III. Inner membrane is convoluted infoldings.
IV. Enzymes of electron transport are embedded in outer membrane.
V. Mitochondria divide by fragmentation.

(a) I and III (b) II and V
(c) IV and V (d) Only II

146. Broca's area present in the left frontal lobe of the human brain controls
(a) learning and reasoning
(b) movement of tongue
(c) breathing and hiccups
(d) reflex actions

147. Simple, rarely compound, alternate, sessile exstipulate reticulate venation are the characteristics of leaves belonging to family
(a) Fabaceae (b) Brassicaceae
(c) Graminae (d) Malvaceae

148. Golden rice is a successful transgenic crop. When released for cultivation, it will help in
(a) herbicide tolerance
(b) pest resistance
(c) alleviation of vitamin-A deficiency
(d) producing biofuel

149. Electrons from NADH produced in the mitochondrial matrix during citric acid cycle are oxidised by complex I, i.e.
(a) cytochrome-bc_1
(b) succinate dehydrogenase
(c) NADH dehydrogenase
(d) cytochrome-*c* oxidase

150. Pituitary gland or hypophysis is a pea-shaped gland which lies in the cavity called tursica of
(a) ethmoid (b) sphenoid
(c) nasal (d) vomer

151. Which one of the following four glands is incorrectly matched with the accompanying description?
(a) Thyroid - Hyposecretion in children causes cretinism
(b) Parathyroid - Secretes parathormone that regulates amount of calcium and phosphate between blood and other tissues
(c) Pineal - Secretes three groups of steroid hormone from cholesterol
(d) Thymus - Starts undergoing atrophy after puberty

152. Match List I with List II.

List I	List II
A. Chemosynthetic bacteria	1. Chlorophyll-*a*
B. Photosynthetic bacteria	2. Silica
C. Dinoflagellate	3. Nitrates and nitrites
D. Chrysophytes	4. Cellulose

Codes

	A	B	C	D		A	B	C	D
(a)	3	1	4	2	(b)	1	2	4	3
(c)	1	4	3	2	(d)	4	1	2	3

153. Given below are two statements; one is labelled as Assertion (A) and other is labelled as Reason (R).
Assertion (A) Aldosterone helps in the maintenance of electrolytes, osmotic pressure and blood pressure.
Reason (R) Small amounts of androgenic steroids are also secreted by the adrenal cortex.
In the light of the above statements, choose the correct answer from the options given below.
(a) A is false, but R is true
(b) Both A and R are true and R is the correct explanation of A
(c) Both A and R are true, but R is not the correct explanation of A
(d) A is true, but R is false

154. The first phase of translation is
(a) recognition of anti-codon
(b) recognition of DNA molecule
(c) binding of *m*RNA to ribosome
(d) aminoacylation of *t*RNA

155. Haemodialysis is associated with ....
(a) removal of excess water only
(b) blood drained from heart
(c) blood drained from convenient artery
(d) removal of impurities in liver

156. Which one of the following symbols and their representation, used in human pedigree analysis is incorrect?
(a) 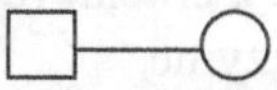 = mating
(b) 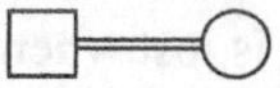 = mating between relatives
(c)  = unaffected male
(d) 

= five affected offsprings

157. The hypercalcaemic hormone that plays a significant role in calcium balance in the body is
(a) thymosins (b) parathyroid hormone
(c) thyroxine (d) epinephrine

158. A type of aneuploidy where unmasking of a recessive lethal allele that is otherwise tolerated in heterozygotes carrying the corresponding wild-type allele, may lead to failure of individual to survive is
(a) trisomy (b) monosomy
(c) disomy (d) amphidiploidy

159. Identify the incorrectly matched pair.
(a) Chitinase – Fungal cell wall
(b) Vector – Vehicles of DNA transfer
(c) Upstream processing – Separation and purification
(d) *Hind* II – First restriction endonulease

160. Choose the correct set of statements for the diagram given below.

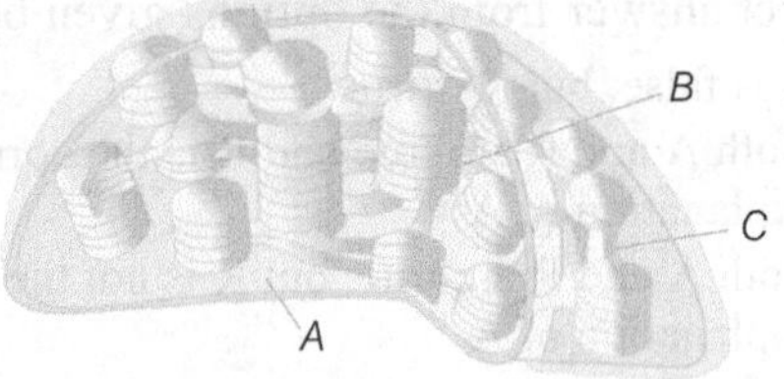

I. *A* contains enzymes required for the synthesis of carbohydrates and proteins.
II. *B* is the site of the location of the enzymes for the biosynthetic phase of photosynthesis in higher plants.
III. C lacks PS-II as well as NADP reductase enzyme.

Codes
(a) I and II (b) II and III
(c) I and III (d) I, II and III

161. Given below are two statements; one is labelled as Assertion (A) and the other is labelled as Reason (R).
Assertion (A) Cofactors have a crucial role to play in catalytic activity of enzyme.
Reason (R) Catalytic activity is lost when cofactor is removed from enzyme.
In the light of the above statements, choose the correct answer from the options given below.
(a) A is false, but R is true
(b) Both A and R are true and R is the correct explanation of A
(c) Both A and R are true, but R is not the correct explanation of A
(d) A is true, but R is false

162. Identify the correct sequences based on progressive evolution.
(a) *Chara, Ulva, Selaginella, Cedrus*
(b) *Agaricus, Chlamydomonas, Pteris, Pinus*
(c) Lichens, *Agaricus, Cedrus, Marchantia*
(d) *Ulva, Funaria, Equisetum, Cedrus*

163. The recent illegal introduction of the African catfish *Clarias gariepinus* for aquaculture purposes is posing a threat to indigenous catfishes in rivers. This is an example of
(a) habitat loss
(b) over-exploitation
(c) alien species invasions
(d) fragmentation

164. The ……… fibres taper at both ends (fusiform) and do not show striations.
(a) skeletal muscle (b) smooth muscle
(c) sardiac muscle (d) neural tissue

165. Eyes of *Octopus* are analogous to………… thus, showing …………
(a) eyes of poriferans ; convergent evolution
(b) eyes of annelids ; adaptive radiation
(c) eyes of mammals ; convergent evolution
(d) eyes of aves ; divergent evolution

166. X-ray diffraction studies were critical evidence indicating that DNA has a double-helix structure. These studies were done by
(a) Watson and Crick
(b) Chargaff
(c) Rosalind Franklin and Maurice Wilkins
(d) Meselson and Stahl

167. What is a polysome?
(a) Initiation site for transcription
(b) Initiation complex for translation
(c) A number of ribosomes on the same transcript
(d) Elongation factor in DNA synthesis or replication

168. Given below are two statements.
Statement I Besides acting as conduits for energy transfer across trophic levels, parasites also play other important roles.
Statement II In the rocky intertidal communities of the American Pacific Coast the starfish *Pisaster* is an important predator.
In the light of the above statements, choose the correct answer from the options given below.
(a) Statement I is incorrect, but statement II is correct
(b) Both statement I and statement II are correct
(c) Both statement I and statement II are incorrect
(d) Statement I is correct, but statement II is incorrect

169. What is the function of centrosome?
(a) Duplication of chromosomes
(b) Formation of spindle fibres
(c) Duplication of DNA
(d) Duplication of RNA

170. Narrow utilitarian aspect of biodiversity conservation includes all of the following, except
(a) pine resin
(b) gums and tannin sources
(c) dyes
(d) pollination

171. Which of the following statements are incorrect with respect to the structural and functional unit of kidney?
I. Inner wall of Bowman's capsule is in close contact with glomerular capillaries.
II. Bowman's capsule and glomerulus together form renal corpuscle.
III. Basement membrane of capillary wall is a discontinuous layer between glomerular capillaries and Bowman's capsule.
IV. PCT starts from Bowman's capsule and lies in the medulla region of kidney.
V. DCT is similar to PCT, but lies in renal cortex.
Choose the correct answer from the options given below.
(a) I and V (b) III and IV
(c) II and IV (d) II and III

172. Match List I with List II

	List I		List II
A.	*Haemophilus influenzae*	1.	Filariasis
B.	*P. falciparum*	2.	Amoebiasis
C.	*W. malayi*	3.	Pneumonia
D.	*Entamoeba histolytica*	4.	Malaria

Codes

	A	B	C	D
(a)	2	3	4	1
(b)	2	1	4	3
(c)	1	4	2	3
(d)	3	4	1	2

173. A person was suffering from a disorder '*X*' usually observed in middle age where a part of his/her heart does not get enough blood and oxygen. Name the disorder '*X*'.
(a) Atherosclerosis (b) Angina pectoris
(c) Hypertension (d) Heart failure

174. Consider the following statements.
I. Spermatogenesis starts at the age of puberty due to significant decrease in secretion of GnRH.
II. All copulations lead to pregnancy.
III. By the end of 12 weeks the foetus begins to show movements.
IV. Process of childbirth is induced by a complex neuroendocrine mechanism.
The incorrect set of statements are
(a) I and IV (b) IV only
(c) II and III (d) III and IV

175. Match List I with List II.

	List I		List II
A.	Plasmid	1.	Cuts at extreme ends
B.	*ori*	2.	Transfer or collection of separated DNA fragments
C.	Restriction exonuclease	3.	Initiation of replication
D.	Elution	4.	Autonomous replication

Choose the correct answer from the options given below.

	A	B	C	D
(a)	3	2	4	1
(b)	4	3	1	2
(c)	1	3	4	2
(d)	2	1	3	4

176. Identify the incorrect statement.
(a) Human Genome Project can identify approx. 40,000 – 15,000 genes in human DNA.
(b) HGP was coordinated by the US department of energy.
(c) *Caenorhabditis elegans, Arabidopsis* can also be sequenced using HGP.
(d) Human genome contains 3164.7 million bp.

177. Which of the following correctly defines phylum-Coelenterata?

(a) Diploblastic, mostly marine and radially symmetrical
(b) Diploblastic, unsegmented body and acoelomate condition
(c) Triploblastic, mostly marine and radially symmetrical
(d) Triploblastic, free-swimming and bilaterally symmetrical

178. Given below are two statements.

Statement I Some aquatic ecosystems have inverted biomass pyramids.

Statement II Pyramid of biomass is always upright.

In the light of the above statements, choose the correct answer from the options given below.

(a) Statement I is incorrect, but statement II is correct
(b) Both statement I and statement II are correct
(c) Both statement I and statement II are incorrect
(d) Statement I is correct, but statement II is incorrect

179. Match List I with List II.

	List I		List II
A.	Tendon	1.	Contractile protein
B.	Smooth muscle	2.	Connective tissue
C.	Myosin	3.	Globular protein
D.	Troponin	4.	Involuntary

Choose the correct answer from the options given below.

	A	B	C	D		A	B	C	D
(a)	1	2	3	4	(b)	3	2	1	4
(c)	2	4	1	3	(d)	1	2	4	3

180. Which of the following statement is incorrect about stem?

(a) In some plants, stems contain chlorophyll and carry out photosynthesis
(b) Stems also act as organs of perennation to tide over unfavourable growth conditions
(c) In *Euphorbia,* stems are modified into flattened structures
(d) Thorns protect plants from browsing animals

Answers

Physics

1.	(d)	2.	(b)	3.	(b)	4.	(a)	5.	(c)	6.	(b)	7.	(d)	8.	(b)	9.	(a)	10.	(c)
11.	(a)	12.	(a)	13.	(a)	14.	(c)	15.	(a)	16.	(a)	17.	(c)	18.	(d)	19.	(a)	20.	(c)
21.	(a)	22.	(c)	23.	(c)	24.	(d)	25.	(a)	26.	(b)	27.	(a)	28.	(a)	29.	(b)	30.	(c)
31.	(d)	32.	(c)	33.	(c)	34.	(d)	35.	(b)	36.	(b)	37.	(c)	38.	(a)	39.	(a)	40.	(a)
41.	(d)	42.	(b)	43.	(c)	44.	(a)	45.	(b)										

Chemistry

46.	(a)	47.	(b)	48.	(b)	49.	(a)	50.	(a)	51.	(d)	52.	(b)	53.	(a)	54.	(b)	55.	(d)
56.	(b)	57.	(d)	58.	(b)	59.	(c)	60.	(c)	61.	(c)	62.	(d)	63.	(a)	64.	(b)	65.	(d)
66.	(a)	67.	(b)	68.	(b)	69.	(b)	70.	(d)	71.	(b)	72.	(c)	73.	(a)	74.	(d)	75.	(b)
76.	(b)	77.	(c)	78.	(a)	79.	(a)	80.	(c)	81.	(b)	82.	(c)	83.	(c)	84.	(b)	85.	(b)
86.	(d)	87.	(d)	88.	(a)	89.	(c)	90.	(a)										

Biology

91	(b)	92	(d)	93	(a)	94	(c)	95	(c)	96	(b)	97	(a)	98	(c)	99	(b)	100	(c)
101	(b)	102	(c)	103	(d)	104	(c)	105	(c)	106	(c)	107	(c)	108	(b)	109	(a)	110	(a)
111	(d)	112	(c)	113	(d)	114	(d)	115	(b)	116	(a)	117	(b)	118	(c)	119	(b)	120	(d)
121	(b)	122	(b)	123	(c)	124	(d)	125	(b)	126	(a)	127	(b)	128	(d)	129	(a)	130	(c)
131	(b)	132	(d)	133	(a)	134	(d)	135	(d)	136	(d)	137	(d)	138	(d)	139	(a)	140	(b)
141	(d)	142	(a)	143	(a)	144	(a)	145	(c)	146	(b)	147	(b)	148	(c)	149	(c)	150	(b)
151	(c)	152	(a)	153	(c)	154	(d)	155	(c)	156	(d)	157	(b)	158	(b)	159	(c)	160	(c)
161	(b)	162	(d)	163	(c)	164	(b)	165	(c)	166	(c)	167	(c)	168	(a)	169	(b)	170	(d)
171	(b)	172	(d)	173	(b)	174	(c)	175	(b)	176	(a)	177	(a)	178	(d)	179	(c)	180	(c)

Scan this QR code from your mobile phone to get the explanations of this paper.

SECTION II

Mastery Builders

PRACTICE SET 12

Maximum Marks : 720	Time : 3 hrs	No. of Questions : 180

Instructions

1. This question paper contains **180** multiple-choice questions (four options with a single correct answer) from **Physics**, **Chemistry** and **Biology**.
2. These questions are distributed as 45 questions, each from Physics and Chemistry and 90 questions in Biology. These are to be compulsorily attempted by the candidate.
3. Each question carries 4 marks. For each correct response, the candidate will get 4 marks. For each incorrect response, one mark will be deducted from the total scores.

PHYSICS

1. The centripetal acceleration of a satellite of mass 1000 kg orbiting at 1600 km above the earth's surface is
(Take, radius of earth $= 6.4 \times 10^6$ m and $g = 9.8\ \text{ms}^{-2}$)

(a) $6.272\ \text{ms}^{-2}$ (b) $2.563\ \text{ms}^{-2}$
(c) $4.525\ \text{ms}^{-2}$ (d) $6.562\ \text{ms}^{-2}$

2. An electromagnetic wave is propagating in a medium with a velocity $v = -a\,\hat{\mathbf{j}}$. Magnetic field oscillates in the direction of $+X$-axis, then the direction of oscillating electric field of electromagnetic wave will be

(a) along $-x$-direction (b) along $+y$-direction
(c) along $-z$-direction (d) along $+z$-direction

3. The dominant mechanism for motion of charge carriers in forward and reverse biased silicon p-n junction are

(a) diffusion in forward biased, drift in reverse bias
(b) drift in forward biased, drift in reverse biased
(c) diffusion in both forward and reverse bias
(d) drift in both forward and reverse bias

4. A resonance air column shows resonance with a tuning fork of frequency 256 Hz at column lengths 32.5 cm and 112.9 cm. The end correction and speed of sound in air are

(a) 4.1 cm, $77.7\ \text{ms}^{-1}$ (b) 7.7 cm, $411.65\ \text{ms}^{-1}$
(c) 5 cm, $224.5\ \text{ms}^{-1}$ (d) 6.7 cm, $352.7\ \text{ms}^{-1}$

5. A monkey is descending from the branch of a tree with constant acceleration. If the breaking strength is 25% of the weight of the monkey, then the maximum acceleration with which monkey can slide down without breaking the branch is

(a) g (b) $\frac{3g}{4}$
(c) $\frac{g}{4}$ (d) $\frac{g}{2}$

6. In Young's double slit experiment, the fringe width is found to 0.5 mm. If the whole apparatus is immersed in liquid of refractive index $\frac{5}{3}$, without disturbing the geometrical arrangement, then new fringe width will be

(a) 0.35 m (b) 0.6 mm
(c) 0.45 mm (d) 0.3 mm

7. In the circuit shown below, current flowing through 25 V cell is

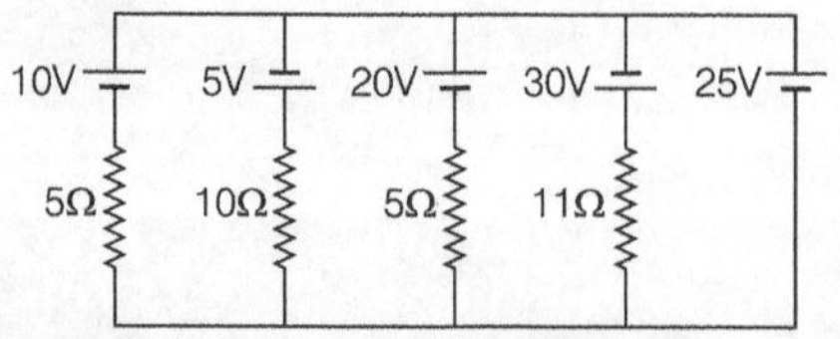

(a) 10 A (b) 7.2 A
(c) 12 A (d) 14.2 A

8. The value of current in the following diagram will be

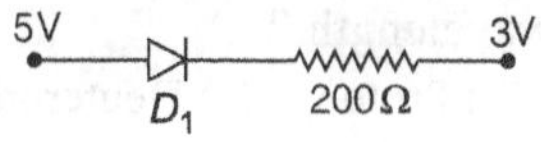

(a) 10 mA (b) 1 mA (c) 0.1 mA (d) zero

9. For an *L-C-R* series resonance circuit, which graph shows the correct relation between frequency (f) of AC source and impedance (Z) ?
[Here, $f_0 \rightarrow$ resonant frequency]

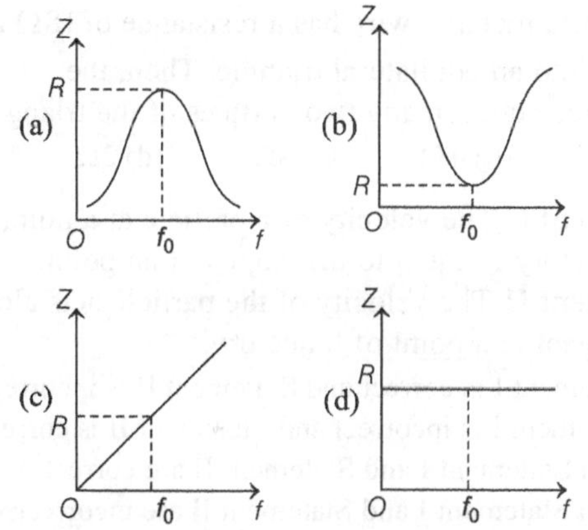

10. A particle is thrown at an angle of θ with velocity u in vertical direction. It just crosses the top of two poles each of height h after 1s and 3s, respectively. The maximum height of the projectile is

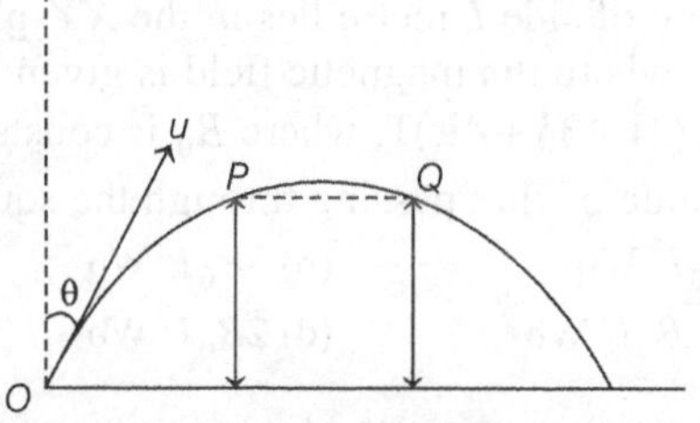

(a) 39.2 m (b) 19.6 m
(c) 9.8 m (d) 4.9 m

11. In the given (V-T) graph, what is the relation between p_1 and p_2?

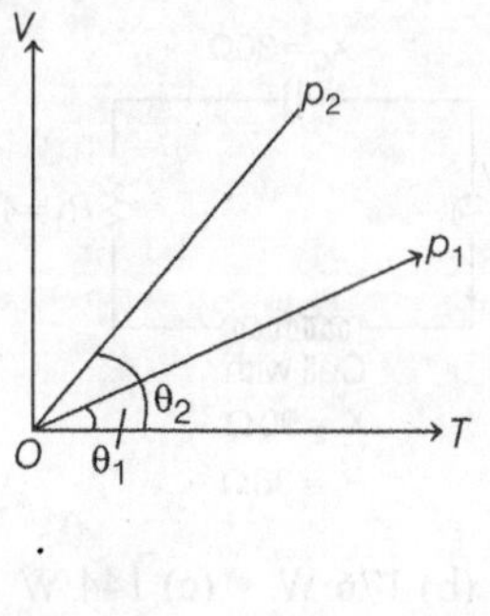

(a) $p_1 = \frac{3}{2} p_2$ (b) $p_2 = p_1$
(c) $p_2 > p_1$ (d) $p_2 < p_1$

12. Given below are two statements

Statement I If two unlike charges are brought nearer, then potential energy of system increases.

Statement II If two charges q_1 and q_2 are separated by a distance r, then potential energy of the system is given by $U = \frac{1}{4\pi\varepsilon_0} \frac{q_1 q_2}{r^2}$.

(a) Both Statement I and Statement II are correct.
(b) Both Statement I and Statement II are incorrect.
(c) Statement I is correct but Statement II is incorrect.
(d) Statement I is incorrect but Statement II is correct.

13. The radius of gyration k of a solid sphere of mass M and radius R about a certain axis is equal to $\sqrt{2}\,R$. Find the distance of that axis from the centre of the sphere.

(a) $\frac{\sqrt{2}}{5} R$ (b) $\frac{2\sqrt{2}}{\sqrt{5}} R$
(c) $\frac{2}{\sqrt{5}} R$ (d) $\sqrt{\frac{2}{5}} R$

14. When a gas expands adiabatically,

(a) no energy is required for expansion
(b) energy is required and it comes from the container wall
(c) internal energy of the gas is used in performing work
(d) law of conservation of energy is violated

15. A beam of light composed of red and green rays is incident obliquely at a point on the face of a rectangular glass slab. When coming out on the opposite parallel face, then the red and green rays emerge from

(a) two points propagating in two different non-parallel directions.
(b) two points propagating in two different parallel directions.
(c) one point propagating in two different directions.
(d) one point propagating in the same direction.

16. The frequency of a light wave in a material is 2×10^{14} Hz and wavelength is 5000Å. The refractive index of material will be

(a) 1.40 (b) 1.50
(c) 3 (d) 1.33

17. The following observations were taken for determining surface tension T of water by capillary method. Diameter of capillary, $D = 1.25 \times 10^{-2}$ m

Rise of water, $h = 1.45 \times 10^{-2}$ m

Using $g = 9.80$ ms^{-2} and the simplified relation, $T = \frac{rhg}{2} \times 10^3$ Nm^{-1}, the possible error in surface tension is closest to

(a) 0.15 % (b) 1.5 % (c) 2.4 % (d) 10 %

18. An isotropic material has coefficient of linear expansion α_1, α_2 and α_3 along X, Y and Z axes, respectively. If γ is coefficient of cubical expansion of its material, then

(a) $3\gamma = \alpha_1 + 2\alpha_2 + \alpha_3$ (b) $\gamma = \alpha_1 + \alpha_2 + \alpha_3$

(c) $2\gamma = 2\alpha_1 + \alpha_2 + \alpha_3$ (d) $\gamma = \alpha_1 + \alpha_2 + \frac{\alpha_1^2}{\alpha_3}$

19. If a stone is hit a point at a distance d away and height h above the point from where the stone starts as shown in the figure. The initial velocity of stone is

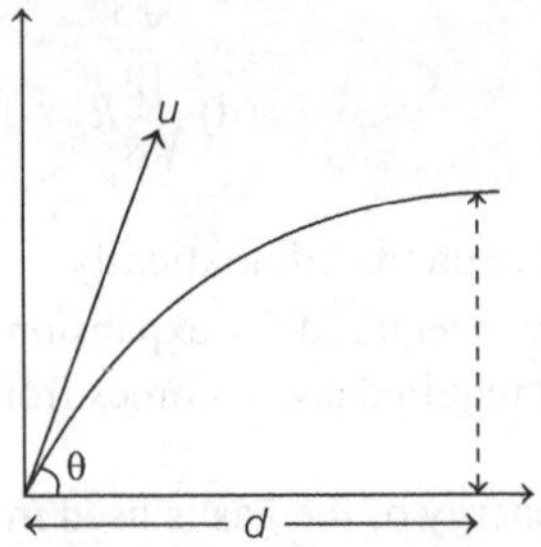

(a) $\sqrt{\frac{gd^2}{d-h}}$ (b) $\frac{d}{\cos\theta}\sqrt{\frac{g}{2(d\tan\theta - h)}}$

(c) $\sqrt{\frac{gd^2}{h\cos^2\theta}}$ (d) $\frac{g}{\cos\theta}\sqrt{\frac{d}{2(d\tan\theta - h)}}$

20. A charge q is enclosed in a cube at its centre, then electric flux associated with two opposite faces of the cube is

(a) $q/6\varepsilon_0$ (b) zero (c) $q/3\varepsilon_0$ (d) $2q/3\varepsilon_0$

21. The copper wire is stretched to make it 0.5% longer. The percentage change in its electrical resistance, if its volume remain unchanged is

(a) 2.0% (b) 1.0% (c) 0.5% (d) 2.5%

22. The magnetic field of an electromagnetic wave is given by $B_y = 3 \times 10^{-7} \sin(10^3 x + 6.28 \times 10^{12} t)$.

The wavelength of the electromagnetic wave is

(a) 0.32 cm (b) 0.63 cm (c) 6.28 cm (d) 3.14 cm

23. If the particles listed below all have the same kinetic energy, which one would possess the shortest de-Broglie wavelength ?

(a) Electron (b) Proton (c) Deuteron (d) α-particle

24. A bar magnet is cut into four equal parts such that each part has cross-sectional area and length equal to half of the original values the pole strength of each part is

(a) half of the initial (b) remains same

(c) one-fourth of the initial (d) None of these

25. A uniform metallic wire has a resistance of 18Ω and is bent into an equilateral triangle. Then, the resistance between any two vertices of the triangle is

(a)12Ω (b) 4Ω (c) 8Ω (d) 2Ω

26. **Statement I** The velocity of a particle at a point on its trajectory is equal to the slope at that point.

Statement II The velocity of the particle acts along the tangent at a point of trajectory.

(a) Statement I is correct and Statement II is incorrect.
(b) Statement I is incorrect and Statement II is correct.
(c) Both Statement I and Statement II are correct.
(d) Both Statement I and Statement II are incorrect.

27. A stone of mass 0.3 kg attached to a 1.5 m long string is whirled around in a horizontal circle at a speed of 6 m/s. The tension in the string is

(a) 10 N (b) 30 N (c) 7.2 N (d) 5.5 N

28. A square of side L metre lies in the XY-plane in a region, where the magnetic field is given by $\mathbf{B} = B_0(2\hat{\mathbf{i}} + 3\hat{\mathbf{j}} + 4\hat{\mathbf{k}})$T, where B_0 is constant. The magnitude of flux passing through the square is

(a) $4B_0L^2$ Wb (b) $3B_0L^2$ Wb

(c) $\sqrt{29}B_0L^2$ Wb (d) $2B_0L^2$ Wb

29. A series circuit consists of a capacitor of capacitive reactance 30Ω, a non-inductive resistor of 44Ω and a coil of inductive reactance 90Ω and a resistance of 36Ω connected across 200 V, 60 H line as shown in the figure. Find the power dissipated in the coil.

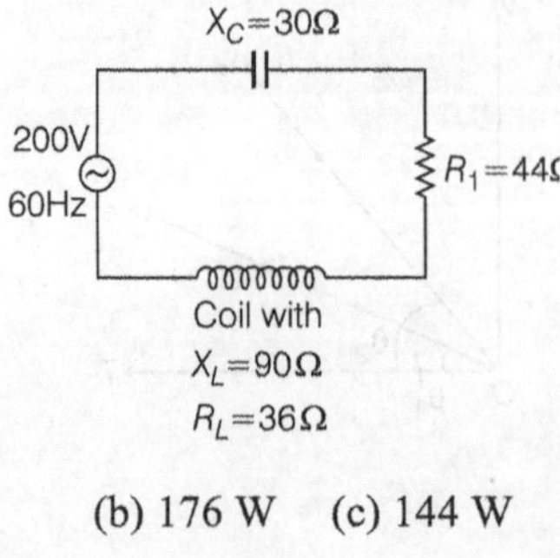

(a) 0 W (b) 176 W (c) 144 W (d) 320 W

30. If voltage across a bulb rated 220 V-100 W drop by 2.5% of its rated value, the percentage of the rated value by which the power would decrease is
(a) 2.5% (b) 10%
(c) 20% (d) 5%

31. An AC voltage source has an output of $\Delta V = (200\text{ V})\sin 2\pi ft$. The source is connected to a 100Ω resistor. The rms current in the resistance is
(a) 0.71 A (b) 2.41 A
(c) 1.41 A (d) 3.41 A

32. The de-Broglie wavelength of neutron at 27°C is λ, what will be its wavelength at 927°C?
(a) $\frac{\lambda}{2}$ (b) $\frac{\lambda}{3}$ (c) $\frac{\lambda}{9}$ (d) $\frac{\lambda}{4}$

33. A solid cylinder of radius 5 cm and mass 300 g rolls down an inclined plane (1 in 20). The velocity of cylinder after 5s will be
(a) 1.63 ms^{-1} (b) 1.56 ms^{-1}
(c) 2 ms^{-1} (d) 3.26 ms^{-1}

34. Radius of an air bubble at certain depth of Indian ocean is r and it becomes $18r$, when air bubble rises to the top surface of the ocean. If pressure due to t cm depth in the ocean is equal to the atmospheric pressure, then the depth of the ocean is
(a) $3835\,t$ cm (b) $3400\,t$ cm
(c) $4852\,t$ cm (d) $5831\,t$ cm

35. The gravitational field due to a mass distribution is $I = k / r^3$ in the x-direction (k is a constant). The gravitational potential is taken to be zero at infinity, then its value at a distance x is
(a) k/x (b) $k/2x$ (c) k/x^2 (d) $k/2x^2$

36. Two polaroids are crossed. If now one of them is rotate through 30° and unpolarised light of intensity I_0 is incident on the first polaroid, then the intensity of transmitted light will be
(a) $\frac{I_0}{4}$ (b) $\frac{3I_0}{4}$ (c) $\frac{3I_0}{8}$ (d) $\frac{I_0}{8}$

37. A body of mass m_1 moving with a velocity 3 ms^{-1} collides with another body at rest of mass m_2. After collision, the velocities of the two bodies are 2 ms^{-1} and 5 ms^{-1} respectively, along the direction of motion of m_1. The ratio of $\frac{m_1}{m_2}$ is
(a) $\frac{5}{12}$ (b) 5 (c) $\frac{1}{5}$ (d) $\frac{12}{5}$

38. Three long, straight parallel wires carrying currents are placed in a plane as shown in the fig. The force acting on half metre length of wire C will be

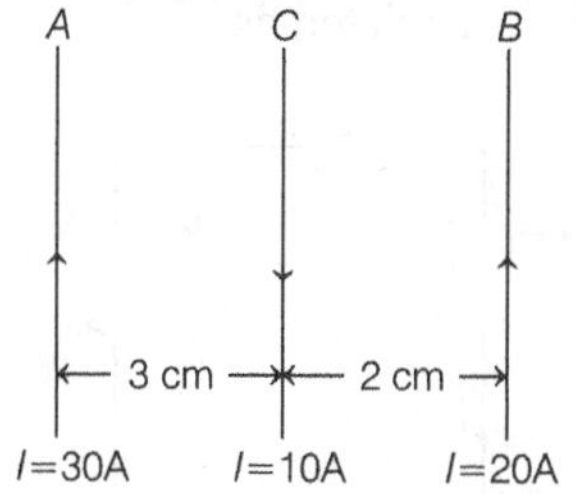

(a) 2.5×10^{-4} N (b) 1.4×10^{-5} N
(c) 3.7×10^{-3} N (d) zero

39. A free nucleus of mass 2 amu emits a gamma photon (when initially at rest) the wavelength of gamma photon is 0.01 Å. Find recoil speed of the nucleus.
(a) 2×10^5 m/s
(b) 5×10^4 m/s
(c) 6×10^4 m/s
(d) 12×10^5 m/s

40. Three rods A, B and C made of same material and having cross-section in ratio 1 : 2 : 3 are joined as shown in the figure. Each rod is of same length. The temperature at the junction of the three rods (in °C) is

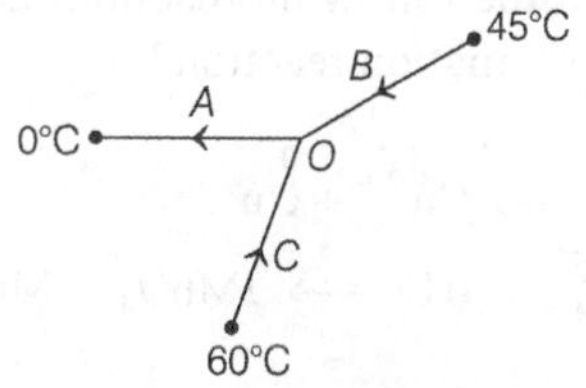

(a) 45 (b) 60
(c) 80 (d) 35

41. When a weight of 1 kg is suspended from a weightless spring, its length increases by 2 cm. The weight is pulled down by 10 cm and released, then the period of oscillation of spring and its kinetic energy are (take, $g = 10\text{ ms}^{-2}$)
(a) 2.5 s, 0.28 J
(b) 0.5 s, 5 J
(c) 0.28 s, 2.5 J
(d) 5 s, 0.5 J

42. An electron is orbiting in 4th orbit of H-atom. If radius of this orbit is r, then de-Broglie wavelength associated with electron is
(a) πr (b) $2\pi r$
(c) $8\pi r$ (d) $12\pi r$

43. A charge Q is fixed at each of two opposite corners of square. A charge q is placed at each of the other corners. If the resultant electric force on Q is zero, then Q and q are related as

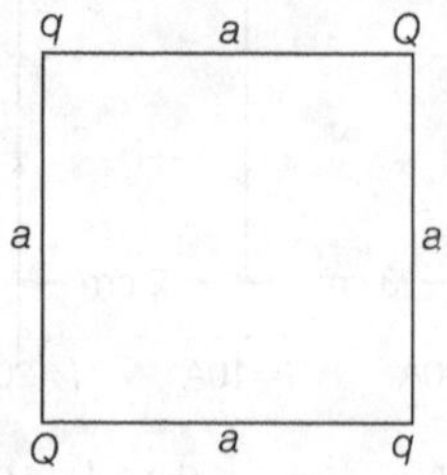

(a) $Q=-2\sqrt{2}q$
(b) $Q=2\sqrt{2}q$
(c) $Q=\sqrt{2}q$
(d) $Q=-\sqrt{2}q$

44. In the circuit below, capacitors A and B have identical geometry but a material of dielectric constant 3 is present between the plate of B. The potential differences across A and B are, respectively

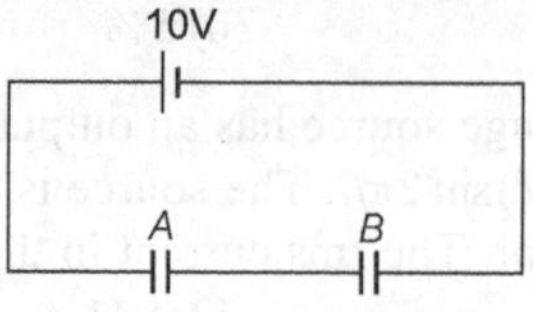

(a) 2.5V, 0.5V (b) 8V, 2V
(c) 2V, 8V (d) 7.5V, 2.5 V

45. A current of 2 A flows through a 2Ω resistor, when connected across a battery. The same battery supplies a current of 0.5 A when connected across a 9Ω resistor. The internal resistance of the battery is

(a) 0.5Ω (b) 1Ω
(c) $(1/3)\Omega$ (d) $(1/4)\Omega$

CHEMISTRY

46. One litre of pond water contains 20 mg of Ca^{+2} and 12 mg of Mg^{+2} ions, what is the volume of 0.2 N. Na_2CO_3 required to soften 5000 liters of pond water.

(a) 0.5 L (b) 25 L (c) 75 L (d) 50 L

47. Which of the following reactions are disproportionation reaction?

A. $2Cu^+ \longrightarrow Cu^{2+} + \overset{0}{Cu}$

B. $3MnO_4^{2-} + 4H^+ \longrightarrow 2MnO_4^- + MnO_2 + 2H_2O$

C. $2KMnO_4 \xrightarrow{\Delta} K_2MnO_4 + MnO_2 + O_2$

D. $2MnO_4^- + 3Mn^{2+} + 2H_2O \longrightarrow 5MnO_2 + 4H^+$

E. $2H_2O_2^{-1} \longrightarrow H_2\overset{-2}{O} + \overset{0}{O_2}$

In the light of the above statements. Choose the correct statements.

(a) A, C, D (b) C and B
(c) D, C, B (d) A, B and E

48. Given below are two statements.

Statement I Boron is extremely hard indicating its high lattice energy.

Statement II Boron has highest melting and boiling point compared to its other group members.

In the light of the above statements, choose the most appropriate answer from the options given below.

(a) Both Statement I and Statement II are false.
(b) Statement I is true but Statement II is false.
(c) Statement I is false but Statement II is true.
(d) Both Statement I and Statement II are true.

49. Match List-I with List-II.

List-I	List-II
A. Kolbe's reaction	I. $RX + NaI \xrightarrow{Acetone} RI + NaX \; (X = Cl, Br)$
B. Swart's reaction	II. 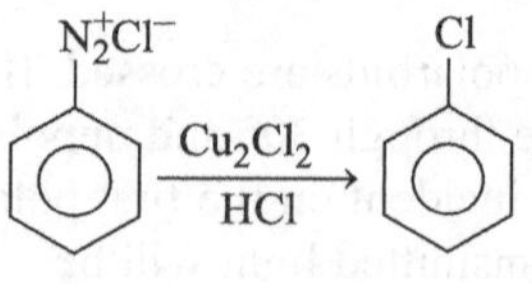
C. Finkelstein reaction	III. 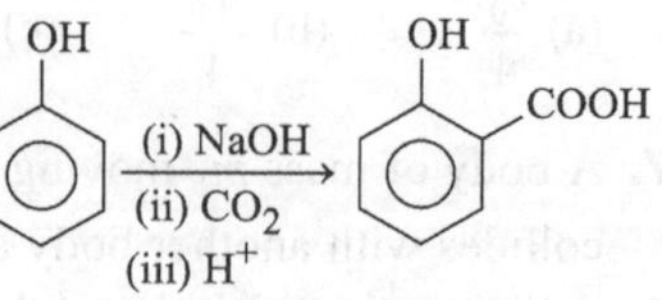
D. Sandmeyer's reaction	IV. $CH_3Br + AgF \longrightarrow H_3CF + AgBr$

Choose the correct answer from the options given below:
(a) A-II, B-I, C-III, D-IV (b) A-III, B-I, C-IV, D-II
(c) A-III, B-IV, C-I, D-II (d) A-I, B-II, C-III, D-IV

50. The given graph is a representation of kinetics of a reaction. The y and x axes for zero and first order reactions, respectively are

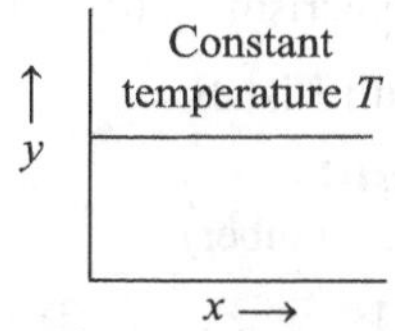

(a) (Zero order $x =$ concentration, $y =$ time, (1st order $x =$ concentration, $y = t_{1/2}$)
(b) (Zero order $x =$ concentration, $y =$ time), (1st order $x =$ rate, $y = t_{1/2}$)
(c) (Zero order $x =$ concentration, $y =$ rate), (1st order $x =$ concentration, $y = t_{1/2}$)
(d) (Zero order $y =$ concentration, $x =$ rate), (1st order $x = t_{1/2}$, $y =$ rate)

51. Which of the following reaction is appropriate for converting acetamide to methanamine?
(a) Stephen's reaction
(b) Hoffmann bromamide synthesis
(c) Carbylamine reaction
(d) Phthalimide reaction

52. A first order reaction has a specific reaction rate of $10^{-2}\ s^{-1}$. How much time (in seconds) will it take for 20 g of the reactant to reduce 5 g? [Given : $\log 4 = 0.602$]
(a) 138.65 s (b) 238.65 s
(c) 693.0 s (d) 346.56 s

53. Among the following identify an incorrect statement.
(a) An increase in temperature increases the collision frequency of molecules.
(b) The rate of reaction increases generally by 2 to 3 times for every 10°C rise in temperature.
(c) For $aA + bB \longrightarrow$ product, the order of reaction is equal to $(a + b)$.
(d) The probability that more than three molecules can collide and react simultaneously is very small, hence the molecularity greater than three is rare.

54. The correct statement regarding electrophile is
(a) It is a negatively charged species and can form a bond by accepting a pair of electrons from another electrophile.
(b) It is a negatively charge species and can form a bond by accepting a pair of electrons from a nucleophile.
(c) They are generally neutral species and can form a bond by donating a pair of electrons from a nucleophile.
(d) It can be either neutral or positively charged species and can form a bond by accepting a pair of electrons from a nucleophile.

55. During the electrolysis of molten sodium chloride, the time required to produce 0.10 mol of chlorine gas using a current of 3 amperes is
(a) 107.22 min (b) 360 min
(c) 720 min (d) 180 min

56. Match List-I with List-II.

	List-I		List-II
A.	Coke	(i)	Carbon atoms are sp^3-hybridised.
B	Diamond	(ii)	Used as a dry lubricant.
C.	Fullerene	(iii)	Used as a reducing agent.
D.	Graphite	(iv)	Cage like structures.

Choose the correct answer from the options given below.
(a) A-(iii), B-(i), C-(iv), D-(ii)
(b) A-(iv), B-(iii), C-(ii), D-(i)
(c) A-(i), B-(ii), C-(iii), D-(iv)
(d) A-(ii), B-(iv), C-(i), D-(iii)

57. Given below are two statements, one is labelled as Assertion (A) and the other is labelled as Reason (R)
Assertion (A) I—Cl is more reactive than I_2.
Reason (R) I—Cl bond is weaker than I—I bond.
In the light of the above statements, choose the correct answer from the options given below.
(a) Both (A) and (R) are true but (R) not the correct explanation of (A).
(b) Both (A) and (R) are true and (R) is the correct explanation of (A).
(c) (A) is false but (R) is true.
(d) (A) is true but (R) is false.

58. Given below are two statements.
Statement I The electron gain enthalpy of F is more negative than that of Cl.
Statement II Ionisation enthalpy decreases in a group of periodic table.
In the light of the above statements, choose the most appropriate answer from the options given below.
(a) Both Statement I and Statement II are false.
(b) Statement I is true but Statement II is false.
(c) Statement I is false but Statement II is true.
(d) Both Statement I and Statement II are true.

59. Which among the following statement is incorrect for bimolecular nucleophilic substitution reaction (S_N2)?
(a) S_N2 reaction occurs in single step without forming intermediate.
(b) The rate of S_N2 reaction does not depends on concentration of both substrate and nucleophilic reagent.
(c) It is a second order reaction.
(d) In S_N2 reaction the substrate does not undergo homolytic fission.

60. Which one is the correct order of acidity?
(a) $CH{\equiv}CH > CH_3{-}C{\equiv}CH > CH_2{=}CH_2 > CH_3{-}CH_3$
(b) $CH{\equiv}CH > CH_2{=}CH_2 > CH_3{-}C{\equiv}CH > CH_3{-}CH_3$
(C) $CH_3{-}CH_3 > CH_2{=}CH_2 > CH_3{-}C{\equiv}CH > CH{\equiv}CH$
(d) $CH_2{=}CH_2 > CH_3{-}CH{=}CH_2 > CH_3{-}C{\equiv}CH > CH{\equiv}CH$

61. Select the incorrect statement.
(a) Phosphonic acid is a dibasic acid.
(b) In phosphonic acid 2P—H bonds are present.
(c) $H_4P_2O_5$ is a tetrabasic acid.
(d) In pyrophosphoric acid, P—O—P linkage is present.

62. Match List - I with List - II.

List-I	List-II
A. PCl_5	(i) Square pyramidal
B. SF_6	(ii) Trigonal planar
C. BrF_5	(iii) Octahedral
D. BF_3	(iv) Trigonal bipyramidal

Choose the correct answer from the options given below.
(a) A-(iii), B-(i), C-(iv), D-(ii)
(b) A-(iv), B-(iii), C-(i), D-(ii)
(c) A-(i), B-(ii), C-(iii), D-(iv)
(d) A-(ii), B-(iv), C-(i), D-(iii)

63. The incorrect statement among the following is
(a) Lanthanoids are good conductors of heat and electricity
(b) Actinoid contraction is greater for element than lanthanoid contraction.
(c) Most of the trivalent lanthanoid ions are colourless in the solid state.
(d) Actinoids are highly reactive metals, especially when finely divided.

64. Decreasing order of stability of O_2, O_2^-, O_2^+ and O_2^{2-} is
(a) $O_2 > O_2^+ > O_2^{2-} > O_2^-$ (b) $O_2^- > O_2^{2-} > O_2 > O_2^+$
(c) $O_2^+ > O_2 > O_2^- > O_2^{2-}$ (d) $O_2^{2-} > O_2 > O_2 > O_2^+$

65. The type of isomerism shown by the complex $[CoCl_2(en)_2]$ is
(a) geometrical isomerism (b) coordination isomerism
(c) ionisation isomerism (d) linkage isomerism

66. Match List-I with List-II.

List-I (Quantum number)		List-II (Orbital)	
A.	$n=2, l=1$	(i)	2s
B.	$n=3, l=2$	(ii)	3s
C.	$n=3, l=0$	(iii)	2p
D.	$n=2, l=0$	(iv)	3d

Choose the correct answer from the options given below.
(a) A-(iii), B-(iv), C-(ii), D-(i)
(b) A-(iii), B-(iv), C-(i), D-(ii)
(c) A-(iv), B-(iii), C-(i), D-(ii)
(d) A-(iv), B-(iii), C-(ii), D-(i)

67. Given below are two statements.
Statement I Treatment of chloroethane with saturated solution of AgCN give ethyl isocyanide as major product.
Statement II Cyanide ion (CN^-) is an ambident nucleophile.
In the light of the above statements, choose the correct answer from the options given below.
(a) Both Statement I and Statement II are false.
(b) Statement I is true but Statement II is false.
(c) Statement I is false but Statement II is true.
(d) Both Statement I and Statement II are true.

68. Match the following

	Complex		Colour
A.	$[Ni(H_2O)_6]^{+2}(aq)$	I.	Green
B.	$[Ni(H_2O)_4(en)]^{+2}(aq)$	II.	Violet
C.	$[Ni(H_2O)_2(en)_2]^{+2}(aq)$	III.	Purple
D.	$[Ni(en)_3]^{+2}(aq)$	IV.	Pale blue

Choose the correct answer from the options given below:
(a) A-III, B-I, C-IV, D-II (b) A-I, B-IV, C-III, D-II
(c) A-I, B-III, C-II, D-IV (d) A-I, B-II, C-III, D-IV

69. Match List-I with List-II.

List-I (Oxoacids of sulphur)	List-II (Bonds)
A. Peroxodisulphuric acid	(i) Two S—OH, Four S=O, One S—O—S
B. Sulphuric acid	(ii) Two S—OH, One S=O
C. Pyrosulphuric acid	(iii) Two S—OH, Four S=O, One S—O—O—S
D. Sulphurous acid	(iv) Two S—OH, Two S=O

Choose the correct answer from the options given below.

(a) A-(iii), B-(iv), C-(i), D-(ii)
(b) A-(i), B-(iii), C-(iv), D-(ii)
(c) A-(iii), B-(iv), C-(ii), D-(i)
(d) A-(i), B-(iii), C-(ii), D-(iv)

70. Amount of oxalic acid present in a solution can be determined by its titration with $KMnO_4$ solution in the presence of H_2SO_4. The titration gives unsatisfactory result when carried out in the presence of HCl, because HCl

(a) furnishes H^+ ions in addition to those from oxalic acid.
(b) reduces permanganate to Mn^{2+}.
(c) oxidises oxalic acid to carbon dioxide and water.
(d) gets oxidised by oxalic acid to chlorine..

71. Which of the following reagents would distinguish *cis*-cyclopenta-1-2-diol from the *trans*-isomer?

(a) MnO_2 (b) Aluminium isopropoxide
(c) Acetone (d) Ozone

72. Ratio of spin only magnetic moment of the ions Fe^{+2} and Ti^{+2} is

(a) $\sqrt{15}$ (b) 1 (c) 3 (d) 1.73

73. Which of the following is incorrect statement?

(a) GeF_4 is more stable than GeF_2.
(b) SnF_4 is ionic in nature.
(c) PbF_4 is covalent in nature.
(d) $SiCl_4$ is easily hydrolysed.

74. Given below are two statements, one is labelled as Assertion (A) and the other is labelled as Reason (R).

Assertion (A) Ionisation enthalpy increases along each series of the transition elements from left to right. However, small variations occur.

Reason (R) There is corresponding increase in nuclear charge which accompanies the filling of electrons in the inner *d*-orbitals.

In the light of the above statements, choose the most appropriate answer from the options given below.

(a) Both (A) and (R) are correct and (R) is the correct explanation of (A).
(b) Both (A) and (R) are true but (R) is not the correct explanation of (A).
(c) (A) is true but (R) is false.
(d) (A) is false but (R) is true.

75. Given below are two statements.

Statement I The acidic strength of mono-substituted nitrophenol is higher than phenol because of electron withdrawing nitro-group.

Statement II *o*-nitrophenol, *m*-nitrophenol and *p*-nitrophenol will have same acidic strength as they have one nitro-group attached to the phenolic ring.

In the light of the above statements, choose the most appropriate answer from the options given below:

(a) Both Statement I and Statement II are false.
(b) Statement I is true but Statement II is false.
(c) Statement I is false but Statement II is true.
(d) Both Statement I and Statement II are true.

76. The correct statement regarding the basicity of arylamines is

(a) Arylamines are generally less basic than alkylamines because lone-pair electrons in nitrogen are delocalised by interaction with the aromatic ring π-electron system.
(b) Arylamines are generally more basic than alkylamines because the nitrogen lone-pair electrons are not delocalised by interaction with the aromatic ring π-electron system.
(c) Arylamines are generally more basic than alkylamines because of aryl group.
(d) Arylamines are generally more basic than alkylamine because the nitrogen atom in arylamine is *sp*-hybridised.

77. In the reaction,the electrophile involved is

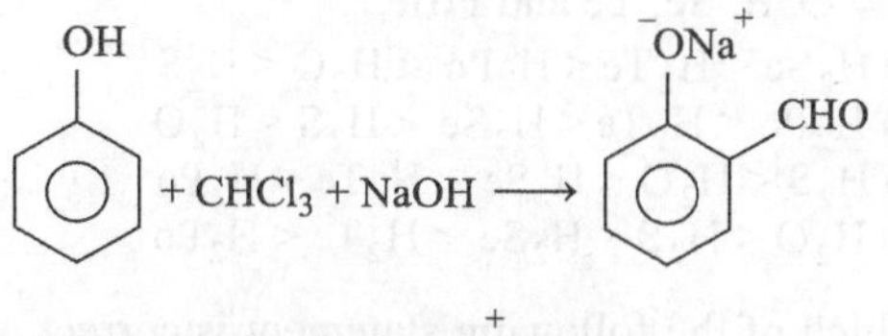

(a) dichloromethyl cation ($\overset{+}{C}HCl_2$)
(b) formyl cation ($\overset{+}{C}HO$)
(c) dichloromethyl anion ($\overset{-}{C}HCl_2$)
(d) dichlorocarbene ($:CCl_2$)

78. Which of the following given alkane doesn't undergo Wurtz reaction?

(a) 2, 3-dimethylbutane (b) *n*-heptane
(c) *n*-butane (d) *n*-hexane

79. For the following reaction
$FeO(s) + CO(g) \rightleftharpoons Fe(s) + CO_2(g)$
Initial partial pressure of CO, CO_2 are 1.4 atm, 0.8 atm respectively. The equilibrium partial pressures of CO and CO_2 at 1050 K and K_p at 0.265 atm is

(a) 0.461 atm, 0.339 atm (b) 1.739 atm, 0.461 atm
(c) 0.339 atm, 0.339 atm (d) 0.461 atm, 2.7 atm

80. Correct statement regarding dioxygen

(a) In formation of dioxgen from oxygen atoms ten molecular orbitals will be formed.
(b) Total no. of bonding molecular orbitals will not be same as total number of antibonding orbitals in dioxygen.
(c) No. of filled bonding orbitals will be same as no. of filled antibonding molecular orbitals.
(d) All molecular orbitals in dixoygen molecule are completely filled.

81. At 100°C the vapour pressure of a solution of 6.5 g of a solute in 100 g water is 732 mm of Hg. If $K_b = 0.52$, the boiling point of this solution will be

(a) 102.21°C (b) 102°C
(c) 100°C (d) 101.06°C

82. Which of the following relation is correct thermodynamic conditions for the spontaneous reaction at all temperatures ?

(A) $\Delta H < 0$ and $\Delta S > 0$ (B) $\Delta H < 0$ and $\Delta S = 0$
(C) $\Delta H < 0$ and $\Delta S < 0$ (D) $\Delta H > 0$ and $\Delta S < 0$
(E) $\Delta H = 0$ and $\Delta S < 0$

(a) A, B, C (b) A and B
(c) A, C, D (d) B, D and E

83. Which is the correct thermal stability order for H_2E (E = O, S, Se, Te and Po)?

(a) $H_2Se < H_2Te < H_2Po < H_2O < H_2S$
(b) $H_2Po < H_2Te < H_2Se < H_2S < H_2O$
(c) $H_2S < H_2O < H_2Se < H_2Te < H_2Po$
(d) $H_2O < H_2S < H_2Se < H_2Te < H_2Po$

84. Which of the following statement is correct regarding chirality?

A. Chiral compounds are those compounds which have a chiral centre.
B. Enantiomers are non-superimposable mirror images of each other.
C. A racemic mixture shows zero optical rotation.
D. Enantiomers does not differ with respect to the rotation of plane polarised light.
E. Stereoisomers related as superimposable mirror image of each other are enantiomers.

(a) A, B and C
(b) B and C
(c) B and D
(d) C, D and E

85. Which of the following has longest C—O bond length? (Free C—O bond length in CO is 1.128 A)

(a) $[Fe(CO)_4]^{2-}$ (b) $[Mn(CO)_6]^+$
(c) $[Ni(CO_4)]$ (d) $[Co(CO)_4]^{1-}$

86. Given below are two statements.

Statement I Glycerol is purified by distillation under reduced pressure.

Statement II Refining of petroleum involves fractional distillation.

In the light of the above statements, choose the correct answer from the options given below.

(a) Both Statement I and Statement II are false.
(b) Statement I is true, but Statement II is false.
(c) Statement I is false, but Statement II is true.
(d) Both Statement I and Statement II are true.

87. Which amongst the following aqueous solution of electrolytes will have minimum elevation in boiling point?

(a) 0.05 m NaCl (b) 0.1 m KCl
(c) 0.1 m $MgSO_4$ (d) 1 m NaCl

88. The density of 1 M solution of a compound 'X' is 1.25 g mL^{-1}. The correct option for the molality of solution is (Molar mass of compound X = 85g mol^{-1})

(a) 0.705 m (b) 1.208 m
(c) 1.165m (d) 0.839 m

89. Which of the following compounds can form a Zwitter ion?

(a) Aniline (b) Acetanilide
(c) Benzoic acid (d) Glycine

90. Consider the following reaction and identify the missing reagent/chemical.

$$CH_3CH_2COO^-Na^+ \xrightarrow[\text{Heat}]{\text{NaOH, + ?}} CH_3CH_3 + Na_2CO_3$$

(a) DIBAL-H (b) B_2H_6
(c) Red phosphorus (d) CaO

BIOLOGY

91. The marine protozoan that have silica shells on their surface is
(a) *Paramecium*
(b) *Plasmodium*
(c) *Entamoeba*
(d) *Trypanosoma*

92. Bleeding and cramps of menstruation begins due to
(a) increase in level of progesterone
(b) decrease in level of progesterone
(c) increase in level of LH
(d) decrease in level of FSH

93. While constructing the first recombinant DNA molecule, Stanley Cohen and Herbert Boyer isolated plasmid from ...I... while ...II... acted as host for the recombinant plasmid.

	I	II
(a)	*E. coli*	*Salmonella typhimurium*
(b)	*Salmonella typhimurium*	*E. coli*
(c)	*Haemophilus influenzae*	*Agrobacterium tumefaciens*
(d)	*Agrobacterium tumefaciens*	*Haemophilus influenzae*

94. Which of the following statements is not true?
(a) Auxin is synthesised from amino acid tryptophan
(b) Methionine is the precursor of ethylene
(c) Kinetin is the most prevalent natural cytokinin in plants
(d) Root apical meristem is the main site for cytokinin synthesis

95. If the internal body temperature of Shyam is 40°C, what will be the temperature required for spermatogenesis?
(a) 38°C (b) 36°C
(c) 42°C (d) 48°C

96. The heart wood of *Acacia* is rich in
(a) gums
(b) resins
(c) tannins
(d) mucilages

97. Find the incorrectly matched pair.

(a)	Sap vacuole	Store and concentrate mineral salt and nutrients
(b)	Contractile vacuole	Osmoregulation
(c)	Food vacuole	Stores digestive enzymes
(d)	Sphaerosomes	Stores metabolic gases

98. When the correction of infertility is not possible in infertility clinics then the couples could be assisted to have children through certain special techniques commonly called as
(a) AST (b) ART (c) MTP (d) RTI

99. Which one of the following statement is not correct regarding Leguminosae family?
(a) The stems are erect or climber
(b) They show racemose inflorescence
(c) Flowers are unisexual and actinomorphic
(d) Pulses like mung, soybean belong to this family

100. With reference to species diversity, identify the incorrect statement.
(a) Species diversity means species richness in any habitat
(b) Greater the species richness, greater will be their diversity
(c) Species diversity is same as species abundance
(d) Example of species diversity includes Western ghats that have a greater amphibian species diversity than Eastern ghats

101. The lock and key model of enzyme action illustrates that particular enzyme molecule
(a) may be destroyed and resynthesised several times
(b) interacts with a specific type of substrate molecule
(c) reacts at identical rates under all conditions
(d) forms a permanent enzyme substrate complex

102. Following double fertilisation, events of endosperm and embryo development, maturation of ovules into seeds and ovary into fruits are collectively termed as
(a) pollen-pistil interaction
(b) artificial hybridisation
(c) embryogenesis
(d) post-fertilisation events

103. Given below are some statements. Choose which of the following is incorrect?

(a) Units of life called spores were transferred to different planets including earth according to theory of spontaneous generation.
(b) Oparin and Haldane proposed that life arises from non-living organic molecule by chemical evolution.
(c) *Psilophyton* can be considered as ancestor of conifers.
(d) Coelacanth possibly evolved into the first amphibians.

104. Which of the following structure or material is incorrectly matched with a tissue?

(a)	Collagen fibres	Bone
(b)	Fibroblast	Skeleton muscle
(c)	Chondrin	Cartilage
(d)	Basement membrane	Epithelium

105. Which of the following is/are formed by vascular cambium and pass through secondary xylem and phloem as radiating strips?

(a) Interfascicular cambium
(b) Bulliform cells
(c) Secondary medullary rays
(d) Bundle sheath cells

106. Both mitosis and meiosis are independent processes with individual significances. Which of the following is unique to mitosis, but not a part of meiosis?

(a) Homologous chromosomes behave independently
(b) Chromatids separate during anaphase
(c) Homologous chromosomes pair up and form bivalents
(d) Homologous chromosomes cross over

107. In frog, there are ……… pairs of cranial nerves and brain is divided into ……… parts.

(a) 11, 2 (b) 9, 3
(c) 10, 3 (d) 11, 4

108. Bones are rich in ……… and the bone cells are present in the spaces called ……… .

(a) potassium, chondrion
(b) sodium, lacunae
(c) calcium salts, lacunae
(d) calcium, chondrion

109. Given below are two statements.

Statement I In grass family, the cotyledon called scutellum is situated towards one side of embryonal axis.

Statement II At the lower end of dicot seed, the embryonal axis has the radical and root cap enclosed in a differentiated sheath called coleoptile.

In the light of the above statements, choose the correct answer from the options given below.

(a) Statement I is incorrect, but statement II is correct
(b) Both statement I and statement II are correct
(c) Both statement I and statement II are incorrect
(d) Statement I is correct, but statement II is incorrect

110. In which of the following methods a probe is allowed to hybridise to its complementary DNA in the clone of cells?

(a) Gene therapy (b) Autoradiography
(c) PCR (d) ELISA

111. A system of classification in which a large number of traits are considered is

(a) artificial system (b) natural system
(c) synthetic system (d) phylogenetic system

112. The procedure in which we separate fragments of DNA by the technique of gel electrophoresis followed by transferring those short fragments for radioactive probing is included under

(a) gene mapping (b) gene cloning
(c) PCR (d) Southern blotting

113. Consider the following statements regarding reptiles and choose the incorrect statement.

(a) They are poikilothermic animals
(b) An endoskeleton of horny epidermal scales is always present
(c) They are oviparous with direct development
(d) Heart is incompletely four-chambered with two auricles and partly divided ventricles

114. Match List I with List II.

List I	List II
A. Monocistronic	1. No effect on mice after injection
B. Polycistronic	2. Mice dies after injection
C. Heat killed S-strain	3. *m*RNA in prokaryotes
D. Heat killed S-strain with live R-strain	4. *m*RNA in eukaryotes

Choose the correct answer from the options given below.

	A	B	C	D		A	B	C	D
(a)	3	4	1	2	(b)	4	3	2	1
(c)	4	3	1	2	(d)	3	1	2	4

115. Which of the following statements is incorrect?
(a) WM Stanley showed that viruses could be crystallised
(b) Mosaic disease in tobacco is caused by fungi
(c) The viroids were discovered by TO Diener
(d) The term *Contagium vivum fluidum* was coined by MW Beijerinck

116. Given below are two statements.
Statement I The conducting part of the respiratory system is the site of actual diffusion.
Statement II The thoracic chamber is formed dorsally by vertebral column.
In the light of the above statements, choose the correct answer from the options given below.
(a) Statement I is incorrect, but statement II is correct
(b) Both statement I and statement II are correct
(c) Both statement I and statement II are incorrect
(d) Statement I is correct, but statement II is incorrect

117. Given below are two statements.
Statement I Second step of Calvin cycle involves utilisation of 2 molecules of ATP for reduction and 2 molecules of NADPH for phosphorylation per CO_2 molecule fixed.
Statement II The regeneration step requires one ATP for phosphorylation to form RuBP.
In the light of the above statements, choose the correct answer from the options given below.
(a) Statement I is incorrect, but statement II is correct
(b) Both statement I and statement II are correct
(c) Both statement I and statement II are incorrect
(d) Statement I is correct, but statement II is incorrect

118. The male cones and megasporophylls borne on different trees is seen in
(a) *Pinus* (b) *Cycas*
(c) *Selaginella* (d) *Salvinia*

119. From the given situation, choose the one which can prevent autogamy and geitonogamy?
(a) Monoecious plant bearing unisexual flowers
(b) Dioecious plants bearing only male or female flowers
(c) Monoecious plants with bisexual flowers
(d) Dioecious plants with bisexual flower

120. Four vaccines, assigned with codes A-D are listed below. DPT, Cholera, Hepatitis-B, Salk's polio vaccine
A B C D
Which of the above is a second generation vaccine?
(a) B (b) D (c) A (d) C

121. In *E. coli*, the *lac* operon gets switched on when
(a) lactose is present and it binds to the repressor
(b) repressor binds to operator
(c) RNA polymerase binds to the operator
(d) lactose is present and it binds to RNA polymerase

122. Read the following statements and identify the correct statements.
I. Prokaryotic and eukaryotic flagella are structurally similar.
II. Cilia work like oars and are comparatively smaller than flagella.
III. The core of cilium or flagellum is called axoneme.
IV. Central tubules are connected by spokes and is enclosed by central sheath.
V. Central sheath is connected to one of the tubules of each peripheral doublets by a radial spoke. There are nine radial spokes.

Choose the correct answer from the options given below.
(a) III, IV and V (b) II, IV and V
(c) I, II and III (d) II, III and V

123. Consider the given diagrammatic representation of cell cycle.

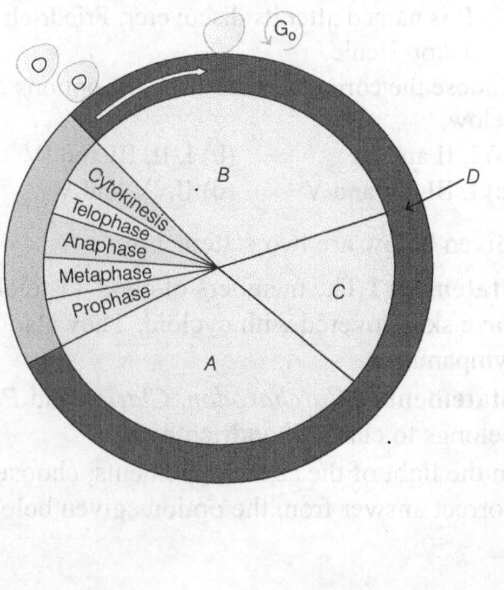

During which of the above labels A, B, C or D, will the amount of DNA per cell double?

(a) A (b) C (c) B (d) D

124. A restriction enzymes breaks bonds between

(a) base pair of DNA molecule
(b) base pair of DNA-RNA hybrid molecule
(c) sugar and phosphate components of a nucleic acid molecule
(d) exons and introns of a DNA molecule

125. Consider the following statements about incomplete dominance and identify the incorrect statements.

I. In incomplete dominance, F_1 phenotype does not resemble either of the two parents.
II. *Antirrhinum* sp. is a good example to understand incomplete dominance.
III. In a cross between true breeding red and white flowered plants, the F_1 was pink.
IV. When the F_1 was self-pollinated the F_2 resulted in red (RR), white (rr) and Pink (Rr) flowers in the ratio of 1:2:1.
V. It is also known as partial dominance.

Choose the incorrect statement (s) from the options given below.

(a) I and III (b) I and V
(c) II and IV (d) Only IV

126. Identify the correct statements with reference to loop of Henle.

I. It is also called as pars recta.
II. It is bell-shaped.
III. It can be divided into two regions.
IV. It is the main site for urine concentration.
V. It is named after its discoverer, Friedrich Gustar Jakob Henle.

Choose the correct answer from the options given below.

(a) I, II and III (b) I, II, III and IV
(c) I, III, IV and V (d) II, IV and V

127. Given below are two statements.

Statement I The members of class–Osteichthyes, have skin covered with cycloid. They also have tympanum.

Statement II *Carcharodon, Clarias* and *Pristis* belongs to class–Chondrichthyes.

In the light of the above statements, choose the correct answer from the options given below.

(a) Statement I is incorrect, but statement II is correct
(b) Both statement I and statement II are correct
(c) Both statement I and statement II are incorrect
(d) Statement I is correct, but statement II is incorrect

128. DNA precipitation from a mixture of biomolecules can be achieved by treating it with

(a) chilled chloroform
(b) isopropanol
(c) chilled ethanol
(d) methanol at room temperature

129. Volume of air that will accommodate in the lungs at the end of a forced inspiration is about

(a) 8000 mL (b) 6000 mL
(c) 4000 mL (d) 2000 mL

130. The reduced ubiquinone is oxidised with the transfer of electrons to cytochrome-*c via*

(a) complex-I (b) complex-II
(c) complex-III (d) complex-IV

131. Given below are two statements; one is labelled as Assertion (A) and others is labelled as Reason (R).

Assertion (A) Sebaceous glands help to provide a protective oily covering for the skin.

Reason (R) Sebaceous glands produce sweat containing NaCl, urea, etc.

In the light of the above statements, choose the correct answer from the options given below.

(a) A is false, but R is true
(b) Both A and R are true and R is the correct explanation of A
(c) Both A and R are true, but R is not the correct explanation of A
(d) A is true, but R is false

132. Given below are two statements.

Statement I Carboxylation is the fixation of CO_2 into a stable organic intermediate.

Statement II The carboxylation reaction is catalysed by the enzyme PEPCase.

In the light of the above statements, choose the correct answer from the options given below.

(a) Statement I is incorrect, but statement II is correct
(b) Both statement I and statement II are correct
(c) Both statement I and statement II are incorrect
(d) Statement I is correct, but statement II is incorrect

133. In which of the following reactions of Krebs' cycle, substrate level phosphorylation takes place?
(A) Malic acid $\rightarrow$ Oxalosuccinic acid
(B) Succinyl Co-A $\rightarrow$ Succinic acid + Co-A
(C) PEP $\rightarrow$ Pyruvate
(D) 3PGA $\rightarrow$ 2 PGA
Codes
(a) A and D (b) B only
(c) B and C (d) A, B and D

134. The ventricular systole involves the closure of
(a) semilunar valve and aortic valve
(b) tricuspid and bicuspid valves
(c) pulmonary valve and vena cava
(d) semilunar valve and pulmonary valve

135. Match List I with List II.

	List I		List II
A.	Abscisic acid	1.	Coleoptile of oat seedling
B.	Ethylene	2.	Volatile
C.	Gibberellic acid	3.	Dormin
D.	Auxin	4.	Bakane

Choose the correct answer from the options given below.

	A	B	C	D
(a)	3	2	4	1
(b)	2	4	3	1
(c)	1	3	4	2
(d)	1	2	4	3

136. Name a trematode parasite whose life cycle depends on snail and a fish as host.
(a) Helminthes
(b) Liver fluke
(c) *Entamoeba histolytica*
(d) Tapeworm

137. A compound that allows free diffusion of protons across the membrane is added to cells that actively undergo cellular respiration. This addition would
(a) stop glycolysis
(b) inhibit ATP synthesis
(c) stop electron transport system
(d) prevent chemiosmotic synthesis of ATP

138. The prickly pear cactus which caused havoc in Australia was brought under control after the introduction of cactus feeding moth. This is an example of
(a) competition (b) predation
(c) parasitism (d) mutualism

139. In sickel-cell anaemia the sequence of amino acid from the first to the seventh position of the β-chain of haemoglobin –S(Hb^s) is
(a) His, Leu, Thr, Pro, Glu, Val, Val
(b) Val, His, Leu, Val, Pro, Val, Gul
(c) Thr, His, Pro, Thr, Pro, Gul, Gul
(d) Val, His, Leu, Thr, Pro, Val, Glu

140. The sarcoplasmic reticulum of skeletal muscle is a
(a) form of smooth endoplasmic reticulum
(b) site where calcium is released during muscle relaxation
(c) site of potassium binding protein storage
(d) site where calcium is inhibited

141. Given below are two statements; one is labelled as Assertion (A) and other is labelled as Reason (R).
Assertion (A) Chalaza represents the junction between ovule and funicle.
Reason (R) The chalazal pole is characterised by the presence of three haploid cells.
In the light of the above statements, choose the correct answer from the options given below.
(a) A is false, but R is true
(b) Both A and R are true and R is the correct explanation of A
(c) Both A and R are true, but R is not the correct explanation of A
(d) A is true, but R is false

142. The phenomenon of co-evolved plant-pollinator mutualism is a classic example of
(a) fragmentation (b) over-exploitation
(c) co-extinction (d) alien-species invasion

143. Meiosis holds much importance in the life of living organisms. This may be due to the fact that
(a) it produces new daughter cells which resemble to their parents
(b) it produces two daughter cells, each from one parent
(c) it allows organisms to produce identical copies of themselves
(d) it brings survived features along

144. Match List I with List II.

	List I		List II
A.	Echinoderms	1.	Air bladder
B.	Hemichordata	2.	Placoid scale
C.	Chondrichthyes	3.	Water vascular system
D.	Osteichthyes	4.	Proboscis gland

Choose the correct answer from the options given below.

	A	B	C	D		A	B	C	D
(a)	3	4	2	1	(b)	2	4	3	1
(c)	1	2	4	3	(d)	2	1	3	4

145. Given below are two statements; one is labelled as Assertion (A) and other is labelled as Reason (R).

Assertion (A) In bacteria, DNA is circular and associated with non-histone basic protein.

Reason (R) Histone protein is basic in nature due to rich lysine and arginine residues.

In the light of the above statements, choose the correct answer from the options given below.

(a) A is false, but R is true
(b) Both A and R are true and R is the correct explanation of A
(c) Both A and R are true, but R is not the correct explanation of A
(d) A is true, but R is false

146. Lysosomes are sometimes included in microbodies. However, they differ in

(a) their mode of formation
(b) their small size
(c) presence of enzymes
(d) their large size

147. A research student wanted to perform a biochemical analysis of mitochondria. For accurate analysis, he would opt for

(a) plasmolysing the cell first, filtering it and then taking the debris
(b) selecting cells having large mitochondria
(c) grinding out the cell and filtering out the mixture
(d) subjecting the cells to centrifuge and obtaining mitochondria

148. During protein denaturation, which of the following is disrupted?

(a) Peptide bond sequence of amino acid
(b) Secondary and tertiary structures
(c) Primary structures
(d) Tertiary structures

149. Consider the given statements regarding muscle protein.

I. Thick filaments mainly constitute of myosin protein.
II. Myosin is splitted by an enzyme trypsin into LMM and HMM.
III. ATPase requires Na^+ for its functioning.
IV. Number of mitochondria are more in white fibres.
V. The endoplasmic reticulum is the store house of calcium ion.

Which of the above statements is/are correct?

(a) Only I
(b) I, II and V
(c) II, III and IV
(d) Only IV

150. Suppose in an ecosystem following are the dry weights of different consumers, i.e. secondary consumer (11 kg/m^2), tertiary consumer (1.5 kg/m^2), primary consumer (37 kg/m^2) and primary producer (809 kg/m^2).

On the basis of above data choose the correct type of ecological pyramid from the options below.

(a) Upright pyramid of biomass
(b) Inverted pyramid of biomass
(c) Inverted pyramid of energy
(d) Inverted pyramid of number

151. Read the following statements and identify the incorrect statements.

I. Ovules generally differentiate a single Megaspore Mother Cell (MMC) in the chalazal region of the nucellus.
II. The MMC undergoes reduction division and produces four megaspores.
III. In a majority of angiosperms, one of the megaspore gets degenerated while the other three remains functional.
IV. The nucleus of the functional megaspore divides mitotically three times and form 2-nucleate, 4-nucleate and later 8-nucleate stages of the embryo sac.
V. The mitotic division are strictly free nuclear, that is nuclear division are immediately followed by cell wall formation.

Choose the correct answer from the options given below.

(a) I, II and III
(b) II, III and IV
(c) III and IV
(d) I, III and V

152. Consider the given figure. Which alkaloid is obtained from it?

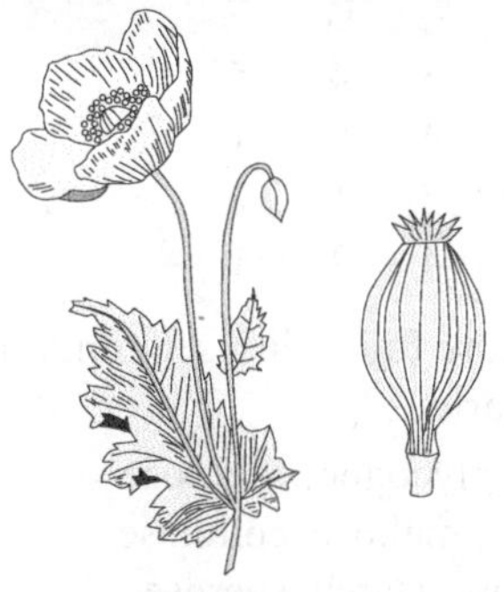

(a) Psilocybin (b) Morphine
(c) LSD (d) Atropine

153. Given below are two statements; one is labelled as Assertion (A) and other is labelled as Reason (R).

Assertion (A) Synthesis of daughter or new strand occurs continuously along the parent $3' \rightarrow 5'$ strand.

Reason (R) DNA polymerase can polymerise nucleotides in $3' \rightarrow 5'$ directions on $5' \rightarrow 3'$ strand.

(a) A is false, but R is true
(b) Both A and R are true and R is the correct explanation of A
(c) Both A and R are true, but R is not the correct explanation of A
(d) A is true, but R is false

154. Given below are two statements; one is labelled as Assertion (A) and other is labelled as Reason (R).

Assertion (A) Meiosis-II is similar to mitosis.

Reason (R) Meiosis-I cannot occur in haploid cells.

In the light of the above statements, choose the correct answer from the options given below.

(a) A is false, but R is true
(b) Both A and R are true and R is the correct explanation of A
(c) Both A and R are true, but R is not the correct explanation of A
(d) A is true, but R is false

155. Arrange the following events of meiosis in correct order.

I. Appearance of bivalent as tetrads.
II. Chromosomes compaction.
III. Terminalisation of chiasmata.
IV. Recombination between homologous chromosomes.

Choose the correct answer from the options given below.

(a) II→III→IV→I (b) II→I→IV→III
(c) IV→III→II→I (d) I→II→IV→III

156. Given below are two statements.

Statement I Squamous epithelium are found in the walls of blood vessels and air sacs of lungs.

Statement II Columnar epithelium are found in the lining of stomach and in intestine for secretion and absorption.

In the light of the above statements, choose the correct answer from the options given below.

(a) Statement I is incorrect, but statement II is correct
(b) Both statement I and statement II are correct
(c) Both statement I and statement II are incorrect
(d) Statement I is correct, but statement II is incorrect

157. Given below are two statements.

Statement I Anaerobic digestion of activated sludge produce biogas inside the sludge digester.

Statement II Penicillin was discovered, while working on *Streptococcous* bacteria.

In the light of the above statements, choose the correct answer from the options given below.

(a) Statement I is incorrect, but statement II is correct
(b) Both statement I and statement II are correct
(c) Both statement I and statement II are incorrect
(d) Statement I is correct, but statement II is incorrect

158. In plants that shed pollen grain at two celled condition, the generative cell divides and form two male gametes during the

(a) entry of pollen tube in the ovule
(b) entry of pollen tube in the synergid
(c) growth of pollen tube in the stigma
(d) growth of pollen tube in the style

159. Match List I with List II.

List I	List II
A. Multipolar	1. Granular bodies in cytoplasm
B. Nissl's granules	2. Connect the hemispheres
C. Nodes of Ranvier	3. Gaps between myelin sheath
D. Corpus callosum	4. One axon, two or more dendrites

Choose the correct answer from the options given below.

	A	B	C	D
(a)	1	2	4	3
(b)	4	1	3	2
(c)	4	1	2	3
(d)	3	4	2	1

160. Given below are two statements; one is labelled as Assertion (A) and others is labelled as Reason (R).

Assertion (A) The spongy of *Pinus* shows no distinction as spongy and palisade.

Reason (R) Parenchymatous cells are present in mesophyll of *Pinus*.

In the light of the above statements, choose the correct answer from the options given below.

(a) A is false, but R is true
(b) Both A and R are true and R is the correct explanation of A
(c) Both A and R are true, but R is not the correct explanation of A
(d) A is true, but R is false

161. Given below are two statements.

Statement I The pituitary is located in a bony cavity called sella tursica.

Statement II The adenohypophysis is known as posterior pituitary which stores and releases two hormones, i.e. oxytocin and vasopressin.

In the light of the above statements, choose the correct answer from the options given below.

(a) Statement I is incorrect, but statement II is correct
(b) Both statement I and statement II are correct
(c) Both statement I and statement II are incorrect
(d) Statement I is correct, but statement II is incorrect

162. Match List I with List II.

List I (Stem modification)		List II (Found in)	
A.	Underground stem	1.	*Euphorbia*
B.	Stem tendril	2.	*Opuntia*
C.	Stem thorns	3.	Potato
D.	Flattened stem	4.	*Citrus*
E.	Fleshy cylindrical stem	5.	Cucumber

Choose the correct answer from the options given below.

	A	B	C	D	E
(a)	1	2	3	4	5
(b)	2	3	4	5	1
(c)	3	4	5	1	2
(d)	3	5	4	2	1

163. Which of the following set contains polysaccharides?

(a) Starch, glycogen, cellulose
(b) Sucrose, maltose, cellulose
(c) Galactose, starch, sucrose
(d) Glucose, fructose, lactose

164. Among the given characteristic feature of chordata which is incorrect?

(a) Notochord is a solid, rod-like structure present on the dorsal side of the body
(b) Nerve cord is a hollow tube-like structure present on the dorsal side of the body
(c) Pharyngeal gill slits are like paired openings formed on the lateral sides of the pharynx
(d) A ventral heart and open circulatory system is present

165. Read the following statements and identify the incorrect statement.

I. A large sized tree may support and provide nourishment to several frugivorous birds. The graph for this will be upright.
II. During transfer of energy at any trophic level only 10% of the energy present in one trophic becomes part of next tropic level.
III. Measurement of biomass in terms of dry weight is more preferred to avoid variations in weight due to seasonal moisture difference.
IV. In a particular climatic condition, decomposition rate is faster if detritus is rich in lignin and chitin.
V. Warm and moist environment favour decomposition.

Choose the correct answer from the options given below.

(a) II and V
(b) III and IV
(c) Only I
(d) Only IV

166. Match List I with List II.

	List I		List II
A.	Eosinophils	1.	Coagulation
B.	RBCs	2.	Universal recipient
C.	AB group	3.	Resist infection
D.	Platelets	4.	Contraction of heart
E.	Systole	5.	Gas transport

Choose the correct answer from the options given below.

	A	B	C	D	E
(a)	2	3	5	4	1
(b)	1	2	3	4	5
(c)	3	5	2	1	4
(d)	3	4	2	5	1

167. The diseases, Bovine Spongiform Encephalopathy (BSE) and Cr-Jacob disease are caused by

(a) viroids (b) prions (c) lichens (d) fungi

168. Which one of the following bacteria has found extensive use in genetic engineering work in plants?

(a) *Clostridium septicum*
(b) *Xanthomonas citri*
(c) *Bacillus coagulens*
(d) *Agrobacterium tumefaciens*

169. Read the following statements and identify the correct statement.

I. Temperature lower than the normal internal body is necessary for spermatogenesis.
II. In some animals testis remain permanently in the abdomen.
III. Each testis is covered by a dense sheath enclosing it in a capsule of connective tissue.
IV. Each testis has testicular lobules and each lobule contains one seminiferous tubule.
V. Secretions of epididymis, vas deferens, seminal vesicle and prostate are essential for maturation and motility of sperms.

Choose the correct answer from the options given below.

(a) I, III and IV
(b) I and II only
(c) I, II, III and V
(d) III and V only

170. In a certain plant, red colour flower (R) is dominant over white colour flower (r). When a heterozygous Rr plant is crossed 64 offspring are obtained. The number of white offspring is

(a) 64 (b) 0 (c) 16 (d) 32

171. Given below are two statements; one is labelled as Assertion (A) and other is labelled as Reason (R).

Assertion (A) Restriction enzymes cut the strand of DNA to produce sticky ends.

Reason (R) Stickiness of the ends facilitates the action of the enzyme DNA polymerase.

In the light of the above statements, choose the correct answer from the options given below.

(a) A is false, but R is true
(b) Both A and R are true and R is the correct explanation of A
(c) Both A and R are true, but R is not the correct explanation of A
(d) A is true, but R is false

172. Consider the following statements and choose the correct one.

I. The cell wall helps in cell-to-cell interaction and provides barrier.
II. The secondary wall is formed on the inner side of the cell.
III. Amyloplasts are the colourless plastids.
IV. Leucoplast stores food in the form of starch.
V. Elaioplast store oils and fats.

Choose the correct answer from the options given below.

(a) I and II (b) I, II and V
(c) III and V (d) III, IV and V

173. Consider the following statements and mark the incorrect statements.

(a) Phenylketonuria is an autosomal recessive trait
(b) Thalassemia is an autosomal recessive trait
(c) Down's syndrome is due to the trisomy of chromosome number 21
(d) Turner's syndrome is caused due to the absence of one of the Y-chromosomes

174. Consider the following statements about innate immunity.

I. B-lymphocytes produce immunoglobulins in response to pathogen attack.
II. PMNL, macrophages, lymphocytes in tissues can phagocytose and destroy microbes.

III. Saliva in the mouth prevents microbial growth.
IV. Mucous in urogenital tracts helps in trapping microbes entering our body.
V. Interferons stimulates the synthesis of enzyme which inhibits the synthesis of protein required for replication of virus.

Choose the correct answer from the options given below.

(a) I and III (b) II, III, IV and V
(c) II, IV and V (d) I, II and III

175. A ring of meristematic cells that divides and forms cork on outside and secondary cortex on the inner side is

(a) phellogen
(b) phelloderm
(c) intrafascicular cambium
(d) interfascicular cambium

176. Which is not true with respect to transgenic animals and their contribution towards human welfare?

(a) Transgenic mice are being used to test safety of polio vaccine
(b) Rosie cow's milk contained human gene insulin
(c) Transgenic cows give milk with less fat
(d) Transgenic sheep produce more wool

177. The protein hormone secreted by thyroid gland that regulates the blood calcium levels is called

(a) thyroxine (b) tetraiodothyronine
(c) triiodothyronine (d) thyrocalcitonin

178. A women with two genes for haemophilia and one gene for colour blindness on one of the 'X' chromosomes marries a normal man. How will the progeny be?

(a) 50% haemophilic colourblind sons and 50% haemophilic sons
(b) 50% haemophilic daughters and 50% colour blind daughters
(c) All sons and daughters haemophilic and colour blind
(d) Haemophilic and colourblind daughters

179. Match List I with List II.

List I	List II
A. Bryophytes	1. Dorsiventral thallus
B. Pteridophytes	2. Soil binders
C. Gymnosperms	3. Bear strobilli
D. Algae	4. Moist stones and wood

Choose the correct answer from the options given below.

	A	B	C	D
(a)	1	2	4	3
(b)	2	1	4	3
(c)	1	2	3	4
(d)	2	1	3	4

180. While conducting an experiment, an *E. coli* was placed in a medium containing radioactive thymidine for some time to replicate. Then it is again allowed to replicate, but in a normal medium. Among the given options which will be the correct observation?

(a) Both the strands of DNA will be radioactive
(b) Each half strand radioactive
(c) One strand radioactive
(d) None of the strands are radioactive

Answers

Physics

1.	(a)	2.	(c)	3.	(a)	4.	(b)	5.	(b)	6.	(d)	7.	(c)	8.	(a)	9.	(b)	10.	(b)
11.	(d)	12.	(d)	13.	(b)	14.	(c)	15.	(a)	16.	(c)	17.	(b)	18.	(b)	19.	(b)	20.	(c)
21.	(b)	22.	(b)	23.	(d)	24.	(a)	25.	(b)	26.	(b)	27.	(c)	28.	(a)	29.	(c)	30.	(d)
31.	(c)	32.	(a)	33.	(a)	34.	(d)	35.	(d)	36.	(d)	37.	(b)	38.	(d)	39.	(a)	40.	(a)
41.	(c)	42.	(c)	43.	(a)	44.	(d)	45.	(c)										

Chemistry

46.	(d)	47.	(d)	48.	(d)	49.	(c)	50.	(c)	51.	(b)	52.	(a)	53.	(c)	54.	(d)	55.	(a)
56.	(a)	57.	(b)	58.	(c)	59.	(b)	60.	(a)	61.	(c)	62.	(b)	63.	(c)	64.	(c)	65.	(a)
66.	(a)	67.	(d)	68.	(b)	69.	(a)	70.	(b)	71.	(c)	72.	(d)	73.	(c)	74.	(a)	75.	(b)
76.	(a)	77.	(d)	78.	(b)	79.	(b)	80.	(b)	81.	(d)	82.	(b)	83.	(b)	84.	(a)	85.	(a)
86.	(d)	87.	(a)	88.	(d)	89.	(d)	90.	(d)										

Biology

91	(c)	92	(b)	93	(b)	94	(c)	95	(a)	96	(c)	97	(d)	98	(b)	99	(c)	100	(c)
101	(b)	102	(d)	103	(a)	104	(b)	105	(c)	106	(a)	107	(c)	108	(c)	109	(d)	110	(b)
111	(b)	112	(d)	113	(b)	114	(c)	115	(b)	116	(a)	117	(a)	118	(b)	119	(b)	120	(d)
121	(a)	122	(d)	123	(b)	124	(c)	125	(d)	126	(c)	127	(c)	128	(c)	129	(b)	130	(c)
131	(d)	132	(d)	133	(b)	134	(b)	135	(a)	136	(b)	137	(d)	138	(b)	139	(d)	140	(a)
141	(a)	142	(c)	143	(a)	144	(a)	145	(c)	146	(a)	147	(d)	148	(b)	149	(b)	150	(a)
151	(d)	152	(b)	153	(d)	154	(c)	155	(b)	156	(b)	157	(d)	158	(c)	159	(b)	160	(c)
161	(d)	162	(d)	163	(a)	164	(d)	165	(d)	166	(c)	167	(b)	168	(d)	169	(c)	170	(c)
171	(d)	172	(b)	173	(d)	174	(b)	175	(a)	176	(b)	177	(d)	178	(a)	179	(c)	180	(c)

Scan this QR code from your mobile phone to get the explanations of this paper.

SECTION II

Mastery Builders

PRACTICE SET 13

Maximum Marks : 720 | Time : 3 hrs | No. of Questions : 180

Instructions

1. This question paper contains **180** multiple-choice questions (four options with a single correct answer) from **Physics, Chemistry** and **Biology**.
2. These questions are distributed as 45 questions, each from Physics and Chemistry and 90 questions in Biology. These are to be compulsorily attempted by the candidate.
3. Each question carries 4 marks. For each correct response, the candidate will get 4 marks. For each incorrect response, one mark will be deducted from the total scores.

PHYSICS

1. Electrons of mass m with de-Broglie wavelength λ fall on the target in an X-rays tube. The cut-off wavelength (λ_0) of the emitted X-rays is

(a) $\lambda_0 = \lambda$ (b) $\lambda_0 = \frac{2mc\lambda^2}{h}$

(c) $\lambda_0 = \frac{2h}{ml}$ (d) $\lambda_0 = \frac{2m^2c^2\lambda^3}{h^2}$

2. Two bodies of mass 4 kg and 6 kg are tied to ends of a massless string. The string passes over a pulley which is frictionless shown in figure. The acceleration of the system in terms of acceleration due to gravity (g) is

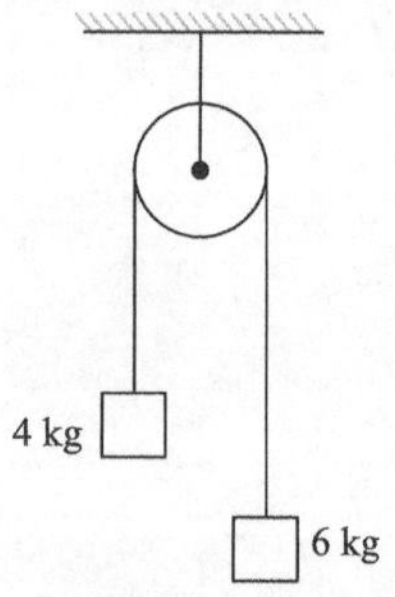

(a) $g/2$
(b) $g/5$
(c) $g/10$
(d) g

3. The surface tension of a soap solution is 2×10^{-2} Nm^{-2}. To blow a bubble of radius 1 cm, the work done is

(a) $4\pi\times10^{-6}$ J (b) $8\pi\times10^{-6}$ J
(c) $12\pi\times10^{-6}$ J (d) $16\pi\times10^{-6}$ J

4. An experiment measured quantities a, b, c and then X is calculated from $X = ab^2/c^3$. If the percentage errors in a, b, c are $\pm1\%$, $\pm3\%$ and $\pm2\%$, respectively, then the percentage error in X can be

(a) $\pm7\%$ (b) $\pm4\%$ (c) $\pm13\%$ (d) $\pm1\%$

5. A magnet of magnetic moment $50\hat{\mathbf{i}}$ A-m^2 placed along X-axis, where magnetic field is $\mathbf{B} = (0.5\hat{\mathbf{i}} + 3.0\hat{\mathbf{j}})$ T. The torque acting on magnet is

(a) $175\hat{\mathbf{k}}$ N-m (b) $150\hat{\mathbf{k}}$ N-m
(c) $75\hat{\mathbf{k}}$ N-m (d) $25\sqrt{37}\,\hat{\mathbf{k}}$ N-m

6. Bohr model is applied to singly ionised helium He^+. Consider the lines that lie in the visible region of the spectrum. Which of the following transitions can give a photon of visible light?

(a) $n=5$ to $n=4$ (b) $n=7$ to $n=4$
(c) $n=2$ to $n=1$ (d) $n=8$ to $n=3$

7. A long solenoid has 1000 turns. When a current of 4 A flows through it, the magnetic flux linked with each turn of the solenoid is 4×10^{-3} Wb. The self-inductance of the solenoid is

(a) 2 H (b) 4 H (c) 1 H (d) 3 H

8. An ideal gas is initially at p_1, V_1 is expanded to p_2, V_2, isothermally and then compressed adiabatically to the same volume V_1 and pressure p_3. If W is the net work done by the gas in complete process, which of the following is true?

(a) $W > 0$; $p_3 > p_1$ (b) $W < 0$; $p_3 > p_1$
(c) $W > 0$; $p_3 < p_1$ (d) $W < 0$; $p_3 < p_1$

9. In the circuit, the potential difference between A and B is

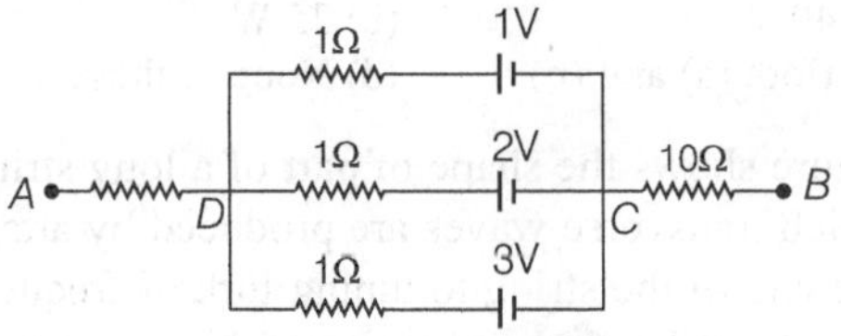

(a) 6 V (b) 1 V (c) 3 V (d) 2 V

10. A small mass executes linear SHM about O with amplitude a and period T. Its displacement from O at time $T/8$ after passing through O is

(a) $\frac{a}{8}$ (b) $\frac{a}{2}$ (c) $\frac{a}{\sqrt{2}}$ (d) $\frac{a}{2\sqrt{2}}$

11. A capacitor stores 10 μC charge when connected across a battery. When the gap between the plates is filled with a dielectric, a charge of 30 μC flows through the battery. Find the dielectric constant of the dielectric.

(a) $K = 2$ (b) $K = 3$
(c) $K = 4$ (d) $K = 1$

12. The electromagnetic wave travelling in a medium has relative permeability 1.3 and relative permittivity 2.14. The speed of EM wave in that medium will be

(a) 13.6×10^6 m/s (b) 1.8×10^6 m/s
(c) 3.6×10^8 m/s (d) 1.8×10^8 m/s

13. The pressure and density of a diatomic gas $\left[\gamma = \frac{7}{5}\right]$ change adiabatically from (P, d) to (P', d'). If $\frac{d'}{d} = 243$, then ratio of $\frac{P'}{P}$ should be

(a) 1 : 243 (b) 2187 : 1
(c) 1 : 2187 (d) 243 : 1

14. The truth table for the following logic circuit is

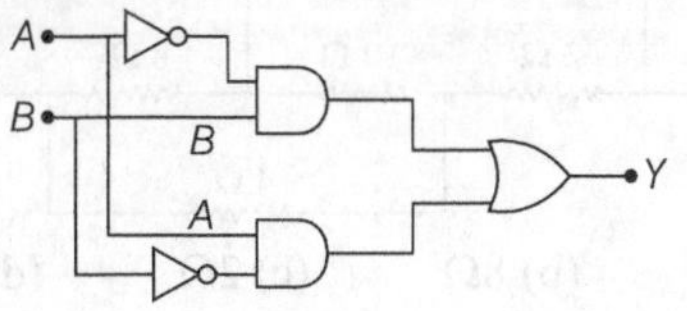

(a)

A	B	Y
0	0	0
0	1	1
1	0	1
1	1	0

(b)

A	B	Y
0	0	1
0	1	1
1	0	1
1	1	1

(c)

A	B	Y
0	0	1
0	1	0
1	0	1
1	1	0

(d)

A	B	Y
0	0	1
0	1	1
1	0	0
1	1	1

15. A car moving on a straight road covers one-third of a certain distance with 20 km/h and the rest with 60 km/h. The average speed is

(a) 40 km/h (b) $46\frac{2}{3}$ km/h (c) 36 km/h (d) 80 km/h

16. A body rotating with uniform angular acceleration covers 100 π (radian) in the first 5 s after the start. Its angular speed (in rad/s) at the end of 5 s is

(a) 30 π (b) 10 π (c) 40 π (d) 20 π

17. A hollow metal sphere of radius 5 cm is charged such that the potential on its surface is 10 V. The potential at the centre of the sphere will be

(a) 10 V (b) 0.2 V (c) 5 V (d) zero

18. When a thin film of thickness t is placed in the path of light wave emerging out of the slit, then increase in the length of optical path will be

(a) μt (b) $\frac{\mu}{t}$ (c) $(\mu - 1)t$ (d) $(\mu + 1)t$

19. A wire of resistance R is bent to form a square $ABCD$ as shown in the figure. The effective resistance between E and C is (E is mid-point of arm CD)

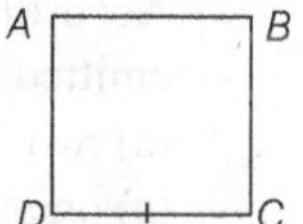

(a) R (b) $\frac{1}{16}R$ (c) $\frac{7}{64}R$ (d) $\frac{3}{4}R$

20. Initially body was at rest, calculate the distance travelled by body in its 6th second, if the acceleration of body is 4 m/s^2.

(a) 23 m (b) 22 m
(c) 21 m (d) 20 m

21. **Statement I** A narrow pulse of light is sent through a medium. The pulse will retain its shape as it travels through the medium.

Statement II A narrow pulse is made of harmonic waves with a large range of wavelengths.

In the light of above statemens, choose the most appropriate answer from the option given below

(a) Both Statement I and Statement II are correct.
(b) Both Statement I and Statement II are incorrect.
(c) Statement I is correct and Statement II is incorrect.
(d) Statement I is incorrect and Statement II is correct.

22. If v_e is escape velocity and v_o is orbital velocity of a satellite for orbit close to the earth's surface, then these are related by

(a) $v_e = \sqrt{2}v_o$ (b) $v_o = \sqrt{2}v_e$
(c) $v_e = \sqrt{2v_o}$ (d) $v_o = v_e$

23. If the planes of two identical concentric coils are perpendicular and the magnetic moment of each coil is M, then the resultant magnetic moment of the two coils will be

(a) $3M$ (b) $\sqrt{2}M$ (c) $2M$ (d) M

24. An alternating voltage E (in volts) $= 200\sqrt{2}\sin(100t)$ is connected to a $1\mu F$ capacitor through an AC ammeter. The reading of the ammeter will be

(a) 80 mA (b) 40 mA (c) 20 mA (d) 10 mA

25. The barrier potential in a p-n junction is 0.3 V. The current required is 6 mA. The emf of the cell required for use in the circuit, if a resistance of 200Ω is connected in series with junction is

(a) 1.5 V (b) 2 V (c) 3 V (d) 5 V

26. Ionisation potential of hydrogen atom is 13.6 eV. Hydrogen atom in the ground state are excited by monochromatic radiation of photon energy 12.1 eV. According to Bohr's theory, the spectral lines emitted by hydrogen will be

(a) two (b) three
(c) one (d) six

27. If there is a positive error of 50% in the measurement of velocity of a body, then the error in the measurement of kinetic energy is

(a) 25% (b) 50% (c) 100% (d) 125%

28. A convex lens of focal length 0.12 m produces a virtual image which is thrice the size of the object. Find the distance between the object and the lens.

(a) 0.12 m (b) 0.24 m (c) 0.08 m (d) 0.04 m

29. Statement I Lenz's law violates the principle of conservation of energy.

Statement II Induced emf always opposes the change in magnetic flux responsible for its production.

In the light of above statemens, choose the most appropriate answer from the option given below

(a) Statement I is correct and Statement II is incorrect.
(b) Statement I is incorrect and Statement II is correct.
(c) Both Statement I and Statement II are correct.
(d) Both Statement I and Statement II are incorrect.

30. If two bulbs of power 25 W and 100 W, respectively each rated at 220 V are connected in series with the supply of 440 V. Which bulb will fuse ?

(a) 40 W (b) 25 W
(c) Both (a) and (b) (d) None of these

31. Figure shows the shape of part of a long string in which transverse waves are produced by attaching one end of the string to tuning fork of frequency 250 Hz. What is the velocity of the waves ?

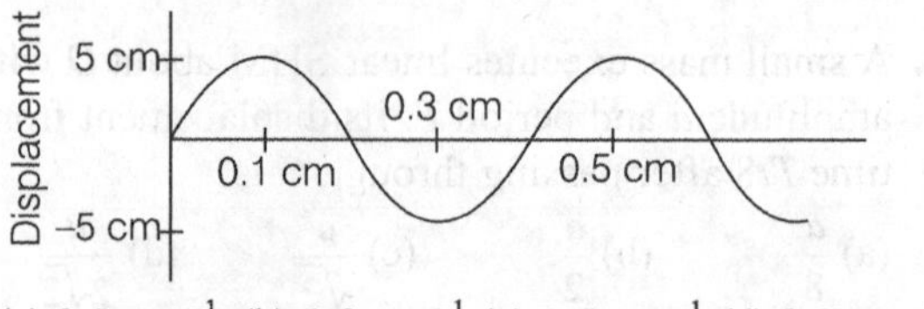

(a) $2.5\ ms^{-1}$ (b) $1.0\ ms^{-1}$ (c) $1.5\ ms^{-1}$ (d) $2.0\ ms^{-1}$

32. A sphere has a charge of +50 C. The absolute potential at a point at distance of 10^{-12} m from centre of the sphere is
(Radius of the sphere is $< 10^{-12}$ m)

(a) 4.5×10^{23} V (b) 45×10^{24} V
(c) 45×10^{23} V (d) 4500 V

33. 200 g of a solid ball at 20° C is dropped in an equal amount of water at 80° C. The resulting temperature is 60° C. This means that specific heat of solid is

(a) four times of water (b) twice of water
(c) one-half of water (d) one-fourth of water

34. The position of x of a particle with respect to time t along x-axis is given by $x = 9t^2 - t^3$, where x is in metres and t in seconds. What will be the position of this particle when it achieves maximum speed along the +x-direction ?

(a) 32 m (b) 24 m (c) 81 m (d) 54 m

35. Find the equivalent resistance between the points A and B.

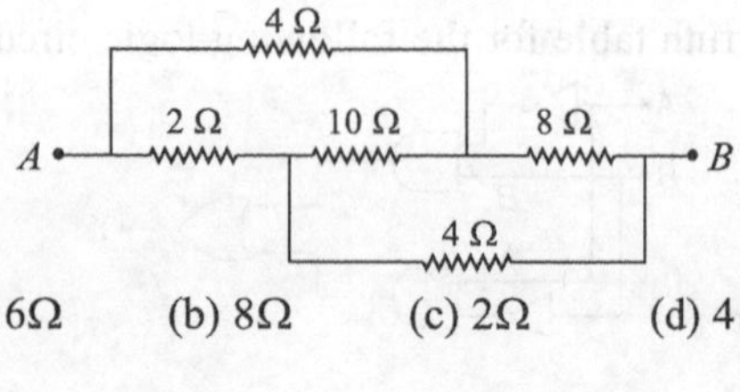

(a) 16Ω (b) 8Ω (c) 2Ω (d) 4Ω

36. With the increase in principal quantum number, the energy difference between the two successive energy levels

(a) remains constant
(b) increases
(c) decreases
(d) sometimes increases and sometimes decreases

37. At time $t = 0$ s, particle starts moving along the x-axis. If its kinetic energy increased uniformly with time t, the net force acting on it must be proportion to

(a) constant (b) t (c) $\sqrt{t}$ (d) $\frac{1}{\sqrt{t}}$

38. The rms value of potential difference V shown in the figure is

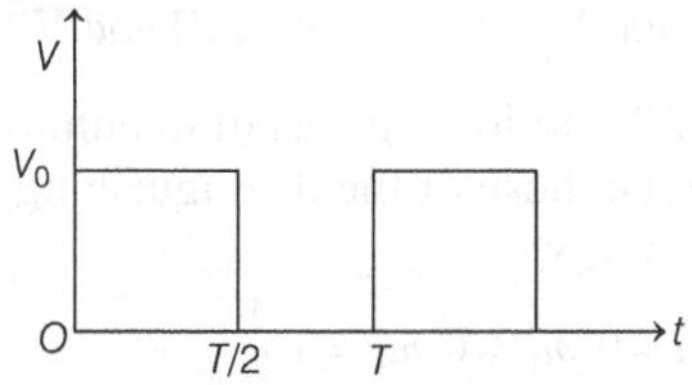

(a) V_0 (b) $\frac{V_0}{\sqrt{2}}$ (c) $\frac{V_0}{2}$ (d) $\frac{V_0}{\sqrt{3}}$

39. A stone of mass 2 kg is tied to a string of length 0.5 m. If the breaking tension of the string is 900 N, then the maximum angular velocity, the stone can have in uniform circular motion is

(a) 40 rad s^{-1} (b) 10 rad s^{-1}
(c) 20 rad s^{-1} (d) 30 rad s^{-1}

40. A wheel starting from rest is uniformly accelerated at 2 rad s^{-2} for 20 s. It is allowed to rotate uniformly for the next 10 s and is finally brought to rest in next 20 s. The total angle rotated by the wheel (in rad) is

(a) 300 (b) 1800 (c) 1200 (d) 600

41. At what height from the surface of the earth, the total energy of the satellite is equal to its potential energy at a height of $2R$ from the surface of earth ? (R = radius of earth)

(a) $4R$ (b) $2R$ (c) $\frac{R}{2}$ (d) $\frac{R}{4}$

42. Two free parallel wires carrying currents in opposite direction,

(a) attract each other.
(b) repel each other.
(c) neither attract nor repel.
(d) get rotated to be perpendicular to each other.

43. The energy of the electromagnetic waves is of the order of 15 keV. To which part of the spectrum, does it belong ?

(a) Ultraviolet rays (b) γ-rays
(c) Infrared rays (d) X-rays

44. If the screw on a screw gauge is given 8 rotations, then it moves by 4 mm on main scale. If there are 100 divisions on the circular scale, then the least count of the screw gauge is

(a) 0.05 mm (b) 0.0005 mm
(c) 0.005 mm (d) 0.500 mm

45. A wire of resistance $12\Omega\ m^{-1}$ is bent to form a complete circle of radius 10 cm. The resistance between its two diametrically opposite points A and B as shown in the figure

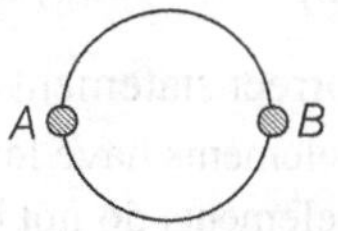

(a) $0.6\pi\Omega$ (b) 3Ω (c) $6\pi\Omega$ (d) 6Ω

CHEMISTRY

46. Match List-I with List-II.

	List-I		List-II
A.	Mathematical expression for rate of reaction.	I.	Rate constant
B.	Units of rate constant for zero order reaction is same as that of	II.	Rate law
C.	Order of a complex reaction is determined by	III.	Order of slowest step
D.	Rate of reaction for zero order reaction is equal to	IV.	Rate of reaction

Choose the correct answer from the options given below.

(a) A-II, B-IV, C-III, D-I (b) A-I, B-II, C-IV, D-III
(c) A-III, B-IV, C-II, D-I (d) A-II, B-I, C-IV, D-III

47. Which of the following is false?

(a) Sucrose is a non-reducing sugar.
(b) Glucose is oxidised by bromine water.
(c) Glucose rotates plane polarised light in clock-wise direction.
(d) Fructose is oxidised by bromine water.

48. The number of structural isomers for C_6H_{14} is

(a) 4 (b) 3 (c) 6 (d) 5

49. Choose the correct statement for transition elements.

(a) Transition elements have low melting points.
(b) Transition elements do not have catalytic activity.
(c) Transition elements exhibit variable oxidation states.
(d) Transition elements exhibit inert pair effect.

50. Which of the following statements are correct?

A. Wilkinson's catalyst $[(Ph_3P)_3RhCl]$ is used for the hydrogenation of alkenes.
B. EDTA is used in the treatment of lead poisoning.
C. *cis*-platin stimulate the growth of tumor.
D. Hardness of water is estimated by simple titration with Na_2EDTA.
E. EDTA combines with cations to form clathrates.

Choose the correct answer from the options given below.

(a) A, B, C (b) A, B, D (c) A, C, D (d) B, C, D

51. Which statement is correct for an electron that has $n = 4$ and $m = -2$?

(a) The electron may be in a *d*-orbital.
(b) The electron is in the 3rd-orbit.
(c) The electron may be in a *p*-orbital.
(d) The electron must have a spin quantum number + 1/2.

52. Which of the following species results in electron pair up in the lower energy *d*-orbitals before occupying high energy orbitals in 3*d* series.

I. CN^- II. H_2O
III. CO IV. Cl^-
V. $C_2O_4^{2-}$

Choose the most appropriate answer from the options given below.

(a) I, II, III and IV (b) I, III and IV
(c) II, IV and V (d) I, III and V

53. Which of the following sets of quantum numbers could not be those of the distinguishing (last) electron of Mo?

A. $n = 4, l = 0, m_l = 0, m_s = +\frac{1}{2}$

B. $n = 5, l = 1, m_l = 9, m_s = -\frac{1}{2}$

C. $n = 4, l = 2, m_l = -1, m_s = +\frac{1}{2}$

D. $n = 5, l = 2, m_l = +2, m_s = -\frac{1}{2}$

E. $n = 3, l = 2, m_l = 0, m_s = +\frac{1}{2}$

(a) A, B and C (b) B, C and D
(c) A, B, D and E (d) C and D

54. For given carbanion,

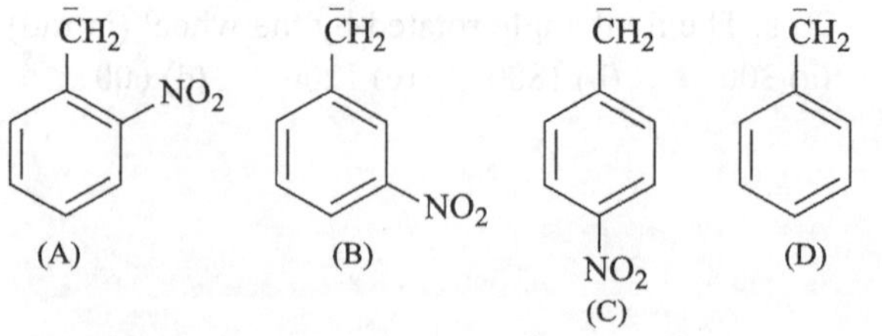

Stability order will be

(a) A > B > C > D (b) D > B > C > A
(c) A > C > B > D (d) D > C > B > A

55. The product (*D*) of the following reaction is

$$CH_3Cl \xrightarrow{KCN} (A) \xrightarrow{H_2O/H^+} (B) \xrightarrow{NH_3} (C) \xrightarrow{\Delta} (D)$$

(a) $CH_3CH_2NH_2$
(b) CH_3CN
(c) $HCONH_2$
(d) CH_3CONH_2

56. Correct IUPAC name of $[Ni(en)Br_2(PPh_3)_2]$ is
(a) Dibromidoethyleneditriphenylnickel (II)
(b) Dibromido*bis*(ethylenediamine) *bis*(triphenylphosphine) nickel (II)
(c) Dibromoethylenediamine*bis* (triphenylphosphine) nickel (II)
(d) Dibromoethylenebromidophosphinenickel (II)

57. For a certain process, $\Delta H = 280\ kJ\ mol^{-1}$ and $\Delta S = 140\ JK^{-1} mol^{-1}$. What is the minimum temperature at which the process will be spontaneous?
(a) 2000 K
(b) 200 K
(c) 140 K
(d) 420 K

58. Which of the following statement is not correct?
(a) Aliphatic amines are stronger bases than ammonia.
(b) Aromatic amines are stronger bases than ammonia.
(c) The alkyl group in alkyl ammonium ion stabilises the ion more relative to the amine.
(d) The aryl group in aryl ammonium ion stabilises the ion less relative to the amine.

59. Indicate the organic structure for product expected when 2-methylpropene is heated with acetyl chloride in the presence of anhydrous $ZnCl_2$.
(a) 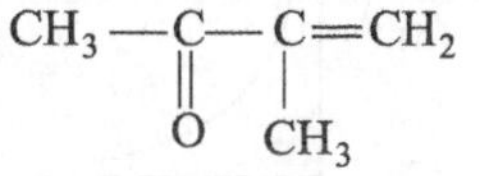
(b) 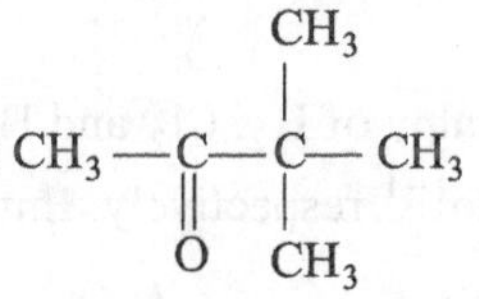
(c) 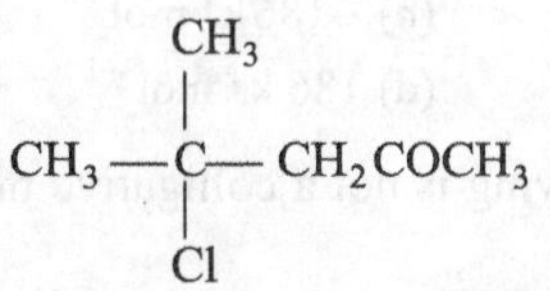
(d) 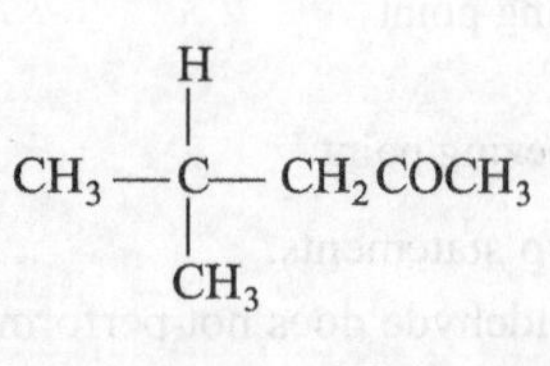

60. Benzene reacts with 2-methyloxirane in the presence of anhy. $AlCl_3$. It gives a product of molecular formula $C_9H_{12}O$. Identify the product from the following.
(a) 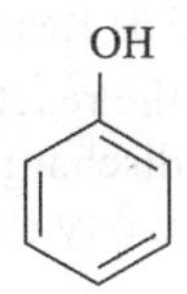
(b) 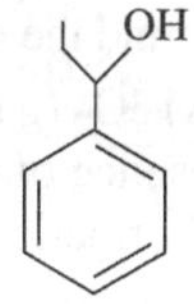
(c) 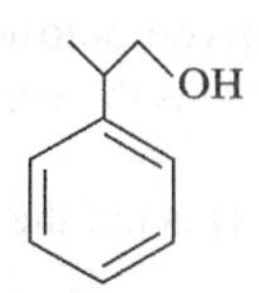
(d) 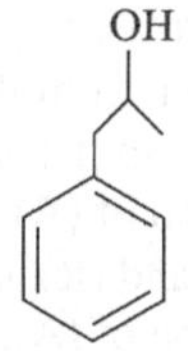

61. Consider the following reaction sequence.
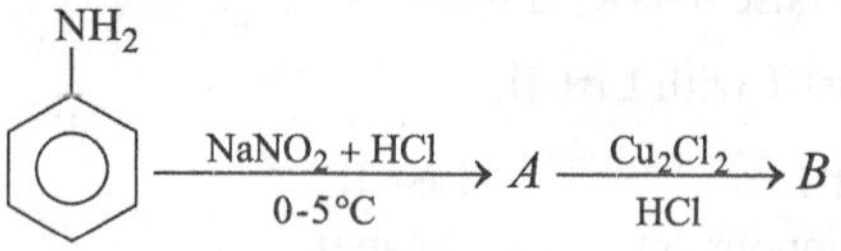

Product *B* is
(a) 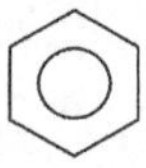
(b) 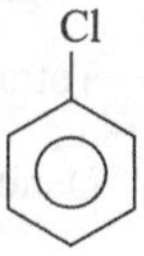
(c) 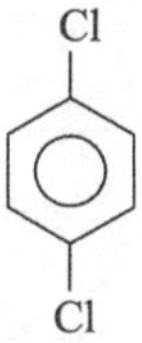
(d) 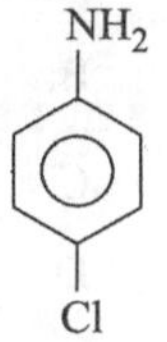

62. The decreasing order of reactivity towards electrophilic substitution of the following compounds is
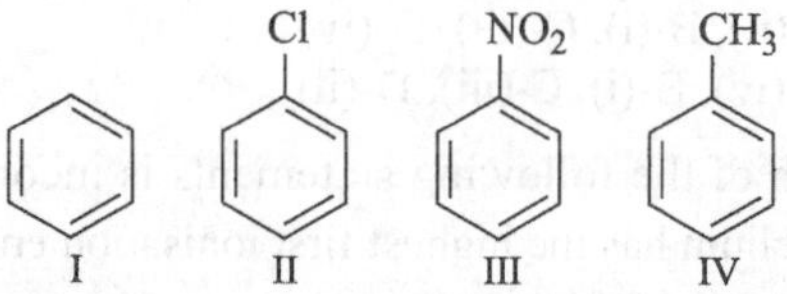
(a) I > III > IV > II
(b) IV > I > III > II
(c) IV > I > II > III
(d) I > IV > III > II

63. 2g of a mixture of CO and CO_2 on reaction with excess I_2O_5 produced 2.54 g of I_2. What would be the mass % of CO_2 in the original mixture?
(a) 60
(b) 30
(c) 70
(d) 35

64. Which of the following is incorrect?
(a) Ionisation energy of noble gas is highest in respective period.
(b) Ionisation energy of group-I metals is lowest in respective period.
(c) Ionisation energy of Al and Ga is almost same.
(d) Subsequent ionisation energy generally decreases.

65. Given below are two statements, one is labelled as Assertion (A) and the other is labelled as Reason (R).

Assertion (A) $3O_2(g) \longrightarrow 2O_3(g)$ the reaction occurs in presence of silent electric discharge.

Reason (R) Formation of ozone from oxygen is an exothermic process.

In the light of the above statements, choose the correct answer from the options given below.

(a) Both (A) and (R) are true and (R) is the correct explanation of (A).
(b) Both (A) and (R) are true but (R) is not the correct explanation of (A).
(c) (A) is true but (R) is false.
(d) (A) is false but (R) is true.

66. Match List-I with List-II.

	List-I (Compounds)		List-II (Shape)
A.	XeF_4	(i)	Trigonal pyramidal
B.	$SnCl_6^{2-}$	(ii)	Tetrahedral
C.	XeO_3	(iii)	Octahedral
D.	CCl_4	(iv)	Square planar

Choose the correct answer from the options given below.

(a) A-(iv), B-(iii), C-(i), D-(ii)
(b) A-(i), B-(ii), C-(iii), D-(iv)
(c) A-(ii), B-(i), C-(iii), D-(iv)
(d) A-(iv), B-(i), C-(iii), D-(ii)

67. Which of the following statements is incorrect?

(a) Helium has the highest first ionisation enthalpy in the periodic table.
(b) In any period, atomic radius of alkali metal is the highest.
(c) Mercury and bromine are liquids at room temperature.
(d) Chlorine has less negative electron gain enthalpy than fluorine.

68. Match the List-I with List-II.

	List-I (Compound)		List-II (Oxidation state of nitrogen)
A.	N_2O_5	(i)	-2
B.	NaN_3	(ii)	$+5$
C.	NO	(iii)	$-\frac{1}{3}$
D.	N_2H_4	(iv)	$+2$

Choose the correct answer from the options given below.

(a) A-(ii), B-(iii), C-(iv), D-(i)
(b) A-(i), B-(ii), C-(iii), D-(iv)
(c) A-(iv), B-(i), C-(ii), D-(iii)
(d) A-(iii), B-(i), C-(iv), D-(ii)

69. Given below are two statements.

Statement I Boric acid is a weak dibasic and protonic acid.

Statement II Ammonia and diborane mix with 2 : 1 ratio at 200°C to produce inorganic graphite.

In the light of the above statements, choose the correct answer from the options given below.

(a) Both Statement I and Statement II are true.
(b) Both Statement I and Statement II are false.
(c) Statement I is true but Statement II is false.
(d) Statement I is false but Statement II is true.

70. Which of the following curve gives the variation of Λ_m with $\sqrt{C}$ for CH_3COOH?

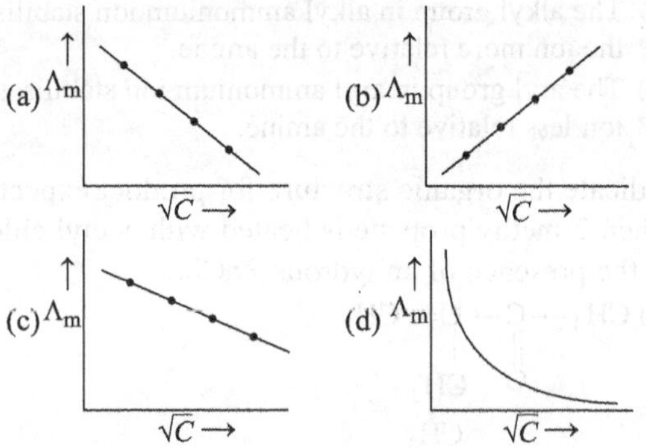

71. Bond dissociation enthalpy of H_2, Cl_2 and HCl are 434, 242 and 431 kJ mol^{-1} respectively. Enthalpy of formation of HCl is

(a) -93 kJ mol^{-1}
(b) -186 kJ mol^{-1}
(c) 93 kJ mol^{-1}
(d) 186 kJ mol^{-1}

72. Which of the following is not a colligative property?

(a) Osmotic pressure
(b) Elevation in boiling point
(c) Vapour pressure
(d) Depression in freezing point

73. Given below are two statements.

Statement I Formaldehyde does not perform aldol condensation.

Statement II Aldol is formed as an intermediate product during aldol condensation.

In the light of the above statements, choose the correct answer from the options given below.
(a) Both Statement I and Statement II are true.
(b) Both Statement I and Statement II are false.
(c) Statement I is true but Statement II is false.
(d) Statement I is false but Statement II is true.

74. The potential energy diagram for the reaction $R \rightarrow P$ is given below.

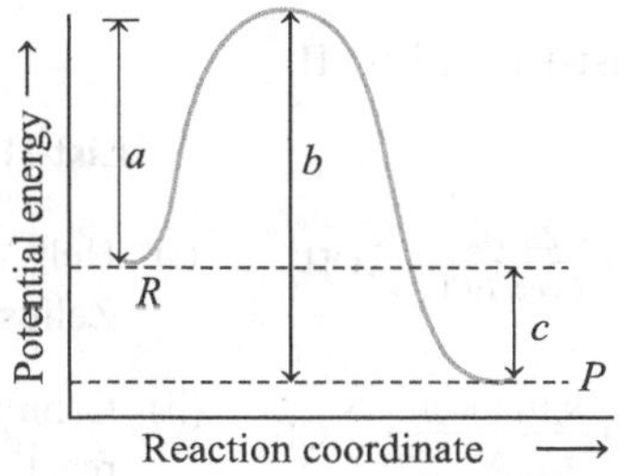

$\Delta H°$ of the reaction corresponds to the energy
(a) a (b) b (c) c (d) $a + b$

75. Consider the following reaction sequence

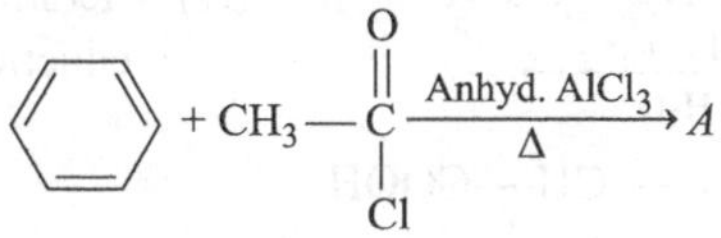

Product A is

(a) 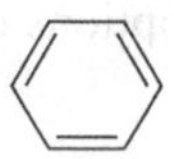

(b) 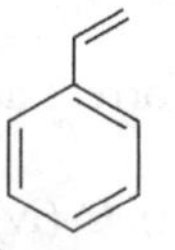

(c) 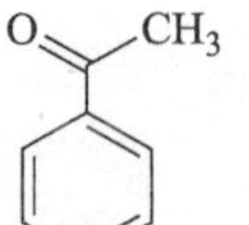

(d) 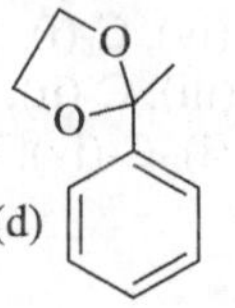

76. Given below are two statements.
Statement I Be_2 molecule does not exists.
Statement II O_2 molecule is paramagnetic in nature.
In the light of the above statements, choose the correct answer from the options given below.
(a) Both Statement I and Statement II are true.
(b) Both Statement I and Statement II are false.
(c) Statement I is true but Statement II is false.
(d) Statement I is false but Statement II is true.

77. When SO_2 is passed through acidified $K_2Cr_2O_7$ solution
(a) the solution turns blue.
(b) the solution is decolourised.
(c) SO_2 is reduced.
(d) green $Cr_2(SO_4)_3$ is formed.

78. A given quantity of PCl_5 was heated in a 10 dm^3 vessel at 250°C,

$$PCl_5(g) \rightleftharpoons PCl_3(g) + Cl_2(g)$$

At equilibrium, the vessel contains 0.1 mole of PCl_5 and 0.2 mole of Cl_2. The equilibrium constant of the reaction is
(a) 0.05 (b) 0.04
(c) 0.02 (d) 0.025

79. Given below are two statements.
Statement I Copper sulphate cannot be stored in zinc vessel.
Statement II Zinc is less reactive than copper.
In the light of the above statements, choose the correct answer from the options given below.
(a) Both Statement I and Statement II are false.
(b) Statement I is true Statement II is false.
(c) Statement I is false but Statement II is true.
(d) Both Statement I and Statement II are true.

80. Cyclopentene on treatment with alkaline $KMnO_4$ gives
(a) cyclopentanol
(b) *trans*-1, 2-cyclopentanediol
(c) *cis*-1, 2-cyclopentanediol
(d) 1 : 1 mixture of *cis*- and *trans*-1, 2-cyclopentanediol

81. In the reaction of *p*-chlorotoluene with KNH_2 in liq. NH_3, the major product is
(a) *o*-toluidine (b) *p*-toluidine
(c) *m*-toluidine (d) *p*-chloroaniline

82. The vapour pressure of CCl_4 at 25°C is 143 mm Hg, if 0.5 g of a non-volatile solute (mol. weight = 65) is dissolved in 100 g of CCl_4, the vapour pressure of the solution will be
(a) 99.39 mm Hg (b) 199.34 mm Hg
(c) 141.31 mm Hg (d) 143.99 mm Hg

83. Time required to deposit one millimole of aluminium metal by the passage of 9.65 amperes through molten electrolyte containing aluminium ion is
(a) 30 s (b) 10 s
(c) 30,000 s (d) 10,000 s

84. If 75% of a first order reaction was completed in 32 minutes then 50% of the reaction was complete in
(a) 4 min (b) 8 min
(c) 16 min (d) 24 min

85. Solid XeF_6 exists as
(a) XeF_4^+ and F_2^- (b) XeF_5^+ and F^-
(c) XeF_7^- and F^+ (d) Xe_4^+ and F_4^-

86. One mole of calcium phosphide on reaction with excess water gives
(a) one mole of phosphine
(b) two moles of phosphoric acid
(c) two moles of phosphine
(d) one mole of phosphorus pentoxide

87. Increasing order of reactivity of the following alkyl halides in the Williamson's synthesis is
I. $CH_2{=}CHCH_2Cl$ II. $CH_3CH_2CH_2Br$
III. $(CH_3)_3CCH_2Br$ IV. $CH_3CH_2CH_2Cl$
(a) II < III < IV < I
(b) III < II < IV < I
(c) IV < III < I < II
(d) III < IV < II < I

88. Given below are two statements.
Statement I The reaction of alkyl chloride with sodium iodide in presence of acetone to produce alkyl iodide is called Fittig reaction.
Statement II Wurtz-Fittig reaction involves one mol each of aryl and alkyl halides.
In the light of the above statements, choose the correct answer from the options given below.
(a) Both Statement I and Statement II are true.
(b) Both Statement I and Statement II are false.
(c) Statement I is true but Statement II is false.
(d) Statement I is false but Statement II is true.

89. Which of the following statements regarding chemical properties of acetophenone are incorrect?
A. It is reduced to methyl phenyl carbinol by sodium and ethanol.
B. It is oxidised to benzoic acid with acidified $KMnO_4$.
C. It does not undergo electrophilic substitution like nitration at *meta*-position.
D. It does not undergo iodoform reaction with iodine and alkali.
E. It is a colourless or pale yellow organic compound.
Choose the correct answer from the options given below.
(a) A and B (b) B and D
(c) C and D (d) B and C

90. Match List-I with List-II.

	List-I	List-II
A.	$>C{=}O \xrightarrow[\text{Conc. HCl}]{\text{Zn, Hg}} >CH_2$	(i) Hell-Volhard Zelinsky
B.	$>C{=}O \xrightarrow[\Delta]{N_2H_4 + KOH} >CH_2$	(ii) Cannizzaro reaction
C.	$HCHO \xrightarrow{\text{Conc. KOH}} HCOOK + CH_3OH$	(iii) Wolff-Kishner reduction
D.	$R{-}CH_2{-}COOH \xrightarrow[H_2O]{\text{Red P} + X_2} R{-}\underset{X}{\underset{\mid}{C}H}{-}COOH$	(iv) Clemmensen's reduction

Choose the correct answer from the options given below.
(a) A-(ii), B-(i), C-(iv), D-(iii)
(b) A-(iii), B-(iv), C-(i), D-(ii)
(c) A-(iv), B-(iii), C-(ii), D-(i)
(d) A-(iii), B-(i), C-(iv), D-(ii)

BIOLOGY

91. The ovulation phase is followed by the luteal phase during which the remaining parts of the Graafian follicle transform into corpus luteum, which secretes large amounts of
(a) leutinizing hormone which is essential for maintenance of the endometrium
(b) oestrogen hormone which is essential for disintegration of endometrium
(c) human chorionic gonadotropin which proliferates the endometrium
(d) progesterone which is essential for maintenance of endometrium

92. Which of the following match pair is incorrect?
(a) *In situ* conservation - It refers to the conservation of biodiversity outside of the normal habitats
(b) Paul Ehrlich - Rivet popper hypothesis
(c) David Tilman - Increased diversity contributes higher productivity
(d) *Ex situ* conservation - Gametes of threatened species can be preserved

93. Which of the following is not the characteristic of an Intra uterine device?
(a) It increases phagocytosis of sperms within the uterus
(b) It suppresses sperm motility and the fertilising capacity of sperms.
(c) It makes the uterus unsuitable for implantation
(d) It suppresses the formation of egg and changes the quality of Fallopian tube

94. What could be the most appropriate reason for lipids, whose molecular weights do not exceed 800 Da, being categorised under acid insoluble fraction ?
(a) They are insoluble in water as water is a non polar molecule
(b) They are a heterogenous group of compounds but are mainly composed of hydrocarbon chains
(c) They are oily or greasy nonpolar molecule that are stored in the adipose tissue of the body
(d) They are present in the structures of cell membranes and other membranes which form acid insoluble vesicles

95. Given below are two statements; one is labelled as Assertion (A) and the other is labelled as Reason (R).
Assertion (A) The primary and secondary immune responses are carried out with the help of B and T lymphocytes, present in our blood.
Reason (R) During the secondary immune response, the immune system can eliminate the antigen, which has been encountered by the individual during primary invasion, more rapidly and efficiently.
In the light of the above statements, choose the correct answer form the options given below.
(a) A is false, but R is true
(b) Both A and R are true and R is the correct explanation of A
(c) Both A and R are true, but R is not the correct explanation of A
(d) A is true, but R is false

96. Which of the following statement is incorrect ?
(a) The pyramid of biomass in sea is generally inverted because the biomass of fishes far exceeds that of phytoplankton because these are microscopic or small organisms
(b) Pyramid of energy is always upright, can never be inverted, because when energy flows from a particular trophic level to the next trophic level some energy is always lost as heat at each step
(c) Each bar in the energy pyramid indicates the amount of energy present at each trophic level in a given time or annually per unit area
(d) Saprophytes play a vital role in the ecosystem, they are placed on second or sometimes third trophic level in energy pyramid

97. What type of ecological pyramid would be obtained from the following given data?
I. Primary consumer - 10,000 in number
II. Primary producer - One in number
III. Secondary consumer - 10 is number
(a) Inverted pyramid of number
(b) Upright pyramid of number
(c) Spindle pyramid of number
(d) Inverted pyramid of number

98. Which of the following group of animals have modified placoid teeth, absence of air bladder, heart is two chambered and lack capacity to regulate their body temperature?
(a) *Ichthyophis* and *Rana*
(b) *Labeo* and *Clarias*
(c) *Scoliodon* and *Trygon*
(d) *Lamprey* and Hagfish

99. Given below are two statements.

Statement I Lactational amenorrhea method is based on the fact that ovulation and therefore the menstrual cycle do not occur during the period of intense lactation following parturition.

Statement II Breastfeeding is accompanied by high levels of LH which remain higher than normal until the frequency and duration of daily sucking decreases and thus, disrupts the menstrual cycle.

In the light of the above statements, choose the correct answer from the options given below.

(a) Statement I is incorrect, but statement II is correct
(b) Both statement I and statement II are correct
(c) Both statement I and statement II are incorrect
(d) Statement I is correct, but statement II is incorrect

100. Given below are two statements.

Statement I Order is a more specific rank than class, assemblage of families which exhibit a few similar characters. The similar characters are more in number as compared to different genera included in a family.

Statement II Family has a group of related genera with less number of similarities compared to genus and species.

In the light of the above statements, choose the correct answer from the options given below.

(a) Statement I is incorrect, but statement II is correct
(b) Both statement I and statement II are correct
(c) Both statement I and statement II are incorrect
(d) Statement I is correct, but statement II is incorrect

101. Which of the following statement is incorrect?

(a) Protein is imagined as a line, the left end represented by the first amino acid and right end represented by the last amino acid first and latter is also known as N-terminal amino acid and C-terminal amino acid, respectively
(b) Adult human haemoglobin consists of 4 subunits, two subunits of α type and two subunits of β type together constitute the human haemoglobin
(c) Co-enzymes are organic compounds and their association with the apoenzyme is only transient, usually occurring during the course of catalysis, serve as cofactors in a number of different enzyme catalysed reactions
(d) A number of enzymes require metal ions for their activity which form hydrogen bonds with side chain at the active site and at the same time form only one hydrogen bonds with the substrate

102. If a foreign DNA ligated at the *Bam*HI site of tetracycline resistance gene in the vector pBR322, it will lose tetracycline resistance but can still be selected out from non-recombinant ones by

(a) growing the transformants on kanameycin plate
(b) plating the transformants on ampicillin plate
(c) plating the transformants on tetracycline plate
(d) plating the transformants on chloramphenicol

103. Chemiosmosis occurs mainly in the thylakoids of chloroplast. It was first presented by D. Mitchell in 1961. The requirements of chemiosmosis are

(a) NADH, CO_2 proton pump, proton gradient and NADPH reductase
(b) a membrane, a proton gradient, a proton pump and ATP synthase
(c) NADPH reductase, a proton pump, PS-I and electron
(d) PS-I, PS-II, cytochrome oxidase and ATP synthase

104. Which of the following statements is/are correct?

I. In all connective tissues except blood, the cells secrete fibres of structural proteins, collagen or elastin.
II. Neuroglial cells protect and support the neurons.
III. Osteocytes are present in spaces called bone matrix osteoid.
IV. Striated muscle fibres are bundled together in parallel fashion.
V. Biceps are involuntary and striated.

Choose the correct answer from the options given below.

(a) II, IV and V (b) I, II and IV
(c) I, II and III (d) III and IV

105. Hatch and Slack pathway is an important photosynthetic pathway in C_4 plants. This pathway takes place in mesophyll cells which are present near the bundle sheath cells. These cells

(a) contain PEP carboxylase and lack RuBisCO enzyme
(b) have large number of chloroplast and lack PEPcase
(c) are thick impervious to gaseous exchange and contain RuBisCO enzyme
(d) contains both the enzymes, i.e PEPcase and RuBisCO enzyme

106. Which of the following structure of a sperm is not correctly matched with their particular feature/function?

(a) Acrosome - Filled with enzymes that help fertilise the ovum
(b) Middle piece - possesses numerous mitochondria, produce energy for the movement of tail
(c) Tail - Facilitate sperm motility
(d) Head - contains an elongated diploid nucleus

107. The cross between tall and dwarf plants produce gametes, by the process of meiosis. The alleles of the parental pair ...*A*... from each other and only one allele is transmitted to a gamete; the segregation of alleles is a ...*B*.... process and so there is a ...*C*... chance of gamete containing either allele. Identify *A*, *B*, and *C* from the following option.

	A	*B*	*C*
(a)	segregate	planned	50 %
(b)	segregate	random	50 %
(c)	segregate	sequential	10 %
(d)	segregate	sequential	40 %

108. Which of the following statements is incorrect?

(a) Most of the cartilages in vertebrate embryos are replaced by bones in adults and are present in the tip of nose, outer ear joints and between adjacent bones of the vertebral column
(b) Muscle fibres are composed of numerous myofibrils, which contract in response to stimulation, then relax and return to their uncontracted state in a coordinated fashion
(c) The smooth muscle fibres taper at both ends and show striations, these are voluntary as their functioning can be directly controlled
(d) Skeletal muscle tissue is closely attached to skeletal bones, they are bundled together in a parallel fashion

109. *Neurospora* is an Ascomycetes fungi, which is widely used in biochemical and genetic work due to the fact that

(a) it is easy to grow and found every where
(b) it has haploid life cycle which makes genetic analysis easy
(c) fungal nature, requires less nutrient medium to grow
(d) its diploid life cycle is comparable to human genetics

110. Which of the following statement is/are incorrect?

I. Electrons from NADH produced in the mitochondrial matrix during citric acid cycle are oxidised by an NADH dehydrogenase and electrons are then transferred to ubiquinone.
II. In fermentation there is a net gain of only one molecule of ATP for each molecule of glucose
degraded to pyruvic acid whereas many more molecule of ATP are generated under aerobic conditions.
III. The F_1 headpiece of ATP synthase is a peripheral membrane protein complex and contains the site for synthesis of ATP from ADP and inorganic phosphasphate.
IV. The NADH synthesised in glycolysis is transferred into the mitochondria and undergoes photophosphorylation.
V. When carbohydrates are used as substrate the RQ will be 0.7, because CO_2 evolved is more than O_2 consumed.

Choose the correct answer from the options given below.

(a) I, II, III and V (b) II, IV and V
(c) II, III, IV and V (d) I and II

111. Given below are two statements; one is labelled as Assertion (A) and the other is labelled as Reason (R).

Assertion (A) The signals for parturition originate from the fully developed foetus and the placenta which induce mild uterine contractions called foetal ejection reflex.
Reason (R) Oxytocin acts on the uterine muscle and causes stronger uterine contractions, which in turn stimulates further secretion of oxytocin.

In the light of the above statements, choose the correct answer form the options given below.

(a) A is false, but R is true
(b) Both A and R are true, but R is not the correct explanation of A

(c) Both A and R are true and R is the correct explanation of A
(d) A is true, but R is false

112. Match List I with List II.

	List I		List II
A.	It is lined by simple cuboidal brush border epithelium which increases surface area for reabsorption	1.	Collecting Duct
B.	It maintains high osmolarity of medullary interstitial fluid	2.	Distal convoluted tubule
C.	Conditional reabsorption of Na^+ and water takes place	3.	Henle's loop
D.	It allows passage of small amounts of urea into the medullary interstitium	4.	Proximal convoluted tubule

Choose the correct answer from the options given below.

	A	B	C	D
(a)	4	3	2	1
(b)	4	2	3	1
(c)	2	3	1	4
(d)	3	4	1	2

113. After penetrating stigmatic and stylar tissue, the pollen tube usually grows downwards towards egg because
(a) there is no other path to follow
(b) it grows under the control of egg nucleus
(c) it is attracted by dissimilar electric charge
(d) the filiform apparatus of synergids is believed to attract the pollen tube

114. Given below are two statements.

Statement I Hemichordata was earlier considered under the phylum chordata, but now is placed in separate phylum under non-chordata due to the presence of a rudimentary structure in the collar region called stomochord, similar to notochord.

Statement II Hemichordata consists of a small group of worm like marine animals which are triploblastic, radially symmetrical and coelomate, excretory system is absent.

In the light of the above statements, choose the correct answer from the options given below.
(a) Statement I is incorrect, but statement II is correct
(b) Both statement I and statement II are correct
(c) Both statement I and statement II are incorrect
(d) Statement I is correct, but statement II is incorrect

115. The microsporogenesis refers to
(a) process of formation of embryo sac from the megaspore mother cell *via* meiotic division
(b) process of formation of microspores from a pollen mother cell through meiosis
(c) process of formation of microspores from a pollen mother cell through mitosis
(d) process of formation of embryo sac from the megaspore mother cell through mitosis

116. Read the following statements and identify the incorrect statements.

I. The squamous epithelium is composed of a single layer of cube-like cells, commonly found in ducts of glands and tubular parts of nephrons in kidneys and its main functions are secretion and absorption.
II. The columnar epithelium is composed of a single layer of tall and slender cells. Their nuclei are located at the base.
III. Gap junctions facilitate the cells to communicate with each other by connecting the cytoplasm of adjoining cells, for rapid transfer of ions, small molecules.
IV. In all connective tissue, the cells secrete fibres of structural proteins called collagen or elastin, these provide strength, elasticity and flexibility to the tissue.
V. In areolar tissue, the cells and fibres are loosely arranged in a semi-fluid ground substance.

Choose the correct answer form the options given below.
(a) I, III and V
(b) II, III and V
(c) I and IV
(d) Only V

117. Match List I with List II.

	List I		List II
A.	First trophic level	1.	Birds, fishes and wolf
B.	Third trophic level	2.	Zooplankton, grasshopper and cow
C.	Fourth trophic level	3.	Phytoplankton, grasses and trees
D.	Second trophic level	4.	Man, lion and vulture

Choose the correct answer from the options given below.

	A	B	C	D		A	B	C	D
(a)	3	1	4	2	(b)	3	2	4	1
(c)	1	4	3	2	(d)	2	4	3	1

118. Match List I with List II.

	List I		List II
A.	It is mostly terrestrial animal and body is covered by dry and cornified skin	1.	*Struthio*
B.	Skin is dry without glands except the oil gland at the base of the tail	2.	*Pristis*
C.	They have four pairs of gills which are covered with operculum	3.	*Calotes*
D.	Gill slits are separate and without operculum	4.	*Pterophyllum*

Choose the correct answer from the options given below.

	A	B	C	D		A	B	C	D
(a)	1	3	4	2	(b)	3	1	4	2
(c)	3	2	1	4	(d)	2	4	3	1

119. Parthenocarpic tomato fruits can be produced by

(a) treating plants with high concentration of ethylene and gibberellic acid
(b) treating the plants with phenyl mercuric acetate
(c) treating plants with low concentrations of gibberellic acid and auxins
(d) removing androecium of flowers before pollen grains are released

120. Which of the following types of joints are found between humerus and pectoral girdle and between the adjacent vertebrae the vertebral column ?

(a) Cartilaginous joint and synovial joint
(b) Fibrous joints and hinge joint
(c) Synovial joint and cartilaginous joint
(d) Cartilaginous joint and saddle joint

121. Identify the incorrect statement with respect to biogas plant.

(a) It consists of a concrete tank, 10-15 feet deep in which bio-waste are collected and a slurry of dung is fed
(b) A floating cover is placed over the slurry, which keeps on rising as the gas is consumed in the tank
(c) It has an outlet, which is connected to pipe to supply biogas to nearby houses
(d) The spent slurry is removed and may be used as fertiliser

122. Which of the following statements is correct about human excretory system ?

I. The tubule begins with a double walled cup-like structure called Bowman's capsule, which encloses the glomerulus, the glomerulus along with Bowman's capsule is called the Malpighian body or renal corpuscle.
II. A hairpin shaped Henle's loop is the next part of the tubule which has descending and an ascending limb, the descending limb continues as another highly coiled tubular region, DCT.
III. The Malpighian corpuscle, PCT and DCT of the nephron are situated in the medulla region of the kidney where as the loop of Henle dips into the cortical region.
IV. The distal convoluted tubule of many nephrons open into a straight tube called collecting duct, many of which converge and open into the renal pelvis through medullary pyramids in the calyces.
V. The peritubular capillaries are a fine capillary network around the renal tubule formed from efferent arteriole which emerges from column of Bertini.

Choose the correct answer from the options given below.

(a) II, IV and V
(b) I and IV
(c) II, III and IV
(d) II, III, IV and V

123. The relationship between species richness and area for a wide variety of taxa turns out to be a rectangular hyperbola. On a logarithm scale, the relationship is a straight line described by the equation

(a) $\log S = \log C + Z \log A$
(b) $N_t = N_o e^{rt}$
(c) $dN/dt = RN\left(\frac{K-N}{K}\right)$
(d) $\log C = \log S + Z \log A$

124. Given below are two statements; one is labelled as Assertion (A) and other is labelled as Reason (R)

Assertion (A) PMNL-neutrophils form a part of cellular barriers which provide innate immunity in humans.

Reason (R) They phagocytose and destroy microbes.

In the light of the above statements, choose the correct answer form the options given below.

(a) A is false, but R is true
(b) Both A and R are true, but R is not the correct explanation of A
(c) Both A and R are true and R is the correct explanation of A
(d) A is true, but R is false

125. Synovial joints are characterised by the presence of a fluid filled synovial cavity. It includes

I. Hinge joint
II. Between carpal and metacarpal of thumb
III. Between atlas and axis
IV. Accumulation of uric acid between joints
V. Joints of vertebral column.

Choose the correct option from the following.

(a) I, II and III (b) I, II, IV and V
(c) IV and V only (d) II, IV and V

126. Given below are two statements; one is labelled as Assertion (A) and the other is labelled as Reason (R).

Assertion (A) Test cross is used to determine an unknown genotype within one breeding generation.

Reason (R) It is a cross between F_1 hybrid and dominant parent.

In the light of the above statements, choose the correct answer form the options given below.

(a) A is false, but R is true
(b) Both A and R are true and R is the correct explanation of A
(c) Both A and R are true, but R is not the correct explanation of A
(d) A is true, but R is false

127. In test tube method, ova from wife and sperms from the husband are collected and are induced to form zygote under simulated conditions in the laboratory. The zygote or early embryos upto 8 blastomeres could be transferred into the

(a) Fallopian tube
(b) uterus
(c) vagina
(d) cervix

128. Which of the following groups of plants shows root-like, leaf-like or stem-like structures, main plant body as haploid, sex organs are multicellular sporophyte dependent on photosynthetic gametophyte?

(a) *Selaginella* and *Equisetum*
(b) *Lycopodium* and *Cycas*
(c) *Funaria* and *Polytrichum*
(d) *Funaria* and *Lycopodium*

129. Given below are two statements.

Statement I Each muscle fibre is lined by the sarcolemma enclosing the sarcoplasm, which is syncitium as it contains many nuclei and sarcoplasmic reticulum is the store house of calcium ions.

Statement II Myofibril has alternate dark and light bands, the dark bands contain actin and is called isotropic band whereas light band is called anisotropic that contains myosin.

In the light of the above statements, choose the correct answer from the options given below.

(a) Statement I is incorrect, but statement II is correct
(b) Both statement I and statement II are correct
(c) Both statement I and statement II are incorrect
(d) Statement I is correct, but statement II is incorrect

130. Given below are two statements; one is labelled as Assertion (A) and the other is labelled as Reason (R).

Assertion (A) The cloning vectors which have very few or single recognition sites for the commonly used restriction enzymes are preferred.

Reason (R) Presence of more than one recognition sites with in the vector will generate several fragments, which will complicate the gene cloning.

In the light of the above statements, choose the correct answer form the options given below.

(a) A is false, but R is true
(b) Both A and R are true and R is the correct explanation of A
(c) Both A and R are true, but R is not the correct explanation of A
(d) A is true, but R is false

131. Consider the given floral diagram and identify the incorrect statement.

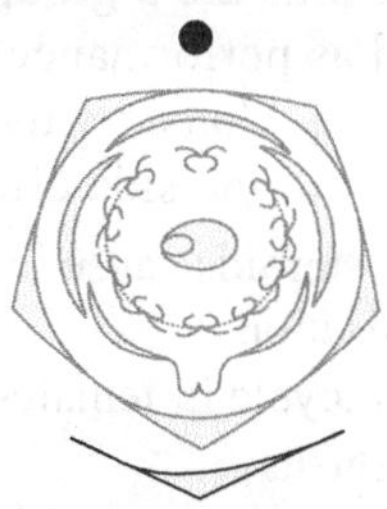

(a) Leaves are alternate and simple
(b) Have 5 united petals with vexillary aestivation
(c) Members of the family are economically important in the fodder as well as medical industries
(d) These are usually climbers

132. The sequential event in the heart which is cyclically repeated is called cardiac cycle. Consider the steps involved in cardiac cycle and arrange them in proper order.

I. SAN generates action potential.
II. All four chambers of the heart are in relaxed state.
III. Ventricles relax and ventricular pressure falls causing closure of semilunar valves.
IV. Ventricular systole causes closure of tricuspid and bicuspid valves.

Choose the correct answer from the options given below.

(a) I→III→II→IV (b) II→I→III→IV
(c) IV→I→III→II (d) II→I→IV→III

133. Which of the following correctly represents the complex IV?

(a) Complex IV is generated during oxidation of succinate in the citric acid cycle
(b) It drives the whole process by removing hydrogen from the ETS
(c) Ubiquinone receives reduced NADPH from complex IV
(d) It is cytochrome *c* oxidase complex containing cytochromes *a* and a_3 and two copper centers

134. Which of the following events causes the ventricular muscles to contract?

(a) The action potential is conducted to the ventricular side by the AVN and AV bundle from where the bundle of His transmits it through the entire ventricular musculature
(b) The ventricular pressure falls causing the closure of semilunar valves, prevents the back flow of blood into the ventricle
(c) The SAN generates an action potential, stimulates both the atria and ventricle
(d) The opening of tricuspid and bicuspid valves allows the blood to move freely in the ventricle

135. Which of the following statements about gymnosperms is correct?

I. Gymnosperms have ovules enclosed by an ovary wall.
II. The seeds in gymnosperms are covered and not exposed.
III. Gymnosperms include trees and shrubs, with unbranched stems in *Cycas*.
IV. Gymnosperms produce spores within sporangia that are borne on sporophylls.
V. The pollen grain in gymnosperms is a multicellular female gametophyte.

Choose the correct answer from the options given below.

(a) III and IV
(b) II and V
(c) I and IV
(d) III and V

136. Given below are two statements; one is labelled as Assertion (A) and the other is labelled as Reason (R).

Assertion (A) Parathyroid hormone is a hypercalcemic hormone as it increases the blood calcium levels in body and works antagonistic to calcitonin.

Reason (R) Parathyroid hormone acts on bones and stimulates the process of bone resorption by dissolution and demineralsation.

In the light of the above statements, choose the correct answer form the options given below.

(a) A is false, but R is true
(b) Both A and R are true, but R is not the correct explanation of A
(c) Both A and R are true and R is the correct explanation of A
(d) A is true, but R is false

137. Read the statements carefully and choose the incorrect option with respect to productivity.

(a) Primary productivity mainly depends upon photosynthesis
(b) NPP may contribute to the secondary productivity
(c) GPP always depends upon NPP
(d) GPP always depends upon temperature, soil moisture and nutrients in soil

138. A TS of a specimen is shown under microscope, it represents sclerenchymatous hypodermis, a large number of scattered vascular bundles, each surrounded by a sclerenchymatous bundle sheath and a large ground tissue. The TS of specimen could be

(a) dicot leaf (b) monocot stem
(c) dicot root (d) monocot root

139. Which of the following process helps in the formation of concentrated urine ?

(a) Suppression of ADH and vasopressin from the hypothalamus and neurohypophysis, respectively
(b) NaCl is returned to the interstitium by the ascending portion of vasa recta
(c) Suppression of release of aldosterone from adrenal cortex
(d) The administration of vasodilating agents

140. Which of the following statement is incorrect ?

I. Stem tendrils developing from terminal buds, are slender and spirally coiled and help plants to climb.
II. In mint and jasmine a slender lateral branch arises from the base of the main axis and after growing aerially for some time arch downwards to touch the ground.
III. In banana, the lateral branches originate from the basal and underground portion of the main stem, grow horizontally beneath the soil and then come out obliquely upward giving rise to leafy shoots.
IV. Leaf is a lateral, generally flattened structure borne on the stem, originating from shoot apical meristems and arranged in basipetal order.
V. Aleurone layer is a proteinous outer covering of endosperm which separates the embryo.

Choose the correct answer from the options given below.

(a) I and IV (b) II and III
(c) II, III and IV (d) V only

141. Alien species are non-native species that have been introduced into a region, either purposefully or accidently. These sometimes become invasive, resulting in the extinction or decline of native species, all of the given species are related to alien species invasion, except,

(a) extinction of Steller's sea cow
(b) extinction of cichlid fish
(c) introduction of *Clarias gariepinus* into Indian rivers
(d) introduction of *Eichhornia* in India

142. Anabolic steroids are a group of synthetic drugs that are used as performance and image enhancing drug. Consider the following statements about the side effects of these drugs.

I. Anabolic steroids cause increase in masculinisation.
II. Menstrual cycle in females is disturbed.
III. Liver cirrhosis
IV. These drugs cause damage to the nervous system.
V. A decreased sperm production is observed in males by their intake.

Choose the correct answer from the options given below.

(a) I, II and V
(b) III and V
(c) I, II, III and IV
(d) II and IV

143. Plasmid and Bacteriophage are considered as the ideal vector because

(a) these have many recognition sites for several restriction enzymes
(b) they are transferred from one bacterial cell to another by the process of conjugation
(c) these have ability to transform the normal cell into tumour cell by inserting a DNA piece
(d) these have very high copy number of their genome within the bacterial cells

144. Match List I with List II.

	List I	List II
A.	It contains centres for respiration, cardiovascular reflexes and gastric secretions	1. Hypothalamus
B.	It forms the connections between the brain and spinal cord	2. Pons
C.	It controls body temperature urge for eating and drinking	3. Brain stem
D.	It consists of fibre tracts that interconnect different regions of the brain	4. Medulla

Choose the correct answer from the options given below.

	A	B	C	D		A	B	C	D
(a)	2	4	3	1	(b)	4	3	1	2
(c)	3	4	1	2	(d)	4	3	2	1

145. Given below are two statements.

Statement I The possibility of a female becoming a haemophilic is extremely rare because mother of such a female has to be at least carrier and the father should be haemophilic.

Statement II In Haemophilic disease, a single protein that is a part of the cascade of proteins involved in the clotting of blood is affected.

In the light of the above statements, choose the correct answer from the options given below.

(a) Statement I is incorrect, but statement II is correct
(b) Both statement I and statement II are correct
(c) Both statement I and statement II are incorrect
(d) Statement I is correct, but statement II is incorrect

146. Which of the following group of biomolecules are protein ?

(a) Vinblastine, Insulin, Inulin and Trypsin
(b) Tyrosine, Abrin, Glucosamine and Guanine
(c) Collagen, GLUT-4, Immunoglobulin A, and Trypsin
(d) Carbonic Anhydrase, Glycogen and Collagen

147. Which of the following is not the key feature of meiosis ?

(a) It involves pairing of homologous chromosomes and recombination between non-sister chromatids of homologous chromosomes
(b) It results in the production of diploid daughter cells with identical genetic complement.
(c) Meiosis-I is initiated after the parental chromosomes have replicated to produce identical sister chromatids at the S phase
(d) It has two sequential cycles of nuclear and cell division but only a single cycle of DNA replication.

148. Given below are two statements.

Statement I The repressor of the operon is synthesised from the p gene, this protein binds to the promoter region of the operon and prevents RNA polymerase from transcribing the operon.

Statement II In presence of an inducer, such as lactose or allolactose, the repressor is inactivated by interaction with the inducer.

In the light of the above statements, choose the correct answer from the options given below.

(a) Statement I is incorrect, but statement II is correct
(b) Both statement I and statement II are correct
(c) Both statement I and statement II are incorrect
(d) Statement I is correct, but statement II is incorrect

149. Identify the correct match pair from the following.

(a) Synapsis aligns homologous chromosomes - Pachytene
(b) Dissolution of the synaptonemal complex - diakinesis
(c) Action of enzyme recombinase - Zygotene
(d) Centromeres do not separate but chromatids move towards opposite poles - Anaphase-I

150. Given below are two statements; one is labelled as Assertion (A) and the other is labelled as Reason (A).

Assertion (A) Divergent evolution represents the evolutionary pattern in which species sharing a common ancestry become more distinct due to differential selection pressure.

Reason (R) Divergent evolution gradually leads to speciation over an evolutionary time period.

In the light of the above statements, choose the correct answer form the options given below.

(a) A is false, but R is true
(b) Both A and R are true and R is the correct explanation of A
(c) Both A and R are true, but R is not the correct explanation of A
(d) A is true, but R is false

151. If two species belong to the same genus, what can be inferred about them?

(a) They belong to different families
(b) They share a high degree of morphological similarities
(c) They are members of different kingdoms
(d) They have no common characteristics

152. Which of the following is not the function of endomembrane system of a cell?

(a) It includes oxidative phosphorylation to produce cellular ATP

(b) They principally perform the function of packaging materials which delivered either intra-cellular or secreted outside the cell
(c) It provides major site for synthesis of lipid and lipid - like steroidal hormones
(d) They produce hydrolytic enzymes such as lipases, proteases and carbohydrates

153. Which of the following methods of pollination is true for the aquatic plant water hyacinth and waterlily?
(a) The female flowers reach the surface of water and pollen grains are carried passively by water currents
(b) The flowers emerge above the level of water and are pollinated by insects or wind
(c) Flowers remain submerged in water and the pollen grains are released inside the water
(d) Pollen grains are long, ribbon like and they are carried passively inside the water

154. Given below are two statements.
Statement I Origin of replication is a sequence, which helps in identifying and eliminating non-transformants and selectively permitting the growth of the transformants.
Statement II Origin of replication is also responsible for controlling the copy number of the linked DNA.
In the light of the above statements, choose the correct answer from the options given below.
(a) Statement I is incorrect, but statement II is correct
(b) Both statement I and statement II are correct
(c) Both statement I and statement II are incorrect
(d) Statement I is correct, but statement II is incorrect

155. Match List I with List II.

	List I		List II
A.	Gynoecium occupies the highest position while the other parts are situated below	1.	*Citrus*
B.	Gynoecium is situated in the centre and other parts are located on the rim of the thalamus	2.	Plum
C.	Stamens united into one bunch or one bundle	3.	Mustard
D.	Stamens united into more than two bundles	4.	China rose

Choose the correct answer from the options given below.

	A	B	C	D		A	B	C	D
(a)	4	3	2	1	(b)	3	4	1	2
(c)	3	2	4	1	(d)	1	3	4	2

156. Which of the following statements is incorrect?
(a) The pulmonary trunk with left and right arteries is part of pulmonary circulation
(b) The aorta is a part of systemic circulation
(c) The aorta receives blood from left ventricle
(d) Pulmonary vein collects deoxygenated blood from body and pour it into right atrium

157. Given below are two statements; one is labelled as Assertion (A) and the other is labelled as Reason (R).
Assertion (A) Evolution is not a directed process in the sense of determinism, but is based on chance events in nature and chance mutation in the organisms.
Reason (R) The excessive and continuous use of pesticides has resulted in the evolution of some new species of pests due to natural selection.
In the light of above statement, choose the correct answer from the options given below.
(a) A is false, but R is true
(b) Both A and R are true and R is the correct explanation of A
(c) Both A and R are true, but R is not the correct explanation of A
(d) A is true, but R is false

158. Which of the following pair of microorganisms is used to produce streptokinase and cyclosporin-A, respectively?
(a) *Monascus purpureus* and *Trichoderma polysporum*
(b) *Streptococcus* and *Trichoderma polysporum*
(c) *Saccharomyces cerevisiae* and *Streptococcus*
(d) *Saccharomyces cerevisiae* and *Monasus purpureus*

159. Carbon dioxide is the major limiting factor for photosynthesis. The C_3 and C_4 plants respond differently to CO_2 concentration. The C_4 plants show
(a) saturation at about 360 μ / L^{-1} while C_3 responds to saturation beyond 550 μ L^{-1}

(b) saturation at about 360 μ / L^{-1} while C_3 get saturated beyond 450 μ / L^{-1}
(c) saturation at 120 μ / L^1 while C_3 get saturated at 360 μ / L^{-1}
(d) saturation at 150 μ / L^{-1} while C_3 get saturated beyond 450 μ / L^{-1}

160. Arrange the following stages in the life cycle of *Plasmodium* in correct order from human to mosquito.

I. Parasites reproduce asexually in RBCs
II. Sporozoites reach the liver
III. Fertilisation in the mosquito intestine
IV. Gametocytes develop in RBCs

Choose the answer from the options given below.
(a) I → III → IV → II
(b) II → I → IV → III
(c) II → IV → III → I
(d) III → I → IV → II

161. Fruit drop is caused by
(a) more auxin in fruit than in stem
(b) less auxin in fruit than in stem
(c) equal distribution of auxin in stem and fruit
(d) absence of auxin in stem and frui.

162. Match List I with List II.

	List I		List II
A.	It is elongated or tube like cell with thick and lignified walls	1.	Xylem fibres
B.	Cells are devoid of protoplasm, interconnected through perforations in their common walls.	2.	Xylem parenchyma
C.	It has highly thickened walls and obliterated central lumens	3.	Tracheid
D.	These are living and thin walled, cell walls are made up of cellulose	4.	Vessel

Choose the correct answer from the options given below.

	A	B	C	D
(a)	3	4	1	2
(b)	1	3	4	2
(c)	2	4	3	1
(d)	4	2	3	1

163. Plants, bacteria, fungi and animals whose genes have been altered by manipulation are called genetically modified organisms. These organisms have been useful in many ways, except
(a) that these are more tolerant to abiotic stresses
(b) providing horizontal gene transfer of pesticide, herbicide resistance to other organisms
(c) that they helped to reduced post harvest losses
(d) that they increased efficiency of mineral usage of plants

164. Match List I with List II.

	List I		List II
A.	Autoimmune disorder affecting neuromuscular junction leading to fatigue	1.	Muscular dystrophy
B.	Progressive degeneration of skeletal muscle	2.	Osteoporosis
C.	Rapid spasms in muscle due to low calcium ions in body fluid	3.	Myasthenia gravis
D.	Decresed levels of oestrogen	4.	Tetany

Choose the correct answer from the options given below.

	A	B	C	D
(a)	2	3	4	1
(b)	4	2	1	3
(c)	3	1	4	2
(d)	3	4	1	2

165. Which of the following is not responsible for the opening of stomatal aperture ?
(a) Change in the turgidity of guard cells
(b) The inner wall of guard cell is thick and elastic
(c) Orientation of cellulosic microfibrils
(d) Position of subsidiary cells

166. Which of the following statements are correct?

I. In human beings, the membrane of the erythrocyte has approximately 52 % protein and 40 % lipids.
II. The pili are elongated tubular structures made of a special protein and fimbriae are small bristle like fibres sprouting out of the cell.
III. Ribosomes are membrane bound organelles found in all cells both eukaryotic and prokaryotic within the cell cytoplasm.

IV. Rudolf Virchow first explained that cells had a thin outer layer and their presence is a unique character of the plant cells.
V. The cytoplasm is the main area of cellular activities in both the plant and animal cells, various chemical reactions occur to keep the cell in the living state.

Choose the correct answer from the options given below.

(a) I, II and IV (b) I, II and V
(c) III, IV and V (d) II, IV and V

167. What is not correct with respect to ETC?
(a) Ubiquinone receives electrons from NADH + H^+ and $FADH_2$
(b) The reduced ubiquinone is called ubiquinol
(c) Cytochrome-*c*, *a* and a_3 is iron containing enzyme
(d) O_2 is terminal electron acceptor generating metabolic water

168. Under the microscope, a cell shows chromosomal material condensed to form compact mitotic chromosomes, seen to be composed of two chromatids attached together at the centromere. Each centromere radiates out microtubules called asters. Identify the stage of cell cycle.
(a) Metaphase (b) Anaphase
(c) Quiescent stage (d) Prophase

169. Which of the following statements is/are correct?
I. Wheat, maize, barley, castor and sunflower seeds are endospermic or albuminous.
II. Most zygotes divide only after certain amount of endosperm is formed.
III. Though the seeds differ greatly, the early stages of embryo development is similar in both monocots and dicots.
IV. The zygote divides to form proembryo and subsequently globular, heart-shaped and mature embryo.
V. Epicotyl and hypocotyl are absent in monocot seeds.

Choose the correct answer from the options given below.

(a) II, IV and V (b) II, III and V
(c) I, II and III (d) I, II, III and IV

170. Match List I with List II.

	List I		List II
A.	Presence of an additional copy of the chromosome number 21	1.	Turner's syndrome
B.	Presence of an additional copy of X-chromosome	2.	Phenylketonuria
C.	Females are sterile as ovaries are rudimentary	3.	Down's syndrome
D.	Inherited as the autosomal recessive trait	4.	Klinefelter's syndrome

Choose the correct answer from the options given below.

	A	B	C	D
(a)	1	3	4	2
(b)	3	4	1	2
(c)	4	1	3	2
(d)	2	3	4	1

171. Identify the correct order of events of cell cycle in which they occur.
I. The cell is metabolically active and continuously grows but does not replicate its DNA
II. The interphase lasts more than 95 % of the duration of cell cycle.
III. Proteins are synthesised in preparation for mitosis
IV. Synthesis of DNA or replication.

Choose the correct answer from the options given below.

(a) II → I → IV → III (b) II → I → III → IV
(c) I → III → IV → II (d) III → I → IV → II

172. Exchange of gases is found to occur between blood and tissues. Identify the statement that does not relate to gaseous exchange in humans.
(a) Alveoli are the major or primary sites in exchange of gases where gaseous exchange occurs by facilitated diffusion
(b) Pressure contributed by an individual gas in a mixture of gases is pX where X denotes the gas
(c) Partial pressure of carbon dioxide is 45 mm Hg in tissues
(d) Solubility of CO_2 is 20-25 times higher than that of O_2

173. Hydrolytic enzymes are the enzymes that catalyse the hydrolysis of various bonds such as peptide, ester, glycosidic, ether, carbon-carbon bonds. All the given reactions are catalysed by hydrolytic enzymes, except

(a) lysosomal lipase digests lipids and cholesterol to free fatty acids
(b) salivary amylase converts starch to maltose
(c) phosphates catalyses the removal of phosphate moiety from the substrate.
(d) amination of fumaric acid to form aspartic acid

174. Match List I with List II.

List I	List II
A. Sexual deceit employed by orchid *Ophrys*	1. Predation
B. Fitness of one species significantly lowers the presence of another species	2. Parasitism
C. Some species of insects are cryptically coloured	3. Mutualism
D. Human liver fluke depends on two hosts	4. Competition

Choose the correct answer from the options given below.

	A	B	C	D		A	B	C	D
(a)	1	3	2	4	(b)	3	1	4	2
(c)	3	4	1	2	(d)	4	3	1	2

175. Eli Lilly, an American company prepared two DNA sequences corresponding to A and B chains of human insulin and introduced them in plasmids of *E. coli*, the two chains were produced separately, extracted and combined by creating

(a) Hydrogen bonds (b) disulphide bonds
(c) N-glycosidic bonds (d) phophate bond

176. Consider the following floral formulas of two different families *A* and *B*.

A – EBr. ⊕ ⚥ $K_{2+2}C_4A_{2+4}\underline{G}_{(2)}$

B – Br % ⚥ $K_{(5)}C_{1+2+(2)}$

Which of the following pairs of plants represent both *A* and *B* correctly?

(a) Cotton, pea
(b) *Cherianthus cheiri*, sunhemp
(c) Pea, groundnut
(d) Gram, *Brassica campestris*

177. Which of the following statements are incorrect?

I. A specialised centre present in the pons region of the brain called pneumotaxic centre can moderate the functions of the respiratory rhythm centre, neural signal from this centre can reduce the duration of inspiration.
II. An increase in pulmonary volume decreases the intra-pulmonary pressure to less than the atmosphere pressure which forces the air from outside to move into the lungs.
III. Contraction of the diaphragm and the inter-costal muscles returns the diaphragm and sternum to their normal positions and increase the thoracic volume and thereby the pulmonary volume.
IV. The volume of air involved in breathing movements can be estimated by using a spirometer which helps in clinical assessment of pulmonary functions.
V. The solubility of O_2 is 20-25 times higher than that of CO_2, the amount of O_2 that can diffuse through the diffusion membrane per unit difference in partial pressure is much higher compared to that of CO_2.

Choose the correct answer from the options given below.

(a) III and V (b) I, II and III
(c) II, III, IV and V (d) II, IV and V

178. Which of the following step is not included in the recombinant DNA technology ?

(a) Karyotyping of host DNA
(b) Isolation of desired DNA
(c) Fragmentation of DNA by restriction endonuclease
(d) Culturing the host cell in a medium

179. Which of the following statements are correct ?

I. A nitrogenous base is linked to the pentose sugar through N-glycosidic linkage to form a nucleotide.
II. Adenine forms two hydrogen bonds with thymine from opposite strand and vice-versa, guanine is bonded with cytosine with three hydroden bonds.
III. The promoter and terminator flank the structural gene in a transcription unit, promoter is located towards 3′ end of the structural gene.
IV. Different types of DNA dependent RNA polymerase are needed to catalyse the transcription of all types of RNA in bacteria.

V. The RNA polymerase associates transiently with initiation factor (σ) and termination factor (ρ) to initiate and terminate the transcription, respectively.

Choose the correct answer from the options given below.

(a) I, III and IV (b) II and V
(c) I, II, III and V (d) II and IV

180. Which of the following statements is incorrect ?

(a) Restriction enzymes cut the strand of DNA a little away from the centres of the palindrome sites, but between the same two bases on the opposite strands
(b) DNA fragments are positively charged molecules that can be separated by forcing them to move towards the cathode under an electric field through a medium
(c) The DNA fragments separate according to their size through sieving effect provided by the agarose gel
(d) A stirred - tank reactor is usually cylindrical or with a curved base to facilitate the mixing of the reactor content

Answers

Physics

1.	(b)	2.	(b)	3.	(d)	4.	(c)	5.	(b)	6.	(b)	7.	(c)	8.	(b)	9.	(d)	10.	(c)
11.	(b)	12.	(d)	13.	(b)	14.	(a)	15.	(c)	16.	(c)	17.	(a)	18.	(c)	19.	(c)	20.	(b)
21.	(d)	22.	(a)	23.	(b)	24.	(c)	25.	(a)	26.	(b)	27.	(c)	28.	(c)	29.	(b)	30.	(b)
31.	(b)	32.	(a)	33.	(c)	34.	(d)	35.	(d)	36.	(c)	37.	(d)	38.	(b)	39.	(d)	40.	(c)
41.	(c)	42.	(b)	43.	(d)	44.	(c)	45.	(a)										

Chemistry

46.	(a)	47.	(d)	48.	(d)	49.	(c)	50.	(b)	51.	(a)	52.	(d)	53.	(c)	54.	(c)	55.	(d)
56.	(c)	57.	(a)	58.	(b)	59.	(c)	60.	(c)	61.	(b)	62.	(c)	63.	(b)	64.	(d)	65.	(c)
66.	(a)	67.	(d)	68.	(a)	69.	(b)	70.	(d)	71.	(a)	72.	(c)	73.	(c)	74.	(c)	75.	(c)
76.	(a)	77.	(d)	78.	(b)	79.	(b)	80.	(c)	81.	(c)	82.	(c)	83.	(a)	84.	(c)	85.	(b)
86.	(c)	87.	(d)	88.	(d)	89.	(c)	90.	(c)										

Biology

91	(d)	92	(a)	93	(d)	94	(d)	95	(c)	96	(d)	97	(c)	98	(c)	99	(d)	100	(a)
101	(d)	102	(b)	103	(b)	104	(b)	105	(a)	106	(d)	107	(b)	108	(c)	109	(b)	110	(b)
111	(b)	112	(a)	113	(d)	114	(d)	115	(b)	116	(c)	117	(a)	118	(b)	119	(c)	120	(c)
121	(b)	122	(b)	123	(a)	124	(c)	125	(a)	126	(d)	127	(a)	128	(c)	129	(d)	130	(b)
131	(b)	132	(d)	133	(d)	134	(a)	135	(a)	136	(c)	137	(c)	138	(b)	139	(b)	140	(a)
141	(a)	142	(a)	143	(d)	144	(b)	145	(b)	146	(c)	147	(b)	148	(a)	149	(d)	150	(b)
151	(b)	152	(a)	153	(b)	154	(a)	155	(c)	156	(d)	157	(c)	158	(b)	159	(b)	160	(b)
161	(b)	162	(a)	163	(b)	164	(c)	165	(d)	166	(b)	167	(c)	168	(d)	169	(d)	170	(b)
171	(a)	172	(a)	173	(d)	174	(c)	175	(b)	176	(b)	177	(a)	178	(a)	179	(b)	180	(b)

Scan this QR code from your mobile phone to get the explanations of this paper.

NEET
TEST DRIVE

SECTION III
Achiever's Section

This section contains **2 Practice Sets** having a slightly higher difficulty level than NEET. These practice sets will help you achieve mastery over advanced concepts and give you an edge in the competitive landscape.

SECTION III
Achiever's Section

PRACTICE SET 14

Maximum Marks : 720	Time : 3 hrs	No. of Questions : 180

Instructions

1. This question paper contains **180** multiple-choice questions (four options with a single correct answer) from **Physics**, **Chemistry** and **Biology**.
2. These questions are distributed as 45 questions, each from Physics and Chemistry and 90 questions in Biology. These are to be compulsorily attempted by the candidate.
3. Each question carries 4 marks. For each correct response, the candidate will get 4 marks. For each incorrect response, one mark will be deducted from the total scores.

PHYSICS

1. Light of frequency 1.9 times the threshold frequency is incident on a photosensitive material. If the frequency is halved and intensity is doubled, the photocurrent becomes

(a) quadrupled (b) doubled
(c) halved (d) zero

2. A particle moves in a straight line such that its displacement time graph in a straight line inclined at an angle of 45° with the time axis. The particle is undergoing

(a) uniform velocity (b) uniform acceleration
(c) variable velocity (d) variable acceleration

3. The magnifying power of a telescope is M. If the focal length of the eyepiece is halved, the magnifying power will become

(a) $M/2$ (b) $4M$ (c) $M/4$ (d) $2M$

4. An ideal gas undergoes an state change according to p-V diagram. What is the value of V_x?

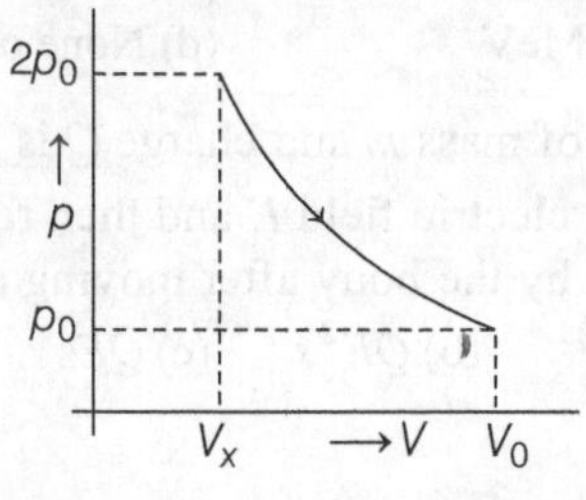

(a) $V_0/2$ (b) V_0 (c) $2V_0$ (d) $V_0/4$

5. How much work has to be done to transfer a charge of 3 C across two points having a potential difference of 10 V ?

(a) −30A (b) 30 A (c) −30J (d) 30J

6. A body is moving under the action of two forces $\mathbf{F_1} = 3\hat{i} - 6\hat{j}$, $\mathbf{F_2} = 4\hat{i} - 5\hat{j}$, its velocity will become uniform under a third force $\mathbf{F_3}$ given by

(a) $5\hat{i} - \hat{j}$ (b) $5\hat{i} + \hat{j}$ (c) $7\hat{i} + 11\hat{j}$ (d) $-7\hat{i} + 11\hat{j}$

7. Which one of the following light is completely polarised, when light is incident at polarising angle?

(a) Refracted light (b) Reflected light
(c) Both (a) and (b) (d) Neither (a) nor (b)

8. Calculate the current i in the given figure.

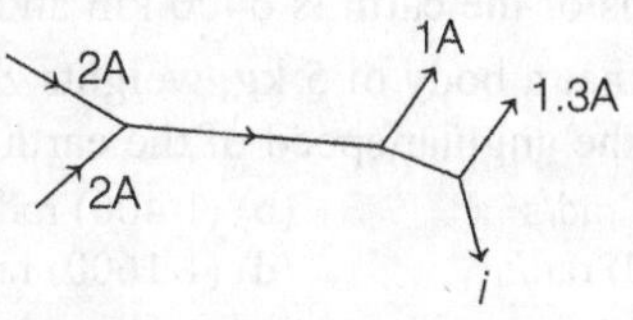

(a) 1.7 A (b) 3.7 A (c) 1.3 A (d) 1 A

9. A bus travelling with a speed of 30 m/s is braked and it slows down with uniform retardation. It covers a distance of 90 m as its velocity reduces to 24 m/s. If the bus continues to slow down with the

same rate, after what further distance will it be brought to stop ?
(a) 24.5 m (b) 25 m
(c) 160 m (d) 200 m

10. If a source is transmitting electromagnetic wave of frequency 8.2×10^6 Hz, then wavelength of the electromagetic waves transmitted from the source will be
(a) 36.5 m (b) 40.8 m (c) 50 m (d) 53.4 m

11. The earth and the satellite are subjected to the sun's gravitational force. What does the orbit of the satellite look like from the sun ?
(a) Elliptical (b) Some what elliptical
(c) Parabola (d) Hyperbola

12. The magnetic field of an electromagnetic wave is given by $B_y = 4 \times 10^{-7} \sin(10^4 x + 5.28 \times 10^{12} t)$. The wavelength of the electromagnetic wave is
(a) 6.28×10^{-4} m (b) 5.78×10^3 m
(c) 6.3×10^4 m (d) 2.5×10^{-7} m

13. A body is released from the top of an incline of height *h*,
(a) its KE at the bottom of the incline depends on angle of incline.
(b) its KE at the bottom will depends on angle of incline only if the incline is not smooth.
(c) its KE of bottom of the incline will not depend on angle of incline irrespective of whether incline is smooth or rough.
(d) Cannot say unless mass is given.

14. Crude oil at a pressure of 4×10^4 Nm^{-2} flows at 2 ms^{-1} through a pipe of 0.02 m^2 cross-sectional area which reduces to 0.01 m^2. The pressure in the smaller cross-section of the pipe is (density of crude oil is 1000 kg/m^3)
(a) 3.4×10^4 Nm^{-2} (b) 4.4×10^4 Nm^{-2}
(c) 5.4×10^4 Nm^{-2} (d) None of these

15. The radius of the earth is 6400 km and $g = 10$ m/s^2. In order that a body of 5 kg, weights zero at the equator, the angular speed of the earth is
(a) (1/80) rad/s (b) (1/400) rad/s
(c) (1/800) rad/s (d) (1/1600) rad/s

16. An engine uses 30 A of current and the resistance offered is 15 Ω. Calculate the power consumed by the engine (in HP).
(a) 18 (b) 19 (c) 17 (d) 13500

17. Given below are two statements.
Statement I To hear different beats, difference of frequencies of two sources should be less than 10.
Statement II More the number of beats more is the confusion.
In the above statements, choose the correct options given below.
(a) Both Statement I and Statement II are true.
(b) Both Statement I and Statement II are false.
(c) Statement I is true, but Statement II is false.
(d) Statement I is false but Statement II is true.

18. A straight wire carrying current $2I$ is turned into a circular loop. If the magnitude of magnetic moment associated with it is *M*, the length of wire will be
(a) $\sqrt{\frac{4\pi M}{I}}$ (b) $\sqrt{\frac{2M\pi}{I}}$ (c) $\sqrt{\frac{M\pi}{I}}$ (d) $\sqrt{\frac{3\pi}{MI}}$

19. Four silicon diodes are connected as shown in figure. Assume the diodes to be ideal. The current through the resistance *R* is

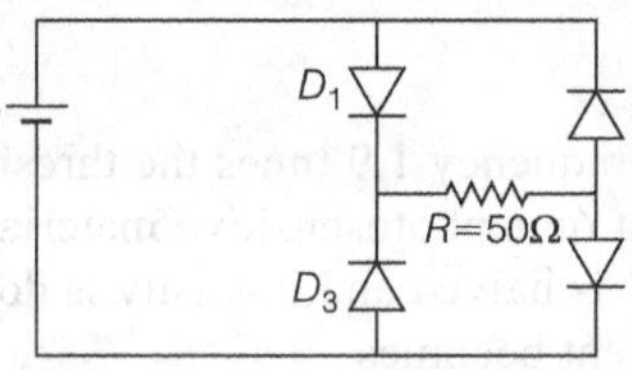

(a) 0.2 A (b) 0.1 A (c) 0.3 A (d) 0.5 A

20. The potential difference between points *A* and *B* of adjoining figure is

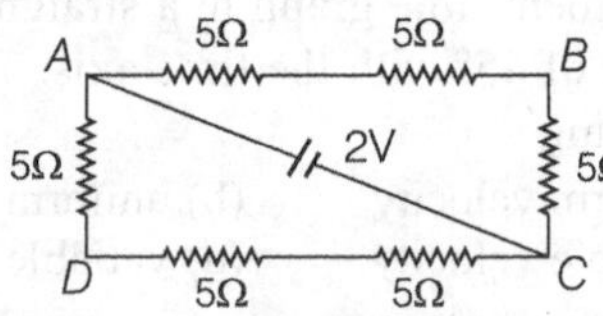

(a) (2/3) V (b) (8/9) V
(c) (4/3) V (d) 2 V

21. The mass of proton, neutron and helium nucleus are respectively 1.00734, 1.00874 and 4.00154. The binding energy of helium nucleus is
(a) 14.2 MeV (b) 10.46 MeV
(c) 28.4 MeV (d) None of these

22. A body of mass *m* and charge *Q* is placed at rest in a uniform electric field *E* and then released. The KE attained by the body after moving a distance *s* is
(a) QEs^2 (b) QE^2s (c) QEs (d) Q^2Es

23. A sinusoidal voltage of peak value 284 V and frequency 50 Hz is applied to a series L-C-R circuit in which $R = 3\Omega$, $L = 25.48$ mH and $C = 780\ \mu$F. The impedance of the circuit is
(a) $\sqrt{26.7}\Omega$ (b) 5Ω (c) $\sqrt{37}\Omega$ (d) $\sqrt{68.7}\Omega$

24. The reading of the ammeter as per the given figure

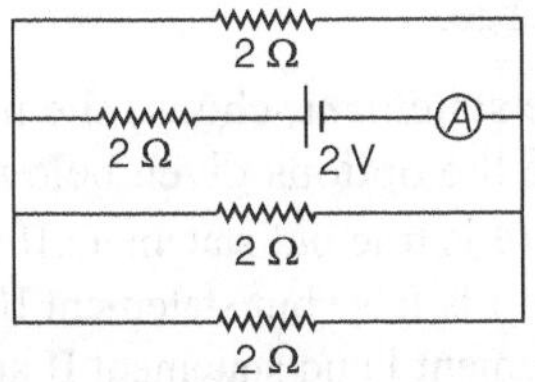

(a) (1/8) A (b) (3/4) A (c) (1/2) A (d) 2 A

25. A charge particle moving with velocity 3×10^5 m/s enters in a magnetic field of 0.3 T, at an angle of 30°. The radius of curvature of its path will be ($m = 1.67 \times 10^{-27}$ kg, $q = 1.6 \times 10^{-19}$ C)
(a) 0.5 cm (b) 0.5 m (c) 0.2 m (d) 1.25 cm

26. Two waves represented by $y = a \sin(\omega t - kx)$ and $y = a \sin(\omega t - kx + 2\pi/3)$ are superposed, then the amplitude of the resultant wave will be
(a) a (b) a^2 (c) $2a$ (d) $a^{1/3}$

27. A copper rod of length 0.19 m is moving parallel to a long wire with a uniform velocity of 10 m/s. The long wire carries 5 A current and is perpendicular to the rod. The ends of the rod are at distances 0.01 m and 0.2 m from the wire. The emf induced in the rod will be
(a) 10 μV (b) 20μV (c) 30μV (d) 40μV

28. What are dimensions of E/B ?
(a) $[LT^{-1}]$ (b) $[LT^{-3}]$ (c) $[MLT^{-2}]$ (d) $[M^{-1}L^2T^{-1}]$

29. The x and y-coordinates of the particle at any time are $x = 5t - 2t^2$ and $y = 10t$ respectively, where x and y are in metre and t in second. The acceleration of the particle at $t = 2$ s is
(a) 0 (b) 5 ms^{-2} (c) 4 ms^{-2} (d) -8 ms^{-2}

30. Calculate the effective capacitances between the points a and b in the given figure.

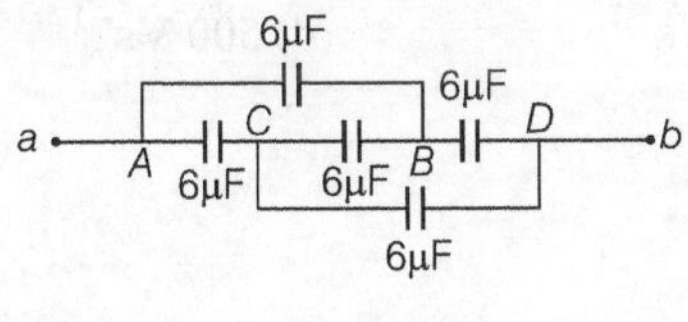

(a) 6μF (b) 12μF (c) 18μF (d) 24μF

31. The inward and outward electric flux for a closed surface in units of N-m^2/C are 8×10^3 and 4×10^3 respectively, then the total charge inside the surface is
(a) 4×10^3 C (b) -4×10^3 C
(c) $\dfrac{-4 \times 10^3}{\varepsilon}$ C (d) $-4 \times 10^3 \varepsilon_0$ C

32. A car of mass 5000 kg accelerates uniformly from rest to 30 m/s in 10 s. Calculate its acceleration and average power of the engine during the period (neglect friction).
(a) 3 m/s^2, 225 kW (b) 2 m/s^2, 2250 W
(c) 3 m/s^2, 22.5 kW (d) 2 m/s^2, 228 kW

33. An electron changes its position from orbit $n = 1$ to $n = 3$ of an atom. The wavelength of the emitted radiations is (R = Rydberg's constant)
(a) $\dfrac{16}{3R}$ (b) $\dfrac{12}{11R}$ (c) $\dfrac{9}{8R}$ (d) $\dfrac{7}{6R}$

34. Two identical conducting rods are first connected independently to two vessels, one containing water at 100°C and the other containing ice at 0°C. In the second case, the rods are joined end-to-end and connected to the same vessels. Let q_1 and q_2 gram per second be the rate of melting of ice in the two cases, respectively. The ratio of $\dfrac{q_1}{q_2}$ is
(a) $\dfrac{1}{2}$ (b) $\dfrac{2}{1}$ (c) $\dfrac{4}{1}$ (d) $\dfrac{1}{4}$

35. A body executes SHM with amplitude A and time period T, when the displacement from the equilibrium position is half the amplitude, what fractions of the total energy are kinetic and potential ?
(a) 75% of E and 25% of E
(b) 60% of E and 28% of E
(c) 25% of E and 30% of E
(d) 85% of E and 40% of E

36. A coil of one turn is made of a wire of certain length and then from the same length another coil of two turns is made. If the same current is passed in both the cases, then the ratio of the magnetic induction at their centres will be
(a) 2:1 (b) 1:4 (c) 4:1 (d) 1:2

37. If a medium has a critical angle for total internal reflection from the medium to vacuum as 60°, what is the velocity of light in the medium ?
(a) 0.5×10^8 m/s (b) $2\sqrt{3} \times 10^8$ m/s
(c) $1.5\sqrt{3} \times 10^8$ m/s (d) 0.2×10^8 m/s

38. There are two vernier calipers both of which have 1 cm divided into 10 equal divisions on the main scale. The vernier scale of one of the calipers (C_1) has 10 equal divisions that correspond to 9 main scale divisions. The vernier scale of the other caliper (C_2) has 10 equal divisions that correspond to 11 main scale divisions. The readings of the two calipers are shown in the figure. The measured values (in cm) by calipers C_1 and C_2, respectively are

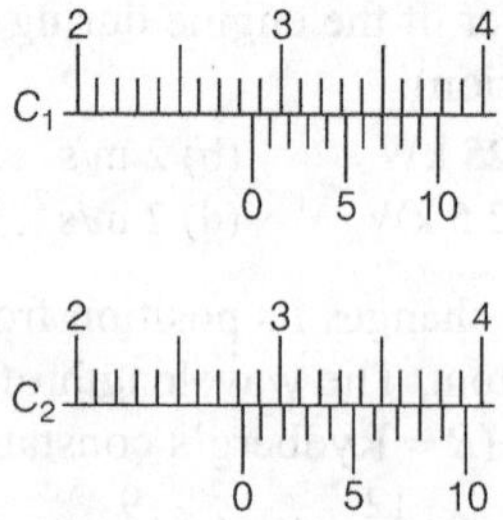

(a) 2.87 and 2.87 (b) 2.87 and 2.83
(c) 2.85 and 2.82 (d) 2.87 and 2.86

39. A rectangular coil is 20 turns and area of cross-section 25 cm^2 has a resistance of 100Ω. If a magnetic field which is perpendicular to the plane of coil changes at a rate of 1000 T/s, the current in the coil is

(a) 1A (b) 50 A (c) 0.5 A (d) 5 A

40. Two long parallel wires are at a distance of 1 m. Both of them carry 1 A of current in the same direction. The force of attraction per unit length between the two wires is

(a) 2×10^{-7} N/m (b) 8×10^{-7} N/m
(c) 4×10^{-7} N/m (d) None of these

41. The current in the network is

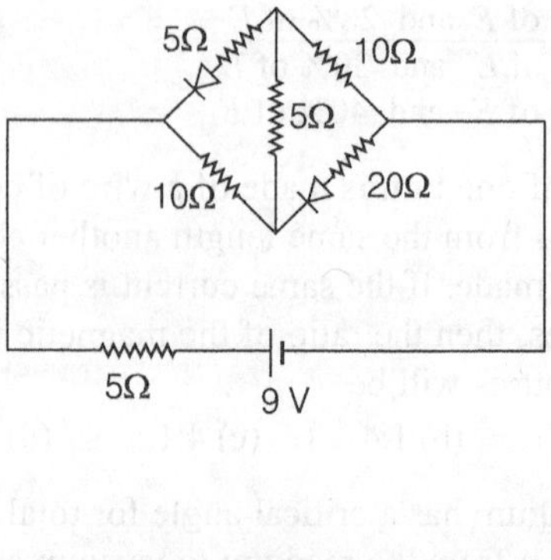

(a) 0.2 A (b) 0 A
(c) 0.6 A (d) 0.3 A

42. Given below are two statements

Statements I By doping silicon semiconductor with pentavalent material, the electrons density increases.

Statement II The *n*-type semiconductor has net negative charge.

In the above statement, choose the most appropriate answer from the options given below.

(a) Statement I is true but statement II is false.
(b) Statement I is false but statement II is true.
(c) Both statement I and statement II are true.
(d) Both statement I and statement II are false.

43. In the given circuit for ideal diode, the current through the battery is

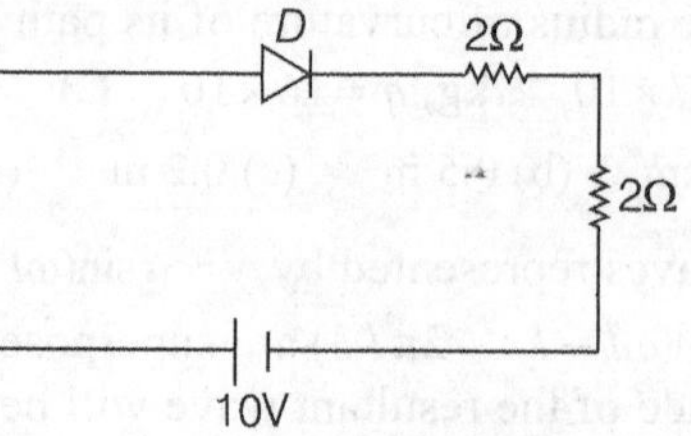

(a) 1.5 A (b) 2.5 A
(c) 3 A (d) 3.5 A

44. Four charges are placed on the corners of a square as shown in figure having side of 5 cm. If Q is 1μC then electric field intensity at centre will be

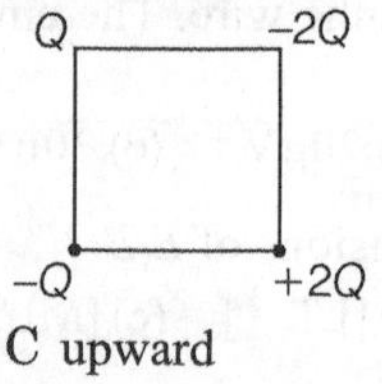

(a) 1.02×10^7 N/C upward
(b) 2.04×10^7 N/C downward
(c) 2.04×10^7 N/C upward
(d) 1.02×10^7 N/C downward

45. In order to establish an instantaneous displacement current of 1 mA in the space between the plates of 2μF parallel plate capacitor, the potential difference need to apply is

(a) 200 Vs^{-1} (b) 800 Vs^{-1}
(c) 300 Vs^{-1} (d) 500 Vs^{-1}

CHEMISTRY

46. Given below are two statements one is labelled as Assertion (A) and other is labelled as Reason (R).

Assertion (A) BF_3 is weaker Lewis acid than BCl_3.

Reason (R) $p\pi$-$p\pi$ back bonding is stronger in BF_3 than in BCl_3.

In the light of the above statements choose the most appropriate answer from the options given below.

(a) Both (A) and (R) are true but (R) is not the correct explanation of (A).
(b) (A) is true but (R) is false.
(c) (A) is false but (R) are true.
(d) Both (A) and (R) are true and (R) is the correct explanation of (A).

47. Match the List-I with List-II.

List-I	List-II
A. Bromine	(i) Transition element
B. Germanium	(ii) Chalcogens
C. Oxygen	(iii) Metalloid
D. Copper	(iv) Non-metal

Choose the correct answer from the options given below.

(a) A-(iv), B-(iii), C-(ii), D-(i)
(b) A-(i), B-(iii), C-(iv), D-(ii)
(c) A-(iv), B-(ii), C-(iii), D-(i)
(d) A-(ii), B-(iv), C-(iii), D-(i)

48. The IUPAC name of α-methoxy propionaldehyde is

(a) 2-methyl propanal
(b) 2-methoxy propanal
(c) 3-methoxy propanal
(d) 3-methyl propanal

49. An electron has a speed of 50 m/s with uncertainty of 0.02%. The uncertainty in locating its position is

(a) 1.1×10^{-1} m
(b) 3.2×10^{-7} m
(c) 1.2×10^{-5} m
(d) 5.8×10^{-3} m

50. Predict the effect of increased pressure on the following reaction equilibrium.

$$N_2(g) + 3H_2(g) \rightleftharpoons 2NH_3(g)$$

(a) Equilibrium will shift to left side.
(b) Equilibrium will shift to right side.
(c) No effect on equilibrium.
(d) Reaction will stop.

51. Match List-I with List-II.

List-I		List-II	
A.	SF_4	I.	sp
B.	IF_5	II.	sp^3d
C.	NO_2^+	III.	sp^3d^2
D.	NH_4^+	IV.	sp^3

Choose the correct answer from the options given below.

(a) A-II, B-III, C-I, D-IV
(b) A-I, B-III, C-II, D-IV
(c) A-III, B-II, C-IV, D-I
(d) A-IV, B-I, C-II, D-III

52. Major products obtained when *n*-hexane is heated in the presence of anhydrous $AlCl_3$ and HCl gas are

(a) 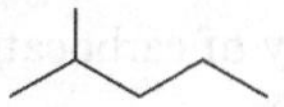 and 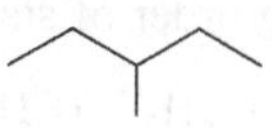

(b) 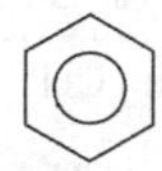 and 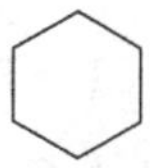

(c) 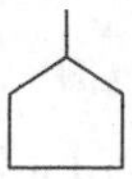 and 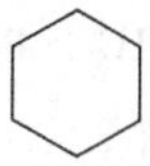

(d) 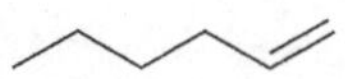 and 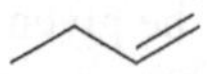

53. Which of the following carboxylic acids is highly insoluble in water?

(a) Butanoic acid (b) Propanoic acid
(c) Decanoic acid (d) Pentanoic acid

54. The reagents 'X' and 'Y' respectively for the given conversion is

$$CH_3COCl \xrightarrow{(X)} CH_3CHO \xrightarrow{(Y)} CH_3-\underset{\text{OH}}{\overset{|}{C}H}-CH_2CHO$$

(a) CrO_3 and CO_2
(b) Pd / $BaSO_4$ and dil. NaOH
(c) I_2/NaOH and H_3O^+
(d) NaOH and $LiAlH_4$

55. Which of the following hydrocarbon is solid at room temperature?

(a) Ethane (b) Octadecane
(c) Pentane (d) Octane

56. Hybridisation of Ni(II) in $K_2[NiBr_4]$ is

(a) sp^3d^2 (b) dsp^2 (c) sp^3 (d) sp^3d

57. Which of the following is not a characteristic of alcohol?

(a) Lower alcohols are colourless liquids with pleasant smell.
(b) The boiling points of alcohols increases with increase in the number of carbon atoms.
(c) Solubility of alcohols increases with increase in branching.
(d) They are non-flammable and produce light yellow flame.

58. Secondary structure of protein refers to

(a) the pattern in which the polypeptide chains are arranged.
(b) bonding between NH_3^+ and COO^- of two peptides.
(c) bonds between alternate polypeptide chains.
(d) folding patterns of polypeptide chains.

59. The decreasing order of stability of carbocation is

(a) $Ph_2\overset{+}{C}H > Ph\overset{+}{C}H_2 > (CH_3)_2\overset{+}{C}H > C_6H_5^+$
(b) $C_6H_5^+ > (CH_3)_2\overset{+}{C}H > Ph\overset{+}{C}H_2 > Ph_2\overset{+}{C}H$
(c) $Ph_2\overset{+}{C}H > Ph\overset{+}{C}H_2 > C_6H_5^+ > (CH_3)_2\overset{+}{C}H$
(d) $(CH_3)_2\overset{+}{C}H > C_6H_5^+ > Ph\overset{+}{C}H_2 > Ph_2\overset{+}{C}H$

60. Relative stability of +1 oxidation state of group 13 elements may be given as

(a) $Al^+ > B^+ > Ga^+ > Tl^+ > In^+$
(b) $Tl^+ > In^+ > Ga^+ > Al^+ > B^+$
(c) $B^+ > Al^+ > Ga^+ > In^+ > Tl^+$
(d) $Al^+ > Ga^+ > Tl^+ > In^+ > B^+$

61. Match the List-I with List-II.

List-I	List-II
A. Sulphanilic acid	(i) Lewis base
B. Aniline	(ii) Colourless crystalline solid
C. N-methyl amine	(iii) Zwitter ion
D. Benzene diazonium	(iv) Secondary amine

Choose the correct answer from the options given below.

(a) A-(iv), B-(i), C-(ii), D-(iii)
(b) A-(ii), B-(iv), C-(iii), D-(i)
(c) A-(i), B-(iii), C-(ii), D-(iv)
(d) A-(iii), B-(i), C-(iv), D-(ii)

62. The rate constant for a first order reaction is $19 \times 10^{-3}\ s^{-1}$. How long will 4.0 g of this reactant take to reduce to 2.0 g? [Given : $\log 2 = 0301$]

(a) 72.97 s (b) 8.45 s
(c) 36.48 s (d) 48.50 s

63. Consider the following reaction.

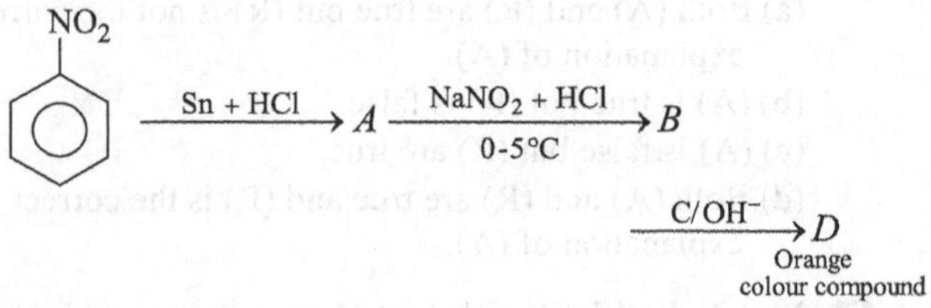

The compounds *C* and *D* respectively are

(a) 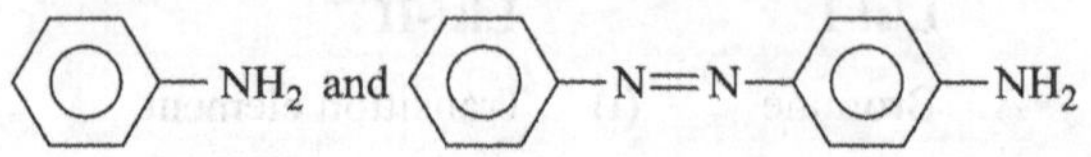

(b) 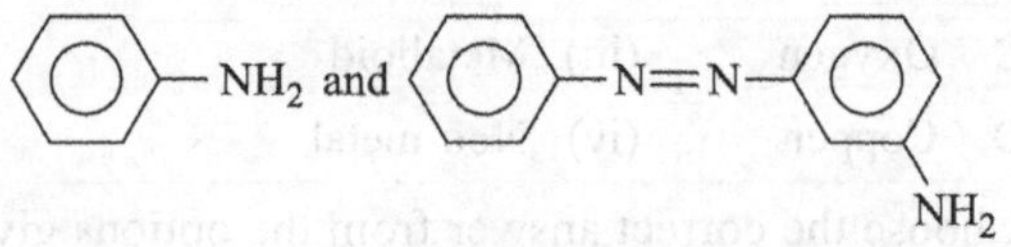

(c) 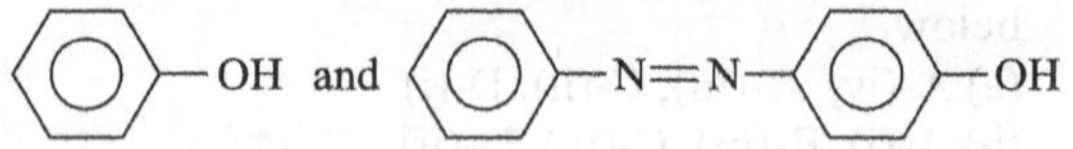

(d) 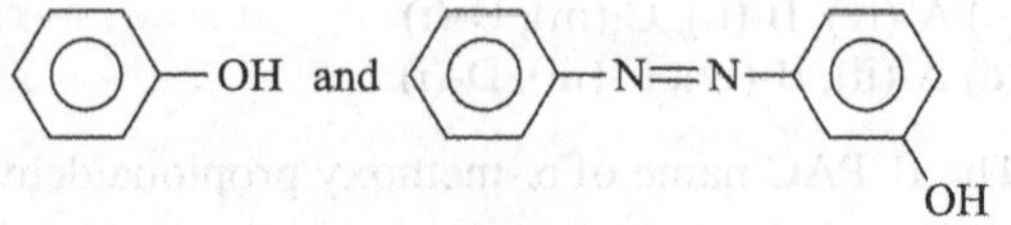

64. Match the List-I with List-II.

List-I	List-II
A. $\Delta S_{(Total)}$	(i) Non-spontaneous process
B. $dU = 0$	(ii) $-RT \ln K$
C. $\Delta G°$	(iii) Cyclic process
D. $\Delta G° > 0$	(iv) $nR \ln \frac{V_2}{V_1}$

Choose the correct answer from the options given below.

(a) A-(iv), B-(iii), C-(ii), D-(i)
(b) A-(iv), B-(ii), C-(i), D-(iii)
(c) A-(iii), B-(ii), C-(i), D-(iv)
(d) A-(i), B-(iii), C-(iv), D-(ii)

65. Study the given graph and choose the correct option.

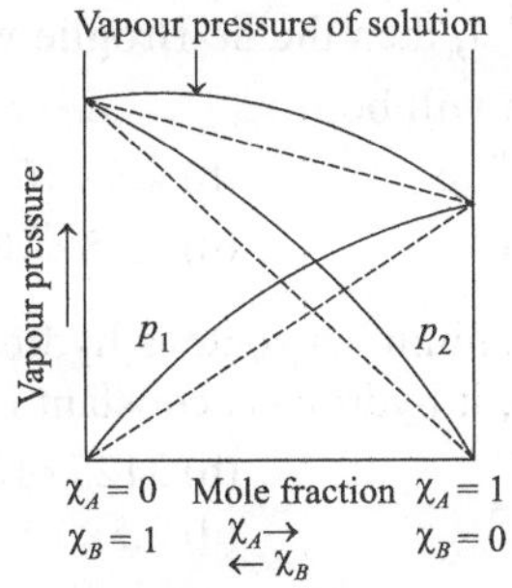

The best suitable example for the given graph is
(a) phenol and aniline
(b) chloroform and benzene
(c) water and HNO_3
(d) carbon disulphide and acetone

66. An organic compound gave 0.4895 g of CO_2 on complete combustion. If the mass of the compound taken was 0.2429 g, then the percentage of C in it will be
(a) 15.84%
(b) 11.45%
(c) 26.67%
(d) 54.96%

67. Given below are two statements one is labelled as Assertion (A) and other is labelled as Reason (R).

Assertion (A) Cr^{6+} is colourless in nature.

Reason (R) The electronic configuration of chromium is $[Ar]3d^5 4s^1$.

In the light of the above statements choose the most appropriate answer from the options given below
(a) (A) is false but (R) is true.
(b) Both (A) and (R) are true and (R) is a correct explanation of (A).
(c) Both (A) and (R) are true but (R) is not a correct explanation of (A).
(d) (A) is true but (R) is false.

68. Given below are two statements

Statement I Ethene's molecular mass is half its empirical mass.

Statement II The empirical formula represents the simplest whole-number ratio of the various atoms present in a compound.

In the light of the above statements, choose the most appropriate answer from the options given below
(a) Both statement I and statement II are true.
(b) Both Statement I and statement II are false.
(c) Statement I is true but statement II is false.
(d) Statement I is false but statement II is true.

69. Which of the following reaction represents Dow's process?

(a) 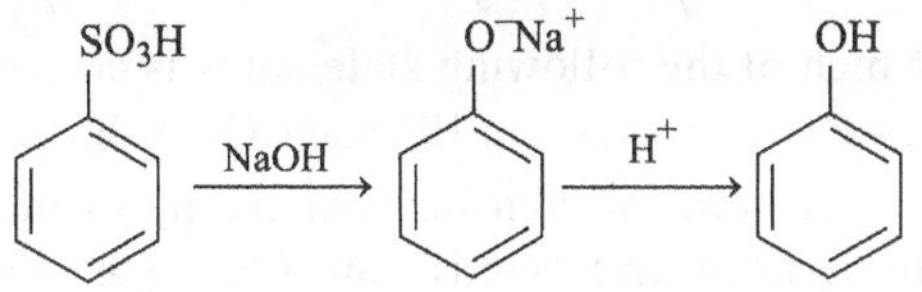

(b) 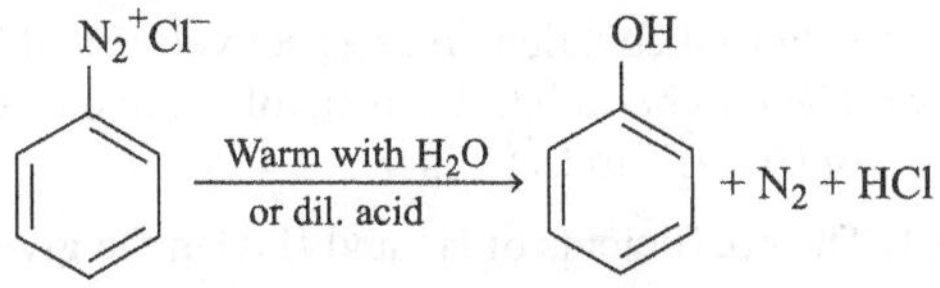

(c) 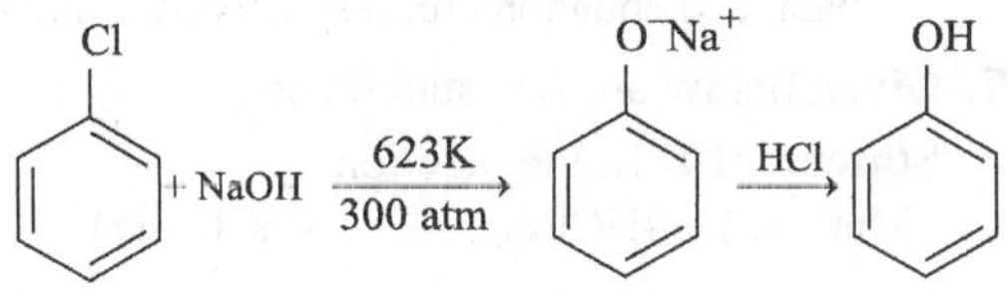

(d) 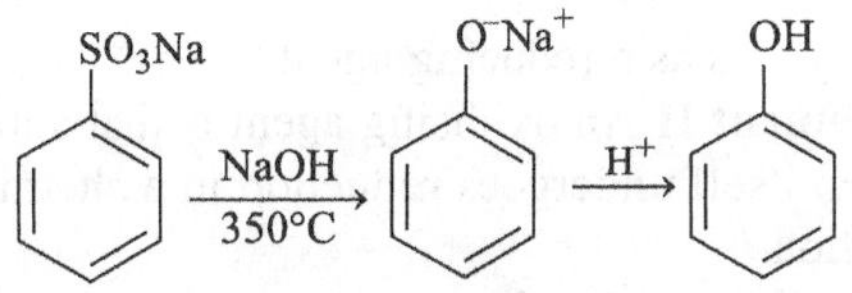

70. Given below are two statements

Statement I Methane cannot be obtained by Wurtz reaction.

Statement II Wurtz reaction leads to the formation of symmetrical alkanes having an even number of carbon atoms.

In the light of the above statements, choose the correct answer from the options given below.
(a) Both statement I and Statement II are false.
(b) Statement I is true, but Statement II is false.
(c) Statement I is false, but Statement II is true.
(d) Both Statement I and Statement II are true.

71. The structure of white phosphorus is
(a) octahedral
(b) trigonal bipyramidal
(c) linear
(d) tetrahedral

72. The dipole moment of HBr is 0.8×10^{-30} cm and interatomic spacing is 1 Å. The % ionic character of HBr is
(a) 7% (b) 5% (c) 20% (d) 10%

73. An alkali is titrated against an acid with methyl orange as indicator, which of the following is a correct combination?

	Base	Acid	End point
(a)	Weak	Strong	Pink to yellowish brown
(b)	Strong	Strong	Pinkish red to yellow
(c)	Weak	Strong	Yellow to pinkish red
(d)	Strong	Strong	Pink to colourless

74. In the reaction,

$H^{\oplus} + Cr_2O_7^{2-} + C_2O_4^{2-} \longrightarrow Cr^{3+} + CO_2 + H_2O$

Which of the following statements is correct?

(a) The coefficients of $H^{\oplus}$ and CO_2 in the given balanced equation are, respectively 14 and 6.

(b) The coefficients of $H^{\oplus}$ and CO_2 in the given balanced equation are, respectively 7 and 2.

(c) The number of electrons involved in the conversion of $Cr_2O_4^{2-}$ to Cr^{3+} is 4.

(d) The coefficients of $H^{\oplus}$ and H_2O in the given balanced equation are, respectively 7 and 6.

75. Given below are two statements.

Statement I In the reaction,

$MnO_2(s) + 4HCl(aq) \longrightarrow MnCl_2(aq) + Cl_2(g) + 2H_2O(l)$

MnO_2 acts as a reducing agent.

Statement II An oxidising agent is that substance which itself undergoes reduction in a chemical reaction.

In the light of the above statements, choose the correct answer from the options given below.

(a) Both Statement I and Statement II are true.
(b) Both Statement I and Statement II are false.
(c) Statement I is true but Statement II is false.
(d) Statement I is false but Statement II is true.

76. Given below are two statements.

Statement I $[Fe(CN)_6]^{3-}$ has d^2sp^3 type hybridisation.

Statement II $[Fe(CN)_6]^{3-}$ ion shows magnetic moment corresponding to two unpaired electrons.

In the light of the above statements, choose the correct answer from the options given below.

(a) Both Statement I and Statement II are false.
(b) Statement I is true, but Statement II is false.
(c) Statement I is false, but Statement II is true.
(d) Both statement I and Statement II are true.

77. In S_N2 mechanism the sequence of bond breaking and bond formation follows the trend.

(a) Bond breaking and bond formation takes place simultaneously.
(b) Bond breaking is followed by bond formation.
(c) Bond formation is followed by bond breaking.
(d) Bond breaking and bond formation takes place randomly.

78. Which of the following statement is incorrect regarding transition metals?

(a) They do not form alloys.
(b) Generally, they are coloured in aqueous state.
(c) They form interstitial compounds.
(d) Their enthalpy of atomisation is high.

79. If an electron is moving with a kinetic energy of 4.55×10^{-23} J, then the de-Broglie wavelength for this electron will be

(a) 8.5×10^{-9} m (b) 4.8×10^{-10} m
(c) 6×10^4 m (d) 7.25×10^{-8} m

80. 0.5 M ammonium benzoate is hydrolysed to 0.25 per cent. Hence, it hydrolysis constant is

(a) 6.25×10^{-6} (b) 3.125×10^{-6}
(c) 1.25×10^{-5} (d) 2.5×10^{-5}

81. The value of $\Delta G°$ for the reaction,

$Cu^{2+} + Fe \longrightarrow Fe^{2+} + Cu$ is

(Given : $E^{\circ}_{Cu^{2+}/Cu} = +0.34$ V, $E^{\circ}_{Fe^{2+}/Fe} = -0.44$ V)

(a) − 48.5 kJ (b) − 150.5 kJ
(c) − 98.45 kJ (d) − 115.6 kJ

82. Consider the following cell reaction.

$2Fe(s) + O_2(g) + 4H^+(aq) \longrightarrow 2Fe^{2+}(aq) + 2H_2O(l);\ E° = 1.67$ V

At, $[Fe^{2+}] = 10^{-3}$ M, $P(O_2) = 0.1$ atm and pH = 3, the cell potential at 25°C is

(a) 1.47 V (b) 1.77 V (c) 1.87 V (d) 1.57 V

83. Which of the following order of arrangement agree with the variation of property indicated against it.

I. $Al^{3+} < Mg^{2+} < Na^+ < F^-$ (Increasing ionic size)
II. B < C < N < O (Increasing I[st] ionisation enthalpy)
III. I < Br < Cl < F (Increasing electron gain enthalpy)
IV. Li < Na < K < Rb (Increasing metallic radius)
V. O < N < C < B (Increasing I[st] ionisation enthalpy)

Choose the correct answer from the following option.

(a) I and IV (b) I, III and V
(c) II, III and IV (d) I, II and III

84. Consider the reaction,

$2NO(g) + O_2(g) \longrightarrow 2NO_2(g)$

If $\frac{-d[O_2]}{dt} = 0.026$ M/s, then $\frac{d[NO_2]}{dt}$ will be

(a) 0.016 M/s (b) 0.052 M/s
(c) 0.114 M/s (d) 0.084 M/s

85. Match the List-I with List-II.

List-I	List-II
A. Conductance	(i) $S\ cm^2\ mol^{-1}$
B. Molar conductivity	(ii) Siemens
C. Cell constant	(iii) $S\ m^{-1}$
D. Conductivity	(iv) cm^{-1}

Choose the correct answer from the options given below.

(a) A-(iii), B-(iv), C-(i), D-(ii)
(b) A-(i), B-(iv), C-(iii), D-(ii)
(c) A-(ii), B-(i), C-(iv), D-(iii)
(d) A-(iv), B-(iii), C-(ii), D-(i)

86. Which of the following statement is correct about ethers?

A. Ethers form peroxides by free radical oxidation.
B. Ethers are flammable.
C. Ethers are widely used as an extraction solvents.
D. An ethereal oxygen can act as Lewis acid.
E. Ethers are insoluble in water.

Choose the correct answer from the options given below.

(a) A, B and C only (b) B, C and D only
(c) C, D and E only (d) A, D and E only

87. In a zero order reaction, for every 10°C rise of temperature, the rate is doubled. If the temperature is increased from 10°C to 60°C, the rate of the reaction becomes.

(a) 32 times (b) 16 times
(c) 64 times (d) 128 times

88. When $KMnO_4$ solution is added to oxalic acid solution, the decolourisation is slow in the begining but becomes instantaneous after sometime because

(a) H^+ catalyses the reaction.
(b) $C_2O_4^{2-}$ acts as auto catalyst.
(c) Mn^{2+} acts as auto catalyst.
(d) MnO_4^- catalyses the reaction.

89. The correct order of increasing basic nature of the following amines is

(a) $C_6H_5NH_2 < C_6H_5NH_2CH_3 < C_6H_5NH_2NO_2$
(b) $C_6H_5NH_2NO_2 < C_6H_5NH_2 < C_6H_5NH_2CH_3$
(c) $C_6H_5NH_2CH_3 < C_6H_5NH_2 < C_6H_5NH_2NO_2$
(d) $C_6H_5NH_2CH_3 \approx C_6H_5NH_2 < C_6H_5NH_2NO_2$

90. If 9.08 g of $BaCl_2$ is present in 10^5 g of solution, then the concentration of solution will be

(a) 0.908 ppm (b) 90.8 ppm
(c) 908 ppm (d) 0.0908 ppm

BIOLOGY

91. A novel strategy was adopted to prevent the nematode infection in the roots of tobacco plants, this strategy involves ....

(a) *Meloidegyne incognita;* silencing of a specific *m*RNA due to a complementary *ds*RNA
(b) *Rhizobium;* silencing of a DNA replication by the introduction of some chemical
(c) *Azotobacter;* spraying of nematocide chemical extracted from transgenic bacteria
(d) *Agrobacterium;* spraying of insecticidal protein on the tobacco plant

92. The age pyramid with small base indicates

(a) less population growth and high fecundity rate
(b) population of young members are more than old members
(c) more sterility in females
(d) declining population growth and low fecundity rate

93. The oviducts, uterus and vagina constitute the female accessory ducts. Each Fallopian tube is about 10-12 cm long and extends from the periphery of each ovary to the uterus, the part closer to the ovary is the funnel-shaped known as

(a) fimbriae (b) ampulla
(c) uterine fundus (d) infundibulum

94. Which of the following set of hormones is released only during pregnancy in women?

(a) Oestrogens, hCG and relaxin
(b) Human placental lactogen, oestrogens and progestogens
(c) Human placental lactogen, human chorionic gonadotropin and relaxin
(d) Prolactin, thyroxine and human placental lactogen

95. Which one of the following pairs is incorrectly matched?

(a) Trichomes – Multicellular
(b) Bulliform cells – Sunflower
(c) Lenticels – Gases exchange
(d) Bark – Dead tissue

96. Self-incompatibility is a genetic mechanism, it represents

(a) negative interaction which inhibit the germination of self pollen
(b) positive interaction which inhibit the germination of incompatible pollen
(c) negative interaction which inhibit the germination of compatible pollen
(d) positive interaction which enhance the pollen compatibility

97. Which of the following matching pairs is incorrect?

(a) *Antedon*—Endoskeleton is made up of calcareous ossicles
(b) Corals—Endoskeleton is composed of calcium carbonate
(c) *Pleurobrachia*—They exhibit metagenesis
(d) *Nereis*—Blood vascular system is closed type

98. Which of the following proceses is not involved in the coagulation of blood?

(a) Thrombokinase is an enzyme complex, which initiate the blood coagulation
(b) A dark reddish brown scum is formed at the site of a cut
(c) Fibrins are formed by the conversion of inactive fibrinogens in the plasma by the enzyme thrombin
(d) Heparin stimulate the cellular cascade of blood clot and release thrombin

99. Sclerenchymatous fibres are greatly elongated and tapering at both the ends. These cells are

(a) always dead, polygonal and walls are lignified
(b) living, polygonal and walls are made up of pectin
(c) always living, contain protoplasm without intercellular spaces
(d) always dead, isodiametric and having well developed intercellular spaces

100. Gregor Mendel, conducted artificial pollination /cross pollination experiments using several true-breeding pea lines. He selected 14-true breeding pea plant varieties, as pairs which were

(a) heterozygous in F_1-generation and homozygous in F_2-generation
(b) recessive for all the 7 characters
(c) similar except for one character with contrasting traits
(d) similar for all the characters

101. According to '*X*' model of plasma membrane, the quasi fluid nature of lipid enables lateral movement of proteins within the overall bilayer. This ability to move within the membrane is measured as its '*Y*'. Identify '*X*' and '*Y*' from the given options.

	X	*Y*
(a)	Singer and Nicolson model	Plasticity
(b)	Sandwich model	Liquidity
(c)	Fluid mosaic model	Fluidity
(d)	Unit membrane model	Plasticity

102. The axoneme possesses a number of microtubules running parallel to the long axis, it has usually

(a) two pairs of doublets of radially arranged peripheral microtubules and a pair of centrally located microtubules
(b) two pairs of centrally located microtubules and a pair of doublets of radially arranged peripheral microtubules
(c) nine doublets of radially arranged peripheral microtubules and a pair of centrally located microtubules
(d) nine pairs of centrally located microtubules and a pair of radially arranged pheripheral microtubules

103. Which of the following are considered as the properties of heartwood?

I. Region of heartwood comprises of dead cells.
II. It is involved in conduction of water and minerals.
III. It provides mechanical support to stem.
IV. It is lighter in colour.
V. The region has highly lignified walls.

Choose the correct answer from the options given below.

(a) I, III and V only (b) III and IV only
(c) II, III and V (d) II, III, IV only

104. Each seminiferous tubule is lined on its inside by two types of cells, i.e. male germ cells and Sertoli cells. The functions of these cells are respectively

(a) synthesise and secrete testicular hormone and provide nutrition to the germ cells
(b) facilitate insemination and lubrication of the penis
(c) sperm formation and providing nutrition to the germ cells
(d) sperm formation and maintaining the low temperature of germ cell

105. Given below are two statements; one is labelled as Assertion (A) and other one is labelled as Reason (R).

Assertion (A) Nucleo-cytoplasmic ratio in eukaryotes is restored by meiosis.

Reason (R) When the cell grows, the cytoplasm content increases and thus the volume of

cytoplasm is more than the nucleus, it disturbs the ratio in terms of volume between nucleus and cytoplasm.
In the light of the above statements, choose the correct answer form the options given below.
(a) A is false, but R is true
(b) Both A and R are true and R is the correct explanation of A
(c) Both A and R are true, but R is not the correct explanation of A
(d) A is true, but R is false

106. Which of the following is the characteristic of compound epithelium?
(a) The cells of this tissue are specialised to store fats
(b) They are found in the walls of blood vessels and air sacs of lungs
(c) It is composed by single layer of tall and slender cells
(d) Their main function is to provide protection against chemical and mechanical stresses

107. Given below are two statements.
Statement I Positive and negative assertive mating might result in deviations from Hardy Weinberg equation due to heterozygote deficiency or excess of it, respectively.
Statement II If a population consists of several subpopulation and individuals randomly mate within, but not between subpopulations, then homozygous alleles in the overall population will be constant according to the Hardy-Weinberg equation.
In the light of the above statements, choose the correct answer from the options given below.
(a) Statement I is incorrect, but statement II is correct
(b) Both statement I and statement II are correct
(c) Both statement I and statement II are incorrect
(d) Statement I is correct, but statement II is incorrect

108. In the electron transport chain, the electrons pass from one carrier to another *via* complex-I to IV, they are
(a) coupled to cytochrome-*c* oxidase for the production of electron
(b) coupled to ATP synthase for the production of ATP
(c) coupled to complex-II for the production of H_2O
(d) coupled to complex-II for the production of ATP

109. What is the correct sequence of events during fertilisation?
(a) Capacitation of sperm → acrosomal reaction → agglutination → slow block → fast block
(b) Acrosomal reaction → capacitation → agglutination → prevention of polyspermy
(c) Capacitation → approximation → acrosomal reaction → cone of reception formation → prevention of polyspermy
(d) Acrosomal reaction → agglutination → capacitation → prevention of polyspermy → cone of reception formation

110. The enzymes having mutliple molecular forms, occuring in some organism and having a similar substrate activity are known as
(a) endoenzymes (b) apoenzymes
(c) isoenzymes (d) allosteric enzymes

111. Given below are two statements.
Statement I In molluscs, body is covered by calcareous shell and is unsegmented with a distinct head, muscular foot and visceral hump.
Statement II Excretion in molluscs takes place through Malpighian tubules.
In the light of the above statements, choose the correct answer from the options given below.
(a) Statement I is incorrect, but statement II is correct
(b) Both statement I and statement II are correct
(c) Both statement I and statement II are incorrect
(d) Statement I is correct, but statement II is incorrect

112. Which of the following statements are incorrect?
I. The most important fact of biological systems is that all living organisms exist in an equilibrium steady-state to perform work.
II. Inorganic catalysts work efficiently at high temperatures and high pressure, while enzymes get damaged at high temperatures.
III. Prosthetic groups are organic compounds distinguished from other cofactors in that they are permanently bound to the apoenzymes.
IV. Lyases enzymes catalyse the hydrolysis of ester.
V. An active site of an enzyme is a crevice or pocket into which the substrate fits.
Choose the correct answer from the options given below.
(a) I and IV (b) II, IV and V
(c) II and III (d) I, II, III and IV

113. The graphical representation of population growth curve is given below.

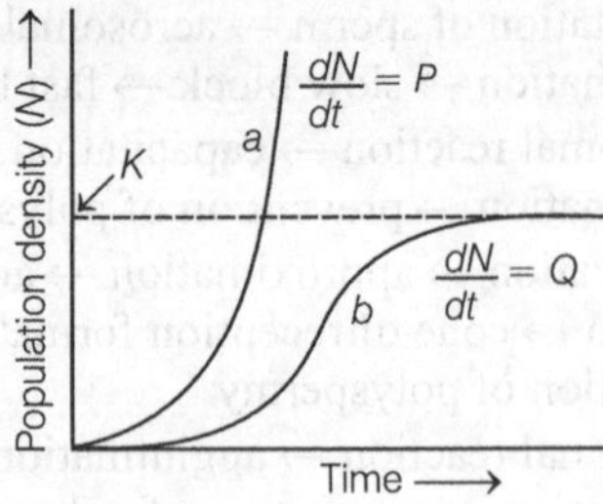

Identify P and Q from the following.

	P	Q
(a)	N	$r\left(\frac{K+N}{K}\right)$
(b)	rN	$rN\left(\frac{K-N}{K}\right)$
(c)	tN	$t\left(\frac{K-N}{K}\right)$
(d)	rN	$t\left(\frac{K-N}{N}\right)$

114. Which of the following statements is correct regarding anatomy of frog?

I. Male reproductive organs consists of a pair of yellowish ovoid testes, which are found adhered to the upper part of kidneys by a double fold of peritoneum called mesorchium.

II. Vasa efferentia are 20-22 in number that arise from testes, enter the kidneys on their side and open into cloacal aperture.

III. The thin-walled urinary bladder is present lateral to the rectum which also opens in the cloaca.

IV. The prominent endocrine glands found in frog are pituitary, thyroid, parathyroid, thymus, pineal body, pancreatic islets, adrenal and gonads.

V. The bidder's canal is a small, median chamber which is used to pass faecal matter, urine and sperms to the outside.

Choose the correct answer from the options given below.

(a) I and IV only
(b) II, III and V only
(c) I, II and III only
(d) III, IV and V only

115. Secondary growth in dicot root differ from secondary growth in dicot stem in

(a) being confined in stelar zone only
(b) forming wavy ring of cambium initially
(c) having contribution of pericycle
(d) formation of wave like vascular cambium in extra stelar region

116. Mucosa-associated lymphoid tissue is located within the lining of the major tracts, i.e. respiratory, digestive and urogenital tracts. It

(a) provides micro-environments for the development and maturation of T-lymphocytes
(b) acts as filter of the blood by trapping blood borne microorganisms
(c) is a large reservoir of lymphocytes
(d) constitutes about 50% of the lymphoid tissue in human body

117. Find the correctly matched pair.

(a)	Birds	—	Oxygenated and deoxygenated blood gets mixed up in the single ventricle
(b)	Mammals	—	Blood flows in two pathways
(c)	Single circulation	—	Blood flows at a high pressure
(d)	Crocodile	—	Incomplete double circulation

118. Carefully examine the following structure given below.

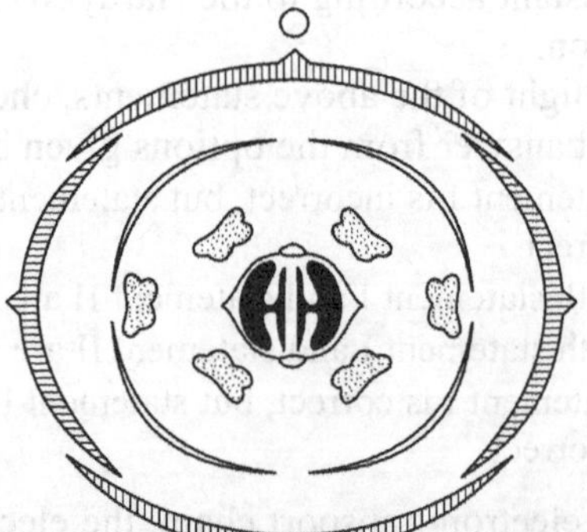

Which of the following is incorrect w.r.t the given family representing the floral diagram?

(a) It exhibits corymose, racemose or corymb inflorescence
(b) Gynoecium is bicarpellary, syncarpous and has superior with parietal placentation

(c) Calyx are five, gamosepalous imbricate or valvate

(d) Corolla are four, polypetalous and reduced

119. *E. coli* is grown in a medium containing $^{15}NH_4Cl$ as the only nitrogen source for many generations. Then it is transferred into a medium with normal $^{14}NH_{14}Cl$. What could be the possible ratio of light and hybrid DNA after 60 min?

(a) 6 : 3 (b) 3 : 1

(c) 4 : 1 (d) 1 : 1

120. Given below are two statements; one is labelled as Assertion (A) and other one is labelled as Reason (R).

Assertion (A) Glomerulus is a tuft of capillaries formed by the afferent arteriole.

Reason (R) Blood from the glomerulus is carried away by an afferent arteriole.

In the light of the above statements, choose the correct answer from the options given below.

(a) A is false, but R is true

(b) Both A and R are true and R is the correct explanation of A

(c) Both A and R are true, but R is not the correct explanation of A

(d) A is true, but R is false

121. The human evolved from *Homo habilis* about 1.5 mya in the Pleistocene, who made more elaborate tools and had a brain volume around 900 cc is

(a) *Homo erectus* (b) *Homo neanderthalensis*

(c) *Homo sapiens* (d) Cro-Magnon man

122. Which of the following epithelial tissue found in the lining of stomach and intestine helps in secretion and absorption?

(a) Cuboidal epithelium (b) Squamous epithelium

(c) Columnar epithelium (d) Ciliated epithelium

123. Given below are two statements, one is labelled as Assertion (A) and the other one is labelled as Reason (R).

Assertion (A) The conventional taxonomic methods are not suitable for identifying microbial species.

Reason (R) Many microbial species are simply not culturable under laboratory conditions.

In the light of the above statements, choose the correct answer from the options given below.

(a) A is false, but R is true

(b) Both A and R are true and R is the correct explanation of A

(c) Both A and R are true, but R is not the correct explanation of A

(d) A is true, but R is false

124. Which of the following properties correctly represent differences between sieve element and companion cells?

(a) Sieve element contain nucleus and are living in nature

(b) Nucleus is not found in mature cells of companion cells

(c) Companion cells are found in pteridophytes and gymnosperm

(d) Companion cells are living and contain nucleus

125. In a mutant strain of *E. coli*, the operator region of the *lac* operon has been deleted. What is most likely to happen to the transcription of the structural genes (*lac z, lac y, lac a*) in the absence of lactose?

(a) Transcription will be constitutive, as the repressor can no longer bind

(b) Transcription will be repressed, as the repressor can bind directly to the promoter

(c) Transcription will be inducible in the presence of lactose as normal regulation is unaffected

(d) Transcription will not occur due to a loss of RNA polymerase binding to the promoter

126. Given below is an imaginary pyramid of numbers. Identify the correct possibility about certain organisms at some of the different levels?

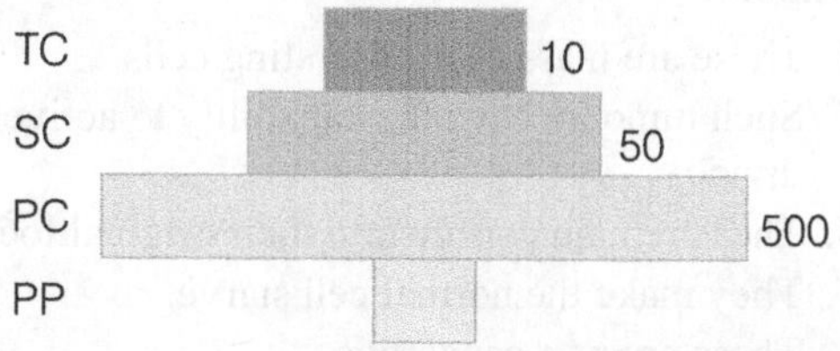

(a) Level PC is insects and level SC is small insectivorous birds

(b) Level PP is phytoplanktons in sea and whale on top level TC

(c) Level PP represents peepal tree and the level SC is sheep

(d) Level PC is rat and SC is cat

127. How many plants belong to family-Leguminosae in the given box?

Soyabean, Gram, Brinjal, Lily, Mustard, Lupin, Muliathi, *Indigofera*, *Aloe*

(a) Four (b) Eight
(c) Three (d) Five

128. Given below are two statements; one is labelled as Assertion (A) and other one is labelled as Reason (R).

Assertion (A) Coenzymes are organic molecules that bind to active sites of certain enzymes and help in catalysing reactions.

Reason (R) Coenzymes serves as cofactors in a number of different enzyme catalysed reactions.

In the light of the above statements, choose the correct answer from the options given below.

(a) A is false, but R is true
(b) Both A and R are true and R is the correct explanation of A
(c) Both A and R are true, but R is not the correct explanation of A
(d) A is true, but R is false

129. When a person encounters HIV, the person becomes so immuno deficient that he/she is unable to protect herself/himself against various infections. The person's immunity is deficient due to

(a) decrease in the number of helper T-lymphocytes
(b) increase in the amount of interferons
(c) decrease in the number of macrophage cells
(d) increase in the certain types of leukocytes

130. Identify the correct statements related to malignant tumours.

I. These are mass of proliferating cells.
II. Such tumours have the capability to actively divide.
III. These remain confined to their original location.
IV. They make the normal cell starve.
V. These are non-cancerous.

Choose the correct answer from the options given below.

(a) I and II only (b) I, II and IV only
(c) III, IV and V (d) II and IV only

131. Arrange the following events of menstrual cycle from beginning to end of the cycle.

I. Ovulation is controlled by the increased level of LH in the blood.
II. The level of progesterone in the blood declines.
III. Corpus luteum begins to secrete hormone called progesterone.
IV. FSH stimulates the change of a primary follicle of the ovary into a Graafian follicle.

Choose the correct answer from the options given below.

(a) IV $\rightarrow$ I $\rightarrow$ III $\rightarrow$ II
(b) I $\rightarrow$ IV $\rightarrow$ III $\rightarrow$ II
(c) I $\rightarrow$ III $\rightarrow$ IV $\rightarrow$ II
(d) IV $\rightarrow$ III $\rightarrow$ I $\rightarrow$ II

132. Match List I with List II.

List I	List II
A. Plants show different pathways in response to environment	1. Geometric growth
B. Sum of growth and differentiation	2. Arithmetic growth
C. Type of growth in which the rate of growth is constant	3. Plasticity
D. It is common in unicellular organisms when grown in nutrient rich medium	4. Development

Choose the correct answer from the options given below.

	A	B	C	D		A	B	C	D
(a)	3	4	2	1	(b)	4	3	1	2
(c)	1	2	3	4	(d)	2	1	4	3

133. Given below are two statements, one is labelled as Assertion (A) and the other one is labelled as Reason (R).

Assertion (A) PCR is based on using the ability of DNA polymerase to synthesise new strand of DNA complementary to the template strand.

Reason (R) DNA polymerase can add nucleotide only on a pre-existing 3′- OH group, and needs a primer to which it can add the first nucleotide.

In the light of the above statements, choose the correct answer from the options given below.
(a) A is false, but R is true
(b) Both A and R are true and R is the correct explanation of A
(c) Both A and R are true, but R is not the correct explanation of A
(d) A is true, but R is false

134. Given below are two statements.
Statement I In Urochordata, notochord is present only in larval tail, while in cephalochordata, it extends from head to tail region and is persistent throughout their life.
Statement II The vertebrates possess notochord during the embryonic period which is replaced by a cartilaginous or bony vertebral column in the adult.
In the light of the above statements, choose the correct answer from the options given below.
(a) Statement I is incorrect, but statement II is correct
(b) Both statement I and statement II are correct
(c) Both statement I and statement II are incorrect
(d) Statement I is correct, but statement II is incorrect

135. Match List I with List II.

List I	List II
A. ANF (Atrial Natriuretic factor)	1. It activates the JG cells to release renin.
B. GFR (Glomerular Filtration Rate)	2. Impermeable to electrolytes
C. Proximal convoluted tubule	3. It maintain the pH
D. Henle's loop	4. Vasodilation

Choose the correct answer from the options given below

	A	B	C	D
(a)	4	1	3	2
(b)	3	4	1	2
(c)	2	4	1	3
(d)	3	2	4	1

136. Match List I with List II.

List I	List II
A. Autotrophic component of lichen	1. Heterocyst
B. It is found in cyanobacteria, which fix atmospheric nitrogen	2. Mycobiont
C. These are the simplest and smallest unicellular organism	3. Diatoms
D. Chief producers in the oceans	4. Mycoplasm
	5. Phycobiont

Choose the correct answer from the options given below.

	A	B	C	D		A	B	C	D
(a)	1	3	4	2	(b)	5	1	4	3
(c)	2	3	4	1	(d)	1	2	5	3

137. Which of the following statements are correct?
I. Bacteriophages are usually double-stranded DNA viruses having protein coat, called capsid made up of small subunits of capsomeres arranged in helical or polyhedral form which protects the nucleic acid.
II. The mode of asexual reproduction in fungi is through conidia, sporangiophores and zoospores and sexual reproduction takes place *via* oospores, ascospores and basidiospores.
III. Ciliated protozoans are aquatic, actively moving organisms because of the presence of cilia. They have a cavity (gullet) that opens to the outside of the cell surface.
IV. The euglenoids have two flagella, usually both are long. Each flagellum arises from cytopharynx.
V. Slime moulds are saprophytic protists, their body moves along decaying twigs and leaves engulfing organic material.

Choose the correct answer from the options given below.
(a) III and IV (b) IV and V
(c) I, II, III and V (d) II, III and V

138. The two main neurotransmitters in nervous system are
(a) adrenaline and acetylcholine
(b) histamine and choline
(c) adrenaline and epinephrine
(d) acetyl choline and histamine

139. Given below are two statements; one is labelled as Assertion (A) and other one is labelled as Reason (R).
Assertion (A) Saheli is the oral contraceptive for the females that contains a non-steroidal preparation.
Reason (R) It has to be taken daily for a period of 21 days starting preferably within the first five days of menstrual cycle.
In the light of the above statements, choose the correct answer from the options given below.
(a) A is false, but R is true
(b) Both A and R are true and R is the correct explanation of A
(c) Both A and R are true, but R is not the correct explanation of A
(d) A is true, but R is false

140. Match List I with List II.

List I	List II
A. It hydrolyses internal phosphodiester bonds in a polynucleotide chain	1. RNA polymerase-III
B. Catalyses the synthesis of *m*RNA	2. DNA polymerase
C. It catalyses the polymerisation of deoxynucleotides	3. Endonuclease
D. It catalyses the synthesis of *t*RNA	4. RNA polymerase-II

Choose the correct answer from the options given below

	A	B	C	D		A	B	C	D
(a)	3	4	2	1	(b)	4	3	1	2
(c)	1	2	3	4	(d)	2	3	4	1

141. If two persons with 'AB' blood group marry and have sufficient large number of children; these children could be classified as 'A' blood group; AB blood group and B blood group in 1 : 2 : 1 ratio. Modern technique of protein electrophoresis reveals presence of both 'A' and 'B' type of proteins in 'AB' blood group individuals. This is an example of
(a) incomplete dominance (b) partial dominance
(c) codominace (d) complete dominance

142. Match List I with List II.

List I	List II
A. Pectinase	1. Clot buster
B. Lipase	2. Clarification of juice
C. Streptokinase	3. Immunosuppressive agent
D. Cyclosporin-A	4. Detergent formulation

Choose the correct answer from the options given below

	A	B	C	D		A	B	C	D
(a)	2	3	1	4	(b)	4	1	2	3
(c)	2	4	1	3	(d)	3	2	1	4

143. Which of the following statements is not correct?
I. In proteins, amino acids are linked by peptide bond, which is formed when the carboxyl group of one amino acid reacts with the amino group of the next amino acid.
II. Exoskeleton of arthropods have a complex polysaccharide called chitin.
III. Cellulose is made up of unbranched chain of fructose units linked by 1-4 glycosidic linkage. It produces red colour with iodine as it holds I_2.
IV. Collagen is the most abundant protein in animal world and Ribulose Bisphosphate Carboxylase-Oxygenase (RuBisCO) is the most abundant protein in the whole biosphere.
V. Proteins are heteropolymers containing strings of amino acids.

Choose the correct answer from the options given below.
(a) I and II (b) III, IV and V
(c) II, IV and I (d) III only

144. Which of the following is not a correct statement w.r.t ecosystem, and its components?
(a) The structural component of ecosystem includes all living organisms and their inter-relationships
(b) Interaction of biotic and abiotic components results in a chemical structure that forms backbone of each living being

(c) Decomposers are called reducers and include fungi
(d) Decomposition given rise to humus

145. Read the following statements carefully and choose the correct option.

Statement I Heterospory condition is present in *Selaginella*, still seed is not formed in it.

Statement II Female gametophyte is not retained permanently inside megasporangium in heterosporous species of pteridophytes.

(a) Both statements I and statement II are incorrect
(b) Statement I is correct, but statement II is incorrect
(c) Both statement I and statement II are correct
(d) Statement I is incorrect, but statement II is correct

146. Given below are two statements.

Statement I Deoxyribonucleic acid is a hydrophilic molecule and cannot pass directly through cell membrane. Certain treatments are made in host cells, so that they became competent.

Statement II The DNA solution is injected directly inside the cell using capillary glass or microsyringe.

In the light of the above statements, choose the correct answer from the options given below.

(a) Statement I is incorrect, but statement II is correct
(b) Both statement I and statement II are correct
(c) Both statement I and statement II are incorrect
(d) Statement I is correct, but statement II is incorrect

147. The double-stranded actin filaments are covered by tropomyosin, which blocks the interaction between

(a) myosin and actin when the muscle is inactive
(b) troponin and F-actin when the muscle is active
(c) light chain and heavy chain when muscle is contracted
(d) light chain and heavy chain when muscle is relaxed

148. Consider the following statements.

I. Restriction enzymes cut the strand of DNA a little away from the centre of the palindrome sites, but between the same two bases on the opposite strands.
II. DNA are negatively charged molecules, they can be separated by forcing them to move towards the anode under an electric field through a medium.
III. Cloning sites are a sequence from where replication starts and any piece of DNA when linked to this sequence can be made to replicate within the host cells.
IV. The genes encoding resistance to antibiotics such as ampicillin, tetracycline, etc. are considered useful selectable marker for *E. coli*.
V. Selection of recombinants due to inactivation of antibiotics depends on their ability to produce blue colour in the presence of a chromogenic substrate.

Choose the correct answer from the options given below.

(a) Statements I, II and V are true and III and IV is false
(b) Statements I, II and III are true and IV and V are false
(c) Statements III and V are false and I, II and IV are true
(d) Statements II and III are false and I, IV and V are true

149. Organelle '*B*' is membrane bound vesicular structure formed by the process of packaging in the Golgi apparatus. Identify the incorrect statement considering the '*B*' organelle.

(a) These are absent in prokaryotes, but present in all eukaryotic animal cells, except mammalian RBCs
(b) It can occupy up to 90 % of the volume of the animal cell
(c) It is rich in hydrolytic enzymes
(d) They release enzymes for digesting carbohydrates, proteins, lipids and nucleic acids.

150. Which of the following statements are correct regarding binomial nomenclature?

I. In binomial nomenclature, first word denoting the genus starts with a small letter while the specific epithet starts with a capital letter.
II. All the scientific names of organisms are usually Latin. Hence, they are written in Italics.
III. Name of the author appears after the genus, i.e. at the end of the biological name and is written in Italics.
IV. The first word in a biological name represents the specific epithet, while the second component denotes the genus.
V. Both the words in a biological name, when handwritten, are separately underlined, or printed in Italics to indicate their Latin origin.

Choose the correct answer from the options given below.

(a) I and II (b) III, IV and V
(c) II and V (d) I, II and III

151. Match List I with List II.

	List I		List II
A.	Viral diseases	1.	Typhoid
B.	Bacterial diseases	2.	Common cold
C.	Protozoan disease	3.	Filariasis
D.	Helminthic disease	4.	Malaria

Choose the correct answer from the options given below.

	A	B	C	D		A	B	C	D
(a)	2	3	1	4	(b)	2	1	4	3
(c)	1	2	4	3	(d)	4	3	1	2

152. Which of the following statements are incorrect?

I. The shoulder girdle and pelvis provide connection points between the appendicular skeleton and the axial skeleton to where mechanical loads transfer.

II. Out of 206 bones in the adult human body, a total of 126 bones form the appendicular skeleton.

III. The sternum of the axial skeleton articulates with the clavicle of the appendicular skeleton with the help of sternoclavicular joint.

IV. Scapula is a large triangular flat bone situated in the dorsal part of the thorax between the third and the sixth ribs.

V. In human 12 pairs of ribs are found, each rib is a thin flat bone connected dorsally to the sternum and ventrally to the vertebral column.

Choose the correct answer from the options given below.

(a) IV and V (b) II and V
(c) I, III and V (d) II, III and IV

153. The flippers of penguins and dolphins and bones of forelimbs of bats and human are the examples of

(a) homologous and divergent evolution, respectively
(b) divergent evolution and adaptive radiation, respectively
(c) convergent evolution and divergent evolution respectively
(d) divergent evolution and convergent evolution, respectively

154. Sacred groves have a significant role in conservation of biodiversity. They are found in

I. Khasi and Jaintia Hills in Meghalaya
II. Aravalli Hills of Rajasthan
III. Chanda and Bastar area of MP
IV. Indo-Burma and Himalaya

Choose the correct answer from the options given below.

(a) I, II and III
(b) I and III only
(c) I, II and IV
(d) III and IV only

155. Given below are two statements.

Statement I In the solar system of the milky way galaxy, earth was supposed to have been formed about 4.5 billion years ago and there was no atmosphere on early earth.

Statement II The surface of the early earth was covered by water vapour, methane, carbon dioxide and ammonia, which is released from the molten mass of earth.

In the light of the above statements, choose the correct answer from the options given below.

(a) Statement I is incorrect, but statement II is correct
(b) Both statement I and statement II are correct
(c) Both statement I and statement II are incorrect
(d) Statement I is correct, but statement II is incorrect

156. The members of Rhodophyceae are commonly called red algae because of the predominance of the red pigment in their body, these pigments are

(a) chlorophyll-*a* and fucoxanthin
(b) phycoerythrin and chlorophyll-*d*
(c) mannitol and phycocyanin
(d) floridean starch and phycoerythrin

157. The separated DNA fragments can be visualised only after staining the DNA with a compound known as

(a) triaryl methane followed by exposure to sunlight
(b) ethidium bromide followed by exposure to UV radiation
(c) nitrocellulose followed by exposure to UV radiation
(d) ethidium bromide followed by exposure to gamma (γ) radiation

158. Match List I with List II.

List I	List II
A. Erythropoietin	1. Stimulates secretion of water and bicarbonate ions from pancreas
B. Secretin	2. Stimulates the secretion of pancreatic enzymes
C. Cholecystokinin	3. Stimulates the formation of RBC
D. Gastric Inhibitory Peptide (GIP)	4. It inhibits gastric secretion and motility

Choose the correct answer from the options given below.

	A	B	C	D		A	B	C	D
(a)	3	1	2	4	(b)	1	3	4	2
(c)	2	4	1	3	(d)	4	2	1	3

159. Which of the following statements is correct?

(a) The apical bud always suppresses the growth of axillary buds present beneath it, due to the presence of relatively higher quantities of auxin near the stem apex
(b) Gibberellins are strong acidic growth hormones having gibbane ring structure, which cause cell elongation of intact plants
(c) Auxin cause fruits like apple to elongate and improve its shape
(d) Some naturally occurring cytokinins are 2, 4 D

160. Match List I with List II.

List I	List II
A. Euglenoids	1. Red tide
B. *Gonyaulax*	2. Saprophytes
C. Chrysophytes	3. Stagnant fresh water
D. Slime moulds	4. Golden algae

Choose the correct answer from the options given below.

	A	B	C	D
(a)	2	1	4	3
(b)	3	4	1	2
(c)	3	1	4	2
(d)	2	3	1	4

161. Each trophic level has a certain mass of living material at a particular time called as the standing crop, it is measured as the

(a) mass of living organisms and used energy in a unit area
(b) number of trophic level and mass of non-living material
(c) number and weight of the organic material
(d) mass of living organism or the number in a unit area

162. Match List I with List II.

List I (Types of placentation)	List I (Examples)
A. Marginal	1. China rose, lemon
B. Axile	2. Mustard, *Argemone*
C. Parietal	3. Pea, moong
D. Basal	4. Sunflower, marigold

Choose the correct answer from the options given below.

	A	B	C	D		A	B	C	D
(a)	3	1	2	4	(b)	3	4	2	1
(c)	2	4	1	3	(d)	4	3	2	1

163. Thyrotropin releasing hormone from the hypothalamus causes the anterior pituitary to release thyrotropin which stimulates thyroid gland to release

(a) T_3 and T_4 (b) ADH and T_4
(c) thyrocalcitonin and ADH
(d) thyrocalcitonin and T_3

164 Given below are two statements; one is labelled as Assertion (A) and other is labelled as Reason (R).

Assertion (A) Chewing tobacco increases the heart rate and may lead to cancer of oral cavity.

Reason (R) It increases CO content in blood and reduce the concentration of haem bound oxygen.

In the light of the above statements, choose the correct answer from the options given below.

(a) A is false, but R is true
(b) Both A and R are true and R is the correct explanation of A
(c) Both A and R are true, but R is not the correct explanation of A
(d) A is true, but R is false

165. Match List I with List II.

List I	List II
A. Non-reducing sugar	1. Glucose
B. Grape sugar	2. Fructose
C. Inulin	3. Sucrose
D. Dairy sugar	4. Galactose

Codes

	A	B	C	D		A	B	C	D
(a)	3	1	4	2	(b)	1	3	2	4
(c)	3	1	2	4	(d)	2	4	1	3

166. Which of the following is true regarding pollination in *Vallisneria*?

(a) Pollination occurs in submerged condition by water
(b) Flowers emerge above surface of water and pollination occurs by insects
(c) Flowers emerge above water and pollen is carried by wind
(d) Male flowers are carried by water currents to female flowers at the surface of water

167. PCR is a revolutionary method developed by Kary Mullis in the 1980s. The reactions of PCR are sometimes limited due to certain limitations. These limitations include all, except

(a) self annealing of primers
(b) *Taq* polymerase limitation
(c) self-annealing of the accumulating product
(d) accumulation of deoxyribonucleotide

168. Given below are two statements; one is labeled as Assertion (A) and other one is labelled as Reason (R).

Assertion (A) Most endonucleases optimally digest the target DNA at 37°C.

Reason (R) *Taq* I optimally digests the target DNA at temperature 65°C.

In the light of the above statements, choose the correct answer from the options given below.

(a) A is false, but R is true
(b) Both A and R are true and R is the correct explanation of A
(c) Both A and R are true, but R is not the correct explanation of A
(d) A is true, but R is false

169. ...*A*... uses X-rays to generate a three-dimensional image of the internals of an object whereas ...*B*... uses strong magnetic field and non-ionising radiations to accurately detect pathological and physiological changes in the living tissue. Identify *A* and *B* from the following.

	A	*B*
(a)	Computed tomography	MRI
(b)	X-ray	CT
(c)	CT	Autoradiography
(d)	Biopsy	CT

170. Every chromosome essentially has a primary constriction or the centromere on the side of which disc shaped structures is present, these structure is called as

(a) perinuclear space (b) kinetochores
(c) histones (d) chromatin

171. Which of the following pairs of animals correctly represent characteristics like bilateral symmetry, triploblastic, acoelomate, organ level of organisation and flame cells that help in osmoregulation and excretion?

(a) *Taenia* and *Fasciola*
(b) *Pleurobrachia* and *Ctenoplana*
(c) *Adamsia* and *Taenia*
(d) *Schistosoma* and *Ascaris*

172. A student is looking through a light microscope in her biology class and is asked to identify the cell on the slide as either a plant or animal cell. Which of the following organelle's presence would help her to identify the type of cell?

(a) The presence of a centrosome
(b) The presence of a rough endoplasmic reticulum
(c) The presence of a nucleus
(d) The presence of a Golgi apparatus

173. How many genera show the retention of the female gametophyte on the parental sporophyte?

Spirogyra, Cycas, Lycopodium, Funaria, Marchantia, Selaginella

(a) 4 (b) 3
(c) 2 (d) 5

174. Given below are two statements.

Statement I Pyruvate formed by the glycolytic catabolism of carbohydrates in the cytosol, undergoes photodecarboxylation by a complex set of reactions catalysed by succinate dehydrogenase in the mitochondrial matrix.

Statement II The condensation of acetyl group in the TCA cycle is catalysed by the enzyme citrate synthase and a molecule of Co-A is released.

In the light of the above statements, choose the correct answer from the options given below.

(a) Statement I is incorrect, but statement II is correct
(b) Both statement I and statement II are correct
(c) Both statement I and statement II are incorrect
(d) Statement I is correct, but statement II is incorrect

175. The intrafascicular cambium and interfascicular cambium joins together and form cambium ring, these cambium rings are

(a) primary and secondary in origin, respectively
(b) secondary and primary in origin, respectively
(c) primary in origin
(d) secondary in origin

176. Match List I with List II.

List I	List II
A. It is used to detect very low concentration of pathogen	1. Adenosine deaminase deficiency
B. It detects the antibodies synthesised against the pathogen	2. Probe
C. The first clinical gene therapy was given in 1990 to a 4 year old girl	3. PCR
D. A single-stranded DNA or RNA, tagged with a radioactive molecule	4. ELISA

Choose the correct answer from the options given below.

	A	B	C	D
(a)	3	2	1	4
(b)	3	4	1	2
(c)	2	1	3	4
(d)	4	1	3	2

177. Match List I with List II.

List I	List II
A. Competition	1. Lion and deer
B. Parasitism	2. Abingdon tortoise and goat
C. Mutualism	3. Cuckoo and crow
D. Predation	4. *Rhizobium* and legumes

Choose the correct answer from the options given below.

	A	B	C	D
(a)	1	3	4	2
(b)	2	3	4	1
(c)	2	3	1	4
(d)	4	1	2	3

178. Which of the following statements is not correct?

(a) Down's syndrome arises due to the failure of separation of 21st pair of autosomes during meiosis.
(b) Grasshopper is an example of XO type of sex-determination in which the males have only one type X-chromosome besides the autosome, whereas females have both of X-chromosomes
(c) More than two alternative forms of a gene in a population occupying the same locus on a chromosome or its homologous are known as multiple alleles
(d) In *Drosophila*, the two different sex chromosomes Z and W are found in female, whereas males have a pair of Z-chromosomes besides the autosomes

179. Given below are two statements.

Statement I PS-I with reaction center P_{700} lies on the inner surface of the thylakoid and results in the photolysis of water molecule,

Statement II The cyclic flow results only in the synthesis of ATP, but not of $NADPH + H^+$, it involves only PS-I.

In the light of the above statements, choose the correct answer from the options given below.

(a) Statement I is correct, but statement II is incorrect
(b) Both statement I and statement II are incorrect

(c) Statement I is incorrect, but statement II is correct
(d) Both statement I and statement II are correct

180. Given below are two statements.

Statement I A fully processed *m*RNA, has cap of methylated guanine at 3′ end followed successively by an initiation codon, a long coding region, a termination codon and a poly-A tail of adenine at 5′ end.

Statement II In eukaryotes, *m*RNA is polycistronic as it is transcribed from many cistron.

In the light of the above statements, choose the correct answer from the options given below.

(a) Statement I is incorrect, but statement II is correct
(b) Both statement I and statement II are correct
(c) Both statement I and statement II are incorrect
(d) Statement I is correct, but statement II is incorrect

Answers

Physics

1.	(d)	2.	(b)	3.	(b)	4.	(a)	5.	(c)	6.	(b)	7.	(d)	8.	(a)	9.	(b)	10.	(b)
11.	(d)	12.	(d)	13.	(b)	14.	(c)	15.	(a)	16.	(c)	17.	(b)	18.	(b)	19.	(b)	20.	(c)
21.	(b)	22.	(b)	23.	(d)	24.	(a)	25.	(a)	26.	(a)	27.	(c)	28.	(a)	29.	(c)	30.	(a)
31.	(d)	32.	(a)	33.	(c)	34.	(c)	35.	(a)	36.	(b)	37.	(c)	38.	(b)	39.	(c)	40.	(a)
41.	(d)	42.	(a)	43.	(b)	44.	(a)	45.	(d)										

Chemistry

46.	(d)	47.	(a)	48.	(b)	49.	(d)	50.	(b)	51.	(a)	52.	(a)	53.	(c)	54.	(b)	55.	(b)
56.	(c)	57.	(d)	58.	(d)	59.	(a)	60.	(b)	61.	(d)	62.	(c)	63.	(c)	64.	(a)	65.	(d)
66.	(d)	67.	(c)	68.	(d)	69.	(c)	70.	(d)	71.	(d)	72.	(b)	73.	(c)	74.	(a)	75.	(d)
76.	(b)	77.	(a)	78.	(a)	79.	(d)	80.	(b)	81.	(b)	82.	(d)	83.	(a)	84.	(b)	85.	(c)
86.	(a)	87.	(a)	88.	(c)	89.	(b)	90.	(b)										

Biology

91	(a)	92	(d)	93	(d)	94	(c)	95	(b)	96	(a)	97	(c)	98	(d)	99	(a)	100	(c)
101	(c)	102	(c)	103	(a)	104	(c)	105	(a)	106	(d)	107	(d)	108	(b)	109	(c)	110	(c)
111	(d)	112	(a)	113	(b)	114	(a)	115	(b)	116	(d)	117	(b)	118	(c)	119	(b)	120	(d)
121	(a)	122	(c)	123	(b)	124	(d)	125	(a)	126	(a)	127	(c)	128	(c)	129	(a)	130	(b)
131	(a)	132	(a)	133	(c)	134	(b)	135	(a)	136	(b)	137	(c)	138	(a)	139	(d)	140	(a)
141	(c)	142	(c)	143	(d)	144	(b)	145	(c)	146	(b)	147	(a)	148	(c)	149	(b)	150	(c)
151	(b)	152	(a)	153	(c)	154	(a)	155	(b)	156	(b)	157	(b)	158	(a)	159	(a)	160	(c)
161	(d)	162	(a)	163	(a)	164	(c)	165	(c)	166	(d)	167	(d)	168	(c)	169	(a)	170	(b)
171	(a)	172	(a)	173	(b)	174	(a)	175	(a)	176	(b)	177	(b)	178	(d)	179	(c)	180	(c)

Scan this QR code from your mobile phone to get the explanations of this paper.

SECTION III

Achiever's Section

PRACTICE SET 15

Maximum Marks : 720 | Time : 3 hrs | No. of Questions : 180

Instructions

1. This question paper contains **180** multiple-choice questions (four options with a single correct answer) from **Physics, Chemistry** and **Biology**.
2. These questions are distributed as 45 questions, each from Physics and Chemistry and 90 questions in Biology. These are to be compulsorily attempted by the candidate.
3. Each question carries 4 marks. For each correct response, the candidate will get 4 marks. For each incorrect response, one mark will be deducted from the total scores.

PHYSICS

1. Mass m_2 is hanged using a uniform string whose other end is attached to a mass m_1. A string connects m_1 to ground as shown in figure. Tension in this string is

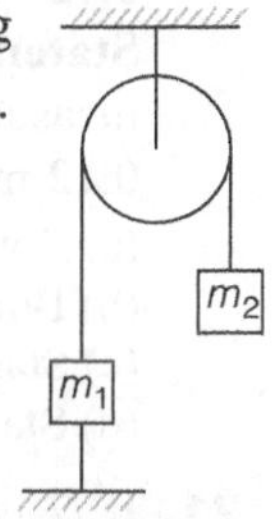

(a) zero (b) $m_1 g$
(c) $m_2 g$ (d) $(m_2 - m_1)g$

2. A solid cylinder rolls without slipping down an inclined plane at an angle 60° with the horizontal. The acceleration of the cylinder is

(a) $\frac{g}{3}$ (b) $3g$ (c) $\frac{g}{\sqrt{3}}$ (d) $\frac{2}{3}g$

3. A progressive wave of frequency 500 Hz is travelling with velocity of 360 m/s. How far apart are two points 60° out of phase ?

(a) 0.42 m (b) 0.32 m (c) 0.22 m (d) 0.12 m

4. A body under the action of a force $\mathbf{F} = 6\hat{\mathbf{i}} - 8\hat{\mathbf{j}} + 10\hat{\mathbf{k}}$, acquires an acceleration of 1 m/s^2. The mass of this body must be

(a) $10\sqrt{2}$ kg (b) 15 kg (c) $2\sqrt{2}$ kg (d) 30 kg

5. A thin steel rod of length l, area of cross-section A and Young's modulus Y is clamped between two fixed supports. If it is heated such that its temperature increases by ΔT and its change in length is zero, then the thermal compressive force exerted on the rod is

(a) $\frac{AY}{\alpha \Delta T}$ (b) $AY\alpha\Delta T$ (c) $lAY\alpha\Delta T$ (d) $\frac{lAY}{\alpha \Delta T}$

6. A particle of mass M is situated at the centre of a spherical shell of same mass and radius a. The gravitational potential at a point situated at $a/2$ distance from the centre will be

(a) $-\frac{4GM}{a}$ (b) $-\frac{3GM}{a}$ (c) $-\frac{2GM}{a}$ (d) $-\frac{GM}{a}$

7. The frequencies of X-rays, γ-rays and ultraviolet rays are respectively a, b and c, then

(a) $a > b, b < c$ (b) $a < b, b > c$
(c) $a < b, b < c$ (d) $a > b, b > c$

8. A ball is projected with a velocity 20 ms^{-1}, at an angle of 60° with the vertical direction. Its speed (in m/s) at the highest point of its trajectory will be

(a) $5\sqrt{3}$ (b) $10\sqrt{3}$ (c) $15\sqrt{3}$ (d) $20\sqrt{3}$

9. A monochromatic light of wavelength 6000Å is incident on a thin glass plate of refractive index $\sqrt{2}$, such that the angle of refraction in the plate is 45°, then smallest thickness of the plate which will make it dark by reflection

(a) 3000 Å (b) 1500 Å (c) 4000 Å (d) 45(

10. A student performs an experiment to determine the Young's modulus of a wire, exactly 2 m long. In a particular reading, the student measures the extension in the length of the wire to be 0.8 mm with an uncertainty of ±0.05 mm at a load of exactly 1.0 kg. The student also measures the diameter of the wire to be 0.4 mm with an uncertainty of ±0.01 mm. Take, $g = 9.8\ m/s^2$ (exact). The Young's modulus obtained from the reading is close to

(a) $(2.0 \pm 0.3)10^{11}\ N/m^2$
(b) $(2.0 \pm 0.2) \times 10^{11}\ N/m^2$
(c) $(2.0 \pm 0.1) \times 10^{11}\ N/m^2$
(d) $(2.0 \pm 0.05) \times 10^{11}\ N/m^2$

11. The electric field at a distance $3R/2$ from the centre of a charged conducting spherical shell of radius R is E. The electric field at a distance $R/2$ from the centre of the sphere is

(a) $\frac{E}{4}$ (b) $\frac{E}{2}$ (c) E (d) zero

12. The temperature of inversion of a thermocouple is 620° C and the neutral temperature is 300° C. What is the temperature of cold junction ?

(a) 40° C (b) 20° C
(c) −20° C (d) 320° C

13. A square loop of side 20 cm having resistance 50Ω is placed in an uniform magnetic field of 2.5 T to the plane of loop. If we attempt to pull it out of the field with a constant velocity 25 m/s, then the power requirement is

(a) 2.75 W (b) 3.75 W
(c) 3.125 W (d) 5.125 W

14. The dimensions of universal gravitational constant is

(a) $[M^{-2}L^2T^{-1}]$ (b) $[M^{-1}L^3T^{-2}]$
(c) $[M^{-2}L^3T^{-2}]$ (d) $[ML^2T^{-1}]$

15. A monoatomic gas at a pressure p, having a volume V expands isothermally to a volume $2V$ and then adiabatically to a volume $16V$. The final pressure of the gas is (take $\gamma = \frac{5}{3}$)

(a) $\frac{p}{64}$ (b) $30\ p$ (c) $70\ p$ (d) $18\ p$

16. **Statement I** When an object is placed between two plane parallel mirrors, then all the images found are of equal intensity.

Statement II In case of plane parallel mirrors, only two images are possible.

(a) Both Statement I and Statement II are correct.
(b) Both Statement I and Statement II are incorrect.
(c) Statement I is correct and Statement II is incorrect.
(d) Statement I is incorrect and Statement II is correct.

17. Which of the following is a dimensional constant ?

(a) Relative density (b) Strain
(c) Refractive index (d) Gravitational constant

18. A ball is thrown vertically upward. It has a speed of 10 m/s, when it has reached one-half of its maximum height. How high does the ball rise ? (Take, $g = 10\ m/s^2$)

(a) 20 m (b) 10 m
(c) 5 m (d) 15 m

19. The chromatic aberration in lenses is due to

(a) dissimilarity of main axis of rays.
(b) variation of focal length of lenses with wavelength.
(c) dissimilarity of radii of curvature.
(d) None of the above.

20. Given below are two statements

Statement I If 8th vernier scale division of a vernier caliper coincide with its 7th main scale division, then the least count of the vernier caliper is 0.125 mm.

Statement II Using above vernier caliper, the measurement of diameter of an object can be 0.12 mm.

(a) Both Statement I and Statement II are correct.
(b) Both Statement I and Statement II are incorrect.
(c) Statement I is correct but Statement II is incorrect.
(d) Statement I is incorrect but Statement II is correct.

21. If N is the number of turns in a coil, the value of self-inductance varies as

(a) N^0 (b) N
(c) N^{-2} (d) N^2

22. A car battery has emf 12 V and internal resistance $5 \times 10^{-2}\ \Omega$. If it draws 60 A current, the terminal voltage of the battery will be

(a) 10 V (b) 9 V
(c) 12 V (d) 8 V

23. In a parallel plate capacitor, the distance between the plates is d and potential difference across the plates is V. Energy stored per unit volume between the plates of capacitor is

(a) $\frac{1}{2}\varepsilon_0 \frac{V^2}{d}$ (b) $\frac{1}{2}\frac{V^2}{\varepsilon_0 d^2}$
(c) $\frac{Q^2}{2V^2}$ (d) $\frac{1}{2}\varepsilon_0 \frac{V^2}{d^2}$

24. If the input waveform is as shown, express the output waveform at load resistance.

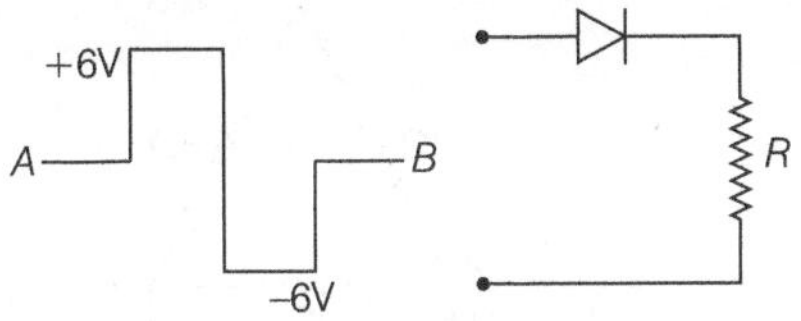

(a) 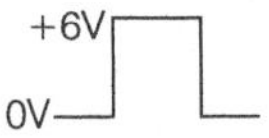

(b) 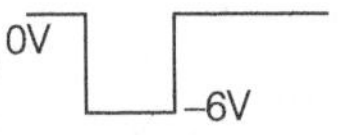

(c) 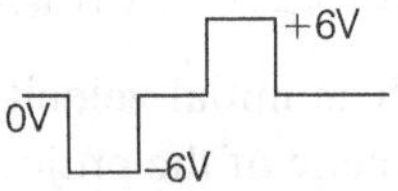

(d) 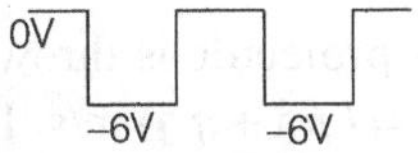

25. In an AC circuit, an alternating voltage $e = 200\sqrt{2} \sin 100\,t$ volts is connected to a capacitor of capacity 1 μF. The rms value of the current in the circuit is

(a) 25 mA (b) 80 mA (c) 20 mA (d) 50 mA

26. A diode shown in the diagram is connected to a battery of external resistance and an electromotive force. Suppose a diode layer of 0.5 V is produced in the diode, then find the value of current (in mA).

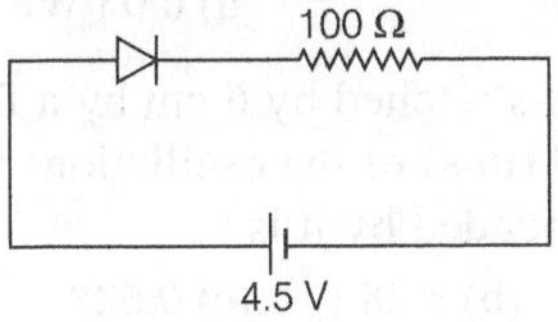

(a) 45 (b) 40
(c) 20 (d) 10

27. The mean free path for a gas, with molecular diameter d and number density n can be expressed as

(a) $\dfrac{1}{\sqrt{2}\, n\pi d}$ (b) $\dfrac{1}{\sqrt{2} n^2 \pi^2 d^2}$

(c) $\dfrac{1}{\sqrt{2} n\pi d^2}$ (d) $\dfrac{1}{\sqrt{2} n^2 \pi^2 d^2}$

28. Sand is being dropped on a conveyor belt at the rate of $2M$ kg/s. The force (in newton) necessary to keep the belt moving with a constant velocity v m/s will be

(a) $2\,Mv$ (b) Mv (c) $\dfrac{2M}{v}$ (d) $\dfrac{v}{2M}$

29. Two condensers of capacities 1 μF and 2 μF are connected in series and the system is charged by 120 V, then the potential difference on 1 μF capacitor (in V) will be

(a) 80 (b) 60 (c) 40 (d) 140

30. What will be the formula of the mass in terms of g, R and G ? (R = radius of the earth)

(a) $g\dfrac{R^2}{G}$ (b) $G\dfrac{R}{g}$ (c) $g^2\dfrac{R}{G}$ (d) $G\dfrac{R^2}{g}$

31. The internal resistance of a 2.1 V cell which gives a current of 0.2 A through a resistance of 10Ω is

(a) 0.5Ω (b) 0.8Ω (c) 1.0Ω (d) 0.2Ω

32. Photoelectric emission occurs only when the incident light has more than a certain minimum

(a) intensity (b) frequency
(c) power (d) wavelength

33. The resistance of a wire is R ohm. If it is melted and stretched to n times of its original length, its new resistance will be

(a) $n^2 R$ (b) $\dfrac{R}{n^2}$ (c) $\dfrac{R}{n}$ (d) nR

34. If an orbital radius of the electron in a hydrogen atoms is 4.7×10^{-11} m, compute the kinetic energy of the electron in hydrogen atom.

(a) 15.3 eV (b) –15.3 eV
(c) 13.6 eV (d) –13.6 eV

35. The mean free path of electrons in a metal is 4×10^{-8} m. The electric field which can give on an average 2eV energy to an electron in the metal will be (in V/m)

(a) 5×10^7 (b) 6×10^{-11} (c) 7×10^7 (d) 9×10^7

36. The energy of a hydrogen atom in the ground state is –13.6 eV. The energy of a He^+ ion in the first excited state will be

(a) –1.51 eV (b) –13.6 eV
(c) –0.85 eV (d) –3.4 eV

37. A sinusoidal voltage of peak value 200 V is connected to a diode and resistance R in the circuit shown in figure, so that half-wave rectification occurs. If the forward resistance of the diode is negligible compared to R, the rms voltage (in V) across R approximately

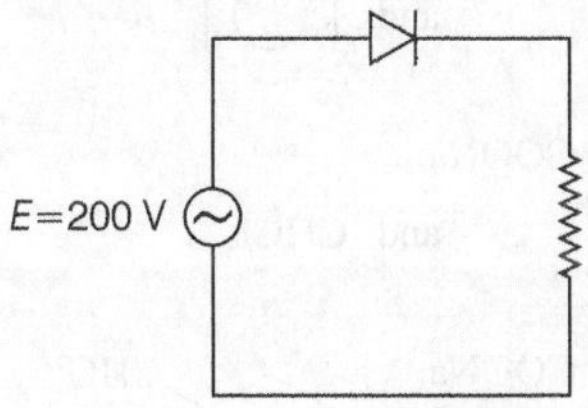

(a) 200 (b) 100 (c) $\dfrac{200}{\sqrt{2}}$ (d) 280

38. A 220 V input is supplied to a transformer. The output circuit draws a current of 2.0A at 440V. If the efficiency of the transformer is 80%, the current drawn by the primary windings of the transformer is

(a) 4 A (b) 3 A (c) 2.5 A (d) 5 A

39. According to Einstein's photoelectric equation, the graph between the kinetic energy of ejected photoelectrons and frequency of incident radiation is

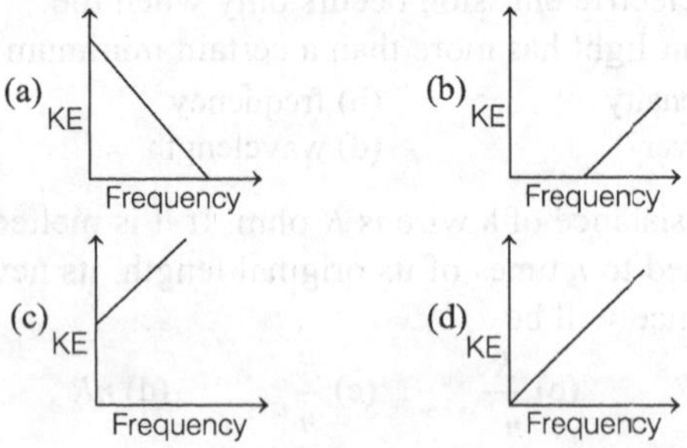

40. The ratio of KE to the total energy of an electron in a Bohr orbit of the hydrogen atom is

(a) 1 : 1 (b) 2 : −1 (c) 1:−1 (d) 1:−2

41. For a process of a ideal gas, $dW = 0$ and $dQ < 0$. Then for the gass.

(a) The temperature will decrease
(b) The volume will increase
(c) The pressure will remian constant
(d) The temperature will increase

42. The current I in the following circuit is

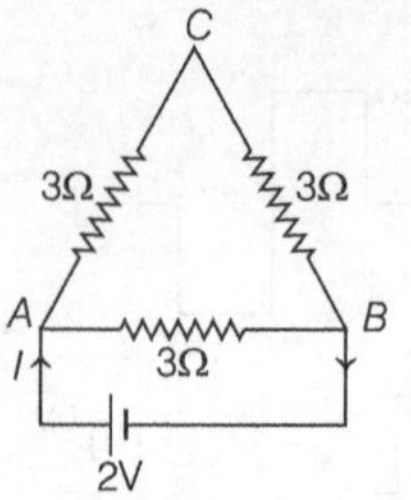

(a) 2 A (b) 4 A (c) 5/2 A (d) 1 A

43. A projectile is thrown with an initial velocity of $v = (p\hat{i} + q\hat{j})$ m/s. If the range of the projectile is double the maximum height reached by it, then

(a) $q = p$ (b) $q = 2p$ (c) $p = 2q$ (d) $q = 4p$

44. A rectangular bar magnet of area 20 cm^2 has ability to produce a magnetic field of 2.5 T at a point 30 cm away from its mid-point on axial line. If it is assumed that dipole is surrounded by a spherical region in space, then net magnetic flux passes through the sphere is

(a) 0 (b) 0.005 Wb
(c) 0.15 Wb (d) 0.05 Wb

45. A spring is stretched by 6 cm by a force 12 N. The time period (in s) of the oscillations when a mass of 2 kg is suspended by it is

(a) 6.008 (b) 6.28 (c) 0.628 (d) 0.0628

CHEMISTRY

46. Consider the following reaction.

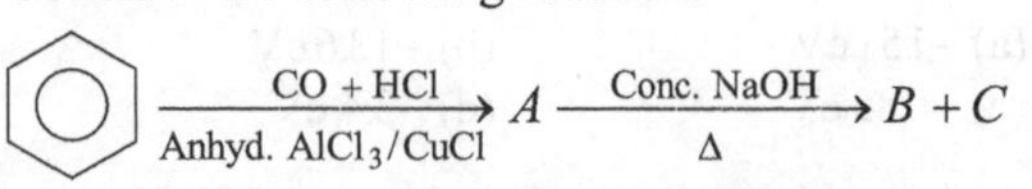

Products B and C are

(a) 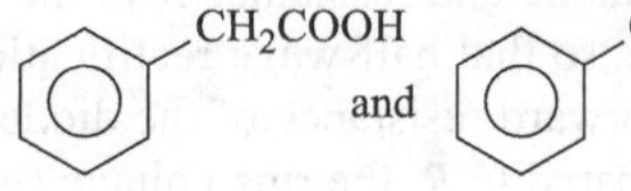

(b) 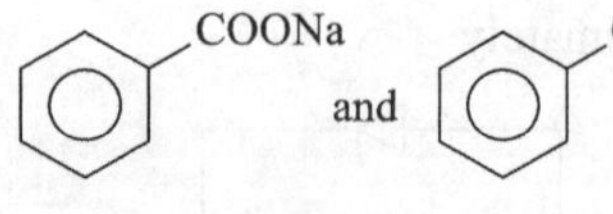

(c) 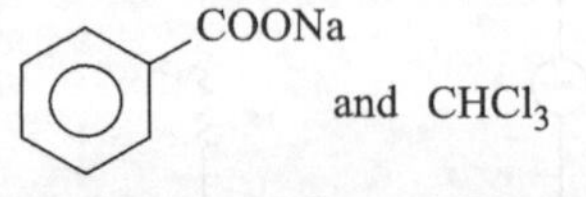

(d) 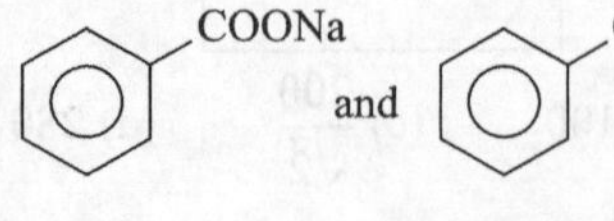

47. Which of the following statement is incorrect?

(a) Sucrose is a dextrorotatory sugar.
(b) Sucrose has a pyranose and furanose ring linked together by 1, 1'- glycosidic linkage.
(c) Maltose has one glycosidic linkage and a free hemiacetal end.
(d) Sucrose is a reducing sugar.

48. Match List-I with List-II.

	List-I		List-II
A.	Benzene sulphonyl chloride	I.	Test for primary amines
B.	Hofmann bromamide reaction	II.	Anti-Saytzeff
C.	Carbylamine reaction	III.	Hinsberg reagent
D.	Hofmann elimination	IV.	Known reaction of isocyanates

Choose the correct answer from the options given below.
(a) A-IV, B-III, C-I, D-II (b) A-III, B-IV, C-I, D-II
(c) A-IV, B-II, C-I, D-III (d) A-IV, B-III, C-II, D-I

49. All the following statements about the 3*d*-series elements are true except that
(a) scandium has lowest melting point.
(b) enthalpy of atomisation of zinc is lowest.
(c) first ionisation energy of Sc is lowest and zinc is highest .
(d) scandium has lowest density.

50. Which of the following statements are correct regarding VBT?
I. It does not explain the colour of coordination compounds.
II. It can distinguish between strong and weak ligands.
III. It does not explain the kinetic stabilities of coordination compounds.
IV. It is unreliable in the prediction of geometries of 4-coordinate complexes.
V. It explain the colour of coordination compounds.
(a) I and II only (b) Only III
(c) II, III and IV (d) I, III and IV

51. Which one is an incorrect statement?
(a) Principal quantum number gives the average distance of an electron from the nucleus.
(b) Azimuthal quantum number gives the information of angular momentum of an electron present in an subshell.
(c) The value of m for p_z-orbital is +1.
(d) Five *d*-orbitals of a particular *d*-subshell are degenerate.

52. Compound *P* reacts with $CHCl_3$ and KOH to give an offensive smelling compound. The original compound *P* can be
A. 1° aliphatic amine B. 2° amine
C. 3° amine D. 1° aromatic amine
Choose the correct answer from the options given below.
(a) A, D (b) B, C (c) C, D (d) A, C

53. Given below are two statements.
Statement I In the highest oxidation states, the transition metals show basic character and form cationic complexes.
Statement II In transition elements, once the d^5 configuration is exceeded, the tendency to involve all the 3*d* electrons in bonding decreases.
In the light of the above statements, choose the correct answer from the options given below.
(a) Both Statement I and Statement II are incorrect.
(b) Statement I is correct but Statement II is incorrect.
(c) Statement I is incorrect but Statement II is correct.
(d) Both Statement I and Statement II are correct.

54. IUPAC name of

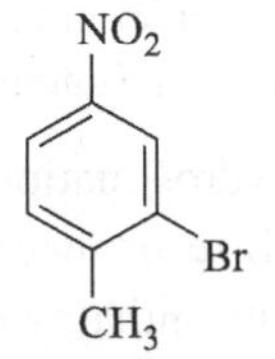

(a) 3-bromo-4 methylnitrobenzene
(b) 2-bromo-1-methyl-4-nitrobenzene
(c) 6-bromo-4-nitrotoluene
(d) 2-methyl-5-nitrobromobenzene

55. Arrange the following carbanions in decreasing order of stability.

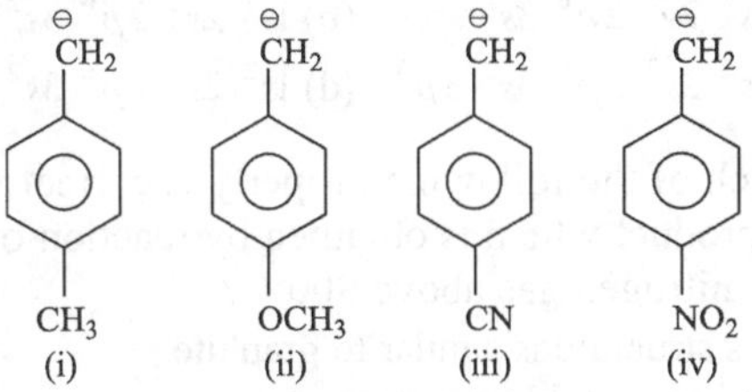

Choose the correct option.
(a) (iv) > (iii) > (i) > (ii)
(b) (iii) > (iv) > (ii) > (i)
(c) (i) > (iii) > (ii) > (iv)
(d) (ii) > (i) > (iii) > (iv)

56. In a set of reactions, acetic acid yielded a product *S* as follows

$$CH_3COOH \xrightarrow{SOCl_2} P \xrightarrow[\text{anhy. } AlCl_3]{\text{Benzene}} Q \xrightarrow{HCN} R \xrightarrow{H_2O} S$$

Here, *S* is

(a) 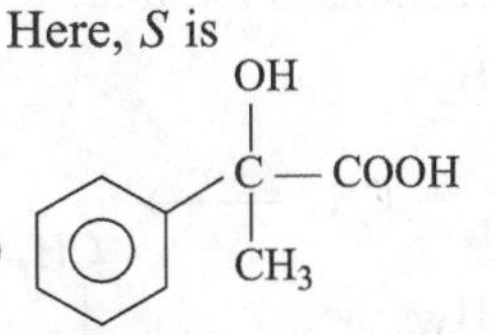

(b) 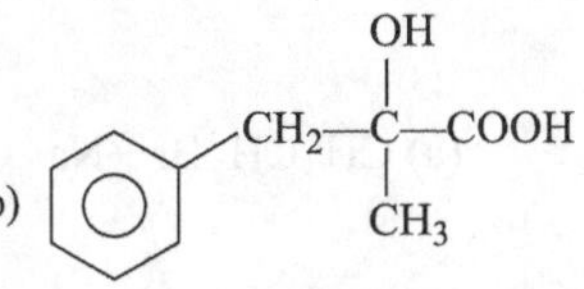

(c) 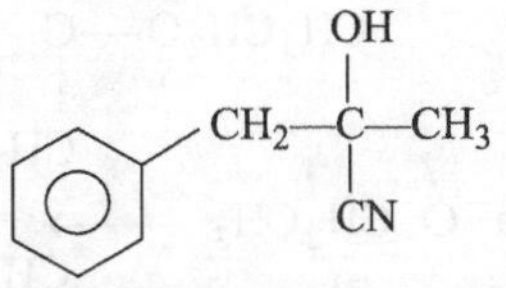

(d) 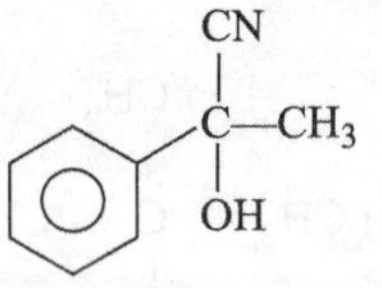

57. Consider the following statements.
Statement I The rate of a reaction typically increases with an increase in temperature due to rise in the kinetic energy of the molecules.

Statement II The rate constant of a reaction increases with an increase in temperature of an endothermic reaction.
In the light of the above statements, choose the most appropriate answer from the options given below.
(a) Statement I is correct but Statement II is incorrect.
(b) Both Statement I and Statement II are correct.
(c) Statement I is incorrect but Statement II is correct.
(d) Both Statement I and Statement II are incorrect.

58. The enthalpy of hydrogenation of cyclohexene is $-119.5\ \text{kJ mol}^{-1}$. If resonance energy of benzene is $-150.4\ \text{kJ mol}^{-1}$, its enthalpy of hydrogenation would be
(a) $-269.9\ \text{kJ mol}^{-1}$ (b) $-358.5\ \text{kJ mol}^{-1}$
(c) $-508.9\ \text{kJ mol}^{-1}$ (d) $-208.1\ \text{kJ mol}^{-1}$

59. A sudden jump between the values of second and third ionisation energies of an element would be associated with the electronic configuration
(a) $1s^2\ 2s^2\ 2p^6\ 3s^1$ (b) $1s^2\ 2s^2\ 2p^6\ 3s^2\ 3p^1$
(c) $1s^2\ 2s^2\ 2p^6\ 3s^2\ 3p^3$ (d) $1s^2\ 2s^2\ 2p^6\ 3s^2$

60. Which of the following property is correct regarding the product which is obtained by reaction of boron with nitrogen gas above 900°C?
(a) Its structure is similar to graphite.
(b) It has unstable structure.
(c) Boron and nitrogen atoms are bound by ionic bonds.
(d) It is isomorphous with diamond.

61. The $t_{75\%}$ for a zero order reaction having 0.07 M initial concentration of reactant is 120 s. The rate constant (in mol $L^{-1}\ s^{-1}$) for the reaction is
(a) 2.8×10^{-4} (b) 1.4×10^{-4}
(c) 1.1×10^{-3} (d) 1.7×10^{-5}

62. Which of the following reactions is feasible?

(a) 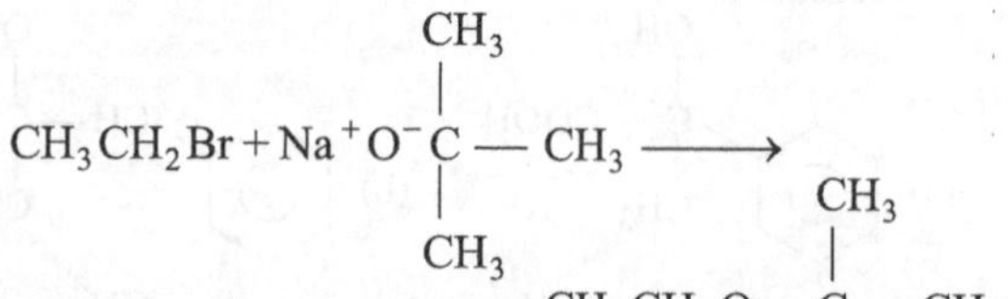

(b) 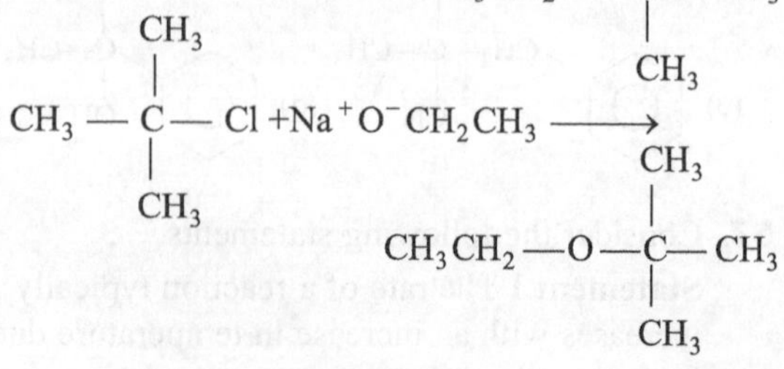

(c) Secondary amine react with $CHCl_3$ and KOH gives isocyanide.
(d) Tertiary amine reacts with $CHCl_3$ and KOH gives isocyanide.

63. 20 g of naphthoic acid ($C_{11}H_8O_2$) dissolved in 50 g of benzene ($K_f = 1.72\ \text{K kg mol}^{-1}$) shows a depression in freezing point of 2 K. The van't Hoff factor is
(a) 0.5 (b) 0.1
(c) 2 (d) 3

64. Arrange the following carbonyl compounds in decreasing order of their reactivity in nucleophilic addition reaction.

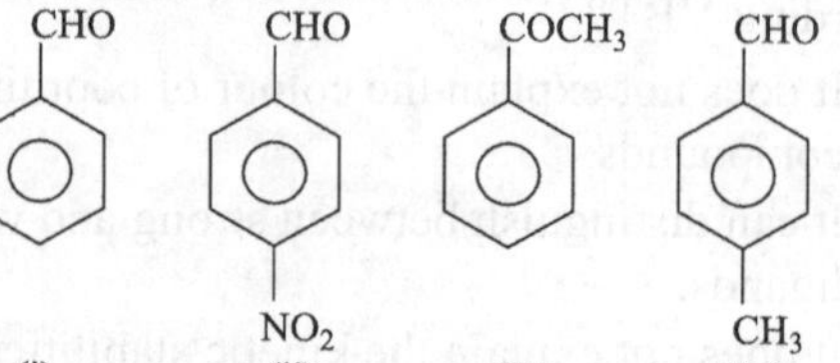

(i) (ii) (iii) (iv)

(a) (ii) > (iii) > (i) > (iv)
(b) (ii) > (i) > (iv) > (iii)
(c) (iii) > (ii) > (i) > (iv)
(d) (iii) > (i) > (iv) > (ii)

65. The electron gain enthalpies of halogens in kJ mol^{-1} are as given below.
F = −332, Cl = −349, Br = −324, I = −295.
The less negative value for F as compared to that of Cl is due to
(a) strong electron-electron repulsion in the compact $2p$-subshell of F.
(b) weak electron-electron repulsion in the bigger $3p$-subshell of Cl.
(c) smaller electronegativity value of F than Cl.
(d) Both (a) and (b)

66. Given below are two statements, one is labelled as Assertion (A) and other is labelled as Reason (R).
Assertion (A) N_2O is represented by (i) $\overset{-}{N}=\overset{+}{N}=O$ and (ii) $N\equiv N\rightarrow O$ but later is more stable.
Reason (R) The form (ii) shows resonance.
In the light of the above statements, choose the most appropriate answer from the options given below.
(a) (A) is false but (R) is true.
(b) Both (A) and (R) are true and (R) is a correct explanation of (A).
(c) Both (A) and (R) are true and (R) is not a correct explanation of (A).
(d) (A) is true but (R) is false.

67. Match the List-I with List-II

List-I (Species)		List-II (Lone pair of electrons on central atom)	
A.	Cl^-	(i)	3
B.	XeF_4	(ii)	1
C.	SF_4	(iii)	2
D.	$(I_3)^-$	(iv)	4

Choose the correct answer from the options given below.
(a) A-(iv), B-(iii), C-(ii), D-(i)
(b) A-(iv), B-(iii), C-(i), D-(ii)
(c) A-(i), B-(iii), C-(ii), D-(iv)
(d) A-(i), B-(ii), C-(iii), D-(iv)

68. Match Column I with Column II.

Column I	Column II
A. $CH_3C\equiv CH \xrightarrow[CH_3COOH]{BH_3, THF}$	I. $CH_3-\overset{O}{\overset{\parallel}{C}}-CH_3$
B. Toluene $\xrightarrow{KMnO_4/NaOH}$	II. Acetophenone
C. $CH_3-C\equiv CH + H_2O \xrightarrow[1\%\ HgSO_4]{42\%\ H_2SO_4}$	III. Benzoic acid
D. Benzene + $CH_3Cl \xrightarrow{\text{Anhyd. } AlCl_3}$	IV. $CH_3-CH_2-\overset{O}{\overset{\parallel}{C}}-H$

Choose the correct answer from the options given below.
(a) A-IV, B-III, C-I, D-II
(b) A-III, B-II, C-IV, D-I
(c) A-II, B-IV, C-III, D-I
(d) A-IV, B-I, C-II, D-III

69. Match the List-I with List-II.

List-I	List-II
A. $Na_2O_2 + H_2SO_4 \longrightarrow Na_2SO_4 + H_2O_2$	(i) Redox reaction
B. $H_2 + Cl_2 \longrightarrow 2HCl$	(ii) Oxidation reaction
C. $Cr(OH)_3 \longrightarrow CrO_4^{2-}$	(iii) Not a redox reaction
D. $IO_3^- \longrightarrow I^-$	(iv) Reduction reaction

Choose the correct answer from the options given below.
(a) A-(iii), B-(i), C-(ii), D-(iv)
(b) A-(iii), B-(ii), C-(i), D-(iv)
(c) A-(i), B-(iii), C-(ii), D-(iv)
(d) A-(iii), B-(i), C-(iv), D-(ii)

70. Consider the following substance.
A. Na_2O B. Na_2SO_4
C. Al_2O_3 D. NaCl
E. Silica gel
Which of the following substances are used as an adsorbent in the column chromatography?
(a) C and E (b) A and B
(c) C and D (d) A, C and E

71. Given below are two statements.
Statement I A tertiary acid (R_3CCOOH) usually fail in sodalime catalysed decarboxylation reaction to produce alkane, rationalise.
Statement II Tertiary carbanion is highly unstable,very less likely to be formed.
In the light of the above statements, choose the correct answer from the options given below.
(a) Both Statement I and Statement II are true.
(b) Both Statement I and Statement II are false.
(c) Statement I is true but Statement II is false.
(d) Statement I is false but Statement II is true.

72. The molecule in which an atom is associated with more than $8e^-$ is known as hyper valent molecule. All hypervalent molecules must have $d\pi$-$p\pi$ bonding but the molecule having back bonding need not have always $d\pi$-$d\pi$ bonding. Which of the molecule is not hypervalent but completes its octet?
(a) $AlCl_3$ (b) $AlBr_3$
(c) AlF_3 (d) BF_3

73. If the solubility product of AB_2 is 3.2×10^{-11} M^3, then the solubility of AB_2 in pure water is (mol L^{-1}) [Assuming that neither kind of ion reacts with water]
(a) $\left(\frac{3.2\times10^{-11}}{4}\right)^{\frac{1}{3}}$ (b) $(3.2\times10^{-11})^{\frac{1}{3}}$
(c) $\left(\frac{3.2\times10^{-11}}{2}\right)^{\frac{1}{3}}$ (d) $\left(\frac{3.2\times10^{-11}}{4}\right)^{3}$

74. Which of the following equimolar solution have highest vapour pressure?
(a) Glucose (b) NaCl
(c) K_2SO_4 (d) $K_4[Fe(CN)_6]$

75. 20 mL of KOH solution was titrated with 0.20 M H_2SO_4 solution in a conductivity cell. The data obtained were plotted to give the graph shown below. The concentration of the KOH solution was

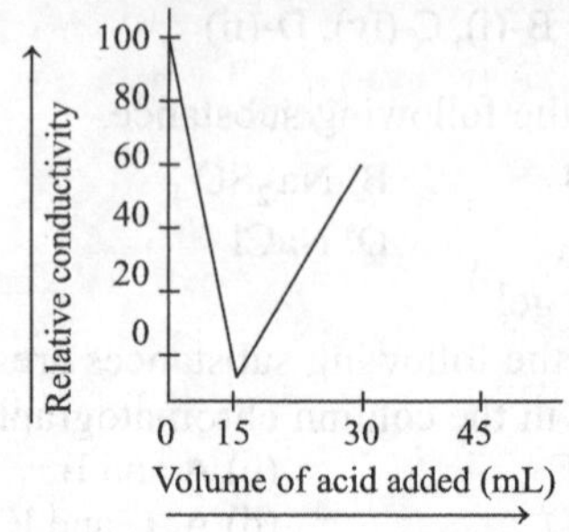

(a) 0.30 mol L^{-1} (b) 0.15 mol L^{-1}
(c) 0.12 mol L^{-1} (d) 0.075 mol L^{-1}

76. The energy of activation for the backward reaction is

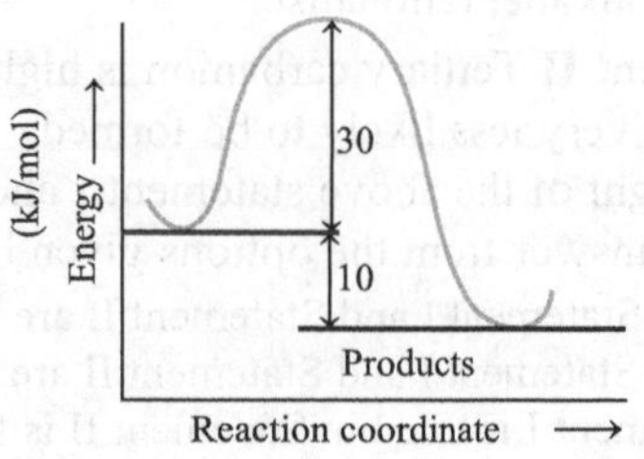

(a) 30 kJ mol^{-1} (b) 20 kJ mol^{-1}
(c) 10 kJ mol^{-1} (d) 40 kJ mol^{-1}

77. Which of the following set contain all extensive property?
(a) Mass, volume, internal energy
(b) Enthalpy, temperature, density
(c) Mass, pressure, density
(d) Internal energy, temperature, pressure

78. Given below are two statements.
Statement I XeO_3 has 4 σ-bonds and 4π-bonds.
Statement II The hybridisation of Xe in XeF_4 is sp^3d^2.
In the light of the above statements, choose the correct answer from the options given below.
(a) Both Statement I and Statement II are true.
(b) Both Statement I and Statement II are false.
(c) Statement I is true but Statement II is false.
(d) Statement I is false but Statement II is true.

79. The spin only magnetic moment of $[Fe(CN)_6]^{3-}$ will be
(a) 2.98 BM (b) 8.96 BM
(c) 5.92 BM (d) 1.732 BM

80. Compound $C_7H_8O(A)$ gives colour with neutral $FeCl_3$ and can be nitrated to form three types of nitro compound *A* can be

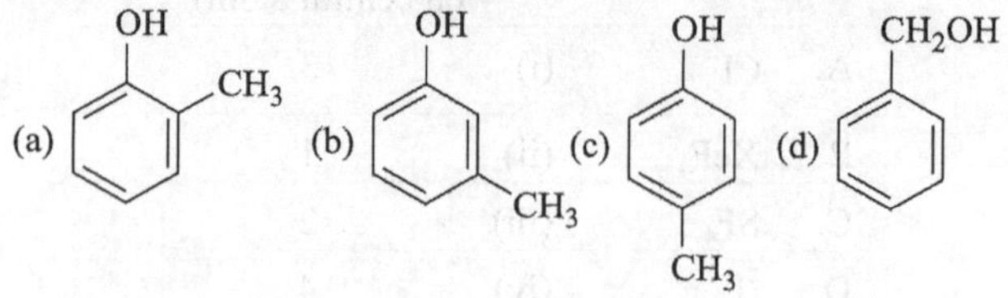

81. Choose the correct product among four options regarding following reaction.

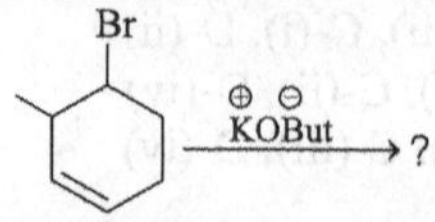

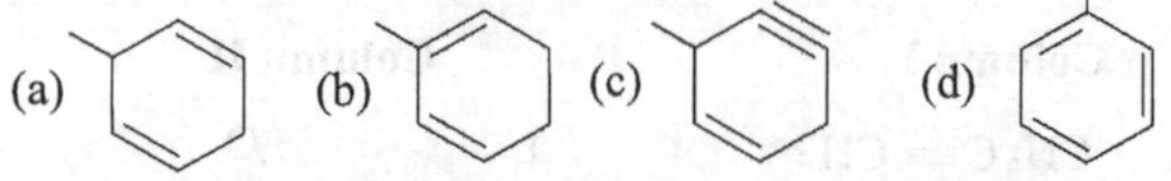

82. 12g of a non-volatile solute dissolved in 108 g of water produces the relative lowering of vapour pressure of 0.1. The molecular mass of the solute is
(a) 80 (b) 40 (c) 20 (d) 120

83. A solution of sodium chloride discharges 6.1×10^{16} Na^+ ions and 4.6×10^{16} Cl^- ions in 10 seconds. Find the current passing through the solution.
(a) 1.7 mA (b) 1.8 mA
(c) 1.9 mA (d) 1.6 mA

84. Consider the following statements.
Statement I The value of equilibrium constant is independent of initial concentrations of the reactants and products.
Statement II The reaction will proceed in the direction of reactant of $Q < K_c$ (Q is reaction quotient)
In the light of the above statements, choose the most appropriate answer from the options given below.
(a) Statement I is correct but Statement II is incorrect.
(b) Both Statement I and Statement II are correct.
(c) Statement I is incorrect but Statement II is correct.
(d) Both Statement I and Statement II are incorrect.

85. The crystal field stabilisation energy (CFSF) and the spin-only magnetic moment in Bohr Magneton (BM) for the complex $K_3[Fe(CN)_6]$ are respectively.
(a) $0.0\Delta_0$ and $\sqrt{35}$ BM (b) $2.0\Delta_0$ and $\sqrt{3}$ BM
(c) $1.6\Delta_0$ and $\sqrt{24}$ BM (d) $-2.4\Delta_0$ and 0 BM

86. Which is not correct reaction ?

(a) $XeF_6 + NaF \longrightarrow [XeF_5]^+ [2F^-][Na^+]$

(b) $XeF_6 + PF_5 \longrightarrow [XeF_5^+][PF_6^-]$

(c) $XeF_6 + SbF_5 \longrightarrow [XeF_5^+][SbF_6^-]$

(d) $XeF_2 + PF_5 \longrightarrow [XeF^+][PF_6^-]$

87. For the compounds phenol (I) *p*-cresol (II) *m*-nitrophenol (III) and *p*-nitrophenol (IV) the order of acidity is

(a) III > IV > I > II (b) I > IV > III > II

(c) II > I > III > IV (d) IV > III > I > II

88. Given below are two statements.

Statement I C_2H_5Br on treating with sodium ethoxide forms diethylether.

Statement II Benzyl chloride with sodium cyanide followed by reduction gives β-phenylethylamine.

In the light of the above statements, choose the correct answer from the options given below:

(a) Both Statement I and Statement II are true.

(b) Both Statement I and Statement II are false.

(c) Statement I is true but Statement II is false.

(d) Statement I is false but Statement II is true.

89. Which of the following cannot be used to form CH_3COOH from C_2H_5OH?

I. PCC II. PDC

III. $K_2Cr_2O_7$ / H^+ IV. $KMnO_4/H^+$

V. $LiAlH_4$

(a) I and II only (b) III and IV only

(c) Only I (d) I, II, III and IV

90. Match the List-I with List-II:

List-I (Aldehyde)	List-II (Oxidised product of aldehyde)
A. Formaldehyde	(i) Acetic acid
B. Acetaldehyde	(ii) Propanoic acid
C. Propionaldehyde	(iii) Isobutyric acid
D. Isobutylaldehyde	(iv) Methanoic acid

Choose the correct answer from the options given below.

(a) A-(iv), B-(i), C-(ii), D-(iii)

(b) A-(i), B-(iv), C-(iii), D-(ii)

(c) A-(i), B-(iii), C-(iv), D-(ii)

(d) A-(iv), B-(ii), C-(iii), D-(i)

BIOLOGY

91. An operon is considered to regulate a/an

(a) translational unit (b) genetic unit

(c) protein unit (d) enzymatic unit

92. Find out the correct order of the family of plants muliathi, turnip and daisies.

(a) Leguminosae, Cruciferae, Compositae

(b) Compositae, Leguminosae, Cruciferae

(c) Cruciferae, Leguminosae, Compositae

(d) Leguminosae, Compositae, Cruciferae

93. The Sertoli cells play very important roles in male reproductive system. The characteristic features of Sertoli cells are all, except that

(a) they synthesise and secrete testicular hormones, i.e. androgens which regulate the internal environment of the seminiferous tubules by secreting paracrine factors

(b) form intercellular tight junctions at the base

(c) disturbances in these cells can result in smaller testes

(d) number of Sertoli cells determines the ultimate spermatogenic output of the testes

94. Oogenesis is initiated during the embryonic development stage. When a couple of million gametes mother cells are formed within each foetal ovary, no more oogonia are formed and added after birth. These cells starts division and enter into

(a) metaphase-I of the meiotic division and temporarily arrested

(b) prophase-II of the meiotic division and get arrested at this stage

(c) prophase-I of the meiotic division and get arrested at this stage

(d) anaphase-I of the meiotic division and get arrested

95. Which of the following is not the feature of cell wall?

(a) The middle lamella is mainly made up of cellulose, which holds the different neighbouring cells

(b) Algal cell wall is made up of cellulose, galactans, mannans and calcium carbonate

(c) Plant cell wall consists of cellulose, hemicellulose, pectins and proteins
(d) Secondary cell wall is formed on the inner side of the cell

96. Which of the following characteristics is common in both humans and adult frogs?
(a) Ureotelic mode of excretion
(b) Four-chambered heart
(c) Internal fertilisation
(d) Nucleated RBCs

97. In a stable population of a country,
(a) Reproductive and pre-reproductive individuals are equal in number
(b) Reproductive individuals are less than the post-reproductive individuals
(c) Pre-reproductive individuals are more than the reproductive individuals
(d) Pre-reproductive individuals are less than the reproductive individuals

98. When Morgan hybridised yellow-bodied, white-eyed females to brown bodied, red-eyed males and intercrossed their progeny, the F_2 ratio deviate very significantly from 9 : 3 : 3 : 1 ratio. This can be attributed to the fact that.
(a) the gene exhibits incomplete dominance
(b) the genes are locaed on X and Y-chromosomes
(c) fruitfly has abnormal chromosomes
(d) the genes are located on X-chromosomes

99. Which of the following statements is incorrect?
(a) A true-breeding line is one that, having undergone continuous self-pollination, shows the stable trait inheritance and expression for several generations
(b) The law of dominance is used to explain the expression of both the parental characters in a monohybrid cross in the F_1-generation in snapdragon
(c) Law of segregation states that alleles do not show any blending and both the characters are recovered in the F_2-generation, while one of the character is not seen in the F_1-stage
(d) A homozygous parent produces all gametes that are similar while a heterozygous one produces two kinds of gametes each having one allele with equal proportion

100. What are the constituents of mitotic apparatus?
(a) Chromatids, centrosomes
(b) Chromatids, spindle fibres
(c) Asters, spindle fibres
(d) Kinetochores, centrosomes

101. Which of the following statements is incorrect?
(a) Parthenocarpy can be induced by application of IAA in a paste form to the stigma of a flower or by spraying the flowers with a dilute solution of IAA
(b) In maize, application of NAA during the period of inflorescence differentiation can induce formation of hermaphrodite or female flowers in a male inflorescence
(c) Abscisic acid promotes cold hardiness and inhibits growth of pathogens
(d) In low concentration, abscisic acid stimulates root initiation and growth of lateral roots and root hair.

102. What type of vascular bundle is commonly found in stem and leaves?
(a) Xylem and phloem are jointly situated along the same radius of vascular bundles
(b) The phloem lies in the centre and remains completely surrounded by xylem
(c) In vascular bundle, the xylem lies towards outer side and phloem towards inner side
(d) The xylem lies in the centre and remains completely surrounded by phloem

103. Match List-I with List-II

	List-I		List-II
A.	Mycoplasma	1.	Cell wall forms two thin overlapping shell
B.	Diatoms	2	Cell wall contains stiff cellulose plates on the outer surface
C.	*Gonyaulax*	3.	Protein rich layer
D.	*Euglena*	4.	Cell wall is absent

Choose the correct answer from the options given below.

	A	B	C	D		A	B	C	D
(a)	4	1	3	2	(b)	4	1	2	3
(c)	1	2	3	4	(d)	2	3	1	4

104. Organelle '*X*' is found in all the animal cell, except mature mammalian RBCs. It is also found in most of protists and motile plant cells like antherozoids of ferns. It is without unit membrane structure. Identify the organelle '*X*' from the options given below.

(a) Flagella (b) Centrosome
(c) Glyoxysomes (d) Lysosome

105. Given below are two statements.

Statement I Frederich Griffith hypothesised that a chemical component from the virulent R cells had somehow transformed the S cell into the more virulent R form.

Statement II Avery, MacLeod and McCarty purified biochemicals from the heat-killed R cells to see which ones could transform live S-cells into R cells.

In the light of the above statements, choose the correct answer from the options given below.

(a) Statement I is incorrect, but statement II is correct
(b) Both statement I and statement II are correct
(c) Both statement I and statement II are incorrect
(d) Statement I is correct, but statement II is incorrect

106. Which of the following statements is incorrect?

(a) A dihybrid genotye is heterozygous at two gene loci, whereas monohybrid genotype is heterozygous at one gene loci only
(b) A dihybrid cross considers the inheritance of two traits, each of which is specified by a different pair of genes on same chromosomes
(c) When F_1 progeny is back crossed to the parent with dominant phenotype, no recessive individuals are obtained in the progeny, but when F_1 progeny is back crossed with its recessive parent, both phenotypes are obtained
(d) The phenotypes of the offspring produced by a test cross reveal the number of different gametes formed by the parental genotype

107. Connective tissue connects and supports all the other tissues. Which of the following is the not the function of connective tissue?

I. Skeletal connective tissue like bones and cartilages provide the body with a supporting skeletal frame work, protects various organ and help in locomotion.
II. The jelly-like ground substance of connective tissues acts as shock absorber around some organs such as eye balls and kidneys.
III. Their main function is to provide protection against chemical and mechanical stresses, they cover the dry surface of the skin and the moist surface of buccal cavity.
IV. It produces or secretes histamine, serotonin and heparin. Histamine dilate the blood vessels in allergic and inflammatory conditions, it checks the clotting of blood inside the blood vessels.
V. It serves as insulating layer of neurons, preventing loss of energy during nerve impulse conductive conduct nerve impulses to the effector organs which responds to the stimuli.

Choose the correct answer from the options given below.

(a) III and V (b) I, II and III
(c) III, IV and V (d) I, III and V

108. Match List I with List II.

	List I		List II
A.	Fragments of *m*RNA sequences derived through single sequencing reaction performed on randomly selected clones from *c*DNA libraries.	1.	VNTR
B.	Short nucleotide sequence organised as a tandem repeat.	2.	Expressed sequence tags
C.	It contributes to the formation of crucial chromosome structures, heterochromatic establishment, genome stability and development.	3.	Single nucleotide polymorphism
D.	It represents a difference in a single DNA	4.	Satellite DNA

Choose the correct answer from the options given below.

	A	B	C	D
(a)	1	2	3	4
(b)	2	1	4	3
(c)	3	4	1	2
(d)	4	3	2	1

109. Human beings have a significant ability to maintain and moderate the respiratory rhythm to suit the demands of the body tissues. The primary regulator of respiration in the human body is

(a) oxygen level in the blood
(b) pH levels in the blood
(c) carbon dioxide levels in the blood
(d) blood glucose level

110. Given below are two statements.

Statement I The members of vertebrate possess notochord during the embryonic period of development.

Statement II In Hemichordata, the notochord is replaced by a cartilaginous or bony vertebral column in the adult.

In the light of the above statements, choose the correct answer from the options given below.

(a) Statement I is incorrect, but statement II is correct
(b) Both statement I and statement II are correct
(c) Both statement I and statement II are incorrect
(d) Statement I is correct, but statement II is incorrect

111. Match List I with List II.

	List I		List II
A.	It is the point of attachment of funicle with the body	1.	Tegmen
B.	Sometimes funicle fuses with the body of the ovule on one side and forms ridge	2.	Integument
C.	It is a protective envelope covering the ovule	3.	Raphe
D.	Lie inner to testa	4.	Hilum

Choose the correct answer from the options given below.

	A	B	C	D		A	B	C	D
(a)	4	3	2	1	(b)	3	4	1	2
(c)	2	4	1	3	(d)	1	4	3	2

112. Which of the following statements is not correct?

(a) A given species in an ecosystem may occupy more than one trophic level at the same time and contribute in the energy transfer
(b) Plants capture only 2-10% of the PAR and this small amount of energy sustains the entire living world
(c) An ecosystem can be visualised as a functional unit of nature, where living organisms interact among themselves and also with the surrounding physical environment
(d) The annual net primary productivity of the whole biosphere is approximately 170 billion tons of organic matter, oceans occupy 70% of the surface and their contribution in productivity is also very high

113. Match List I with List II.

	List I	List II
A.	They are dorso-ventrally flattened like leaf	1. Deuterostomia
B.	It includes true multicellular organisms	2. *Euspongia*
C.	The blastopore develops into the anus	3. Platyhelminthes
D.	Their skeleton is formed of spicules or spongin fibres	4. Coelenterata

Choose the correct answer from the options given below.

	A	B	C	D		A	B	C	D
(a)	3	4	1	2	(b)	4	3	1	2
(c)	2	4	3	1	(d)	3	2	1	4

114. The ability of the pistil to recognise the pollen followed by its acceptance or rejection is

(a) a chance factor only
(b) due to certain protein factors of petals
(c) the result of a continuous dialogue between the pistil and pollen grain
(d) is mediated physically, but not chemically

115. The size of a population for any species is not a static parameter which keeps changing with time. The process of any population which results in instant increase in population density is

(a) natality (b) mortality
(c) immigration (d) emigration

116. *Eco*RI is a type II restriction enzyme, which is isolated from *E. coli* while *Hind* II is also type II restriction enzyme, which is isolated from *Haemophilus influenzae*. The recognition sequences of *Eco*RI and *Hind* II are

(a) GAATTC and GTPyPuAC, respectively
(b) CAPuPyTC and GAATTC, respectively
(c) AATTCG and CCGAAT, respectively
(d) CCGGTT and TTAGGG, respectively

117. Given below are two statements; one is labelled as Assertion (A) and other is labelled as Reason (R).

Assertion (A) The skeleton of sponges is made up of spicules.

Reason (R) Composition of spicules help in classification of sponges.

In the light of the above statements, choose the correct answer from the options given below.

(a) A is false, but R is true
(b) Both A and R are true and R is the correct explanation of A
(c) Both A and R are true, but R is not the correct explanation of A
(d) A is ture, but R is false

118. Which of the following is not a physiological effect/property of cytokinins?

(a) It is produced in actively growing tissue
(b) It is transported through xylem elements
(c) It enhances the expansion of leaf cell in leaf discs and cotyledons
(d) It enhances the senescence of leaves

119. Given below are two statements.

Statement I Energy released from biological oxidation is used in the formation of high energy phosphate bond of ATP, NAD and FAD.

Statement II NADP is a universal hydrogen acceptor, produced only in aerobic respiration, work as coenzyme in ATP generation through ETS.

In the light of the above statements, choose the correct answer from the options given below.

(a) Statement I is incorrect, but statement II is correct
(b) Both statement I and statement II are correct
(c) Both statement I and statement II are incorrect
(d) Statement I is correct, but statement II is incorrect

120. PCR is a test-tube reaction and does not involve the use of living cells. Its reaction is based on the temperature change, Δt 94° C, at this temperature

(a) primers are allowed to attach to their annealing positions
(b) hydrogen bonds between two polynucleotides of the double helix are broken
(c) long products is synthesised from each strand of the target DNA
(d) DNA synthesis begins with the attachment of *Taq* polymerase

121. Given below are two statements; one is labelled as Assertion (A) and other is labelled as Reason (R).

Assertion (A) Restriction endonucleases are used in genetic engineering to form recombinant molecules of DNA, which are composed of DNA from different sources.

Reason (R) When DNA is cut by the same restriction enzyme, the resultant DNA fragments have the same kind of sticky ends, these can be joined together using DNA ligases.

In the light of the above statements, choose the correct answer from the options given below.

(a) A is false, but R is true
(b) Both A and R are true and R is the correct explanation of A
(c) Both A and R are true, but R is not the correct explanation of A
(d) A is true, but R is false

122. Convergent evolution occurs when species occupy similar ecological niches and adapt in similar ways in response to similar selective pressure. It is represented by all, except

(a) the wings of butterfly and the wings of birds
(b) the flippers of penguins and the flippers of dolphins
(c) sweet potato and potato
(d) thorn of *Bougainvillea* and tendrils of *Cucurbita*

123. Given below are two statements.

Statement I A nematocyst is a small, cylindrical, venom-filled capsule that is fired from the surface of nematode cells.

Statement II The nematocyst is composed of a coiled tubule that is attached to a disc-like structure at one end. The tubule is filled with venom and the disc contains barbs that anchor the nematocyst in prey.

In the light of the above statements, choose the correct answer from the options given below.

(a) Statement I is incorrect, but statement II is correct
(b) Both statement I and statement II are correct
(c) Both statement I and statement II are incorrect
(d) Statement I is correct, but statement II is incorrect

124. Given below are two statements.

Statement I Long distance flow of photoassimilates in plants occurs through the sieve tubes.

Statement II Sieve tubes are the conducting elements of phloem, which are elongated tubular channels formed by end-to-end union of numerous cells.
In the light of the above statements, choose the correct answer from the options given below.
(a) Statement I is incorrect, but statement II is correct
(b) Both statement I and statement II are correct
(c) Both statement I and statement II are incorrect
(d) Statement I is correct, but statement II is incorrect

125. In grasses, certain adaxial epidermal cells along the veins modify themselves into large, empty, colourless cells. These are called ...*A*.... When these cells absorb water and are turgid the leaf surface is ...*B*.... Identity *A* and *B* from the following

	A	*B*
(a)	bulliform cell	exposed
(b)	mesophyll cell	curl
(c)	spongy parenchyma	exposed
(d)	connective tissue	curl

126. Given below are two statements; one is labelled as Assertion (A) and other is labelled as Reason (R).
Assertion (A) The enzyme controlled reactions are always reversible. The enzymes affect only the rate of biochemical reactions, not the direction.
Reason (R) Lipase can catalyse the splitting of fat molecules into fatty acid and glycerol as well as synthesis of fatty acid and glycerol into fats.
In the light of the above statements, choose the correct answer from the options given below.
(a) A is false, but R is true
(b) Both A and R are true and R is the correct explanation of A
(c) Both A and R are true, but R is not the correct explanation of A
(d) A is ture, but R is false

127. Due to some catastrophic events, decomposers get completely removed from an ecosystem. What will be the future consequences among those given below?
(a) Net primary productivity reduced
(b) Soil becomes fertile
(c) Mineral movement will be blocked
(d) Number of herbivores increased

128. Given below are two statements.
Statement I The final stage of meiotic prophase-I is marked by terminalisation of chiasmata.
Statement II In metaphase-I, the bivalent chromosomes align on the equatorial plate.
In the light of the above statements, choose the correct answer from the options given below.
(a) Statement I is incorrect, but statement II is correct
(b) Both statement I and statement II are correct
(c) Both statement I and statement II are incorrect
(d) Statement I is correct, but statement II is incorrect

129. Identify the incorrect statements from the following.
I. The two kingdom classification is based on cell structure, body organisation, mode of nutrition, reproduction and phylogenetic relationship.
II. The two kingdom system did not distinguish between the eukaryotes and prokaryotes, unicellular and multicellular and photosynthetic and non-photosynthetic organisms.
III. Kingdom–Monera has brought together *Chlamydomonas*, *Chlorella* both having cell walls with *Paramecium* and *Amoeba* both lacking cell wall.
IV. Methanogens are present in the gut of several ruminant animals such as cows and buffaloes and they are responsible for the production of methane from the dung.
V. Kingdom–Monera includes all the simplest prokaryotic organisms, they lack a nuclear membrane and membrane bound organelles.

Choose the correct answer from the options given below.
(a) I, III and IV (b) II, III, IV and V
(c) I and III (d) I, II and IV

130. Which of the following toxic substance is responsible for the chill and high fever recurring every three to four days in malaria?
(a) Haemotoxin (b) Haemoglobin
(c) Haemozoin (d) Sporozoites

131. Given below are two statements; one is labelled as Assertion (A) and other is labelled as Reason (R).

Assertion (A) Decrease in species diversity occur as we ascend a high mountain.

Reason (R) Only deliberate introduction of non-native species leads to a decline in the population of local species.

In the light of the above statements, choose the correct answer from the options given below.

(a) A is false, but R is true
(b) Both A and R are true and R is the correct explanation of A
(c) Both A and R are true, but R is not the correct explanation of A
(d) A is true, but R is false

132. Which of the following statements is false for uterus?

(a) It is also called womb and its shape is like an inverse pear
(b) It is supported by ligaments attached to the pelvic wall
(c) It opens into oviducts through cervix whose cavity called cervical canal
(d) It is bounded by three layers, outer perimetrium, middle myometrium and inner endometrium.

133. Arrange the following process of spermatogenesis in the sequence in which they occur

I. The secondary spermatocytes undergo the second meiotic division to produce four haploid spermatids.
II. The spermatogonia present on the inside wall of seminiferous tubules multiply by mitotic division.
III. A primary spermatocyte undergoes meiotic division, leading to formation of secondary spermatocytes.
IV. Sperm heads become embedded in the Sertoli cells.
V. The spermatids are transformed into spermatozoa.

Choose the correct answer from the options given below.

(a) I $\rightarrow$ III $\rightarrow$ V $\rightarrow$ IV $\rightarrow$ II
(b) II $\rightarrow$ III $\rightarrow$ I $\rightarrow$ V $\rightarrow$ IV
(c) IV $\rightarrow$ III $\rightarrow$ I $\rightarrow$ II $\rightarrow$ V
(d) I $\rightarrow$ II $\rightarrow$ III $\rightarrow$ IV $\rightarrow$ V

134. What is common between the algal species *Polysiphonia, Porphyra* and *Gracilaria*?

(a) The vegetative cells have a cellulosic wall usually covered on the outside by a gelatinous coating
(b) The cell wall of red algae contains mucopolysaccharides like carrageenan
(c) The chloroplasts may be discoid, reticulate, cup-shaped or spiral in different species
(d) Food is stored as complex carbohydrates, which may be in the form of laminarin or mannitol

135. Which of the following statements are correct?

I. The blood transports CO_2 comparatively easily due to its high solubility.
II. Approximately, 8.9% of CO_2 is transported being dissolved in the plasma of blood.
III. The CO_2 produced by the tissues diffuses passively into the bloodstream and into the red blood corpuscles and reacts with water to form H_2CO_3.
IV. The oxyhaemoglobin (HbO_2) in erythrocytes is basic in nature.
V. The chloride ions diffuse from the plasma into the erythrocytes to maintain the ionic balance.

Choose the correct answer from the options given below.

(a) II, IV and V (b) II, III, IV and V
(c) IV and V (d) I, III and V

136. Which of the following statements are incorrect?

I. The most obvious and technically complicated feature of all living organisms is the ability to sense their surroundings.
II. An isolated metabolic reaction outside the body of an organism, performed in a test tube is neither living nor non-living, but these reactions are surely living reactions.
III. External and internal structures, along with the structure of cell, developmental process and ecological information of organisms are essential and form the basis of modern taxonomic studies.
IV. Taxonomic hierarchy includes identification, nomenclature and classification, it takes into account evolutionary relationships between organisms.
V. All organisms, including plant and animal kingdoms have species as the second last category, these category include related individuals able to produce fertile offspring.

Choose the correct answer from the options given below.

(a) I, II and III (b) III, IV and V
(c) I, III and IV (d) IV and V

137. Enzyme-Linked Immuno Sorbent Assay (ELISA) is a heterogenous EIA (Enzyme Immuno Assays) technique used in clinical analyses. In this type of assay, one of the reaction components is

(a) non-specifically absorbed to the surface of a solid phase
(b) non-covalently bound to the surface of a plastic bead
(c) quantified and allowed to bind non-covalently
(d) hybridised with the fluorescent material

138. Which of the following cell organelles play significant role in photorespiration, respiration and photosynthesis?

(a) Peroxisomes, mitochondria and chloroplast, respectively
(b) Chloroplast, mitochondria and peroxisome, respectively
(c) Centerosome, mitochondria and glyoxysome, respectively
(d) Sphaerosomes, chloroplast and glyoxysome, respectively

139. Which of the following stages of malarial parasite in human gives clinical manifestations of the disease?

(a) Parasites differentiate into sexual erythrocytic stages
(b) Rupture of RBCs and release of haemozoin
(c) Multiplication in the erythrocytes
(d) Replication of parasite in the liver cell

140. Which of the following features are not related to chloroplast?

I. Chloroplasts possess double-stranded circular DNA.
II. The plastids contain ribosomes.
III. These play an important role in cell movement.
IV. Chloroplasts were first observed by Garnier.
V. They are absent in case of bryophytes.

Choose the correct answer from the options given below.

(a) I, III and V
(b) I, II and IV
(c) III, IV and V
(d) I, II and III

141. A person's alveoli is infected and filled with fluid which is leading to severe problems in respiration. His lips and finger nails turns grey to bluish in colour. The person could be infected with

(a) Rhino virus
(b) *Plasmodium falciparum*
(c) *Streptococcus pneumoniae*
(d) *Salmonella typhi*

142. Which of the following statements are correct?

I. Inorganic chemicals are present mostly in aqueous phase while organic in both, aqueous and non-aqueous. Cellular pool comprises of both crystalloid and colloidal particles.
II. Water is universal solvent, as it can dissolve both polar and non-polar solutes, it has high boiling point due to hydrogen bonding.
III. Some proteins are an assembly of more than one polypeptide. The manner in which these individual subunits arrange forms the architecture of protein.
IV. In protein's tertiary structure, the coils and folds are so arranged as to hide polar side chains inside and expose the non-polar side chains.
V. The conformation of protein is easily changed by pH, temperature and chemical substances and hence, its function is labile and subject to regulation.

Choose the correct answer from the options given below.

(a) I, II, III and V (b) III and IV
(c) III, IV and V (d) I, II, IV and V

143. The rate of prokaryotic bacterium *E. coli* and eukaryotic human DNA replication is

(a) 1000 nucleotides and 50 nucleotides per second, respectively
(b) 50 nucleotides and 100 nucleotides per second, respectively
(c) 40 nulceotides and 50 nucleotides per second, respectively
(d) 1000 nucleotides and 100 nucleotides per second, respectively

144. Which of the following is not the step of pollen-pistil interaction?

(a) The pistil recognise the pollen followed by its acceptance or rejection
(b) Compatible pollen grain germinates on the stigma to produce a pollen tube through one of the germ pores

(c) One of the male gamete moves towards the egg cell and fuses with its nucleus
(d) The generative cell divides and forms two male gametes during the growth of pollen tube in the stigma in some angiosperms

145. The megaspore mother cells is the progenitor of embryo sac. It undergoes several changes to become functional embryo sac. The number of meiotic and mitotic divisions required for the production of mature embryo sac are
(a) one and four, respectively
(b) one and three, respectively
(c) two and three, respectively
(d) three and three, respectively

146. Consider the following statements.
I. Chrysophytes group includes diatoms and golden algae. They have no common cell wall structure, some lack cell walls, others have cell walls, primarily made of cellulose and contain significant amounts of silica.
II. *Alternaria* is referred to as imperfect fungi, because their only known reproduction mechanism is asexual; but a parasexual cycle generally operates in their life.
III. Basidiomycetes are mushrooms, bracket fungi or puffballs, they reproduce only by means of conidia. Conidia are produced in more complex structure such as pycnidia, sporodochia or synnemata.
IV. The name virus that means venom or poisonous fluid was given by DJ Iwanowsky, these viruses are smaller than bacteria because they can pass through bacteria proof filters.
V. In the species of Ascomycetes, the asexual reproduction takes place by zoospores or by aplanospores, their mycelium is aseptate and coenocytic.

Choose the correct set of statements from the options given below.
(a) I, II and IV
(b) III, IV and V
(c) I, II, IV and V
(d) II, III and IV

147. Which of the following matching pairs is incorrect?

(a)	Intercalary meristem	–	Found in grasses and regenerated parts are removed by the grazing herbivore
(b)	Lateral meristem	–	They are cylindrical and produce secondary tissues
(c)	Sclereids	–	Thickened walls with wide central lumen
(d)	Parenchyma	–	Their cells are isodiametric

148. Hugo de Vries is known as a proponent of the mutation theory of evolution, in which new species are believed to arise by single mutational events. This theory is based on the breeding experiment conducted for 13 years with the
(a) *Oenothera lamarckiana* (b) *Catharanthus roseus*
(c) Marsupial mouse (d) *Euphorbia mili*

149. The fibres which are made up of sclerenchymatous cells, are absent in the primary phloem, but are found in secondary phloem. These are elongated, unbranched and have pointed, needle-like apices and are called as
(a) bast fibres (b) xylem fibres
(c) husk fibres (d) leaf fibres

150. Which of the following sets does not correctly depict the enzymes used in replication and their function?
(a) DNA gyrase—Reduces the torsional strain created by the unwinding of DNA
(b) DNA polymerase delta—The catalytic subunit of polymerase delta contains a 3′ to 5′ exonuclease activity, functioning in proof reading
(c) Helicase—It separates the strands at the forks, using one ATP molecule for each base split
(d) Primase—It aids in the fusion of DNA strands

151. Which of the following statements is correct?
I. *Agrobacterium tumefaciens,* a pathogen of several dicot plants is able to deliver a piece of DNA known as T-DNA to transfer normal plant cells into a tumour and direct these tumour cells to produce the chemicals required by the pathogen.

II. Restriction enzyme digestions are performed by incubating purified DNA molecules with restriction enzymes, at the optimal conditions for that specific enzyme.
III. The first and most commonly used DNA polymerase is *Pfu* DNA polymerase, whereas *Taq* DNA polymerase from *Thermus aquatics* is widely used because of its higher fidelity of copying DNA.
IV. Primers are short stretch of single-stranded DNA, usually around 40-100 nucleotides in length. To many primers are used in each PCR reaction and they are designed, so that they flank the target region.
V. Primers bind to the DNA during annealing process of PCR. They require 55-65°C of temperature to bind their complementary sequences.

Choose the correct answer from the options given below.

(a) I, II and V only (b) III and IV
(c) I, III and IV (d) II, III and V

152. To maintain pH balance, the respiratory system regulates the amount of CO_2 in the body by

(a) increasing the rate and depth of breathing when blood pH is too high
(b) decreasing the rate and depth of breathing when blood pH is too low
(c) decreasing the amount of oxygen in the air we breathe
(d) increasing the amount of water vapour in the air we breathe

153. Given below are two statements.

Statement I Eastern ghats have a greater amphibian species diversity than Western ghats.
Statement II More than 70 per cent of all the species recorded are animals, while plants comprise not more than 22% of total.

In the light of the above statements, choose the correct answer from the options given below.

(a) Statement I is incorrect, but statement II is correct
(b) Both statement I and statement II are correct
(c) Both statement I and statement II are incorrect
(d) Statement I is correct, but statement II is incorrect

154. Pineal gland is a small, whitish flattened gland situated at the tip of a small fibrous stalk that arises from dorsal wall of dienceptation. It is known to secrete one hormone, which

(a) causes dilation of blood vessels
(b) retards glucose consumption and protein synthesis
(c) causes demineralisation of bones
(d) helps in maintaining the normal rhythms of sleep wake cycle

155. Carefully analyse the following structure given below.

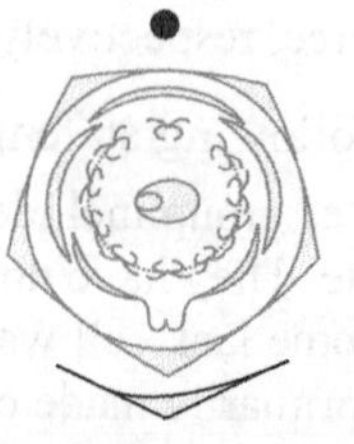

Which of the folowing is correct regarding the given floral diagram?

(a) Br% ⚥ $K_{(5)}C_{1+2+(2)}A_{(9)}+{}_1\underline{G}_1$
(b) ⊕ ⚥ $K_{(5)}C_{(5)}A_{(5)}\underline{G}_{(2)}$
(c) Br ⊕ ⚥ $P_{(3+3)}\overparen{A_{3+3}\underline{G}}_{(3)}$
(d) Ebr ⊕ ⚥ $K_{2+2}C_4A_{2+4}\underline{G}_{(2)}$

156. A small, median chamber that is used to pass faecal matter, urine and sperms to the exterior in frogs is called as

(a) mesorchium (b) bidder's canal
(c) cloaca (d) ureter

157. Match List I with List II.

	List I		List II
A.	Auxin	1.	It induces the hydrolytic enzymes in the aleurone layer of endosperm
B.	Gibberellin	2.	It inhibits abscission of leaves and fruits
C.	Cytokinin	3.	It increases the number of female flowers
D.	Ethylene	4.	It acts antagonistically to auxin

Choose the correct answer from the options given below.

	A	B	C	D		A	B	C	D
(a)	2	1	4	3	(b)	2	1	3	4
(c)	1	2	4	3	(d)	4	3	1	2

158. Which of the following statements is incorrect?

(a) The major function of thymus is to secrete thymosin hormone, thymic humoral factor, thymic factor, thymopoietin; they induce not only the proliferation of lymphocytes, but also their differentiation

(b) Glucagon is secreted by β-cells of islets of langerhans, which reduce glucose level in blood when glucose is more in blood

(c) The secretion of insulin and glucagon is regulated by a limit control feedback or push and pull feedback control system

(d) Low aldosterone and gluco-corticoids level in blood, initiates the excretion of sodium ions and water in urine, leading to dehydration, low blood pressure and weakness

159. The genetic code is a set of three letter combinations of nucleotides called codons, each of which corresponds to a specific amino acid or stop signal, they possess some special features, these are all, except

(a) the genetic code is universal

(b) the genetic codes are unambiguous

(c) some amino acids are coded by more than one codon

(d) the codon in *m*RNA is read in a non-contiguous fashion

160. Angina pectoris is the medical term for acute chest pain, it appears

(a) due to the deposition of calcium, fat, cholesterol, etc.

(b) when no enough oxygen is reaching the heart muscle

(c) when alveoli of lungs become rigid

(d) when the heart muscle is suddenly damaged

161. The centre controlling the heart rate is present in medulla oblongata of brain and possess chemoreceptors sensitive for CO_2, O_2 and blood pressure. Heart rate is affected by several factors.

These factors include all, except

(a) decrease in thyroxine hormone

(b) increase in K^+ ions in heart muscles

(c) increase in Ca^{+2} ions in blood

(d) increase in oxytocin level

162. Given below is the diagrammatic representation of cyclic photophosphorylation. Identify the function of '*A*' element from the options given below.

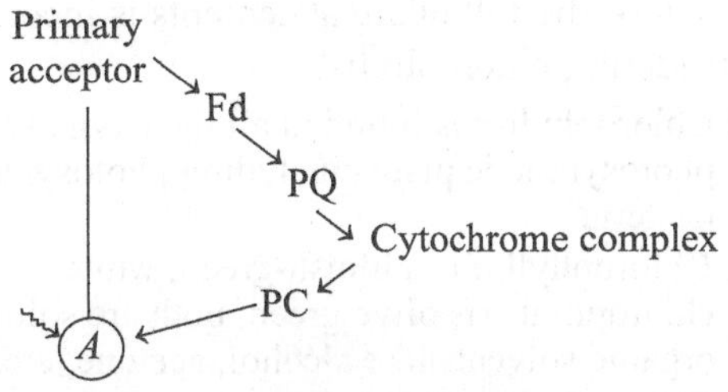

(a) It utilises H_2O for evolution of O_2

(b) It absorb wavelength shorter than 680 nm

(c) It generates ATP molecules

(d) It produces a strong oxidant

163. The Z-disc is a protein structure found in the sarcomere of skeletal and cardiac muscle fibres. It serves as

(a) the stretching of the sarcomere and maintain its flexibility

(b) an anchor for the actin filaments and helps to maintain the structural integrity of the sarcomere

(c) a energy releasing point which helps in muscle contraction

(d) connection between A-band and H-zone

164. Among the following characters how many are associated with family-Malvaceae in the given box?

Schizocarp fruit, Twisted aestivation; bracteate; stipulate reticulate venation; bithecous anther; monocarpellary

(a) 2 (b) 3 (c) 4 (d) 5

165. Match List I with List II.

	List I		List II
A.	The cell wall has stiff cellulose plates on the outer surface.	1.	Chrysophytes
B.	It is the connecting link between plant and animal.	2.	*Mycoplasma*
C.	They are chief producers in the ocean.	3.	*Euglena*
D.	They completely lack a cell wall.	4.	Dinoflagellates

Choose the correct answer from the options given below.

	A	B	C	D		A	B	C	D
(a)	1	2	4	3	(b)	3	2	4	1
(c)	4	3	1	2	(d)	3	4	2	1

166. Which of the following statements is incorrect considering chlorophylls?

(a) Chlorophyll-*a* is found in all the oxygen evolving photosynthetic plants including photosynthetic bacteria

(b) Chlorophyll-*a* is a bluish-green, while chlorophyll-*b* is olive green, both are soluble in organic solvents like alcohol, acetone, etc.

(c) Chlorophyll molecule is made up of a squarish tetrapyrrolic ring known as head and a phytol alcohol called tail

(d) The magnesium atom is present in the central position of tetrapyrrolic ring, four pyrrole rings of porphyrin head are linked together by methine group

167. Given below are two statements; one is labelled as Assertion (A) and other is labelled as Reason (R).

Assertion (A) An alternative selectable marker is used which differentiates recombinants from non-recombinants on the basis of their ability to produce colour in the presence of a chromogenic substrate.

Reason (R) The presence of a chromogenic substrate gives blue coloured colonies of the plasmid in the bacteria which have an insert and bacteria which do not have insert, produce white colonies.

In the light of the above statements, choose the correct answer form the options given below.

(a) A is false, but R is true

(b) Both A and R are true and R is the correct explanation of A

(c) Both A and R are true, but R is not the correct explanation of A

(d) A is true, but R is false

168. Which of the following factors/features is not related to allergies?

(a) The body is able to differentiate self and non-self and the cell-mediated immune response is responsible for the reaction of allergy

(b) Symptoms of allergic reactions are sneezing, watery eyes, running nose and difficulty in breathing

(c) It is due to the release of chemicals like histamine and serotonin from the mast cells

(d) It can be reduced by the use of anti-histamine, adrenalin and steriods

169. Which of the following pair of animals have tympanum in ear, 3-chambered heart, separate sexes, internal fertilisation and ovipary?

(a) *Corvus* and *Columba* (b) *Testudo* and *Bangarus*

(c) *Alligator* and *Neophron*

(d) *Clarias* and *Betta*

170. Given below are two statements; one is labelled as Assertion (A) and other is labelled as Reason (R).

Assertion (A) Both male and female can be infertile.

Reason (R) Infertile couple can have children with the help of ARTs.

In the light of the above statements, choose the correct answer from the options given below.

(a) A is false, but R is true

(b) Both A and R are true and R is the correct explanation of A

(c) Both A and R are true, but R is not the correct explanation of A

(d) A is true, but R is false

171. Bones have a hard and non-pliable ground substance rich in

(a) calcium and phosphorus salts, which gives bone strength

(b) calcium salts and collagen fibres, which gives bone strength

(c) actin and myosin, which built framework

(d) plasma and collagen fibres, which built framework

172. Given below are two statements.

Statement I Stirred tank bioreactors provide suitable environment in which an organisms can efficiently produce a target product that may be cell biomass, metabolite or bioconversion product.

Statement II The sparge ring is located below the agitator and used to break the incoming air into small bubbles.

In the light of the above statements, choose the correct answer from the options given below.

(a) Statement I is incorrect, but statement II is correct

(b) Both statement I and statement II are correct

(c) Both statement I and statement II are incorrect
(d) Statement I is correct, but statement II is incorrect

173. Which of the following pair of biomolecules is mainly present in the structure of cell membrane?
(a) Lipids and carbohydrates
(b) Lipids and proteins
(c) Proteins and carbohydrates
(d) Carbohydrates and nucleic acid

174. Match List I with List II.

	List I		Lust II
A.	IgA	1.	Antibody responsible for allergic reactions
B.	Humoral immune response	2.	It is present in colostrum, which secreted during initial days of lactation
C.	IgE	3.	It is mediated by T-lymphocyte
D.	Cell-mediated immunity	4.	It is mediated by antibodies

Choose the correct answer from the options given below.

	A	B	C	D		A	B	C	D
(a)	2	4	1	3	(b)	4	2	1	3
(c)	1	4	3	2	(d)	2	3	1	4

175. Which of the following statements is incorrect about chromosomal theory of inheritance?
(a) Each parent synthesises gametes which constitute only half of their chromsomal complement
(b) The gametic chromsomes fuse during fertilisation to produce offspring with the same number of a chromosome as their parents
(c) In somatic cell, the chromosome or gene occurs in pair because one chromosome is from father and other from mother to form homologous pair
(d) The sorting of chromosomes from each homologous pair into pre-gametes appears to be non-random

176. Which of the following statements is/are correct about mechanism of muscle contraction?

I. Muscle contraction is initiated by a signal sent by the peripheral neural system *via* a motor neuron. A motor neuron alongwith the muscle fibres connected to it constitute a motor unit.
II. The junction between a motor neuron and the sarcolemma of the muscle fibre is called the neuromuscular junction or motor-end plate.
III. A neural signal reaching the neuromuscular junction releases a neurotransmitter which generates and action potential in the sarcolemma.
IV. The release of Ca^{+} ions into the sarcoplasm leads to the calcium binding with a subunit of troponin on actin filaments and thereby remove the masking of active sites for myosin.
V. The myosin head binds to the exposed sites on actin to form a cross bridge with the utilisation of energy from ATP hydrolysis.

Choose the correct answer from the options given below.
(a) Only I
(b) II, III, IV and V
(c) III, IV and V
(d) III and V

177. Match List I with List II.

	List I		List II
A.	Make decision regarding the validity of GM research	1.	Gene therapy
B.	Use of bio-resources by multinational companies and other organisations without proper authorisation from the concerned countries.	2.	Second amendment of Indian patent bill
C.	It takes issues including patent terms emergency provisions and research and development initiative.	3.	Biopiracy
D.	The use of bioengineered cells or other biotechnology techniques to treat human genetic disorder.	4.	GEAC

Choose the correct answer from the options given below.

	A	B	C	D		A	B	C	D
(a)	3	4	2	1	(b)	2	3	4	1
(c)	4	3	2	1	(d)	4	3	1	2

178. Which of the following statements is incorrect about biotic interaction?
(a) The two symbionts or partners may be in close contact with their tissue intermingled or one partner may live within the cavity of the other or attached to its surface
(b) The lichens are composed of a matrix formed by a fungus within which cells of alga are embedded. The alga depends upon the fungus for water, minerals and protection and fungus receives food from alga

(c) Predation provides energy to prolong the life and promote the reproduction of the organisms to the predator and determine to the prey
(d) The interaction among individuals of the same species is known as inter-specific and among the organisms of different species is termed as intra-specific relationship

179. The golgi apparatus remain in close association with endoplasmic reticulum. The Golgi complex plays a major role
(a) in trapping the light and transforming it into chemical energy
(b) in digesting proteins and carbohydrates
(c) as energy transferring organelles
(d) in post-translational modification of proteins and glycosidation of lipids

180. Consider the following statements.
I. Biogas is produced by the activity of anaerobic bacteria on animal waste.
II. Methanobacterium is an aerobic bacterium found in rumen of cattle.
III. Biogas, commonly called gobar gas, is a pure methane.
IV. Activated sludge sediment in settlement takes of sewage treatment plant is rich source of aerobic bacteria.
V. The technoloy of biogas production was developed in India mainly due to the efforts of Indian Council of Agriculture Research.

Choose the correct statements from the options given below.
(a) I, III and IV (b) II, IV and V
(c) I, II and IV (d) I, II and III

Answers

Physics

1.	(d)	2.	(c)	3.	(d)	4.	(a)	5.	(b)	6.	(b)	7.	(b)	8.	(b)	9.	(a)	10.	(b)
11.	(d)	12.	(c)	13.	(c)	14.	(b)	15.	(a)	16.	(b)	17.	(d)	18.	(b)	19.	(b)	20.	(c)
21.	(d)	22.	(b)	23.	(d)	24.	(a)	25.	(c)	26.	(b)	27.	(c)	28.	(a)	29.	(a)	30.	(a)
31.	(a)	32.	(b)	33.	(a)	34.	(a)	35.	(a)	36.	(b)	37.	(b)	38.	(d)	39.	(b)	40.	(c)
41.	(a)	42.	(d)	43.	(b)	44.	(a)	45.	(c)										

Chemistry

46.	(b)	47.	(d)	48.	(b)	49.	(a)	50.	(d)	51.	(c)	52.	(a)	53.	(c)	54.	(a)	55.	(a)
56.	(a)	57.	(b)	58.	(d)	59.	(d)	60.	(a)	61.	(b)	62.	(a)	63.	(a)	64.	(b)	65.	(d)
66.	(d)	67.	(a)	68.	(a)	69.	(a)	70.	(a)	71.	(a)	72.	(c)	73.	(a)	74.	(a)	75.	(a)
76.	(d)	77.	(a)	78.	(d)	79.	(d)	80.	(b)	81.	(b)	82.	(c)	83.	(a)	84.	(a)	85.	(b)
86.	(a)	87.	(d)	88.	(a)	89.	(a)	90.	(a)										

Biology

91	(b)	92	(a)	93	(a)	94	(c)	95	(a)	96	(a)	97	(a)	98	(d)	99	(b)	100	(c)
101	(d)	102	(a)	103	(b)	104	(b)	105	(c)	106	(b)	107	(a)	108	(b)	109	(c)	110	(d)
111	(a)	112	(d)	113	(a)	114	(c)	115	(c)	116	(a)	117	(c)	118	(d)	119	(d)	120	(b)
121	(c)	122	(d)	123	(a)	124	(b)	125	(a)	126	(a)	127	(c)	128	(b)	129	(c)	130	(c)
131	(d)	132	(c)	133	(b)	134	(b)	135	(d)	136	(d)	137	(a)	138	(a)	139	(b)	140	(c)
141	(c)	142	(a)	143	(a)	144	(c)	145	(b)	146	(a)	147	(c)	148	(a)	149	(a)	150	(d)
151	(a)	152	(b)	153	(a)	154	(d)	155	(a)	156	(c)	157	(a)	158	(b)	159	(d)	160	(b)
161	(d)	162	(c)	163	(b)	164	(c)	165	(c)	166	(a)	167	(d)	168	(a)	169	(b)	170	(c)
171	(b)	172	(b)	173	(b)	174	(a)	175	(d)	176	(b)	177	(c)	178	(d)	179	(d)	180	(c)

Scan this QR code from your mobile phone to get the explanations of this paper.

NEET

TEST DRIVE

SECTION IV

Conquer the Competition

This section contains **Past Year exam paper** of NEET. Solving this authentic paper assess your readiness, identify areas for improvement and helps in enhancing your overall exam performance.

SECTION IV

Conquer the Competition

NEET Solved Paper 2024

Maximum Marks : 720	Time : 3 hrs 20 Min	No. of Questions : 200

Instructions

- This question paper contains 200 Multiple Choice Question from the subjects **Physics, Chemistry & Biology** (Botany & Zoology). There are 50 questions in each subject, divided into two Sections : Section-A and Section B.
- **Section A** contains 35 questions in each subject (Q. Nos. 1 to 35, 51 to 85, 101 to 135 and 151 to 185) and all questions are compulsory.
- **Section B** contains 15 questions from each subject (Q. Nos. 36 to 50, 86 to 100, 136 to 150 and 186 to 200) out of which 10 questions are to be attempted.
- Each question carries 4 Marks. For each correct response, the candidate will get 4 marks. For each incorrect response 1 mark will be deducted from the total scores.

PHYSICS

Section-A (Q. No. 1 to 35)

1. A bob is whirled in a horizontal plane by means of a string with an initial speed of ω rpm. The tension in the string is T. If speed becomes 2ω while keeping the same radius, the tension in the string becomes

(a) T (b) $4T$ (c) $T/4$ (d) $\sqrt{2}T$

2. A particle moving with uniform speed in a circular path maintains

(a) constant velocity
(b) constant acceleration
(c) constant velocity but varying acceleration
(d) varying velocity and varying acceleration

3. A logic circuit provides the output Y as per the following truth table.

A	B	Y
0	0	1
0	1	0
1	0	1
1	1	0

The expression for the output Y is

(a) $A.B + \overline{A}$ (b) $A.\overline{B} + \overline{A}$ (c) $\overline{B}$ (d) B

4.

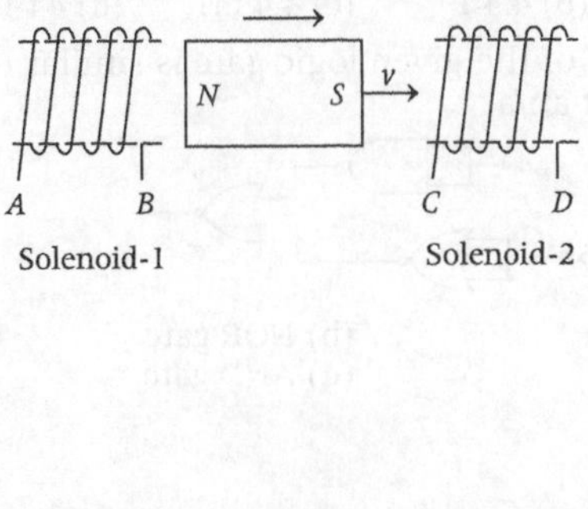

In the above diagram, a strong bar magnet is moving towards solenoid-2 from solenoid-1. The direction of induced current in solenoid-1 and that in solenoid-2, respectively, are through the directions.

(a) AB and DC (b) BA and CD
(c) AB and CD (d) BA and DC

5. Given below are two statements. One is labelled as Assertion (A) and the other is labelled as Reason (R).

Assertion (A) The potential V at any axial point, at 2 m distance r from the centre of the dipole of dipole moment vector **p** of magnitude, 4×10^{-6} C m, is $\pm 9\times10^{3}$ V.

(Take, $\frac{1}{4\pi\varepsilon_0} = 9\times10^9$ SI units)

Reason (R) $V = \pm\frac{2p}{4\pi\varepsilon_0 r^2}$, where r is the distance of any axial point, situated at 2 m from the centre of the dipole.

In the light of the above statements, choose the correct answer from the options given below.

(a) Both A and R are true and R is the correct explanation of A.
(b) Both A and R are true but R is not the correct explanation of A.
(c) A is true but R is false.
(d) A is false but R is true.

6. Match List-I with List-II.

List-I (Material)		**List-II** (Susceptibility (χ))	
A	Diamagnetic	I.	$\chi = 0$
B	Ferromagnetic	II.	$0 > \chi \geq -1$
C	Paramagnetic	III.	$\chi >> 1$
D	Non-magnetic	IV.	$0 < \chi < \varepsilon$ (a small positive number)

Choose the correct answer from the options given below.
(a) A-II, B-III, C-IV, D-I (b) A-II, B-I, C-III, D-IV
(c) A-III, B-II, C-I, D-IV (d) A-IV, B-III, C-II, D-I

7. In a uniform magnetic field of 0.049 T, a magnetic needle performs 20 complete oscillations in 5 s as shown. The moment of inertia of the needle is 9.8×10^{-6} kg m^2. If the magnitude of magnetic moment of the needle is $x \times 10^{-5}$ Am^2, then the value of x is

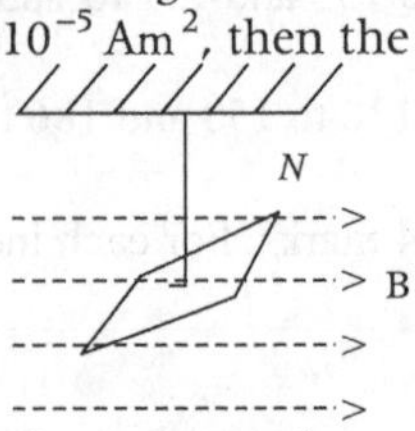

(a) $5\pi^2$ (b) $128\pi^2$ (c) $50\pi^2$ (d) $1280\pi^2$

8. In an ideal transformer, the turns ratio is $\frac{N_p}{N_s} = \frac{1}{2}$. The ratio $V_s : V_p$ is equal to (the symbols carry their usual meaning)
(a) 1 : 2 (b) 2 : 1 (c) 1 : 1 (d) 1 : 4

9. In a vernier callipers, $(N + 1)$ divisions of vernier scale coincide with N divisions of main scale. If 1 MSD represents 0.1 mm, the vernier constant (in cm) is
(a) $\frac{1}{10N}$ (b) $\frac{1}{100(N+1)}$ (c) $100N$ (d) $10(N + 1)$

10. A horizontal force 10 N is applied to a block A as shown in figure. The mass of blocks A and B are 2 kg and 3 kg, respectively. The blocks slide over a frictionless surface. The force exerted by block A on block B is

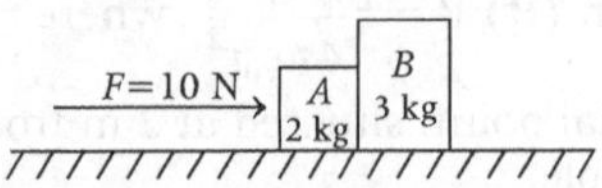

(a) zero (b) 4 N
(c) 6 N (d) 10 N

11. If $x = 5 \sin\left(\pi t + \frac{\pi}{3}\right)$ m represents the motion of a particle executing simple harmonic motion, the amplitude and time period of motion, respectively, are
(a) 5 cm, 2 s (b) 5 m, 2 s (c) 5 cm, 1 s (d) 5 m, 1 s

12. The terminal voltage of the battery, whose emf is 10 V and internal resistance 1Ω when connected through an external resistance of 4 Ω as shown in the figure is

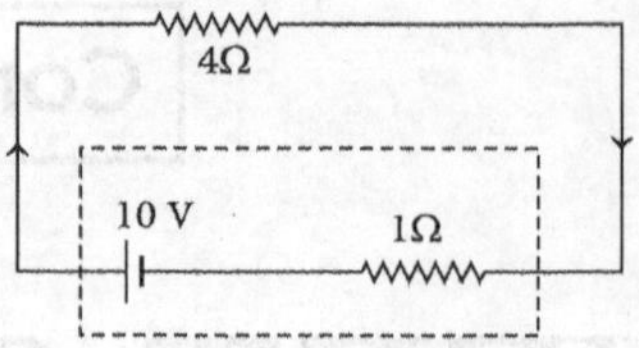

(a) 4 V (b) 6 V (c) 8 V (d) 10 V

13. Given below are two statements.
Statement I Atoms are electrically neutral as they contain equal number of positive and negative charges.
Statement II Atoms of each element are stable and emit their characteristic spectrum.
In the light of the above statements, choose the most appropriate answer from the options given below.
(a) Both Statement I and Statement II are correct.
(b) Both Statement I and Statement II are incorrect.
(c) Statement I is correct but Statement II is incorrect.
(d) Statement I is incorrect but Statement II is correct.

14. If c is the velocity of light in free space, the correct statements about photon among the following are
A. The energy of a photon is $E = h\nu$.
B. The velocity of a photon is c.
C. The momentum of a photon, $p = \frac{h\nu}{c}$
D. In a photon-electron collision, both total energy and total momentum are conserved.
E. Photon possesses positive charge.
Choose the correct answer from the options given below
(a) A and B only (b) A, B, C and D only
(c) A, C and D only (d) A, B, D and E only

15. Match List I with List II.

List I (Spectral lines of Hydrogen for transitions from)	**List II** (Wavelengths (nm))
A. $n_2 = 3$ to $n_1 = 2$	I. 410.2
B. $n_2 = 4$ to $n_1 = 2$	II. 434.1
C. $n_2 = 5$ to $n_1 = 2$	III. 656.3
D. $n_2 = 6$ to $n_1 = 2$	IV. 486.1

Choose the correct answer from the options given below.
(a) A-II, B-I, C-IV, D-III (b) A-III, B-IV, C-II, D-I
(c) A-IV, B-III, C-I, D-II (d) A-I, B-II, C-III, D-IV

16. A tightly wound 100 turns coil of radius 10 cm carries a current of 7 A. The magnitude of the magnetic field at the centre of the coil is (Take, permeability of free space as $4\pi \times 10^{-7}$ SI units)
(a) 44 mT (b) 4.4 T (c) 4.4 mT (d) 44 T

17. The output Y of the given logic gate is similar to the output of an/a

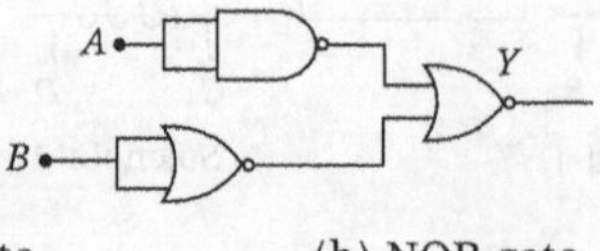

(a) NAND gate (b) NOR gate
(c) OR gate (d) AND gate

18. A wire of length l and resistance 100 Ω is divided into 10 equal parts. The first 5 parts are connected in series while the next 5 parts are connected in parallel. The two combinations are again connected in series. The resistance of this final combination is

(a) 26 Ω (b) 52 Ω (c) 55 Ω (d) 60 Ω

19. $^{290}_{82}X \xrightarrow{\alpha} {}^{286}_{80}Y \xrightarrow{e^+} Z \xrightarrow{\beta^-} P \xrightarrow{e^-} Q$

In the nuclear emission stated above, the mass number and atomic number of the product Q respectively are

(a) 280, 81 (b) 286, 80 (c) 288, 82 (d) 286, 81

20. The maximum elongation of a steel wire of 1 m length if the elastic limit of steel and its Young's modulus, respectively, are 8×10^8 Nm^{-2} and 2×10^{11} Nm^{-2}, is

(a) 4 mm (b) 0.4 mm (c) 40 mm (d) 8 mm

21. If the monochromatic source in Young's double slit experiment is replaced by white light, then

(a) interference pattern will disappear
(b) there will be a central dark fringe surrounded by a few coloured fringes
(c) there will be a central bright white fringe surrounded by a few coloured fringes
(d) all bright fringes will be of equal width

22. At any instant of time t, the displacement of any particle is given by $2t - 1$ (SI unit) under the influence of force of 5 N. The value of instantaneous power is (in SI unit)

(a) 10 (b) 5 (c) 7 (d) 6

23. Consider the following statements A and B and identify the correct answer.

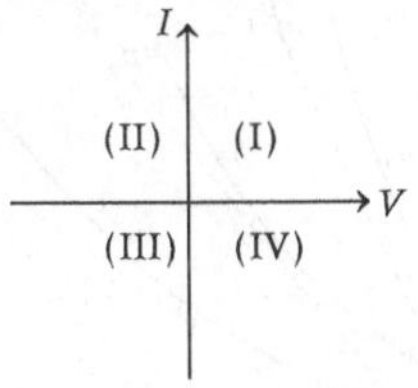

A. For a solar-cell, the I-V characteristics lies in the (IV) quadrant of the given graph.

B. In a reverse biased p-n junction diode, the current measured in (μA), is due to majority charge carriers.

(a) A is correct but B is incorrect.
(b) A is incorrect but B is correct.
(c) Both A and B are correct.
(d) Both A and B are incorrect.

24. Two bodies A and B of same mass undergo completely inelastic one dimensional collision. The body A moves with velocity v_1 while body B is at rest before collision. The velocity of the system after collision is v_2. The ratio is

(a) 1 : 2 (b) 2 : 1 (c) 4 : 1 (d) 1 : 4

25. A light ray enters through a right angled prism at point P with the angle of incidence 30° as shown in figure. It travels through the prism parallel to its base BC and emerges along the face AC. The refractive index of the prism is

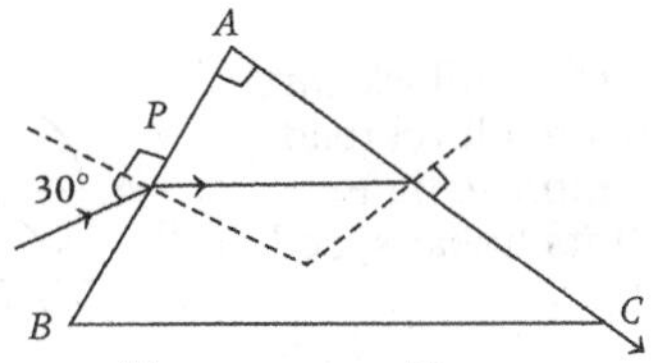

(a) $\frac{\sqrt{5}}{4}$ (b) $\frac{\sqrt{5}}{2}$ (c) $\frac{\sqrt{3}}{4}$ (d) $\frac{\sqrt{3}}{2}$

26. The graph which shows the variation of $\frac{1}{\lambda^2}$ and its kinetic energy, E is (where, λ is de-Broglie wavelength of a free particle)

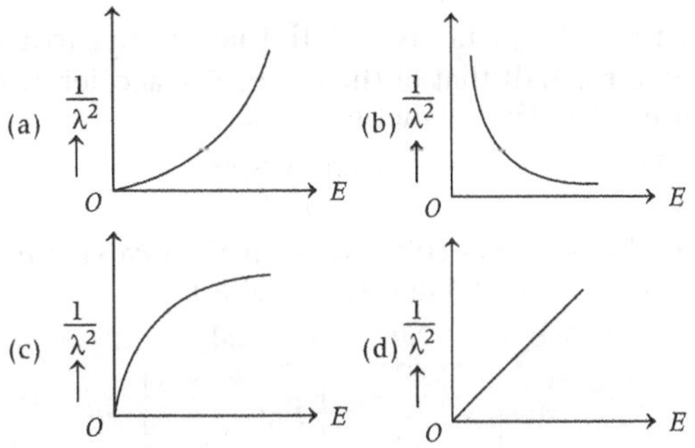

27. The quantities which have the same dimensions as those of solid angle are

(a) strain and angle (b) stress and angle
(c) strain and arc (d) angular speed and stress

28. An unpolarised light beam strikes a glass surface at Brewster's angle. Then

(a) the reflected light will be partially polarised.
(b) the refracted light will be completely polarised.
(c) both the reflected and refracted light will be completely polarised.
(d) the reflected light will be completely polarised but the refracted light will be partially polarised.

29. The moment of inertia of a thin rod about an axis passing through its mid-point and perpendicular to the rod is 2400 g cm^2. The length of the 400 g rod is nearly

(a) 8.5 cm (b) 17.5 cm (c) 20.7 cm (d) 72.0 cm

30. A thin flat circular disc of radius 4.5 cm is placed gently over the surface of water. If surface tension of water is 0.07 Nm^{-1}, then the excess force required to take it away from the surface is

(a) 19.8 mN (b) 198 N (c) 1.98 mN (d) 99 N

31. A thermodynamic system is taken through the cycle $abcda$. The work done by the gas along the path bc is

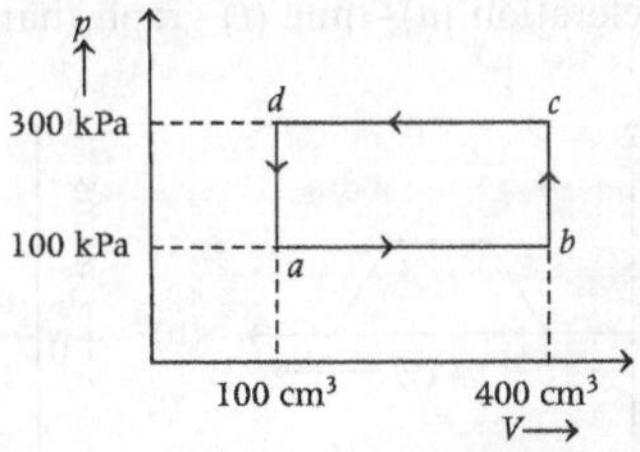

(a) zero (b) 30 J (c) −90 J (d) −60 J

32. A wheel of a bullock cart is rolling on a level road as shown in the figure below. If its linear speed is v in the direction shown, which one of the following options is correct (P and Q are any highest and lowest points on the wheel, respectively)?

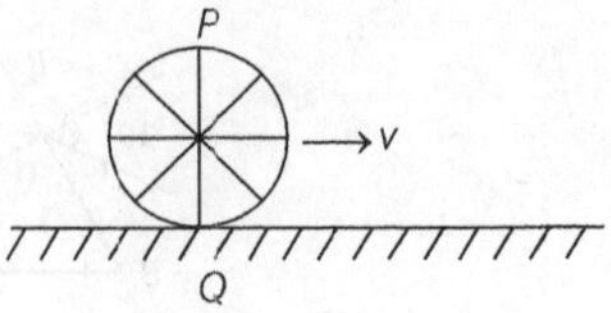

(a) Point P moves slower than point Q
(b) Point P moves faster than point Q
(c) Both the points P and Q move with equal speed
(d) Point P has zero speed

33. The mass of a planet is 1/10 th that of the earth and its diameter is half that of the earth. The acceleration due to gravity on that planet is

(a) 19.6 ms^{-2} (b) 9.8 ms^{-2}
(c) 4.9 ms^{-2} (d) 3.92 ms^{-2}

34. In the following circuit, the equivalent capacitance between terminal A and terminal B is

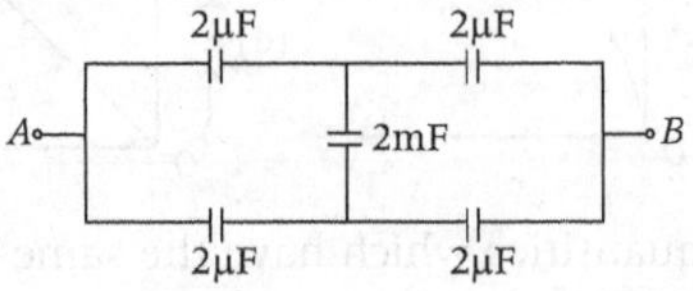

(a) 2 μF (b) 1 μF
(c) 0.5 μF (d) 4 μF

35. A thin spherical shell is charged by some source. The potential difference between the two points C and P (in V) shown in the figure is

(Take, $\frac{1}{4\pi\varepsilon_0} = 9 \times 10^9$ SI units)

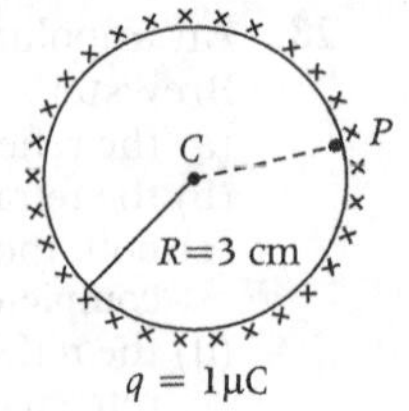

(a) 3×10^5 (b) 1×10^5
(c) 0.5×10^5 (d) zero

Section-B (Q. No. 36 to 50)

36. The velocity (v)-time (t) plot of the motion of a body is shown below

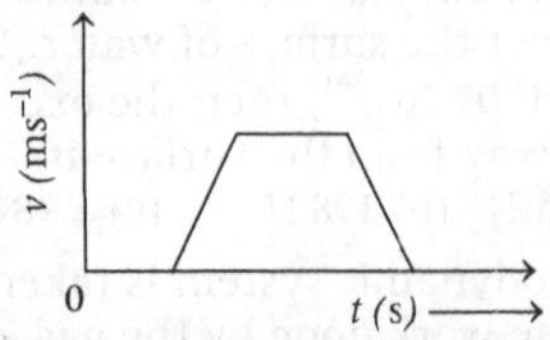

The acceleration (a)- time (t) graph that best suits this motion is

(a)
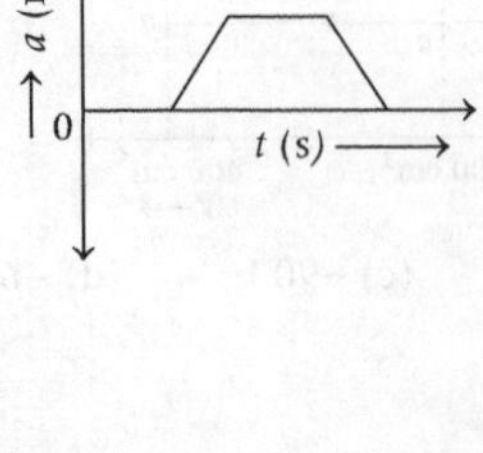

(b)
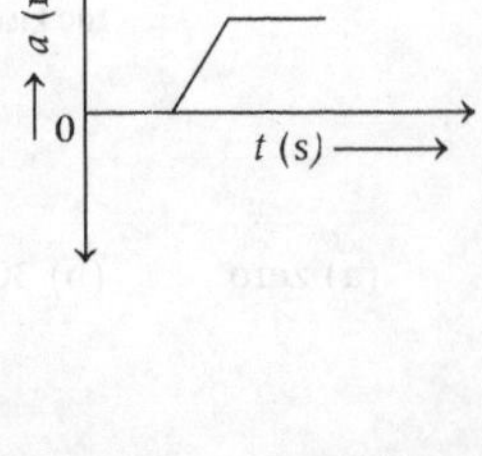

(c)
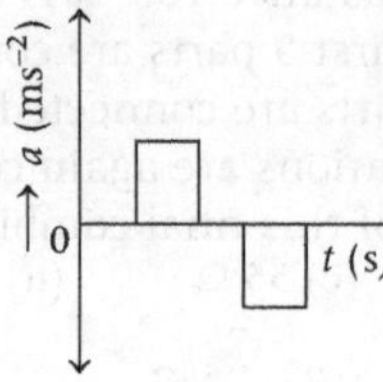

(d)
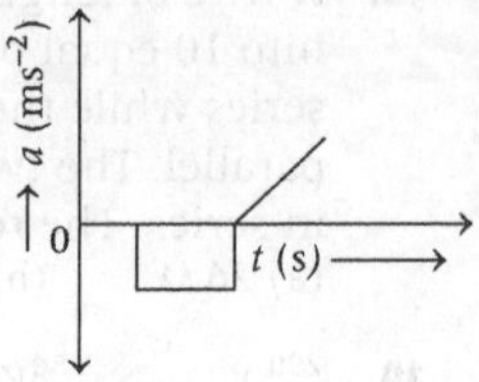

37. If the mass of the bob in a simple pendulum is increased to thrice its original mass and its length is made half its original length, then the new time period of oscillation is $x/2$ times its original time period. Then, the value of x is

(a) $\sqrt{3}$ (b) $\sqrt{2}$ (c) $2\sqrt{3}$ (d) 4

38. A 10 μF capacitor is connected to a 210 V, 50 Hz source as shown in figure. The peak current in the circuit is nearly ($\pi = 3.14$).

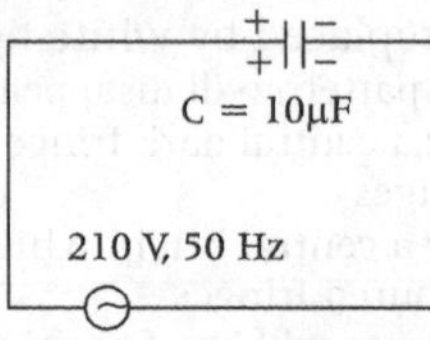

(a) 0.58 A (b) 0.93 A
(c) 1.20 A (d) 0.35 A

39. The following graph represents the T-V curves of an ideal gas (where T is the temperature and V the volume) at three pressures p_1, p_2 and p_3 compared with those of Charles's law represented as dotted lines.

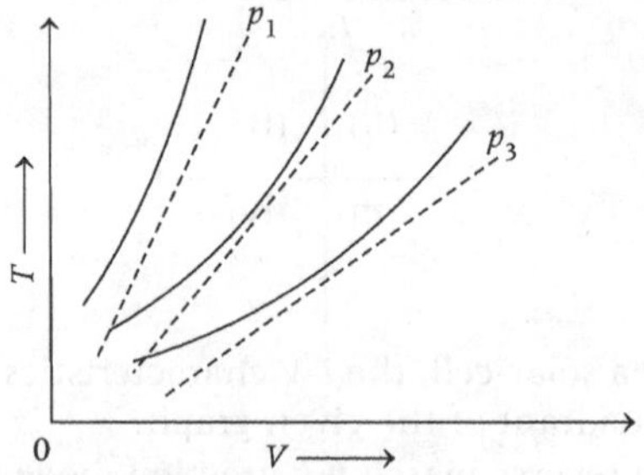

Then the correct relation is.

(a) $p_3 > p_2 > p_1$ (b) $p_1 > p_3 > p_2$
(c) $p_2 > p_1 > p_3$ (d) $p_1 > p_2 > p_3$

40. An iron bar of length L has magnetic moment M. It is bent at the middle of its length such that the two arms make an angle 60° with each other. The magnetic moment of this new magnet is

(a) M (b) $\frac{M}{2}$ (c) $2M$ (d) $\frac{M}{\sqrt{3}}$

41. The minimum energy required to launch a satellite of mass m from the surface of earth of mass M and radius R in a circular orbit at an altitude of $2R$ from the surface of the earth is

(a) $\frac{5GmM}{6R}$ (b) $\frac{2GmM}{3R}$ (c) $\frac{GmM}{2R}$ (d) $\frac{GmM}{3R}$

42. A parallel plate capacitor is charged by connecting it to a battery through a resistor. If I is the current in the circuit, then in the gap between the plates.
(a) There is no current.
(b) Displacement current of magnitude equal to I flows in the same direction as I.
(c) Displacement current of magnitude equal to I flows in a direction opposite to that of I.
(d) Displacement current of magnitude greater than I flows but can be in any direction.

43. The property which is not of an electromagnetic wave travelling in free space is that
(a) They are transverse in nature
(b) The energy density in electric field is equal to energy density in magnetic field
(c) They travel with a speed equal to $\frac{1}{\sqrt{\mu_0 \varepsilon_0}}$
(d) They originate from charges moving with uniform speed

44. A metallic bar of Young's modulus, 0.5×10^{11} N m^{-2} and coefficient of linear thermal expansion 10^{-5} °C^{-1}, length 1 m and area of cross-section 10^{-3} m^2 is heated from 0°C to 100°C without expansion or bending. The compressive force developed in it is
(a) 5×10^3 N (b) 50×10^3 N
(c) 100×10^3 N (d) 2×10^3 N

45. Choose the correct circuit which can achieve the bridge balance.

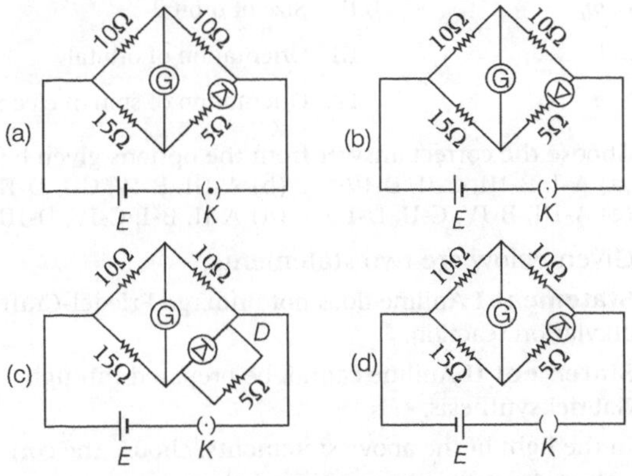

46. A sheet is placed on a horizontal surface in front of a strong magnetic pole. A force is needed to
A. hold the sheet there if it is magnetic.
B. hold the sheet there if it is non-magnetic.
C. move the sheet away from the pole with uniform velocity if it is conducting.
D. move the sheet away from the pole with uniform velocity if it is both, non-conducting and non-polar.
Choose the correct statement(s) from the options given below
(a) B and D only (b) A and C only
(c) A, C and D only (d) C only

47. If the plates of a parallel plate capacitor connected to a battery are moved close to each other, then
A. the charge stored in it, increases.
B. the energy stored in it, decreases.
C. its capacitance increases.
D. the ratio of charge to its potential remains the same.
E. the product of charge and voltage increases.
Choose the most appropriate answer from the options given below
(a) A, B and E only (b) A, C and E only
(c) B, D and E only (d) A, B and C only

48. Two heaters A and B have power rating of 1 kW and 2 kW, respectively. Those two are first connected in series and then in parallel to a fixed power source. The ratio of power outputs for these two cases is
(a) 1 : 1 (b) 2 : 9 (c) 1 : 2 (d) 2 : 3

49. A small telescope has an objective of focal length 140 cm and an eyepiece of focal length 5.0 cm. The magnifying power of telescope for viewing a distant object is
(a) 34 (b) 28 (c) 17 (d) 32

50. A force defined by $F = \alpha t^2 + \beta t$ acts on a particle at a given time t. The factor which is dimensionless, if α and β are constants, is
(a) $\frac{\beta t}{\alpha}$ (b) $\frac{\alpha t}{\beta}$ (c) $\alpha\beta t$ (d) $\frac{\alpha\beta}{t}$

CHEMISTRY

Section-A (Q. No. 51 to 85)

51. 'Spin only' magnetic moment is same for which of the following ions?
A. Ti^{3+} B. Cr^{2+}
C. Mn^{2+} D. Fe^{2+}
E. Sc^{3+}
Choose the most appropriate answer from the options given below.
(a) B and D only (b) A and E only
(c) B and C only (d) A and D only

52. The most stable carbocation among the following is

(a) 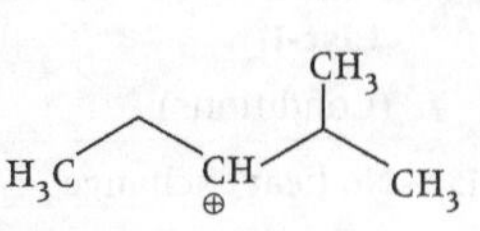

(b) 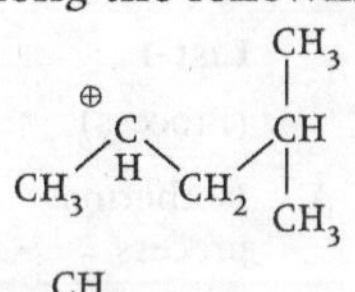

(c) 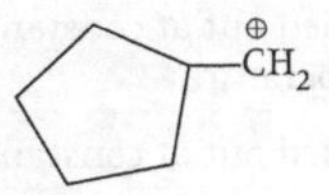

(d) 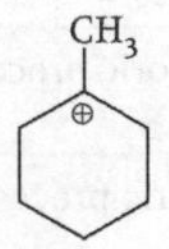

53. Given below are two statements:

Statement I The boiling point of hydrides of group 16 elements follow the order

$H_2O > H_2Te > H_2Se > H_2S$

Statement II On the basis of molecular mass, H_2O is expected to have lower boiling point than the other members of the group but due to the presence of extensive H-bonding in H_2O, it has higher boiling point.

In the light of the above statements, choose the correct answer from the options given below.

(a) Both Statement I and Statement II are true.
(b) Both Statement I and Statement II are false.
(c) Statement I is true but Statement II is false.
(d) Statement I is false but Statement II is true.

54. Match List I with List II.

	List I (Compound)		List II (Shape/geometry)
A.	NH_3	I.	Trigonal pyramidal
B.	BrF_5	II.	Square planar
C.	XeF_4	III.	Octahedral
D.	SF_6	IV.	Square pyramidal

Choose the correct answer from the options given below:

(a) A-I, B-IV, C-II, D-III (b) A-II, B-IV, C-III, D-I
(c) A-III, B-IV, C-I, D-II (d) A-II, B-III, C-IV, D-I

55. The highest number of helium atoms is in

(a) 4 moles of helium
(b) 4 u of helium
(c) 4 g of helium
(d) 2.271098 L of helium at STP

56. Identify the correct reagents that would bring about the following transformation.

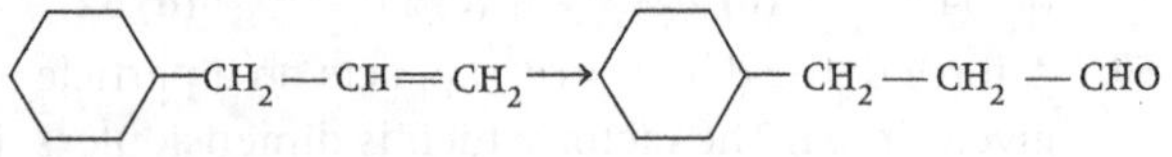

(a) (i) $H_2O/H^{\oplus}$ (ii) CrO_3
(b) (i) BH_3 (ii) $H_2O_2/\overset{\ominus}{O}H$ (iii) PCC
(c) (i) BH_3 (ii) $H_2O_2/\overset{\ominus}{O}H$ (iii) Alk. $KMnO_4$ (iv) $H_3O^{\oplus}$
(d) (i) $H_2O/H^{\oplus}$ (ii) PCC

57. Match List I with List II.

	List-I (Process)		List-II (Conditions)
A.	Isothermal process	I.	No heat exchange
B.	Isochoric process	II.	Carried out at constant temperature
C.	Isobaric process	III.	Carried out at constant volume
D.	Adiabatic process	IV.	Carried out at constant pressure

Choose the correct answer from the options given below:

(a) A-IV, B-III, C-II, D-I
(b) A-IV, B-II, C-III, D-I
(c) A-I, B-II, C-III, D-IV
(d) A-II, B-III, C-IV, D-I

58. Which one of the following alcohols reacts instantaneously with Lucas reagent?

(a) $CH_3CH_2CH_2CH_2OH$ (b) $CH_3-CH_2-CH(CH_3)-OH$
(c) $CH_3-CH(CH_3)-CH_2OH$ (d) $CH_3-C(CH_3)_2-OH$

59. In which of the following equilibria, K_p and K_c are not equal?

(a) $PCl_5(g) \rightleftharpoons PCl_3(g) + Cl_2(g)$
(b) $H_2(g) + I_2(g) \rightleftharpoons 2HI(g)$
(c) $CO\ (g) + H_2O\ (g) \rightleftharpoons CO_2(g) + H_2(g)$
(d) $2BrCl(g) \rightleftharpoons Br_2(g) + Cl_2(g)$

60. Match List I with List II.

List I (Quantum Number)		List II (Information provided)
A. m_l	I.	Shape of orbital
B. m_s	II.	Size of orbital
C. l	III.	Orientation of orbital
D. n	IV.	Orientation of spin of electron

Choose the correct answer from the options given below :

(a) A-I, B-III, C-II, D-IV (b) A-III, B-IV, C-I, D-II
(c) A-III, B-IV, C-II, D-I (d) A-II, B-I, C-IV, D-III

61. Given below are two statements.

Statement I Aniline does not undergo Friedel-Crafts alkylation reaction.

Statement II Aniline cannot be prepared through Gabriel synthesis.

In the light of the above statements, choose the correct answer from the options given below:

(a) Both statement I and statement II are true.
(b) Both statement I and statement II are false.
(c) Statement I is true but statement II is false.
(d) Statement I is false but Statement II is true.

62. Intramolecular hydrogen bonding is present in

(a)
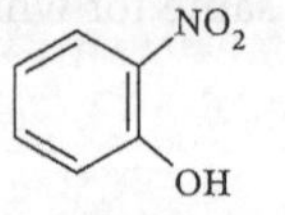

(b)
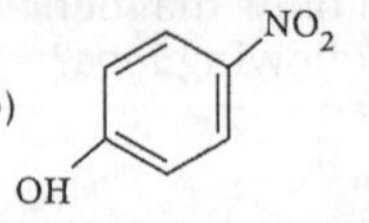

(c)
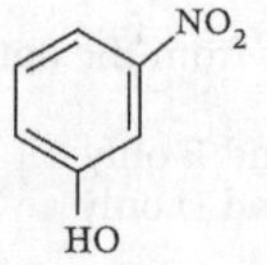

(d) HF

63. On heating, some solid substances change from solid to vapour state without passing through liquid state. The technique used for the purification of such solid substances based on the above principle is known as
(a) crystallisation (b) sublimation
(c) distillation (d) chromatography

64. In which of the following processes entropy increases?
A. A liquid evaporates to vapour.
B. Temperature of a crystalline solid lowered from 130 K to 0 K.
C. $2NaHCO_3(s) \longrightarrow Na_2CO_3(g) + CO_2(g) + H_2O(g)$
D. $Cl_2(g) \longrightarrow 2Cl(g)$
Choose the correct answer from the options given below:
(a) A and C (b) A, B and D
(c) A, C and D (d) C and D

65. Among group 16 elements, which one does not show –2 oxidation state?
(a) O (b) Se (c) Te (d) Po

66. Match List I with List II.

List I (Conversion)		List II (Number of Faraday required)
A. 1 mole of H_2O to O_2	I.	3F
B. 1 mole of MnO_4^- to Mn^{2+}	II.	2F
C. 1.5 mole of Ca from molten $CaCl_2$	III.	1F
D. 1 mole of FeO to Fe_2O_3	IV.	5F

Choose the correct answer from the options given below:
(a) A-II, B-IV, C-I, D-III (b) A-III, B-IV, C-I, D-II
(c) A-II, B-III, C-I, D-IV (d) A-III, B-IV, C-II, D-I

67. Arrange the following elements in increasing order of electronegativity:
N, O, F, C, Si
Choose the correct answer from the options given below:
(a) $Si < C < N < O < F$ (b) $Si < C < O < N < F$
(c) $O < F < N < C < Si$ (d) $F < O < N < C < Si$

68. A compound with a molecular formula of C_6H_{14} has two tertiary carbons. Its IUPAC name is
(a) *n*-hexane (b) 2-methylpentane
(c) 2,3-dimethylbutane (d) 2,2-dimethylbutane

69. Fehling's solution '*A*' is
(a) aqueous copper sulphate
(b) alkaline copper sulphate
(c) alkaline solution of sodium potassium tartrate (Rochelle's salt)
(d) aqueous sodium citrate

70. Activation energy of any chemical reaction can be calculated if one knows the value of
(a) rate constant at standard temperature
(b) probability of collision
(c) orientation of reactant molecules during collision
(d) rate constant at two different temperatures

71. Which plot of ln *k* *vs* 1/*T* is consistent with Arrhenius equation?

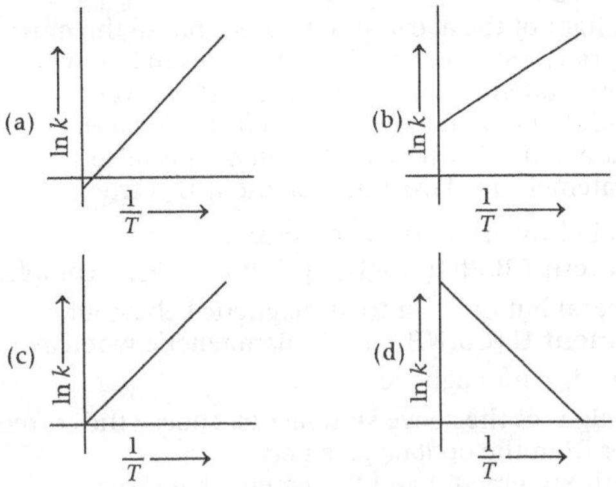

72. Match List I with List II.

List I (Reaction)	List II (Reagents/Condition)
A. 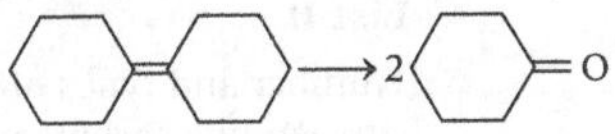	I. 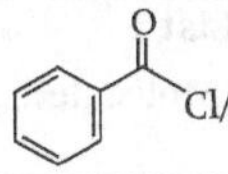 Cl/Anhyd. $AlCl_3$
B. 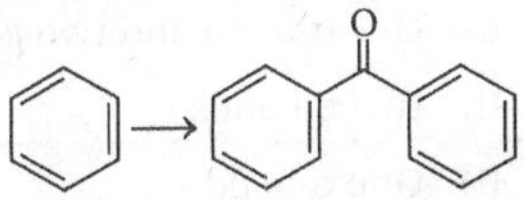	II. CrO_3
C. 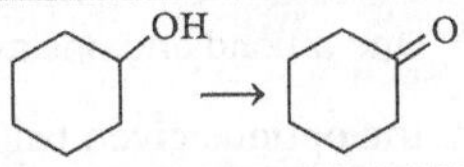	III. $KMnO_4$ /KOH,Δ
D. 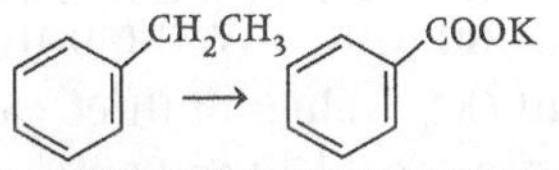	IV. (i) O_3 (ii) Zn-H_2O

Choose the correct answer from the options given below:
(a) A-IV, B-I, C-III, D-II (b) A-III, B-I, C-II, D-IV
(c) A-IV, B-I, C-II, D-III (d) A-I, B-IV, C-II, D-III

73. The compound that will undergo S_N1 reaction with the fastest rate is
(a) 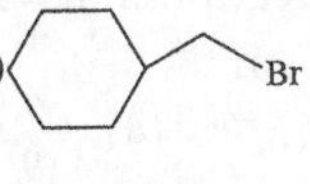 (b) 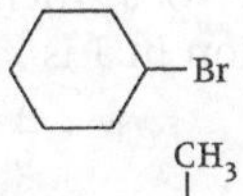
(c) 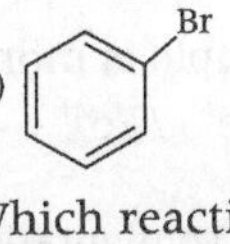 (d) 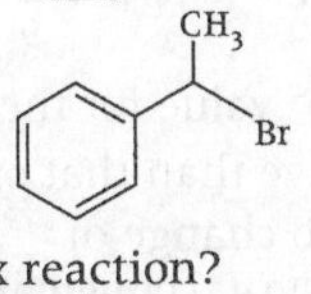

74. Which reaction is not a redox reaction?
(a) $Zn + CuSO_4 \longrightarrow ZnSO_4 + Cu$
(b) $2KClO_3 + I_2 \longrightarrow 2KIO_3 + Cl_2$
(c) $H_2 + Cl_2 \longrightarrow 2HCl$
(d) $BaCl_2 + Na_2SO_4 \longrightarrow BaSO_4 + 2NaCl$

75. Given below are two statements:
Statement I The boiling point of three isomeric pentanes follows the order
n-pentane > isopentane > neopentane
Statement II When branching increases, the molecule attains a shape of sphere. This results in smaller surface

area for contact, due to which the intermolecular forces between the spherical molecules are weak, thereby lowering the boiling point.

In the light of the above statements, choose the most appropriate answer from the options given below:
(a) Both Statement I and Statement II are true.
(b) Both Statement I and Statement II are false.
(c) Statement I is true but Statement II is false.
(d) Statement I is false but Statement II is true.

76. Given below are two statements :
Statement I Both $[Co(NH_3)_6]^{3+}$ and $[CoF_6]^{3-}$ complexes are octahedral but differ in their magnetic behaviour.
Statement II $[Co(NH_3)_6]^{3+}$ is diamagnetic whereas $[CoF_6]^{3-}$ is paramagnetic.
In the light of the above statements, choose the correct answer from the options given below:
(a) Both Statement I and Statement II are true.
(b) Both Statement I and Statement II are false.
(c) Statement I is true but Statement II is false.
(d) Statement I is false but Statement II is true.

77. Match List I with List II.

List I (Molecule)	List II (Number and types of bond/s between two carbon atoms)
A. Ethane	I. One σ-bond and two π-bonds
B. Ethene	II. two π-bonds
C. Carbon molecule, C_2	III. One σ-bond
D. Ethyne	IV. One σ-bond and one π-bond

Choose the correct answer from the options given below:
(a) A-I, B-IV, C-II, D-III (b) A-IV, B-III, C-II, D-I
(c) A-III, B-IV, C-II, D-I (d) A-III, B-IV, C-I, D-II

78. The Henry's law constant (K_H) values of three gases (A, B, C) in water are 145, 2×10^{-5} and 35 kbar, respectively. The solubility of these gases in water follow the order:
(a) $B > A > C$ (b) $B > C > A$
(c) $A > C > B$ (d) $A > B > C$

79. The energy of an electron in the ground state ($n = 1$) for He^+ ion is $-x$ J, then that for an electron in $n = 2$ state for Be^{3+} ion in J is
(a) $-x$ (b) $-\frac{x}{9}$ (c) $-4x$ (d) $-\frac{4}{9}x$

80. The $E°$ value for the Mn^{3+}/Mn^{2+} couple is more positive than that of Cr^{3+}/Cr^{2+} or Fe^{3+}/Fe^{2+} due to change of
(a) d^5 to d^4 configuration (b) d^5 to d^2 configuration
(c) d^4 to d^5 configuration (d) d^3 to d^5 configuration

81. The reagents with which glucose does not react to give the corresponding tests/products are
A. Tollen's reagent B. Schiff's reagent
C. HCN D. NH_2OH
E. $NaHSO_3$
Choose the correct options from the given below:
(a) B and C (b) A and D
(c) B and E (d) E and D

82. Match List I with List II.

List I (Complex)	List II (Type of isomerism)
A. $[Co(NH_3)_5(NO_2)]Cl_2$	I. Solvate isomerism
B. $[Co(NH_3)_5(SO_4)]Br$	II. Linkage isomerism
C. $[Co(NH_3)_6][Cr(CN)_6]$	III. Ionisation isomerism
D. $[Co(H_2O)_6]Cl_3$	IV. Coordination isomerism

Choose the correct answer from the options given below:
(a) A-II, B-III, C-IV, D-I (b) A-I, B-III, C-IV, D-II
(c) A-I, B-IV, C-III, D-II (d) A-II, B-IV, C-III, D-I

83. Arrange the following elements in increasing order of first ionisation enthalpy:
Li, Be, B, C, N
Choose the correct answer from the options given below:
(a) Li < Be < B < C < N (b) Li < B < Be < C < N
(c) Li < Be < C < B < N (d) Li < Be < N < B < C

84. 1 g of sodium hydroxide was treated with 25 mL of 0.75 M HCl solution, the mass of sodium hydroxide left unreacted is equal to
(a) 750 mg (b) 250 mg
(c) zero mg (d) 200 mg

85. For the reaction, $2A \rightleftharpoons B + C, K_C = 4\times10^{-3}$. At a given time, the composition of reaction mixture is: $[A]=[B]=[C]=2\times10^{-3}$M.
Then, which of the following is correct?
(a) Reaction is at equilibrium.
(b) Reaction has a tendency to go in forward direction.
(c) Reaction has a tendency to go in backward direction.
(d) Reaction has gone to completion in forward direction.

Section-B (Q. No. 86 to 100)

86. Given below are certain cations. Using inorganic qualitative analysis, arrange them in increasing group number from 0 to VI.
A. Al^{3+} B. Cu^{2+} C. Ba^{2+} D. Co^{2+}
E. Mg^{2+}
Choose the correct answer from the options given below.
(a) B, A, D, C, E (b) B, C, A, D, E
(c) E, C, D, B, A (d) E, A, B, C, D

87. The products A and B obtained in the following reactions, respectively are

$$3ROH + PCl_3 \longrightarrow 3RCl + A$$
$$ROH + PCl_5 \longrightarrow RCl + HCl + B$$

(a) $POCl_3$ and H_3PO_3 (b) $POCl_3$ and H_3PO_4
(c) H_3PO_4 and $POCl_3$ (d) H_3PO_3 and $POCl_3$

88. Mass in grams of copper deposited by passing 9.6487 A current through a voltmeter containing copper sulphate solution for 100 seconds is (Given : Molar mass of Cu : 63 mol^{-1}, 1 F = 96487 C)
(a) 3.15 g (b) 0.315 g (c) 31.5 g (d) 0.0315

89. The plot of osmotic pressure (π) *vs* concentration (mol L^{-1}) for a solution gives a straight line with slope 25.73 L bar mol^{-1}. The temperature at which the osmotic pressure measurement is done is
(Use, $R = 0.083$ L bar $mol^{-1}K^{-1}$)
(a) 37°C (b) 310°C (c) 25.73°C (d) 12.05°C

90. Identify the major product *C* formed in the following reaction sequence:

$$CH_3—CH_2—CH—I \xrightarrow{NaCN} A \xrightarrow[\text{Partial hydrolysis}]{OH^-} B \xrightarrow[Br_2]{NaOH} \underset{\text{(major)}}{C}$$

(a) propylamine (b) butylamine
(c) butanamide (d) α-bromobutanoic acid

91. Identify the correct answer.
(a) Three resonance structures can be drawn for ozone.
(b) BF_3 has non-zero dipole moment.
(c) Dipole moment of NF_3 is greater than that of NH_3.
(d) Three canonical forms can be drawn for CO_3^{2-} ion.

92. Given below are two statements :
Statement I $[Co(NH_3)_6]^{3+}$ is a homoleptic complex whereas $[Co(NH_3)_4Cl_2]^+$ is a heteroleptic complex.
Statement II Complex $[Co(NH_3)_6]^{3+}$ has only one kind of ligands but $[Co(NH_3)_4Cl_2]^+$ has more than one kind of ligands.
In the light of the above statements, choose the correct answer from the options given below.
(a) Both Statement I and Statement II are true.
(b) Both Statement I and Statement II are false.
(c) Statement I is true but Statement II is false.
(d) Statement I is false but Statement II is true.

93. For the given reaction

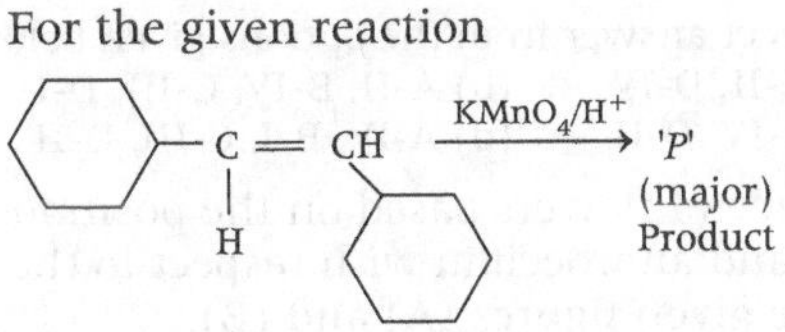

'*P*' is

(a) 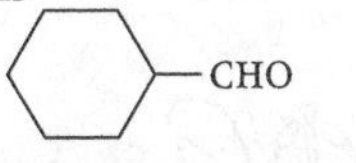

(b) 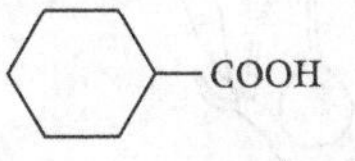

(c) 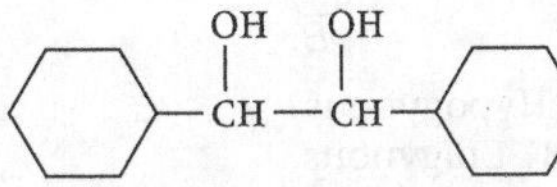

(d) 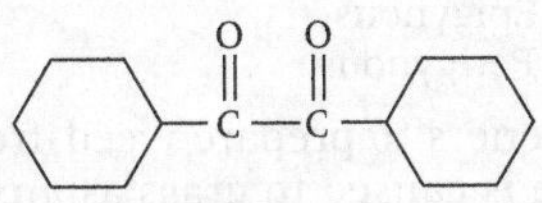

94. The pair of lanthanoid ions which are diamagnetic is
(a) Ce^{4+} and Yb^{2+} (b) Ce^{3+} and Eu^{2+}
(c) Gd^{3+} and Eu^{3+} (d) Pm^{3+} and Sm^{3+}

95. Consider the following reaction in a sealed vessel at equilibrium with concentrations of
$N_2 = 3.0 \times 10^{-3}$ M, $O_2 = 4.2 \times 10^{-3}$ M
and $NO = 2.8 \times 10^{-3}$ M

$$2NO(g) \rightleftharpoons N_2(g) + O_2(g)$$

If 0.1 mol L^{-1} of NO (g) is taken in a closed vessel, what will be degree of dissociation (α) of NO(g) at equilibrium?
(a) 0.00889 (b) 0.0889 (c) 0.8889 (d) 0.717

96. A compound *X* contains 32% of *A*, 20% of *B* and remaining percentage of *C*. Then, the empirical formula of *X* is
(Given, atomic masses of $A = 64; B = 40; C = 32$u)
(a) A_2BC_2 (b) ABC_3 (c) AB_2C_2 (d) ABC_4

97. The work done during reversible isothermal expansion of one mole of hydrogen gas at 25°C from pressure of 20 atmosphere to 10 atmosphere is
(Given, $R = 2.0$ cal $K^{-1}mol^{-1}$)
(a) 0 calorie (b) −413.14 calories
(c) 413.14 calories (d) 100 calories

98. During the preparation of Mohr's salt solution (Ferrous ammonium sulphate), which of the following acid is added to prevent hydrolysis of Fe^{2+} ion?
(a) Dilute hydrochloric acid (b) Concentrated sulphuric acid
(c) Dilute nitric acid (d) Dilute sulphuric acid

99. The rate of a reaction quadruples when temperature changes from 27°C to 57°C. Calculate the energy of activation.
Given, $R = 8.314$ J $K^{-1}mol^{-1}$, log4 = 0.6021
(a) 38.04 kJ/mol (b) 380.4 kJ/mol
(c) 3.80 kJ/mol (d) 3804 kJ/mol

100. Major products *A* and *B* formed in the following reaction sequence are

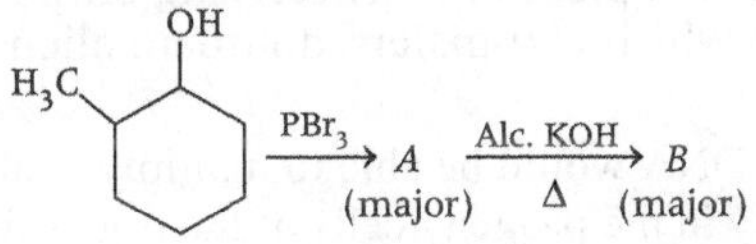

(a) A= 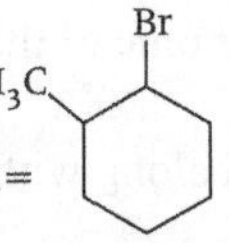 ; B= 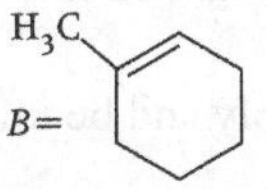

(b) A= 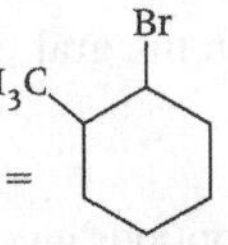 ; B= 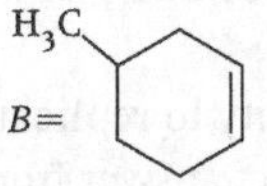

(c) A= 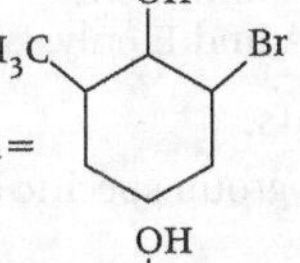 ; B= 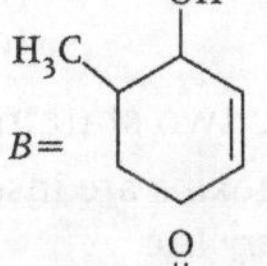

(d) A= 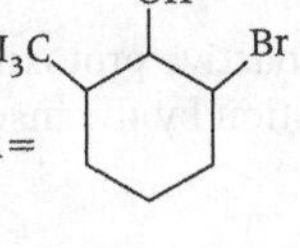 ; B= 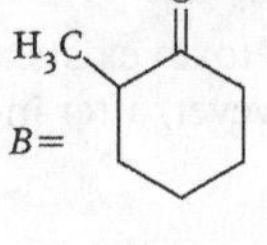

BIOLOGY

Botany

Section-A (Q. No. 101 to 135)

101. Lecithin, a small molecular weight organic compound found in living tissues, is an example of
(a) amino acids (b) phospholipids
(c) glycerides (d) carbohydrates

102. Which of the following are required for the dark reaction of photosynthesis?
A. Light B. Chlorophyll
C. CO_2 D. ATP
E. NADPH
Choose the correct answer from the options given below.
(a) A, B and C only (b) B, C and D only
(c) C, D and E only (d) D and E only

103. Spindle fibres attach to kinetochores of chromosomes during
(a) prophase (b) metaphase (c) anaphase (d) telophase

104. Bulliform cells are responsible for
(a) inward curling of leaves in monocots.
(b) protecting the plant from salt stress.
(c) increased photosynthesis in monocots.
(d) providing large spaces for storage of sugars.

105. In the given figure, which component has thin outer walls and highly thickened inner walls?

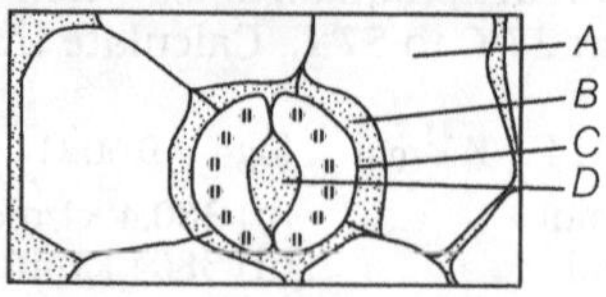

(a) C (b) D (c) A (d) B

106. What is the fate of a piece of DNA carrying only gene of interest which is transferred into an alien organism?
A. The piece of DNA would be able to multiply itself independently in the progeny cells of the organism.
B. It may get integrated into the genome of the recipient.
C. It may multiply and be inherited along with the host DNA.
D. The alien piece of DNA is not an integral part of chromosome.
E. It shows ability to replicate.
Choose the correct answer from the options given below.
(a) A and B only (b) D and E only
(c) B and C only (d) A and E only

107. Given below are two statements.
Statement I *Bt* toxins are insect group specific and coded by a gene *cry* IAc.
Statement II *Bt* toxin exists as inactive protoxin in *B. thuringiensis*. However, after ingestion by the insect the inactive protoxin gets converted into active form due to acidic pH of the insect gut.
In the light of the above statements, choose the correct answer from the options given below.
(a) Both Statement I and Statement II are true
(b) Both Statement I and Statement II are false
(c) Statement I is true but Statement II is false
(d) Statement I is false but Statement II is true

108. List of endangered species was released by
(a) GEAC (b) WWF (c) FOAM (d) IUCN

109. Identify the part of the seed from the given figure which is destined to form root when the seed germinates.

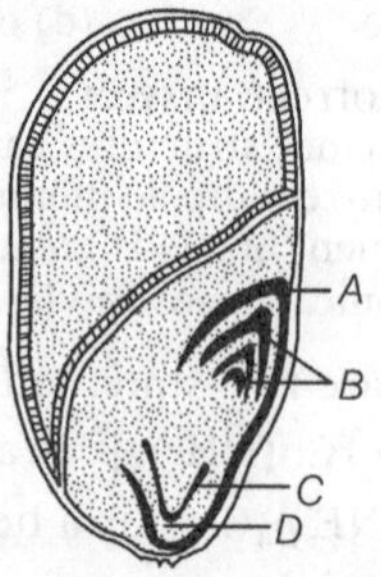

(a) A (b) B (c) C (d) D

110. Match List I with List II.

	List I		List II
A.	*Clostridium butylicum*	I.	Ethanol
B.	*Saccharomyces cerevisiae*	II.	Streptokinase
C.	*Trichoderma polysporum*	III.	Butyric acid
D.	*Streptococcus* sp.	IV.	Cyclosporin-A

Choose the correct answer from the options given below:
(a) A-III, B-I, C-II, D-IV (b) A-II, B-IV, C-III, D-I
(c) A-III, B-I, C-IV, D-II (d) A-IV, B-I, C-III, D-II

111. Identify the type of flowers based on the position of calyx, corolla and androecium with respect to the ovary from the given figures (A) and (B).

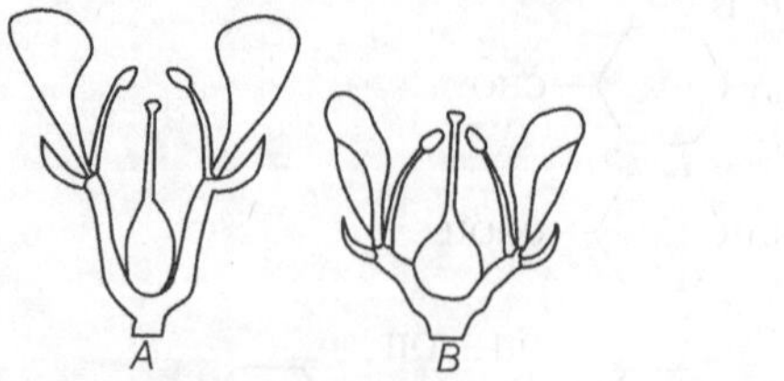

(a) (A) Epigynous; (B) Hypogynous
(b) (A) Hypogynous; (B) Epigynous
(c) (A) Perigynous; (B) Epigynous
(d) (A) Perigynous; (B) Perigynous

112. Auxin is used by gardeners to prepare weed-free lawns. But no damage is caused to grass as auxin
(a) promotes apical dominance.
(b) promotes abscission of mature leaves only.
(c) does not affect mature monocotyledonous plants.
(d) can help in cell division in grasses, to produce growth.

113. A pink flowered snapdragon plant was crossed with a red flowered Snapdragon plant. What type of phenotype/s is/are expected in the progeny?
(a) Only red flowered plants
(b) Red flowered as well as pink flowered plants
(c) Only pink flowered plants
(d) Red, pink as well as white flowered plants

114. Which one of the following is not a criterion for classification of fungi?
(a) Morphology of mycelium
(b) Mode of nutrition
(c) Mode of spore formation
(d) Fruiting body

115. The lactose present in the growth medium of bacteria is transported to the cell by the action of
(a) beta-galactosidase (b) acetylase
(c) permease (d) polymerase

116. In a plant, black seed colour (BB/Bb) is dominant over white seed colour (bb). In order to find out the genotype of the black seed plant, with which of the following genotype will you cross it?
(a) BB (b) bb (c) Bb (d) BB/Bb

117. Given below are two statements.
Statement I Parenchyma is living, but collenchyma is dead tissue.
Statement II Gymnosperms lack xylem vessels, but presence of xylem vessels is the characteristic of angiosperms.
In the light of the above statements, choose the correct answer from the options given below.
(a) Both Statement I and Statement II are true
(b) Both Statement I and Statement II are false
(c) Statement I is true but Statement II is false
(d) Statement I is false but Statement II is true

118. How many molecules of ATP and NADPH are required for every molecule of CO_2 fixed in the Calvin cycle?
(a) 2 molecules of ATP and 3 molecules of NADPH
(b) 2 molecules of ATP and 2 molecules of NADPH
(c) 3 molecules of ATP and 3 molecules of NADPH
(d) 3 molecules of ATP and 2 molecules of NADPH

119. A transcription unit in DNA is defined primarily by the three regions in DNA and these are with respect to upstream and down stream end;
(a) Repressor, operator gene, structural gene
(b) Structural gene, transposons, operator gene
(c) Inducer, repressor, structural gene
(d) Promoter, structural gene, terminator

120. Tropical regions show greatest level of species richness because
A. tropical latitudes have remained relatively undisturbed for millions of years, hence more time was available for species diversification.
B. tropical environments are more seasonal.
C. more solar energy is available in tropics.
D. constant environments promote niche specialisation.
E. tropical environments are constant and predictable.
Choose the correct answer from the options given below.
(a) A, C, D and E only (b) A and B only
(c) A, B and E only (d) A, B and D only

121. The equation of Verhulst-Pearl logistic growth is $\frac{dN}{dt} = rN\left[\frac{K-N}{K}\right]$.
From this equation, K indicates
(a) intrinsic rate of natural increase
(b) biotic potential
(c) carrying capacity
(d) population density

122. Inhibition of succinic dehydrogenase enzyme by malonate is a classical example of
(a) cofactor inhibition (b) feedback inhibition
(c) competitive inhibition (d) enzyme activation

123. Which one of the following can be explained on the basis of Mendel's law of dominance?
A. Out of one pair of factors one is dominant and the other is recessive.
B. Alleles do not show any expression and both the characters appear as such in F_2-generation.
C. Factors occur in pairs in normal diploid plants.
D. The discrete unit controlling a particular character is called factor.
E. The expression of only one of the parental characters is found in a monohybrid cross.
Choose the correct answer from the options given below.
(a) A, B and C only (b) A, C, D and E only
(c) B, C and D only (d) A, B, C, D and E

124. Match List I with List II.

List-I	List-II
A. Nucleolus	I. Site of formation of glycolipid
B. Centriole	II. Organisation like the cartwheel
C. Leucoplasts	III. Site for active ribosomal RNA synthesis
D. Golgi apparatus	IV. For storing nutrients

Choose the correct answer from the options given below:
(a) A-III, B-II, C-IV, D-I (b) A-II, B-III, C-I, D-IV
(c) A-III, B-IV, C-II, D-I (d) A-I, B-II, C-III, D-IV

125. Identify the set of correct statements.
A. The flowers of *Vallisneria* are colourful and produce nectar.
B. The flowers of water lily are not pollinated by water.
C. In most of water-pollinated species, the pollen grains are protected from wetting.
D. Pollen grains of some hydrophytes are long and ribbon like.
E. In some hydrophytes, the pollen grains are carried passively inside water.

Choose the correct answer from the options given below.
(a) C, D and E only
(b) A, B, C and D only
(c) A, C, D and E only
(d) B, C, D and E only

126. Match List I with List II.

	List-I		List-II
A.	*Rhizopus*	I.	Mushroom
B.	*Ustilago*	II.	Smut fungus
C.	*Puccinia*	III.	Bread mould
D.	*Agaricus*	IV.	Rust fungus

Choose the correct answer from the options given below.
(a) A-III, B-II, C-IV, D-I
(b) A-I, B-III, C-II, D-IV
(c) A-III, B-II, C-I, D-IV
(d) A-IV, B-III, C-II, D-I

127. *Hind* II always cuts DNA molecules at a particular point called recognition sequence and it consists of
(a) 8 bp (b) 6 bp
(c) 4 bp (d) 10 bp

128. Which of the following is an example of actinomorphic flower?
(a) *Datura* (b) *Cassia* (c) *Pisum* (d) *Sesbania*

129. The type of conservation in which the threatened species are taken out from their natural habitat and placed in special setting where they can be protected and given special care is called
(a) *in-situ* conservation
(b) biodiversity conservation
(c) semi-conservative method
(d) sustainable development

130. Given below are two statements.
Statement I Chromosomes become gradually visible under light microscope during leptotene stage.
Statement II The beginning of diplotene stage is recognised by dissolution of synaptonemal complex.
In the light of the above statements, choose the correct answer from the options given below.
(a) Both Statement I and Statement II are true
(b) Both Statement I and Statement II are false
(c) Statement I is true but Statement II is false
(d) Statement I is false but Statement II is true

131. Formation of interfascicular cambium from fully developed parenchyma cells is an example for
(a) differentiation
(b) redifferentiation
(c) dedifferentiation
(d) maturation

132. The capacity to generate a whole plant from any cell of the plant is called
(a) totipotency
(b) Micropropagation
(c) differentiation
(d) Somatic hybridisation

133. Match List I with List II.

List I	List II
A. Two or more alternative forms of a gene	I. Back cross
B. Cross of F_1 progeny with homozygous recessive parent	II. Ploidy
C. Cross of F_1 progeny with any of the parents	III. Allele
D. Number of chromosome sets in plant	IV. Test cross

Choose the correct answer from the options given below:
(a) A-I, B-II, C-III, D-IV (b) A-II, B-I, C-III, D-IV
(c) A-III, B-IV, C-I, D-II (d) A-IV, B-III, C-II, D-I

134. The cofactor of the enzyme carboxypeptidase is
(a) zinc (b) niacin (c) flavin (d) haem

135. These are regarded as major causes of biodiversity loss:
A. Overexploitation
B. Co-extinction
C. Mutation
D. Habitat loss and fragmentation
E. Migration
Choose the correct option:
(a) A, C and D only (b) A, B, C and D only
(c) A, B and E only (d) A, B and D only

Section-B (Q. No. 136 to 150)

136. Match List I with List II.

	List I (Types of Stamens)		List II (Example)
A.	Monoadelphous	I.	Citrus
B.	Diadelphous	II.	Pea
C.	Polyadelphous	III.	Lily
D.	Epiphyllous	IV.	China rose

Choose the correct answer from the options given below.
(a) A-IV, B-II, C-I, D-III (b) A-IV, B-I, C-II, D-III
(c) A-I, B-II, C-IV, D-III (d) A-III, B-I, C-IV, D-II

137. Match List I with List II.

	List I		List II
A.	GLUT-4	I.	Hormone
B.	Insulin	II.	Enzyme
C.	Trypsin	III.	Intercellular ground substance
D.	Collagen	IV.	Enables glucose transport into cells

Choose the correct answer from the options given below.
(a) A-IV, B-I, C-II, D-III (b) A-I, B-II, C-III, D-IV
(c) A-II, B-III, C-IV, D-I (d) A-III, B-IV, C-I, D-II

138. Identify the step in tricarboxylic acid cycle, which does not involve oxidation of substrate.
(a) Malic acid → Oxaloacetic acid
(b) Succinic acid → Malic acid
(c) Succinyl-Co-A → Succinic acid
(d) Isocitrate → Ñ-ketoglutaric acid

139. Match List I with List II.

	List I		List II
A.	Citric acid cycle	I.	Cytoplasm
B.	Glycolysis	II.	Mitochondrial matrix
C.	Electron transport system	III.	Intermembrane space of mitochondria
D.	Proton gradient	IV.	Inner mitochondrial membrane

Choose the correct answer from the options given below.
(a) A-I, B-II, C-III, D-IV
(b) A-II, B-I, C-IV, D-III
(c) A-III, B-IV, C-I, D-II
(d) A-IV, B-III, C-II, D-I

140. Match List I with List II.

	List I		List II
A.	Frederick Griffith	I.	Genetic code
B.	Francois Jacob and Jacque Monod	II.	Semi-conservative mode of DNA replication
C.	Har Gobind Khorana	III.	Transformation
D.	Meselson and Stahl	IV.	*Lac* operon

Choose the correct answer from the options given below.
(a) A-III, B-II, C-I, D-IV
(b) A-III, B-IV, C-I, D-II
(c) A-II, B-III, C-IV, D-I
(d) A-IV, B-I, C-II, D-III

141. Given below are two statements.
Statement I In C_3 plants, some O_2 binds to RuBisCO, hence CO_2 fixation is decreased.
Statement II In C_4 plants, mesophyll cells show very little photorespiration, while bundle sheath cells do not show photorespiration.
In the light of the above statements, choose the correct answer from the options given below.
(a) Both Statement I and Statement II are true
(b) Both Statement I and Statement II are false
(c) Statement I is true but Statement II is false
(d) Statement I is false but Statement II is true

142. Identify the correct description about the given figure.

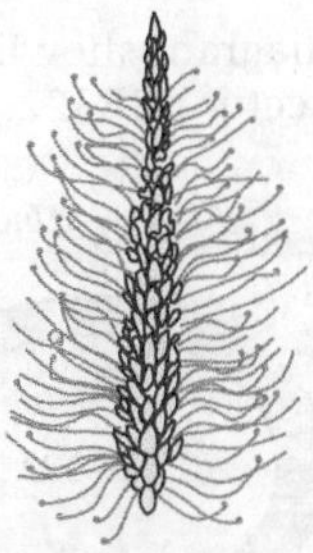

(a) Wind pollinated plant inflorescence showing flowers with well exposed stamens.
(b) Water pollinated flowers showing stamens with mucilaginous covering.
(c) Cleistogamous flowers showing autogamy.
(d) Compact inflorescence showing complete autogamy

143. Match List I with List II.

	List I		List II
A.	Rose	I.	Twisted aestivation
B.	Pea	II.	Perigynous flower
C.	Cotton	III.	Drupe
D.	Mango	IV.	Marginal placentation

Choose the correct answer from the options given below.
(a) A-II, B-IV, C-I, D-III
(b) A-I, B-II, C-III, D-IV
(c) A-IV, B-III, C-II, D-I
(d) A-II, B-III, C-IV, D-I

144. Read the following statements and choose the set of correct statements.
In the members of Phaeophyceae,
A. asexual reproduction occurs usually by biflagellate zoospores.
B. sexual reproduction is by oogamous method only.
C. Stored food is in the form of carbohydrates which is either mannitol or laminarin.
D. the major pigments found are chlorophyll-*a*, *c* and carotenoids and xanthophyll.
E. vegetative cells have a cellulosic wall, usually covered on the outside by gelatinous coating of algin.
Choose the correct answer from the options given below.
(a) A, B, C and D only
(b) B, C, D and E only
(c) A, C, D and E only
(d) A, B, C and E only

145. In an ecosystem if the Net Primary Productivity (NPP) of first trophic level is $100 \times (\text{kcal m}^{-2})\text{yr}^{-1}$. What will be the GPP (Gross Primary Productivity) of the third trophic level of the same ecosystem
(a) $\frac{x}{10}(\text{kcal m}^{-2})\text{yr}^{-1}$
(b) $x(\text{kcal m}^{-2})\text{yr}^{-1}$
(c) $10x(\text{kcal m}^{-2})\text{yr}^{-1}$
(d) $\frac{100x}{3x}(\text{kcal m}^{-2})\text{yr}^{-1}$

146. Which of the following statement is correct regarding the process of replication in *E. coli*?
(a) The DNA-dependent DNA polymerase catalyses polymerisation in one direction that is $3' \rightarrow 5'$
(b) The DNA-dependent RNA polymerase catalyses polymerization in one direction, that is $5' \rightarrow 3'$
(c) The DNA-dependent DNA polymerase catalyses polymerisation in $5' \rightarrow 3'$ as well as $3' \rightarrow 5'$ direction
(d) The DNA-dependent DNA polymerase catalyses polymerisation in $5' \rightarrow 3'$ direction

147. Which of the following are fused in somatic hybridisation involving two varieties of plants?
(a) Callus
(b) Somatic embryos
(c) Protoplasts
(d) Pollens

148. Spraying sugarcane crop with which of the following plant growth regulators, increases the length of stem, thus increasing the yield?
(a) Auxin
(b) Gibberellin
(c) Cytokinin
(d) Abscisic acid

149. Match List I with List II.

	List I		List II
A.	Robert May	I.	Species-area relationship
B.	Alexander von Humboldt	II.	Long term ecosystem experiment using outdoor plots
C.	Paul Ehrlich	III.	Global species diversity at about 7 million
D.	David Tilman	IV.	Rivet popper hypothesis

Choose the correct answer from the options given below.

(a) A-II, B-III, C-I, D-IV (b) A-III, B-I, C-IV, D-II
(c) A-I, B-III, C-II, D-IV (d) A-III, B-IV, C-II, D-I

150. The DNA present in chloroplast is

(a) linear, double-stranded
(b) circular, double-stranded
(c) linear, single-stranded
(d) circular, single-stranded

ZOOLOGY

Section-A (Q. No. 151 to 185)

151. Match List I with List II.

	List I		List II
A.	Common cold	I.	*Plasmodium*
B.	Haemozoin	II.	Typhoid
C.	Widal test	III.	Rhinoviruses
D.	Allergy	IV.	Dust mites

Choose the correct answer from the options given below.

(a) A-II, B-IV, C-III, D-I (b) A-I, B-III, C-II, D-IV
(c) A-III, B-I, C-II, D-IV (d) A-IV, B-II, C-III, D-I

152. Match List I with List II.

	List I		List II
A.	Cocaine	I.	Effective sedative in surgery
B.	Heroin	II.	*Cannabis sativa*
C.	Morphine	III.	*Erythroxylum*
D.	Marijuana	IV.	*Papaver somniferum*

Choose the correct answer from the options given below:

(a) A-IV, B-III, C-I, D-II
(b) A-I, B-III, C-II, D-IV
(c) A-II, B-I, C-III, D-IV
(d) A-III, B-IV, C-I, D-II

153. Match List I with List II.

	List I		List II
A.	Fibrous joints	I.	Adjacent vertebrae, limited movement
B.	Cartilaginous joints	II.	Humerus and pectoral girdle, rotational movement
C.	Hinge joints	III.	Skull, do not allow any movement
D.	Ball and socket joints	IV.	Knee, help in locomotion

Choose the correct answer from the options given below.

(a) A-IV, B-II, C-III, D-I
(b) A-I, B-III, C-II, D-IV
(c) A-II, B-III, C-I, D-IV
(d) A-III, B-I, C-IV, D-II

154. Which of the following are autoimmune disorders?

A. Myasthenia gravis
B. Rheumatoid arthritis
C. Gout
D. Muscular dystrophy
E. Systemic Lupus Erythematosus (SLE)

Choose the most appropriate answer from the options given below.

(a) A, B and D only (b) A, B and E only
(c) B, C and E only (d) C, D and E only

155. Which of the following is not a component of Fallopian tube?

(a) Uterine fundus (b) Isthmus
(c) Infundibulum (d) Ampulla

156. The flippers of the penguins and dolphins are the example of the

(a) adaptive radiation (b) natural selection
(c) convergent evolution (d) divergent evolution

157. Match List I with List II.

	List I		List II
A.	$\alpha-1$ antitrypsin	I.	Cotton bollworm
B.	*cry* IAb	II.	ADA deficiency
C.	*cry* IAc	III.	Emphysema
D.	Enzyme replacement therapy	IV.	Corn borer

Choose the correct answer form the options given below.

(a) A-II, B-I, C-IV, D-III (b) A-III, B-I, C-II, D-IV
(c) A-III, B-IV, C-I, D-II (d) A-II, B-IV, C-I, D-III

158. The following diagram showing restriction sites in *E. coli* cloning vector pBR322. Find the role of *'X'* and *'Y'* genes.

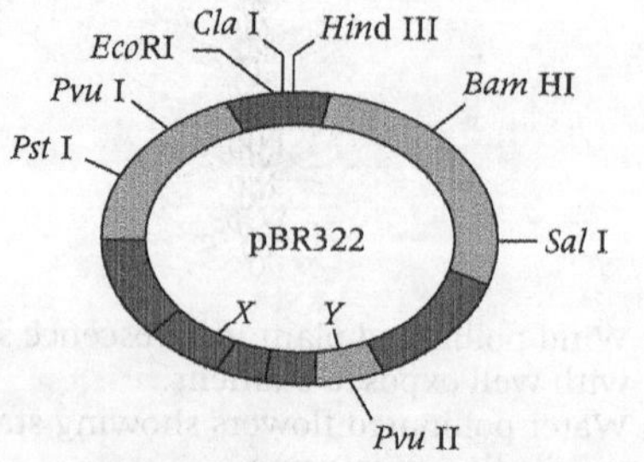

(a) The gene 'X' is responsible for resistance to antibiotics and 'Y' for protein involved in the replication of plasmid.
(b) The gene 'X' is responsible for controlling the copy number of the linked DNA and 'Y' for protein involved in the replication of plasmid.
(c) The gene 'X' is for protein involved in replication of plasmid and 'Y' for resistance to antibiotics.
(d) Gene 'X' is responsible for recognitions sites and 'Y' is responsible for antibiotic resistance.

159. Given below are two statements; one is labelled as Assertion (A) and the other is labelled as Reason (R).
Assertion (A) Breast-feeding during initial period of infant growth is recommended by doctors for bringing a healthy baby.
Reason (R) Colostrum contains several antibodies absolutely essential to develop resistance for the new born baby.
In the light of the above statements, choose the most appropriate answer from the options given below.
(a) Both A and R are correct and R is the correct explanation of A
(b) Both A and R are correct, but R is not the correct explanation of A
(c) A is correct but R is not correct
(d) A is not correct but R is correct

160. The Ti-plasmid of *Agrobacterium tumefaciens* stands for
(a) Tumour inhibiting plasmid
(b) Tumour independent plasmid
(c) Tumour inducing plasmid
(d) Temperature independent plasmid

161. Match List I with List II.

	List I		List II
A.	*Pleurobrachia*	I.	Mollusca
B.	Radula	II.	Ctenophora
C.	Stomochord	III.	Osteichthyes
D.	Air bladder	IV.	Hemichordata

Choose the correct answer from the options given below.
(a) A-IV, B-II, C-III, D-I (b) A-II, B-I, C-IV, D-III
(c) A-II, B-IV, C-I, D-III (d) A-IV, B-III, C-II, D-I

162. Given below are some stages of human evolution. Arrange them in correct sequence. (Past to Recent)
A. *Homo habilis* B. *Homo sapiens*
C. *Homo neanderthalensis* D. *Homo erectus*
Choose the correct sequence of human evolution from the options given below.
(a) D-A-C-B (b) B-A-D-C
(c) C-B-D-A (d) A-D-C-B

163. Which of the following is not a steroid hormone?
(a) Cortisol (b) Testosterone
(c) Progesterone (d) Glucagon

164. In both sexes of cockroach, a pair of jointed filamentous structures called anal cerci are present on
(a) 5th segment (b) 10th segment
(c) 8th and 9th segment (d) 11th segment

165. Which one of the following factors will not affect the Hardy-Weinberg equilibrium?
(a) Genetic recombination (b) Genetic drift
(c) Gene migration (d) Constant gene pool

166. Match List I with List II.

List I		List II
A. Pons	I.	Provides additional space for neurons, regulates posture and balance.
B. Hypothalamus	II.	Controls respiration and gastric secretions.
C. Medulla	III.	Connects different regions of the brain.
D. Cerebellum	IV.	Neuro secretory cells

Choose the correct answer from the options given below.
(a) A-II, B-III, C-I, D-IV
(b) A-III, B-IV, C-II, D-I
(c) A-I, B-III, C-II, D-IV
(d) A-II, B-I, C-III, D-IV

167. Match List I with List II.

	List I		List II
A.	Down's syndrome	I.	11th chromosome
B.	α-thalassemia	II.	X-chromosome
C.	β-thalassemia	III.	21st chromosome
D.	Klinefelter's syndrome	IV.	16th chromosome

Choose the correct answer from the options given below.
(a) A-I, B-II, C-III, D-IV (b) A-II, B-III, C-IV, D-I
(c) A-III, B-IV, C-I, D-II (d) A-IV, B-I, C-II, D-III

168. Which one is the correct product of DNA dependent RNA polymerase to the given template?
3'TACATGGCAAATATCCATTCA5'
(a) 5'AUGUACCGUUUAUAGGUAAGU3'
(b) 5'AUGUAAAGUUUAUAGGUAAGU3'
(c) 5'AUGUACCGUUUAAGGGAAGU3'
(d) 5'ATGTACCGTTTATAGGTAAGT3'

169. Given below are two statements; one is labelled as Assertion A and the other is labelled as Reason (R).
Assertion (A) FSH acts upon ovarian follicles in female and Leydig cells in male.
Reason (R) Growing ovarian follicles secrete oestrogen in female while interstitial cells secrete androgen in male human being.
In the light of the above statements, choose the correct answer from the options given below .
(a) Both A and R are true and R is the correct explanation of A
(b) Both A and R are true, but R is not the correct explanation of A
(c) A is true, but R is false
(d) A is false, but R is true

170. Which of the following is not a natural/traditional contraceptive method?
(a) Coitus interruptus (b) Periodic abstinence
(c) Lactational amenorrhea (d) Vaults

171. Match List I with List II.

	List I		List II
A.	Non-medicated IUD	I.	Multiload 375
B.	Copper releasing IUD	II.	Progestogens
C.	Hormone releasing IUD	III.	Lippes loop
D.	Implants	IV.	LNG-20

Choose the correct answer from the option given below:
(a) A-III, B-I, C-II, D-IV
(b) A-I, B-III, C-IV, D-II
(c) A-IV, B-I, C-II, D-III
(d) A-III, B-I, C-IV, D-II

172. Consider the following statements.
A. Annelids are true coelomates
B. Poriferans are pseudocoelomates
C. Aschelminthes are acoelomates
D. Platyhelminthes are pseudocoelomates
Choose the correct answer from the options given below.
(a) B only (b) A only
(c) C only (d) D only

173. Three types of muscles are given as (i), (ii) and (iii). Identify the correct matching pair along with their location in human body:

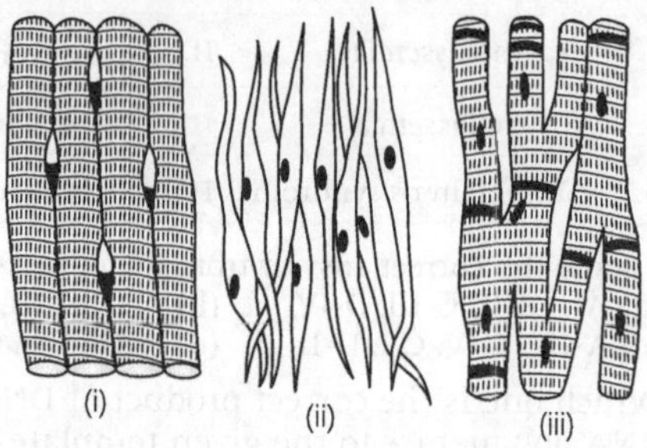

Name of muscle/location
(a) (i) Smooth - Toes
(ii) Skeletal - Legs
(iii) Cardiac - Heart
(b) (i) Skeletal - Triceps
(ii) Smooth - Stomach
(iii) Cardiac - Heart
(c) (i) Skeletal - Biceps
(ii) Involuntary-Intestine
(iii) Smooth - Heart
(d) (i) Involuntary - Nose tip
(ii) Skeletal - Bone
(iii) Cardiac - Heart

174. Following are the stages of pathway for conduction of an action potential through the heart.
A. AV bundle B. Purkinje fibres
C. AV node D. Bundle branches
E. SA node
Choose the correct sequence of pathway from the options given below.
(a) E-C-A-D-B (b) A-E-C-B-D
(c) B-D-E-C-A (d) E-A-D-B-C

175. Match List I with List II.

	List I		List II
A.	Lipase	I.	Peptide bond
B.	Nuclease	II.	Ester bond
C.	Protease	III.	Glycosidic bond
D.	Amylase	IV.	Phosphodiester bond

Choose the correct answer from the options given below.
(a) A-IV, B-II, C-III, D-I (b) A-III, B-II, C-I, D-IV
(c) A-II, B-IV, C-I, D-III (d) A-IV, B-I, C-III, D-II

176. Match List I with List II.

	List I		List II
A.	Axoneme	I.	Centriole
B.	Cartwheel pattern	II.	Cilia and flagella
C.	Crista	III.	Chromosome
D.	Satellite	IV.	Mitochondria

Choose the correct answer from the options given below.
(a) A-IV, B-III, C-II, D-I
(b) A-IV, B-II, C-III, D-I
(c) A-II, B-IV, C-I, D-III
(d) A-II, B-I, C-IV, D-III

177. Match List I with List II.

	List I (Sub-phases of Prophase-I)		List II (Specific Characters)
A.	Diakinesis	I.	Synaptonemal complex formation
B.	Pachytene	II.	Completion of terminalisation of chiasmata
C.	Zygotene	III.	Chromosomes look like thin threads
D.	Leptotene	IV.	Appearance of recombination nodules

Choose the correct answer from the options given below
(a) A-IV, B-II, C-III, D-I
(b) A-I, B-II, C-IV, D-III
(c) A-II, B-IV, C-I, D-III
(d) A-IV, B-III, C-II, D-I

178. Which of the following factors are favourable for the formation of oxyhaemoglobin in alveoli?
(a) High pO_2 and high pCO_2
(b) High pO_2 and lesser H^+ concentration
(c) Low pCO_2 and high H^+ concentration
(d) Low pCO_2 and High temperature

179. Match List I with List II.

	List I		List II
A.	*Pterophyllum*	I.	Hag fish
B.	*Myxine*	II.	Saw fish
C.	*Pristis*	III.	Angel fish
D.	*Exocoetus*	IV.	Flying fish

Choose the correct answer from the options given below.
(a) A-II, B-I, C-III, D-IV
(b) A-III, B-I, C-II, D-IV
(c) A-IV, B-I, C-II, D-III
(d) A-III, B-II, C-I, D-IV

180. Match List I with List II.

	List I		List II
A.	Typhoid	I.	Fungus
B.	Leishmaniasis	II.	Nematode
C.	Ringworm	III.	Protozoa
D.	Filariasis	IV.	Bacteria

Choose the correct answer from the options given below.
(a) A-I, B-III, C-II, D-IV
(b) A-IV, B-III, C-I, D-II
(c) A-III, B-I, C-IV, D-II
(d) A-II, B-IV, C-III, D-I

181. Which of the following statements is incorrect?
(a) A bio-reactor provides optimal growth conditions for achieving the desired product.
(b) Most commonly used bio-reactors are of stirring type.
(c) Bio-reactors are used to produce small scale bacterial cultures.
(d) Bio-reactors have an agitator system, an oxygen delivery system and foam control system.

182. Given below are two statements
Statement I In the nephron, the descending limb of loop of Henle is impermeable to water and permeable to electrolytes.
Statement II The proximal convoluted tubule is lined by simple columnar brush border epithelium and increases the surface area for reabsorption.
In the light of the above statements, choose the correct answer from the option given below.
(a) Both Statement I and Statement II are true
(b) Both Statement I and Statement II are false
(c) Statement I is true but Statement II is false
(d) Statement I is false but Statement II is true

183. Given below are two statements.
Statement I The presence or absence of hymen is not a reliable indicator of virginity.
Statement II The hymen is torn during the first coitus only.
In the light of the above statements, choose the correct answer from the options given below.
(a) Both Statement I and Statement II are true
(b) Both Statement I and Statement II are false
(c) Statement I is true, but Statement II is false
(d) Statement I is false, but Statement II is true

184. Match List I with List II.

	List I		List II
A.	Expiratory capacity	I.	Expiratory reserve volume + Tidal volume + Inspiratory reserve volume
B.	Functional residual capacity	II.	Tidal volume + Expiratory reserve volume
C.	Vital capacity	III.	Tidal volume + Inspiratory reserve volume
D.	Inspiratory capacity	IV.	Expiratory reserve volume + Residual volume

Choose the correct answer from the options given below.
(a) A-II, B-IV, C-I, D-III
(b) A-III, B-II, C-IV, D-I
(c) A-II, B-I, C-IV, D-III
(d) A-I, B-III, C-II, D-IV

185. Following are the stages of cell division
A. Gap 2 phase
B. Cytokinesis
C. Synthesis phase
D. Karyokinesis
E. Gap 1 phase
Choose the correct sequence of stages from the options given below.
(a) C-E-D-A-B
(b) E-B-D-A-C
(c) B-D-E-A-C
(d) E-C-A-D-B

Section-B (Q. No. 186 to 200)

186. Given below are two statements.
Statement I Mitochondria and chloroplasts both are double membranes bound organelles.
Statement II Inner membrane of mitochondria is relatively less permeable, as compared to chloroplast.
In the light of the above statements, choose the most appropriate answer from the options given below.
(a) Both Statement I and Statement II are true
(b) Both Statement I and Statement II are false
(c) Statement I is true, but Statement II is false
(d) Statement I is false, but Statement II is true

187. Match List I with List II.

	List I		List II
A.	Mesozoic Era	I.	Lower invertebrates
B.	Proterozoic Era	II.	Fish and Amphibia
C.	Cenozoic Era	III.	Birds and reptiles
D.	Paleozoic Era	IV.	Mammals

Choose the correct answer from the options given below.
(a) A-II, B-I, C-III, D-IV
(b) A-III, B-I, C-II, D-IV
(c) A-I, B-II, C-IV, D-III
(d) A-III, B-I, C-IV, D-II

188. Given below are two statements.
Statement I Gause's competitive exclusion principle states that two closely related species competing for different resources cannot exist indefinitely.
Statement II According to Gause's principle, during competition, the inferior will be eliminated. This may be true if resources are limiting.
In the light of the above statements, choose the correct answer from the options given below.
(a) Both Statement I and Statement II are true.
(b) Both Statement I and Statement II are false.
(c) Statement I is true but Statement II is false.
(d) Statement I is false but Statement II is true.

189. Match List I with List II.

	List I		List II
A.	Unicellular glandular epithelium	I.	Salivary glands
B.	Compound epithelium	II.	Pancreas
C.	Multicellular glandular epithelium	III.	Goblet cells of alimentary canal
D.	Endocrine glandular epithelium	IV.	Moist surface of buccal cavity

Choose the correct answer from the options given below.
(a) A-II, B-I, C-III, D-IV
(b) A-IV, B-III, C-I, D-II
(c) A-III, B-IV, C-I, D-II
(d) A-II, B-I, C-IV, D-III

190. Match List I with List II related to digestive system of cockroach.

	List I		List II
A.	The structures used for storing of food	I.	Gizzard
B.	Ring of 6-8 blind tubules at junction of foregut and midgut.	II.	Gastric caeca
C.	Ring of 100-150 yellow coloured thin filaments at junction of midgut and hindgut.	III.	Malpighian tubules
D	The structures used for grinding the food.	IV.	Crop

Choose the correct answer from the options given below.
(a) A-IV, B-II, C-III, D-I (b) A-I, B-II, C-III, D-IV
(c) A-IV, B-III, C-II, D-I (d) A-III, B-II, C-IV, D-I

191. Choose the correct statement given below regarding juxta medullary nephron.
(a) Juxta medullary nephrons are located in the columns of Bertini.
(b) Renal corpuscle of juxta medullary nephron lies in the outer portion of the renal medulla.
(c) Loop of Henle of juxta medullary nephron runs deep into medulla.
(d) Juxta medullary nephrons outnumber the cortical nephrons.

192. Match List I with List II.

	List I		List II
A.	RNA polymerase	I.	*sn*RNPs
B.	Termination of transcription	II.	Promotor
C.	Splicing of exons	III.	*rho* factor
D.	TATA box	IV.	*sn*RNAs, *t*RNA

Choose the correct answer from the options given below :
(a) A-II, B-IV, C-I, D-III
(b) A-III, B-II, C-IV, D-I
(c) A-III, B-IV, C-I, D-II
(d) A-IV, B-III, C-I, D-II

193. Given below are two statements.
Statement I The cerebral hemispheres are connected by nerve tract known as corpus callosum.
Statement II The brain stem consists of the medulla oblongata, pons and cerebrum.
In the light of the above statements, choose the most appropriate answer from the options given below.
(a) Both Statement I and Statement II are true
(b) Both Statement I and Statement II are false
(c) Statement I is true, but Statement II is false
(d) Statement I is false, but Statement II is true

194. Identify the correct option (A), (B), (C), (D) with respect to spermatogenesis.

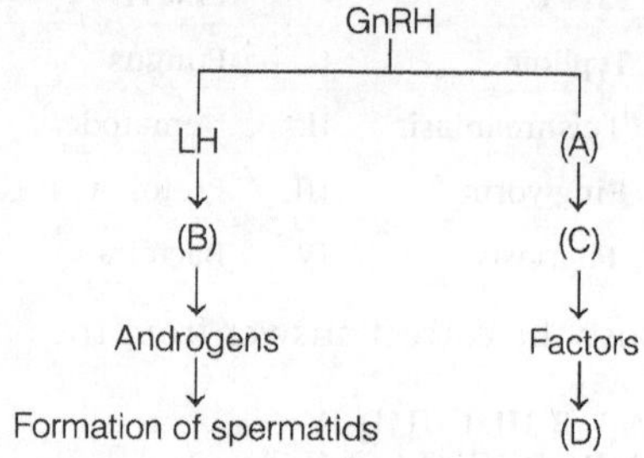

Formation of spermatids
(a) FSH, Leydig cells, Sertoli cells, Spermiogenesis
(b) ICSH, Interstitial cells, Leydig cells, spermiogenesis
(c) FSH, Sertoli cells, Leydig cells, Spermatogenesis
(d) ICSH, Leydig cells, Sertoli cells, Spermatogenesis

195. As per ABO blood grouping system, the blood group of father is B^+, mother is A^+ and child is O^+. Their respective genotype can be
A. $I^Bi / I^Ai / ii$ B. $I^BI^B / I^AI^A / ii$
C. $iI^B / iI^A / I^AI^B$ D. $I^Ai / I^Bi / I^Ai$
E. $iI^B / iI^A / I^AI^B$
Choose the most appropriate answer from the options given below.
(a) A only (b) B only
(c) C and B only (d) D and E only

196. Given below are two statements :
Statement I Bone marrow is the main lymphoid organ where all blood cells including lymphocytes are produced.
Statement II Both bone marrow and thymus provide micro environments for the development and maturation of T-lymphocytes.
In the light of above statements, choose the most appropriate answer from the options given below
(a) Both Statement I and Statement II are true
(b) Both Statement I and Statement II are false
(c) Statement I is true, but Statement II is false
(d) Statement I is false, but Statement II is true

197. Regarding catalytic cycle of an enzyme action, select the correct sequential steps.
A. Substrate enzyme complex formation.
B. Free enzyme ready to bind with another substrate.
C. Release of products.
D. Chemical bonds of the substrate broken.
E. Substrate binding to active site.
Choose the correct answer from the options given below.
(a) E, A, D, C, B (b) A, E, B, D, C
(c) B, A, C, D, E (d) E, D, C, B, A

198. Match List I with List II.

	List I		List II
A.	P-wave	I.	Heart muscles are electrically silent.
B.	QRS-complex	II.	Depolarisation of ventricles.
C.	T-wave	III.	Depolarisation of atria.
D.	T-P gap	IV.	Repolarisation of ventricles.

Choose the correct answer from the options given below.

(a) A-I, B-III, C-IV, D-II (b) A-III, B-II, C-IV, D-I
(c) A-II, B-III, C-I, D-IV (d) A-IV, B-II, C-I, D-III

199. Match List I with List II.

	List I		List II
A.	Exophthalmic goitre	I.	Excess secretion of cortisol, moon face and hypergylcemia.
B.	Acromegaly	II.	Hyposecretion of thyroid hormone and stunted growth.
C.	Cushing's syndrome	III.	Hypersecretion of thyroid hormone and protruding eye balls.
D.	Cretinism	IV.	Excessive secretion of growth hormone.

Choose the correct answer from the options given below.

(a) A-I, B-III, C-II, D-IV
(b) A-IV, B-II, C-I, D-III
(c) A-III, B-IV, C-II, D-I
(d) A-III, B-IV, C-I, D-II

200. The following are the statements about non-chordates.

A. Pharynx is perforated by gill slits.
B. Notochord is absent.
C. Central nervous system is dorsal.
D. Heart is dorsal if present.
E. Post anal tail is absent.

Choose the most appropriate answer from the options given below.

(a) A and C only (b) A, B and D only
(c) B, D and E only (d) B, C and D only

Answers

Physics

1. (b)	2. (d)	3. (c)	4. (a)	5. (c)	6. (a)	7. (d)	8. (b)	9. (b)	10. (c)
11. (b)	12. (c)	13. (c)	14. (b)	15. (b)	16. (c)	17. (d)	18. (b)	19. (d)	20. (a)
21. (c)	22. (a)	23. (a)	24. (b)	25. (b)	26. (d)	27. (a)	28. (d)	29. (a)	30. (a)
31. (a)	32. (b)	33. (d)	34. (a)	35. (d)	36. (c)	37. (b)	38. (b)	39. (d)	40. (b)
41. (a)	42. (b)	43. (d)	44. (b)	45. (a)	46. (b)	47. (b)	48. (b)	49. (b)	50. (b)

Chemistry

51. (a)	52. (d)	53. (a)	54. (a)	55. (a)	56. (b)	57. (d)	58. (d)	59. (a)	60. (b)
61. (a)	62. (a)	63. (b)	64. (c)	65. (d)	66. (a)	67. (a)	68. (c)	69. (a)	70. (d)
71. (d)	72. (c)	73. (d)	74. (d)	75. (a)	76. (a)	77. (c)	78. (b)	79. (a)	80. (c)
81. (c)	82. (a)	83. (b)	84. (b)	85. (c)	86. (a)	87. (d)	88. (b)	89. (a)	90. (a)
91. (d)	92. (a)	93. (b)	94. (a)	95. (d)	96. (b)	97. (b)	98. (d)	99. (a)	100. (a)

Botany

101. (b)	102. (c)	103. (b)	104. (a)	105. (a)	106. (c)	107. (c)	108. (d)	109. (c)	110. (c)
111. (d)	112. (c)	113. (b)	114. (b)	115. (c)	116. (b)	117. (d)	118. (d)	119. (d)	120. (a)
121. (c)	122. (c)	123. (b)	124. (a)	125. (d)	126. (a)	127. (b)	128. (a)	129. (b)	130. (a)
131. (c)	132. (a)	133. (c)	134. (a)	135. (d)	136. (a)	137. (a)	138. (c)	139. (b)	140. (b)
141. (c)	142. (a)	143. (a)	144. (c)	145. (c)	146. (d)	147. (c)	148. (b)	149. (b)	150. (b)

Zoology

151. (c)	152. (d)	153. (d)	154. (b)	155. (a)	156. (c)	157. (c)	158. (b)	159. (a)	160. (c)
161. (b)	162. (d)	163. (d)	164. (b)	165. (d)	166. (b)	167. (c)	168. (a)	169. (d)	170. (d)
171. (d)	172. (b)	173. (b)	174. (a)	175. (c)	176. (d)	177. (c)	178. (b)	179. (b)	180. (b)
181. (c)	182. (b)	183. (c)	184. (a)	185. (d)	186. (c)	187. (d)	188. (d)	189. (c)	190. (a)

Explanations

Physics

1. *(b)* The tension in the string will be equal to centripetal force is,

$$F_c = \frac{mv^2}{r} = m\omega^2 r$$

According to question, $T = m\omega^2 r$

and $\quad T' = m(2\omega)^2 r$

$$\frac{T'}{T} = \frac{m(4\omega^2)r}{m\omega^2 r} \Rightarrow T' = 4T$$

2. *(d)* The direction of motion changes continuously in a circular motion, therefore circular motion is an accelerated motion.

So, uniform circular motion have varying velocity as well as varying acceleration.

3. *(c)* Output from the truth table

$$Y = \overline{A}\overline{B} + A\overline{B} = \overline{B}(A + \overline{A})$$
$$Y = \overline{B}$$

So, correct option is (c).

4. *(a)* The direction of induced current is always such that it opposes the cause which created it. For solenoid-1, the magnet is moving away. Thus, near the *B*-point, *S*-pole will be generated.

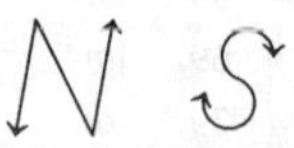

Thus, the current in solenoid-1 will be from *A* to *B*.

Similarly, the current in the solenoid-2 will be from *D* to *C*.

5. *(c)* We know that, potential at point due to an ideal point at any point on axial line is given

$$V = \pm \frac{1}{4\pi\varepsilon_0}\frac{p}{r^2}$$

Putting the values of *p* and *r*, we get

$$V = \pm\, 9 \times 10^9 \times \frac{4 \times 10^{-6}}{(2)^2} = \pm\, 9 \times 10^3 \text{ V}$$

Hence, A is true but R is false.

6. *(a)* For a diamagnetic material magnetic susceptibility χ is small and negative, is, $0 > \chi \geq -1$.

For a ferromagnetic material, $\chi >> 1$.

For a paramagnetic material, $0 < \chi < \varepsilon$ (ε is a small positive number) and for non-magnetic material, $\chi = 0$.

Hence, correct option is (a).

7. *(d)* Given, magnetic field $B = 0.049$ T

Time period, $T = \frac{5}{20} = \frac{1}{4}$ s

Moment of inertia, $I = 9.8 \times 10^{-6}$ kg m^2

The time period of oscillation of a magnetic needle in a magnetic field is given by $T = 2\pi\sqrt{\frac{I}{MB}}$

where, *M* is the magnetic moment of the needle.

Thus, $T = 2\pi\sqrt{\frac{9.8 \times 10^{-6}}{M \times 0.049}}$

$$\Rightarrow \left(\frac{1}{4}\right)^2 = (2\pi)^2\left(\frac{9.8 \times 10^{-6}}{M \times 4.9 \times 10^{-2}}\right)$$

$$\Rightarrow \frac{1}{16} = \frac{4\pi^2 \times 2 \times 10^{-4}}{M}$$

$$\Rightarrow M = 16 \times 8 \times \pi^2 \times 10^{-4}$$
$$= 128\pi^2 \times 10^{-4} \text{Am}^2$$
$$= 1280\pi^2 \times 10^{-5} \text{Am}^2$$

8. *(b)* We know that, transformation ratio,

$$r = \frac{N_s}{N_p} = \frac{V_s}{V_p}$$

$$\because \quad \frac{N_p}{N_s} = \frac{1}{2} = \frac{V_p}{V_s}$$

$$\Rightarrow \quad V_s : V_p = 2 : 1$$

9. *(b)* Given, 1 MSD = 0.1 mm

$(N+1)$ VSD $= N$ MSD

$$\therefore \quad 1 \text{ VSD} = \left(\frac{N}{N+1}\right) \text{MSD}$$

Least count or vernier constant,

$$1 \text{MSD} - 1 \text{VSD} = \left[1 - \frac{N}{N+1}\right] \text{MSD}$$

$$= \left(\frac{1}{N+1}\right) \text{MSD} = \left(\frac{0.1}{N+1}\right) \text{mm}$$

$$= \frac{1}{100(N+1)} \text{cm}$$

10. *(c)* Net force on *A* and *B* = 10 N

Acceleration of both *A* and $B = \frac{F}{m}$

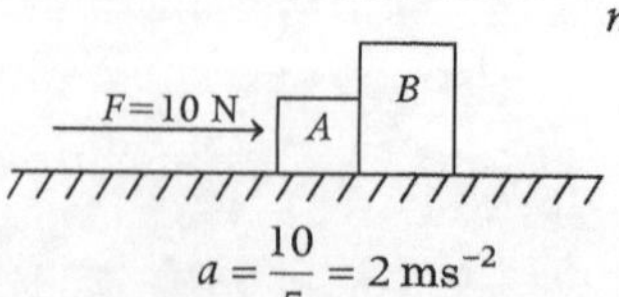

$$a = \frac{10}{5} = 2 \text{ ms}^{-2}$$

For block *A*,

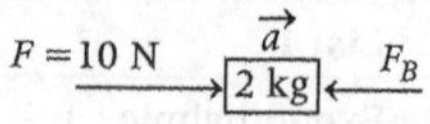

F_B = force exerted by block *B* on block *A*.

$$F - F_B = 2 \times a$$
$$\Rightarrow \quad 10 - F_B = 2 \times 2 \Rightarrow F_B = 6\text{N}$$

For block *B*,

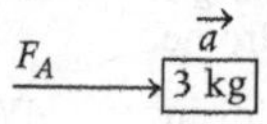

Force exerted by *A* on B,

$$F_A = 3a = 6 \text{ N}$$

11. *(b)* Given, $x = 5\sin\left(\pi t + \frac{\pi}{3}\right)$ m $\quad$ ...(i)

The standard Eq. for SHM is

$$x = A\sin(\omega t + \phi) \quad \text{...(ii)}$$

Thus, comparing Eqs. (i) and (ii), we get

$$A = 5 \text{ m and } \omega = \pi$$

$$\Rightarrow \quad \frac{2\pi}{T} = \pi \Rightarrow T = 2\text{s}$$

Hence, option (b) is correct.

12. *(c)* Given,

EMF, $\varepsilon = 10$ V

Internal resistance, $r = 1\,\Omega$

External resistance, $R = 4\,\Omega$

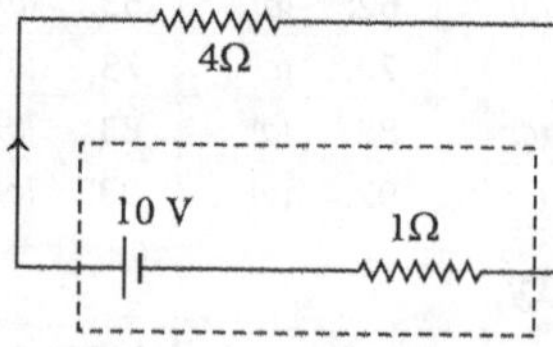

Terminal voltage, $V = \varepsilon - Ir$

and $\quad I = \frac{\varepsilon}{R + r} = \frac{10}{4+1} = 2$ A

Thus, $V = 10 - 2 \times 1 = 8$ V

13. *(c)* Atoms are electrically neutral as they contain equal number of protons and electrons. Statement II is incorrect because atom of radioactive elements are not stable.

So, option (c) is correct.

14. *(b)* Photon is quanta of energy. It is a massless and chargeless particle. The rest mass of photon is zero. In free space, it moves with velocity *c* and energy of photon is equal to $h\nu$. The momentum of the photon is given as $p = \frac{E}{c} = \frac{h\nu}{c}$.

15. *(b)* The wavelength of spectral line is given by

$$\frac{1}{\lambda} = R\left[\frac{1}{n_1^2} - \frac{1}{n_2^2}\right]$$

A. $\frac{1}{\lambda} = 1.09737 \times 10^7\left[\frac{1}{2^2} - \frac{1}{3^2}\right]$

$= 1.09737 \times 10^7\left[\frac{1}{4} - \frac{1}{9}\right]$

$= 1.09737 \times 10^7\left[\frac{5}{36}\right]$

$\Rightarrow \lambda = \frac{36 \times 10^{-7}}{5 \times 1.09737}$

$= 6.56114 \times 10^{-7}$

$\simeq 656.3$ nm

B. $\lambda = \frac{10^{-7}}{1.09737\left[\frac{1}{2^2} - \frac{1}{4^2}\right]}$

$= \frac{10^{-7} \times 16}{1.09737 \times 3} = 4.8601 \times 10^{-7}$ m

$\simeq 486.1$ nm

C. $\lambda = \frac{10^{-7}}{1.09737 \times \left[\frac{1}{2^2} - \frac{1}{5^2}\right]}$

$= \frac{10^{-7} \times 100}{1.09737 \times 21} = 4.3393 \times 10^{-7}$ m

$\simeq 434.1$ nm

D. $\lambda = \frac{10^{-7}}{1.09737 \times \left[\frac{1}{2^2} - \frac{1}{6^2}\right]}$

$= \frac{10^{-7} \times 144}{1.09737 \times 32} \simeq 410.2$ nm

Hence, A - III, B - IV, C - II, D - I

16. *(c)* Given, number of turns $N = 100$

radius, $r = 10$ cm $= 10 \times 10^{-2}$ m

current, $I = 7$A

Magnetic field at the centre of a solenoid,

$$B = \frac{\mu_0 NI}{2r} = \frac{4\pi \times 10^{-7} \times 100 \times 7}{2 \times 10 \times 10^{-2}}$$

$= 44 \times 10^{-4} = 4.4 \times 10^{-3}$ T

$= 4.4$ mT

17. *(d)* The given combination of gates can be taken as

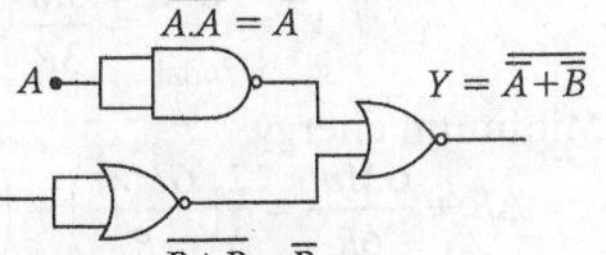

$Y = \overline{\overline{A} + \overline{B}} = \overline{\overline{A}} \cdot \overline{\overline{B}} = A \cdot B$

Hence, the output Y of the given logic gate is similar to AND gate.

18. *(b)* Given,

wire of length l is divided into 10 parts

each having $\frac{100}{10}\,\Omega = 10\,\Omega$ resistance.

According to question, 5 parts are connected in series

i.e., $R_1 = 5 \times 10 = 50\,\Omega$

5 parts are connected in parallel

i.e., $R_2 = \frac{R}{5} = \frac{10}{5} = 2\,\Omega$

Then, both R_1 and R_2 are connected in series

Thus, $R_{net} = R_1 + R_2$

$= 50 + 2 = 52\,\Omega$

19. *(d)* Given,

$$^{290}_{82}X \xrightarrow{\alpha} Y \xrightarrow{e^+} Z \xrightarrow{\beta^-} P \xrightarrow{e^-} Q$$

From $X \to Y$, α-particle is emitted thus $^{286}_{80}Y$.

Now, $Y \to Z$, e^+ is emitted, thus $^{286}_{79}Z$.

Again $Z \to P$, β^- is emitted thus $^{286}_{80}P$.

Again $P \to Q$, e^- is emitted thus $^{286}_{81}Q$.

20. *(a)* Length of wire $= 1$ m

Elastic limit, $E = 8 \times 10^8$ Nm^{-2}

Young's modulus $Y = 2 \times 10^{11}$ Nm^{-2}

We know that, $Y = \frac{F}{A}\frac{l}{\Delta l}$

Here, $\frac{F}{A}$ = Elastic limit E

$\Rightarrow Y = E\frac{l}{\Delta l} \Rightarrow \Delta l = \frac{E}{Y}l$

$\Rightarrow \Delta l = \frac{8 \times 10^8}{2 \times 10^{11}} \times 1 = 4 \times 10^{-3}$ m

$= 4$ mm

21. *(c)* When YDSE is performed in white light instead of monochromatic light, all wavelengths shows their maxima and minima in order of their wavelength. Thus, a central bright is observed along with few fringes that will be different colours.

22. *(a)* Given,

$x = 2t - 1$ unit

Force, $F = 5$ N

Instantaneous power, $P = F.v$

Thus, $P = F\frac{dx}{dt} = 5 \times \frac{d(2t-1)}{dt}$

$= 5 \times 2 = 10$ unit

23. *(a)* A is correct but B is incorrect.

In reverse biased p-n junction, the current is due to minority charge carriers, which is very small and hence measured in terms of μA.

24. *(b)* Let both masses be m

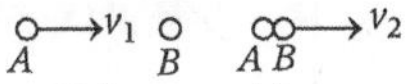

Thus, applying conservation of momentum, we get

$m_1u_1 + m_2u_2 = m_1v_1 + m_2v_2$

Both masses A and B stick together as a system.

So, $mv_1 = 2mv_2$ $\quad [\because u_2 = 0]$

$v_1 = 2v_2 \Rightarrow \frac{v_1}{v_2} = \frac{2}{1}$

Hence, option (b) is correct.

25. *(b)* Given, the rays in the prism is parallel to base.

$A = r_1 + r_2$

i.e., $r_2 = 90 - r_1$ ...(i)

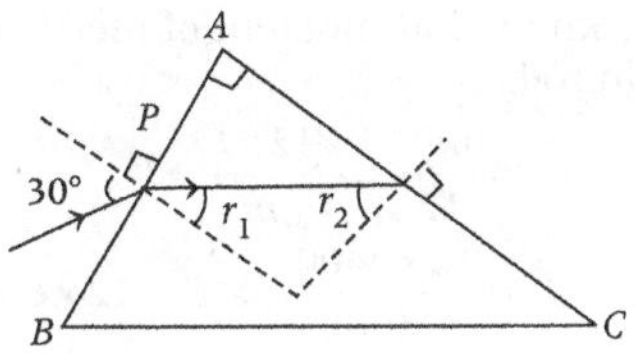

For AB interface,

$\sin 30° = \mu \sin r_1$

$\Rightarrow \sin r_1 = \frac{1}{2\mu}$ ...(ii)

For AC interface,

$\mu \sin r_2 = 1 \sin 90° \Rightarrow \sin r_2 = \frac{1}{\mu}$

$\Rightarrow \sin(90 - r_1) = \frac{1}{\mu}$

$\cos r_1 = \frac{1}{\mu}$ ...(iii)

We know that, $\sin^2\theta + \cos^2\theta = 1$

From Eqs. (ii) and (iii), we get

$\sin^2 r_1 + \cos^2 r_1 = 1$

$\Rightarrow \left(\frac{1}{2\mu}\right)^2 + \left(\frac{1}{\mu}\right)^2 = 1 \Rightarrow \frac{1}{4\mu^2} + \frac{1}{\mu^2} = 1$

$\Rightarrow \frac{1}{\mu^2}\left(\frac{1}{4} + \frac{1}{1}\right) = 1$

$\Rightarrow \mu^2 = \frac{5}{4} \Rightarrow \mu = \frac{\sqrt{5}}{2}$

26. *(d)* We know that $\lambda = \frac{h}{p} = \frac{h}{\sqrt{2mE}}$

Here, E = kinetic energy

Thus, $\lambda^2 = \frac{h^2}{2mE} \Rightarrow \frac{1}{\lambda^2} = \frac{2mE}{h^2}$

$\propto E$

Hence, option (d) is correct.

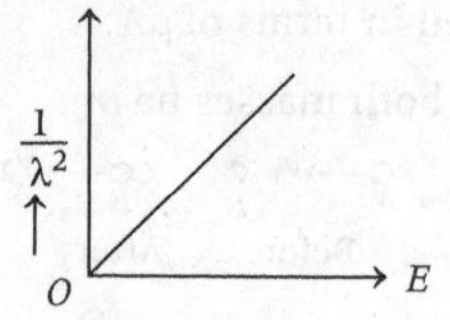

27. (a) Strain and angle are dimensionless quantities as solid angle.
Arc has dimension of length.
Stress has dimension of pressure.

28. (d) At Brewster's angle, the angle between refracted and reflected rays is 90°. The reflected ray is completely linearly polarised and the refracted rays is partially polarised.

29. (a) Given, moment of inertia
$I = 2400 \text{ g cm}^2$
mass of rod, $m = 400 \text{ g}$
We know that moment of inertia of a thin rod,

$$I = \frac{ml^2}{12} \Rightarrow \frac{12\times I}{m} = l^2$$

$$\Rightarrow \quad l^2 = \frac{12\times 2400}{400} \Rightarrow l^2 = 12\times 6$$

$$\Rightarrow \quad l = \sqrt{72} = 8.48 \simeq 8.5 \text{ cm}$$

30. (a) Radius of disc, $r = 4.5$ cm
$= 4.5\times 10^{-2}$ m
Surface tension, $S = 0.07 \text{ Nm}^{-1}$
The force required to take away circular disc from the surface of water,

$$F = S\times 2\pi r$$
$$= 0.07\times 2\times 3.14\times 4.5\times 10^{-2}$$
$$= 1.9782\times 10^{-2} \text{ N} = 19.8 \text{ mN}$$

31. (a) Work done in an isochoric process is always zero.

32. (b) In rolling motion, wheel is rolling with velocity v. All the points move with different velocity as shown

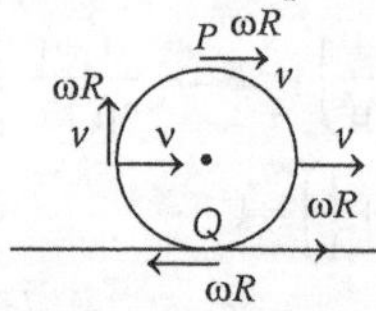

Thus, the velocity of P is greater than velocity at Q.

33. (d) We know that, $g = \frac{GM}{R^2}$

According to question,

$$g = \frac{G\left(\frac{M}{10}\right)}{\left(\frac{R}{2}\right)^2} = \frac{GM\times 4}{R^2\times 10} = \frac{GM}{R^2}\times\frac{2}{5}$$

$$\text{Hence, } \frac{g'}{g} = \frac{\frac{GM}{R^2}\times\frac{2}{5}}{\frac{GM}{R^2}}$$

$$\Rightarrow \quad g' = \frac{2}{5}\times g = \frac{2}{5}\times 9.8 = 3.92 \text{ ms}^{-2}$$

34. (a) Given combination of capacitors represent Wheatstone bridge, thus central capacitor can be removed.

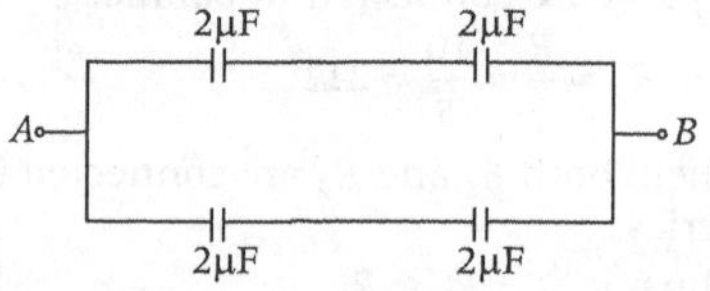

Capacitance of each branch,

$$C = \frac{2}{2} = 1 \mu\text{F}$$

Capacitance between A and B,
$C_{\text{net}} = 1 + 1 = 2\mu\text{F}$

35. (d) Since, there is no electric field inside the shell the potential at any point inside the shell is equal to the potential on the surface of the shell is

$$V = \frac{1}{4\pi\varepsilon_0}\frac{q}{r}$$

$$V_C - V_P = 0$$

36. (c) We know that

$$a = \frac{dv}{dt}$$

For v = constant, $a = 0$
Thus, for v - t graph when v is positive and linearly increasing a will be positive constant and if v is decreasing linearly a will be negative constant.
Hence, option (c) is correct.

37. (b) Time period of a bob is given by,

$$T = 2\pi\sqrt{\frac{l}{g}}$$

According to question, $T' = 2\pi\sqrt{\frac{l}{2g}}$

$$= \frac{2\pi\sqrt{l}}{\sqrt{2g}}$$

Thus, $\frac{T'}{T} = \frac{T}{\sqrt{2}} = \frac{x}{2}T$

Hence, $x = \sqrt{2}$

38. (b) Given, $C = 10\mu\text{F} = 10\times 10^{-6}$ F
Potential, $V = 210$ V
Frequency, $f = 50$ Hz
Reactance of circuit, $X_C = \frac{1}{\omega C} = \frac{1}{2\pi f C}$

$$= \frac{1}{2\times 3.14\times 50\times 10\times 10^{-6}} = \frac{10^3}{3.14}$$

Peak current, $I_m = \frac{V\sqrt{2}}{X_C} = \frac{210\times\sqrt{2}}{\frac{10^3}{3.14}}$

$$= \frac{3.14\times 210\times\sqrt{2}}{1000} \simeq 0.93 \text{ A}$$

39. (d) Charle's law states that volume of a gas is proportional to its temperature on Kelvin scale at constant pressure.
It is clear for p_1, T is higher.
Thus, $p_1 > p_2 > p_3$.

Alternate Solution

We know that $pV = nRT$

$$\frac{T}{V} = \frac{p}{nR}$$

$$\text{Slope} = \frac{p}{nR}$$

i.e., slope $\propto p$
Hence, $p_1 > p_2 > p_3$

40. (b)

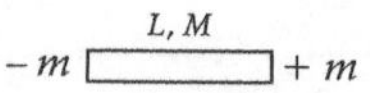

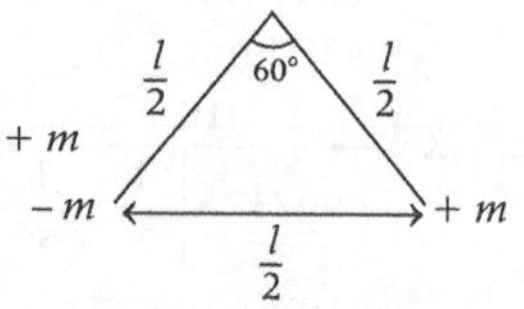

The magnetic moment is given by
$M = m\cdot L$
New magnetic moment, $M' = m\cdot L'$

$$= m\cdot\frac{l}{2} = \frac{ml}{2}$$

Thus, $M' = \frac{M}{2}$

41. (a) Given altitude, $h = 2R$
From surface, $r_1 = R$
and $r_2 = 2R + R = 3R$
Then, energy required to launch a satellite from orbit r_1 to r_2 is sum of difference in energies in the orbit (ΔE) and energy on the surface of the earth.

$$\Delta E = GMm\left(\frac{1}{r_1} - \frac{1}{r_2}\right) = GMm\left(\frac{1}{R} - \frac{1}{3R}\right)$$

$$= \frac{2}{3}\left(\frac{GMm}{R}\right)$$

Energy on surface $= \frac{1}{2}mv^2$

$$v^2 = \frac{GM}{r_{\text{orbit}}} = \frac{GM}{3R}$$

∴ Minimum energy

$$= \Delta E + \frac{GMm}{6R} = \frac{2}{3}\left(\frac{GMm}{R}\right) + \left(\frac{GMm}{6R}\right)$$

$$= \frac{5}{6}\frac{GMm}{R}$$

42. *(b)* When a capacitor is charged through a battery, its opposite plates are charged to a maximum value. There is displacement current as the capacitor is being charged, $I_d = \varepsilon \cdot \frac{d\phi_E}{dt}$

Due to charging, ϕ_E changes and hence displacement current equal to conduction current arises while charging. When capacitor gets fully charged, the displacement current became zero.

43. *(d)* Electromagnetic waves are generated by accelerated charged particles.

Hence, option (d) is incorrect.

44. *(b)* Given,

Young's modulus, $Y = 0.5 \times 10^{11}\ \text{Nm}^{-2}$

Coefficient of liner thermal expansion,

$$\alpha = 10^{-5}\ {}^\circ\text{C}^{-1}$$

Length, $l = 1\ \text{m}$

Area of cross-section, $A = 10^{-3}\text{m}^2$

$$\Delta T = 100^\circ\text{C}$$

We know that, stress $= Y \cdot \frac{\Delta l}{l}$

Here, $\Delta l = l\alpha\Delta T = 1 \times 10^{-5} \times 100 = 10^{-3}$

$$\Rightarrow \frac{F}{A} = Y \cdot \frac{10^{-3}}{1}$$

Compressive force,

$$F = 0.5 \times 10^{11} \times 10^{-3} \times 10^{-3}$$
$$= 0.5 \times 10^5 = 50 \times 10^3\ \text{N}$$

45. *(a)* For a diode to be active it must be forward biased. In option (b) and (d), diode is reverse biased.

Hence, option (b) and (d) cannot achieve bridge balance.

For option (a) :

Balance bridge condition is $\frac{10}{15} = \frac{10}{5+r}$

If $r = 10\Omega$, bridge can be balanced.

For option (c) : $\frac{10}{15} = \frac{10}{5||r}$

In this case, the resistance of 5Ω branch can only decrease.

$\therefore$ This circuit can not achieve balance condition.

46. *(b)* If the sheet is magnetic in nature, then the flux will be linked through the sheet and a small amount of force will be needed to held the sheet. The pole will apply a force on the sheet.

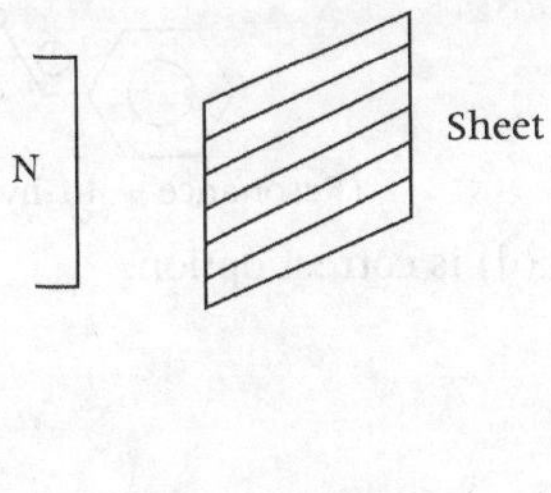

Also, to move the sheet towards or away from the magnetic pole, a force will be required.

If sheet is non-magnetic then no force will be required either to hold it or move it when the sheet is non-conducting.

47. *(b)* We know that,

$$C = \frac{\varepsilon_0 A}{d}$$

$$E = \frac{1}{2}CV^2 \text{ and } Q = C.V$$

As the distance between the plates decreases capacitance increases, therefore energy increases and also charge stored is increased.

Hence, A, C, and E are correct.

48. *(b)* Given,

$$P_1 = 1\ \text{kW}$$
$$P_2 = 2\ \text{kW}$$

$$P_{\text{Series}} = \frac{P_1P_2}{P_1 + P_2} \text{ and } P_{\text{Parallel}} = P_1 + P_2$$

According to question,

$$\frac{P_{\text{Series}}}{P_{\text{Parallel}}} = \frac{\frac{1 \times 2}{1+2}}{1+2} = \frac{2}{3 \times 3} = \frac{2}{9}$$

49. *(b)* Given,

Focal length of objective, $f_0 = 140\ \text{cm}$

Focal length of eyepiece, $f_e = 5\ \text{cm}$

Magnifying power, $M = \left[\frac{f_0}{f_e}\right]$

$$= \left[\frac{140}{5}\right] = 28$$

50. *(b)* Given, $F = \alpha t^2 + \beta t$

We know that dimensions on the both sides will be the same, i.e.,

$$[\text{F}] = [\alpha t^2] = [\beta t]$$

$$\Rightarrow [\alpha]\,[\text{T}^2] = [\text{M}^1\text{L}^1\text{T}^{-2}] \Rightarrow \alpha = [\text{M}^1\text{L}^1\text{T}^{-4}]$$

and $[\beta][\text{T}] = [\text{M}^1\text{LT}^{-2}] \Rightarrow \beta = [\text{M}^1\text{L}^1\text{T}^{-3}]$

(a) $\frac{[\beta t]}{[\alpha]} = \frac{[\text{M}^1\text{L}^1\text{T}^{-2}]}{[\text{M}^1\text{L}^1\text{T}^{-4}]} = [\text{T}^{+2}]$

(b) $\frac{[\alpha t]}{[\beta]} = \frac{[\text{M}^1\text{L}^1\text{T}^{-4}][\text{T}]}{[\text{M}^1\text{L}^1\text{T}^{-3}]} = [\text{M}^0\text{L}^0\text{T}^0]$

Hence, option (b) is correct.

Chemistry

51. *(a)* Spin only magnetic moment is given by, $\mu_s = \sqrt{n(n+2)}$

where, n = number of unpaired electrons

A. $Ti^{3+} \longrightarrow 3d^1, n = 1$

$$\mu_s = \sqrt{1(1+2)} = \sqrt{3}$$

B. $Cr^{2+} \longrightarrow 3d^4, n = 4$

$$\mu_s = \sqrt{4(4+1)} = \sqrt{20}$$

C. $Mn^{2+} \longrightarrow 3d^5, n = 5$

$$\mu_s = \sqrt{5(5+1)} = \sqrt{30}$$

D. $Fe^{2+} \longrightarrow 3d^6, n = 4$

$$\mu_s = \sqrt{4(4+1)} = \sqrt{20}$$

E. $Sc^{3+} \longrightarrow 3d^0,\ \mu_s = 0$

Hence, B and D have same value of magnetic moment.

52. *(d)* The stability of carbocation is depending on number of α-hydrogen. The more the number of alpha hydrogen atoms, more is the stability of the carbocation.

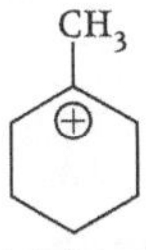

has 7 α-hydrogen, which is highest among all given structures.

53. *(a)* Both statement I and statement II are true.

54. *(a)* The correct match is

A-I, B-IV, C-II, D-III.

A. $NH_3 \longrightarrow sp^3$ hybridised with 1 lone pair $\longrightarrow$ trigonal pyramidal.

B. $BrF_5 \longrightarrow sp^3d^2$ hybridised with 1 lone pair $\longrightarrow$ square pyramidal

C. $XeF_4 \longrightarrow sp^3d^2$ hybridised with 2 lone pairs $\longrightarrow$ square planar

D. $SF_6 \longrightarrow sp^3d^2$ hybridised with zero lone pair $\longrightarrow$ octahedral

55. *(a)* In 4 moles of He, number of He atom $= 4 \times N_A$

In 4u of He, number of He atom = 1

In 4g of He, number of He atom = N_A

In 2.271098 L of He, number of He atom $= \frac{2.27}{22.7} \times N_A = 0.1 N_A$

Hence, option (a) is correct.

56. *(b)* The complete reaction is as follows,

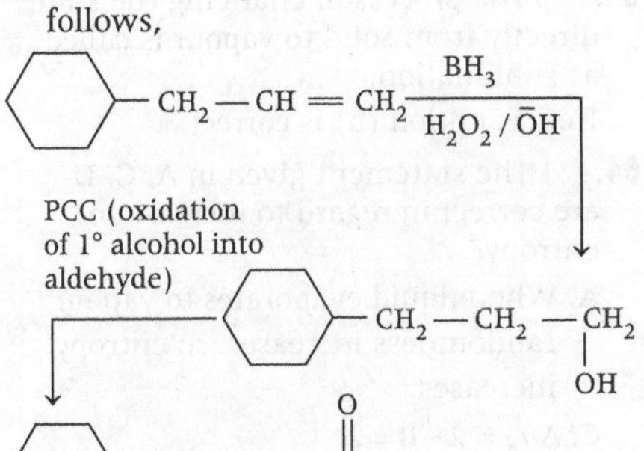

57. *(d)* The correct match is A-II, B-III, C-IV, D-I.

58. *(d)* The reactivity order of alcohols toward Lucas' reagent is 3° alcohols > 2° alcohols > 1° alcohol.

(a) $CH_3—CH_2—CH_2—CH_2—OH$
(1° alcohol)

(b) $CH_3—CH_2—CH(CH_3)—OH$
(2° alcohol)

(c) $CH_3—CH(CH_3)—CH_2—OH$
(1° alcohol)

(d) $CH_3—C(CH_3)_2—OH$
(3° alcohol)

Hence, option (d) is correct.

59. *(a)* In

$PCl_5(g) \rightleftharpoons PCl_3(g) + Cl_2(g)$

$K_p = K_C(RT)^{\Delta n_g}$

when $\Delta n_g = 0$ then $K_p = K_C$

$\Delta n_g \neq 0$ then $K_p \neq K_C$

In $PCl_5(g)$,

$\Delta n_g \neq 0 \quad \therefore \quad K_p \neq K_C$

Rest all options has $\Delta n_g = 0$.

So $K_p = K_C$ for them.

60. *(b)* The correct match is A-III, B-IV, C-I, D-II.

61. *(a)* Both statement I and statement II are true.

62. *(a)* Intramolecular hydrogen bonding is present in *o*-nitrophenol.

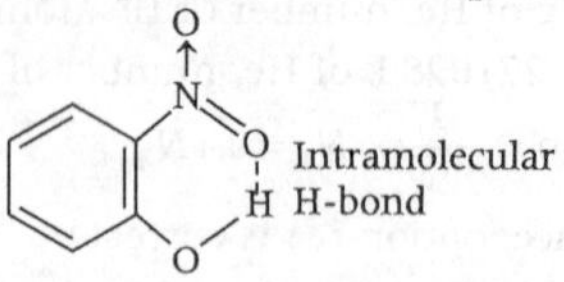

63. *(b)* The process of changing the state directly from solid to vapour is called as sublimation.

Hence, option (b) is correct.

64. *(c)* The statement given in A, C, D are correct in regard to increase in entropy.

A. When liquid evaporates to vapour, randomness increases, so entropy increases.

C. $\Delta n_g = 2 - 0 = 2$

$\Delta n_g = +ve \longrightarrow \Delta S = +ve$

$\Rightarrow$ Entropy increases.

D. $\Delta n_g = 2 - 1 = 1$

$\Delta n_g = +ve \longrightarrow \Delta S = +ve$

$\Rightarrow$ Entropy increases.

Statement given in B is incorrect, because, when temperature decreases, entropy decreases.

65. *(d)* Among the given elements, only Po does not show –2 oxidation state due to its highly metallic nature.

66. *(a)* The correct match is A-II, B-IV, C-I, D-III.

A. $2H_2O \longrightarrow O_2 + 4H^+ + 4e^-$

2 mol H_2O require 4F charge

1 mol H_2O will require 2F charge.

B. $8H^+ + MnO_4^- + 5e^- \longrightarrow Mn^{2+} + 4H_2O$

1 mole of MnO_4^- will require 5F charge.

C. $CaCl_2 + 2e^- \longrightarrow Ca + 2Cl^{-1}$

1 mole of Ca will require 2F charge.

1.5 moles of Ca will require 3F charge.

D. $FeO + H_2O \longrightarrow Fe_2O_3 + 2H^+ + 2e^-$

2 moles of FeO will require 2F charge.

1 mole of FeO will require 1 F charge.

67. *(a)* Electronegativity increases in period from left to right. The electronegativity values of given elements are,

Si = 1.8, C = 2.5

N = 3.0, O = 3.5

F = 4

Hence, the correct sequence is

Si < C < N < O < F.

68. *(c)* The correct IUPAC name and structure is,

$CH_3—\overset{3°}{CH}(CH_3)—\overset{3°}{CH}(CH_3)—CH_3$

2, 3-dimethylbutane

[2 tertiary (3°) carbon]

69. *(a)* Fehling reagent comprises of two solutions.

Fehling *A* → Aqueous solution of $CuSO_4$.

Fehling *B* → Alkaline sodium potassium tartrate (Rochelle's salt).

70. *(d)* Formula for calculating activation energy is given by

$$\log_{10}\left(\frac{k_2}{k_1}\right) = \frac{E_a}{2.303R}\left[\frac{1}{T_1} - \frac{1}{T_2}\right]$$

Here, k_1 is rate constant at T_1

k_2 is rate constant at T_2.

Hence, rate constant at two different temperatures should be known to calculate the activation energy of any chemical reaction.

71. *(d)* According to Arrhenius equation,

$k = A.e^{-E_a/RT} \Rightarrow \ln k = \ln A - \frac{E_a}{RT}$

$\ln k = \frac{-E_a}{R}\left(\frac{1}{T}\right) + \ln A$

Compare it with $y = mx + c$

$\ln k \rightarrow y$ and $1/T \rightarrow x$

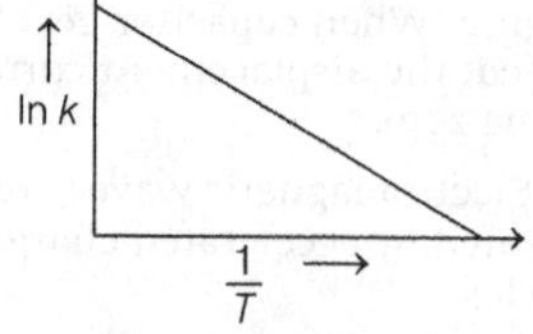

Hence, option (d) match the correct graph.

72. *(c)* The correct match is A-IV, B-I, C-II, D-III.

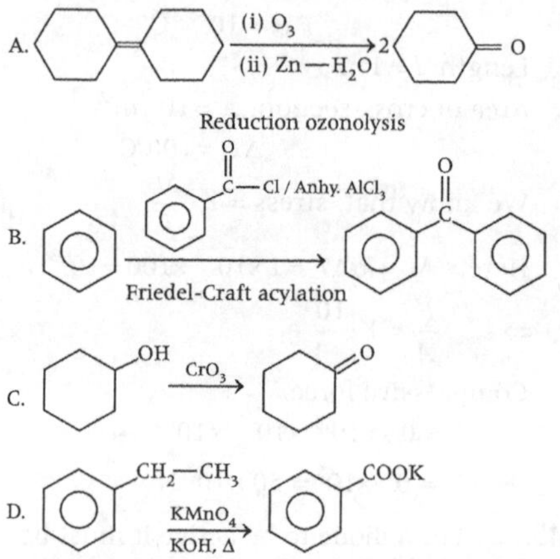

73. *(d)* Reactivity toward $S_N1 \propto$ stability of carbocation, and stability of carbocation depends on number of α-hydrogen.

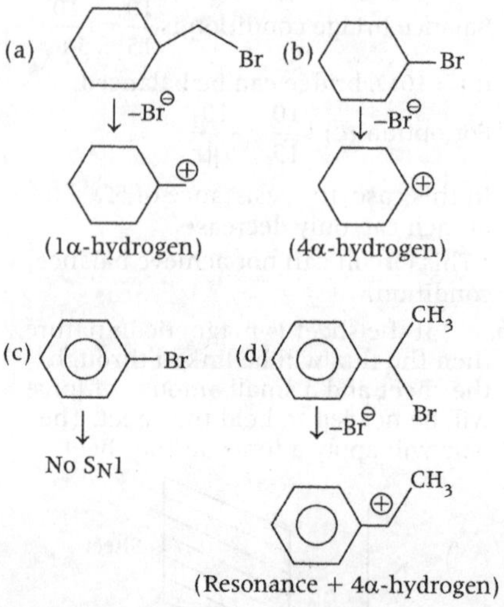

Hence, (d) is correct option.

74. (*d*) $\overset{+2\ -1}{BaCl_2} + \overset{+1\ +6-2}{Na_2SO_4} \longrightarrow \overset{+2\ +6\ -2}{BaSO_4} + \overset{+1\ -1}{2NaCl}$

As there is no change in oxidation state of any element, hence it is not a redox reaction.

75. (*a*) Both statement I and statement II are true.

76. (*a*) Both statement I and statement II are true.

77. (*c*) The correct match is A-III, B-IV, C-II, D-I.

Molecule	Structure	(Type of bonds between two carbon atoms)
A. Ethane	H_3C-CH_3	1σ
B. Ethene	$H_2C=CH_2$	1 σ, 1 π
C. C_2	C=C	2π (as per MOT)
D. Ethyne	H—C≡C—H	1 σ, 2π

78. (*b*) The relation between solubility and Henry's law constant is

Solubility $\propto \dfrac{1}{K_H}$

if K_H decreases then solubility increases. K_H for gas *B* is lowest (2×10^{-5}kbar) and *A* has highest (145 k bar).

Hence, the order of solubility is given by $B > C > A$.

79. (*a*) $E \propto \dfrac{Z^2}{n^2} \Rightarrow \dfrac{E_1}{E_2} = \dfrac{Z_1^2}{n_1^2} \times \dfrac{n_2^2}{Z_2^2}$

$He^+ \longrightarrow n_1 = 1$ and $Z_1 = 2$

$Be^{3+} \longrightarrow n_2 = 2$ and $Z_2 = 4$

$\dfrac{E_1}{E_2} = \dfrac{2^2}{1^2} \times \dfrac{2^2}{4^2} = 1 \Rightarrow E_1 = E_2$

Hence, it will be same as $-xJ$ for Be^{3+} ion.

80. (*c*) $E° = +ve$ for Mn^{3+}/Mn^{2+}

$Mn = 25 \longrightarrow 3d^5 4s^2$

$Mn^{2+} \longrightarrow 3d^5$

$Mn^{3+} \longrightarrow 3d^4$

Mn^{2+} has half-filled ($3d^5$) stable configuration.

Thus, Mn^{3+} has very high tendency to gain an electron due to this it has high +ve value of electrode potential ($E°$) while in other case, they does not gain electron easily.

Hence, the reason is change of d^4 to d^5-configuration.

81. (*c*) Glucose does not react with Schiff's reagent and $NaHSO_3$.

Glucose + Tollen's reagent ⟶ silver mirror

Glucose + HCN ⟶ cyanohydin formation

Glucose + NH_2OH ⟶ oxime formation

82. (*a*) The correct match is A-II, B-III, C-IV, D-I.

83. (*b*) First ionisation enthalpy is the energy required to remove the first most loosely bound electron from an isolated atom in its ground state.

The electronic configuration is,

$Li \rightarrow 2s^1$, $Be \rightarrow 2s^2$, $B \rightarrow 2s^2, 2p^1$

$C \rightarrow 2s^2 2p^2$, $N \rightarrow 2s^2 2p^3$

The correct increasing order is,

$Li < B < Be < C < N$

84. (*b*) $NaOH + HCl \longrightarrow NaCl + H_2O$

Given, mass of NaOH = 1g

Mole of NaOH $= \dfrac{1}{40}$ mol $= 0.025$ mol

Mole of HCl $= \dfrac{0.75 \times 25}{1000} = 0.01875$ mol

Now finding the limiting reagent (LR)

value $= \dfrac{\text{Given amount}}{\text{Stiochiometry coefficient}}$

NaOH : HCl, $\dfrac{0.025}{1} > \dfrac{0.01875}{1}$

So, limiting reagent (LR) will be HCl

Unreacted moles of NaOH

$= 0.025 - 0.01875 = 0.00625$ mol

Unreacted mass $= 0.00625 \times 40$ g $= 0.25$ g $= 250$ mg

85. (*c*) For the given reaction,

$2A \rightleftharpoons B + C$, $K_C = 4 \times 10^{-3}$

At a given time

$[A] = [B] = [C] = 2 \times 10^{-3}$ M

$Q_C = \dfrac{[B][C]}{[A]^2} \Rightarrow Q_C = 1$

As $Q_C > K_C$, reaction has tendency to go in backward direction.

86. (*a*)

Basic radical	Group number	
(B) Cu^{2+}	II	Group number increases ↓
(A) Al^{3+}	III	
(D) Co^{2+}	IV	
(C) Ba^{2+}	V	
(E) Mg^{2+}	VI	

Hence, the correct order is B, A, D, C, E.

87. (*d*) The reaction involves are,

$3R{-}OH + PCl_3 \longrightarrow 3RCl + H_3PO_3(A)$

$R{-}OH + PCl_5 \longrightarrow R{-}Cl + HCl + POCl_3(B)$

Hence, products *A* and *B* are

$A = H_3PO_3$; $B = POCl_3$

88. (*b*) Given, current (i) = 9.6487 A

1F = 96487 C

$t = 100$ s

$w = \dfrac{E(it)}{96487} \Rightarrow w = \dfrac{\frac{63}{2} \times 9.6487 \times 100}{96487}$

$w = 0.315$ g of Cu

89. (*a*) Osmotic pressure is given by,

$\pi = CRT$

Plot is of between osmotic pressure and concentration, i.e. π *vs* *C*.

On comparing with $y = mx + C$

Slope $m = RT$

$25.73 = 0.083 \times T$

$T = 310\,K = 37°C$

90. (*a*) The complete reaction is as follow,

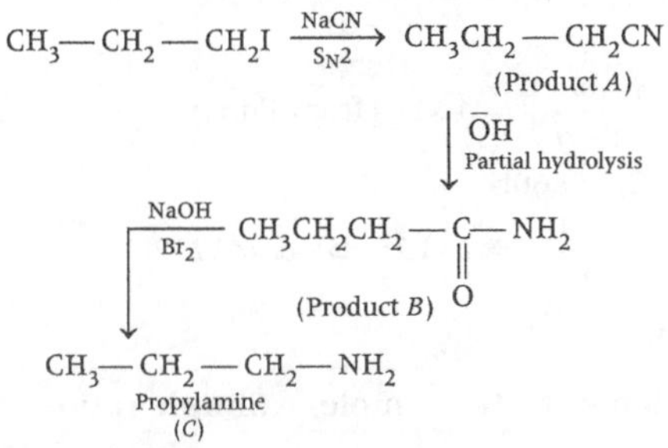

91. (*d*) Three canonical form can be drawn for CO_3^{2-} ion.

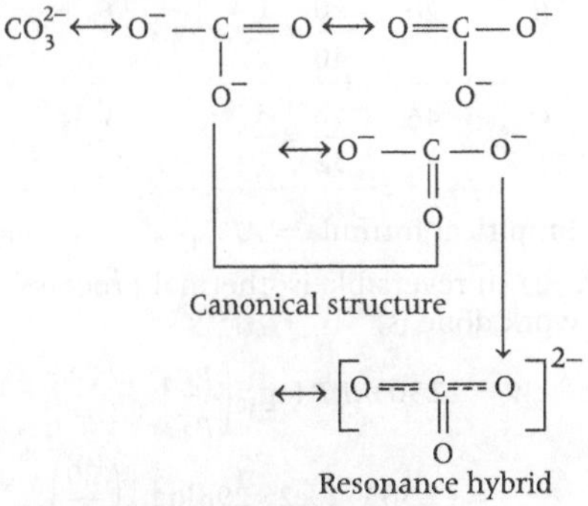

Other corrected forms are

(a) Ozone has only two resonating structure.

(b) BF_3 has zero dipole moment.

(c) Dipole moment of NH_3 is greater than NF_3.

92. *(a)* Both statement I and statement II are true.

93. *(b)* The complete reaction is as follows,

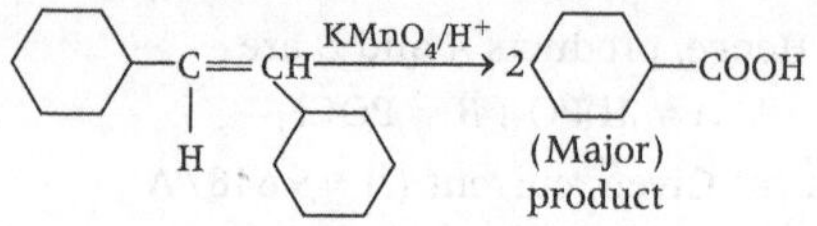

(Major) product

94. *(a)* $Ce^{4+} = [Xe]\,4f^0\,5d^0$

$Yb^{2+} = [Xe]4f^{14}\,5d^0$

Both ions does not contain any unpaired electrons.

Hence, they are diamagnetic.

95. *(d)* $\underset{(2.8\times10^{-3}M)}{2NO(g)} \rightleftharpoons \underset{(3\times10^{-3}M)}{N_2(g)} + \underset{(4.2\times10^{-3}M)}{O_2(g)}$

$$K_C = \frac{[N_2][O_2]}{[NO]^2}$$

$$= \frac{3\times10^{-3}\times4.2\times10^{-3}}{(2.8\times10^{-3})^2} = 1.60 \quad .... \text{(i)}$$

$$\underset{t=t_{eq}\ (C-C\alpha)}{2NO(g)} \rightleftharpoons \underset{\frac{C\alpha}{2}}{N_2(g)} + \underset{\frac{C\alpha}{2}}{O_2(g)}$$

$$K_C = \frac{(C\alpha)^2}{4C^2(1-\alpha)^2}$$

$$\left(\frac{\alpha}{1-\alpha}\right)^2 = 4\times1.6 \text{ [from Eq.(i)}$$

$K_C = 1.60]$

$$\frac{\alpha}{1-\alpha} = 2\times1.26 \Rightarrow \alpha = 0.717$$

96. *(b)*

Element	%	mole	Simple ratio
A	32	$\frac{32}{64}=\frac{1}{2}$	1
B	20	$\frac{20}{40}=\frac{1}{2}$	1
C	46	$\frac{48}{32}=\frac{3}{2}$	3

Empirical formula = ABC_3

97. *(b)* In reversible isothermal process, work done is,

$$W = -2.303nRT\log_{10}\left(\frac{p_1}{p_2}\right)$$

$$= -2.303\times1\times2\times298\log_{10}\left(\frac{20}{10}\right)$$

$= -413.14$ calories

98. *(d)* Dilute H_2SO_4 do not act as oxidising agent which prevent oxidation of Fe^{2+} into Fe^{3+} while concentrated H_2SO_4 will oxidise Fe^{2+} into Fe^{3+}.

99. *(a)* Given, rate is quadruples, i.e. $r_2 = 4r_1$

We know, $\frac{r_2}{r_1} = 4 = \frac{k_2}{k_1}$

Now, $\log_{10}\left(\frac{k_2}{k_1}\right) = \frac{E_a}{2.303R}\left[\frac{1}{T_1} - \frac{1}{T_2}\right]$

[where, $T_1 = 27°C = 300K$,

$T_2 = 57°C = 330K$]

$$\log_{10}(4) = \frac{E_a\times1000}{2.303\times8.314}\left(\frac{1}{300} - \frac{1}{330}\right)$$

$E_a = 38.04$ kJ/mol

100. *(a)* The complete reaction is as follow,

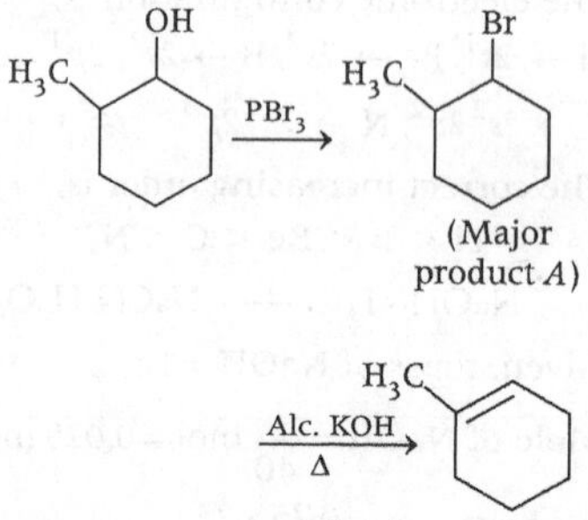

(Major product *A*)

(Major product *B*)

Botany

101. *(b)* Lecithin is a type of phospholipid which is a class of lipids. These are the major components of cell membranes. Lecithin specifically contains a phosphate group, a glycerol backbone, two fatty acid chains and a choline molecule.

102. *(c)* The dark reaction of photosynthesis, also known as biosynthetic phase, occurs in the stroma of chloroplasts. It does not require direct light, instead it utilises the products of the light dependent reaction, i.e. ATP and NADPH, along with CO_2, to produce glucose. These molecules provide the necessary energy and carbon source for the synthesis of glucose during the dark reaction of photosynthesis.

Therefore, the correct option is (c).

103. *(b)* During metaphase, the chromosomes are aligned at the metaphase plate, which is the equitorial plane of the cell. At this stage, spindle fibres, also known as microtubules, attach to the kinetochores, which are specialised protein structures located at the centromeres of the chromosomes. These spindle fibres help to align the chromosomes properly along the metaphase plate. It also ensures that each chromatid will be pulled to opposite poles of the cell during anaphase.

104. *(a)* In grasses (monocots), certain adaxial epidermal cells along the veins modify themselves into large, empty, colourless cells. These are called bulliform cells. When the bulliform cells in the leaves have absorbed water and become turgid, the leaf surface is exposed. When they are flaccid due to water stress, they make the leaves curl inwards to minimise water loss.

105. *(a)* Component *c* represents guard cells.

Guard cells are kidney-shaped, specialised cells in plants that control the opening and closing of the stomata. The outer walls of guard cells are thin and inner walls are highly thickened.

Rest components can be identified as

A-**Epidermal cells** are parenchymatous with a small amount of cytoplasm lining the cell wall and a large vacuole.

B-**Subsidiary cells** are specialised epidermal cell, in the vicinity of the guard cells.

D-**Stomatal pores** are tiny openings on the surface of leaves that control gaseous exchange in plants.

106. *(c)* Statements B and C are correct regarding the piece of DNA carrying only gene of interest, transferred into an alien organism.

Rest statements are incorrect and these can be corrected as

- DNA typically requires host cellular machinery to replicate. It cannot multiply independently in progeny cells without the help of the host organism.
- When the DNA integrates into the host genome, it becomes an integral part of the chromosome.
- While the transferred DNA indeed have the ability to replicate if it contains appropriate regulatory sequences, replication alone does not guarantee its inheritance or integration into the host genome.

107. *(c)* Statement I is true, but statement II is false. The incorrect statement can be corrected as

The *Bt* toxin protein exists as inactive protoxins in *B. thuringiensis*, but once an insect ingest the inactive toxin, it is converted into an active form of toxin due to the alkaline pH of the gut.

108. *(d)* The International Union for Conservation of Nature and Natural Resources (IUCN) is a global organisation dedicated to assessing the conservation status of species and ecosystems. It releases lists of endangered species in Red Data Book. The IUCN Red List of threatened species is the most comprehensive source of information on the list of extinction for animal, plant and fungus species.
As of 2023, the IUCN Red List includes more than 157,100 species, with more than 44,000 threatened with extinction.

109. *(c)* Based on the given figure of a seed, the part destined to form the root when the seed germinates is the embryonic root or radicle *(C)*.
It is the first part of the embryo to develop into the plant's root system. The radicle grows downward into the soil, anchoring the seedling and allowing it to absorb water and nutrients.
Rest parts can be identified as
A-**Coleoptile** is a cylindrical, rigid, protective sheath that covers the first leaf and shoot apex of a grass seedling.
B-**Plumule** is the embryonic shoot of a plant.
D-**Coleorhiza** is a protective layer of tissue that surrounds the embryonic root or radicle of monocot seeds.

110. *(c)* A-III, B-I, C-IV, D-II
- ***Clostridium butylicum*** is a bacterium known for its ability to produce butyric acid through fermentation.
- ***S. cerevisiae*** is a yeast commonly used in fermentation process, such as brewing and baking, where it produces ethanol as a metabolic byproduct.
- ***Trichoderma polysporum*** is a fungus that produces cyclosporin-A, a potent immunosuppressive agent.
- ***Streptococcus* sp.** produces streptokinase, a thrombolytic agent.

111. *(d)* Both of the given figures *A* and *B* represent perigynous condition. In this condition gynoecium is situated in the centre and other parts of the flower are located on the rim of the thalamus almost at the same level. The ovary in these flowers is said to be half inferior, e.g. plum, rose, peach, etc.

112. *(c)* Auxin is a plant hormone that regulates various aspects of plant development. They are commonly used by gardeners to prepare weed free lawns, it does not affect mature monocotyledonous plants (grass). Auxin primarily promotes the abscission of mature leaves, particularly in broad leaf weeds, i.e. dictoyledonous weeds.
Rest other options are correct regarding auxin, but not relevant to the scenario described.

113. *(b)* The inheritance of flower colour in snapdragon shows incomplete dominance.
The cross between pink flower and red flower is as follows

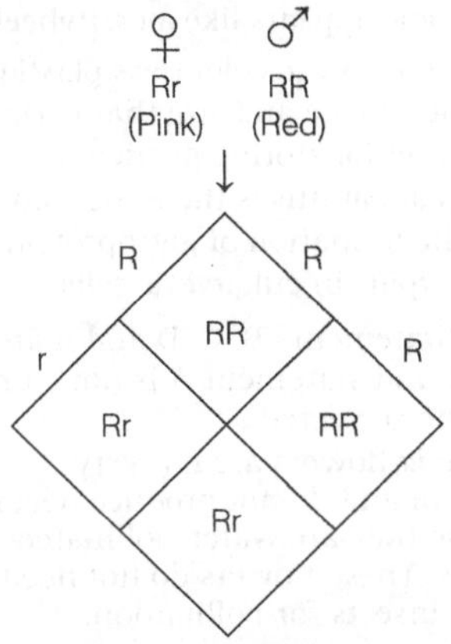

Genotypic ratio—(Red) : Pink
1 1
Phenotypic ratio—RR : Rr
1 : 1
Thus, the expected progeny will be red as well as pink flowered plants.

114. *(b)* The morphology of the mycelium, mode of spore formation and fruiting bodies form the basis for the division of the kingdom into various classes. It does not depend on the mode of nutrition. Fungi are heterotrophs, they can not make their own food.

115. *(c)* Permease is a type of transporter protein that facilitates the movement of molecules such as lactose, across the cell membrane.
Other options can be explained as
In *E. coil*, it is coded by gene *Y*.
Inside the bacterial cell, the enzyme β-galactosidase catalyses the hydrolysis of lactose into its constituent monosaccharides, i.e., glucose and galactose.
This enzymatic reaction enables the bacterium to utilise lactose as a carbon source for energy and growth.
- Acetylase is involved in acetylation reactions. It speeds up the production of acetic acid esters.
- Polymerase is an enzyme involved in DNA replication and RNA transcription.

116. *(b)* To determine the genotype of the black seed plant, one needs to perform a test cross by crossing it with a plant that has the homozygous recessive genotype (bb)
It can be explained through the following crosses
Case I If parent is homozygous dominant.
Gametes from homozygous dominant parent (BB)

Gametes from recessive parent (bb)		B	B
	b	Bb	Bb
	b	Bb	Bb

All of the progeny will be of dominant phenotype.
Case II If parent is heterozygous dominant.
Gametes from heterozygous parent (Bb)

Gametes from recessive parent (bb)		B	b
	b	Bb	bb
	b	Bb	bb

It will results into 1 : 1 ratio of black and white seed.

117. *(d)* Statement I is false, but Statement II is true. Incorrect statement can be corrected as
Both parenchyma and collenchyma cells are living tissue. The collenchyma occurs in layers below the epidermis in most of the dicotyledonous plants. It consists of cells which are more thickened at the corners due to the deposition of cellulose, hemicellulose and pectin.

118. *(d)* Each turn of Calvin cycle requires a certain number of molecules of ATP and NADPH to provide energy and reducing power, respectively, for the various chemical reactions involved.
For every CO_2 molecule entering the Calvin cycle, 3 molecules of ATP and 2 molecules of NADPH are required.

119. *(d)* A transcription unit is a segment of DNA that takes part in transcription. It has three components.

(i) **Promoter** It is located towards 5′ end of the structural gene and provides binding site for RNA polymerase.

(ii) **Structural gene** It codes for an RNA.

(iii) **Terminator** : It is located towards 3′-end of the coding strand and usually defines the end of the process of transcription.

120. *(a)* Statements A, C, D and E are the correct explanation for the species richness in tropical regions because

- tropical latitudes have remained relatively undisturbed for millions of years and thus had a long evolutionary time for species diversification.
- these environments are less seasonal, relatively more constant and predictable. Such constant environments promote niche specialisation. It leads to a greater species diversity.
- more solar energy is available in the tropics, which contributes to higher productivity. This, in turn might contribute indirectly to greater diversity.

121. *(c)* In the Verhulst-Pearl logistic growth equation, K represents the carrying capacity of the environment for a particular species. Carrying capacity is the maximum population size that the environment can sustainably support over the long term. It is determined by factors such as the availability of resources, space and other environmental conditions.

122. *(c)* Competitive inhibition occurs when a molecule, known as the inhibitor, competes with the substrate for binding to the active site of the enzyme. In the case of succinic dehydrogenase, malonate competes with the substrate for binding to the active site of the enzyme. Malonate structurally resembles succinate, the substrate for succinate dehydrogenase, and can therefore bind to the enzyme's active site.

Rest options can be explained as

- **Cofactor inhibition** involves the inhibition of an enzyme by binding to its cofactor, not the active site.
- **Feedback inhibition** occurs when the end product of a metabolic pathway inhibits an enzyme earlier in the pathway.
- **Enzyme activation** refers to processes that increase the activity of an enzyme.

123. (b) Statements A, C, D, and E can be explained on the basis of Mendel's law of dominance.

Statement B contradicts Mendel's law of dominance because, in the F_2-generation, the recessive alleles can still be expressed if present in the genotype, although they may be masked in the F_1-generation due to dominance.

124. *(a)* A-III, B-II, C-IV, D-I

- Nucleolus is the site for active ribosomal RNA synthesis.
- Centrioles are the two cylindrical structures in the centrosome. Each centriole appears like a cartwheel.
- Leucoplasts are colourless plastids of various shape and size that perform function for storing nutrients.

  Golgi apparatus is the important site for the formation of glycoproteins and glycolipids in eukaryotic cells.

125. *(d)* Statements B, C, D and E are correct and statement A is not correct, it can be corrected as

Vallisneria flowers are not very colourful and do not produce nectar because they are water-pollinated flowers. These flowers do not need to attract insects for pollination.

126. *(a)* A-III, B-II, C-IV, D-I.

- *Rhizopus* is commonly known as bread mould. It belongs to Class-Phycomycetes of kingdom of Fungi.
- *Ustilago* is commonly known as smut. It belongs to Class-Basidiomycetes of kingdom of Fungi.
- *Puccinia* is commonly known as rust fungi.

  It belongs to Class-Basidiomycetes of kingdom of Fungi.
- *Agaricus* is commonly called mushroom. It belongs to Class-Basidiomycetes of kingdom Fungi.

127. *(b)* *Hind* II is a restriction endonuclease that cuts DNA molecules at a specific point by recognising a sequence of 6 base pairs. This specific base sequence is known as the recognition sequence. *Hind* II specifically recognises 5′–AAGCTT - 3′ -sequence.

128. *(a)* An actinomorphic flower is one that can be divided into symmetrical halves in any plane, typically through the center, resulting in multiple lines of symmetry. In the given example, *Datura* flower shows actinomorphic symmetry.

In *Cassia*, *Pisum* and *Sesbania*, zygomorphic flowers are seen.

129. *(b)* The type of conservation in which threatened animals and plants are taken out from their natural habitat and placed in special setting where they can be protected and given special care is called *ex situ* conservation. It is a type of biodiversity conservation.

The biodiversity conservation is a broad term that encompasses various conservation strategies, including both *in situ* and *ex situ* conservation.

130. *(a)* Both statement I and statement II are true.

131. *(c)* Dedifferentiation is a cellular process in plants where differentiated cells revert to a less differentiated or stem cell-like state. This process allows the cells to regain their ability to divide and re-enter the cell cycle.

In the case of the formation of interfascicular cambium from fully developed parenchyma cells, these parenchyma cells undergo dedifferentiation to become meristematic cells that are capable of division. These meristematic cells then differentiate into cambial cells, which give rise to secondary growth in plants.

Other options can be explained as

- Differentiation refers to the process by which undifferentiated cells become specialised into specific cell types.
- Redifferentiation is a process by which dedifferentiated cells regain their specialised characteristics.

132. *(a)* Totipotency refers to the capacity of a single plant cell to give rise to an entire new plant. Totipotent cells have the ability to regenerate into all types of cell and tissues. It plays crucial role in various aspects of plant biology, including regeneration, tissue culture and plant propagation.

Rest options can be explained as

- Micropropagation is a technique used to produce large numbers of genetically identical plants from a single parent plant using tissue culture methods.

- Somatic hybridisation involves the fusion of protoplasts from different plant species to produce hybrids with combined traits.

133. *(c)* A-III, B-IV, C-I, D-II.
- Two or more alternative forms of gene are called alleles.
- Cross of F_1-progeny with homozygous recessive parent is a test cross.
- Cross of F_1-progeny with any of the parents is a back cross.
- Number of chromosome sets in plant is called ploidy.

134. *(a)* Zinc is a cofactor for the proteolytic enzyme carboxypeptidase. A cofactor is a non-protein part of an enzyme that is made up of metal ions. In carboxypeptidase, the zinc cofactor is located in the active site of the enzyme and is essential for its catalytic ativity.
- Niacin is associated with coenzyme NAD and NADP.
- Haem is the prosthetic group in peroxidase and catalase.
- Flavin as a cofactor catalyses the oxidation of nucleophilic nitrogen, sulphur and phosphate.

135. *(d)* The accelerated rates of sepcies extinctions that the world is facing now are largely due to human activities.
These are four major causes ('The Evil Quartet' is the sobriquet used to describe them)
(i) Habitat loss and fragmentation
(ii) Overexploitation
(iii) Alien-species invasions
(iv) Co-extinctions
Hence, the correct option is (d).

136. *(a)* A-IV, B-II, C-I, D-III.
- In China rose monoadelphous androecium is present.
- Diadelophous androecium is found in pea plant.
- Polyadelphous androecium is found is citrus.
- Epiphyllous androecium is found in lily.

137. *(a)* A-IV, B-I, C-II, D-III.
- GLUT-4 is a glucose transporter protein found in the membrane of certain cells.
- Insulin is a hormone produced by the pancreas that regulates glucose metabolism.
- Trypsin is an enzyme involved in the digestion of proteins.
- Collagen is a structural protein found in the extracellular matrix of various tissues.

138. *(c)* In the tricarboxylic acid cycle, most of the steps involve the oxidation of substrates, leading to the generation of reducing equivalents, i.e., NADH and $FADH_2$ and ATP. However, the conversion of succinyl Co-A to succinic acid by the enzyme succinyl Co-A synthetase, does not directly involve oxidation.
Rest other conversions involve oxidation.

139. *(b)* A-II, B-I, C-IV, D-III.
- The citric acid cycle occurs in the mitochondrial matrix.
- The glycolysis occurs in the cytoplasm of the cell.
- The electron transport system takes place in the inner mitochondrial membrane.
- The proton gradient is established across the intermembrane space of mitochondria.

140. *(b)* A-III, B-IV, C-I, D-II.
- Frederick Griffith's in a series of experiment with *Streptococcus pneumoniae* witness miraculous transformation in the bacteria.
- The elucidation of *lac* operon was a result of a close association between geneticist, Francois Jacob and a biochemist, Jacque Monod.
- Har Gobind Khorana developed chemical method to define combination of bases in genetic code.
- Meselson and Stahl provide proof of the semi-conservative mode of DNA replication.

141. *(c)* Statement I is true, but Statement II is false. It can be corrected as
Photorespiration does not occur in C_4 plants as they lack RuBisCO in mesophyll cells. Additionally, bundle sheath cells in C_4-plants do not show photorespiration due to the Kranz anatomy.

142. *(a)* The correct description about the given figure is given in option (a). Wind pollinated flowers possess well exposed stamens. This is an adaptation to maximise pollen dispersal by wind. Having well exposed stamens ensures that the pollen is readily available for dispersal.

143. *(a)* A-II, B-IV, C-I, D-III.
- In rose, gynoecium is said to be perigynous.
- In pea, placenta forms a ridge along the ventral suture of the ovary and the ovules are borne on this ridge forming two rows. This type of placentation is known as marginal.
- In twisted aestivation, margin of the appendage overlaps that of the next one, e.g. cotton.
- In mango, fruit is drupe.

144. *(c)* Statements A, C, D and E are correct w.r.t the members of Phaeophyceae. Statement B is not correct, it can be corrected as
In members of Phaeophyceae, sexual reproduction can be isogamous, anisogamous and oogamous. They produce motile gametes that are biflagellate, with two laterally attached flagella.

145. *(c)* The NPP of the first trophic level is the GPP of the second trophic level and the NPP of the second trophic level is GPP of the third trohpic level.
According to the 10% law, 90% is the respiratory loss at each trophic level.
$NPP = GPP - R$
At the first trophic level NPP is $100x$ which is GPP of second trophic level.
At second trophic level NPP is 10% of $GPP = 10x$. Since, the GPP of the 3rd trophic level is the same as the NPP of the second trophic level, it is equal to $10x$.

146. *(d)* Statement in option (d) is correct regarding the process of replication in *E. coli*. It can be explained as
In living cells, such as E. coli, the process of replication requires a set of catalysts .or enzymes. The main enzyme is referred to as DNA-dependent DNA polymerase. These enzymes use a DNA template to catalyse the polymerisation of deoxynucleotides. The enzyme DNA-dependent DNA polymerase catalyses polymerisation only in one direction, i.e. $5' \rightarrow 3'$.

147. *(c)* In somatic hybridisation, protoplasts of two varieties of plants are fused. During this process, protoplasts are isolated and brought together and fused using techniques such as chemical treatment or electric fields. This fusion combines the genetic material from the two parent plants, leading to the formation of somatic hybrids.

148. *(b)* Spraying sugarcane crop with gibberellin increases the length of the stem, thus increasing the yield by as much as 20 tonnes per acre.

Gibberellins are plant hormones that promote stem elongation, cell division and cell expansion. Applying gibberellin to sugarcane crops, stimulate the elongation of the internodes. This increased stem length allows for more space for sugar accumulation and ultimately leads to higher yields.

Other options can be corrected as

- Auxin primarily regulates plant growth by promoting cell elongation and is not responsible for stem elongation in sugarcane.
- Cytokinin is involved in cell division and lateral bud development, whereas abscisic acid acts as stress hormone.

149. *(b)* A-III, B-I, C-IV, D-II.

- Robert May places the global species diversity at about 7 million.
- Alexander von Humboldt provided species-area relationship.
- Paul Ehrlich used an analogy "rivet popper hypothesis" to explain the role of species in the ecosystem.
- David Tilman performed long term ecosystem experiments using outdoor plots.

150. *(b)* Chloroplasts are organelles found in plant cells, responsible for photosynthesis. They contain their own genome, which is typically a circular molecule of DNA. This DNA is double stranded.

The circular nature of chloroplast DNA is a characteristic feature shared with bacterial DNA, reflecting the endosymbiotic theory.

Zoology

151. *(c)* A-III, B-I, C-II, D-IV.

- Common cold is caused by rhinoviruses.
- Haemozoin is a chemical released due to the rupturing of RBC by *Plasmodium*.
- Widal test is used to diagnose typhoid.
- Allergy is caused by allergens like dust, mites.

152. *(d)* A-III, B-IV, C-I, D-II.

- Cocaine is derived from coca plant, i.e. *Erythroxylum*.
- Heroin is an opioid obtained from latex of poppy plant, *Papaver somniferum*.
- Morphine is an effective sedative used for treating patients who have undergone surgery.
- Marijuana is a cannabinoid obtained from the plant *Cannabis sativa*.

153. *(d)* A-III, B-I, C-IV, D-II.

- Fibrous joints are present in skull. They do not allow any movement.
- Cartilaginous joints are present in adjacent vertebrae. They provide limited movement.
- Hinge joint is present in knee and helps in locomotion.
- Ball and socket joints are present between humerus and pectoral girdle and provide rotational movement.

154. *(b)* Among the given options myasthenia gravis, rheumatoid arthritis and Systemic Lupus Erythematosus (SLE) are autoimmune disorders. The autoimmune disease is a type of disease in which the body's immune system attacks healthy tissues of the body. Other options can be explained as

Gout is an inflammatory disorder and muscular dystrophy is a progressive degeneration of skeletal muscles in which mutated genes interfere with healthy muscle function.

155. *(a)* Uterine fundus is not a component of Fallopian tube. It is the part of uterus that is farthest away from its opening, the cervix. On the other hand isthmus, infundibulum and ampulla are the parts of Fallopian tube.

156. *(c)* The flippers of the penguins and dolphins are the examples of convergent evolution. The convergent evolution can be defined as a process in which unrelated organisms evolve similar body forms, colourations and adaptations. However, they do not belong to a common ancestor.

157. *(c)* A-III, B-IV, C-I, D-II.

- α-1 antitrypsin is used for treatment of emphysema.
- *cry* I Ab gene controls corn borer.
- *cry* I Ac controls cotton bollworm.
- Enzyme replacement therapy can be used as treatment in ADA deficiency.

158. *(b)* In the given figure of pBR322, *X* represents *'ori'* region, while *Y* represent *'rop'* region. The *'ori'* site is the origin of replication that controls the copy number of the linked DNA. Whereas *rop* codes for proteins which are involved in the process of replication of the plasmid.

159. *(a)* Both A and R are correct and R is the correct explanation of A.

Doctors recommend breast-feeding during initial period of infant growth because it contains IgA antibodies that provide passive immunity to the new born baby.

160. *(c)* The 'Ti-plasmid' of *Agrobacterium tumefaciens* stands for tumour inducing plasmid. It induces crown gall disease in plants by transferring crucial regions from the plasmid.

161. (b) A-II, B-I, C-IV, D-III.

- *Pleurobrachia* is a member of phylum-Ctenophora.
- Radula is a rasping or feeding organ present in phylum-Mollusca.
- Stomochord is rudimentary structure similar to notochord found in collar region of members of phylum-Hemichordata.
- Air bladder is found in Osteichthyes, which regulates buoyancy.

162. (d) The correct sequence of human evolution from past to recent is as follows

Homo habilis → *Homo erectus* → *Homo neanderthalensis* → *Homo sapiens*

Homo habilis appeared around 3.2 mya. They were capable of making sharpened tools and their cranial capacity was 650-800 cc.

Homo erectus appeared around 1.5 mya. They had erect body posture and cranial capacity was 900 cc.

Homo neanderthalensis appeared around 40,000 to 1,00,000 years ago. They had cranial capacity of 1400 cc.

Homo sapiens is the modern man evolved somewhere between 75,000 to 10,000 years ago. Their cranial capacity is 1450 cc.

163. *(d)* Glucagon is a peptide hormone. It is produced by α-cells of the pancreas. It raises the concentration of glucose and fatty acids in the blood stream. On the other hand, cortisol, testosterone and progesterone are the examples of steroid hormones.

164. *(b)* Anal cerci, a pair of jointed filamentous structures are present on 10th segment in both sexes of cockroach. These are sense organs that are sensitive to wind and also detect vibration.

165. *(d)* Among the given options, a constant gene pool will not affect the Hardy-Weinberg equilibrium. It was proposed by GH Hardy and W Weinberg independently in 1908. According to this, a stable population has constant allelic frequencies in sexually reproducing organisms from generations to generations. The factors which cause change in allelic frequencies in a population are recombination, mutation, gene migration, genetic drift and natural selection.

166. *(b)* A-III, B-IV, C-II, D-I.
- Pons connects different regions of the brain.
- Hypothalamus also have neuro secretory cells which secrete hormone.
- Medulla controls respiration and gastric secretion.
- Cerebellum provides additional space for neurons, regulates posture and balance.

167. *(c)* A-III, B-IV, C-I, D-II.
- Down's syndrome is caused due to trisomy of 21st chromosome.
- α-thalassemia is controlled by two closely linked genes HBA1 and HBA2 on chromosome 16 of each parent and occurs due to mutation or deletion of one or more of the four genes.
- β-thalassemia is controlled by a single gene HBB on chromosome 11 of each parent and occurs due to mutation of one or both genes.
- Klinefelter's syndrome is caused due to the presence of an additional copy of X chromosome resulting into a karyotype of 47, XXY.

168. *(a)* The strand of DNA which is copied into *m*RNA and subsequently translated, possesses complementary sequence to the *m*RNA. It is called as template strand. During transcription, RNA polymerase binds to the template strand and synthesis RNA. However, due to the complementarity rule, in RNA uracil is present in place of thyamine. Therefore, the correct product will be determined as follows :

3′ TACATGGCAAATATCCATTCA5′
5′ AUGUACCGUUUAUAGGUAAGU3′

169. *(d)* A is false, but R is true. A can be corrected as
LH and FSH both are secreted by anterior pituitary. In females, FSH acts upon ovarian follicles; while LH stimulates Leydig's cells of testis to secrete androgen.

170. *(d)* Among the given options, vaults are not the natural contraceptive methods instead, they are barrier methods. The vaults are disposable cup like structures made of rubber that are inserted into the vaginal tract to cover the cervix before coitus. They prevent the entry of sperms through cervix to prevent fertilisation.

171. *(d)* A-III, B-I, C-IV, D-II.
- Example of non-medicated IUD is lippes loop.
- Example of copper releasing IUD is Multiload 375.
- Example of hormone releasing IUD is LNG-20.
- Example of implants is progestogens.

172. *(b)* Among the given statements, only statement A is correct. Rest of the statements are incorrect and can be corrected as follows
- Poriferans and Platyhelminthes are acoelomate as they lack coelom.
- Aschelminthes are pseudocoelomates.

173. *(b)* (i) represents skeletal muscles which is present in triceps. These are voluntary muscles and show striations.
(ii) represents smooth muscles which are involuntary in action and are present in stomach, whereas (iii) represents cardiac muscles which are exclusively found in heart.

174. *(a)* The correct sequence of pathway for conduction of an action potential through the heart is as follows

SA node → AV node → AV bundle → Bundle branches → Purkinje fibres

175. *(c)* A-II, B-IV, C-I, D-III.
- Lipase helps in digestion of ester bond.
- Nuclease helps in digestion of phosphodiester bond.
- Protease helps in digestion of peptide bond.
- Amylase helps in digestion of glycosidic bond.

176. (d) A-II, B-I, C-IV, D-III.
- Axoneme is seen in cilia and flagella.
- Centriole shows cartwheel appearance.
- Crista is found in mitochondria.
- Few chromosomes have secondary constrictions at a constant location. This gives the appearance of a small fragment called satellite.

177. *(c)* A-II, B-IV, C-I, D-III.
- In diakinesis, completion of terminalisation of chiasmata takes place.
- In pachytene, appearance of recombination nodule takes place.
- In zygotene, synaptonemal complex formation takes place.
- In leptotene, chromosomes look like thin threads.

178. *(b)* Among the given factors, high pO_2 and lesser H^+ concentration are favourable for the formation of oxyhaemoglobin in alveoli. The higher the partial pressure of oxygen. The more efficiently haemoglobin binds to O_2.

179. *(b)* A-III, B-I, C-II, D-IV.
- *Pterophyllum* is the scientific name for angel fish.
- *Myxine* is the scientific name for hag fish.
- *Pristis* is the scientific name for saw fish.
- *Exocoetus* is the scientific name for flying fish.

180. *(b)* A-IV, B-III, C-I, D-II.
- Typhoid is caused by *Salmonella typhimurium* (Bacteria).
- Leishmaniasis is caused by protozoan i.e. *Leishmania donovani*.
- Ringworm is caused by fungi belonging to genera-*Microsporum*.
- Filariasis is caused by *Wuchereria bancrofti* (Nematode).

181. *(c)* All the statements are correct except (c), which can be corrected as. Bio-reactors are used to produce large scale bacterial cultures.

182. *(b)* Both statement I and II are incorrect. These can be corrected as
- In the nephron, the decending limb of loop of Henle is permeable to water, but almost impermeable to electrolytes.
- The PCT is lined by simple cuboidal brush border epithelium which

increases the surface area for reabsorption.

183. *(c)* Statement I is true, but statement II is false. Statement II can be corrected as

The hymen is often torn during first coitus. However, it may get torn due to a sudden fall or a jolt during horse-riding, cycling, gymnastics and dance movements, etc.

184. *(a)* A-II, B-IV, C-I, D-III.

• Expiratory capacity	Total volume + Expiratory reserve volume.
• Functional residual capacity	Expiratory reserve volume + Residual volume
• Vital capacity	Expiratory reserve volume + Tidal volume + Inspiratory reserve volume
• Inspiratory capacity	Tidal volume + Inspiratory reserve volume

185. *(d)* The correct sequence of different stages of cell division is as follows

Gap 1 phase → Synthesis phase → Gap 2 phase → Karyokinesis → Cytokinesis

In Gap 1 and Gap 2 phases, cell prepares itself for cell division; while actual division occurs in synthesis phase. Karyokinesis is division of nucleus that is followed by cytokinesis.

186. *(c)* Statement I is true, but Statement II is false. The incorrect statement can be corrected as

The inner membrane of chloroplast is relatively less permeable; as compared to mitochondria.

187. *(d)* A-III, B-I, C-IV, D-II.

- Birds and reptiles evolved in mesozoic era.
- Lower invertebrates evolved in Proterozoic era.
- Mammals evolved in Cenozoic era.
- Fish and amphibians evolved in Palozoic era.

188. *(d)* Statement I is false, but statement II is true. Statement I can be corrected as.

Gause's competitive exclusion theory states that two closely related species competing for the same resources cannot co-exist indefinitely.

189. *(c)* A-III, B-IV, C-I, D-II.

- Unicellular glandular epithelium is present in goblet cells of alimentary canal.
- Compound epithelium is present in moist surface of buccal cavity.
- Multicellular glandular epithelium is present in salivary glands.
- Endocrine glandular epithelium is present in pancreas.

190. *(a)* A-IV, B-II, C-III, D-I.

- The structures used for storing of food are crop.
- Ring of 6-8 blind tubules at junction of foregut and midgut is gastric caeca.
- Ring of 100-150 yellow coloured thin filaments at the junction of midgut and hindgut are called Malpighian tubules.
- The structures used for grinding the food are gizzard.

191. *(c)* Statement (c) is correct, while rest of the statements are incorrect. These can be corrected as follows.

- Juxta medullary nephrons are not present in columns of Bertini.
- Renal corpuscle of juxta medullary nephron lies in the inner cortical region.
- Juxta medullary nephrons are lesser in number than cortical nephrons.

192. *(d)* A-IV, B-III, C-I, D-II.

- In eukaryotes, RNA polymerase-III is responsible for transcription of *sn*RNAs, *t*RNA and 5*sr*RNA
- rho factor is responsible for termination of transcription.
- Splicing of exons is performed by *sn*RNPs.
- TATA box is present in promoter region of transcription unit.

193. *(c)* Statement I is true, but statement II is false. Statement II can be corrected as

The brain stem consist of the medulla oblongata, pons and midbrain.

Hence, option (c) is the correct answer.

194. *(a)* In the given question A, B, C and D are respectively FSH, leydig cells, Sertoli cells and Spermiogenesis. LH and FSH both are secreted by anterior pituitary. LH stimulates Leydig's cells to secrete androgens. FSH stimulates Sertoli cells that release some factors which help in spermiogenesis.

195. *(a)* If the blood group of father is B^+, mother is A^+ and child is O^+ their respective genotypes will be

$I^Bi / I^Ai / ii$

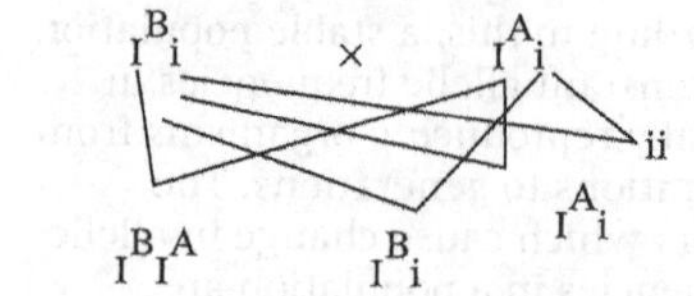

196. *(a)* Both Statement I and Statement II are true.

197. *(a)* The catalytic cycle of an enzyme action occurs in the following steps

Substrate binding to active site (E)

↓

Substrate enzyme complex formation (A)

↓

Chemical bonds of the substrate broken (D)

↓

Release of products (C)

↓

Free enzyme ready to bind with another substrate (B)

Thus, the correct answer is option (a).

198. *(b)* A-III, B-II, C-IV, D-I.

- P-wave–Depolarisation of atria.
- QRS complex–Depolarisation of ventricles.
- T-wave–Repolarisation of ventricles.
- T-P gap–Heart muscles are electrically silent.

199. *(d)* A-III, B-IV, C-I, D-II.

- Exophthalmicgoitre – Hypersecretion of thyroid hormone and protruding eye balls.
- Acromegaly – Excessive secretion of growth hormone.
- Cushing's syndrome – Excess secretion of cortisol, moon face and hyperglycemia.
- Cretinism – Hyposecretion of thyroid hormone and stunted growth.

200. *(c)* Statements B, D and E are true for non-chordates, while statements A and C are incorrect. These can be corrected as

- Pharynx is not perforated by gill slits in non-chordates.
- In non-chordates, the central nervous system is ventral and solid.